T-50724

**610 Statistical record of
STA health and medicine**

DATE DUE	BORROWER'S NAME	

**610 Statistical record of
STA health and medicine**

Statistical Record
OF Health &
Medicine

2nd Edition

ISSN 1078-6961

Statistical Record

Record

^{OF} Health &

Medicine

2nd Edition

Arsen J. Darnay, Editor

GALE

DETROIT • NEW YORK • TORONTO • LONDON

Helen S. Fisher and Arsen Darnay, *Editors*

Editorial Code & Data Inc. Staff

Robert S. Lazich, Annemarie Muth, Susan M. Turner and David Smith, *Contributing Editors*
Kenneth J. Muth, *Manager, Technical Operations*

Gale Research Staff

Nicole Beatty, *Coordinating Editor*
Mary Beth Trimper, *Production Director*
Cynthia Baldwin, *Product Design Manager*
Barbara J. Yarrow, *Graphic Services Supervisor*
C. J. Jonik, *Desktop Publisher*

The paper used in this publication meets the minimum requirements of American National Standard for Information Sciences—Permanence Paper for Printed Library Materials, ANSI Z39.48-1984.

ISBN 0-7876-0093-8
ISSN 1078-6961
10 9 8 7 6 5 4 3 2 1

Printed in the United States of America

TABLE OF CONTENTS

CHAPTER 2 - HEALTH STATUS OF AMERICANS continued:

Features of This Edition

Statistical Record of Health and Medicine (SRHM), now in its second edition, provides a comprehensive compilation of national, state, and municipal health and medical statistics drawn from government, academic, association, trade, technical, and media sources. *SRHM* provides broad subject coverage of the field with data on contemporary health-related issues and concerns. Highlights of this edition include:

- 950 statistical tables.
- Approximately 300 sources.
- National, state, and local data.
- Comparative statistics from selected foreign countries.
- Summary indicator tables.
- Explanations of health and medical acronyms and abbreviations.
- Annotated source listings.
- Comprehensive keyword index, with extensive cross-references.

Locate Hard-to-Find Data Easily and Quickly

Locating timely and accurate statistical data on health-related matters can be troublesome. Consumers of professional journals and trade periodicals often discard their personal copies only to find that they need to reference a chart or graph from last month's or last year's issue—if indeed the consumer can recall the correct issue in which to locate the material. Libraries (particularly small or specialized ones) cannot purchase every source or retain unlimited back issues of material owing to budget and space constraints, so relevant statistical tables may not be available among the holdings. Frequently charts, graphs, and tables are omitted from online versions of material. *SRHM,* however, provides substantial and detailed coverage of statistics related to major areas of health and medicine. Here are statistics useful to a variety of individuals; for example,

- The student preparing a report or speech.
- The health care practitioner compiling a patient information brochure or journal article.
- The job seeker identifying employment possibilities throughout the United States.
- The consumer of medical services comparing costs of treatments or procedures.

SRHM tables are arranged conveniently by subject for quick access. Related tables are located easily through the Keyword Index and its many cross-references.

Universal Coverage

SRHM covers the health arena comprehensively. Topics include long-standing concerns such as leading causes of death, occupational health and safety, costs of medical care, compensation of health professionals, industry data, trends and projections regarding Social Security's future, detailed data on Medicare and Medicaid, medical malpractice, etc. In addition, *SRHM* presents a wide range of data on contemporary issues, notably assisted suicide, AIDS, violence, women's health, mergers and acquisitions, etc. Valuable information is provided for the student, the parent, the analyst, the jobseeker, the administrator, litigator, legislator, and others.

Introduction

Statistical Record of Health and Medicine (SRHM) is a comprehensive compilation of national, state, and municipal health and medical statistics profiling health in the United States. Data in *SRHM* are drawn from about 300 government, academic, association, trade, technical, and media sources, thus providing broad subject coverage of health and medical fields. *SRHM* provides statistics on:

- The health status and lifestyle of Americans;

- Specific health care and medical establishments such as hospitals and nursing homes;

- Occupational health and safety;

- Insurance;

- Health care costs and expenditures of consumers, governments, and businesses;

- Health care programs, including Medicaid and Medicare;

- Health care industries, including companies, products, and market trends;

- Medical professions and occupations;

- The medical establishment—from the physician in solo private practice to the largest hospital chains;

- Political issues, opinions and attitudes, and the laws related to health care and medicine; and

- International rankings and comparisons.

This edition, like the first, also features summary indicator tables, a comprehensive keyword index, annotated source listings, and explanations of acronyms and abbreviations.

Scope and Coverage

Subjects Covered. *SRHM* provides a comprehensive overview of the health arena. Chapters include:

Summary Indicators. The tables in this chapter summarize important facts and trends for rapid review. Data for each line of each table are drawn from other tables throughout *SRHM*.

Health Status of Americans. This chapter profiles the health status of Americans by presenting 275 tables on such topis as aging; children; death; dental health; disabilities and handicaps; diseases and illnesses; environmental health; injuries and accidents; life expectancy; men's and women's health; mental health; pregnancy and childbirth; and a variety of other subjects.

Health Care Establishment. This chapter features 205 tables profiling health care providers, establishments, treatments, practices, and procedures. Topics include centers, drugs and medicine, establishment data and ratios, HMOs, home health care, hospices, hospitals, insurance carriers, mergers and acquisitions, and nursing homes. A notable new feature is establishment data and ratios from the most recent *1992 Economic Census*, upgrading the last edition's coverage from 1987.

Lifestyles and Health. Healthy habits lead to healthy outcomes. In this chapter, factors that contribute to health or harm it are profiled in 76 tables under such topics as diets, fitness, obesity, safety, sex, smoking and tobacco, and substance abuse.

Health in the Workplace. This brief chapter presents seven tables on occupational health and safety. Topics include occupational health and safety, injuries, and illnesses.

Health Expenditures and Funding. The 45 tables in this chapter present data on expenditures, prices, trends, and projections. Some expenditure data are also presented, separately, in the chapter on Health Care Programs, most notably data on Medicare and Medicaid—presented later so that major subjects will be grouped together.

Health Care Programs. This chapter is largely devoted to major programs under the auspices of which health care is actually delivered. In 108 tables children's programs, health insurance coverage, HMOs, Medicaid, and Medicare are covered. Special emphasis has been given, in this edition, to Medicaid and Medicare data.

Medical Professions. The medical field is described in this chapter from the viewpoint of its workers in 169 tables—the doctors, nurses, technicians, and other occupations engaged in the delivery of health care services to us. Topics include compensation, education, employment, health personnel, physicians, and work-place issues. As a special feature of this edition, detailed compensation tables, by locality, are provided from the U.S. Department of Labor's *Area Wage Survey*.

Medical Practices and Procedures. This chapter presents 19 tables on such topics as cosmetic procedures, inpatient discharges, medication errors, organ transplants, surgery, technology, and treatment options and alternatives.

Politics, Opinion, and Law. Issues that relate to politics, law, and opinion are shown in the 24 tables of this chapter. Topics include controversies (assisted suicide, smoking), disciplinary actions, discrimination, Family and Medical Leave Act, lost work time, malpractice, and some tables on opinion.

International Comparisons. Tables in this chapter compare and rank health care performance of other nations with that of the United States. Topics include expenditures, children, diseases, and women.

Geographic Area Covered. *SRHM* covers health and medicine in the United States. Depending on the table, data presented may reflect the national, state, or local level. Chapter 11 profiles health care on a worldwide basis. Tables in this chapter offer comparisons and rankings of foreign countries in the subject areas profiled for the United States elsewhere in this edition. Nations selected usually are similar to the United States in economic development.

Period Covered. Most of the material in *SRHM* dates from the early 1990s or later. If the only data available pre-dated 1990, then that material was included to ensure comprehensive coverage of the field. Some of the tables also present earlier data for historical purposes; for example, to illustrate changes—growth or decline—over time. Whenever possible, projections have been provided to indicate trends and forecasts. In any case, the most recent data available at the time of compilation have been included in this edition.

Sources

Thousands of health-related statistics are produced by a variety of reliable sources each year. Data were selected for inclusion in *SRHM* on the basis of their timeliness, interest, or value to researchers and the general public, and their ability to contribute to the comprehensive coverage of the field.

Much of the statistical material included in *SRHM* comes from the U.S. federal government or from state and other government levels under federal mandate. Many of the tables were drawn from statistical services or special reports of major federal departments; for example, the Department of Health and Human Services, the body that administers programs and collects statistics on health and medicine in the United States. Statistics from departments of Commerce, Labor, Education, and Justice frequently are cited, as is material from Congressional hearings.

SRHM also features data from media sources, including newspapers, business periodicals, trade magazines, professional journals, and association publications. These media often rely on the government or other sources for the information they provide. Nevertheless, presentation of material in current literature is indicative of issues, anxieties, and aspirations occupying the American consciousness. In addition, *SRHM* offers statistics collected by associations, special surveys and studies, opinion polls, and elections.

Acknowledgments

Many people and organizations contributed data, suggestions, permission, and advice in the compilation of *SRHM.* The editorial staff thanks them all for their help and guidance.

Comments and Suggestions

Although every effort has been made to ensure the accuracy and timeliness of the data in *SRHM,* errors and omissions may occur. Notification of changes or additions deemed appropriate by users of this edition are appreciated. Comments and suggestions for the improvement of *SRHM* are welcome. Please contact:

Statistical Record of Health and Medicine
Gale Research
835 Penobscot Building
Detroit, MI 48226-4094
Phone: (313) 961-2242
Toll-free: 800-347-GALE
Fax: (313) 961-6815

How to Use This Book

Statistical Record of Health and Medicine (SRHM) is organized into 11 chapters, the first of which contains summary indicators. (See the Table of Contents or the Introduction in the preceding pages for a list of chapters.) Each chapter begins with notes that explain its contents and reference related material elsewhere in *SRHM.* To facilitate browsing through 950 *SRHM* tables, the chapter titles also appear in the upper right- or upper left-hand corners of pages.

SRHM chapters are subdivided by alphabetically arranged topics. Topic notations are placed above the first table in subject groupings for easy identification. The topic is shown again in italic type below each subsequent table's reference number.

Organization of Tables

Tables are arranged alphabetically by title within each topic grouping. In addition, each table is numbered sequentially, beginning with the first table in the first chapter. Hence, data may be accessed through table reference numbers or alphabetically by topic and table title.

Tables appear in the Sources list by table number. Tables can be accessed by reference number or by page number using the Table of Contents or the Keyword Index.

Some tables display graphic presentations such as bar graphs and pie charts. If the table has more than one column of data, the number of the column represented by the graphic is identified. Complete tabular data follow each graphic.

A selection of material in *SRHM* is of a textual nature. Nevertheless, these entries contain predominantly statistical data. Occasionally, such entries offer explanatory material.

Special Features

Abbreviations and Acronyms. This list shows all the abbreviations, acronyms, and initialisms that appear in tables throughout *SRHM.* While explanations and translations of abbreviations will be found within the text of tables, a general listing is provided here for the convenience of *SRHM* users. Abbreviations and acronyms are listed in alphabetic order, with explanations following.

Summary Indicators. A brief introductory chapter provides quick access to some of the more conventional material included in the body of *SRHM.* These graphic summaries contain data extracted from one or more tables located elsewhere in the text to offer a convenient overview of health issues such as causes of death or political clout of the medical establishment.

Sources. An appendix lists all the sources cited in tables included in *SRHM.* Sources are arranged alphabetically by author name or title as appropriate. In the case of periodicals, dates of issues consulted are shown. The list provides table references, showing all data citing a particular source.

Keyword Index. This index allows users to access all subjects, issues, diseases, medical specialties, industries, companies, programs, insurance carriers, associations, schools, educational programs, occupations, personal names, and locations cited in the tables of *SRHM.* Each citation is followed by table and page reference numbers. Page references do not necessarily identify the page on which a table begins. In the cases where tables span two or more pages, references point to the page on which the index term appears—which may be the second or subsequent page of a table. Frequent cross-references have been added to index citations to facilitate the location of related topics and tables.

Sample Table

The following sample table shows elements commonly included in *SRHM* tables. Each numbered paragraph corresponds to the numbered item in the sample.

2		1

620

Occupational Health and Safety: Fatalities

3

Death Rates for Work-Related Injuries: 1983-2000

4

The table below shows death rates for work-related injuries among full-time workers in the United States for selected years. Data are provided by selected occupations.

5

[Deaths per 100,000 population]

6

Occupation	1983-1987 average	1988	1989	1990	Year 2000 target
All full-time workers	5.9	5.0	5.4	4.3	4.0
Mine workers	30.5	33.8	17.3	[1]	21.0
Construction workers	25.0	24.5	22.4	20.6	17.0
Transportation workers	15.2	13.5	12.2	10.0	10.0
Farm workers	14.0	13.8	13.9	23.8	9.5

7

Source: National Center for Health Statistics. "Healthy People 2000 Review." *Health United States, 1992.* Hyattsville, MD: Public Health Service, 1993, p. 293. Primary source: Bureau of Labor Statistics. *Annual Summary of Occupational Injuries and Illnesses.* Remarks: "Healthy People 2000" is a national prevention initiative that presents the strategy for improving health in the United States. *Notes:* Death rates are crude death rates. 1. Data not available.

8		9

1	**Table reference number.**

2	**Topic within chapter.**

3	**Table title.**

4	**Headnote.** Provides a brief explanation of the table, or explains unusual terminology. Note that this material, unless enclosed within quotes, has been prepared by the editors and is not taken from the original source unless otherwise stated.

5	**Quantifying information.** Indicates measurement or units used within the table.

6	**Table.**

7	**Source.** Identifies the material from which table originated. If data for the table were not compiled by the source cited, a **primary source** notation will follow.

8	**Remarks.** In some instances, additional remarks appear for clarification of source notations or other reasons.

9	**Footnotes**. Footnotes or other explanations help to clarify data in the table (for example, missing information or special criteria for reported information) or to explain and clarify as in the case of translating acronyms and abbreviations.

Abbreviations and Acronyms

Abbreviations and acronyms used in tables or notes are explained within the context of the data presented. The listing below includes all abbreviations, acronyms, and initialisms used in the *Statistical Record of Health and Medicine*, together with their full translations or meanings. One abbreviation may represent multiple items or organizations. Where more than one use is possible, all explanations of the term are provided. Abbreviations and acronyms in this list appear in alphabetic order.

AAHSLD	Association of Academic Health Sciences Library Directors		**AR**	Arkansas
AAMC	Association of American Medical Colleges		**ASHA**	American Speech-Language-Hearing Association
AAP	American Academy of Pediatrics		**ATV**	All-terrain vehicle
ADA	American Dental Association		**AZ**	Arizona
	American Dietetic Association		**BA**	Bachelor of Arts
	Americans With Disabilities Act		**BAC**	Blood alcohol content
ADL	Activities of daily living		**BATF**	Bureau of Alcohol, Tobacco, and Firearms
AFDC	Aid to Families With Dependent Children		**BLS**	Bureau of Labor Statistics
AHCA	American Health Care Association		**BPH**	Benign prostatic hypertrophy
AHIMA	American Health Information Management Association		**BS**	Bachelor of Science
			BSN	Bachelor of Science in Nursing
AIDS	Acquired immunodeficiency syndrome		**CA**	California
AK	Alaska		**CAD**	Computer-assisted design
AL	Alabama		**CAM**	Computer-assisted manufacture
ALHS	Archivists and Librarians in the Health Sciences (formerly Association of Librarians in the History of Health Sciences)		**CAT**	Computerized axial tomography (CAT scan)
			CBO	Congressional Budget Office
			CC	Child and Adult Care
ALS	Amyotropic lateral sclerosis		**CCC-A**	Certificate of Clinical Competence — Audiology
AMA	American Medical Association			
AMHL	Association of Mental Health Librarians		**CCC-SLP**	Certificate of Clinical Competence — Speech-Language Pathology
APA	American Psychological Association			
			CDC	Centers for Disease Control and Prevention

CE	Consumer Expenditure Survey		DT	Diphtheria, tetanus
CEO	Chief executive officer		DTP	Diphtheria, tetanus, pertussis
CFOI	Census of Fatal Occupational Injuries		DVT	Deep-vein thrombosis
CHAMPUS	Civilian Health and Medical Program of the Uniformed Services		EAP	Employee Assistance Program
			EEOC	Equal Employment Opportunity Commission
CI	Cumulative incidence			
CIA	Clinical Investigator Awards		EEG	Electroencephalograph
cm	Centimeter		EEO	Equal Employment Opportunity
CMSA	Consolidated Metropolitan Statistical Area		EKG	Electrocardiograph
			EPSDT	Early and periodic screening, diagnosis, and treatment
CO	Colorado			
COBRA	Consolidated Omnibus Reconciliation Act		ESA	Economics and Statistics Administration
			ESOP	Employee stock option plan
COPD	Chronic obstructive pulmonary disease			Employee stock ownership plan
COTH	Council of Teaching Hospitals		ESRD	End-stage renal disease
CPI	Consumer Price Index		FADHPS	Financial Aid for Disadvantaged Health Professions Students
CPR	Cardiopulmonary resuscitation			
CPS	Current Population Survey		FARS	Fatal Accident Reporting System
CQI	Continuous quality improvement		FAS	Financial accounting standard
CRS	Congenital rubella syndrome		FCoA	Federal Council on the Aging
CSA	Community Services Administration		FDA	U.S. Food and Drug Administration
CT	Connecticut		FDC	Families with Dependent Children
CTS	Carpal Tunnel Syndrome		FL	Florida
DC	District of Columbia		FMG	Foreign medical graduates
DE	Delaware		FMI	Food Marketing Institute
DFTERN	Demand for full-time equivalent registered nurses		FNS	Food and Nutrition Service
			FSMB	Federal State Medical Board
DHHS	U.S. Department of Health and Human Services		FTE	Full-time equivalent
			FY	Fiscal year
DI	Disability insurance		g	gram(s)
dl	deciliter			
DO	Doctor of Osteopathy		GA	Georgia
DOS	Disk operating system		GAO	U.S. General Accounting Office
DPT	Diphtheria, pertussis, and tetanus		GDP	Gross Domestic Product
DRG	Diagnosis-related group		GERD	Gastroesophageal reflux disease
			GF	Government finances

GNP	Gross National Product
GOP	Grand Old Party; Republican Party
HCFA	Health Care Financing Administration
HCPP	Health care prepayment plan
HCV	Hepatitis C virus
HEAL	Health Education Assistance Loan
HHANES	Hispanic Health and Nutrition Examination Survey
HI	Hawaii
	Hospital Insurance
HIV	Human immunodeficiency virus
HMO	Health Maintenance Organization
HR	Human Resources
IA	Iowa
IADL	Instrumental activities for daily living
IAQ	Indoor air quality
ICF	Intermediate care facility
ID	Idaho
IL	Illinois
IMG	International medical graduate
IN	Indiana
IPA	Independent Practice Association
IPEDS	Integrated Postsecondary Education Data System
IRA	Individual retirement account
IUD	Intrauterine device
IVDA	Intravenous drug abuse
JAMA	Journal of the American Medical Association
JAVMA	Journal of American Veterinary Medicine Association
JTPA	Job Training Partnership Act
KS	Kansas
KY	Kentucky
LA	Louisiana
LCME	Liaison Committee on Medical Education

LIHEAP	Low-Income Home Energy Assistance Program
LPN	Licensed practical nurse
LSC	Life Safety Code
LSD	Lysergic acid diethylamide
LTC	Long-term care
MA	Massachusetts
	Master of Arts
MAA	Medical Assistance for the Aged
MD	Doctor of Medicine
	Maryland
ME	Maine
MERIT	Method to Extend Research in Time
MFS	Medicare Fee Schedule
MI	Michigan
	Myocardial infarction
MLA	Medical Library Association
MLA-MHLS	Medical Library Association-Mental Health Librarians Section
MMR	Measles-mumps-rubella
MN	Minnesota
MO	Missouri
MRI	Magnetic resonance imager or imaging
MS	Master of Science
	Mississippi
MSA	Metropolitan Statistical Area
MSHA	Mine Safety and Health Administration
MT	Montana
MeSH	Medical subject headings
NA	Not available; not applicable
NC	North Carolina
NCHS	National Center for Health Statistics
NCIPC	National Center for Injury Prevention and Control
ND	North Dakota

NE	Nebraska		PCP	Phencyclidine
NEISS	National Electronic Injury Surveillance System		PHS	Public Health Service
NETS	Network of Employers for Traffic Safety		PID	Pelvic inflammatory disease
NH	New Hampshire		POS	Point-of-service plan
NHA	National Health Accounts		PSA	Physician Scientist Awards
NHLBI	National Heart, Lung, and Blood Institute		PPO	Preferred Provider Organization
NIA	National Institute on Aging		PPS	Prospective Payment System
NIH	National Institutes for Health		PR	Puerto Rico
NIJ	National Institute of Justice		PRK	Photorefractive keratectomy
NJ	New Jersey		PhD	Doctor of Philosophy
NM	New Mexico		R&D	Research and development
no.	Number		RCA	Research Career Awards
NSLP	National School Lunch Program		RN	Registered nurse
NV	Nevada		RPG	Research Project Grant
NY	New York		RR	Relative risk
OASDHI	Old-Age, Survivors, and Disability Health Insurance		RSI	Repetitive strain injury
OASDI	Old-Age, Survivors, and Disability Insurance		SB	School Breakfast
			SBIR	Small Business Innovation Research
OASI	Old-Age, Survivors Insurance		SBS	Sick building syndrome
OB	Obstetrics; obstetrician		SC	South Carolina
OECD	Organization for Economic Cooperation and Development		SCOR	Specialized Centers for Research
			SD	South Dakota
OH	Ohio		SES	Socioeconomic status
OHD	Other health doctorates		SF	School Funding
OK	Oklahoma		SGLI	Servicemen's Group Life Insurance
OR	Oregon		SMA	State Mental Health Agency
OSHA	Occupational Safety and Health Administration		SMI	Supplementary Medical Insurance
			SNF	Skilled nursing facility
PA	Pennsylvania		SOA	Survey on Aging
PAA	Pulmonary Academic Awards		SPF	Sun protection factor
PAC	Political action committee		SPVDAA	Systemic Pulmonary and Vascular Disease Academic Awards
PBGC	Pension Benefit Guaranty Corporation		SSA	Social Security Administration
PCAA	Preventive Cardiology Academic Awards		SSI	Supplemental Security Income

STD	Sexually transmitted disease
TB	Tuberculosis
TMAA	Transfusion Medicine Academic Awards
TN	Tennessee
TQM	Total quality management
TX	Texas
UAP	Unlicensed assistive personnel
UCLA	University of California, Los Angeles
UN	United Nations
UR	Utilization review
USC	University of Southern California
UT	Utah
VA	U.S. Department of Veterans Affairs
	U.S. Veterans Administration
	Virginia

VI	Virgin Islands
VMLS/MLA	Veterinary Medical Libraries Section/Medical Library Association
VN	Vocational nurse
VT	Vermont
WA	Washington
WHO	World Health Organization
WI	Wisconsin
WIC	Special Supplemental Food Program for Women, Infants, and Children
WV	West Virginia
WY	Wyoming

Statistical Record
OF Health &
Medicine

2nd Edition

Chapter 1
SUMMARY INDICATORS

The 10 tables in this chapter show summaries of the material included in this edition of *Statistical Record of Health and Medicine.* Each table features data included elsewhere in *SRHM,* highlighting major aspects of health or medicine. The tables from which data were taken are shown in the column headed "Source Table". Numbers in this column reference table (not page) numbers.

★ 1 ★

Leading Causes of Death

This table shows that heart disease is the leading cause of death followed by cancer. Deaths from AIDS may be caused by a variety of diseases.

Item	Value	Denomination	Date	Source Table
Leading Cause of Death				
Heart disease	734.1	Thousands	1994	40
Malignancies	536.9	Thousands	1994	40
Accidents	90.1	Thousands	1994	40
Pulmonary disease	101.9	Thousands	1994	40
Pneumonia and Influenza	82.1	Thousands	1994	40
Diabetes mellitus	55.4	Thousands	1994	40
Other infections and parasitic causes	48.5	Thousands	1994	40
Suicide	32.4	Thousands	1994	40
HIV	37.3	Thousands	1993	45

Source: Data are drawn from tables in the rest of *Statistical Record of Health and Medicine.* Columns headed by the phrase Source Table show the source of the data in this book.

★ 2 ★

Leading Causes of Death by Age Groups

This table shows the three leading causes of death and the death rates for the youngest and oldest age groups.

Segment of Population	Value	Denomination	Date	Source Table
All Causes	2,268,553	Number	1993	45
Heart Disease				
Under 1 year	20.4	Per 100,000	1994	51
15-24 years	2.4	Per 100,000	1994	51
55-64	327.6	Per 100,000	1994	51
65-74	817.7	Per 100,000	1994	51
75-84	2,120.6	Per 100,000	1994	51
85 years and older	6,521.3	Per 100,000	1994	51
Malignant Neoplasms				
Under 1 year	-			
15-24 years	4.8	Per 100,000	1994	51
55-64	430.3	Per 100,000	1994	51
65-74	882.5	Per 100,000	1994	51
75-84	1,375.8	Per 100,000	1994	51
85 years and older	1,786.8	Per 100,000	1994	51
Cerebrovascular Diseases				
Under 1 year	2.8	Per 100,000	1994	51
15-24 years	0.4	Per 100,000	1994	51
55-64	46.2	Per 100,000	1994	51
65-74	137.6	Per 100,000	1994	51
75-84	484.9	Per 100,000	1994	51
85 years and older	1,609.0	Per 100,000	1994	51

Source: Data are drawn from tables in the rest of *Statistical Record of Health and Medicine.* Columns headed by the phrase Source Table show the source of the data in this book.

★3★

Suicide

This table shows that men are more prone to commit suicide than women and white men more than African American men.

Item	Value	Denomination	Date	Source Table
Suicide rates				
Total	12.1	Per 100,000	1993	55
Men				
White	21.4	Per 100,000	1993	55
Black	12.5	Per 100,000	1993	55
Women				
White	5.0	Per 100,000	1993	55
Black	2.1	Per 100,000	1993	55

Source: Data are drawn from tables in the rest of *Statistical Record of Health and Medicine.* Columns headed by the phrase Source Table show the source of the data in this book.

★4★

AIDS

This table profiles acquired immunodeficiency syndrome (AIDS), showing changes between 1984 and 1995 and modes of transmission.

Item	Value	Denomination	Date	Source Table
Deaths recorded in 1989				
Total	26,355	Number	1989	105
Male	23,742	Number	1989	105
Female	2,613	Number	1989	105
Deaths recorded in 1995				
Total	31,256	Number	1995	105
Male	26,375	Number	1995	105
Female	4,881	Number	1995	105
New diagnoses	6,161	Number	1984	121
New diagnoses	35,052	Number	1988	121
New diagnoses	57,667	Number	1994	121
Profile 1995				
Total cases	513,486	Number	1995	122
Total deaths	319,849	Number	1995	122
Male top 3 modes of transmission				
Male-to-male sex	259,672	Number	1995	122
Intravenous drug use	95,244	Number	1995	122

[Continued]

★ 4 ★

AIDS
[Continued]

Item	Value	Denomination	Date	Source Table
Both	33,195	Number	1995	122
Female top 3 modes of transmission				
Intravenous drug use	33,452	Number	1995	122
Heterosexual sex	26,516	Number	1995	122
Transfusion or transplant	3,106	Number	1995	122
Children				
Birth	6,256	Number	1995	122
Transfusion or transplant	366	Number	1995	122
Hemophilia treatment	227	Number	1995	122

Source: Data are drawn from tables in the rest of *Statistical Record of Health and Medicine*. Columns headed by the phrase Source Table show the source of the data in this book.

★ 5 ★

Cancer

This table shows new cases of cancer in 1996. The leading types of cancer are prostate, breast, and lung cancer. In 1994, 536,900 people died of cancer.

Item	Value	Denomination	Date	Source Table
New Cases of Cancer				
Bladder	52,900	Number	1996	124
Breast	185,700	Number	1996	125
Cervical	15,700	Number	1996	128
Colorectal	133,500	Number	1996	130
Endometrial	34,000	Number	1996	133
Kidney	30,600	Number	1996	134
Leukemia	27,600	Number	1996	135
Lung	177,000	Number	1996	136
Melanoma of the skin	38,300	Number	1996	137
Ovarian	26,700	Number	1996	138
Pancreatic	26,300	Number	1996	139
Prostate	317,100	Number	1996	140

Source: Data are drawn from tables in the rest of *Statistical Record of Health and Medicine*. Columns headed by the phrase Source Table show the source of the data in this book.

★ 6 ★

Disability

Slightly more than 24 million Americans suffer from a severe disability. Arthritis/rheumatism and back/spinal injuries account for more than half of all disabilities.

Item	Value	Denomination	Date	Source Table
Severely disabled				
Number	24.117	Million	1996	77
Percent of population	9.6	Percent	1996	77
White	5.4	Percent of population	1996	87
Black	11.8	Percent of population	1996	87
Hispanic	7.1	Percent of population	1996	87
Other Races	5.6	Percent of population	1996	87
People with a functional limitation	17.5	Percent of population	1996	85
People with severe functional limitation	7.8	Percent of population	1996	85
Leading causes of disability				
Arthritis/rheumatism	27	Percent of causes	1995	90
Back/spinal injury	21	Percent of causes	1995	90
Heart problem	17	Percent of causes	1995	90
Respiratory problem	10	Percent of causes	1995	90

Source: Data are drawn from tables in the rest of *Statistical Record of Health and Medicine.* Columns headed by the phrase Source Table show the source of the data in this book.

★ 7 ★

Health Habits and Living Conditions

Item	Value	Denomination	Date	Source Table
People who:				
Have exercise videos	33	Percent	1995	495
Currently use tobacco	29.1	Percent	1991	520
Smoke cigarettes	25.0	Percent	1993	525
Drank coffee in the last month	130,000,000	Number	1996	565
Lack health insurance	15.4	Percent	1995	640
Have hypertension	23.1	Percent	1988-91	151
Became infected with sexually				
transmitted diseases	12,000,000	Number	1996	178
Alcohol consumption:				
Beer	32.0	Gal. per capita	1994	493

[Continued]

★ 7 ★

Health Habits and Living Conditions
[Continued]

Item	Value	Denomination	Date	Source Table
Wine	2.5	Gal. per capita	1994	493
Distilled spirits	1.8	Gal. per capita	1994	493

Source: Data are drawn from tables in the rest of *Statistical Record of Health and Medicine*. Columns headed by the phrase Source Table show the source of the data in this book.

★ 8 ★

Medicaid and Medicare

Please note that medical coverage categories, e.g., Medicaid and Medicare, may overlap.

Item	Value	Denomination	Date	Source Table
Medicaid medical assistance payment				
1975	2,343	$ per beneficiary	1975	663
1994	4,087	$ per beneficiary	1994	663
Medicaid total expenditures				
1975	51.559	bil. 1994 dollars	1975	663
1994	143.265	bil. 1994 dollars	1994	663
Medicaid recipients as percent of population	14	% of population	1995	694
Medicare outlays				
1992	135,845	$ mil.	1992	703
1995	184,203	$ mil.	1995	703
Number covered by government health insurance				
Medicaid	31,877	Thousands	1995	640
Medicare	34,655	Thousands	1995	640
Military	9,375	Thousands	1995	640
Number covered by private health insurance	185,881	Thousands	1995	640
Number not covered by any health insurance	40,582	Thousands	1995	640

Source: Data are drawn from tables in the rest of *Statistical Record of Health and Medicine*. Columns headed by the phrase Source Table show the source of the data in this book.

★ 9 ★

Medical Establishment

This table shows the Medical Establishment in the U.S. as measured by the Economic Census (1992) conducted by the U.S. Bureau of the Census. More detail is available in the body of the book.

Category	Establishments	Revenues ($ mil)	Employment	Payroll per Employee ($)	Source Table
Offices of Dentists	108,200	35,172	549,357	23,483	373
Offices of Doctors of Medicine	192,965	128,839	1,231,342	51,699	374
General Medical Clinics	4,736	12,590	125,343	40,466	340
Clinics of Doctors and Dentists - tax exempt	3,302	16,622	157,758	33,569	310
Dental Clinics	604	351.2	5,232	26,408	324
General Medical and Surgical Hospitals	704	24,162	323,141	24797	332
Specialty Hospitals	699	6,921	105,009	24,222	396
Psychiatric Hospitals	492	4,396	69,669	23,105	384
Skilled Nursing Care Facilities	10,242	28,798	937,907	14,416	392

Source: Data are drawn from tables in the rest of *Statistical Record of Health and Medicine.* Columns headed by the phrase Source Table show the source of the data in this book.

★ 10 ★

Medical Professions

Item	Value	Denomination	Date	Source Table
Doctors				
Number in 1994	428,642	Number	1994	875
Number in 2005	562,701	Number	2005	875
How they work				
Self-employed solo practitioners	29.3	Percent	1994	876
Self-employed group practitioners	28.4	Percent	1994	876
Employed by others	42.3	Percent	1994	876
Number of first enrollments (medicine)	15,554	Number	1993	833
Number of first enrollments (osteopathy)	1,609	Number	1993	833
Compensation:				
Family practice	122,000	$ a year	1994	815
Cardiology (invasive)	313,000	$ a year	1994	815
Dentists				
Number in 1994	84,452	Number	1994	848
Number in 2005	89,018	Number	2005	848
Number of first enrollments (dentistry)	4,029	Number	1993	833
Registered Nurses				
Number in 1994	1,887,055	Number	1994	882

[Continued]

★ 10 ★

Medical Professions
[Continued]

Item	Value	Denomination	Date	Source Table
Number in 2005	2,355,863	Number	2005	882
Number of graduates (nursing)	88,144	Number	1993	833

Source: Data are drawn from tables in the rest of *Statistical Record of Health and Medicine*. Columns headed by the phrase Source Table show the source of the data in this book.

Chapter 2
HEALTH STATUS OF AMERICANS

This chapter presents tables that, collectively, provide the health status of Americans. Major categories covered are diseases and illnesses, deaths, births, life expectancy, injuries and accidents. In addition, there are a number of tables on a wide variety of subjects, including aging, physician contacts, dental health, environmental health, and health status of groups, e.g., children, men, and women. Somewhat related tables, but from a workplace perspective, may be found in Chapter 5 - Health in the Workplace and from an international perspective in Chapter 11 - International Comparisons. Data in Chapter 4 - Lifestyles and Health are also relevant to this broad subject.

Aging

★ 11 ★

Pain and Older Americans

"Nearly 1 in 5 Americans over age 60 regularly takes pills for pain. And a quarter of them suffer side effects such as drowsiness, dizziness and gastrointestinal complications."

Source: Cronin, Brian. "Health Report: The Bad News." *Time,* 23 June 1997, p. 23. Primary source: National Council on the Aging.

Allergies

★ 12 ★

Allergies in Children

"Researchers find that 95% of kids who develop allergies to nuts—a potentially life-threatening problem—suffer from asthma, eczema, or hay fever. They warn children with any of these problems to lay off peanut butter and other nutty foods."

Source: Cronin, Brian. "Health Report: The Bad News." *Time,* 6 May 1996, p. 21. Primary source: *British Medical Journal.*

★ 13 ★
Allergies

Allergy Prescriptions

Table shows cities which had the most prescriptions written for allergy medications in 1996.

City	Millions
New York-Newark, NY-NJ	2.67
Dallas, TX	1.59
Gary-Chicago, IN-IL	1.44
Philadelphia, PA	1.42
Los Angeles, CA	1.33

Source: "'Gesundheit' Cities." *USA TODAY,* 20 March 1997, p. 1A. Primary source: IMS America for Hoechst Marion Roussel.

Births

★ 14 ★

Births to Teenage Mothers, by State: 1985 and 1994

[In number of births per 100,000 females age 15-19]

State	1985	1994
District of Columbia	72	115
Mississippi	76	83
Arizona	67	79
Texas	72	78
New Mexico	73	77
Arkansas	73	76
Louisiana	72	75
Nevada	55	74
Alabama	64	72
Georgia	68	72
California	53	71
Tennessee	61	71
South Carolina	63	67
North Carolina	57	66
Oklahoma	69	66
Kentucky	63	65
Florida	58	64
Illinois	51	63
Delaware	51	60
Missouri	54	59
Indiana	52	58
Alaska	56	55
Ohio	50	55
Colorado	48	54
Hawaii	48	54
Kansas	52	54
West Virginia	54	54
Michigan	43	52
Oregon	43	51
Virginia	46	51
Maryland	46	50
Rhode Island	36	48
Washington	45	48
Wyoming	59	48
Idaho	47	47
New York	36	46
Pennsylvania	40	44
Nebraska	40	43
South Dakota	46	43
Utah	50	43
Montana	44	41
Connecticut	31	40
Iowa	35	40

[Continued]

★ 14 ★

Births to Teenage Mothers, by State: 1985 and 1994
[Continued]

State	1985	1994
New Jersey	34	39
Wisconsin	39	39
Massachusetts	29	37
Maine	42	36
North Dakota	36	35
Minnesota	31	34
Vermont	36	33
New Hampshire	32	30

Source: "American Pie: Teen Moms." *U.S. News & World Report,* 11 November 1996, p. 14.

★ 15 ★

Births

Cesarean Section Deliveries, by Age of Mother: 1990 to 1993

AGE OF MOTHER	1990	1991	1992	1993
Number of cesarean deliveries (1,000)	945	905	921	917
Rate: Mothers, all ages[1]	23.5	22.6	22.3	22.8
Under 20 years	16.6	16.4	17.5	15.6
20 to 24 years	21.0	19.9	21.4	19.9
25 to 29 years	23.3	23.3	23.2	23.0
30 to 34 years	27.8	25.7	27.1	26.3
35 years and over	31.4	29.4	30.1	30.3

Source: 1996 Statistical Abstract of the United States on CD-ROM [machine-readable datafiles]. CD-8A-97. Washington, DC: U.S. Department of Commerce, Economics and Statistics Administration, Bureau of the Census, Data User Services Division, January 1997. Primary source: U.S. National Center for Health Statistics, *Vital Statistics of the United States,* annual. *Notes:* 1. Cesarean rates are the number of cesarean deliveries per 100 total deliveries for specified category.

★ 16 ★
Births

Live Births, by Place of Delivery; Median and Low-Birth Weight; and Prenatal Care: 1970 to 1993

Represents registered births. Excludes births to nonresidents of the United States.

Year	Births attended (1,000)			Median birth weight[3]			Percent of births with low birth weight[5]			Percent of births by period in which prenatal care began	
	In hospital[1]	Not in hospital		Total[4]	White	Black[6]	Total[4]	White	Black[6]	1st trimester	3d trimester or no prenatal care
		Physician	Midwife and other[2]								
1970	3,708	5	18	7 lb.-4 oz	7 lb.-5 oz	6 lb.-14 oz	7.9	6.8	13.9	68.0	7.9
1980	3,576	12	24	7 lb.-7 oz	7 lb.-8 oz	7 lb.-0 oz	6.8	5.7	12.5	76.3	5.1
1990	4,110	14	21	7 lb.-7 oz	7 lb.-8 oz	7 lb.-0 oz	7.0	5.7	13.3	74.2	6.0
1993	3,959	8	20	7 lb.-7 oz	7 lb.-8 oz	7 lb.-0 oz	7.2	6.0	13.3	78.9	4.8

Source: 1996 Statistical Abstract of the United States on CD-ROM [machine-readable datafiles]. CD-8A-97. Washington, DC: U.S. Department of Commerce, Economics and Statistics Administration, Bureau of the Census, Data User Services Division, January 1997. Primary source: U.S. National Center for Health Statistics, *Vital Statistics of the United States*, annual; *Monthly Vital Statistics Report*; and unpublished data. *Notes:* 1. Includes all births in hospitals or institutions and in clinics. 2. Includes births with attendant not specified. 3. Beginning 1989, median birth weight based on race of mother; prior to 1989, based on race of child. 4. Includes other races not shown separately. 5. Through 1975, births of 2,500 grams (5 lb.- 8 oz.) or less at birth; thereafter, less than 2,500 grams. 6. For 1970 represents Black and other races.

Children's Health

★ 17 ★

Causes of Asthma in Children

"Asthma-related illnesses are especially prevalent among inner-city children, for reasons that have long proved elusive. Physicians typically blamed bad air quality, inadequate health care and increased exposure to dust mites, animal dander and mold spores. But in the May 8 issue of the *New England Journal of Medicine,* a research group reported that another allergen is largely at work. They found that among 476 urban children with asthma, 37 percent were allergic to cockroaches. And when they sampled the dust in the children's bedrooms, they found that half had high levels of cockroach allergen; only 10 percent or so had similarly high levels of the other irritants."

Source: Leutwyler, Kristin. "In Brief: Bad News Bugs." *Scientific American* (July 1997), p. 26.

★ 18 ★

Children's Health

Nearsightedness in Children, by Age Group

Age	Percent nearsighted
5-9	3
10-12	8
Teenagers	16

Source: "Science & Society: Rethinking Eyeglasses for Kids." *U.S. News & World Report,* 14 August 1995, p. 10. Primary source: American Optometric Association.

★ 19 ★

Children's Health

Vaccinations of Children Age 19-35 Months for Selected Diseases, by Race, Poverty Status, and Residence in MSA: 1994

[In percentages]

Vaccination	Total	Race		Poverty status[1]		Location of residence		
						Inside MSA[7]		Outside MSA
		White	Black	Below poverty	At or above poverty	Central city	Remaining areas	
DTP[2,3]	89.5	90.6	84.4	88.8	90.3	87.7	90.4	90.0
Polio[3]	79.2	80.3	73.2	79.4	79.9	76.4	80.9	79.5
Measles-containing[4]	90.3	91.7	86.0	88.3	91.8	87.9	91.7	91.0
HIB[5]	75.0	76.6	67.2	72.1	76.6	70.6	76.7	77.6
Combined series[6]	67.5	68.4	61.2	64.9	68.8	63.5	69.7	68.3

Source: U.S. Department of Health and Human Services. Public Health Service. Centers for Disease Control and Prevention. National Center for Health Statistics. *Health, United States, 1995.* Hyattsville, MD: Public Health Service, 1996, p. 163. *Notes:* Refusals and unknowns were omitted (14 percent for DTP and polio; 16 percent for MMR; 19 percent for HIB). 1. Poverty status is based on family income and family size using Bureau of the Census poverty thresholds. 2. Diphtheria-tetanus-pertussis. 3. Three doses or more. 4. Respondents were asked about measles-containing or MMR (Measles-Mumps-Rubella) vaccines. 5. Haemophilus b, 3 or more doses. 6. The combined series consists of 4 doses of DTP vaccine, 3 doses of polio vaccine, and 1 dose of a measles-containing vaccine. 7. MSA stands for Metropolitan Statistical Area.

★ 20 ★
Children's Health

Whooping Cough: 1997

"The incidence of children with whooping cough—a serious, sometimes fatal disease that's preventable with a vaccination—has shot up 83% so far this year, compared with the same period in 1996."

Source: Cronin, Brian. "Health Report: The Bad News." *Time,* 28 April 1997, p. 26. Primary source: Centers for Disease Control and Prevention.

Chronic Conditions

★ 21 ★

Activity Limitations Caused by Chronic Conditions, by Selected Characteristics: 1994

[In percent of population]

Characteristic	Total with limitation of activity	Limited but not in major activity	Limited in amount or kind of major activity	Unable to carry on major activity
Total[1,2]	14.3	4.4	5.6	4.4
Age				
Under 15 years	6.4	1.6	4.1	0.7
Under 5 years	3.1	0.8	1.6	0.7
5-14 years	8.1	2.0	5.4	0.7
15-44 years	10.1	3.1	4.0	3.0
45-64 years	22.6	5.5	7.9	9.2
65 years and over	38.2	15.6	11.9	10.7
65-74 years	34.1	13.2	10.0	10.8
75 years and over	44.1	18.9	14.5	10.7
Sex and age				
Male[1]	14.3	4.2	5.3	4.8
Under 15 years	7.6	1.8	5.0	0.8
15-44 years	10.1	2.8	3.9	3.4
45-64 years	21.3	4.6	6.9	9.9
65-74 years	34.7	13.3	8.5	12.8
75 years and over	40.7	21.6	10.2	8.9
Female[1]	14.3	4.6	5.7	4.0
Under 15 years	5.1	1.4	3.1	0.6
15-44 years	10.1	3.5	4.0	2.6

[Continued]

★ 21 ★

Activity Limitations Caused by Chronic Conditions, by Selected Characteristics: 1994
[Continued]

Characteristic	Total with limitation of activity	Limited but not in major activity	Limited in amount or kind of major activity	Unable to carry on major activity
45-64 years	23.9	6.4	8.8	8.6
65-74 years	33.5	13.2	11.2	9.2
75 years and over	46.2	17.3	17.1	11.7
Race and age				
White[1]	14.0	4.4	5.5	4.0
Under 15 years	6.0	1.5	3.9	0.6
15-44 years	10.0	3.3	4.1	2.7
45-64 years	21.9	5.6	7.8	8.5
65-74 years	33.2	13.3	9.8	10.2
75 years and over	43.5	19.0	14.2	10.3
Black[1]	18.0	4.2	6.7	7.1
Under 15 years	8.5	1.9	5.6	1.0
15-44 years	11.4	2.6	4.1	4.8
45-64 years	30.7	5.3	9.5	15.8
65-74 years	44.4	13.8	13.1	17.6
75 years and over	52.5	18.5	18.1	15.9
Family income[1]				
Less than $14,000	26.4	5.7	9.2	11.5
$14,000-$24,999	16.5	4.5	6.5	5.5
$25,000-$34,999	13.6	4.3	5.9	3.5
$35,000-$49,999	11.5	4.2	4.6	2.6
$50,000 or more	9.2	3.7	3.8	1.7
Geographic region[1]				
Northeast	13.1	3.8	5.3	4.0
Midwest	13.9	4.2	6.0	3.7
South	15.2	4.5	5.8	5.0
West	14.5	4.9	5.0	4.5
Location of residence[1]				
Within MSA	13.9	4.3	5.4	4.2
Outside MSA	15.8	4.8	6.1	4.8

Source: U.S. Department of Health and Human Services. Public Health Service. Centers for Disease Control and Prevention. National Center for Health Statistics. *Health, United States, 1995.* Hyattsville, MD: Public Health Service, 1996, p. 171. Primary source: Centers for Disease Control and Prevention, National Center for Health Statistics, Division of Health Interview Statistics. Data from the National Health Interview Survey. *Notes:* 1. Age adjusted. 2. Includes all other races not shown separately and unknown family income.

Contact With Health Care Providers

★ 22 ★

Interval Since Last Physician Contact: 1994

The table below shows the percent distribution and persons contacting physicians at specified intervals. Percent distribution includes persons who never have visited a physician.

Characteristic	Less than 1 year	1 year-less than 2 years	2 years or more[1]
Total[2,4]	79.2	9.5	11.3
Age			
Under 15 years	84.8	9.6	5.7
Under 5 years	94.8	4.3	0.9
5-14 years	79.5	12.4	8.2
15-44 years	73.1	11.4	15.4
45-64 years	78.8	8.0	13.1
65 years and over	89.3	4.2	6.5
65-74 years	87.9	4.7	7.4
75 years and over	91.4	3.4	5.2
Sex and age			
Male[2]	74.2	10.7	15.2
Under 15 years	84.8	9.5	5.7
5-14 years	63.8	13.7	22.6
45-64 years	73.5	9.3	17.2
65-74 years	85.9	5.2	8.9
75 years and over	90.5	3.5	6.0
Female[2]	84.1	8.3	7.5
Under 15 years	84.7	9.7	5.6
5-14 years	82.2	9.2	8.5
45-64 years	83.8	6.8	9.3
65-74 years	89.5	4.3	6.2
75 years and over	92.0	3.3	4.7
Race and age			
White[2]	79.6	9.2	11.2
Under 15 years	85.5	9.0	5.4
5-14 years	73.5	11.2	15.3
45-64 years	78.7	8.1	13.2
65-74 years	88.0	4.6	7.5
75 years and over	91.3	3.5	5.3
Black[2]	79.5	10.6	9.9
Under 15 years	82.4	12.2	5.3

[Continued]

★ 22 ★

Interval Since Last Physician Contact: 1994
[Continued]

Characteristic	Less than 1 year	1 year-less than 2 years	2 years or more[1]
5-14 years	73.5	12.7	13.7
45-64 years	82.2	7.2	10.6
65-74 years	87.8	5.0	7.2
75 years and over	93.3	2.8[4]	3.9[4]
Family income[2]			
Less than $14,000	78.0	9.2	12.7
$14,000-$24,999	76.0	10.2	13.8
$25,000-$34,999	78.5	9.9	11.6
$35,000-$49,999	79.8	9.4	10.8
$50,000 or more	83.7	8.3	8.0
Geographic region[2]			
Northeast	83.4	8.1	8.6
Midwest	79.5	9.4	11.1
South	77.3	10.5	12.2
West	78.4	9.2	12.4
Location of residence[2]			
Within MSA	80.0	9.2	10.8
Outside MSA	76.3	10.5	13.2

Source: U.S. Department of Health and Human Services. Public Health Service. Centers for Disease Control and Prevention. National Center for Health Statistics. *Health, United States, 1995.* Hyattsville, MD: Public Health Service, 1996, p. 190. Primary source: Centers for Disease Control and Prevention, National Center for Health Statistics, Division of Health Interview Statistics. Data from National Health Interview Survey. *Notes:* 1. Includes persons who never visited a physician. 2. Age adjusted. 3. Includes all other races not shown separately and unknown family income. 4. Relative standard error greater than 30 percent.

★ 23 ★

Contact With Health Care Providers

Physician Contacts, by Method of Contact and Selected Patient Characteristics: 1994

[In percentages]

Characteristic	Doctor's office	Hospital outpatient department[1]	Telephone	Home	Other[2]
Total[3,4]	56.8	13.6	13.2	3.5	12.8
Age					
Under 15 years	60.6	13.1	14.3	0.8	11.1
Under 5 years	59.2	12.7	15.4	0.9[5]	11.8
5-14 years	62.1	13.5	13.1	0.8[5]	10.5
15-44 years	55.7	14.1	13.1	1.8	15.2
45-64 years	55.1	15.0	14.2	3.6	12.2
65 years and over	53.4	10.1	8.6	18.6	9.3
65-74 years	55.4	11.9	9.4	12.4	10.9
75 years and over	51.1	7.9	7.8	25.8	7.4
Sex[3]					
Male	55.4	15.6	11.7	3.5	13.9
Female	57.7	12.2	14.3	3.5	12.2
Race[3]					
White	58.4	12.5	14.1	3.3	11.8
Black	47.9	20.3	8.1	4.2	19.4
Family income[3]					
Less than $14,000	43.9	19.0	11.9	5.7	19.5
$14,000-$24,999	53.8	16.6	13.0	3.9	12.7
$25,000-$34,999	61.5	12.1	12.7	2.0	11.6
$35,000-$49,999	56.9	11.6	16.3	3.9	11.2
$50,000 or more	63.8	9.4	15.5	1.6	9.8
Geographic region[3]					
Northeast	59.0	13.0	12.8	4.0	11.2
Midwest	55.8	14.0	15.1	2.2	12.9
South	58.4	14.0	12.5	4.3	10.8
West	54.1	13.5	12.8	3.2	16.5

[Continued]

★ 23 ★

Physician Contacts, by Method of Contact and Selected Patient Characteristics: 1994
[Continued]

Characteristic	Doctor's office	Hospital outpatient department[1]	Telephone	Home	Other[2]
Location of residence[3]					
Within MSA	57.1	13.4	13.2	3.0	13.3
Outside MSA	55.7	14.6	13.3	5.2	11.2

Source: U.S. Department of Health and Human Services. Public Health Service. Centers for Disease Control and Prevention. National Center for Health Statistics. *Health, United States, 1995.* Hyattsville, MD: Public Health Service, 1996, p. 188. Primary source: Centers for Disease Control and Prevention, National Center for Health Statistics, Division of Health Interview Statistics. Data from National Health Interview Survey. *Notes:* 1. Includes hospital outpatient clinic, emergency room, and other hospital contacts. 2. Includes clinics or other places outside a hospital. 3. Age adjusted. 4. Includes all other races not shown separately and unknown family income. 5. Relative standard error greater than 30 percent.

★ 24 ★

Contact With Health Care Providers

Physician Contacts by Place and Patient Characteristics: 1990 and 1994

Data are based on household interviews of a sample of the civilian noninstitutionalized population. Data shown by percent distribution.

Characteristic	Total	Place of contact									
		Doctor's office		Hospital outpatient department[1]		Telephone		Home		Other[2]	
		1990	1994	1990	1994	1990	1994	1990	1994	1990	1994
Total[3,4]	100.0	59.9	56.8	13.7	13.6	12.7	13.2	2.1	3.5	11.6	12.8
Age											
Under 15 years	100.0	60.7	60.6	13.6	13.1	14.9	14.3	0.9	0.8	9.9	11.1
Under 5 years	100.0	59.1	59.2	14.0	12.7	15.9	15.4	1.1[5]	0.9[5]	9.8	11.8
5-14 years	100.0	62.6	62.1	13.1	13.5	13.7	13.1	0.6[5]	0.8[5]	10.0	10.5
15-44 years	100.0	59.4	55.7	14.3	14.1	12.0	13.1	0.6	1.8	13.7	15.2
45-64 years	100.0	60.4	55.1	14.1	15.0	12.2	14.2	2.0	3.6	11.4	12.2
65 years and over	100.0	58.7	53.4	11.1	10.1	9.9	8.6	11.8	18.6	8.4	9.3
65-74 years	100.0	60.2	55.4	13.7	11.9	9.7	9.4	7.0	12.4	9.4	10.9
75 years and over	100.0	56.8	51.1	7.8	7.9	10.2	7.8	18.1	25.8	7.0	7.4
Sex[3]											
Male	100.0	57.6	55.4	16.1	15.6	11.3	11.7	2.1	3.5	12.9	13.9
Female	100.0	61.6	57.7	12.2	12.2	13.4	14.3	2.0	3.5	10.9	12.2
Race[3]											
White	100.0	61.7	58.4	12.3	12.5	13.1	14.1	1.9	3.3	11.0	11.8
Black	100.0	48.2	47.9	24.3	20.3	9.1	8.1	2.8	4.2	15.6	19.4

[Continued]

★ 24 ★

Physician Contacts by Place and Patient Characteristics: 1990 and 1994

[Continued]

Characteristic	Total	Place of contact									
		Doctor's office		Hospital outpatient department[1]		Telephone		Home		Other[2]	
		1990	1994	1990	1994	1990	1994	1990	1994	1990	1994
Family Income[3]											
Less than $14,000	100.0	48.9	43.9	19.9	19.0	11.5	11.9	3.2	5.7	16.4	19.5
$14,000-$24,999	100.0	56.9	53.8	16.0	16.6	11.8	13.0	17	3.9	13.5	12.7
$25,000-$34,999	100.0	60.9	61.5	13.8	12.1	13.2	12.7	1.6	2.0	10.4	11.6
$35,000-$49,999	100.0	62.0	56.9	11.5	11.6	14.6	16.3	1.1	3.9	10.9	11.2
$50,000 or more	100.0	66.1	63.8	8.9	9.4	14.1	15.5	1.5	1.6	9.5	9.8
Geographic region[3]											
Northeast	100.0	62.6	59.0	13.0	13.0	11.7	12.8	1.9	4.0	10.8	11.2
Midwest	100.0	55.8	55.8	14.7	14.0	15.4	15.1	1.9	2.2	12.3	12.9
South	100.0	61.1	58.4	13.6	14.0	11.3	12.5	2.6	4.3	11.3	10.8
West	100.0	60.4	54.1	13.6	13.5	12.8	12.8	1.4	3.2	12.0	16.5
Location of residence[3]											
Within MSA	100.0	59.6	57.1	13.7	13.4	13.1	13.2	1.9	3.0	11.7	13.3
Outside MSA	100.0	61.4	55.7	14.1	14.6	10.7	13.3	2.6	5.2	11.2	11.2

Source: U.S. Department of Health and Human Services. Public Health Service. Centers for Disease Control and Prevention. National Center for Health Statistics. *Health, United States, 1995.* Hyattsville, MD: Public Health Service, 1995, p. 188. Primary source: Centers for Disease Control and Prevention, National Center for Health Statistics, Division of Health Interview Statistics. Data from the National Health Interview Survey. *Notes:* 1. Includes hospital outpatient clinic, emergency room, and other hospital contacts. 2. Includes clinics or other places outside a hospital. 3. Age adjusted. 4. Includes all other races not shown separately and unknown family income. 5. Relative standard error greater than 30 percent.

★ 25 ★

Contact With Health Care Providers

Physician Contacts, by Selected Patient Characteristics: 1994

Data are based on household interviews of a sample of the civilian noninstitutionalized population.

[In number of contacts per person]

Characteristic	1994
Total[1,2]	6.0
Age	
Under 15 years	4.6
Under 5 years	6.8
5-14 years	3.4
15-44 years	5.0
45-64 years	7.3

[Continued]

★ 25 ★

Physician Contacts, by Selected Patient Characteristics: 1994
[Continued]

Characteristic	1994
65 years and over	11.3
65-74 years	10.3
75 years and over	12.7
Sex and age	
Male[1]	5.2
Under 5 years	7.0
5-14 years	3.5
15-44 years	3.7
45-64 years	6.3
65-74 years	10.1
75 years and over	11.6
Female[1]	6.7
Under 5 years	6.5
5-14 years	3.3
15-44 years	6.2
45-64 years	8.3
65-74 years	10.5
75 years and over	13.4
Race and age	
White[1]	6.1
Under 5 years	7.1
5-14 years	3.7
15-44 years	5.1
45-64 years	7.4
65-74 years	10.5
75 years and over	12.4
Black[1]	5.7
Under 5 years	5.2
5-14 years	2.5
15-44 years	4.8
45-64 years	7.7
65-74 years	9.3
75 years and over	16.3
Family income[1]	
Under 5 years	7.6
5-14 years	5.9

[Continued]

★ 25 ★

Physician Contacts, by Selected Patient Characteristics: 1994

[Continued]

Characteristic	1994
15-44 years	5.8
45-64 years	6.2
65-74 years	6.0
75 years and over	
Geographic region[1]	
Northeast	5.9
Midwest	6.0
South	5.6
West	6.4
Location of residence[1]	
Within MSA	6.0
Outside MSA	5.7

Source: U.S. Department of Health and Human Services. Public Health Service. Centers for Disease Control and Prevention. National Center for Health Statistics. *Health, United States, 1995.* Hyattsville, MD: Public Health Service, 1996, p. 187. Primary source: Centers for Disease Control and Prevention, National Center for Health Statistics, Division of Health Interview Statistics. Data from National Health Interview Survey. *Note:* 1. Age adjusted.

Deaths

★ 26 ★

Causes of Death for American Indian or Alaska Native Females: 1993

The table shows the number of deaths from leading causes for American Indian or Alaska Native females in the United States.

Cause	Deaths
All causes	4,145
Heart disease	932
Malignant neoplasms	720
Injuries (unintentional)	377
Diabetes mellitus	275
Cerebrovascular diseases	256
Chronic liver disease and cirrhosis	181
Pneumonia and influenza	152
Chronic obstructive pulmonary diseases	142

[Continued]

★ 26 ★

Causes of Death for American Indian or Alaska Native Females: 1993
[Continued]

Cause	Deaths
Nephritis, nephrotic syndrome, and nephrosis	64
Suicide	58

Source: U.S. Department of Health and Human Services. Public Health Service. Centers for Disease Control and Prevention. National Center for Health Statistics. *Health, United States, 1995.* Hyattsville, MD: Public Health Service, 1996. p. 114. Primary source: Centers for Disease Control and Prevention, National Center for Health Statistics, Vital Statistics of the United States, vol. II, Mortality, part A, for data year 1993.

★ 27 ★

Deaths

Causes of Death for American Indian or Alaska Native Males: 1993

The table shows the number of deaths from leading causes for American Indian or Alaska Native males in the United States.

Cause	Deaths
All causes	5,434
Heart disease	1,283
Injuries (unintentional)	850
Malignant neoplasms	771
Chronic liver disease and cirrhosis	222
Suicide	198
Pneumonia and influenza	196
Cerebrovascular diseases	186
Diabetes mellitus	185
Homicide and legal intervention	182
Chronic obstructive pulmonary diseases	145

Source: U.S. Department of Health and Human Services. Public Health Service. Centers for Disease Control and Prevention. National Center for Health Statistics. *Health, United States, 1995.* Hyattsville, MD: Public Health Service, 1996. p. 114. Primary source: Centers for Disease Control and Prevention, National Center for Health Statistics, Vital Statistics of the United States, vol. II, Mortality, part A, for data year 1993.

★ 28 ★

Deaths

Causes of Death for Asian or Pacific Islander Females: 1993

The table shows the number of deaths from leading causes for Asian or Pacific Islander females in the United States.

Cause	Deaths
All causes	10,854
Malignant neoplasms	3,011
Heart disease	2,832
Cerebrovascular diseases	1,074
Injuries (unintentional)	519
Pneumonia and influenza	430
Diabetes mellitus	307
Chronic obstructive pulmonary diseases	239
Suicide	172
Congenital anomalies	139
Homicide and legal intervention	133

Source: U.S. Department of Health and Human Services. Public Health Service. Centers for Disease Control and Prevention. National Center for Health Statistics. *Health, United States, 1995.* Hyattsville, MD: Public Health Service, 1996. p. 114. Primary source: Centers for Disease Control and Prevention, National Center for Health Statistics, Vital Statistics of the United States, vol. II, Mortality, part A, for data year 1993.

★ 29 ★

Deaths

Causes of Death for Asian or Pacific Islander Males: 1993

The table shows the number of deaths from leading causes for Asian or Pacific Islander males in the United States.

Cause	Deaths
All causes	14,532
Heart disease	4,037
Malignant neoplasms	3,625
Cerebrovascular diseases	1,043
Injuries (unintentional)	852
Pneumonia and influenza	598
Chronic obstructive pulmonary diseases	501
Homicide and legal intervention	414
Suicide	380

[Continued]

★ 29 ★

Causes of Death for Asian or Pacific Islander Males: 1993

[Continued]

Cause	Deaths
Diabetes mellitus	286
HIV infection	226

Source: U.S. Department of Health and Human Services. Public Health Service. Centers for Disease Control and Prevention. National Center for Health Statistics. *Health, United States, 1995.* Hyattsville, MD: Public Health Service, 1996. p. 114. Primary source: Centers for Disease Control and Prevention, National Center for Health Statistics, Vital Statistics of the United States, vol. II, Mortality, part A, for data year 1993.

★ 30 ★

Deaths

Causes of Death for Black Females: 1993

The table shows the number of deaths from leading causes for black females in the United States.

Cause	Deaths
All causes	128,649
Heart disease	40,654
Malignant neoplasms	26,802
Cerebrovascular diseases	9,958
Diabetes mellitus	5,732
Injuries (unintentional)	3,807
Pneumonia and influenza	3,673
HIV infection	2,995
Perinatal conditions	2,582
Chronic obstructive pulmonary diseases	2,522
Homicide and legal intervention	2,297

Source: U.S. Department of Health and Human Services. Public Health Service. Centers for Disease Control and Prevention. National Center for Health Statistics. *Health, United States, 1995.* Hyattsville, MD: Public Health Service, 1996. p. 114. Primary source: Centers for Disease Control and Prevention, National Center for Health Statistics, Vital Statistics of the United States, vol. II, Mortality, part A, for data year 1993.

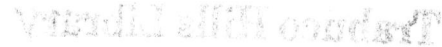

★ 31 ★

Deaths

Causes of Death for Black Males: 1993

The table shows the number of deaths from leading causes for black males in the United States.

Cause	Deaths
All causes	153,502
Heart disease	38,357
Malignant neoplasms	33,071
Homicide and legal intervention	10,640
HIV infection	10,324
Injuries (unintentional)	8,900
Cerebrovascular diseases	7,599
Pneumonia and influenza	4,051
Chronic obstructive pulmonary diseases	3,913
Diabetes mellitus	3,648
Perinatal conditions	3,309

Source: U.S. Department of Health and Human Services. Public Health Service. Centers for Disease Control and Prevention. National Center for Health Statistics. *Health, United States, 1995.* Hyattsville, MD: Public Health Service, 1996. p. 114. Primary source: Centers for Disease Control and Prevention, National Center for Health Statistics, Vital Statistics of the United States, vol. II, Mortality, part A, for data year 1993.

★ 32 ★

Deaths

Causes of Death for Hispanic Females: 1993

The table shows the number of deaths from leading causes for Hispanic females in the United States.

Cause	Deaths
All causes	34,758
Heart disease	9,567
Malignant neoplasms	7,253
Congenital anomalies	7,012
Cerebrovascular diseases	2,222
Diabetes mellitus	1,872
Injuries (unintentional)	1,680
Pneumonia and influenza	1,253
Chronic obstructive pulmonary diseases	906

[Continued]

★ 32 ★

Causes of Death for Hispanic Females: 1993
[Continued]

Cause	Deaths
Perinatal conditions	795
HIV infection	784

Source: U.S. Department of Health and Human Services. Public Health Service. Centers for Disease Control and Prevention. National Center for Health Statistics. *Health, United States, 1995.* Hyattsville, MD: Public Health Service, 1996. p. 114. Primary source: Centers for Disease Control and Prevention, National Center for Health Statistics, Vital Statistics of the United States, vol. II, Mortality, part A, for data year 1993.

★ 33 ★

Deaths

Causes of Death for Hispanic Males: 1993

The table shows the number of deaths from leading causes for Hispanic males in the United States.

Cause	Deaths
All causes	52,177
Heart disease	11,227
Malignant neoplasms	8,487
Injuries (unintentional)	5,884
HIV infection	4,045
Homicide and legal intervention	3,680
Cerebrovascular diseases	2,094
Chronic liver disease and cirrhosis	1,895
Suicide	1,513
Diabetes mellitus	1,471
Pneumonia and influenza	1,430

Source: U.S. Department of Health and Human Services. Public Health Service. Centers for Disease Control and Prevention. National Center for Health Statistics. *Health, United States, 1995.* Hyattsville, MD: Public Health Service, 1996. p. 114. Primary source: Centers for Disease Control and Prevention, National Center for Health Statistics, Vital Statistics of the United States, vol. II, Mortality, part A, for data year 1993.

★ 34 ★
Deaths

Causes of Death for White Females: 1993

The table shows the number of deaths from leading causes for white females in the United States.

Cause	Deaths
All causes	963,108
Heart disease	331,563
Malignant neoplasms	219,996
Cerebrovascular diseases	79,772
Chronic obstructive pulmonary diseases	43,803
Pneumonia and influenza	40,569
Injuries (unintentional)	25,703
Diabetes mellitus	24,150
Atherosclerosis	10,052
Nephritis, nephrotic syndrome, and nephrosis	9,685
Septicemia	9,609

Source: U.S. Department of Health and Human Services. Public Health Service. Centers for Disease Control and Prevention. National Center for Health Statistics. *Health, United States, 1995.* Hyattsville, MD: Public Health Service, 1996. p. 114. Primary source: Centers for Disease Control and Prevention, National Center for Health Statistics, Vital Statistics of the United States, vol. II, Mortality, part A, for data year 1993.

★ 35 ★
Deaths

Causes of Death for White Males: 1993

The table shows the number of deaths from leading causes for white males in the United States.

Cause	Deaths
All causes	988,329
Heart disease	323,802
Malignant neoplasms	241,908
Cerebrovascular diseases	50,220
Chronic obstructive pulmonary diseases	49,812
Injuries (unintentional)	49,515
Pneumonia and influenza	33,151
Suicide	22,524
HIV infection	21,455

[Continued]

★ 35 ★

Causes of Death for White Males: 1993

[Continued]

Cause	Deaths
Diabetes mellitus	19,311
Chronic liver disease and cirrhosis	13,621

Source: U.S. Department of Health and Human Services. Public Health Service. Centers for Disease Control and Prevention. National Center for Health Statistics. *Health, United States, 1995.* Hyattsville, MD: Public Health Service, 1996. p. 114. Primary source: Centers for Disease Control and Prevention, National Center for Health Statistics, Vital Statistics of the United States, vol. II, Mortality, part A, for data year 1993.

★ 36 ★

Deaths

Death Rates, by Age, Sex, and Race: 1970 to 1994

Number of deaths per 100,000 population in specified group. Excludes deaths of nonresidents of the U.S. (except as noted) and fetal deaths. The standard population for this table is the total population of the U.S. enumerated in 1940.

SEX, YEAR, AND RACE	All ages[1]	Under 1 year	1-4 years	5-14 years	15-24 years	25-34 years	35-44 years	45-54 years	55-64 years	65-74 years	75-84 years	85 years and over
MALE, TOTAL[2]												
1970	1,090	2,410	93	51	189	215	403	959	2,283	4,874	10,010	17,822
1980	977	1,429	73	37	172	196	299	767	1,815	4,105	8,817	18,801
1985	949	1,220	59	32	139	180	279	672	1,711	3,856	8,502	18,614
1986	945	1,174	58	32	149	195	289	656	1,670	3,787	8,360	18,351
1987	939	1,150	58	32	143	195	292	648	1,649	3,717	8,241	18,212
1988	945	1,145	57	31	147	200	302	633	1,635	3,682	8,237	18,711
1989	926	1,133	55	31	142	204	308	622	1,596	3,558	7,957	18,019
1990	918	1,083	52	29	147	204	310	610	1,553	3,492	7,889	18,057
1991	912	1,024	52	29	148	204	312	605	1,525	3,439	7,689	17,801
1992	902	957	48	27	142	202	319	592	1,482	3,374	7,483	17,740
1993	924	946	50	27	146	209	329	596	1,480	3,395	7,653	18,257
1994	919	899	52	26	151	207	337	585	1,467	3,347	7,490	17,936
White male												
1970	1,087	2,113	84	48	171	177	344	883	2,203	4,810	10,099	18,552
1980	983	1,230	66	35	167	171	257	699	1,729	4,036	8,830	19,097
1985	964	1,057	53	30	134	159	243	612	1,626	3,771	8,486	18,980
1988	958	964	52	29	136	173	260	569	1,547	3,588	8,197	19,021
1989	937	941	48	28	129	177	263	556	1,504	3,455	7,913	18,242
1990	931	896	46	26	131	176	268	549	1,467	3,398	7,845	18,268
1991	926	861	46	27	128	176	269	545	1,444	3,350	7,642	18,021
1992	917	781	43	25	122	176	277	533	1,399	3,287	7,441	17,956
1993	939	773	43	25	123	181	283	534	1,395	3,307	7,597	18,443
1994	934	732	44	23	130	179	289	523	1,382	3,261	7,434	18,127
Black male												
1970	1,187	4,299	151	67	321	560	957	1,778	3,257	5,803	9,455	12,222
1980	1,034	2,587	111	47	209	407	690	1,480	2,873	5,131	9,232	16,099

[Continued]

★ 36 ★

Death Rates, by Age, Sex, and Race: 1970 to 1994
[Continued]

SEX, YEAR, AND RACE	All ages[1]	Under 1 year	1-4 years	5-14 years	15-24 years	25-34 years	35-44 years	45-54 years	55-64 years	65-74 years	75-84 years	85 years and over
1985	989	2,220	90	42	174	352	630	1,293	2,780	5,172	9,262	15,774
1988	1,026	2,190	92	44	222	417	707	1,297	2,713	5,148	9,455	16,643
1989	1,027	2,172	90	44	235	426	718	1,312	2,700	5,130	9,163	16,752
1990	1,008	2,112	86	41	252	431	700	1,261	2,618	4,946	9,130	16,955
1991	999	1,957	88	42	278	426	702	1,257	2,534	4,851	9,013	16,664
1992	978	1,958	78	41	269	413	697	1,223	2,494	4,747	8,745	16,717
1993	1,006	1,922	86	41	289	429	730	1,266	2,518	4,791	9,013	17,033
1994	994	1,831	87	43	274	411	759	1,227	2,460	4,717	8,915	16,645
FEMALE, TOTAL[2]												
1970	808	1,864	75	32	68	102	231	517	1,099	2,580	6,678	15,518
1980	785	1,142	55	24	58	76	159	413	934	2,145	5,440	14,747
1985	809	951	45	21	50	69	139	375	926	2,097	5,162	14,554
1986	812	923	46	20	52	72	140	368	914	2,096	5,088	14,494
1987	817	919	46	19	51	75	139	364	909	2,069	5,045	14,514
1988	831	921	46	21	52	75	140	355	916	2,064	5,091	14,851
1989	819	917	46	21	51	76	139	345	894	2,020	4,967	14,395
1990	812	856	41	19	49	74	138	343	879	1,991	4,883	14,274
1991	811	804	43	18	50	74	139	339	873	1,977	4,801	14,067
1992	807	771	39	18	47	74	141	326	855	1,971	4,731	13,901
1993	839	759	40	19	49	76	144	330	861	2,001	4,899	14,417
1994	839	719	37	19	47	76	144	326	843	1,989	4,921	14,301
White female												
1970	813	1,615	66	30	62	84	193	463	1,015	2,471	6,699	15,980
1980	806	963	49	23	56	65	138	373	876	2,067	5,402	14,980
1985	840	799	40	20	48	59	122	342	869	2,027	5,112	14,745
1988	865	754	41	19	49	63	120	320	859	1,996	5,040	15,019
1989	852	740	39	19	48	63	119	311	838	1,949	4,911	14,526
1990	847	690	36	18	46	62	117	309	823	1,924	4,839	14,401
1991	848	659	38	17	47	62	117	306	822	1,909	4,753	14,188
1992	844	619	33	16	44	61	117	294	799	1,909	4,696	14,016
1993	879	618	34	17	44	63	120	297	811	1,938	4,845	14,558
1994	883	608	31	17	43	63	120	291	789	1,929	4,878	14,460
Black female												
1970	829	3,369	129	44	112	231	533	1,044	1,986	3,861	6,692	10,707
1980	733	2,124	84	31	71	150	324	768	1,561	3,057	6,212	12,367
1985	734	1,821	71	29	60	138	277	668	1,533	2,968	6,078	12,703
1988	765	1,834	71	31	69	158	305	655	1,513	2,948	5,991	13,461
1989	763	1,840	73	29	68	161	299	641	1,478	2,936	5,930	13,509
1990	748	1,736	68	28	69	160	299	639	1,453	2,866	5,688	13,310
1991	745	1,581	71	26	73	159	304	633	1,400	2,854	5,707	13,259
1992	736	1,610	69	26	68	159	314	621	1,405	2,797	5,483	13,264

[Continued]

★ 36 ★

Death Rates, by Age, Sex, and Race: 1970 to 1994

[Continued]

SEX, YEAR, AND RACE	All ages[1]	Under 1 year	1-4 years	5-14 years	15-24 years	25-34 years	35-44 years	45-54 years	55-64 years	65-74 years	75-84 years	85 years and over
1993	760	1,543	72	30	73	165	317	632	1,364	2,857	5,887	13,351
1994	750	1,308	74	27	68	158	320	630	1,358	2,827	5,806	13,138

Source: 1996 Statistical Abstract of the United States on CD-ROM [machine-readable datafiles]. CD-8A-97. Washington, DC: U.S. Department of Commerce, Economics and Statistics Administration, Bureau of the Census, Data User Services Division, January 1997. Primary source: U.S. National Center for Health Statistics, *Vital Statistics of the United States,* annual; *Monthly Vital Statistics Report;* and unpublished data. *Notes:* 1. Includes unknown age. 2. Includes other races not shown separately.

★ 37 ★

Deaths

Death Rates from Accidents and Violence, by Race and Sex: 1980 to 1993

Rates are per 100,000 population. Excludes deaths of nonresidents of the United States. Deaths classified according to the ninth revision of the *International Classification of Diseases*.

CAUSE OF DEATH AND AGE	WHITE						BLACK					
	MALE			FEMALE			MALE			FEMALE		
	1980	1990	1993	1980	1990	1993	1980	1990	1993	1980	1990	1993
Total[1]	97.1	81.2	77.0	36.3	32.1	31.5	154.0	142.0	140.6	42.6	38.6	38.2
Motor vehicle accidents	35.9	26.1	22.7	12.8	11.4	10.3	31.1	28.1	24.6	8.3	9.4	8.7
All other accidents	30.4	23.6	24.3	14.4	12.4	13.2	46.0	32.7	33.7	18.6	13.4	13.8
Suicide	19.9	22.0	21.4	5.9	5.3	5.0	10.3	12.0	12.5	2.2	2.3	2.1
Homicide	10.9	9.0	8.6	3.2	2.8	3.0	66.6	69.2	69.7	13.5	13.5	13.6
15 to 24 years old	138.6	107.3	99.1	37.3	30.5	28.2	162.0	208.0	242.2	35.0	34.9	39.9
25 to 34 years old	118.4	97.4	92.0	29.0	26.0	24.8	256.9	218.1	197.3	49.4	48.1	46.2
35 to 44 years old	94.1	82.3	82.9	29.2	24.4	24.9	218.1	176.6	169.9	43.2	38.5	40.1
45 to 54 years old	90.8	73.5	70.5	31.8	25.3	24.3	207.3	138.5	137.2	40.2	30.7	28.7
55 to 64 years old	92.3	79.5	71.7	33.8	29.4	26.7	188.5	129.9	112.1	47.3	36.1	31.9
65 years old and over	163.9	150.7	157.1	87.2	80.1	78.6	215.8	175.5	164.3	102.9	81.6	70.8
65 to 74 years old	116.7	99.7	91.1	46.4	40.5	39.0	182.2	141.8	136.3	68.7	50.4	47.1
75 to 84 years old	209.2	195.7	187.3	101.5	89.4	87.1	261.4	206.1	185.9	137.5	95.8	94.9
85 years old and over	438.5	428.3	449.1	268.1	232.4	236.2	379.2	359.1	399.2	235.7	213.0	190.3

Source: 1996 Statistical Abstract of the United States on CD-ROM [machine-readable datafiles]. CD-8A-97. Washington, DC: U.S. Department of Commerce, Economics and Statistics Administration, Bureau of the Census, Data User Services Division, January 1997. Primary source: National Center for Health Statistics, *Vital Statistics of the United States,* annual; and unpublished data. *Note:* 1. Includes persons under 15 years old, not shown separately.

★ 38 ★
Deaths

Death Rates of Men, by Age and Race: 1970 to 1994

Number of deaths per 100,000 population in specified group. Excludes deaths of nonresidents of the U.S. (except as noted) and fetal deaths. The standard population for this table is the total population of the U.S. enumerated in 1940.

YEAR, RACE	All ages[1]	Under 1 year	1-4 years	5-14 years	15-24 years	25-34 years	35-44 years	45-54 years	55-64 years	65-74 years	75-84 years	85 years and over
TOTAL[2]												
1970	1,090	2,410	93	51	189	215	403	959	2,283	4,874	10,010	17,822
1980	977	1,429	73	37	172	196	299	767	1,815	4,105	8,817	18,801
1985	949	1,220	59	32	139	180	279	672	1,711	3,856	8,502	18,614
1986	945	1,174	58	32	149	195	289	656	1,670	3,787	8,360	18,351
1987	939	1,150	58	32	143	195	292	648	1,649	3,717	8,241	18,212
1988	945	1,145	57	31	147	200	302	633	1,635	3,682	8,237	18,711
1989	926	1,133	55	31	142	204	308	622	1,596	3,558	7,957	18,019
1990	918	1,083	52	29	147	204	310	610	1,553	3,492	7,889	18,057
1991	912	1,024	52	29	148	204	312	605	1,525	3,439	7,689	17,801
1992	902	957	48	27	142	202	319	592	1,482	3,374	7,483	17,740
1993	924	946	50	27	146	209	329	596	1,480	3,395	7,653	18,257
1994	919	899	52	26	151	207	337	585	1,467	3,347	7,490	17,936
White												
1970	1,087	2,113	84	48	171	177	344	883	2,203	4,810	10,099	18,552
1980	983	1,230	66	35	167	171	257	699	1,729	4,036	8,830	19,097
1985	964	1,057	53	30	134	159	243	612	1,626	3,771	8,486	18,980
1988	958	964	52	29	136	173	260	569	1,547	3,588	8,197	19,021
1989	937	941	48	28	129	177	263	556	1,504	3,455	7,913	18,242
1990	931	896	46	26	131	176	268	549	1,467	3,398	7,845	18,268
1991	926	861	46	27	128	176	269	545	1,444	3,350	7,642	18,021
1992	917	781	43	25	122	176	277	533	1,399	3,287	7,441	17,956
1993	939	773	43	25	123	181	283	534	1,395	3,307	7,597	18,443
1994	934	732	44	23	130	179	289	523	1,382	3,261	7,434	18,127
Black												
1970	1,187	4,299	151	67	321	560	957	1,778	3,257	5,803	9,455	12,222
1980	1,034	2,587	111	47	209	407	690	1,480	2,873	5,131	9,232	16,099
1985	989	2,220	90	42	174	352	630	1,293	2,780	5,172	9,262	15,774
1988	1,026	2,190	92	44	222	417	707	1,297	2,713	5,148	9,455	16,643
1989	1,027	2,172	90	44	235	426	718	1,312	2,700	5,130	9,163	16,752
1990	1,008	2,112	86	41	252	431	700	1,261	2,618	4,946	9,130	16,955
1991	999	1,957	88	42	278	426	702	1,257	2,534	4,851	9,013	16,664
1992	978	1,958	78	41	269	413	697	1,223	2,494	4,747	8,745	16,717
1993	1,006	1,922	86	41	289	429	730	1,266	2,518	4,791	9,013	17,033
1994	994	1,831	87	43	274	411	759	1,227	2,460	4,717	8,915	16,645

Source: 1996 Statistical Abstract of the United States on CD-ROM [machine-readable datafiles]. CD-8A-97. Washington, DC: U.S. Department of Commerce, Economics and Statistics Administration, Bureau of the Census, Data User Services Division, January 1997. Primary source: U.S. National Center for Health Statistics, *Vital Statistics of the United States*, annual; *Monthly Vital Statistics Report*; and unpublished data. *Notes:* 1. Includes unknown age. 2. Includes other races not shown separately.

★ 39 ★

Deaths

Death Rates of Women, by Age and Race: 1970 to 1994

Number of deaths per 100,000 population in specified group. Excludes deaths of nonresidents of the U.S. (except as noted) and fetal deaths. The standard population for this table is the total population of the U.S. enumerated in 1940.

YEAR, RACE	All ages[1]	Under 1 year	1-4 years	5-14 years	15-24 years	25-34 years	35-44 years	45-54 years	55-64 years	65-74 years	75-84 years	85 years and over
TOTAL[2]												
1970	808	1,864	75	32	68	102	231	517	1,099	2,580	6,678	15,518
1980	785	1,142	55	24	58	76	159	413	934	2,145	5,440	14,747
1985	809	951	45	21	50	69	139	375	926	2,097	5,162	14,554
1986	812	923	46	20	52	72	140	368	914	2,096	5,088	14,494
1987	817	919	46	19	51	75	139	364	909	2,069	5,045	14,514
1988	831	921	46	21	52	75	140	355	916	2,064	5,091	14,851
1989	819	917	46	21	51	76	139	345	894	2,020	4,967	14,395
1990	812	856	41	19	49	74	138	343	879	1,991	4,883	14,274
1991	811	804	43	18	50	74	139	339	873	1,977	4,801	14,067
1992	807	771	39	18	47	74	141	326	855	1,971	4,731	13,901
1993	839	759	40	19	49	76	144	330	861	2,001	4,899	14,417
1994	839	719	37	19	47	76	144	326	843	1,989	4,921	14,301
White												
1970	813	1,615	66	30	62	84	193	463	1,015	2,471	6,699	15,980
1980	806	963	49	23	56	65	138	373	876	2,067	5,402	14,980
1985	840	799	40	20	48	59	122	342	869	2,027	5,112	14,745
1988	865	754	41	19	49	63	120	320	859	1,996	5,040	15,019
1989	852	740	39	19	48	63	119	311	838	1,949	4,911	14,526
1990	847	690	36	18	46	62	117	309	823	1,924	4,839	14,401
1991	848	659	38	17	47	62	117	306	822	1,909	4,753	14,188
1992	844	619	33	16	44	61	117	294	799	1,909	4,696	14,016
1993	879	618	34	17	44	63	120	297	811	1,938	4,845	14,558
1994	883	608	31	17	43	63	120	291	789	1,929	4,878	14,460
Black												
1970	829	3,369	129	44	112	231	533	1,044	1,986	3,861	6,692	10,707
1980	733	2,124	84	31	71	150	324	768	1,561	3,057	6,212	12,367
1985	734	1,821	71	29	60	138	277	668	1,533	2,968	6,078	12,703
1988	765	1,834	71	31	69	158	305	655	1,513	2,948	5,991	13,461
1989	763	1,840	73	29	68	161	299	641	1,478	2,936	5,930	13,509
1990	748	1,736	68	28	69	160	299	639	1,453	2,866	5,688	13,310
1991	745	1,581	71	26	73	159	304	633	1,400	2,854	5,707	13,259
1992	736	1,610	69	26	68	159	314	621	1,405	2,797	5,483	13,264
1993	760	1,543	72	30	73	165	317	632	1,364	2,857	5,887	13,351
1994	750	1,308	74	27	68	158	320	630	1,358	2,827	5,806	13,138

Source: 1996 Statistical Abstract of the United States on CD-ROM [machine-readable datafiles]. CD-8A-97. Washington, DC: U.S. Department of Commerce, Economics and Statistics Administration, Bureau of the Census, Data User Services Division, January 1997. Primary source: U.S. National Center for Health Statistics, *Vital Statistics of the United States*, annual; *Monthly Vital Statistics Report*; and unpublished data. *Notes:* 1. Includes unknown age. 2. Includes other races not shown separately.

★ 40 ★

Deaths

Deaths and Death Rates, by Selected Causes: 1970 to 1994

CAUSE OF DEATH	DEATHS (1,000)					CRUDE DEATH RATE PER 100,000 POPULATION[2]				
	1970	1980	1990	1993[1]	1994[1]	1970	1980	1990	1993[1]	1994[1]
All causes	1,921.0	1,989.8	2,148.5	2,268.6	2,286.0	945.3	878.3	863.8	880.0	876.9
Major cardiovascular diseases	1,008.0	988.5	916.0	948.1	945.2	496.0	436.4	368.3	367.8	362.6
Diseases of heart	735.5	761.1	720.1	743.5	734.1	362.0	336.0	289.5	288.4	281.6
Percent of total	38.3	38.3	33.5	32.8	32.1	38.3	38.3	33.5	32.8	32.1
Rheumatic fever and rheumatic heart disease	14.9	7.8	6.0	5.7	5.5	7.3	3.5	2.4	2.2	2.1
Hypertensive heart disease[3]	15.0	24.8	23.4	23.0	23.8	7.4	10.9	9.5	8.9	9.1
Ischemic heart disease	666.7	565.8	489.2	490.1	487.5	328.1	249.7	196.7	190.1	187.0
Other diseases of endocardium	6.7	7.2	13.0	15.2	14.5	3.3	3.2	5.2	5.9	5.6
All other forms of heart disease	32.3	155.5	188.4	207.0	200.1	15.9	68.7	75.8	80.3	76.8
Hypertension[3]	8.3	7.8	9.2	11.2	11.7	4.1	3.5	3.7	4.4	4.5
Cerebrovascular diseases	207.2	170.2	144.1	150.1	154.4	101.9	75.1	57.9	58.2	59.2
Atherosclerosis	31.7	29.4	18.0	17.3	18.0	15.6	13.0	7.3	6.7	6.9
Other	25.3	20.0	24.6	26.0	27.1	12.5	8.8	9.9	10.1	10.4
Malignancies[4]	330.7	416.5	505.3	529.9	536.9	162.8	183.9	203.2	205.6	206.0
Percent of total	17.2	20.9	23.5	23.4	23.5	17.2	20.9	23.5	23.4	23.5
Of respiratory and intrathoracic organs	69.5	108.5	146.4	154.2	154.3	34.2	47.9	58.9	59.8	59.2
Of digestive organs and peritoneum	94.7	110.6	120.8	124.5	127.2	46.6	48.8	48.6	48.3	48.8
Of genital organs	41.2	46.4	57.5	60.4	62.1	20.3	20.5	23.1	23.4	23.8
Of breast	29.9	35.9	43.7	43.9	43.3	14.7	15.8	17.6	17.0	16.6
Of urinary organs	15.5	17.8	20.7	21.8	22.0	7.6	7.9	8.3	8.4	8.4
Leukemia	14.5	16.5	18.6	19.5	20.1	7.1	7.3	7.5	7.6	7.7
Accidents and adverse effects	114.6	105.7	92.0	90.5	90.1	56.4	46.7	37.0	35.1	34.6
Motor vehicle	54.6	53.2	46.8	41.9	42.2	26.9	23.5	18.8	16.3	16.2
All other	60.0	52.5	45.2	48.6	48.0	29.5	23.3	18.2	18.9	18.4
Chronic obstructive pulmonary diseases and allied conditions[5]	30.9	56.1	86.7	101.1	101.9	15.2	24.7	34.9	39.2	39.1
Bronchitis, chronic and unspecified	5.8	3.7	3.6	3.8	3.6	2.9	1.6	1.4	1.5	1.4
Emphysema	22.7	13.9	15.7	17.6	17.3	11.2	6.1	6.3	6.8	6.6
Asthma	2.3	2.9	4.8	5.2	5.7	1.1	1.3	1.9	2.0	2.2
Other	[6]	35.6	62.6	74.5	75.3	[6]	15.7	25.2	28.9	28.9
Pneumonia and influenza	62.7	54.6	79.5	82.8	82.1	30.9	24.1	32.0	32.1	31.5
Pneumonia	59.0	51.9	77.4	81.8	80.8	29.0	22.9	31.1	31.7	31.0
Influenza	3.7	2.7	2.1	1.0	1.3	1.8	1.2	0.8	0.4	0.5
Diabetes mellitus	38.3	34.9	47.7	53.9	55.4	18.9	15.4	19.2	20.9	21.2
Suicide	23.5	26.9	30.9	31.1	32.4	11.6	11.9	12.4	12.1	12.4
Chronic liver disease and cirrhosis	31.4	30.6	25.8	25.2	25.7	15.5	13.5	10.4	9.8	9.9
Other infectious and parasitic diseases	6.9	5.1	32.2	44.4	48.5	3.4	2.2	13.0	17.2	18.6
Homicide and legal intervention	16.8	24.3	24.9	26.0	23.7	8.3	10.7	10.0	10.1	9.1
Nephritis, nephrotic syndrome, and nephrosis	8.9	16.8	20.8	23.3	23.6	4.4	7.4	8.3	9.0	9.1
Septicemia	3.5	9.4	19.2	20.6	19.9	1.7	4.2	7.7	8.0	7.6
Certain conditions originating in the perinatal period	43.2	22.9	17.7	15.1	14.1	21.3	10.1	7.1	5.9	5.4
Congenital anomalies	16.8	13.9	13.1	12.4	11.9	8.3	6.2	5.3	4.8	4.6
Benign neoplasms[7]	4.8	6.2	6.8	7.4	7.0	2.4	2.7	2.7	2.9	2.7
Ulcer of stomach and duodenum	8.6	6.1	6.2	5.9	6.0	4.2	0.0	2.5	2.3	2.3
Hernia of abdominal cavity and intestinal obstruction[8]	7.2	5.4	5.8	5.9	6.0	3.6	2.4	2.3	2.3	2.3
Anemias	3.4	3.2	4.1	4.3	4.2	1.7	1.4	1.6	1.7	1.6
Cholelithiasis and other disorders of gall bladder	4.0	3.3	3.0	2.8	2.6	2.0	1.5	1.2	1.1	1.0
Nutritional deficiencies	2.5	2.4	3.0	3.5	3.2	1.2	1.0	1.2	1.3	1.2
Tuberculosis	5.2	2.0	1.8	1.6	1.6	2.6	0.9	0.7	0.6	0.6
Infections of kidney	8.2	2.7	1.3	1.0	1.0	4.0	1.2	0.5	0.4	0.4

[Continued]

★ 40 ★

Deaths and Death Rates, by Selected Causes: 1970 to 1994

[Continued]

CAUSE OF DEATH	DEATHS (1,000)					CRUDE DEATH RATE PER 100,000 POPULATION[2]				
	1970	1980	1990	1993[1]	1994[1]	1970	1980	1990	1993[1]	1994[1]
Viral hepatitis	1.0	0.8	1.6	2.5	2.8	0.5	0.4	0.6	1.0	1.1
Meningitis	1.7	1.4	1.0	0.8	0.9	0.8	0.6	0.4	0.3	0.4
Acute bronchitis and bronchiolitis	1.3	0.6	0.6	0.7	0.5	0.6	0.3	0.3	0.3	0.2
Hyperplasia of prostate	2.2	0.8	0.5	0.4	0.5	1.1	0.3	0.2	0.2	0.2
Symptoms, signs, and ill-defined conditions	25.8	28.8	24.1	26.5	26.6	12.7	12.7	9.7	10.3	10.2
All other causes	108.8	120.0	172.9	195.6	206.1	53.5	53.0	69.5	75.9	79.1

Source: 1996 Statistical Abstract of the United States on CD-ROM [machine-readable datafiles]. CD-8A-97. Washington, DC: U.S. Department of Commerce, Economics and Statistics Administration, Bureau of ththe Census, Data User Services Division, January 1997. Primary source: U.S. National Center for Health Statistics, *Vital Statistics of the United States,* annual; *Monthly Vital Statistics Report;* and unpublished data. *Notes:* 1. Based on a 10-percent sample of deaths. Includes deaths of nonresidents. 2. 1970, 1980, and 1990 based on resident population enumerated as of April 1. Other years based on resident population estimated as of July 1. 3. With or without renal disease. 4. Includes other types of malignancies not shown separately. 5. Prior to 1980, data are shown for bronchitis, emphysema, and asthma. 6. Included in "all other causes." Comparable data not available separately. 7. Includes neoplasms of unspecified nature; beginning 1980 also includes carcinoma in situ. 8. Without mention of hernia.

★ 41 ★

Deaths

Deaths and Death Rates, by State: 1980 to 1994

By State of residence. Excludes deaths of nonresidents of the United States, except as noted. Caution should be used in comparing death rates by State; rates are affected by the population composition of the area.

DIVISION AND STATE	1980	1985	1990	1991[1]	1992	1993	1994
NUMBER OF DEATHS (1,000)							
United States	1,990	2,086	2,148	2,165	2,176	2,269	2,286
New England	115	118	115	112	116	120	117
Maine	11	11	11	11	11	12	11
New Hampshire	8	8	8	9	9	9	9
Vermont	5	5	5	5	5	5	5
Massachusetts	55	56	53	51	54	56	55
Rhode Island	9	10	10	9	9	10	9
Connecticut	27	28	28	28	28	29	29
Middle Atlantic	365	367	361	360	361	370	369
New York	173	172	169	167	166	171	168
New Jersey	69	71	70	70	71	73	73
Pennsylvania	124	124	122	124	124	126	128
East North Central	365	370	373	379	373	389	395
Ohio	98	99	99	99	99	103	106
Indiana	47	48	50	52	50	52	53
Illinois	103	102	103	105	102	107	108
Michigan	75	79	79	80	79	83	83
Wisconsin	41	41	43	44	42	45	45
West North Central	159	162	161	164	162	169	170

[Continued]

★ 41 ★

Deaths and Death Rates, by State: 1980 to 1994
[Continued]

DIVISION AND STATE	1980	1985	1990	1991[1]	1992	1993	1994
Minnesota	33	35	35	35	35	36	36
Iowa	27	28	27	26	27	28	26
Missouri	50	50	50	53	51	54	56
North Dakota	6	6	6	6	6	6	6
South Dakota	7	7	6	7	7	7	7
Nebraska	14	15	15	15	15	15	15
Kansas	22	22	22	23	22	24	24
South Atlantic	330	364	392	397	404	423	429
Delaware	5	5	6	6	6	6	6
Maryland	34	37	38	38	39	40	41
District of Columbia	7	7	7	7	7	7	7
Virginia	43	45	48	49	49	52	54
West Virginia	19	19	19	20	20	20	20
North Carolina	48	53	57	59	60	62	65
South Carolina	25	27	30	30	31	32	32
Georgia	44	49	52	53	53	56	56
Florida	105	121	134	135	140	147	148
East South Central	134	140	146	144	146	154	156
Kentucky	34	35	35	35	35	37	37
Tennessee	41	43	46	45	47	49	50
Alabama	36	38	39	38	39	41	42
Mississippi	24	25	25	26	25	26	27
West South Central	195	209	218	222	222	233	237
Arkansas	23	24	25	24	25	27	27
Louisiana	36	37	38	38	38	40	40
Oklahoma	28	30	30	30	31	32	32
Texas	108	118	125	129	129	135	138
Mountain	80	88	97	99	103	110	113
Montana	7	7	7	7	7	7	7
Idaho	7	7	7	8	8	8	9
Wyoming	3	3	3	3	3	3	4
Colorado	19	20	22	22	22	24	24
New Mexico	9	10	11	11	11	12	12
Arizona	21	25	29	29	31	33	35
Utah	8	9	9	9	10	10	11
Nevada	6	7	9	9	10	11	12
Pacific	247	268	286	290	289	300	301
Washington	32	35	37	38	38	40	40
Oregon	22	24	25	25	26	28	27
California	187	202	214	219	216	222	224
Alaska	2	2	2	2	2	2	2
Hawaii	5	6	7	7	7	7	7
RATE PER 1,000 POPULATION [2]							
United States	8.8	8.8	8.6	8.6	8.5	8.8	8.8

[Continued]

★ 41 ★

Deaths and Death Rates, by State: 1980 to 1994
[Continued]

DIVISION AND STATE	1980	1985	1990	1991[1]	1992	1993	1994
New England	9.3	9.3	8.7	8.5	8.8	9.1	8.8
Maine	9.6	9.8	9.0	8.9	9.0	9.3	9.2
New Hampshire	8.3	8.5	7.7	7.7	7.7	7.9	7.8
Vermont	9.0	8.8	8.2	8.0	8.4	8.5	7.9
Massachusetts	9.6	9.5	8.8	8.6	9.0	9.4	9.0
Rhode Island	9.8	10.0	9.5	9.2	9.5	9.7	9.4
Connecticut	8.8	8.8	8.4	8.4	8.6	8.9	8.7
Middle Atlantic	9.9	9.9	9.6	9.5	9.5	9.7	9.7
New York	9.8	9.7	9.4	9.2	9.2	9.4	9.2
New Jersey	9.4	9.4	9.1	9.0	9.1	9.2	9.2
Pennsylvania	10.4	10.5	10.3	10.3	10.3	10.5	10.6
East North Central	8.8	8.9	8.9	8.9	8.7	9.0	9.1
Ohio	9.1	9.2	9.1	9.1	9.0	9.1	9.5
Indiana	8.6	8.8	8.9	9.2	8.8	9.1	9.3
Illinois	9.0	9.0	9.0	9.1	8.8	9.2	9.2
Michigan	8.1	8.7	8.5	8.5	8.4	8.7	8.8
Wisconsin	8.7	8.7	8.7	8.8	8.5	8.7	8.8
West North Central	9.2	9.3	9.1	9.2	9.0	9.6	9.3
Minnesota	8.2	8.3	7.9	8.0	7.8	8.0	8.0
Iowa	9.3	9.8	9.7	9.3	9.5	9.9	9.3
Missouri	10.1	10.1	9.8	10.4	9.8	10.8	10.6
North Dakota	8.6	8.3	8.9	8.9	9.0	9.3	9.6
South Dakota	9.5	9.5	9.1	9.4	9.5	9.6	9.5
Nebraska	9.2	9.4	9.4	9.2	9.2	9.6	9.1
Kansas	9.3	9.1	9.0	9.0	8.8	9.2	9.2
South Atlantic	8.9	9.1	9.0	8.9	9.0	9.3	9.2
Delaware	8.5	8.9	8.7	8.6	8.6	8.7	8.8
Maryland	8.1	8.3	8.0	7.8	7.9	8.7	8.1
District of Columbia	11.1	11.0	12.0	11.7	12.1	11.6	12.1
Virginia	8.0	7.9	7.8	7.8	7.7	8.0	8.2
West Virginia	9.9	10.2	10.8	11.0	10.9	11.0	11.1
North Carolina	8.2	8.5	8.6	8.7	8.7	9.0	9.1
South Carolina	8.1	8.2	8.5	8.4	8.5	8.6	8.6
Georgia	8.1	8.2	8.0	8.0	7.8	8.1	8.0
Florida	10.7	10.7	10.4	10.2	10.4	10.7	10.6
East South Central	9.1	9.4	9.6	9.4	9.4	9.8	9.8
Kentucky	9.2	9.4	9.5	9.5	9.3	9.7	9.8
Tennessee	8.9	9.2	9.5	9.2	9.3	9.7	9.6
Alabama	9.1	9.5	9.7	9.3	9.5	9.9	10.0
Mississippi	9.4	9.5	9.8	9.9	9.7	10.1	10.1
West South Central	8.2	8.0	8.2	8.2	8.1	8.4	8.4
Arkansas	9.9	10.4	10.5	10.2	10.4	10.9	10.9
Louisiana	8.5	8.4	8.9	9.0	8.8	9.3	9.4
Oklahoma	9.3	9.1	9.7	9.6	9.5	10.1	10.0
Texas	7.6	7.3	7.4	7.4	7.3	7.5	7.5
Mountain	7.0	6.9	7.1	7.1	7.2	7.3	7.4

[Continued]

★ 41 ★

Deaths and Death Rates, by State: 1980 to 1994

[Continued]

DIVISION AND STATE	1980	1985	1990	1991[1]	1992	1993	1994
Montana	8.5	8.2	8.6	8.7	8.6	8.9	8.6
Idaho	7.2	7.2	7.4	7.5	7.4	7.6	7.5
Wyoming	6.9	6.6	7.1	6.9	7.1	7.5	7.4
Colorado	6.6	6.3	6.6	6.6	6.5	6.7	6.7
New Mexico	7.0	6.8	7.0	7.2	7.1	7.3	7.4
Arizona	7.9	7.7	7.9	7.8	8.1	8.2	8.5
Utah	5.6	5.5	5.3	5.2	5.4	5.5	5.5
Nevada	7.4	7.6	7.8	7.2	7.7	7.8	8.1
Pacific	7.8	7.6	7.3	7.3	7.1	7.2	7.2
Washington	7.7	7.8	7.6	7.5	7.4	8.0	7.4
Oregon	8.3	8.9	8.8	8.6	8.7	9.0	8.8
California	7.9	7.6	7.2	7.2	7.0	7.0	7.1
Alaska	4.3	3.9	4.0	3.8	3.9	3.8	4.0
Hawaii	5.2	5.6	6.1	5.9	6.0	6.2	6.1

Source: 1996 Statistical Abstract of the United States on CD-ROM [machine-readable datafiles]. CD-8A-97. Washington, DC: U.S. Department of Commerce, Economics and Statistics Administration, Bureau of the Census, Data User Services Division, January 1997. Primary source: U.S. National Center for Health Statistics, *Vital Statistics of the United States*, annual; and *Monthly Vital Statistics Report. Notes:* 1. Includes deaths of nonresidents. 2. Rates based on enumerated resident population as of April 1, for 1980 and 1990; estimated resident population as of July 1, for all other years.

★ 42 ★

Deaths

Deaths and Death Rates from Accidents, by Type: 1970 to 1993

Excludes deaths of nonresidents of the United States. Beginning 1980, deaths classified according to the ninth revision of the *International Classification of Diseases*. For earlier years, classified according to the revision in use at the time.

TYPE OF ACCIDENT	DEATHS (number)					RATE PER 100,000 POPULATION				
	1970	1980	1990	1992	1993	1970	1980	1990	1992	1993
Total	114,638	105,718	91,983	86,777	90,523	56.4	46.7	37.0	34.0	35.1
Motor-vehicle accidents	54,633	53,172	46,814	40,982	41,893	26.9	23.5	18.8	16.1	16.3
Traffic	53,493	51,930	45,827	39,985	40,899	26.3	22.9	18.4	15.7	15.9
Nontraffic	1,140	1,242	987	997	994	0.6	0.5	0.4	0.4	0.4
Water-transport accidents	1,651	1,429	923	837	763	0.8	0.6	0.4	0.3	0.3
Air and space transport accidents	1,612	1,494	941	1,094	859	0.8	0.7	0.4	0.4	0.3
Railway accidents	852	632	663	642	670	0.4	0.3	0.3	0.3	0.3
Accidental falls	16,926	13,294	12,313	12,646	13,141	8.3	5.9	5.0	5.0	5.1
Fall from one level to another	4,798	3,743	3,194	3,091	3,160	2.4	1.7	1.3	1.2	1.2
Fall on the same level	828	415	499	483	529	0.4	0.2	0.2	0.2	0.2
Fracture, cause unspecified, and other and unspecified falls	11,300	9,136	8,620	9,072	9,452	5.6	4.0	3.5	3.6	3.7
Accidental drowning	6,391	6,043	3,979	3,524	3,807	3.1	2.7	1.6	1.4	1.5
Accidents caused by –										
Fires and flames	6,718	5,822	4,175	3,958	3,900	3.3	2.6	1.7	1.6	1.5
Firearms	2,406	1,955	1,416	1,409	1,521	1.2	0.9	0.6	0.6	0.6
Electric current	1,140	1,095	670	525	548	0.6	0.5	0.3	0.2	0.2

[Continued]

★ 42 ★

Deaths and Death Rates from Accidents, by Type: 1970 to 1993

[Continued]

TYPE OF ACCIDENT	DEATHS (number)					RATE PER 100,000 POPULATION				
	1970	1980	1990	1992	1993	1970	1980	1990	1992	1993
Accidental poisoning by –										
Drugs and medicines	2,505	2,492	4,506	5,951	7,382	1.2	1.1	1.8	2.3	2.9
Other solid and liquid substances	1,174	597	549	498	495	0.6	0.3	0.2	0.2	0.2
Gases and vapors	1,620	1,242	748	633	660	0.8	0.5	0.3	0.2	0.3
Complications due to medical procedures	3,581	2437	2,669	2,669	2,724	1.8	1.1	1.1	1.0	1.1
Inhalation and ingestion of objects	2,753	3,249	3,303	3,128	3,160	1.4	1.5	1.3	1.2	1.2

Source: 1996 Statistical Abstract of the United States on CD-ROM [machine-readable datafiles]. CD-8A-97. Washington, DC: U.S. Department of Commerce, Economics and Statistics Administration, Bureau of the Census, Data User Services Division, January 1997. Primary source: U.S. National Center for Health Statistics, *Vital Statistics of the United States*, annual; and unpublished data.

★ 43 ★

Deaths

Deaths from Dog Bites, by Breed: 1979-1996

According to the source, dog attacks increased 37 percent between 1986 and 1994; occur on the dog owner's property 70 percent of the time; account for one-third of homeowners' insurance claims; and involve male dogs six times more often than female dogs.

Dog breed	Number of fatalities
Pit bull	60
Rottweiler	29

Source: Wulf, Steve. "Man's Best Friend?" *Time,* 23 June 1997, p. 58. Primary source: Dr. Jeffrey Sacks, epidemiologist with the National Center for Injury Prevention and Control.

★ 44 ★

Deaths

Homicide Among the Killers

This table shows 1994 death rates (deaths per 100,000 people) for a variety of diseases and homicide.

Cause	Death rate
Heart disease	282
Cancer	206
Stroke/aneurysm	59
Lung diseases	39
Accidents	35
Pneumonia/influenza	32

[Continued]

★ 44 ★

Homicide Among the Killers
[Continued]

Cause	Death rate
Diabetes	21
HIV	16
Suicide	12
Liver disease	10
Homicide	9
Kidney disease	9

Source: "Number of Killings Declines." *USA TODAY,* 24 October 1995, p. 10A. Primary source: Centers for Disease Control and Prevention.

★ 45 ★
Deaths

Leading Causes of Death: 1993

Table shows the number of deaths for top causes in the United States in 1993. Data include all causes and are based on the National Vital Statistics System.

Cause of death	Deaths
All causes	2,268,553
Heart disease	743,460
Malignant neoplasms	529,904
Cerebrovascular diseases	150,108
Chronic obstructive pulmonary diseases	101,077
Injuries (unintentional)	90,523
Pneumonia and influenza	82,820
Diabetes mellitus	53,894
Human immunodeficiency virus infection	37,267
Suicide	31,102
Homicide and legal intervention	26,009

Source: U.S. Department of Health and Human Services. Public Health Service. Centers for Disease Control and Prevention. National Center for Health Statistics. *Health, United States, 1995.* Hyattsville, MD: Public Health Service, 1996, p. 114.

★ 46 ★
Deaths

Motor-Vehicle Fatalities, by State, 1995: Highest Rates

[Rate is per 100,000 population]

State	Number of deaths	Death rate
Wyoming	170	35
Mississippi	868	32
New Mexico	485	29
Alabama	1,113	26
Arkansas	631	25
Montana	215	25
Arizona	1,031	24
South Carolina	881	24
Tennessee	1,259	24
Idaho	262	23
U.S. total	41,798	16

Source: "Speed Traps Focus on Fines, Not Keeping Public Safe." (editorial). *USA TODAY,* 27 November 1996, p. 13A. Primary source: Insurance Institute for Highway Safety.

★ 47 ★
Deaths

Motor-Vehicle Fatalities, by State, 1995: Lowest Rates

[Rate is per 100,000 population]

State	Number of deaths	Death rate
Massachusetts	444	7
Rhode Island	69	7
New York	1,674	9
Connecticut	317	10
New Hampshire	118	10
New Jersey	773	10
Hawaii	130	11
North Dakota	74	12
Ohio	1,366	12
Pennsylvania	1,480	12
Washington	653	12
U.S. total	41,798	

Source: "Speed Traps Focus on Fines, Not Keeping Public Safe." (editorial). *USA TODAY,* 27 November 1996, p. 13A. Primary source: Insurance Institute for Highway Safety.

★ 48 ★

Deaths

Percentage of Patients Admitted to the Hospital by Number of Months Prior to Death

This table shows that cancer patients cared for in hospices are much less likely to be admitted to hospitals before dying than cancer patients treated in other institutional settings.

Time admitted	Percent admitted to hospital from --		
	Hospice	Home care	Other
Last month prior to death	9	68	62
Second month prior to death	13	33	41

Source: Amado, Anthony J., Virginia Grow, and James Nofziger. "An Evaluation of Hospice Care with Terminally Ill Cancer Patients." *Caring Magazine* (November 1995), p. 30.

★ 49 ★

Deaths

Place of Death for Patients, by Type of Care

Location of patients is meaningful, in the context of the source, because costs of hospice care are relatively lower than other forms of terminal care.

Care received	Percent located:			
	Home	Hospice/Other	Hospital	Unknown
Hospice	49	33	14	5
Home Care	22	3	67	8
Other	10	0	75	13

Source: Amado, Anthony J., Virginia Grow, and James Nofziger. "An Evaluation of Hospice Care with Terminally Ill Cancer Patients." *Caring Magazine* (November 1995), p. 30.

★ 50 ★
Deaths

Provisional Death Rates for All Causes, by Race, Sex, and Age: 1994

[Rate is per 100,000 population]

Sex and age	All races	White	Black
Both sexes			
All ages, age adjusted	508.4	480.7	772.0
All ages, crude	876.9	908.0	865.2
Under 1 year	811.1	671.5	1,573.5
1-4 years	44.5	37.4	80.4
5-14 years	22.7	20.1	35.2
15-24 years	99.6	87.7	171.3
25-34 years	141.0	121.6	277.3
35-44 years	239.5	204.4	524.5
45-54 years	452.3	405.6	900.0
55-64 years	1,139.0	1,073.8	1,837.6
65-74 years	2,590.9	2,522.7	3,611.9
75-84 years	5,909.7	5,864.4	6,937.4
85 years and over	15,312.6	15,471.5	14,094.3
Male			
All ages, age adjusted	657.4	620.1	1,034.1
All ages, crude	918.6	934.4	993.5
Under 1 year	898.5	732.1	1,831.2
1-4 years	51.6	43.8	86.8
5-14 years	26.3	22.8	43.2
15-24 years	150.5	129.9	274.3
25-34 years	206.5	179.1	410.9
35-44 years	337.3	288.6	759.0
45-54 years	584.6	523.1	1,227.2
55-64 years	1,466.6	1,382.4	2,459.9
65-74 years	3,346.8	3,260.7	4,717.3
75-84 years	7,490.1	7,433.9	8,915.3
85 years and over	7,935.7	18,126.6	16,644.7
Female			
All ages, age adjusted	384.5	364.5	568.8
All ages, crude	839.3	882.6	749.5
Under 1 year	719.4	607.7	1,308.2
1-4 years	37.1	30.6	73.8
5-14 years	18.9	17.2	26.9
15-24 years	46.5	43.2	68.0
25-34 years	75.5	62.8	157.5
35-44 years	143.5	119.9	319.8
45-54 years	326.0	291.2	629.5
55-64 years	842.6	788.7	1,358.4
65-74 years	1,989.4	1,928.7	2,826.7

[Continued]

★ 50 ★

Provisional Death Rates for All Causes, by Race, Sex, and Age: 1994

[Continued]

Sex and age	All races	White	Black
75-84 years	4,920.7	4,878.4	5,806.1
85 years and over	14,301.3	14,460.4	13,138.3

Source: U.S. Department of Health and Human Services. Public Health Service. Centers for Disease Control and Prevention. National Center for Health Statistics. *Health, United States, 1995.* Hyattsville, MD: Public Health Service, 1996, p. 160. Primary source: Centers for Disease Control and Prevention, National Center for Health Statistics. Annual summary of births, marriages, divorces, and deaths, United States, 1994. Monthly vital statistics report; vols. 42 and 43, no. 13. Hyattsville, Maryland: Public Health Service, 1994 and 1995. *Notes:* Data exclude deaths of persons who were not residents of the 50 States and the District of Columbia. Rates were calculated using 1990's-based postcensal population estimates.

★ 51 ★

Deaths

Provisional Death Rates for the Three Leading Causes of Death, by Age: 1994

[Rate is per 100,000 population]

Cause of death and age	1994
Diseases of heart	
All ages, age adjusted	140.0
All ages, crude	281.6
Under 1 year	20.4
1-14 years	1.1
15-24 years	2.4
25-34 years	7.4
35-44 years	30.4
45-54 years	109.7
55-64 years	327.6
65-74 years	817.7
75-84 years	2,120.6
85 years and over	6,521.3
Malignant neoplasms	
All ages, age adjusted	132.1
All ages, crude	206.0
Under 1 year	[1]
1-14 years	2.9
15-24 years	4.8
25-34 years	12.4
35-44 years	40.3
45-54 years	143.1
55-64 years	430.3

[Continued]

★ 51 ★

Provisional Death Rates for the Three Leading Causes of Death, by Age: 1994

[Continued]

Cause of death and age	1994
65-74 years	882.5
75-84 years	1,375.8
85 years and over	1,786.8
Cerebrovascular diseases	
All ages, age adjusted	26.7
All ages, crude	59.2
Under 1 year	2.8
1-14 years	1
15-24 years	0.4
25-34 years	2.4
35-44 years	6.4
45-54 years	17.5
55-64 years	46.2
65-74 years	137.6
75-84 years	484.9
85 years and over	1,609.0

Source: U.S. Department of Health and Human Services. Public Health Service. Centers for Disease Control and Prevention. National Center for Health Statistics. *Health, United States, 1995.* Hyattsville, MD: Public Health Service, 1996, p. 162. Primary source: Centers for Disease Control and Prevention, National Center for Health Statistics. Annual summary of births, marriages, divorces, and deaths, United States, 1994. Monthly vital statistics report; vols. 42 and 43, no. 13. Hyattsville, Maryland: Public Health Service, 1994 and 1995. *Notes:* Data exclude deaths of persons who were not residents of the 50 States and the District of Columbia. Code numbers for cause of death are based on the International Classification of Diseases, Ninth Revision, described in Appendix II, table V. Rates were calculated using 1990's-based postcensal population estimates. 1. Rates based on 100 or fewer estimated deaths have relative standard errors of 30 percent or more and are not shown.

★ 52 ★

Deaths

States with the Fewest Lung Cancer Deaths: 1996

State	Number of deaths
Alaska	150
Wyoming	200
District of Columbia	320
North Dakota	340
Vermont	380

Source: "Breaking News: Lung Cancer Mortality Highs and Lows." *Patient Care,* 15 June 1997, p. 13. Primary source: American Cancer Society. *Cancer Facts and Figures, 1996.*

★ 53 ★
Deaths

States with the Most Lung Cancer Deaths: 1996

State	Number of deaths
California	13,700
Florida	12,200
New York	10,500
Texas	10,500
Pennsylvania	10,500

Source: "Breaking News: Lung Cancer Mortality Highs and Lows." *Patient Care,* 15 June 1997, p. 13. Primary source: American Cancer Society. *Cancer Facts and Figures, 1996.*

★ 54 ★
Deaths

Suicide Rates of Men, by Race and Age Group: 1980 to 1993

Deaths per 100,000 population in specified group. Excludes deaths of nonresidents of the United States, except as noted. The standard population for this table is the total population of the United States enumerated in 1940. Beginning 1979, deaths classified according to ninth revision of *International Classification of Diseases*; for earlier years, classified according to revision in use at that time.

AGE	TOTAL[1]			MALE					
				WHITE			BLACK		
	1980	1990	1993	1980	1990	1993	1980	1990	1993
All ages	11.9	12.4	12.1	19.9	22.0	21.4	10.3	12.0	12.5
10 to 14 years old	0.8	1.5	1.7	1.4	2.3	2.4	0.5	1.6	2.3
15 to 19 years old	8.5	11.1	10.9	15.0	19.3	18.5	5.6	11.5	14.4
20 to 24 years old	16.1	15.1	15.8	27.8	26.8	27.4	20.0	19.0	25.9
25 to 34 years old	16.0	15.2	15.1	25.6	25.6	25.9	21.8	21.9	21.5
35 to 44 years old	15.4	15.3	15.1	23.5	25.3	25.5	15.6	16.9	16.2
45 to 54 years old	15.9	14.8	14.5	24.2	24.8	23.9	12.0	14.8	14.1
55 to 64 years old	15.9	16.0	14.6	25.8	27.5	25.7	11.7	10.8	9.7
65 to 74 years old	16.9	17.9	16.3	32.5	34.2	31.4	11.1	14.7	11.7
75 to 84 years old	19.1	24.9	22.3	45.5	60.2	52.1	10.5	14.4	16.3
85 years and over	19.2	22.2	22.8	52.8	70.3	73.6	18.9	(B)	(B)

Source: 1996 Statistical Abstract of the United States on CD-ROM [machine-readable datafiles]. CD-8A-97. Washington, DC: U.S. Department of Commerce, Economics and Statistics Administration, Bureau of the Census, Data User Services Division, January 1997. Primary source: U.S. National Center for Health Statistics, *Monthly Vital Statistics Report*; and unpublished data. *Notes:* "B" indicates "Base figure too small to meet statistical standards for reliability of a derived figure." 1. Includes other age groups not shown separately.

★ 55 ★
Deaths

Suicide Rates of Women, by Race and Age Group: 1980 to 1993

Deaths per 100,000 population in specified group. Excludes deaths of nonresidents of the United States, except as noted. The standard population for this table is the total population of the United States enumerated in 1940. Beginning 1979, deaths classified according to ninth revision of *International Classification of Diseases*; for earlier years, classified according to revision in use at that time.

AGE	TOTAL[1]			FEMALE					
				WHITE			BLACK		
	1980	1990	1993	1980	1990	1993	1980	1990	1993
All ages	11.9	12.4	12.1	5.9	5.3	5.0	2.2	2.3	2.1
10 to 14 years old	0.8	1.5	1.7	0.3	0.9	1.0	0.1	(B)	(B)
15 to 19 years old	8.5	11.1	10.9	3.3	4.0	4.2	1.6	1.9	(B)
20 to 24 years old	16.1	15.1	15.8	5.9	4.4	4.4	3.1	2.6	3.9
25 to 34 years old	16.0	15.2	15.1	7.5	6.0	5.5	4.1	3.7	3.1
35 to 44 years old	15.4	15.3	15.1	9.1	7.4	7.1	4.6	4.0	3.0
45 to 54 years old	15.9	14.8	14.5	10.2	7.5	7.8	2.8	3.2	2.2
55 to 64 years old	15.9	16.0	14.6	9.1	8.0	6.8	2.3	2.6	2.6
65 to 74 years old	16.9	17.9	16.3	7.0	7.2	6.2	1.7	2.6	2.2
75 to 84 years old	19.1	24.9	22.3	5.7	6.7	6.1	1.4	(B)	(B)
85 years and over	19.2	22.2	22.8	5.8	5.4	5.4	0.1	(B)	(B)

Source: 1996 Statistical Abstract of the United States on CD-ROM [machine-readable datafiles]. CD-8A-97. Washington, DC: U.S. Department of Commerce, Economics and Statistics Administration, Bureau of the Census, Data User Services Division, January 1997. Primary source: U.S. National Center for Health Statistics, *Monthly Vital Statistics Report*; and unpublished data. *Notes:* "B" indicates "Base figure too small to meet statistical standards for reliability of a derived figure." 1. Includes other age groups not shown separately.

★ 56 ★
Deaths

Suicides, by Sex and Method Used: 1970 to 1993

Excludes deaths of nonresidents of the United States. Beginning 1979, deaths classified according to the ninth revision of the *International Classification of Diseases*. For earlier years, classified according to the revision in use at the time.

METHOD	MALE						FEMALE					
	1970	1980	1985	1990	1992	1993	1970	1980	1985	1990	1992	1993
Total	16,629	20,505	23,145	24,724	24,547	25,007	6,851	6,364	6,308	6,182	6,027	6,095
Firearms[1]	9,704	12,937	14,809	16,285	15,802	16,381	2,068	2,459	2,554	2,600	2,367	2,559
Percent of total	58	63	64	66	65	66	30	39	41	42	39	39
Poisoning[2]	3,299	2,997	3,319	3,221	3,690	3,569	3,285	2,456	2,385	2,203	2,233	2,110

[Continued]

★ 56 ★

Suicides, by Sex and Method Used: 1970 to 1993

[Continued]

METHOD	MALE						FEMALE					
	1970	1980	1985	1990	1992	1993	1970	1980	1985	1990	1992	1993
Hanging and strangulation[3]	2,422	2,997	3,532	3,688	3,822	3,824	831	694	732	756	856	803
Other[4]	1,204	1,574	1,485	1,530	1,571	1,641	667	755	637	623	571	623

Source: 1996 Statistical Abstract of the United States on CD-ROM [machine-readable datafiles]. CD-8A-97. Washington, DC: U.S. Department of Commerce, Economics and Statistics Administration, Bureau of the Census, Data User Services Division, January 1997. Primary source: U.S. National Center for Health Statistics, *Vital Statistics of the United States*, annual; and unpublished data. *Notes:* 1. Includes explosives in 1970. 2. Includes solids, liquids, and gases. 3. Includes suffocation. 4. Beginning 1980, includes explosives.

Dental Health

★ 57 ★

Dental Visits, by Selected Characteristics: 1993

Data refer to percentage of persons age 25 and older who visited a dentist at least once in the past year.

Characteristic	1993
Total[1,2]	60.8
Age	
25-34 years	60.3
35-44 years	66.9
45-64 years	62.0
65 years and over	51.7
65-74 years	56.3
75 years and over	44.9
Sex[2]	
Male	58.2
Female	63.4
Poverty status[2,3]	
Below poverty	35.9
At or above poverty	64.3
Race and Hispanic origin[2]	
White, non-Hispanic	64.0
Black, non-Hispanic	47.3
Hispanic	46.2
Education[2]	
Less than 12 years	38.0
12 years	58.7

[Continued]

★ 57 ★

Dental Visits, by Selected Characteristics: 1993

[Continued]

Characteristic	1993
13 years or more	73.8
Education, race, and Hispanic origin[2] Less than 12 years:	
White, non-Hispanic	41.2
Black, non-Hispanic	33.1
Hispanic	33.0
12 years:	
White, non-Hispanic	60.4
Black, non-Hispanic	48.2
Hispanic	54.6
13 years or more:	
White, non-Hispanic	75.8
Black, non-Hispanic	61.3
Hispanic	61.8

Source: U.S. Department of Health and Human Services. Public Health Service. Centers for Disease Control and Prevention. National Center for Health Statistics. *Health, United States, 1995.* Hyattsville, MD: Public Health Service, 1996. p. 196. Primary source: Centers for Disease Control and Prevention, National Center for Health Statistics, Division of Health Interview Statistics. Data from National Health Interview Survey. *Notes:* Denominators exclude persons with unknown dental data. Estimates for 1993 are based on responses during the last half of the year only. 1. Includes all other races not shown separately and unknown poverty status and education level. 2. Age adjusted. 3. Poverty status is based on family income and family size using Bureau of the Census poverty thresholds.

★ 58 ★

Dental Health

Median Fees Paid for Cosmetic Dental Work: 1995

Data are based on a survey of 130-1600 patients.

Procedure	Median fee ($)
Porcelain crown/jacket	500
Contouring	95
Replacement filling	100
Veneers	350
Braces	2500
Bonding	120
Bleaching	200

Source: "Cosmetic Dental Work." *Consumer Reports* (December 1996), p. 45.

★ 59 ★

Dental Health

National Average Fees for Treatment of Missing Teeth: 1995

Treatment options	National average cost ($)
Three unit bridge	1740-1840
Cantilever fixed bridge	1170-1260
"Maryland" bridge	1180
Implant and crown	2310
Removable partial denture (plastic)	760
Removable partial denture (metal)	890

Source: "Missing Teeth: Comparing Your Options." *Consumer Reports* (December 1996), p. 45. Primary source: Dr. Thomas M. Limoli, Atlanta Dental Consultants.

★ 60 ★

Dental Health

Status of Water Fluoridation in the United States

	Value
Total U.S. Population - 1992 Estimate (million)	258.5
U.S. Population on Public Water Supply Systems (per 1992 EPA data) (million)	232.4
U.S. Population Not Served by Public Water Supply Systems (million)	26.1
Total No. of Public Water Supply Systems (per 1992 EPA data)	59,158
No. of Systems with population less than 100	18,273
No. of Systems with population between 101-500	18,238
No. of Systems with population between 501-1000	6,307
No. of Systems with population over 1,000	15,487
Total No. of Public Water Supply Systems that are Fluoridating	
(1992 Fluoridation Census)	14,351
Adjusted	10,567
Natural	3,784
Total No. of Fluoridated Communities	
(1992 Fluoridation Census)	10,496
Adjusted	8,572
Natural	1,924

[Continued]

★ 60 ★

Status of Water Fluoridation in the United States
[Continued]

	Value
Total U.S. Population on Fluoridated Drinking Water Systems (1992 Fluoridation Census) (millions)	144.6
Adjusted	134.6
Natural	10.0
Percentage of U.S. Population Receiving Fluoridated Water:	55.9
Percentage of Total U.S. Population on Public Water Supply Systems Receiving Fluoridated Water:	62.2

Source: U.S. Department of Health and Human Services. Public Health Service. Centers for Disease Control and Prevention. National Center for Health Statistics. Fluoridation Fact Sheet (FL-141), December 1993.

Disabilities and Handicaps

★ 61 ★

Days of Disability, by Type and Selected Characteristics: 1970 to 1994

Covers civilian noninstitutional population. Beginning 1984, the levels of estimates may not be comparable to estimates for 1970-1980 because the later data are based on a revised questionnaire and field procedures; for further information, see source. Based on National Health Interview Survey.

ITEM	TOTAL DAYS OF DISABILITY (millions)						DAYS PER PERSON					
	1970	1980	1985	1990	1993	1994	1970	1980	1985	1990	1993	1994
Restricted-activity days[1]	2,913	4,165	3,453	3,669	4,346	4,143	14.6	19.1	14.8	14.9	17.1	16.0
Male	1,273	1,802	1,442	1,558	1,844	1,723	13.2	17.1	12.8	13.1	14.9	13.6
Female	1,640	2,363	2,011	2,111	2,502	2,420	15.8	21.0	16.6	16.7	19.2	18.2
White[2]	2,526	3,518	2,899	3,057	3,598	3,375	14.4	18.7	14.5	14.8	17.0	15.7
Black[2]	365	580	489	536	616	608	16.2	22.7	17.4	17.7	19.2	18.4
Under 65 years	2,331	3,228	2,557	2,734	3,289	3,070	12.9	16.6	12.4	12.6	14.7	13.4
65 years and over	582	937	895	936	1,057	1,073	30.7	39.2	33.1	31.4	33.8	34.6
Northeast	709	862	689	656	798	803	14.5	17.9	13.8	13.2	15.9	15.9
Midwest	691	989	744	836	978	879	12.4	17.2	12.7	14.0	15.8	13.9
South	996	1,415	1,308	1,404	1,564	1,443	15.9	19.8	16.3	16.7	18.3	16.4
West	518	899	712	773	1,006	1,017	15.6	22.0	15.7	14.8	17.7	17.6
Family income: Under $10,000	(NA)	(NA)	893	662	741	681	(NA)	(NA)	25.8	27.3	30.2	29.1

[Continued]

★ 61 ★

Days of Disability, by Type and Selected Characteristics: 1970 to 1994
[Continued]

ITEM	TOTAL DAYS OF DISABILITY (millions)						DAYS PER PERSON					
	1970	1980	1985	1990	1993	1994	1970	1980	1985	1990	1993	1994
$10,000 to $19,999	(NA)	(NA)	781	758	857	801	(NA)	(NA)	16.7	19.1	22.3	21.5
$20,000 to $34,999	(NA)	(NA)	791	715	849	825	(NA)	(NA)	12.1	13.5	15.7	15.2
$35,000 or more	(NA)	(NA)	568	912	1,086	1,051	(NA)	(NA)	9.9	10.3	11.2	10.5
Bed-disability days[3]	1,222	1,520	1,436	1,521	1,708	1,603	6.1	7.0	6.1	6.2	6.7	6.2
Male	503	616	583	625	688	623	5.2	5.9	5.2	5.2	5.6	4.9
Female	720	904	852	896	1,020	980	6.9	8.0	7.1	7.1	7.8	7.4
Under 65 years	959	1,190	1,064	1,115	1,286	1,155	5.3	6.1	5.1	5.2	5.8	5.1
65 years and over	263	330	371	406	422	448	13.8	13.8	13.7	13.6	13.5	14.4
Work-loss days[4]	417	485	575	621	666	642	5.4	5.0	5.3	5.3	5.6	5.2
Male	243	271	287	303	315	311	5.0	4.9	4.8	4.7	4.8	4.6
Female	175	215	288	319	351	332	5.9	5.1	6.0	5.9	6.4	5.9
School-loss days[5]	222	204	217	212	250	225	4.9	5.3	4.8	4.6	5.3	4.5
Male	108	95	100	100	121	104	4.7	4.8	4.4	4.3	5.0	4.1
Female	114	109	117	112	129	121	5.1	5.7	5.3	5.0	5.5	5.0

Source: 1996 Statistical Abstract of the United States on CD-ROM [machine-readable datafiles]. CD-8A-97. Washington, DC: U.S. Department of Commerce, Economics and Statistics Administration, Bureau of the Census, Data User Services Division, January 1997. Primary source: U.S. National Center for Health Statistics, *Vital and Health Statistics*, series 10, No. 193; and earlier reports and unpublished data. *Notes:* NA Not available. 1. A day when a person cuts down on his usual activities for more than half a day because of illness or injury. Includes bed-disability, work-loss, and school-loss days. Total includes other races and unknown income, not shown separately. 2. Beginning 1980, race was determined by asking the household respondent to report his race. In earlier years the racial classification of respondents was determined by interviewer observation. 3. A day when a person stayed in bed more than half a day because of illness or injury. Includes those work-loss and school-loss days actually spent in bed. 4. A day when a person lost more than half a workday because of illness or injury. Computed for persons 17 years of age and over (beginning 1984, 18 years of age and over) in the currently employed population, defined as those who were working or had a job or business from which they were not on layoff during the 2-week period preceding the week of interview. 5. Child's loss of more than half a school day because of illness or injury. Computed for children 6-16 years of age. Beginning 1984, children 5-17 years old.

★ 62 ★
Disabilities and Handicaps

Disability: Related to Age

Age group	Percent of people with a severe disability	Percent of people with a non-severe disability
15-24	3.3	6.7
25-34	4.9	7.6
35-44	6.6	10.3
45-54	10.6	12.7
55-64	21.1	15.7

[Continued]

★ 62 ★

Disability: Related to Age
[Continued]

Age group	Percent of people with a severe disability	Percent of people with a non-severe disability
65-74	25.3	19.3
75-84	41.5	22.2

Source: Kraus, Lewis E., Susan Stoddard, and David Gilmartin. *Chartbook on Disability in the United States, 1996.* Washington, DC: U.S. National Institute on Disability and Rehabilitation Research, p. 16.

★ 63 ★

Disabilities and Handicaps

Disabled: Activity Limitation, by Residence

Activity limitations	Percent		
	Not metropolitan statistical area	Metropolitan statistical area-- central cities	Metropolitan statistical area-- not central city
Unable to do major activity	5.4	5.4	3.8
Limited in major activity	6.6	5.9	5.2
Limited in nonmajor activity	5.6	4.5	4.5

Source: Kraus, Lewis E., Susan Stoddard, and David Gilmartin. *Chartbook on Disability in the United States, 1996.* Washington, DC: U.S. National Institute on Disability and Rehabilitation Research, p. 12.

★ 64 ★

Disabilities and Handicaps

Disabled: Activity Limitations

Limitation status	Number	Percent of total
Limited but not in major activity	12,262,000	4.7
Limited in amount or kind of major activity	14,803,000	5.7
Unable to carry on major activity	11,993,000	4.6
With no activity limitation	220,575,000	85.0

Source: Kraus, Lewis E., Susan Stoddard, and David Gilmartin. *Chartbook on Disability in the United States, 1996.* Washington, DC: U.S. National Institute on Disability and Rehabilitation Research, p. 5.

★ 65 ★

Disabilities and Handicaps

Disabled: Activity Limitations, Age 65 and Over

Age	Persons with a disability	Persons with no disability	Persons with an activity limitation	Persons with no activity limitation	Percent disability status	Percent activity limitation status
65-69	4,423,000	10,185,000	3,678,000	9,995,000	43.4	36.8
70-74	3,759,000	8,170,000	2,685,000	8,475,000	46.0	31.7
75-84	6,301,000	9,889,000	4,092,000	9,698,000	63.7	42.2
85 and over	2,058,000	2,445,000	1,486,000	2,624,000	84.2	56.6

Source: Kraus, Lewis E., Susan Stoddard, and David Gilmartin. *Chartbook on Disability in the United States, 1996.* Washington, DC: U.S. National Institute on Disability and Rehabilitation Research, p. 30.

★ 66 ★

Disabilities and Handicaps

Disabled: Activity Limitations, by Educational Attainment

Number of years of education	Percent limited in nonmajor activity	Percent limited in major activity	Percent unable to do major activity
8 years or less	10.0	11.9	16.5
9-11 years	7.3	8.4	9.9
12 years	5.3	6.5	5.3
13-15 years	4.9	5.2	3.8
16 years or more	5.3	3.9	2.3

Source: Kraus, Lewis E., Susan Stoddard, and David Gilmartin. *Chartbook on Disability in the United States, 1996.* Washington, DC: U.S. National Institute on Disability and Rehabilitation Research, p. 23.

★ 67 ★

Disabilities and Handicaps

Disabled: Activity Limitations of Persons Under Age 18, by Family Income

Family income	Percent of children under 18 with activity limitations
Less than $10,000	11.1
$10,000-19,999	8.4
$20,000-34,999	6.5
$35,000 or more	5.3

Source: Kraus, Lewis E., Susan Stoddard, and David Gilmartin. *Chartbook on Disability in the United States, 1996.* Washington, DC: U.S. National Institute on Disability and Rehabilitation Research, p. 33.

★ 68 ★

Disabilities and Handicaps

Disabled: By Race and Ethnicity

Race/ethnicity	Percent with severe disability	Percent with non-severe disability
Asian/Pacific Islander	4.9	5.0
Hispanic origin[1]	8.4	6.9
White	9.4	10.3
Black	12.2	7.8
Native American	9.8	12.1

Source: Kraus, Lewis E., Susan Stoddard, and David Gilmartin. *Chartbook on Disability in the United States, 1996.* Washington, DC: U.S. National Institute on Disability and Rehabilitation Research, p. 19. *Note:* 1. Hispanic origin can be of any race.

★ 69 ★

Disabilities and Handicaps

Disabled: Children with Activity Limitations, by Age

Age group	Percent limited in nonmajor activity	Percent limited in major activity	Percent unable to do major activity
Under age 5	0.7	1.4	0.6
5-13	1.9	5.0	0.6
14-17	2.4	4.5	0.7

Source: Kraus, Lewis E., Susan Stoddard, and David Gilmartin. *Chartbook on Disability in the United States, 1996.* Washington, DC: U.S. National Institute on Disability and Rehabilitation Research, p. 32.

★ 70 ★

Disabilities and Handicaps

Disabled: Children with Special Education Requirements, by Type of Impairment

Impairments	Percentage	Number
Specific learning disabilities	52.1	2,438,147
Orthopedic impairments	1.2	64,110
Serious emotional disturbance	8.7	413,691
Multiple disabilities	2.3	109,203
Hearing impairments	1.3	83,178
Other health impairments	2.7	552,703
Mental retardation	11.6	552,703
Speech or language impairments	21.1	1,007,575
Visual impairments	0.5	24,873
Autism	0.4	18,893
Deaf-blindness	-	5,291
Traumatic brain injury	-	1,315

Source: Kraus, Lewis E., Susan Stoddard, and David Gilmartin. *Chartbook on Disability in the United States, 1996.* Washington, DC: U.S. National Institute on Disability and Rehabilitation Research, p. 34. *Note:* - Represents zero.

★ 71 ★

Disabilities and Handicaps

Disabled: Classroom Arrangements for Children with Special Education Requirements

Type of classroom	Percentage
Regular class	39.8
Public separate facility	2.4
Private separate facility	1.2
Separate class	23.5
Other facility	1.4
Private residential	0.3
Public residential	0.6
Homebound hospital	0.5
Resource room	31.7

Source: Kraus, Lewis E., Susan Stoddard, and David Gilmartin. *Chartbook on Disability in the United States, 1996.* Washington, DC: U.S. National Institute on Disability and Rehabilitation Research, p. 35.

★ 72 ★

Disabilities and Handicaps

Disabled: Limitations in Work Activity, by Race and Ethnicity

Race/ethnicity	Percent of people limited in kind or amount of work activity	Percent of people who are unable to work
Asian or Pacific Islander	2.3	3.4
White Hispanic	3.2	6.3
Other and Unknown	3.1	6.5
White non-Hispanic	5.4	6.2
Black non-Hispanic	4.0	10.3
Black Hispanic	2.7	13.2
Native American	6.9	10.4

Source: Kraus, Lewis E., Susan Stoddard, and David Gilmartin. *Chartbook on Disability in the United States, 1996.* Washington, DC: U.S. National Institute on Disability and Rehabilitation Research, p. 44.

★ 73 ★

Disabilities and Handicaps

Disabled: Median Monthly Earnings Comparison, by Age and Disability Status

[In dollars earned per month]

Age group	Earnings of persons with no disability	Earnings of persons with a non-severe disability	Earnings of persons with a severe disability
Less than age 35	$1,481	$1,281	$1,440
35-64	2,446	2,006	1,562
55 and over	2,137	1,936	1,164

Source: Kraus, Lewis E., Susan Stoddard, and David Gilmartin. *Chartbook on Disability in the United States, 1996.* Washington, DC: U.S. National Institute on Disability and Rehabilitation Research, p. 47.

★ 74 ★

Disabilities and Handicaps

Disabled: Mental Retardation

This table shows that the number of people with mental retardation causing an activity limitation goes down with age.

Years of age	Percent with activity limitation
Under 18	15.8
18-44	3.1
45-69	0.4
70-84	0.1
85 and over	0.1

Source: Kraus, Lewis E., Susan Stoddard, and David Gilmartin. *Chartbook on Disability in the United States, 1996.* Washington, DC: U.S. National Institute on Disability and Rehabilitation Research, p. 8.

★ 75 ★

Disabilities and Handicaps

Disabled: Need for Assistance

Race/ethnicity	Percent of people needing assistance in IADL only	Percent of people needing assistance in ADL
Asian or Pacific Islander	0.9	0.8
Other and unknown	1.5	1.3
White Hispanic	1.5	1.1
Black Hispanic	0.7	1.8
White non-Hispanic	2.6	1.4
Black non-Hispanic	3.0	2.0
Native American	3.0	2.6

Source: Kraus, Lewis E., Susan Stoddard, and David Gilmartin. *Chartbook on Disability in the United States, 1996.* Washington, DC: U.S. National Institute on Disability and Rehabilitation Research, p. 20. *Notes:* ADL stands for activities of daily living. IADL stands for instrumental activities of daily living.

★ 76 ★

Disabilities and Handicaps

Disabled: Need for Assistance Later in Life

Age group	Percent with assistance needs in IADL only	Percent with assistance needs in ADL
5-17	0.0	0.4
18-24	0.6	0.3
25-44	1.3	0.6
45-64	3.3	1.4
65-69	5.0	2.3
70-74	7.5	4.4
75-84	13.9	8.6
85 +	22.3	20.0

Source: Kraus, Lewis E., Susan Stoddard, and David Gilmartin. *Chartbook on Disability in the United States, 1996.* Washington, DC: U.S. National Institute on Disability and Rehabilitation Research, p. 31. *Notes:* ADL stands for activities of daily living. IADL stands for instrumental activities of daily living.

★ 77 ★

Disabilities and Handicaps

Disabled: Number of Disabled

Status	Number	Percent of total
With a disability, not severe	24,819,000	9.9
With a severe disability	24,117,000	9.6
With no disability	202,860,000	80.6

Source: Kraus, Lewis E., Susan Stoddard, and David Gilmartin. *Chartbook on Disability in the United States, 1996.* Washington, DC: U.S. National Institute on Disability and Rehabilitation Research, p. 4.

★ 78 ★

Disabilities and Handicaps

Disabled: People With A Mental Disorder in Any One Year

Mental disorder	Percent having disorder
Any disorder	28.1
Anxiety disorders	12.6
Substance abuse disorders	9.5
Affective disorders	9.5
Cognitive impairment (severe)[1]	2.7
Antisocial personality disorder	1.5
Schizophrenic disorders	1.1
Somatization disorders	0.2

Source: Kraus, Lewis E., Susan Stoddard, and David Gilmartin. *Chartbook on Disability in the United States, 1996.* Washington, DC: U.S. National Institute on Disability and Rehabilitation Research, p. 9. *Notes:* 1. This is a measure of current cognitive status based on the Mini-Mental State Examination.

★ 79 ★

Disabilities and Handicaps

Disabled: Percent Requiring Assistance in Daily Activities

Status	Percentage
People needing assistance in ADL	1.5
People needing assistance in IADL only	2.5
People who are limited in activity but not in ADL or IADL	12.0
People not limited in activity	84.0

Source: Kraus, Lewis E., Susan Stoddard, and David Gilmartin. *Chartbook on Disability in the United States, 1996.* Washington, DC: U.S. National Institute on Disability and Rehabilitation Research, p. 7. *Notes:* ADL stands for activities of daily living. IADL stands for instrumental activities of daily living.

★ 80 ★

Disabilities and Handicaps

Disabled: Persons in Labor Force, by Sex and Disability Status

Sex	Percent with no disability	Percent with disability
Men	91.4	74.9
Women	58.8	45.6

Source: Kraus, Lewis E., Susan Stoddard, and David Gilmartin. *Chartbook on Disability in the United States, 1996.* Washington, DC: U.S. National Institute on Disability and Rehabilitation Research, p. 39.

★ 81 ★

Disabilities and Handicaps

Disabled: Persons Rehabilitated, by Type of Disability

Data refer to the percentage of persons helped by vocational rehabilitation (i.e., those who completed vocational rehabilitation and found work in a variety of jobs).

Disability	Percent of persons rehabilitated
Heart/circulatory	1.7
Deafness	2.9
Other visual impairments	3.9
Hard of hearing	4.9
Blindness	5.5
Learning disabilities	8.0
Substance abuse	10.9
Other disabilities	11.8
Mental illness	16.9
Mental retardation	13.1
Orthopedic impairments	20.5

Source: Kraus, Lewis E., Susan Stoddard, and David Gilmartin. *Chartbook on Disability in the United States, 1996.* Washington, DC: U.S. National Institute on Disability and Rehabilitation Research, p. 48.

★ 82 ★

Disabilities and Handicaps

Disabled: Persons Who Need Assistance with Daily Activities, by Educational Attainment

Years of education attained	Percent of people needing assistance in ADL	Percent of people needing assistance in IADL only	Percent of people limited in activity but not in IADL or ADL
8 years or less	6.1	10.0	22.3
9-11 years	2.4	5.0	18.2
12 years	1.3	2.6	13.1
13-15 years	0.9	1.9	11.1
16 years or more	0.7	1.3	9.5

Source: Kraus, Lewis E., Susan Stoddard, and David Gilmartin. *Chartbook on Disability in the United States, 1996.* Washington, DC: U.S. National Institute on Disability and Rehabilitation Research, p. 24. *Notes:* ADL stands for activities of daily living. IADL stands for instrumental activities of daily living.

★ 83 ★

Disabilities and Handicaps

Disabled: Persons with a Work Disability, by Race and Ethnicity

Race/ethnicity	Percent considered work disabled
White	9.4
Black	15.4
Other races	8.5
Hispanic origin[1]	9.6

Source: Kraus, Lewis E., Susan Stoddard, and David Gilmartin. *Chartbook on Disability in the United States, 1996.* Washington, DC: U.S. National Institute on Disability and Rehabilitation Research, p. 38. *Note:* 1. Persons of Hispanic origin can be of any race.

★ 84 ★

Disabilities and Handicaps

Disabled: Persons with Activity Limitations, by Family Income

Income level	Percent unable to do major activity	Percent limited in amount or kind of major activity	Percent limited in nonmajor activity
Under $10,000	11.2	9.9	6.9
$10,000-19,999	7.3	7.7	6.2
$20,000-34,999	4.1	6.0	4.7
$35,000 or more	1.9	3.9	3.6

Source: Kraus, Lewis E., Susan Stoddard, and David Gilmartin. *Chartbook on Disability in the United States, 1996.* Washington, DC: U.S. National Institute on Disability and Rehabilitation Research, p. 21.

★ 85 ★

Disabilities and Handicaps

Disabled: Population, by Disability Status

Status	Percent
People with no functional limitation	74.8
People with a functional limitation	17.5
People with a severe functional limitation	7.8

Source: Kraus, Lewis E., Susan Stoddard, and David Gilmartin. *Chartbook on Disability in the United States, 1996.* Washington, DC: U.S. National Institute on Disability and Rehabilitation Research, p. 6.

★ 86 ★

Disabilities and Handicaps

Disabled: Ratio of Low Income to Functional Limitations

The poverty threshold for a family of four in 1991 (when the majority of data for this table was collected) was $13,924. In 1992, the poverty threshold for a family of four was $14,335.

Ratio of income to low-income threshold	Percent functional limitation	Percent no functional limitation
Less than 1.00	19.8	12.2
1.00 to 1.49	15.3	8.3
1.50 to 1.99	13.0	9.5
2.0 to 2.99	21.2	19.6
3.0 to 3.99	12.4	16.3
4.00 and over	18.4	34.1

Source: Kraus, Lewis E., Susan Stoddard, and David Gilmartin. *Chartbook on Disability in the United States, 1996.* Washington, DC: U.S. National Institute on Disability and Rehabilitation Research, p. 22.

★ 87 ★

Disabilities and Handicaps

Disabled: Severe Work Disabilities, by Race and Ethnicity

Race/ethnicity	Percent with severe disabilities
White	5.4
Black	11.8
Other races	5.6
Hispanic[1]	7.1

Source: Kraus, Lewis E., Susan Stoddard, and David Gilmartin. *Chartbook on Disability in the United States, 1996.* Washington, DC: U.S. National Institute on Disability and Rehabilitation Research, p. 43. *Note:* 1. Persons of Hispanic origin can be of any race.

★ 88 ★

Disabilities and Handicaps

Disabled: Top Five Chronic Conditions Causing Work Limitation

Chronic conditions	Percent of all conditions causing work limitation
Orthopedic impairment of lower extremity	4.5
Osteoarthritis and allied disorders	6.8
Intervertebral disc disorders	7.8
Orthopedic impairment of back or neck	10.5
Heart disease	10.9

Source: Kraus, Lewis E., Susan Stoddard, and David Gilmartin. *Chartbook on Disability in the United States, 1996.* Washington, DC: U.S. National Institute on Disability and Rehabilitation Research, p. 45.

★ 89 ★

Disabilities and Handicaps

Disabled: Work Disability Status, by Sex and Age

Sex and age	Percent with no work disability	Percent with a work disability
Female		
16-24	25.9	12.0
25-34	57.0	21.5
35-44	58.3	16.5
45-54	62.0	13.8
55-64	42.1	5.7
Male		
16-24	35.1	13.7
25-34	83.9	29.0
35-44	88.4	28.9
45-54	89.3	27.9
55-64	68.5	14.6

Source: Kraus, Lewis E., Susan Stoddard, and David Gilmartin. *Chartbook on Disability in the United States, 1996.* Washington, DC: U.S. National Institute on Disability and Rehabilitation Research, p. 40.

★ 90 ★

Disabilities and Handicaps

Leading Causes of Disability: 1995

Cause	Percentage
Arthritis/rheumatism	27
Back/spinal injury	21
Respiratory problems	10
Heart problems	17

Source: "Americans With Disabilities." *USA TODAY,* 28 August 1995, p. 1A.

Disease Prevalence

★ 91 ★

Disease Prevalence, by Race - Michigan

This chart shows the top 10 causes of death for black men in Michigan; the numbers represent annual deaths per 100,000 people in each category. The Risk Index indicates how many times more likely a black man is to die of each cause than a white man.

Cause of Death	Black male	White male	Risk index
Heart disease	296	203	1.5
Cancer	232	155	1.5
Homicide	101	4	25.3
Stroke	52	28	1.9
Injuries (unintentional)	49	35	1.4
Pneumonia/influenza	31	18	1.7
Obstructive lung diseases	28	27	1.0
Chronic liver diseases	28	10	2.8
Diabetes	23	14	1.6
Suicide	17	19	0.9
All	1,078	614	1.8

Source: Detroit Free Press, 9 April 1996, p. 8F. Primary source: Michigan Department of Public Health.

★ 92 ★

Disease Prevalence

Notifiable Diseases, 1994: Number and Rate

[Rate is cases per 100,000 persons]

Disease	1994
Rate	
Diphtheria	0.00
Hepatitis A	10.29
Hepatitis B	4.81
Mumps	0.60
Pertussis (whooping cough)	1.77
Poliomyelitis, total	---
Paralytic poliomyelitis[1]	---
Rubella (German measles)	0.09
Rubeola (measles)	0.37
Salmonellosis, excluding typhoid fever	16.64
Shigellosis	11.44
Tuberculosis[2]	9.36
Varicella (chicken pox)	135.76
Sexually transmitted diseases:	
Syphilis[3]	32.00
Primary and secondary	8.10
Early latent	12.50
Late and late latent	10.50
Congenital[4]	0.90
Gonorrhea[5]	168.40
Chancroid	0.30
Granuloma inguinale	0.00
Lymphogranuloma venereum	0.10
Number of cases	
Diphtheria	2
Hepatitis A	29,796
Hepatitis B	12,517
Mumps	1,537
Pertussis (whooping cough)	4,617
Poliomyelitis, total	---
Paralytic poliomyelitis[1]	---
Rubella (German measles)	227
Rubeola (measles)	963
Salmonellosis, excluding typhoid fever	43,323
Shigellosis	29,769
Tuberculosis[2]	24,361
Varicella (chicken pox)	151,219
Sexually transmitted diseases:	
Syphilis[3]	81,696
Primary and secondary	20,627
Early latent	32,012
Late and late latent	26,840
Congenital[4]	2,217

[Continued]

★ 92 ★

Notifiable Diseases, 1994: Number and Rate
[Continued]

Disease	1994
Gonorrhea[5]	418,068
Chancroid	773
Granuloma inguinale	3
Lymphogranuloma venereum	235

Source: U.S. Department of Health and Human Services. Public Health Service. Centers for Disease Control and Prevention. National Center for Health Statistics. *Health, United States, 1995*. Hyattsville, MD: Public Health Service, 1996, p. 164. Primary source: Centers for Disease Control and Prevention. Summary of notifiable diseases, United States, 1994. Morbidity and mortality weekly report 43 (53). Atlanta, Georgia. Public Health Service, 1995; National Center for HIV, STD, and TB Prevention, Division of STD Prevention. Sexually transmitted disease surveillance, 1994. Atlanta, Georgia: Public Health Service. Centers for Disease Control and Prevention, 1995. *Notes:* Rates greater than 0 but less than 0.005 are shown as 0.00. The total resident population was used to calculate all rates except those of sexually transmitted diseases, for which the civilian resident population was used prior to 1991. Population data from those states where diseases were not notifiable or where data were not available were excluded from rate calculation. 1. Two suspected cases of paralytic poliomyelitis reported in 1994 are pending confirmation. 2. Data after 1974 are not comparable to prior years because of changes in reporting criteria effective in 1975. 3. Includes stage of syphilis not stated. 4. Data reported for 1989 and later years reflect change in case definition introduced in 1988. 5. Data for 1994 do not include cases from Georgia.

★ 93 ★

Disease Prevalence

Prevalence of Selected Chronic Conditions by Age and Sex: 1994

Covers civilian noninstitutional population. Conditions classified according to ninth revision of *International Classification of Diseases*. Based on National Health Interview Survey.

Chronic condition	Condi-tions (1,000)	Rate[1]							
		Male				Female			
		Under 45 years old	45 to 64 years old	65 to 74 years old	75 years old and over	Under 45 years old	45 to 64 years old	65 to 74 years old	75 years old and over
Arthritis	33,446	27.4	176.8	430.8	424.9	38.2	297.0	513.6	604.4
Dermatitis, including eczema	9,192	29.3	21.8	25.3	17.6[2]	43.6	44.6	38.6	40.2
Trouble with –									
Dry (itching) skin	6,166	17.1	29.6	36.6	46.7	20.5	36.1	30.8	40.5
Ingrown nails	5,987	16.0	32.1	40.9	38.8	16.4	29.7	52.9	61.4
Corns and calluses	4,356	6.9	25.3	21.0	17.8[2]	12.2	32.5	46.5	58.1
Visual impairments	8,601	29.5	52.7	78.4	113.7	12.9	38.0	48.0	110.7
Cataracts	6,473	2.5	12.3	79.0	214.7	2.5	21.9	140.0	259.2
Hearing impairments	22,400	43.2	191.9	298.8	447.1	30.4	87.5	183.3	307.8
Tinnitus	7,033	11.6	60.4	118.1	106.6	9.8	33.2	67.7	79.9
Deformities or orthopedic impairments	31,068	93.5	166.7	144.4	169.3	101.3	173.2	161.8	189.9
Ulcer	4,447	11.3	27.4	27.1	30.9[2]	13.3	23.3	42.8	22.3
Hernia of abdominal cavity	4,778	7.8	31.2	54.7	55.6	5.8	31.3	70.0	72.3
Frequent indigestion	6,957	20.5	42.8	44.6	51.5	18.9	39.0	41.0	45.3

[Continued]

★ 93 ★

Prevalence of Selected Chronic Conditions by Age and Sex: 1994
[Continued]

Chronic condition	Condi-tions (1,000)	Rate[1]							
		Male				Female			
		Under 45 years old	45 to 64 years old	65 to 74 years old	75 years old and over	Under 45 years old	45 to 64 years old	65 to 74 years old	75 years old and over
Frequent constipation	4,040	4.3	6.8	13.8[2]	60.2	15.1	17.3	47.3	102.2
Diabetes	7,766	7.3	63.3	102.4	115.6	8.9	63.0	101.0	91.8
Migraine	11,256	22.0	24.2	17.1[2]	5.2[2]	67.1	78.9	29.9	26.2
Heart conditions	22,279	27.0	162.0	319.3	429.9	33.1	111.0	250.8	361.4
High blood pressure (Hypertension)	28,236	31.9	220.0	307.7	339.2	32.4	224.5	378.7	417.5
Varicose veins of lower extremities	7,260	3.7	17.8	32.5	58.5	23.3	81.0	109.0	83.8
Hemorrhoids	9,321	19.1	68.7	51.0	66.6	29.0	55.8	70.2	58.6
Chronic bronchitis	14,021	43.6	43.8	41.7	68.0	56.5	82.7	79.0	51.7
Asthma	14,562	57.1	32.3	39.3	70.3	60.0	68.0	62.8	34.1
Hay fever, allergic rhinitis without asthma	26,146	98.0	107.3	79.6	56.6	99.2	133.4	92.2	78.8
Chronic sinusitis	34,902	101.9	147.5	118.2	113.9	135.5	210.2	175.5	176.1

Source: 1996 Statistical Abstract of the United States on CD-ROM [machine-readable datafiles]. CD-8A-97. Washington, DC: U.S. Department of Commerce, Economics and Statistics Administration, Bureau of the Census, Data User Services Division, January 1997. Primary source: U.S. National Center for Health Statistics, Vital and Health Statistics, series 10, No. 193, and earlier reports and unpublished data. Notes: 1. Conditions per 1,000 persons. 2. Figure does not meet standards of reliability or precision.

★ 94 ★

Disease Prevalence

Prevalence of Selected Diseases, by Gender

This table shows the ratio of women to men who experience selected diseases, some of which are controversial, i.e., there is no agreement on causal factors (physical, genetic versus psychological). A ratio of 2:1 means that two women experience the disease for every man.

Disease	Ratio of women to men
Chronic fatigue syndrome	9:1
Depression	2:1
Fibromyalgia	9:1
Migraine headaches	3:1
Multiple sclerosis	3:1
Panic disorders	2:1
Rheumatoid arthritis	4:1
Scleroderma	3:1
Systemic lupus erythematosus	9:1

[Continued]

★ 94 ★

Prevalence of Selected Diseases, by Gender

[Continued]

Disease	Ratio of women to men
Graves' disease	7:1
Diabetes, Type I	6:1

Source: Conkling, Winifred. "Women, Men and Illness." *American Health* (July/August 1996), p. 58.

Diseases and Illnesses

★ 95 ★

Acute Conditions, by Type: 1970 to 1994

Covers civilian noninstitutional population. Estimates include only acute conditions which were medically attended or caused at least 1 day of restricted activity. Based on National Health Interview Survey.

YEAR AND CHARACTERISTIC	NUMBER OF CONDITIONS (mil.)					RATE PER 100 POPULATION				
	Infective and parasitic	Respiratory		Diges-tive system	Injuries	Infective and parasitic	Respiratory		Diges-tive system	Injuries
		Common cold	Influ-enza				Common cold	Influ-enza		
1970	48.2	(NA)	(NA)	23.0	59.2	24.1	(NA)	(NA)	11.5	29.6
1975	47.6	(NA)	(NA)	21.6	76.2	22.8	(NA)	(NA)	10.3	36.4
1980	53.6	(NA)	(NA)	24.9	72.7	24.6	(NA)	(NA)	11.4	33.4
1985	47.8	(NA)	(NA)	16.3	64.0	20.5	(NA)	(NA)	7.0	27.4
1990	51.7	61.5	106.8	13.0	60.1	21.0	25.0	43.4	5.3	24.4
1991	46.1	71.2	129.6	16.5	59.7	18.5	28.6	52.1	6.6	24.0
1992	56.2	64.6	107.3	17.6	59.6	22.4	25.7	42.7	7.0	23.7
1993	54.3	68.2	132.6	16.1	62.1	21.3	26.8	52.2	6.3	24.4
1994, total[1]	54.2	66.0	90.4	15.9	61.9	20.9	25.4	34.8	6.1	23.8
Under 5 years old	11.2	14.0	7.6	2.2	5.2	54.7	68.5	37.3	10.5	25.6
5 to 17 years old	20.8	14.6	22.9	4.1	12.9	41.9	29.4	46.3	8.3	26.0
18 to 24 years old	4.7	6.6	9.8	1.9	8.3	18.5	26.1	38.7	7.4	32.7
25 to 44 years old	12.1	18.6	31.4	3.9	20.7	14.6	22.4	37.8	4.7	25.0
45 to 64 years old	3.9	8.4	13.1	2.1	8.7	7.7	16.6	25.9	4.1	17.2
65 years old and over	1.6	3.8	5.7	1.7	6.1	5.2	12.3	18.3	5.6	19.6
Male	23.8	30.3	43.2	6.9	32.6	18.8	24.0	34.1	5.5	25.8
Female	30.4	35.7	47.3	9.0	29.2	22.8	26.8	35.5	6.7	22.0
White	46.4	52.2	78.3	12.1	53.1	21.6	24.3	36.5	5.7	24.8
Black	6.7	9.7	7.7	2.9	6.8	20.2	29.3	23.2	8.9	20.6

[Continued]

★ 95 ★

Acute Conditions, by Type: 1970 to 1994
[Continued]

YEAR AND CHARACTERISTIC	NUMBER OF CONDITIONS (mil.)					RATE PER 100 POPULATION				
	Infective and parasitic	Respiratory		Diges- tive system	Injuries	Infective and parasitic	Respiratory		Diges- tive system	Injuries
		Common cold	Influ- enza				Common cold	Influ- enza		
Northeast	12.4	14.9	13.2	2.6	10.2	24.5	29.4	26.0	5.2	20.2
Midwest	10.5	14.8	26.9	3.3	15.9	16.6	23.3	42.5	5.2	25.2
South	21.5	17.1	22.0	5.9	20.8	24.4	19.4	25.0	6.7	23.6
West	9.8	19.2	28.3	4.1	14.9	17.0	33.3	49.1	7.0	25.8
Family income:										
Under $10,000	3.8	8.0	8.9	2.4	7.9	16.2	34.4	38.0	10.1	33.9
$10,000 to $19,999	6.9	9.7	11.7	3.0	9.3	18.4	26.0	31.3	8.0	25.1
$20,000 to $34,999	11.2	13.6	20.8	3.1	12.5	20.7	25.1	38.5	5.7	23.0
$35,000 or more	24.6	25.5	38.1	5.1	22.1	24.6	25.4	38.0	5.1	22.0

Source: 1996 Statistical Abstract of the United States on CD-ROM [machine-readable datafiles]. CD-8A-97. Washington, DC: U.S. Department of Commerce, Economics and Statistics Administration, Bureau of the Census, Data User Services Division, January 1997. Primary source: U.S. National Center for Health Statistics, *Vital and Health Statistics*, series 10, No. 193, and earlier reports; and unpublished data. *Notes:* NA Not available. 1. Includes other races and unknown income not shown separately.

★ 96 ★

Diseases and Illnesses

Airplane Travel and Blood Clots

"With a typical business-class air ticket costing at least twice the economy fare, company accountants often wonder whether the wider seats and free champagne are really worth it. Some doctors fear that the answer is yes—for safety reasons.

"Not the obvious ones, like crashing into the sea or being buzzed by F-16s. These risks are much the same at either end of the plane. But the lack of legroom in steerage might make middle-aged passengers more likely to develop deep-vein thrombosis (DVT)—potentially lethal blood clots."

Source: "The Torture of Second-Class Travel." Economist, 14 June 1997, p. 91.

★ 97 ★

Diseases and Illnesses

Carpal Tunnel Syndrome and Gardening

"*Physician and Sportsmedicine* magazine regularly ranks gardening in its top 10 list of occupations that promote carpal tunnel syndrome. This debilitating condition and its sister affliction, repetitive strain injuries (RSI), occur when the wrist and/or fingers are repetitively moved out of the neutral position, putting strain on the bones and ligaments of the wrist and hand."

Source: Pipp, Tracy L. "Growing Pains." *Detroit News,* 10 July 1997, p. 1E.

★ 98 ★

Diseases and Illnesses

Illnesses of Long-Term Care Patients, by Percentage of Insurance Claims

[In percentages]

Ailment	Share of insurance claims
Dementia (Alzheimer's)	36
Alzheimer's	36
Bone diseases	17
Joint diseases	17
Cancer	14
Stroke	13
Heart conditions	10
Blood conditions	10
Organ disorders (stomach, liver)	4
Lung disorders	3
Wounds, injuries	2
Diabetes	1

Source: "The List: Health Check." *Business Week,* 19 August 1996, p. 4. Primary source: John Hancock Financial Services.

★ 99 ★

Diseases and Illnesses

Infections: Hospital Charges for Patients With and Without Hospital-Acquired Infections: 1995

Field	With infections	Without infections	Percent increase
Internal medicine	31,267	11,253	178
Family practice medicine	24,456	8,712	181
General surgery	64,363	13,354	382
Cardiac surgery	78,151	33,185	136
Cardiology	43,981	14,485	204

Source: "Workplace Notebook: In-Hospital Infections." *Workplace Vitality* (May 1996), p. 15.

★ 100 ★

Diseases and Illnesses

Leukemia Statistics

Type of Leukemia	Median[1] Age at Diagnosis (Years)	Annual Number of Cases/100,000 people (1985-89)	Percentage of all Childhood Leukemia	Percentage of all Adult Leukemia[2]
Acute lymphocytic	11	1.5	75	6
Acute myeloid	67	2.3	20	54
Chronic lymphocytic	71	2.9	< 1[3]	25
Chronic myeloid	67	1.4	5	15
Hairy cell	53	<1[3]	< 1[3]	2

Source: Leukemia, Research Report, U.S. Department of Health and Human Services, Public Health Service, National Institutes of Health, National Cancer Institute, PHS 94-329, November 1993, modified October 1995. *Notes:* 1. Half of all patients are above this age and half are below. 2. Rounded upwards. 3. Less than one.

★ 101 ★

Diseases and Illnesses

Lyme Disease: Expenditures on Research, FY 1994

Agency	Expenditures ($ mil.)
National Institute of Allergy & Infectious Disease	13.720
National Institute of Arthritis & Musculoskeletal & Skin Diseases	3.112
National Center for Research Resources	.306

Source: Drug Topics, 20 November 1995, p. 74.

★ 102 ★

Diseases and Illnesses

Poisonings: Plants Frequently Implicated

Plant	No. reported exposures
Philodendron	4726
Pepper	3912
Dumb cane	2837
Poinsettia	2798
Holly	2651
Pokeweed or inkberry	2231
Peace lily	2086
Jade plant	1658
Pothos/Devil's ivy	1401
Poison ivy	1308
Umbrella tree	1141
African violet	1137
Rhododendron/Azalea	1029
Yew	969
Eucalyptus	945
Pyracantha	894
Spider plant	787
Christmas cactus	781
English ivy	765
Climbing nightshade	754

Source: U.S. Department of Health and Human Services. Public Health Service. Centers for Disease Control and Prevention. *Morbidity and Mortality Weekly Report,* vol. 44, no. 3, 27 January 1995, p. 43. Primary source: American Association of Poison Control Centers Toxic Exposure Surveillance System.

★ 103 ★

Diseases and Illnesses

Specified Reportable Diseases – Cases Reported: 1970 to 1994

Figures should be interpreted with caution. Although reporting of some of these diseases is incomplete, the figures are of value in indicating trends of disease incidence. Includes cases imported from outside the United States.

DISEASE	1970	1980	1985	1989	1990	1991	1992	1993	1994
AIDS[1]	(NA)	(NA)	8,249	33,722	41,595	43,672	45,472	103,533	78,279
Amebiasis	2,888	5,271	4,433	3,217	3,328	2,989	2,942	2,970	2,983
Aseptic meningitis	6,480	8,028	10,619	10,274	11,852	14,526	12,223	12,848	8,932
Botulism[2]	12	89	122	89	92	114	91	97	143
Brucellosis (undulant fever)	213	183	153	95	85	104	105	120	119
Chicken pox (1,000)	[3]	190.9	178.2	185.4	173.1	147.1	158.4	134.7	151.2
Diphtheria	435	3	3	3	4	5	4	0	2
Encephalitis:									
Primary infectious[4]	1,580	1,362	1,376	981	1,341	1,021	774	919	717
Post infectious[4]	370	40	161	88	105	82	129	170	143
Escherichia coli 0157:H7	[3]	[3]	[3]	[3]	[3]	[3]	[3]	[3]	1,420
Haemophilius influenza	[3]	[3]	[3]	[3]	[3]	2,764	1,412	1,419	1,174
Hepatitis: B (serum) (1,000)	8.3	19.0	26.6	23.4	21.1	18.0	16.1	13.4	12.5
A (infectious) (1,000)	56.8	29.1	23.2	35.8	31.4	24.4	23.1	24.2	29.8
Unspecified (1,000)	[3]	11.9	5.5	2.3	1.7	1.3	0.9	0.6	0.4
Non-A, non-B (1,000)[5]	[3]	[3]	4.2	2.5	2.6	3.6	6.0	4.8	4.4
Legionellosis	[3]	[3]	830	1,190	1,370	1,317	1,339	1,280	1,615
Leprosy (Hansen disease)	129	223	361	163	198	154	172	187	136
Leptospirosis	47	85	57	93	77	58	54	51	38
Lyme disease	[3]	[3]	[3]	[3]	[3]	9,465	9,895	8,257	13,043
Malaria	3,051	2,062	1,049	1,277	1,292	1,278	1,087	1,411	1,229
Measles (1,000)	47.4	13.5	2.8	18.2	27.8	9.6	2.2	0.3	1.0
Meningococcal infections	2,505	2,840	2,479	2,727	2,451	2,130	2,134	2,637	2,886
Mumps (1,000)	105.0	8.6	3.0	5.7	5.3	4.3	2.6	1.7	1.5
Pertussis (1,000)[6]	4.2	1.7	3.6	4.2	4.6	2.7	4.1	6.6	4.6
Plague	13	18	17	4	2	11	13	10	17
Poliomyelitis, acute[7]	33	9	7	9	6	9	6	3	0
Psittacosis	35	124	119	116	113	94	92	60	38
Rabies, animal	3,224	6,421	5,565	4,724	4,826	6,910	8,589	9,377	8,147
Rabies, human	3	0	1	1	1	3	1	3	6
Rheumatic fever, acute[8]	3,227	432	90	144	108	127	75	112	112
Rubella (1,000)[9]	56.6	3.9	0.6	0.4	1.1	1.4	0.2	0.2	0.2
Salmonellosis (1,000)[10]	22.1	33.7	65.3	47.8	48.6	48.2	40.9	41.6	43.3
Shigellosis (1,000)[11]	13.8	19.0	17.1	25.0	27.1	23.5	23.9	32.2	29.8
Tetanus	148	95	83	53	64	57	45	48	51
Toxic-shock syndrome	[3]	[3]	384	400	322	280	244	212	192
Trichinosis	109	131	61	30	129	62	41	16	32
Tuberculosis (1,000)[12]	37.1	27.7	22.2	23.5	25.7	26.3	26.7	25.3	24.4
Tularemia	172	234	177	152	152	193	159	132	96
Typhoid fever	346	510	402	460	552	501	414	440	441
Typhus fever:									
Flea-borne (endemic-murine)	27	81	37	41	50	43	28	25	[3]
Tick-borne (Rocky Mt. spotted fever)	380	1,163	714	623	651	628	502	456	465
Sexually transmitted diseases:									
Gonorrhea (1,000)	600	1,004	911	733	690	620	501	440	418

[Continued]

★ 103 ★

Specified Reportable Diseases – Cases Reported: 1970 to 1994

[Continued]

DISEASE	1970	1980	1985	1989	1990	1991	1992	1993	1994
Syphilis (1,000)	91	69	68	111	134	129	113	101	82
Other (1,000)	2.2	1.0	2.3	4.9	4.6	4.0	2.2	1.7	1.0

Source: 1996 Statistical Abstract of the United States on CD-ROM [machine-readable datafiles]. CD-8A-97. Washington, DC: U.S. Department of Commerce, Economics and Statistics Administration, Bureau of the Census, Data User Services Division, January 1997. Primary source: U.S. Centers for Disease Control and Prevention, Atlanta, GA, *Summary of Notifiable Diseases, United States, Morbidity and Mortality Weekly Report*, vol. 43, No. 53, October 6, 1995. *Notes:* NA Not available. 1. Acquired immunodeficiency syndrome was not a notifiable disease until 1984. Figures are shown for years in which cases were reported to the CDC. Beginning 1993, based on revised classification system and expanded surveillance case definition. 2. Beginning in 1980, includes foodborne, infant, wound, and unspecified cases. 3. Disease was not notifiable. 4. Beginning 1980, reported data reflect new diagnostic categories. 5. Includes some persons positive for antibody to hepatitis C virus who do not have hepatitis. 6. Whooping cough. 7. Revised. Data subject to annual revisions. 8. Based on reports from States: 38 in 1970, 37 in 1980, 38 in 1981, 35 in 1982-1984, 31 in 1985, 29 in 1986 and 1988, 25 in 1987, 28 in 1989, 30 in 1990, 23 in 1991, 26 in 1992 and 1993, and 27 in 1994. 9. German measles. 10. Excludes typhoid fever. 11. Bacillary dysentery. 12. Newly reported active cases. New diagnostic standards introduced in 1980.

★ 104 ★

Diseases and Illnesses

Top Medical Diagnoses in Doctors' Office Visits:
1995

Diagnoses	Percentage
Hypertension	7.2
Acute upper respiratory infection	3.6
Bronchitis	3.0
Chronic sinusitis	2.9
Diabetes mellitus	2.8
Acute pharyngitis	2.8
Otitis media	2.6
Necessary exam	1.5
Depressive disorder	1.4
Routine exam	1.4

Source: "Snapshots of the Workplace Health Industry: What the Doctor Found." *Workplace Vitality* (July/August 1996), p. 15. Primary source: Scott-Levin Associates.

Diseases and Illnesses: AIDS

★ 105 ★

Acquired Immunodeficiency Syndrome (AIDS) Deaths, by Selected Characteristics: Through 1995

Data are shown by year of death and are subject to substantial retrospective changes. Based on reporting by state health departments.

CHARACTERISTIC	NUMBER									DISTRIBUTION	
	Total cases	1985 and before[1]	1989	1990	1991	1992	1993	1994	1995	1995	1993 -1995
Total[2]	305,843	12,493	26,355	29,934	34,651	38,813	41,077	43,975	31,256	100.0	100.0
Age:											
13 to 29 years old	53,632	2,558	4,924	5,427	6,059	6,481	6,815	6,930	5,105	16.3	16.2
30 to 39 years old	138,660	5,714	12,056	13,695	15,582	17,437	18,548	20,037	14,083	45.1	45.3
40 to 49 years old	77,425	2,726	6,205	7,329	8,943	10,339	10,975	11,921	8,543	27.3	27.0
50 to 59 years old	25,383	1,104	2,218	2,433	2,822	3,175	3,389	3,721	2,572	8.2	8.3
60 years old and over	10,743	391	952	1,050	1,245	1,381	1,350	1,366	953	3.0	3.2
Sex:											
Male	268,987	11,553	23,742	26,752	30,725	34,072	35,551	37,360	26,375	84.4	85.4
Female	36,856	940	2,613	3,182	3,926	4,741	5,526	6,615	4,881	15.6	14.6
Race/ethnicity:											
White	159,292	7,267	14,481	16,517	18,693	19,982	20,376	20,733	14,389	46.0	47.7
Black	100,167	3,424	7,950	9,010	10,722	12,839	14,420	16,294	11,879	38.0	36.6
Hispanic	43,154	1,719	3,656	4,120	4,851	5,578	5,820	6,421	4,574	14.6	14.5
Other/unknown	3,230	83	268	287	385	414	461	527	414	1.3	1.2

Source: 1996 Statistical Abstract of the United States on CD-ROM [machine-readable datafiles]. CD-8A-97. Washington, DC: U.S. Department of Commerce, Economics and Statistics Administration, Bureau of the Census, Data User Services Division, January 1997. Primary source: U.S. Centers for Disease Control and Prevention, Surveillance Report, annual. Notes: 1. Includes deaths prior to 1982. 2. Includes other race/ethnicity groups not shown separately.

★ 106 ★

Diseases and Illnesses: AIDS

AIDS Cases: Adults/Adolescents, by Exposure Category and Sex

This table shows AIDS cases for adults/adolescents by exposure category and sex, reported July 1994 through June 1995, July 1995 through June 1996[1] and cumulative totals for both sexes and exposure category, through June 1996, in the United States. AIDS as defined by the Centers for Disease Control and Prevention: "Acquired immunodeficiency syndrome (AIDS) is a specific group of diseases or conditions which are indicative of severe immunosuppression related to infection with the human immunodeficiency virus (HIV)."

Exposure category	Males				Females				Both Sexes Cumul. Total[2]	
	July 1994- June 1995		July 1995- June 1996		July 1994- June 1995		July 1995- June 1996			
	No.	%	No.	%	No.	%	No.	%	No.	%
Men who have sex with men	33,118	54	29,260	51	0	0	0	0	274,192	51
Injecting drug use	14,971	24	13,386	23	5,651	41	5,016	36	137,753	25
Men who have sex with men and inject drugs	3,957	6	3,198	6	-	-	-	-	35,218	7
Hemophilia/ coagulation disorder	432	1	360	1	27	0	20	0	4,280	1
Heterosexual contact:	3,091	5	3,102	5	5,582	41	5,563	40	44,980	8
Sex with injecting drug user	947	-	966	-	2,057	-	1,976	-	20,307	
Sex with bisexual male	-	-	-	-	375	-	377	-	2,425	
Sex with person with hemophilia	6	-	11	-	60	-	35	-	349	
Sex with transfusion recipient with HIV infection	68	-	35	-	63	-	66	-	789	
Sex with HIV-infected person, risk not specified	2,070	-	2,090	-	3,027	-	3,109	-	21,110	
Receipt of blood transfusion, blood components, or tissue[3]	371	1	334	1	312	2	276	2	7,684	1
Other/risk not reported or identified[4]	5,645	9	8,068	14	2,172	16	3,121	22	36,699	7

[Continued]

★ 106 ★

AIDS Cases: Adults/Adolescents, by Exposure Category and Sex
[Continued]

Exposure category	Males				Females				Both Sexes Cumul. Total[2]	
	July 1994-June 1995		July 1995-June 1996		July 1994-June 1995		July 1995-June 1996			
	No.	%	No.	%	No.	%	No.	%	No.	%
Adult/adolescent subtotal	61,585	100	57,708	100	13,744	100	13,996	100	540,806	100

Source: U.S. Department of Health and Human Services. Public Health Service. Centers for Disease Control and Prevention. *HIV/AIDS Surveillance Report, 1996* vol. 8, no. 1. The HIV/AIDS Surveillance Report is now accessible via Internet: www.cdc.gov. The HIV/AIDS Surveillance Report is published semiannually by the Division of HIV/AIDS Prevention, National Center for HIV, STD, and TB Prevention, Centers for Disease Control and Prevention (CDC), Atlanta, GA 30333. All data contained in the Report are provisional. *Notes:* 1. See the primary source for a discussion of the impact of the 1993 AIDS surveillance case definition for adults and adolescents (implemented January 1, 1993) on the number of cases reported annually since 1993. 2. Includes 10 persons known to be infected with human immunodeficiency virus type 2 (HIV-2). 3. Thirty-five adults/adolescents and 3 children developed AIDS after receiving blood screened negative for HIV antibody. Twelve additional adults developed AIDS after receiving tissue, organs, or artificial insemination from HIV-infected donors. Four of the 12 received tissue, organs, or artificial insemination from a donor who was negative for HIV antibody at the time of donation. See *New England Journal of Medicine* 1992; 326:726-32. 4. See table 11 and figure 6 for a discussion of the "other" exposure category. "Other" also includes 39 persons who acquired HIV infection perinatally but were diagnosed with AIDS after age 13. These 39 persons are tabulated under the adult/adolescent, not pediatric, exposure category.

★ 107 ★

Diseases and Illnesses: AIDS

AIDS Cases, by Geographic Division and State: June 30, 1994-1995

[Rate is cases per 100,000 persons][1]

Geographic division and State	12 months ending June 30, 1995
United States[2]	28.48
New England	22.91
Maine	11.21
New Hampshire	10.20
Vermont	5.52
Massachusetts	23.11
Rhode Island	29.19
Connecticut	32.55
Middle Atlantic	52.51
New York	69.23
New Jersey	60.27
Pennsylvania	22.22
East North Central	13.74
Ohio	10.70
Indiana	9.11
Illinois	23.70

[Continued]

★ 107 ★

AIDS Cases, by Geographic Division and State:
June 30, 1994-1995
[Continued]

Geographic division and State	12 months ending June 30, 1995
Michigan	11.28
Wisconsin	7.20
West North Central	9.20
Minnesota	9.04
Iowa	5.13
Missouri	13.19
North Dakota	1.10
South Dakota	2.77
Nebraska	6.84
Kansas	11.12
South Atlantic	41.85
Delaware	44.31
Maryland	58.95
District of Columbia	213.97
Virginia	17.55
West Virginia	6.26
North Carolina	14.36
South Carolina	27.16
Georgia	32.37
Florida	67.21
East South Central	13.68
Kentucky	8.13
Tennessee	17.06
Alabama	13.42
Mississippi	15.51
West South Central	24.05
Arkansas	11.74
Louisiana	26.05
Oklahoma	8.16
Texas	28.04
Mountain	14.23
Montana	2.80
Idaho	5.03
Wyoming	2.73
Colorado	19.64
New Mexico	13.79
Arizona	13.72
Utah	8.02
Nevada	28.35

[Continued]

★ 107 ★

AIDS Cases, by Geographic Division and State: June 30, 1994-1995

[Continued]

Geographic division and State	12 months ending June 30, 1995
Pacific	30.66
Washington	17.46
Oregon	16.40
California	34.96
Alaska	13.03
Hawaii	22.32

Source: U.S. Department of Health and Human Services. Public Health Service. Centers for Disease Control and Prevention. National Center for Health Statistics. *Health, United States, 1995.* Hyattsville, MD: Public Health Service, 1996, p. 168. Primary source: Centers for Disease Control and Prevention, National Center for HIV, STD, and TB Prevention, Division of HIV/AIDS Prevention. *Notes:* The AIDS cases reporting definitions were expanded in 1993. Excludes residents of U.S. territories. Data are updated periodically because of reporting delays. Data have been updated through June 30, 1995. Data as of December 31, 1995 are available in the Centers for Disease Control and Prevention HIV/AIDS Surveillance Report, Year-End Edition, February 1996. 1. Computed using resident population estimates for 1994 based on extrapolation from 1990 census counts from the U.S. Bureau of the Census. 2. Includes unknown State of residence.

★ 108 ★

Diseases and Illnesses: AIDS

AIDS Cases by Metro Area: 1994-1996

Table shows AIDS cases and annual rates per 100,000 population, by metropolitan area with 500,000 or more population, reported July 1994 through June 1995, July 1995 through June 1996; and cumulative totals, by area and age group, through June 1996, United States. AIDS as defined by CDC: "Acquired immunodeficiency syndrome (AIDS) is a specific group of diseases or conditions which are indicative of severe immunosuppression related to infection with the human immunodeficiency virus (HIV)."

Metropolitan area of residence	July 1994 - June 1995		July 1995 - June 1996		Cumulative Totals		
	No.	Rate	No.	Rate	Adults/ adolescents	Children < 13 years	Total
Akron, OH	50	7.4	35	5.2	348	-	348
Albany-Schenectady, NY	170	19.4	213	24.4	1,150	20	1,170
Albuquerque, NM	108	16.7	53	8.0	702	2	704
Allentown, PA	93	15.2	104	17.0	551	7	558
Ann Arbor, MI	34	6.6	39	7.5	282	6	288
Atlanta, GA	1,603	48.1	1,772	51.6	11,308	92	11,400
Austin, TX	387	40.1	296	29.6	2,775	17	2,792
Bakersfield, CA	77	12.6	137	22.2	650	3	653
Baltimore, MD	2,040	83.0	1,518	61.5	9,082	175	9,257
Baton Rouge, LA	166	29.7	221	39.2	1,004	16	1,020
Bergen-Passaic, NJ	612	47.0	491	37.5	3,973	66	4,039
Birmingham, AL	160	18.3	212	24.0	1,233	15	1,248
Boston, MA	1,193	20.8	1,130	19.6	9,852	154	10,006
Buffalo, NY	105	8.8	45	3.8	893	10	903

[Continued]

★ 108 ★

AIDS Cases by Metro Area: 1994-1996

[Continued]

Metropolitan area of residence	July 1994 - June 1995		July 1995 - June 1996		Cumulative Totals		
	No.	Rate	No.	Rate	Adults/ adolescents	Children < 13 years	Total
Charleston, SC	152	29.4	128	25.3	1,043	10	1,053
Charlotte, NC	219	17.4	201	15.6	1,385	18	1,403
Chicago, IL	2,462	32.1	1,809	23.4	15,133	189	15,322
Cincinnati, OH	220	13.9	273	17.1	1,421	13	1,434
Cleveland, OH	473	21.3	249	11.2	2,345	34	2,379
Columbus, OH	193	13.6	196	13.6	1,702	10	1,712
Dallas, TX	1,416	48.8	1,010	34.1	9,123	35	9,158
Dayton, OH	52	5.4	115	12.0	720	15	735
Denver, CO	568	31.6	447	24.4	4,442	19	4,461
Detroit, MI	772	17.9	731	16.9	5,410	61	5,471
El Paso, TX	116	17.4	120	17.7	601	2	603
Ft. Lauderdale, FL	1,589	114.8	1,225	86.7	8,632	197	8,829
Ft. Worth, TX	538	36.7	204	13.7	2,280	23	2,303
Fresno, CA	121	14.5	145	17.2	868	12	880
Gary, IN	97	15.6	66	10.6	465	3	468
Grand Rapids, MI	66	6.7	85	8.5	540	3	543
Greensboro, NC	206	18.6	177	15.7	1,147	17	1,164
Greenville, SC	141	16.2	138	15.6	957	2	959
Harrisburg, PA	92	15.1	94	15.3	580	5	585
Hartford, CT	388	34.7	515	46.2	2,665	41	2,706
Honolulu, HI	193	22.1	140	16.0	1,374	11	1,385
Houston, TX	1,322	36.2	1,334	35.9	13,201	121	13,322
Indianapolis, IN	214	14.6	336	22.8	2,056	12	2,068
Jacksonville, FL	474	49.0	388	39.6	3,100	65	3,165
Jersey City, NJ	880	159.6	634	115.2	4,937	105	5,042
Kansas City, MO	293	17.8	345	20.7	3,076	12	3,088
Knoxville, TN	89	14.1	65	10.1	465	5	470
Las Vegas, NV	337	31.2	376	33.0	2,224	20	2,244
Little Rock, AR	96	17.8	86	15.8	727	10	737
Los Angeles, CA	3,980	43.6	3,922	42.9	32,653	206	32,859
Louisville, KY	143	14.6	151	15.3	888	8	896
Memphis, TN	333	31.5	302	28.3	1,817	14	1,831
Miami, FL	2,961	146.4	2,382	117.3	17,089	422	17,511
Middlesex, NJ	382	35.7	333	30.8	2,396	61	2,457
Milwaukee, WI	209	14.4	162	11.1	1,422	14	1,436
Minneapolis-St. Paul, MN	368	13.7	276	10.1	2,507	16	2,523
Mobile, AL	104	20.3	109	21.1	773	10	783
Monmouth-Ocean City, NJ	350	33.8	288	27.4	2,151	51	2,202
Nashville, TN	286	26.7	294	26.9	1,599	14	1,613
Nassau-Suffolk, NY	550	20.7	641	24.1	4,747	78	4,825
New Haven, CT	581	35.7	865	53.2	4,507	111	4,618
New Orleans, LA	607	46.3	734	55.8	4,831	54	4,885
New York, NY	10,746	125.3	11,309	132.0	85,282	1,695	86,977
Newark, NJ	1,740	90.0	1,531	79.1	12,212	283	12,495
Norfolk, VA	389	25.4	544	35.3	2,190	51	2,241

[Continued]

★ 108 ★

AIDS Cases by Metro Area: 1994-1996
[Continued]

Metropolitan area of residence	July 1994 - June 1995		July 1995 - June 1996		Cumulative Totals		
					Adults/ adolescents	Children < 13 years	Total
	No.	Rate	No.	Rate			
Oakland, CA	747	34.2	667	30.4	6,261	36	6,297
Oklahoma City, OK	108	10.7	113	11.1	1,178	3	1,181
Omaha, NE	77	11.6	64	9.5	518	2	520
Orange County, CA	539	21.2	514	20.0	4,284	25	4,309
Orlando, FL	742	54.4	592	42.6	3,900	64	3,964
Philadelphia, PA	2,015	40.7	1,700	34.3	12,359	182	12,541
Phoenix, AZ	392	15.8	466	18.2	3,371	11	3,382
Pittsburgh, PA	328	13.7	227	9.5	1,822	11	1,833
Portland, OR	399	23.8	354	20.7	3,002	8	3,010
Providence, RI	270	29.6	167	18.4	1,403	15	1,418
Raleigh-Durham, NC	187	19.3	170	17.1	1,374	20	1,394
Richmond, VA	227	24.8	279	30.1	1,703	22	1,725
Riverside-San Bernardino, CA	818	28.1	664	22.5	4,880	44	4,924
Rochester, NY	217	19.9	324	29.8	1,442	8	1,450
Sacramento, CA	351	24.4	275	18.9	2,408	24	2,432
St. Louis, MO	378	14.9	439	17.2	3,357	29	3,386
Salt Lake City, UT	126	10.7	177	14.8	1,119	14	1,133
San Antonio, TX	382	26.7	374	25.6	2,803	23	2,826
San Diego, CA	950	36.1	1,147	43.4	7,892	45	7,937
San Francisco, CA	2,156	131.3	1,807	109.8	23,557	35	23,592
San Jose, CA	298	19.2	298	19.0	2,449	12	2,461
San Juan, PR	1,529	79.4	1,311	67.0	10,703	218	10,921
Sarasota, FL	170	32.8	123	23.4	996	20	1,016
Scranton, PA	48	7.5	31	4.9	299	3	302
Seattle, WA	652	30.0	543	24.7	5,205	14	5,219
Springfield, MA	183	30.8	169	28.5	1,131	21	1,152
Stockton, CA	48	9.3	82	15.6	532	12	544
Syracuse, NY	120	15.9	78	10.4	776	7	783
Tacoma, WA	80	12.5	68	10.5	573	8	581
Tampa-St. Petersburg, FL	820	38.0	755	34.6	5,844	80	5,924
Toledo, OH	48	7.8	64	10.4	414	8	422
Tucson, AZ	118	16.1	146	19.4	1,006	6	1,012
Tulsa, OK	81	10.9	90	12.1	791	6	797
Ventura, CA	71	10.1	89	12.5	597	2	599
Washington, DC	2,142	48.0	2,067	45.8	15,449	218	15,667
West Palm Beach, FL	863	90.4	840	86.4	5,020	172	5,192
Wichita, KS	94	18.6	79	15.5	501	2	503
Wilmington, DE	257	47.6	274	50.2	1,313	9	1,322
Youngstown, OH	34	5.6	28	4.6	236	-	236
Metropolitan areas with 500,000 or more population	63,371	38.9	59,396	36.1	455,954	6,180	462,134
Central counties	62,071	41.7	58,172	38.8	447,649	6,069	453,718
Outlying counties	1,300	9.3	1,224	8.5	8,305	111	8,416

[Continued]

★ 108 ★

AIDS Cases by Metro Area: 1994-1996

[Continued]

Metropolitan area of residence	July 1994 - June 1995		July 1995 - June 1996		Cumulative Totals		
					Adults/ adolescents	Children < 13 years	Total
	No.	Rate	No.	Rate			
Metropolitan areas with 50,000 to 500,000 population	7,876	16.4	7,729	16.0	53,095	689	53,784
Central counties	7,369	17.2	7,248	16.8	49,832	629	50,461
Outlying counties	507	9.6	481	9.0	3,263	60	3,323
Nonmetropolitan areas	4,590	8.6	4,717	8.7	29,358	411	29,769
Total[1]	76,289	28.8	72,416	27.1	540,806	7,296	548,102

Source: U.S. Department of Health and Human Services. Public Health Service. Centers for Disease Control and Prevention. *HIV/AIDS Surveillance Report, 1996* vol. 8, no. 1. The HIV/AIDS Surveillance Report is now accessible via Internet: www.cdc.gov. The HIV/AIDS Surveillance Report is published semiannually by the Division of HIV/AIDS Prevention, National Center for HIV, STD, and TB Prevention, Centers for Disease Control and Prevention (CDC), Atlanta, GA 30333. All data contained in the Report are provisional. *Note:* 1. Totals include persons whose state of residence is unknown.

★ 109 ★

Diseases and Illnesses: AIDS

AIDS Cases by Race and Ethnicity and Exposure Category: Part 1

This table shows AIDS cases for whites and blacks by exposure category, reported July 1995 through June 1996, and cumulative totals (all ethnicities), through June 1996 in the United States. AIDS as defined by the Centers for Disease Control and Prevention: "Acquired immunodeficiency syndrome (AIDS) is a specific group of diseases or conditions which are indicative of severe immunosuppression related to infection with the human immunodeficiency virus (HIV)."

Exposure category	White, not Hispanic				Black, not Hispanic				All Groups Cumul. Total[1]	
	July 1995- June 1996		Cumu- lative Total		July 1995- June 1996		Cumu- lative Total			
	No.	%	No.	%	No.	%	No.	%	No.	%
Men who have sex with men	17,665	70	180,294	76	6,856	33	55,327	39	274,192	59
Injecting drug use	2,783	11	20,664	9	6,845	33	51,143	36	101,714	22
Men who have sex with men and inject drugs	1,614	6	18,670	8	1,077	5	10,869	8	35,218	8
Hemophilia/ coagulation disorder	250	1	3,259	1	57	0	430	0	4,122	1
Heterosexual contact:	566	2	3,234	1	1,765	8	8,527	6	15,268	3
Sex with injecting drug user	183	-	1,351	-	539	-	3,591	-	6,142	-

[Continued]

★ 109 ★

AIDS Cases by Race and Ethnicity and Exposure Category: Part 1
[Continued]

Exposure category	White, not Hispanic				Black, not Hispanic				All Groups Cumul. Total[1]	
	July 1995-June 1996		Cumu-lative Total		July 1995-June 1996		Cumu-lative Total			
	No.	%	No.	%	No.	%	No.	%	No.	%
Sex with person with hemophilia	5	-	20	-	5	-	10	-	37	-
Sex with transfusion recipient with HIV infection	8	-	124	-	15	-	104	-	307	-
Sex with HIV-infected person, risk not specified	370	-	1,739	-	1,206	-	4,822	-	8,872	-
Receipt of blood transfusion, blood components, or tissue	172	1	2,941	1	106	1	907	1	4,449	1
Risk not reported or identified	2,138	8	7,428	3	4,095	20	14,299	10	27,189	6
Total	25,188	100	236,490	100	20,801	100	141,502	100	462,152	100

Source: U.S. Department of Health and Human Services. Public Health Service. Centers for Disease Control and Prevention. *HIV/AIDS Surveillance Report, 1996* vol. 8, no. 1. The HIV/AIDS Surveillance Report is now accessible via Internet: www.cdc.gov. The HIV/AIDS Surveillance Report is published semiannually by the Division of HIV/AIDS Prevention, National Center for HIV, STD, and TB Prevention, Centers for Disease Control and Prevention (CDC), Atlanta, GA 30333. All data contained in the Report are provisional. *Note:* 1. Includes 644 men whose race/ethnicity is unknown.

★ 110 ★

Diseases and Illnesses: AIDS

AIDS Cases by Race and Ethnicity and Exposure Category: Part 2

This table shows AIDS cases for Hispanics by exposure category, reported July 1995 through June 1996, and cumulative totals (all ethnicities), through June 1996, in the United States. AIDS as defined by the Centers for Disease Control and Prevention: "Acquired immunodeficiency syndrome (AIDS) is a specific group of diseases or conditions which are indicative of severe immunosuppression related to infection with the human immunodeficiency virus (HIV)."

Exposure category	Hispanics				All Groups Cumul. Total[2]	
	July 1995- June 1996		Cumu- lative Total			
	No.	%	No.	%	No.	%
Men who have sex with men	4,297	39	34,906	44	274,192	59
Injecting drug use	3,673	33	29,410	37	101,714	22
Men who have sex with men and inject drugs	459	4	5,337	7	35,218	8
Hemophilia/ coagulation disorder	42	0	346	0	4,122	1
Heterosexual contact:	745	7	3,396	4	15,268	3
Sex with injecting drug user	236	-	1,167	-	6,142	
Sex with person with hemophilia	1	-	7	-	37	
Sex with transfusion recipient with HIV infection	9	-	70	-	307	
Sex with HIV-infected person, risk not specified	499	-	2,152	-	8,872	
Receipt of blood transfusion, blood components, or tissue	48	0	491	1	4,449	1

[Continued]

★ 110 ★

AIDS Cases by Race and Ethnicity and Exposure Category: Part 2

[Continued]

Exposure category	Hispanics				All Groups Cumul.	
	July 1995- June 1996		Cumu- lative Total		Total[2]	
	No.	%	No.	%	No.	%
Risk not reported or identified[1]	1,706	16	5,040	6	27,189	6
Total	10,970	100	78,926	100	462,152	100

Source: U.S. Department of Health and Human Services. Public Health Service. Centers for Disease Control and Prevention. *HIV/AIDS Surveillance Report, 1996* vol. 8, no. 1. The HIV/AIDS Surveillance Report is now accessible via Internet: www.cdc.gov. The HIV/AIDS Surveillance Report is published semiannually by the Division of HIV/AIDS Prevention, National Center for HIV, STD, and TB Prevention, Centers for Disease Control and Prevention (CDC), Atlanta, GA 30333. All data contained in the Report are provisional. *Notes:* 1. See primary source for a discussion of the impact of the 1993 AIDS surveillance case definition for adults and adolescents (implemented January 1, 1993) on the number of cases reported annually since 1993. 2. Includes 10 persons known to be infected with human immunodeficiency virus type 2 (HIV-2).

★ 111 ★

Diseases and Illnesses: AIDS

AIDS Cases by Race and Ethnicity and Exposure Category: Part 3

This table shows AIDS cases for Asians/Pacific Islanders and American Indians and Alaskan Natives by exposure category, reported July 1995 through June 1996, and cumulative totals (all ethnicities), through June 1996, in the United States. AIDS as defined by the Centers for Disease Control and Prevention (CDC): "Acquired immunodeficiency syndrome (AIDS) is a specific group of diseases or conditions which are indicative of severe immunosuppression related to infection with the human immunodeficiency virus (HIV)."

Exposure category	Asians/Pacific Islanders				American Indians/Alaskan Natives				All Groups Cumul.	
	July 1995- June 1996		Cumu- lative Total		July 1995- June 1996		Cumu- lative Total		Total[1]	
	No.	%	No.	%	No.	%	No.	%	No.	%
Men who have sex with men	321	67	2,593	77	84	49	726	60	274,192	59
Injecting drug use	33	7	173	5	35	20	175	15	101,714	22
Men who have sex with men and inject drugs	17	4	114	3	26	15	201	17	35,218	8
Hemophilia/ coagulation disorder	7	1	55	2	2	1	26	2	4,122	1
Heterosexual contact:	19	4	78	2	5	3	21	2	15,268	3
Sex with injecting drug user	5	-	22	-	2	-	9	-	6,142	

[Continued]

★ 111 ★

AIDS Cases by Race and Ethnicity and Exposure Category: Part 3
[Continued]

Exposure category	Asians/Pacific Islanders				American Indians/Alaskan Natives				All Groups Cumul. Total[1]	
	July 1995-June 1996		Cumulative Total		July 1995-June 1996		Cumulative Total			
	No.	%	No.	%	No.	%	No.	%	No.	%
Sex with person with hemophilia	-	-	-	-	-	-	-	-	37	
Sex with transfusion recipient with HIV infection	3	-	7	-	-	-	1	-	307	
Sex with HIV-infected person, risk not specified	11	-	49	-	3	-	11	-	8,872	
Receipt of blood transfusion, blood components, or tissue	8	2	96	3	-	-	5	0	4,449	1
Risk not reported or identified	77	16	279	8	20	12	48	4	27,189	6
Total	482	100	3,388	100	172	100	1,202	100	462,152	100

Source: U.S. Department of Health and Human Services. Public Health Service. Centers for Disease Control and Prevention. *HIV/AIDS Surveillance Report, 1996* vol. 8, no. 1. The HIV/AIDS Surveillance Report is now accessible via Internet: www.cdc.gov. The HIV/AIDS Surveillance Report is published semiannually by the Division of HIV/AIDS Prevention, National Center for HIV, STD, and TB Prevention, Centers for Disease Control and Prevention (CDC), Atlanta, GA 30333. All data contained in the Report are provisional. *Notes:* 1. See primary source for a discussion of the impact of the 1993 AIDS surveillance case definition for adults and adolescents (implemented January 1, 1993) on the number of cases reported annually since 1993.

★ 112 ★

Diseases and Illnesses: AIDS

AIDS Cases by State: 1994-1996

Table shows AIDS cases and annual rates per 100,000 population, by state, reported July 1994 through June 1995, July 1995 through June 1996 and cumulative totals, by state and age group, through June 1996, United States[1]. AIDS as defined by the Centers for Disease Control and Prevention (CDC): "Acquired immunodeficiency syndrome (AIDS) is a specific group of diseases or conditions which are indicative of severe immunosuppression related to infection with the human immunodeficiency virus (HIV)."

U.S. state of residence	July 1994 - June 1995		July 1995 - June 1996		Cumulative Totals		
	No.	Rate	No.	Rate	Adults/ adolescents	Children < 13 years	Total
Alabama	565	13.4	666	15.7	3,928	55	3,983
Alaska	79	13.1	37	6.1	337	4	341
Arizona	559	13.7	664	15.7	4,717	19	4,736
Arkansas	287	11.7	286	11.5	2,003	30	2,033
California	10,961	34.9	10,589	33.5	93,240	509	93,749
Colorado	717	19.6	600	16.0	5,509	27	5,536
Connecticut	1,059	32.3	1,532	46.8	7,835	159	7,994
Delaware	310	43.8	320	44.6	1,647	13	1,660

[Continued]

★ 112 ★

AIDS Cases by State: 1994-1996
[Continued]

U.S. state of residence	July 1994 - June 1995		July 1995 - June 1996		Cumulative Totals		
	No.	Rate	No.	Rate	Adults/ adolescents	Children < 13 years	Total
District of Columbia	1,216	214.5	1,045	188.5	8,622	126	8,748
Florida	9,305	66.7	7,741	54.6	54,507	1,183	55,690
Georgia	2,293	32.5	2,503	34.8	15,698	168	15,866
Hawaii	264	22.4	206	17.4	1,870	14	1,884
Idaho	57	5.0	45	3.9	348	2	350
Illinois	2,766	23.5	2,149	18.2	17,374	210	17,584
Indiana	519	9.0	659	11.4	4,187	32	4,219
Iowa	145	5.1	129	4.5	924	8	932
Kansas	264	10.3	263	10.3	1,731	11	1,742
Kentucky	311	8.1	315	8.2	1,984	14	1,998
Louisiana	1,113	25.8	1,374	31.6	8,346	106	8,452
Maine	139	11.2	80	6.4	724	6	730
Maryland	2,915	58.3	2,296	45.5	13,837	245	14,082
Massachusetts	1,371	22.7	1,295	21.3	11,110	177	11,287
Michigan	1,057	11.1	1,040	10.9	7,741	83	7,824
Minnesota	412	9.0	320	6.9	2,843	19	2,862
Mississippi	413	15.5	415	15.4	2,568	38	2,606
Missouri	685	13.0	850	16.0	6,755	49	6,804
Montana	24	2.8	30	3.4	206	2	208
Nebraska	111	6.8	98	6.0	736	8	744
Nevada	412	28.2	459	30.0	2,823	21	2,844
New Hampshire	112	9.9	99	8.6	655	7	662
New Jersey	4,738	60.0	3,995	50.3	30,475	649	31,124
New Mexico	228	13.8	113	6.7	1,288	4	1,292
New York	12,537	69.1	13,251	73.1	99,191	1,858	101,049
North Carolina	1,017	14.4	975	13.6	6,792	95	6,887
North Dakota	6	0.9	9	1.4	72	-	72
Ohio	1,191	10.7	1,117	10.0	8,133	101	8,234
Oklahoma	268	8.2	278	8.5	2,580	18	2,598
Oregon	506	16.4	501	16.0	3,651	14	3,665
Pennsylvania	2,661	22.1	2,270	18.8	16,052	218	16,270
Rhode Island	288	29.0	182	18.4	1,501	16	1,517
South Carolina	992	27.2	970	26.4	5,786	65	5,851
South Dakota	20	2.8	17	2.3	108	4	112
Tennessee	877	16.9	903	17.2	5,112	42	5,154
Texas	5,108	27.7	4,399	23.5	37,025	295	37,320
Utah	153	8.0	199	10.2	1,273	20	1,293
Vermont	30	5.2	39	6.7	280	3	283
Virginia	1,145	17.5	1,513	22.9	8,319	139	8,458
Washington	925	17.3	777	14.3	7,150	26	7,176
West Virginia	113	6.2	146	8.0	680	8	688
Wisconsin	363	7.1	330	6.4	2,647	23	2,670
Wyoming	14	2.9	14	2.9	136	-	136
Subtotal	73,621	28.3	70,103	26.7	523,056	6,943	529,999

[Continued]

★ 112 ★

AIDS Cases by State: 1994-1996

[Continued]

U.S. state of residence	July 1994 - June 1995		July 1995 - June 1996		Cumulative Totals		
					Adults/ adolescents	Children < 13 years	Total
	No.	Rate	No.	Rate			
U.S. dependencies, possessions, and associated nations[1]							
Guam	-	-	4	2.8	17	-	17
Pacific Islands, U.S.	-	-	-	-	2	-	2
Puerto Rico	2,548	69.7	2,153	58.4	17,071	341	17,412
Virgin Islands, U.S.	62	59.7	32	30.6	262	12	274
Total[2]	76,289	28.9	72,416	27.1	540,806	7,296	548,102

Source: U.S. Department of Health and Human Services. Public Health Service. Centers for Disease Control and Prevention. *HIV/AIDS Surveillance Report, 1996* vol. 8, no. 1. The HIV/AIDS Surveillance Report is now accessible via Internet: www.cdc.gov. The HIV/AIDS Surveillance Report is published semiannually by the Division of HIV/AIDS Prevention, National Center for HIV, STD, and TB Prevention, Centers for Disease Control and Prevention (CDC), Atlanta, GA 30333. All data contained in the Report are provisional. *Notes:* 1. U.S. totals presented in this report include data from the United States (50 states and the District of Columbia), and from U.S. dependencies, possessions, and independent nations in free association with the United States. 2. Totals include 398 persons whose state of residence is unknown.

★ 113 ★

Diseases and Illnesses: AIDS

AIDS Cases: Pediatric, by Exposure Category and Sex

This table shows AIDS cases for pediatric level (less than 13 years of age), by exposure category and sex, reported July 1994 through June 1995, July 1995 through June 1996[1] and cumulative totals for both sexes and exposure category, through June 1996, United States. AIDS as defined by the Centers for Disease Control and Prevention (CDC): "Acquired immunodeficiency syndrome (AIDS) is a specific group of diseases or conditions which are indicative of severe immunosuppression related to infection with the human immunodeficiency virus (HIV)."

Exposure category	Males				Females				Both Sexes Cumul. Total[2]	
	July 1994- June 1995		July 1995- June 1996		July 1994- June 1995		July 1995- June 1996			
	No.	%	No.	%	No.	%	No.	%	No.	%
Hemophilia/ coagulation disorder	12	3	2	1	-	-	-	-	228	3
Mother with/at risk for HIV infection[4]:	420	89	328	91	464	95	327	93	6,586	90
Injecting drug use	122	-	97	-	138	-	88	-	2,714	
Sex with injecting drug user	75	-	55	-	70	-	45	-	1,228	
Sex with bisexual male	12	-	3	-	10	-	7	-	140	
Sex with person with hemophilia	1	-	-	-	1	-	1	-	25	

[Continued]

★ 113 ★

AIDS Cases: Pediatric, by Exposure Category and Sex
[Continued]

Exposure category	Males				Females				Both Sexes Cumul.	
	July 1994- June 1995		July 1995- June 1996		July 1994- June 1995		July 1995- June 1996		Total[2]	
	No.	%	No.	%	No.	%	No.	%	No.	%
Sex with transfusion recipient with HIV infection	-	-	-	-	3	-	-	-	25	
Sex with HIV-infected person, risk not specified	102	-	57	-	100	-	60	-	844	
Receipt of blood transfusion, blood components, or tissue	1	-	2	-	5	-	2	-	143	
Has HIV infection, risk not specified	107	-	114	-	137	-	124	-	1,467	
Receipt of blood transfusion, blood components, or tissue[3]	25	5	9	3	15	3	2	1	367	5
Other/risk not reported or identified[4]	13	3	20	6	11	2	24	7	115	2
Pediatric subtotal	470	100	359	100	490	100	353	100	7,296	100
Total	62,055	-	58,067	-	14,234	-	14,349	-	548,102	

Source: U.S. Department of Health and Human Services. Public Health Service. Centers for Disease Control and Prevention. *HIV/AIDS Surveillance Report, 1996* vol. 8, no. 1. The HIV/AIDS Surveillance Report is now accessible via Internet: www.cdc.gov. The HIV/AIDS Surveillance Report is published semiannually by the Division of HIV/AIDS Prevention, National Center for HIV, STD, and TB Prevention, Centers for Disease Control and Prevention (CDC), Atlanta, GA 30333. All data contained in the Report are provisional. *Notes:* 1. See primary source for a discussion of the impact of the 1993 AIDS surveillance case definition for adults and adolescents (implemented January 1, 1993) on the number of cases reported annually since 1993. 2. Includes 10 persons known to be infected with human immunodeficiency virus type 2 (HIV-2). 3. Thirty-five adults/adolescents and 3 children developed AIDS after receiving blood screened negative for HIV antibody. Twelve additional adults developed AIDS after receiving tissue, organs, or artificial insemination from HIV-infected donors. Four of the 12 received tissue, organs, or artificial insemination from a donor who was negative for HIV antibody at the time of donation. See *New England Journal of Medicine* 1992;326:726-32. 4. "Other" also includes 39 persons who acquired HIV infection perinatally but were diagnosed with AIDS after age 13. These 39 persons are tabulated under the adult/adolescent, not pediatric, exposure category.

★ 114 ★

Diseases and Illnesses: AIDS

AIDS: Female Cases by Age at Diagnosis and Race/Ethnicity

This table shows AIDS cases for females by age at diagnosis and race/ethnicity, reported through June 1996, United States. AIDS as defined by the Centers for Disease Control and Prevention (CDC): "Acquired immunodeficiency syndrome (AIDS) is a specific group of diseases or conditions which are indicative of severe immunosuppression related to infection with the human immunodeficiency virus (HIV)."

Age at diagnosis (years)	White not Hispanic		Black not Hispanic		His-panic		Asian Pacific Islander		American Indian Alaska Native		Total[1]	
	No.	%	No.	%	No.	%	No.	%	No.	%	No.	%
Under 5	434	2	1,776	4	648	4	11	3	12	5	2,888	4
5-12	134	1	340	1	173	1	6	1	-	-	656	1
13-19	169	1	605	1	145	1	6	1	1	0	927	1
20-24	1,171	6	2,666	6	1,048	6	24	6	22	10	4,936	6
25-29	3,316	17	6,996	15	2,913	17	45	11	39	17	13,316	16
30-34	4,461	23	10,441	23	4,028	24	82	20	51	22	19,092	23
35-39	3,685	19	9,956	22	3,363	20	75	18	43	19	17,156	21
40-44	2,324	12	6,399	14	2,079	12	59	14	21	9	10,892	13
45-49	1,200	6	2,864	6	1,070	6	39	9	20	9	5,199	6
50-54	676	4	1,489	3	602	4	21	5	8	4	2,799	3
55-59	502	3	845	2	373	2	11	3	5	2	1,738	2
60-64	359	2	536	1	188	1	17	4	3	1	1,103	1
65 or older	794	4	504	1	175	1	19	5	2	1	1,496	2
Female subtotal	19,225	100	45,417	100	16,805	100	415	100	227	100	82,198	100

Source: U.S. Department of Health and Human Services. Public Health Service. Centers for Disease Control and Prevention. *HIV/AIDS Surveillance Report, 1996* vol. 8, no. 1. The HIV/AIDS Surveillance Report is now accessible via Internet: www.cdc.gov. The HIV/AIDS Surveillance Report is published semiannually by the Division of HIV/AIDS Prevention, National Center for HIV, STD, and TB Prevention, Centers for Disease Control and Prevention (CDC), Atlanta, GA 30333. All data contained in the Report are provisional. *Note:* 1. Includes 109 females whose race/ethnicity is unknown.

★ 115 ★

Diseases and Illnesses: AIDS

AIDS in Persons 13 Years Old and Older, by Race/ Ethnicity, Sex, and Transmission Category: January-June 1995

[Data are based on reporting by State Health Departments]

Race, Hispanic origin, Sex, and transmission category	January-June 1995
Race and Hispanic origin	
All races	35,199
Men who have sex with men	15,198
Injecting drug use	8,762
Men who have sex with men and injecting drug use	1,634

[Continued]

★ 115 ★

AIDS in Persons 13 Years Old and Older, by Race/ Ethnicity, Sex, and Transmission Category: January-June 1995
[Continued]

Race, Hispanic origin, Sex, and transmission category	January- June 1995
Hemophilia/coagulation disorder	218
Heterosexual contact[1]	3,496
Sex with injecting drug user	1,198
Transfusion[2]	320
Undetermined[3]	5,571
White, not Hispanic	14,966
Men who have sex with men	9,493
Injecting drug use	1,932
Men who have sex with men and injecting drug use	874
Hemophilia/coagulation disorder	164
Heterosexual contact[1]	840
Sex with injecting drug user	299
Transfusion[2]	161
Undetermined[3]	1,502
Black, not Hispanic	14,367
Men who have sex with men	3,587
Injecting drug use	5,011
Men who have sex with men and injecting drug use	564
Hemophilia/coagulation disorder	33
Heterosexual contact[1]	1,971
Sex with injecting drug user	646
Transfusion[2]	111
Undetermined[3]	3,090
Hispanic	5,413
Men who have sex with men	1,878
Injecting drug use	1,757
Men who have sex with men and injecting drug use	177
Hemophilia/coagulation disorder	17
Heterosexual contact[1]	648
Sex with injecting drug user	245
Transfusion[2]	39
Undetermined[3]	897
Sex	
Male	28,861
Men who have sex with men	15,198
Injecting drug use	6,372
Men who have sex with men and injecting drug use	1,634
Hemophilia/coagulation disorder	209
Heterosexual contact[1]	1,234

[Continued]

★ 115 ★

AIDS in Persons 13 Years Old and Older, by Race/ Ethnicity, Sex, and Transmission Category: January-June 1995
[Continued]

Race, Hispanic origin, Sex, and transmission category	January- June 1995
Sex with injecting drug user	400
Transfusion[2]	185
Undetermined[3]	4,029
Female	6,338
Injecting drug use	2,390
Hemophilia/coagulation disorder	9
Heterosexual contact[1]	2,262
Sex with injecting drug user	798
Transfusion[2]	135
Undetermined[3]	1,542

Source: U.S. Department of Health and Human Services. Public Health Service. Centers for Disease Control and Prevention. National Center for Health Statistics. *Health, United States, 1995.* Hyattsville, MD: Public Health Service, 1996, p. 166. Primary source: Centers for Disease Control and Prevention, National Center for HIV, STD, and TB Prevention, Division of HIV/AIDS Prevention. *Notes:* 1. Includes persons who have had heterosexual contact with a person with human immunodeficiency virus (HIV) infection or risk of HIV infection. 2. Receipt of blood transfusion, blood components, or tissue. 3. Includes persons for whom risk information is incomplete (because of death, refusal to be interviewed, or loss to followup), persons still under investigation, men reported only to have had heterosexual contact with prostitutes, and interviewed persons for whom no specific risk is identified.

★ 116 ★
Diseases and Illnesses: AIDS

AIDS in Teens, by Cause: 1995

Cause	Percentage
Females, ages 13-19	
Contaminated blood or blood products	9
Injecting drugs	18
Risk not reported or not identified	22
Heterosexual sex	52
Males, ages 13-19	
Heterosexual sex	2
Homosexual sex and injecting drugs	5
Risk not reported or not identified	6
Injecting drugs	7
Homosexual sex	32
Contaminated blood or blood products	48

Source: "How Teens Get AIDS." *Current Health* (February 1996), p. 10.

★ 117 ★

Diseases and Illnesses: AIDS

AIDS: Male Cases by Age at Diagnosis and Race/Ethnicity

This table shows AIDS cases for males by age at diagnosis and race/ethnicity, reported through June 1996, United States. AIDS as defined by the Centers for Disease Control and Prevention (CDC): "Acquired immunodeficiency syndrome (AIDS) is a specific group of diseases or conditions which are indicative of severe immunosuppression related to infection with the human immunodeficiency virus (HIV)."

Age at diagnosis (years)	White not Hispanic		Black not Hispanic		His- panic		Asian Pacific Islander		American Indian/ Alaska Native		Total[1]	
	No.	%	No.	%	No.	%	No.	%	No.	%	No.	%
Under 5	443	0	1,763	1	665	1	15	0	9	1	2,899	1
5-12	303	0	322	0	217	0	8	0	1	0	853	0
13-19	726	0	560	0	327	0	19	1	14	1	1,647	0
20-24	6,541	3	5,216	4	3,119	4	113	3	50	4	15,061	3
25-29	32,478	14	19,120	13	12,349	15	438	13	243	20	64,715	14
30-34	55,851	24	31,102	22	19,276	24	741	22	327	27	107,431	23
35-39	53,259	22	32,876	23	17,778	22	736	22	260	21	105,062	23
40-44	38,581	16	24,637	17	12,121	15	602	18	167	14	76,218	16
45-49	22,940	10	13,285	9	6,628	8	349	10	73	6	43,335	9
50-54	12,267	5	7,027	5	3,460	4	182	5	29	2	22,997	5
55-59	6,765	3	3,900	3	1,979	2	112	3	19	2	12,804	3
60-64	3,884	2	2,094	1	1,078	1	46	1	12	1	7,123	2
65 or older	3,198	1	1,685	1	811	1	50	1	8	1	5,759	1
Male subtotal	237,236	100	143,587	100	79,808	100	3,411	100	1,212	100	465,904	100

Source: U.S. Department of Health and Human Services. Public Health Service. Centers for Disease Control and Prevention. *HIV/AIDS Surveillance Report, 1996* vol. 8, no. 1. The HIV/AIDS Surveillance Report is now accessible via Internet: www.cdc.gov. The HIV/AIDS Surveillance Report is published semiannually by the Division of HIV/AIDS Prevention, National Center for HIV, STD, and TB Prevention, Centers for Disease Control and Prevention (CDC), Atlanta, GA 30333. All data contained in the Report are provisional. *Note:* 1. Includes 650 males whose race/ethnicity is unknown.

★ 118 ★

Diseases and Illnesses: AIDS

AIDS: Occupationally Acquired AIDS/HIV Infection

This table shows health care workers with documented and possible occupationally acquired AIDS/HIV infection, by occupation, reported through June 1996, in the United States[1]. AIDS as defined by the Centers for Disease Control and Prevention (CDC): "Acquired immunodeficiency syndrome (AIDS) is a specific group of diseases or conditions which are indicative of severe immunosuppression related to infection with the human immunodeficiency virus (HIV)."

Occupation	Documented occupational transmission[2] No.	Possible occupational transmission[3] No.
Dental worker, including dentist	-	7
Embalmer/morgue technician	-	3
Emergency medical technician/paramedic	-	10
Health aide/attendant	1	12
Housekeeper/maintenance worker	1	7
Laboratory technician, clinical	16	16
Laboratory technician, nonclinical	3	-
Nurse	20	27
Physician, nonsurgical	6	11
Physician, surgical	-	4
Respiratory therapist	1	2
Technician, dialysis	1	2
Technician, surgical	2	1
Technician/therapist, other than those listed above	-	5
Other health care occupations	-	1
Total	51	108

Source: U.S. Department of Health and Human Services. Public Health Service. Centers for Disease Control and Prevention. *HIV/AIDS Surveillance Report, 1996* vol. 8, no. 1. The HIV/AIDS Surveillance Report is now accessible via Internet: www.cdc.gov. The HIV/AIDS Surveillance Report is published semiannually by the Division of HIV/AIDS Prevention, National Center for HIV, STD, and TB Prevention, Centers for Disease Control and Prevention (CDC), Atlanta, GA 30333. All data contained in the Report are provisional. *Notes:* 1. Health care workers are defined as those persons, including students and trainees, who have worked in a health care, clinical, or HIV laboratory setting at any time since 1978. 2. Health care workers who had documented HIV seroconversion after occupational exposure or had other laboratory evidence of occupational infection: 44 had percutaneous exposure, 5 had mucocutaneous exposure, 1 had both percutaneous and mucocutaneous exposures, and 1 had an unknown route of exposure. Forty-six exposures were to blood from an HIV-infected person, 1 to visibly bloody fluid, 1 to an unspecified fluid, and 3 to concentrated virus in a laboratory. Twenty-four of these health care workers developed AIDS. 3. These health care workers have been investigated and are without identifiable behavioral or transfusion risks; each reported percutaneous or mucocutaneous occupational exposures to blood or body fluids, or laboratory solutions containing HIV, but HIV seroconversion specifically resulting from an occupational exposure was not documented.

★ 119 ★

Diseases and Illnesses: AIDS

AIDS: Rates and Cases by State

This table shows AIDS rates per 100,000 population and total cases reported July 1995 through June 1996, in the United States. AIDS as defined by the Centers for Disease Control and Prevention (CDC): "Acquired immunodeficiency syndrome (AIDS) is a specific group of diseases or conditions which are indicative of severe immunosuppression related to infection with the human immunodeficiency virus (HIV)."

State	Rate per 100,000 population		Number of cases	
	Male	Female	Male	Female
Alabama	32.1	7.3	529	134
Alaska	12.7	2.7	31	6
Arizona	36.5	3.9	597	67
Arkansas	24.1	4.6	232	49
California	76.8	8.3	9,501	1,040
Colorado	36.6	3.4	546	53
Connecticut	84.6	30.5	1,086	426
Delaware	87.0	24.0	245	73
District of Columbia	383.6	84.1	822	211
Florida	103.6	30.2	5,787	1,837
Georgia	73.4	14.4	2,045	433
Hawaii	38.9	3.8	187	18
Idaho	9.2	0.6	42	3
Illinois	37.8	7.6	1,735	147
Indiana	25.9	2.7	589	375
Iowa	10.2	1.2	114	15
Kansas	23.1	2.6	233	28
Louisiana	68.5	13.0	1,123	237
Maine	13.6	2.4	67	13
Maryland	85.8	27.6	1,687	587
Massachusetts	41.3	11.4	982	299
Michigan	22.3	5.1	828	204
Minnesota	14.5	2.9	263	55
Mississippi	30.9	8.7	315	99
Missouri	36.0	4.4	743	99
Montana	8.3	0.3	29	1
Nebraska	12.8	2.2	82	15
Nevada	62.7	10.7	393	65
New Hampshire	17.0	4.6	77	22
New Jersey	89.9	34.1	2,788	1,156
New Mexico	16.3	1.2	105	8
New York	139.2	43.1	9,741	3,349
North Carolina	35.8	7.6	728	233
North Dakota	3.5	0.0	9	0
Ohio	22.0	3.1	952	147
Oklahoma	19.2	2.3	246	31
Oregon	36.2	3.4	455	45
Pennsylvania	37.6	8.9	1,778	467
Puerto Rico	122.2	33.0	1,639	486
Rhode Island	32.9	12.6	127	54

[Continued]

★ 119 ★

AIDS: Rates and Cases by State
[Continued]

State	Rate per 100,000 population		Number of cases	
	Male	Female	Male	Female
South Carolina	51.4	14.7	732	231
South Dakota	4.6	1.3	13	4
Texas	52.4	7.9	3,778	594
Utah	24.9	2.4	181	18
Vermont	15.0	1.6	35	4
Virgin Islands	53.7	21.9	20	9
Virginia	46.3	10.0	1,220	280
Washington	31.5	4.0	684	89
West Virginia	17.2	2.2	126	18
Wisconsin	13.8	2.3	280	50
Wyoming	6.7	0.5	13	1

Source: U.S. Department of Health and Human Services. Public Health Service. Centers for Disease Control and Prevention. *HIV/AIDS Surveillance Report, 1996* vol. 8, no. 1. The HIV/AIDS Surveillance Report is now accessible via Internet: www.cdc.gov. The HIV/AIDS Surveillance Report is published semiannually by the Division of HIV/AIDS Prevention, National Center for HIV, STD, and TB Prevention, Centers for Disease Control and Prevention (CDC), Atlanta, GA 30333. All data contained in the Report are provisional.

★ 120 ★

Diseases and Illnesses: AIDS

HIV/AIDS Infection Risk, by Type: 1997
[In estimated risk per episode]

Risk	Percentage
Transfusion of infected blood	89.5
Needle sharing	.67
Needle puncture	.29
Sexual contact:	
Male to male	.06 to 5.1
Male to female	.05 to .23
Female to male	.03 to 5.6

Source: Gorman, Christine. "If the Condom Breaks." *Time,* 23 June 1997, p. 48. Primary source: *New England Journal of Medicine;* Dr. Rachel Royce, U.N.C.

★ 121 ★

Diseases and Illnesses: AIDS

Living with AIDS: 1983 to 1994

Data show new diagnoses, and Americans living with AIDS at year's end.

Year	Deaths	New Diagnoses	Americans Living with AIDS
1983	1,470	3,043	2,523
1984	3,438	6,161	5,246
1985	6,842	11,649	10,053
1986	11,881	18,857	17,029
1987	16,031	28,336	29,334
1988	20,703	35,052	43,683
1989	27,286	41,930	58,327
1990	30,947	47,304	74,684
1991	35,854	57,760	96,590
1992	39,663	75,010	131,937
1993	42,074	72,965	162,828
1994	43,566	57,667	176,929

Source: Gallagher, John. "Fast-Forward." *Advocate,* 19 March 1996, p. 27.

★ 122 ★

Diseases and Illnesses: AIDS

Profile of AIDS: December 1995

Sex and cause	Cases
Total cases	513,486
Total deaths	319,849
Among Men	
Male-to-male sex	259,672
Intravenous drug use	95,244
Male-to-male sex; IV drug use	33,195
Heterosexual sex	13,521
Transfusion or transplant	4,327
Hemophilia treatment	3,970
Other or unknown	24,790
Among women	
Intravenous drug use	33,452
Heterosexual sex	26,516
Transfusion or transplant	3,106
Hemophilia treatment	137
Other or unknown	8,607

[Continued]

★ 122 ★

Profile of AIDS: December 1995
[Continued]

Sex and cause	Cases
Among children	
Birth	6,256
Transfusion or transplant	366
Hemophilia treatment	227
Other or unknown	99

Source: "Latest Statistics." *USA TODAY,* 5 June 1996, p. 1D. Primary source: Centers for Disease Control and Prevention.

Diseases and Illnesses: Cancer

★ 123 ★

Cancer and the Environment

"Half of all fatal cancers are linked to poor diet, smoking and lack of exercise—all factors that individuals can control. Environmental pollution, on the other hand, is responsible for a mere 2% of cancer deaths."

Source: Cronin, Brian. "Health Report: The Good News." *Time,* 2 December 1996, p. 25.

★ 124 ★

Diseases and Illnesses: Cancer

Cancer: Bladder

Data are in number of cases (diagnosed, deaths expected) and in percent for survival rates. Five-year survival means that the percentage of patients shown is expected to be alive five years after discovery of the cancer.

Bladder cancer	Number or Percent
New cases estimated in 1996	52,900
Deaths estimated in 1996	11,700
Five year survival rates	
All stages	80.7
Localized	92.8

[Continued]

★ 124 ★

Cancer: Bladder
[Continued]

Bladder cancer	Number or Percent
Regional spread	48.3
Distant spread	5.9

Source: Scientific American (September 1996), p. 129.

★ 125 ★

Diseases and Illnesses: Cancer

Cancer: Breast

Data are in number of cases (diagnosed, deaths expected) and in percent for survival rates. Five-year survival means that the percentage of patients shown is expected to be alive five years after discovery of the cancer.

Breast cancer	Number or Percent
New cases estimated in 1996	185,700
Deaths estimated in 1996	44,560
Five year survival rates	
All stages	83.2
Localized	96.1
Regional spread	74.9
Distant spread	19.8

Source: Scientific American (September 1996), p. 127.

★ 126 ★

Diseases and Illnesses: Cancer

Cancer: Breast Cancer Risk and Ethnic Origin

This table shows the rate of occurrence of breast cancer by ethnicity. Values are occurrences per 100,000 women.

Race or ethnicity	Age adjusted rate per 100,000 women
White	115.7
Native Hawaiian	105.6
Black	95.4
Japanese	82.3
Alaska Native	78.9
Filipino	73.1
Hispanic	69.8
Chinese	55.0
Vietnamese	37.5
American Indian[1]	31.6
Korean	28.5

Source: Katzenstein, Larry. "Race and Breast Cancer Risk." *American Health* (July/August 1996), p. 15. Primary source: National Cancer Institute. *Note:* 1. New Mexico only.

★ 127 ★

Diseases and Illnesses: Cancer

Cancer Caused by Abnormal P53 Gene: 1995

The table shows the percentage of each cancer believed to have been caused by an abnormal P53 gene and the number of deaths in 1995 attributed to that cancer.

Type	Percentage	Deaths in 1995
Brain	50	13,300
Bladder	35-60	11,200
Breast	30-40	46,240
Cervix[1]	90	4,800
Colon	40-70	47,500
Leukemia	60+	20,400
Liver	10-65	14,200
Lung	50	157,400
Lymphoma	30-35	24,150
Melanoma	50	7,200

[Continued]

★ 127 ★

Cancer Caused by Abnormal P53 Gene: 1995
[Continued]

Type	Percentage	Deaths in 1995
Ovary	40-60	14,500
Stomach	30-60	14,700

Source: "A Good Gene Gone Bad." *Newsweek,* 23 December 1996, p. 45. Primary source: Arnold Levine, National Cancer Institute, Hutchinson Cancer Research Center. *Notes:* 1. Refers to cancer caused by virus. Deaths include all forms of cervical cancer.

★ 128 ★
Diseases and Illnesses: Cancer

Cancer: Cervical

Data are in number of cases (diagnosed, deaths expected) and in percent for survival rates. Five-year survival means that the percentage of patients shown is expected to be alive five years after discovery of the cancer.

Cervical cancer	Number or Percent
New cases estimated in 1996	15,700
Deaths estimated in 1996	4,900
Five year survival rates	
All stages	68.3
Localized	90.9
Regional spread	49.9
Distant spread	8.6

Source: Scientific American (September 1996), p. 130.

★ 129 ★
Diseases and Illnesses: Cancer

Cancer: Chances of Developing Breast Cancer

Table shows the probability that a woman will develop breast cancer.

Age	Probability
By age 25:	1 in 19,608
By age 30:	1 in 2,525
By age 35:	1 in 622
By age 40:	1 in 217
By age 45:	1 in 93

[Continued]

★ 129 ★

Cancer: Chances of Developing Breast Cancer
[Continued]

Age	Probability
By age 50:	1 in 50
By age 55:	1 in 33
By age 60:	1 in 24
By age 65:	1 in 17
By age 70:	1 in 14
By age 75:	1 in 11
By age 80:	1 in 10
By age 85:	1 in 9
Ever:	1 in 8

Source: NCI Surveillance Program. Extracted from *Lifetime Probability of Breast Cancer in American Women*, Cancer Facts, U.S. Department of Health and Human Services, Public Health Service, National Institutes of Health, National Cancer Institute, August 1993.

★ 130 ★

Diseases and Illnesses: Cancer

Cancer: Colorectal

Data are in number of cases (diagnosed, deaths expected) and in percent for survival rates. Five-year survival means that the percentage of patients shown is expected to be alive five years after discovery of the cancer.

Colorectal cancer	Number or Percent
New cases estimated in 1996	133,500
Deaths estimated in 1996	54,900
Five year survival rates	
All stages	61.0
Localized	91.0
Regional spread	62.8
Distant spread	6.9

Source: Scientific American (September 1996), p. 128.

★ 131 ★

Diseases and Illnesses: Cancer

Cancer Deaths of Men, by Cancer Type: 1992 and 1996

The "trend" column shows the percent change in death rates between 1960-62 and 1990-92.

Type	1992	Trend	1996
Lung	91,405	+85	94,400
Prostate	34,240	+29	41,400
Colon and rectum	28,434	-9	27,940
Pancreas	12,672	-5	13,600
Leukemia	10,609	-9	11,600

Source: Nash, J. Madeleine. "The Enemy Within." *Time* (Fall 1996), p. 19.

★ 132 ★

Diseases and Illnesses: Cancer

Cancer Deaths of Women, by Cancer Type: 1992 and 1996

The "trend" column shows the percent change in death rates between 1960-62 and 1990-92.

Type	1992	Trend	1996
Lung	54,538	+438	64,300
Breast	43,068	+4	44,300
Colon and rectum	28,942	-31	28,100
Pancreas	13,399	+12	14,200
Ovary	13,393	-8	14,800

Source: Nash, J. Madeleine. "The Enemy Within." *Time* (Fall 1996), p. 19.

★ 133 ★

Diseases and Illnesses: Cancer

Cancer: Endometrial

Data are in number of cases (diagnosed, deaths expected) and in percent for survival rates. Five-year survival means that the percentage of patients shown is expected to be alive five years after discovery of the cancer.

Endometrial cancer	Number or Percent
New cases estimated in 1996	34,000
Deaths estimated in 1996	6,000
Five year survival rates	
All stages	83.2
Localized	94.9
Regional spread	65.3
Distant spread	26.1

Source: Scientific American (September 1996), p. 130.

★ 134 ★

Diseases and Illnesses: Cancer

Cancer: Kidney

Data are in number of cases (diagnosed, deaths expected) and in percent for survival rates. Five-year survival means that the percentage of patients shown is expected to be alive five years after discovery of the cancer.

Kidney cancer	Number or Percent
New cases estimated in 1996	30,600
Deaths estimated in 1996	12,000
Five year survival rates	
All stages	57.9
Localized	87.5
Regional spread	59.2
Distant spread	9.2

Source: Scientific American (September 1996), p. 131.

★ 135 ★

Diseases and Illnesses: Cancer

Cancer: Leukemia

Data are in number of cases (diagnosed, deaths expected) and in percent for survival rates. Five-year survival means that the percentage of patients shown is expected to be alive five years after discovery of the cancer.

Leukemia	Number or Percent
New cases estimated in 1996	27,600
Deaths estimated in 1996	21,000
Five year survival rates	
Chronic lymphocytic leukemia	68.6
Acute lymphocytic leukemia	55.6
Chronic myelogenous leukemia	27.3
Acute myelogenous leukemia	11.4

Source: Scientific American (September 1996), p. 131.

★ 136 ★

Diseases and Illnesses: Cancer

Cancer: Lung

Data are in number of cases (diagnosed, deaths expected) and in percent for survival rates. Five-year survival means that the percentage of patients shown is expected to be alive five years after discovery of the cancer.

Lung cancer	Number or Percent
New cases estimated in 1996	177,000
Deaths estimated in 1996	158,700
Five year survival rates	
All stages	13.4
Localized	47.4
Regional spread	17.2
Distant spread	1.7

Source: Scientific American (September 1996), p. 128.

★ 137 ★

Diseases and Illnesses: Cancer

Cancer: Melanoma of the Skin

Data are in number of cases (diagnosed, deaths expected) and in percent for survival rates. Five-year survival means that the percentage of patients shown is expected to be alive five years after discovery of the cancer.

Skin melanoma	Number or Percent
New cases estimated in 1996	38,300
Deaths estimated in 1996	7,300
Five year survival rates	
All stages	86.6
Localized	93.8
Regional spread	59.8
Distant spread	15.9

Source: Scientific American (September 1996), p. 130.

★ 138 ★

Diseases and Illnesses: Cancer

Cancer: Ovarian

Data are in number of cases (diagnosed, deaths expected) and in percent for survival rates. Five-year survival means that the percentage of patients shown is expected to be alive five years after discovery of the cancer.

Ovarian cancer	Number or Percent
New cases estimated in 1996	26,700
Deaths estimated in 1996	14,800
Five year survival rates	
All stages	44.1
Localized	90.9
Regional spread	49.5
Distant spread	23.3

Source: Scientific American (September 1996), p. 132.

★ 139 ★

Diseases and Illnesses: Cancer

Cancer: Pancreatic

Data are in number of cases (diagnosed, deaths expected) and in percent for survival rates. Five-year survival means that the percentage of patients shown is expected to be alive five years after discovery of the cancer.

Pancreatic cancer	Number or Percent
New cases estimated in 1996	26,300
Deaths estimated in 1996	27,800
Five year survival rates	
All stages	3.6
Localized	12.0
Regional spread	4.8
Distant spread	1.6

Source: Scientific American (September 1996), p. 132.

★ 140 ★

Diseases and Illnesses: Cancer

Cancer: Prostate

Data are in number of cases (diagnosed, deaths expected) and in percent for survival rates. Five-year survival means that the percentage of patients shown is expected to be alive five years after discovery of the cancer.

Prostate cancer	Number or Percent
New cases estimated in 1996	317,100
Deaths estimated in 1996	41,400
Five year survival rates	
All stages	85.8
Localized	98.6
Regional spread	92.1
Distant spread	29.8

Source: Scientific American (September 1996), p. 127.

★ 141 ★

Diseases and Illnesses: Cancer

Cancer: Sites with Highest and Lowest Survival Rates

Table shows which cancer sites show the highest and lowest five-year relative survival rates (based on all ages combined) for patients diagnosed during the period 1983-1990. A value of 50 means that half of those diagnosed survived for 5 years after diagnosis.

Site	% Survival		
	Age <65	Age 65+	All Ages
All Sites	57.5	50.3	53.9
Highest			
Thyroid Gland	97.0	80.0	94.6
Testis (men)	93.4	80.2	93.3
Melanoma	86.2	82.4	85.1
Corpus Uteri (women)	88.0	78.1	83.9
Breast (women)	79.2	82.2	80.4
Urinary Bladder	85.9	75.4	79.8
Hodgkin's Disease	83.3	40.1	78.9
Lowest			
Chronic Myeloid Leukemia	32.7	12.4	23.7
Stomach	20.3	17.3	18.5
Lung and Bronchus	15.5	11.3	13.4
Acute Myeloid Leukemia	17.3	1.9	10.4
Esophagus	10.3	8.2	9.2
Liver	8.8	3.4	6.0
Pancreas	4.9	2.3	3.2

Source: SEER Cancer Statistics Review 1973-1991, Cancer Facts, U.S. Department of Health and Human Services, Public Health Service, National Institutes of Health, National Cancer Institute, June 1995. SEER stands for Surveillance, Epidemiology, and End Results.

★ 142 ★

Diseases and Illnesses: Cancer

Decrease in Death Rates from Cancer, by Sex and Cancer Type: 1991-96

According to the source, for the first time since 1900, overall cancer death rates in the U.S. are down. Cancer deaths fell from 135 per 100,000 persons in 1990 to 130 deaths per 100,000 persons in 1995—a 3.1% decrease.

Type	Percent of men	Percent of women
All cancers	-4.3	-1.1
Lung	-6.7	+6.4
Breast	0	-6.3
Prostate	-6.2	0
Colorectal	-7	-4.8

Source: Thompson, Dick. "Cancer: the Good News." *Time,* 25 November 1996, p. 98. Primary source: *Cancer.*

★ 143 ★

Diseases and Illnesses: Cancer

Skin Cancer

"Among Caucasians, the incidence of squamous-cell carcinoma is climbing faster than expected. Since the mid-'80s, rates have doubled in women and gone up one quarter in men."

Source: Cronin, Brian. "Health Report: The Bad News." *Time,* 7 July 1997, p. 20. Primary source: *Archives of Dermatology.*

Diseases and Illnesses: Cerebrovascular Disease

★ 144 ★

Heart Attacks and Geography

"A study of New York City's black population finds that blacks who migrated to New York from the South are twice as likely to die of a heart attack as blacks born in the city. Blacks who moved from the Caribbean, however, have just half the risk of a fatal heart attack."

Source: Cronin, Brian. "Health Report: The Bad News." *Time,* 2 December 1996, p. 25.

★ 145 ★

Diseases and Illnesses: Cerebrovascular Disease

Stroke Rate Comparison to National Average, 1996: Southern U.S.

From the source: "For decades, scientists have recognized a distinctive belt of eight Southern states where the incidence of stroke is significantly higher than the national average. But a recent study revealed that in one portion of that region, in an area that parallels the Atlantic seaboard, strokes are even more prevalent. Dubbed the Buckle (of the Stroke Belt, that is), these 153 counties in Georgia and the Carolinas have lower average incomes than the rest of the Belt. Scientists thought there must be a relationship between poverty and stroke mortality, but the study shows that only 5% to 16% of the Belt's excess strokes are due to socio-economic factors. So what's the explanation for the Belt and the Buckle? It's a medical mystery."

The following states have a stroke rate *30% higher* than the national average: Alabama, Arkansas, Louisiana, Mississippi, and Tennessee.

These states have a stroke rate *100% higher* than the national average: Georgia, North Carolina, and South Carolina.

Source: "Notebook: The Belt and the Buckle." *Time,* 26 May 1997, p. 28.

Diseases and Illnesses: Diabetes

★ 146 ★

Complications of Adult-Onset Diabetes, by Type

The table shows the percentage of people with each type of disorder.

Disorder	Percent
Hypertension	41.0
Eye diseases	30.0
Nerve problems	23.0
Heart disease	22.0
Kidney disease	7.0
Amputation	3.0
Bad eyesight	1.0

Source: "Diabetes' Complications." *USA TODAY,* 6 February 1997, p. 1D. Primary source: Wirthlin Worldwide for Bayer Corporation.

★ 147 ★

Diseases and Illnesses: Diabetes

Diabetes in Adults, by Ethnicity: 1996

Ethnicity	Percentage
Mexican American	10.9
Cuban American	9.1
Puerto Rican	9.6
Non-Hispanic	6.2

Source: "Diabetes by Ethnicity." *Hispanic* (August 1996), p. 14. Primary source: American Diabetes Association. *Diabetes Facts: Diabetes Among Hispanic Americans,* January 1996.

★ 148 ★

Diseases and Illnesses: Diabetes

Diabetes Prevalence by Race and Ethnicity

In addition to the data shown, the source reports that from 5-50% of American Indians and from 16-20% of Japanese-Americans have diagnosed and undiagnosed diabetes. Data show percent of each group.

Ethnicity	% of Population
African Americans	9.6
Mexican Americans	9.6
Cuban Americans	9.1
Puerto Rican Americans	10.9
White Americans	6.2

Source: "Spotlight: Adults with Diabetes, by Race, Ethnicity." *Medical Tribune,* 11 January 1996, p. 1. Primary source: National Institute of Diabetes and Digestive and Kidney Diseases.

★ 149 ★

Diseases and Illnesses: Diabetes

New Guidelines for Diabetes

"The National Institutes of Health said new diabetes guidelines, calling for universal testing by age 45, could help identify many of the eight million Americans who have the disease but don't know it. The guidelines, drafted by an international panel, lower the blood-sugar diagnostic standard and list high-risk ethnic groups."

Source: Wall Street Journal, 24 June 1997, p. 1.

Diseases and Illnesses: Hypertension

★ 150 ★

Hypertension Among Persons Age 20 and Older, by Sex, Age: 1988-1991

Data are based on physical examination of a sample of the civilian noninstitutionalized population.

[In percent of population]

Sex, age, race, and Hispanic origin[1]	1988-91
Male	
20-34 years	9.6
35-44 years	19.9
45-54 years	35.5
55-64 years	46.2
65-74 years	59.5
75 years and over	64.4
Female[2]	
20-34 years	2.4
35-44 years	11.5
45-54 years	22.6
55-64 years	46.6
65-74 years	56.6
75 years and over	77.2

Source: U.S. Department of Health and Human Services. Public Health Service. Centers for Disease Control and Prevention. National Center for Health Statistics. Division of Health Examination Statistics. Unpublished data. *Notes:* A person with hypertension is defined by either having elevated blood pressure (systolic pressure of at least 140 mmHg or diastolic pressure of at least 90 mmHg) or taking antihypertensive medication. Percents are based on a single measurement of blood pressure to provide comparable data across the 4 time periods. In 1976-80, 31.3 percent of persons 20-74 years of age had hypertension, based on the average of 3 blood pressure measurements, in contrast to 39.7 percent when a single measurement is used. Some data have been revised and differ from previous editions of *Health, United States.* 1. The race groups, white and black, include persons of Hispanic and non-Hispanic origin. Conversely, persons of Hispanic origin may be of any race. 2. Excludes pregnant women.

★ 151 ★

Diseases and Illnesses: Hypertension

Hypertension Among Persons Age 20 and Older, by Sex, Age, Race, and Ethnicity: 1988-1991

[In percent of population]

Sex, age, race, and Hispanic origin[1]	1988-91
20-74 years, age adjusted	
Both sexes[2]	23.1
Male	26.4
Female[2]	19.7
White male	25.1
White female[2]	18.3
Black male	37.4
Black female[2]	31.0
White, non-Hispanic male	25.3
White, non-Hispanic female[2]	18.3
Black, non-Hispanic male	37.2
Black, non-Hispanic female[2]	31.1
Mexican-American male	26.7
Mexican-American female[2]	21.0

Source: U.S. Department of Health and Human Services. Public Health Service. Centers for Disease Control and Prevention. National Center for Health Statistics. Division of Health Examination Statistics. Unpublished data. *Notes:* A person with hypertension is defined by either having elevated blood pressure (systolic pressure of at least 140 mmHg or diastolic pressure of at least 90 mmHg) or taking antihypertensive medication. medication. Percents are based on a single measurement of blood pressure to provide comparable data across the 4 time periods. In 1976-80, 31.3 percent of persons 20-74 years of age had hypertension, based on the average of 3 blood pressure measurements, in contrast to 39.7 percent when a single measurement is used. Some data have been revised and differ from previous editions of *Health, United States.* 1. The race groups, white and black, include persons of Hispanic and non-Hispanic origin. Conversely, persons of Hispanic origin may be of any race. 2. Excludes pregnant women.

═══

Diseases and Illnesses: Sexually Transmitted Diseases

═══

★ 152 ★

Chancroid, by State

This table shows recorded cases and rates for chancroid by state/area: United States and outlying areas, 1991-1995.

State/Area	Cases					Rates per 100,000 Population				
	1991	1992	1993	1994	1995	1991	1992	1993	1994	1995
Alabama	0	0	23	24	7	0.0	0.0	0.6	0.6	0.2
Alaska	0	0	0	0	0	0.0	0.0	0.0	0.0	0.0
Arizona	8	1	3	3	2	0.2	0.0	0.1	0.1	0.0
Arkansas	0	0	0	0	1	0.0	0.0	0.0	0.0	0.0
California	50	16	12	25	7	0.2	0.1	0.0	0.1	0.0
Colorado	0	0	0	0	0	0.0	0.0	0.0	0.0	0.0
Connecticut	3	0	0	0	0	0.1	0.0	0.0	0.0	0.0
Delaware	3	2	1	0	0	0.4	0.3	0.1	0.0	0.0
Florida	418	96	46	20	24	3.1	0.7	0.3	0.1	0.2
Georgia	76	21	21	0	2	1.1	0.3	0.3	0.0	0.0
Hawaii	0	0	0	0	0	0.0	0.0	0.0	0.0	0.0
Idaho	0	0	0	0	0	0.0	0.0	0.0	0.0	0.0
Illinois	22	135	91	38	21	0.2	1.2	0.8	0.3	0.2
Indiana	2	2	3	0	0	0.0	0.0	0.1	0.0	0.0
Iowa	0	1	0	1	0	0.0	0.0	0.0	0.0	0.0
Kansas	5	3	1	5	2	0.2	0.1	0.0	0.2	0.1
Kentucky	2	4	4	0	0	0.1	0.1	0.1	0.0	0.0
Louisiana	235	341	310	209	129	5.5	8.0	7.2	4.8	3.0
Maine	0	0	0	0	0	0.0	0.0	0.0	0.0	0.0
Maryland	1	4	0	0	0	0.0	0.1	0.0	0.0	0.0
Massachusetts	2	13	2	1	7	0.0	0.2	0.0	0.0	0.1
Michigan	0	0	0	0	0	0.0	0.0	0.0	0.0	0.0
Minnesota	0	0	1	0	0	0.0	0.0	0.0	0.0	0.0
Mississippi	0	0	0	0	0	0.0	0.0	0.0	0.0	0.0
Missouri	22	8	1	2	0	0.4	0.2	0.0	0.0	0.0
Montana	0	0	0	0	0	0.0	0.0	0.0	0.0	0.0
Nebraska	0	0	0	0	0	0.0	0.0	0.0	0.0	0.0
Nevada	0	0	0	0	2	0.0	0.0	0.0	0.0	0.1
New Hampshire	0	2	3	0	0	0.0	0.2	0.3	0.0	0.0
New Jersey	4	4	0	0	4	0.1	0.1	0.0	0.0	0.1
New Mexico	0	0	0	0	0	0.0	0.0	0.0	0.0	0.0
New York	1,227	821	618	365	336	6.8	4.5	3.4	2.0	1.9
North Carolina	25	38	13	10	18	0.4	0.6	0.2	0.1	0.3
North Dakota	0	0	0	0	0	0.0	0.0	0.0	0.0	0.0
Ohio	7	7	21	8	5	0.1	0.1	0.2	0.1	0.0
Oklahoma	0	0	0	0	0	0.0	0.0	0.0	0.0	0.0
Oregon	0	0	0	5	0	0.0	0.0	0.0	0.2	0.0
Pennsylvania	0	0	0	0	0	0.0	0.0	0.0	0.0	0.0
Rhode Island	0	0	0	0	0	0.0	0.0	0.0	0.0	0.0
South Carolina	0	3	0	0	0	0.0	0.1	0.0	0.0	0.0
South Dakota	0	0	0	0	0	0.0	0.0	0.0	0.0	0.0

[Continued]

★ 152 ★

Chancroid, by State
[Continued]

State/Area	Cases					Rates per 100,000 Population				
	1991	1992	1993	1994	1995	1991	1992	1993	1994	1995
Tennessee	70	39	8	3	2	1.4	0.8	0.2	0.1	0.0
Texas	1,273	319	37	51	26	7.3	1.8	0.2	0.3	0.1
Utah	0	1	4	0	0	0.0	0.1	0.2	0.0	0.0
Vermont	0	0	0	0	0	0.0	0.0	0.0	0.0	0.0
Virginia	17	0	3	0	2	0.3	0.0	0.0	0.0	0.0
Washington	3	2	0	1	5	0.1	0.0	0.0	0.0	0.1
West Virginia	0	0	1	0	1	0.0	0.0	0.1	0.0	0.1
Wisconsin	0	1	0	2	3	0.0	0.0	0.0	0.0	0.1
Wyoming	0	1	1	0	0	0.0	0.2	0.2	0.0	0.0
U.S. TOTAL[1]	3,476	1,885	1,229	773	606	1.4	0.7	0.5	0.3	0.2
Guam	1	0	0	0	0	0.7	0.0	0.0	0.0	0.0
Puerto Rico	4	14	25	32	1	0.1	0.4	0.7	0.9	0.0
Virgin Islands	14	6	5	1	2	13.0	5.4	4.5	0.9	1.8
OUTLYING AREAS	19	20	30	33	3	0.5	0.5	0.8	0.8	0.1
TOTAL	3,495	1,905	1,259	806	609	1.4	0.7	0.5	0.3	0.2

Source: U.S. Department of Health and Human Services. Public Health Service. Centers for Disease Control and Prevention. Division of STD Prevention. *Sexually Transmitted Disease Surveillance, 1995.* U.S. Department of Health and Human Services, Public Health Service, September 1996. *Note:* 1. Includes cases reported by Washington, D.C.

★ 153 ★

Diseases and Illnesses: Sexually Transmitted Diseases

Chancroid: Urban Distribution

This table deals with reported cases and rates for chancroid in selected cities of 200,000+ population: United States and outlying areas, 1991-1995.

State/Area	Cases					Rates per 100,000 Population				
	1991	1992	1993	1994	1995	1991	1992	1993	1994	1995
Akron, OH	0	0	0	0	0	0.0	0.0	0.0	0.0	0.0
Albuquerque, NM	0	0	0	0	0	0.0	0.0	0.0	0.0	0.0
Atlanta, GA	27	14	10	0	0	4.1	2.1	1.5	0.0	0.0
Austin, TX	1	0	2	5	0	0.2	0.0	0.3	0.8	0.0
Baltimore, MD	0	0	0	0	0	0.0	0.0	0.0	0.0	0.0
Birmingham, AL	0	0	0	0	0	0.0	0.0	0.0	0.0	0.0
Boston, MA	0	0	0	0	2	0.0	0.0	0.0	0.0	0.4
Buffalo, NY	0	0	0	0	0	0.0	0.0	0.0	0.0	0.0
Charlotte, NC	17	29	10	0	3	3.2	5.4	1.8	0.0	0.5
Chicago, IL	15	132	81	36	21	0.5	4.5	2.7	1.2	0.7
Cincinnati, OH	0	1	2	3	1	0.0	0.1	0.2	0.3	0.1
Cleveland, OH	11	3	0	2	0	0.8	0.2	0.0	0.1	0.0
Columbus, OH	0	0	0	0	0	0.0	0.0	0.0	0.0	0.0

[Continued]

★ 153 ★

Chancroid: Urban Distribution

[Continued]

State/Area	Cases					Rates per 100,000 Population				
	1991	1992	1993	1994	1995	1991	1992	1993	1994	1995
Corpus Christi, TX	2	5	0	0	1	0.7	1.7	0.0	0.0	0.3
Dallas, TX	31	26	0	0	12	1.6	1.4	0.0	0.0	0.6
Dayton, OH	0	1	19	3	1	0.0	0.2	3.3	0.5	0.2
Denver, CO	0	0	0	0	0	0.0	0.0	0.0	0.0	0.0
Des Moines, IA	0	1	0	1	0	0.0	0.3	0.0	0.3	0.0
Detroit, MI	0	0	0	0	0	0.0	0.0	0.0	0.0	0.0
El Paso, TX	0	0	0	1	0	0.0	0.0	0.0	0.1	0.0
Fort Worth, TX	9	3	0	0	0	0.7	0.2	0.0	0.0	0.0
Honolulu, HI	0	0	0	0	0	0.0	0.0	0.0	0.0	0.0
Houston, TX	570	244	34	38	0	19.6	8.2	1.1	1.2	0.0
Indianapolis, IN	1	1	0	0	0	0.1	0.1	0.0	0.0	0.0
Jacksonville, FL	0	0	0	0	0	0.0	0.0	0.0	0.0	0.0
Jersey City, NJ	0	0	0	0	0	0.0	0.0	0.0	0.0	0.0
Kansas City, MO	0	0	0	0	0	0.0	0.0	0.0	0.0	0.0
Los Angeles, CA	20	15	12	20	3	0.2	0.2	0.1	0.2	0.0
Louisville, KY	0	1	1	0	0	0.0	0.1	0.1	0.0	0.0
Memphis, TN	69	39	8	3	2	8.3	4.6	0.9	0.4	0.2
Miami, FL	41	8	1	0	0	2.1	0.4	0.0	0.0	0.0
Milwaukee, WI	0	1	0	0	0	0.0	0.1	0.0	0.0	0.0
Minneapolis, MN	0	0	0	0	0	0.0	0.0	0.0	0.0	0.0
Nashville, TN	0	0	0	0	0	0.0	0.0	0.0	0.0	0.0
New Orleans, LA	208	299	281	201	125	42.4	61.1	57.7	41.5	25.9
New York City, NY	1,220	818	613	357	334	16.7	11.2	8.4	4.9	4.6
Newark, NJ	1	0	0	0	1	0.3	0.0	0.0	0.0	0.3
Norfolk, VA	5	0	0	0	1	2.0	0.0	0.0	0.0	0.4
Oakland, CA	1	0	0	0	2	0.1	0.0	0.0	0.0	0.2
Oklahoma City, OK	0	0	0	0	0	0.0	0.0	0.0	0.0	0.0
Omaha, NE	0	0	0	0	0	0.0	0.0	0.0	0.0	0.0
Philadelphia, PA	0	0	0	0	0	0.0	0.0	0.0	0.0	0.0
Phoenix, AZ	7	0	2	3	0	0.3	0.0	0.1	0.1	0.0
Pittsburgh, PA	0	0	0	0	0	0.0	0.0	0.0	0.0	0.0
Portland, OR	0	0	0	2	0	0.0	0.0	0.0	0.4	0.0
Richmond, VA	0	0	0	0	0	0.0	0.0	0.0	0.0	0.0
Rochester, NY	0	0	0	0	0	0.0	0.0	0.0	0.0	0.0
Sacramento, CA	0	0	0	0	0	0.0	0.0	0.0	0.0	0.0
San Antonio, TX	5	2	0	0	0	0.4	0.2	0.0	0.0	0.0
San Diego, CA	0	0	0	2	2	0.0	0.0	0.0	0.1	0.1
San Francisco, CA	5	1	0	2	0	0.7	0.1	0.0	0.3	0.0
San Jose, CA	0	0	0	0	0	0.0	0.0	0.0	0.0	0.0
Seattle, WA	2	2	0	0	4	0.1	0.1	0.0	0.0	0.3
St. Louis, MO	14	7	1	1	0	3.6	1.8	0.3	0.3	0.0
St. Paul, MN	0	0	0	0	0	0.0	0.0	0.0	0.0	0.0
St. Petersburg, FL	27	0	0	0	0	3.1	0.0	0.0	0.0	0.0
Tampa, FL	47	0	0	0	0	5.6	0.0	0.0	0.0	0.0
Toledo, OH	0	0	0	0	0	0.0	0.0	0.0	0.0	0.0
Tucson, AZ	0	0	0	0	0	0.0	0.0	0.0	0.0	0.0

[Continued]

★ 153 ★

Chancroid: Urban Distribution
[Continued]

State/Area	Cases					Rates per 100,000 Population				
	1991	1992	1993	1994	1995	1991	1992	1993	1994	1995
Tulsa, OK	0	0	0	0	0	0.0	0.0	0.0	0.0	0.0
Washington, DC	1	0	1	0	0	0.2	0.0	0.2	0.0	0.0
Wichita, KS	0	0	0	0	0	0.0	0.0	0.0	0.0	0.0
Yonkers, NY	1	1	0	0	0	0.5	0.5	0.0	0.0	0.0
U.S. CITY TOTAL	2,358	1,654	1,078	680	515	3.5	2.4	1.6	1.0	0.7
San Juan, PR	0	13	7	10	0	0.0	1.5	0.8	1.1	0.0
TOTAL	2,358	1,667	1,085	690	515	3.5	2.4	1.6	1.0	0.7

Source: U.S. Department of Health and Human Services. Public Health Service. Centers for Disease Control and Prevention. Division of STD Prevention. *Sexually Transmitted Disease Surveillance, 1995.* U.S. Department of Health and Human Services, Public Health Service, September 1996.

★ 154 ★
Diseases and Illnesses: Sexually Transmitted Diseases

Chlamydia: Reported Cases

This table shows reported cases and rates of chlamydia by state/area: United States and outlying areas, 1991-1995.

State/Area	Cases					Rates per 100,000 Population				
	1991	1992	1993	1994	1995	1991	1992	1993	1994	1995
Alabama	NR	NR	NR	508	3,188	.	.	.	12.0	75.0
Alaska	NR	NR	NR	NR	NR	.	.	.	.	.
Arizona	11,243	9,464	10,313	9,211	10,061	300.1	246.8	261.5	225.8	238.5
Arkansas	541	684	668	788	680	22.8	28.6	27.5	32.1	27.4
California	51,191	63,416	69,445	69,992	62,501	168.3	205.1	222.4	222.8	197.9
Colorado	7	4	51	9,031	6,650	0.2	0.1	1.4	246.6	177.5
Connecticut	7,840	8,699	7,610	7,146	6,440	238.3	265.3	232.1	218.2	196.7
Delaware	882	778	1,610	2,478	2,701	129.7	112.8	230.3	350.0	376.6
Florida	NR	NR	NR	NR	22,294	.	.	.	.	157.4
Georgia	7,284	9,998	4,217	168	11,193	110.0	147.8	61.1	2.4	155.4
Hawaii	3,260	3,683	2,632	2,484	2,135	287.6	319.4	225.8	210.8	179.9
Idaho	2,418	2,293	1,893	1,752	1,739	232.8	215.1	172.0	154.4	149.5
Illinois	21,826	24,045	23,424	24,605	24,645	189.4	207.1	200.4	209.2	208.3
Indiana	11,897	10,818	10,034	10,346	9,102	212.3	191.4	175.8	179.8	156.8
Iowa	6,638	6,137	5,214	5,413	5,089	237.8	218.6	184.8	191.2	179.1
Kansas	6,786	7,024	5,815	6,391	5,314	272.4	279.3	229.6	250.5	207.1
Kentucky	5,524	5,342	5,479	5,630	6,904	148.7	142.4	144.4	147.1	178.9
Louisiana	1,693	9,835	12,207	10,650	9,111	39.9	230.2	284.6	246.7	209.8
Maine	2,698	2,014	1,580	1,195	1,144	218.3	162.9	127.6	96.4	92.2
Maryland	5,459	5,671	5,157	6,709	8,740	112.3	115.5	104.1	134.2	173.3
Massachusetts	10,898	9,812	8,339	8,066	7,402	181.6	163.6	138.6	133.5	121.9
Michigan	NR	347	4,779	17,686	21,666	.	3.7	50.5	186.3	226.9
Minnesota	8,184	8,543	7,511	7,317	6,032	184.8	191.0	166.0	160.2	130.9

[Continued]

★ 154 ★

Chlamydia: Reported Cases
[Continued]

State/Area	Cases					Rates per 100,000 Population				
	1991	1992	1993	1994	1995	1991	1992	1993	1994	1995
Mississippi	NR	NR	NR	NR	912	.	.	.	.	33.8
Missouri	10,800	11,873	11,624	12,249	12,110	209.4	228.7	222.0	232.0	227.5
Montana	2,177	1,952	1,594	1,403	1,198	269.3	237.1	189.5	163.9	137.7
Nebraska	3,336	3,032	1,733	3,336	2,873	209.6	189.1	107.4	205.4	175.5
Nevada	1,628	3,329	3,385	3,149	3,049	126.7	249.7	244.5	215.4	199.3
New Hampshire	1,929	1,913	1,164	967	898	174.2	171.7	103.7	85.2	78.2
New Jersey	1,716	3,943	2,742	1,831	4,056	22.1	50.5	34.9	23.2	51.0
New Mexico	4,676	4,482	4,747	5,037	4,285	302.2	283.4	293.7	304.3	254.2
New York	10,962	17,043	15,320	26,472	26,686	60.8	94.2	84.4	145.8	147.1
North Carolina	11,927	13,719	15,456	17,796	15,780	176.7	200.7	222.3	251.7	219.3
North Dakota	1,324	1,172	933	1,079	1,324	208.8	184.5	146.5	168.8	206.4
Ohio	32,235	28,647	25,987	32,475	29,124	294.9	260.4	234.9	292.5	261.2
Oklahoma	4,036	5,353	4,737	3,729	5,065	127.4	166.9	146.6	114.5	154.5
Oregon	7,325	5,891	5,527	5,495	5,465	250.9	198.1	182.1	178.0	174.0
Pennsylvania	4,275	23,041	22,552	19,746	22,961	35.8	192.2	187.4	163.7	190.2
Rhode Island	2,071	2,487	2,214	2,095	1,902	206.2	248.3	221.7	210.7	192.2
South Carolina	5,700	5,402	8,063	8,153	8,591	160.3	150.3	222.3	223.8	233.9
South Dakota	2,150	1,925	1,645	1,427	1,313	306.2	271.4	229.5	197.3	180.1
Tennessee	5,360	5,301	5,684	6,787	13,154	108.3	105.6	111.6	131.1	250.3
Texas	32,560	40,791	43,874	46,046	44,627	187.5	230.6	243.1	250.1	238.3
Utah	751	1,613	1,589	1,801	1,676	42.5	89.1	85.4	94.4	85.9
Vermont	859	640	514	522	462	151.1	112.0	89.2	90.0	79.0
Virginia	19,519	12,699	12,582	12,976	12,285	310.5	198.8	194.3	198.1	185.6
Washington	13,299	11,762	10,331	10,577	9,462	265.0	228.6	196.6	198.1	174.2
West Virginia	1,575	1,489	1,935	2,602	2,326	87.6	82.4	106.4	142.7	127.2
Wisconsin	12,374	6,157	11,671	11,769	8,955	250.1	123.2	231.4	231.5	174.8
Wyoming	1,202	992	934	816	703	262.4	213.8	198.8	171.4	146.4
U.S. TOTAL[1]	362,441	405,935	407,312	448,984	477,638	163.1	173.3	172.1	184.7	182.2
Northeast	43,248	69,592	62,035	68,040	71,951	84.9	136.2	121.0	132.4	139.8
Midwest	117,550	109,720	110,370	134,093	127,547	231.4	181.0	180.8	218.4	206.4
South	102,466	117,742	122,466	126,103	169,216	153.0	173.4	177.8	170.2	184.2
West	99,177	108,881	112,441	120,748	108,924	185.3	199.5	202.7	214.7	191.1
Guam	22	54	38	275	461	15.6	38.3	26.9	194.9	326.7
Puerto Rico	74	110	601	2,443	2,305	2.1	3.1	16.6	66.3	62.0
Virgin Islands	256	130	14	50	17	238.1	117.3	12.6	45.1	15.3
OUTLYING AREAS	352	294	653	2,768	2,783	9.3	7.7	16.9	70.3	70.1
TOTAL	362,793	406,229	407,965	451,752	480,421	160.5	170.7	169.6	182.9	180.5

Source: U.S. Department of Health and Human Services. Public Health Service. Centers for Disease Control and Prevention. Division of STD Prevention. *Sexually Transmitted Disease Surveillance, 1995.* U.S. Department of Health and Human Services, Public Health Service, September 1996. *Notes:* NR indicates "no report." 1. Includes cases reported by Washington, D.C.

★ 155 ★

Diseases and Illnesses: Sexually Transmitted Diseases

Chlamydia: Reported Cases - Men

This table shows reported cases and rates of chlamydia in men, by state/area: United States and outlying areas, 1991-1995.

State/Area	Cases					Rates per 100,000 Population				
	1991	1992	1993	1994	1995	1991	1992	1993	1994	1995
Alabama	NR	NR	NR	68	285	.	.	.	3.4	14.0
Alaska	NR	NR	NR	NR	NR	.	.	.	.	.
Arizona	1,710	1,274	1,542	1,531	1,746	92.4	67.2	79.1	75.9	83.7
Arkansas	61	83	94	134	79	5.3	7.2	8.0	11.3	6.6
California	575	2,161	2,118	491	7,343	3.8	14.0	13.6	3.1	46.5
Colorado	NR	NR	1	NR	NR	.	.	0.1	.	.
Connecticut	878	942	827	858	816	55.0	59.2	52.0	54.0	51.3
Delaware	99	130	183	307	406	30.0	38.9	53.9	89.3	116.6
Florida	NR	NR	NR	NR	4,043	.	.	.	.	58.9
Georgia	877	1,309	757	20	930	27.3	39.8	22.6	0.6	26.5
Hawaii	476	605	411	357	257	82.8	103.5	69.7	60.0	42.9
Idaho	584	493	369	341	369	112.9	92.9	67.3	60.3	63.7
Illinois	2,714	2,516	2,769	2,923	4,202	48.5	44.6	48.7	51.1	73.0
Indiana	1,644	1,321	1,617	1,709	1,537	60.5	48.1	58.3	61.1	54.5
Iowa	1,310	1,125	897	1,008	879	96.8	82.6	65.6	73.4	63.7
Kansas	1,485	1,329	1,116	1,166	860	121.5	107.7	89.8	93.1	68.2
Kentucky	574	562	494	621	909	31.9	30.9	26.9	33.4	48.5
Louisiana	283	1,660	2,506	2,110	1,542	13.9	80.6	121.3	101.4	73.7
Maine	329	223	245	147	120	54.6	37.0	40.6	24.3	19.8
Maryland	727	645	612	673	1,094	30.8	27.1	25.5	27.7	44.7
Massachusetts	1,744	1,565	1,298	1,199	1,165	60.5	54.3	44.9	41.3	39.9
Michigan	NR	57	903	2,748	2,916	.	1.2	19.6	59.5	62.8
Minnesota	1,889	1,832	1,503	1,628	1,351	86.9	83.4	67.6	72.5	59.6
Mississippi	NR	NR	NR	NR	63	.	.	.	.	4.9
Missouri	1,216	1,170	1,152	1,050	1,244	48.9	46.7	45.6	41.2	48.4
Montana	292	255	283	260	203	72.9	62.5	67.9	61.2	47.0
Nebraska	687	593	310	647	526	88.5	75.8	39.4	81.6	65.8
Nevada	45	130	525	480	400	6.9	19.2	74.5	64.5	51.3
New Hampshire	332	279	163	149	173	61.2	51.1	29.6	26.8	30.7
New Jersey	153	349	211	98	154	4.1	9.2	5.6	2.6	4.0
New Mexico	549	412	468	501	564	72.1	52.9	58.8	61.4	67.9
New York	1,257	1,207	1,308	2,155	2,086	14.5	13.9	15.0	24.7	23.9
North Carolina	1,558	1,604	2,311	2,889	2,191	47.6	48.4	68.5	84.2	62.7
North Dakota	298	302	224	252	299	94.4	95.4	70.6	79.1	93.5
Ohio	4,032	3,827	3,676	4,594	4,048	76.5	72.1	68.9	85.7	75.1
Oklahoma	705	674	424	418	598	45.7	43.1	26.9	26.3	37.4
Oregon	998	632	1,202	1,472	1,320	69.5	43.2	80.5	96.9	85.3
Pennsylvania	883	3,178	2,702	2,328	2,671	15.4	55.2	46.8	40.2	46.0
Rhode Island	351	432	356	342	304	72.8	89.8	74.2	71.6	63.9
South Carolina	334	353	887	836	813	19.4	20.3	50.5	47.3	45.7
South Dakota	436	386	337	313	274	126.2	110.5	95.5	87.9	76.3
Tennessee	300	291	416	678	2,637	12.6	12.0	16.9	27.1	103.9
Texas	3,367	5,189	6,402	6,732	6,110	39.4	59.5	72.0	74.2	66.2
Utah	238	424	357	398	360	27.1	47.1	38.6	41.9	37.1
Vermont	96	68	44	65	54	34.5	24.3	15.6	22.8	18.8

[Continued]

★ 155 ★

Chlamydia: Reported Cases - Men
[Continued]

State/Area	Cases					Rates per 100,000 Population				
	1991	1992	1993	1994	1995	1991	1992	1993	1994	1995
Virginia	1,564	1,060	1,219	834	989	50.7	33.8	38.3	25.9	30.4
Washington	2,835	2,391	2,238	2,119	1,954	113.9	93.7	85.9	80.0	72.5
West Virginia	249	227	238	323	359	28.8	26.1	27.2	36.8	40.7
Wisconsin	2,357	1,669	2,534	2,683	2,095	97.3	68.2	102.5	107.7	83.4
Wyoming	220	159	176	135	143	95.9	68.4	74.8	56.6	59.4
U.S. TOTAL[1]	43,376	47,181	50,536	52,933	65,697	40.6	41.9	43.7	45.3	52.1
Guam	1	4	1	48	68	1.4	5.5	1.4	66.1	93.6
Puerto Rico	44	63	256	469	400	2.6	3.6	14.6	26.3	22.2
Virgin Islands	76	46	9	11	8	147.3	86.5	16.9	20.7	15.0
OUTLYING AREAS	121	113	266	528	476	6.6	6.1	14.2	27.6	24.7
TOTAL	43,497	47,294	50,802	53,461	66,173	40.0	41.3	43.3	45.0	51.7

Source: U.S. Department of Health and Human Services. Public Health Service. Centers for Disease Control and Prevention. Division of STD Prevention. *Sexually Transmitted Disease Surveillance, 1995.* U.S. Department of Health and Human Services, Public Health Service, September 1996. *Notes:* NR indicates "no report." NG indicates "not reported by gender." Cases and rates underestimated in some areas because of under-reporting or non-reporting by gender. 1. Includes cases reported by Washington, D.C.

★ 156 ★

Diseases and Illnesses: Sexually Transmitted Diseases

Chlamydia: Reported Cases - Women

This table shows reported cases and rates of chlamydia in women, by state/area: United States and outlying areas, 1991-1995.

State/Area	Cases					Rates per 100,000 Population				
	1991	1992	1993	1994	1995	1991	1992	1993	1994	1995
Alabama	NR	NR	NR	425	2,888	.	.	.	19.4	130.6
Alaska	NR	NR	NR	NR	NR	.	.	.	.	.
Arizona	9,533	8,190	8,771	7,680	8,315	502.9	422.3	439.8	372.4	390.1
Arkansas	480	601	574	654	596	39.1	48.5	45.8	51.5	46.4
California	1,780	10,789	10,004	1,724	34,934	11.7	69.9	64.1	11.0	221.2
Colorado	7	4	50	NR	NR	0.4	0.2	2.8	.	.
Connecticut	6,962	7,757	6,783	6,288	5,624	410.7	459.3	401.9	373.0	333.8
Delaware	783	648	1,427	2,171	2,295	223.5	182.5	396.5	595.8	622.0
Florida	NR	NR	NR	NR	18,251	.	.	.	.	250.1
Georgia	6,407	8,689	3,460	148	10,263	187.8	249.8	97.6	4.1	277.5
Hawaii	2,784	3,078	2,221	2,127	1,878	498.4	541.3	385.8	364.6	319.2
Idaho	1,834	1,800	1,524	1,411	1,370	351.6	336.3	275.9	247.8	234.7
Illinois	19,112	21,529	20,655	21,660	20,443	322.6	360.8	343.9	358.5	336.5
Indiana	10,253	9,497	8,417	8,637	7,564	355.4	326.5	286.7	291.9	253.6
Iowa	5,328	5,012	4,317	4,405	4,210	370.3	346.5	297.1	302.3	288.0
Kansas	5,301	5,695	4,699	5,225	4,453	417.6	444.7	364.5	402.5	341.3

[Continued]

★ 156 ★

Chlamydia: Reported Cases - Women
[Continued]

State/Area	Cases					Rates per 100,000 Population				
	1991	1992	1993	1994	1995	1991	1992	1993	1994	1995
Kentucky	4,950	4,780	4,985	5,009	5,995	258.3	247.2	255.1	254.1	301.8
Louisiana	1,410	8,175	9,701	8,540	7,569	64.1	369.3	436.5	381.9	336.5
Maine	2,369	1,791	1,335	1,048	1,024	373.8	282.6	210.3	165.0	160.9
Maryland	4,732	5,026	4,545	6,036	7,646	189.1	198.9	178.3	234.6	294.8
Massachusetts	9,154	8,247	7,041	6,867	6,237	293.6	264.7	225.3	218.9	197.9
Michigan	NR	290	3,876	14,938	18,750	.	6.0	79.8	306.4	382.5
Minnesota	6,295	6,711	5,908	5,689	4,681	279.1	294.7	256.7	244.9	199.8
Mississippi	NR	NR	NR	NR	849	.	.	.	.	60.5
Missouri	9,584	10,703	10,471	11,199	10,866	358.7	398.1	386.4	410.1	394.8
Montana	1,885	1,697	1,311	1,143	995	462.2	408.8	309.2	265.0	227.1
Nebraska	2,649	2,436	1,422	2,661	2,346	324.9	296.6	172.0	319.9	280.0
Nevada	245	673	2,860	2,668	2,649	38.8	102.9	420.7	371.8	352.9
New Hampshire	1,597	1,630	1,001	817	725	282.7	286.9	174.8	141.2	123.9
New Jersey	1,563	3,594	2,531	1,733	3,902	39.0	89.1	62.4	42.5	95.2
New Mexico	4,127	4,070	4,279	4,536	3,721	525.2	507.0	521.7	540.3	435.5
New York	9,705	15,836	14,012	24,317	24,600	103.4	168.3	148.4	257.6	261.0
North Carolina	10,369	12,115	13,145	14,907	13,589	297.9	344.0	367.3	409.6	367.0
North Dakota	1,026	870	709	827	1,025	322.3	272.9	221.9	258.0	318.8
Ohio	28,203	24,820	22,311	27,881	24,883	498.2	435.9	389.8	485.5	431.7
Oklahoma	3,331	4,655	4,266	3,305	4,467	204.9	283.0	257.4	198.0	266.0
Oregon	6,327	5,259	4,325	4,023	4,145	426.5	348.0	280.6	256.7	260.1
Pennsylvania	3,392	19,863	19,850	17,418	20,290	54.6	318.6	317.4	277.9	323.7
Rhode Island	1,720	2,055	1,858	1,753	1,598	329.4	394.9	358.0	339.4	311.0
South Carolina	5,366	4,992	7,077	7,097	6,932	292.7	269.5	378.6	378.1	366.3
South Dakota	1,714	1,539	1,308	1,114	1,039	480.8	427.3	359.5	303.5	280.9
Tennessee	5,060	5,010	5,268	6,109	10,517	197.3	192.7	199.8	228.1	386.9
Texas	29,193	35,602	37,472	39,314	38,517	331.4	396.8	409.3	421.0	405.8
Utah	513	1,189	1,232	1,403	1,316	57.7	130.6	131.8	146.3	134.2
Vermont	763	572	470	457	408	263.1	196.3	160.1	154.6	137.0
Virginia	17,955	11,639	11,363	12,086	11,253	560.7	357.8	344.7	362.5	334.2
Washington	10,464	9,371	8,093	8,458	7,508	413.7	361.4	305.6	314.5	274.5
West Virginia	1,326	1,262	1,697	2,271	1,961	142.0	134.6	180.0	240.3	207.2
Wisconsin	6,944	4,488	9,137	9,086	6,860	274.9	176.0	355.1	350.6	262.8
Wyoming	982	833	758	681	560	429.3	359.6	323.3	286.8	234.0
U.S. TOTAL[1]	265,818	305,670	299,205	318,886	383,956	233.7	255.0	247.1	260.2	290.3
Guam	21	50	37	227	393	30.7	73.0	54.0	331.5	573.9
Puerto Rico	30	47	345	1,974	1,905	1.6	2.5	18.5	103.9	99.3
Virgin Islands	180	84	5	39	9	322.0	145.8	8.7	67.7	15.6

[Continued]

★ 156 ★

Chlamydia: Reported Cases - Women
[Continued]

State/Area	Cases					Rates per 100,000 Population				
	1991	1992	1993	1994	1995	1991	1992	1993	1994	1995
OUTLYING AREAS	231	181	387	2,240	2,307	11.8	9.2	19.4	110.5	112.8
TOTAL	266,049	305,851	299,592	321,126	386,263	229.9	251.1	243.4	257.8	287.6

Source: U.S. Department of Health and Human Services. Public Health Service. Centers for Disease Control and Prevention. Division of STD Prevention. *Sexually Transmitted Disease Surveillance, 1995.* U.S. Department of Health and Human Services, Public Health Service, September 1996. *Notes:* NR indicates "no report." NG indicates "not reported by gender." Cases and rates underestimated in some areas because of under-reporting or non-reporting by gender. 1. Includes cases reported by Washington, D.C.

★ 157 ★

Diseases and Illnesses: Sexually Transmitted Diseases

Chlamydia: Reported Cases, by Major City

This table shows reported cases and rates of chlamydia, by selected cities of 200,000 population: United States and outlying areas, 1991-1995.

State/Area	Cases					Rates per 100,000 Population				
	1991	1992	1993	1994	1995	1991	1992	1993	1994	1995
Akron, OH	1,462	1,632	1,805	2,132	1,457	281.5	312.6	343.7	404.0	274.8
Albuquerque, NM	1,810	1,756	2,145	2,080	1,651	369.8	351.8	423.4	403.2	316.1
Atlanta, GA	1,645	4,407	1,308	NR	4,411	250.9	663.1	193.2	.	629.5
Austin, TX	2,475	1,648	2,060	2,572	2,977	415.9	268.7	326.4	397.5	447.8
Baltimore, MD	3,842	4,223	3,576	3,638	4,000	524.6	582.4	500.1	517.7	578.8
Birmingham, AL	NR	NR	NR	273	992	.	.	.	41.6	150.8
Boston, MA	3,404	3,019	2,668	2,452	2,179	605.0	544.9	482.5	445.6	392.0
Buffalo, NY	NR	NR	NR	NR	NR	.	.	.	.	.
Charlotte, NC	NR	NR	NR	NR	1,063	.	.	.	.	183.4
Chicago, IL	9,739	12,043	11,171	11,984	11,687	331.7	408.5	378.5	406.1	396.4
Cincinnati, OH	2,712	2,339	2,614	2,885	2,846	312.0	268.6	300.0	332.4	329.4
Cleveland, OH	5,399	4,719	3,578	7,036	5,770	382.6	334.6	254.1	501.7	412.7
Columbus, OH	6,829	5,757	5,198	5,380	3,500	698.5	581.8	520.1	535.0	346.2
Corpus Christi, TX	543	444	538	567	1,167	183.1	147.6	175.9	182.2	373.2
Dallas, TX	3,284	3,566	4,528	3,909	5,115	173.6	186.6	234.9	201.2	261.1
Dayton, OH	1,408	1,398	1,344	1,372	869	244.7	242.4	233.2	239.6	152.3
Denver, CO	2	3	17	NR	NR	0.4	0.6	3.4	.	.
Des Moines, IA	694	989	627	692	699	208.7	292.7	183.0	200.1	200.0
Detroit, MI	NR	45	193	4,496	9,026	.	4.2	18.1	425.5	857.6
El Paso, TX	1,065	1,629	2,123	2,238	1,245	173.5	259.2	327.9	335.5	183.5
Fort Worth, TX	1,701	1,407	1,464	2,437	2,540	141.3	115.3	118.5	193.6	198.7
Honolulu, HI	2,643	3,402	2,333	2,147	1,738	311.3	395.1	269.2	245.6	198.1
Houston, TX	7,044	8,919	9,174	9,377	8,075	242.7	301.0	305.3	307.9	262.4
Indianapolis, IN	5,778	5,096	5,092	5,049	4,662	716.8	628.0	625.2	617.8	570.2
Jacksonville, FL	NR	NR	NR	NR	1,611	.	.	.	.	229.6
Jersey City, NJ	31	236	37	83	182	14.2	108.0	17.0	38.1	83.7
Kansas City, MO	2,207	2,246	1,675	1,839	1,997	504.7	513.9	383.2	420.1	455.3
Los Angeles, CA	NR	16,380	19,926	21,664	19,464	.	192.9	233.0	253.3	227.5

[Continued]

★ 157 ★

Chlamydia: Reported Cases, by Major City
[Continued]

State/Area	Cases					Rates per 100,000 Population				
	1991	1992	1993	1994	1995	1991	1992	1993	1994	1995
Louisville, KY	1,376	1,283	1,264	1,130	1,618	206.3	191.6	188.4	168.2	240.4
Memphis, TN	2,675	1,885	1,768	2,489	3,728	320.3	223.8	208.5	290.4	431.0
Miami, FL	NR	NR	NR	NR	2,004	0	0	0	0	98.7
Milwaukee, WI	4,885	1,517	2,940	5,452	4,332	510.6	159.2	310.5	581.3	465.2
Minneapolis, MN	2,456	2,711	2,378	2,394	1,922	650.1	715.7	624.7	626.1	501.2
Nashville, TN	343	835	1,223	1,190	1,926	66.9	161.5	234.3	225.6	362.9
New Orleans, LA	187	1,865	3,144	2,733	3,107	38.1	381.1	645.3	563.7	644.7
New York City, NY	10,962	17,043	15,320	26,472	26,686	150.0	233.3	209.1	361.6	365.0
Newark, NJ	280	1,038	545	292	1,077	95.6	354.7	186.7	100.7	374.6
Norfolk, VA	1,185	1,075	949	944	832	468.2	423.8	378.7	389.0	350.2
Oakland, CA	2,143	2,020	1,284	2,679	3,485	181.3	168.9	106.8	222.2	288.1
Oklahoma City, OK	2,078	2,203	1,855	1,528	1,232	492.0	515.7	429.7	350.4	281.8
Omaha, NE	1,309	1,654	892	1,808	1,335	310.2	388.4	208.3	420.0	307.5
Philadelphia, PA	1,151	8,716	10,053	9,957	8,079	73.5	562.2	653.9	654.6	539.0
Phoenix, AZ	6,529	5,533	5,732	5,218	5,896	301.3	250.1	252.7	222.2	242.4
Pittsburgh, PA	771	3,372	3,195	3,294	2,865	57.8	252.7	240.4	249.4	218.7
Portland, OR	2,834	2,396	2,105	2,072	1,945	603.2	504.6	438.2	429.9	401.4
Richmond, VA	1,773	1,215	1,033	994	2,149	881.7	606.9	517.5	501.7	1083.9
Rochester, NY	NR	NR	NR	NR	NR	0	0	0	0	0
Sacramento, CA	3,527	3,255	1,631	2,443	3,455	326.6	298.0	148.6	222.8	313.1
San Antonio, TX	2,334	3,745	4,447	4,519	4,348	193.2	303.7	353.6	354.3	335.3
San Diego, CA	7,596	6,723	7,250	6,387	4,820	297.2	258.4	277.6	242.8	182.3
San Francisco, CA	2,355	2,167	2,395	2,215	2,008	324.2	297.0	326.9	302.9	274.9
San Jose, CA	4,389	3,245	2,645	3,900	2,588	290.5	212.4	171.3	251.3	165.3
Seattle, WA	4,590	4,066	3,351	3,578	3,286	299.0	260.7	212.5	225.9	206.0
St. Louis, MO	1,948	2,374	2,850	3,013	2,796	497.6	617.0	757.4	819.5	779.5
St. Paul, MN	1,080	1,257	1,133	1,119	1,027	390.3	453.4	410.1	406.5	373.7
St. Petersburg, FL	NR	NR	NR	NR	1,579	0	0	0	0	181.3
Tampa, FL	NR	NR	NR	NR	2,063	0	0	0	0	233.2
Toledo, OH	2,061	1,509	1,767	2,181	968	446.8	327.4	385.0	476.7	212.7
Tucson, AZ	2,121	1,667	2,073	1,847	1,915	313.6	241.0	292.0	252.3	254.5
Tulsa, OK	1,067	1,142	1,191	831	1,028	289.2	305.8	316.8	220.3	271.9
Washington, DC	406	680	797	1,083	1,665	68.3	116.1	137.9	191.0	300.4
Wichita, KS	1,753	1,779	1,362	1,642	1,324	428.4	428.1	325.5	391.7	315.7
Yonkers, NY	NR	NR	NR	NR	NR	0	0	0	0	0
U.S. CITY TOTAL	143,881	177,273	173,766	201,706	210,011	278.8	287.9	280.5	327.2	310.5
San Juan, PR	61	68	377	821	742	7.0	7.8	43.2	94.1	85.1
TOTAL	143,942	177,341	174,143	202,527	210,753	274.3	284.0	277.2	323.9	307.7

Source: U.S. Department of Health and Human Services. Public Health Service. Centers for Disease Control and Prevention. Division of STD Prevention. *Sexually Transmitted Disease Surveillance, 1995.* U.S. Department of Health and Human Services, Public Health Service, September 1996. *Notes:* NR indicates "no report." 1. Includes cases reported by Washington, D.C.

★ 158 ★

Diseases and Illnesses: Sexually Transmitted Diseases

Chlamydia: Reported Cases in Men, by Major City

This table shows reported cases and rates of chlamydia in men, by selected cities of 200,000 population: United States and outlying areas, 1991-1995.

State/Area	Cases					Rates per 100,000 Population				
	1991	1992	1993	1994	1995	1991	1992	1993	1994	1995
Akron, OH	176	244	282	328	191	70.7	97.5	112.0	129.6	75.1
Albuquerque, NM	202	185	250	204	248	84.5	75.9	101.0	80.9	97.1
Atlanta, GA	122	497	273	NR	327	39.0	156.6	84.4	.	97.7
Austin, TX	254	244	244	315	377	85.3	79.5	77.3	97.5	113.5
Baltimore, MD	421	329	326	311	307	123.1	97.1	97.6	94.7	95.0
Birmingham, AL	NR	NR	NR	33	116	.	.	.	10.7	37.7
Boston, MA	705	613	518	486	483	260.6	230.0	194.8	183.7	180.7
Buffalo, NY	NR	NR	NR	NR	NR	.	.	.	.	.
Charlotte, NC	NR	NR	NR	NR	137	.	.	.	.	49.1
Chicago, IL	733	772	1,019	1,057	1,967	51.9	54.4	71.7	74.4	138.6
Cincinnati, OH	307	236	390	515	656	74.6	57.2	94.5	125.3	160.2
Cleveland, OH	592	587	392	873	697	89.3	88.5	59.2	132.3	105.9
Columbus, OH	1,395	1,259	1,054	1,141	617	295.7	263.7	218.6	235.1	126.4
Corpus Christi, TX	64	118	139	137	189	44.1	80.1	92.8	89.9	123.3
Dallas, TX	444	474	505	464	1,165	47.7	50.4	53.2	48.5	120.8
Dayton, OH	140	132	132	128	79	50.8	47.7	47.8	46.6	28.9
Denver, CO	NR	NR	NR	NR	NR	.	.	.	.	.
Des Moines, IA	125	160	107	126	128	78.8	99.2	65.4	76.3	76.7
Detroit, MI	NR	6	24	358	1,017	.	1.2	4.8	71.4	203.6
El Paso, TX	33	196	266	227	133	11.1	64.3	84.5	70.0	40.3
Fort Worth, TX	163	373	518	532	471	27.4	61.8	84.8	85.5	74.5
Honolulu, HI	440	594	397	317	236	102.1	136.0	90.4	71.8	53.3
Houston, TX	612	1,166	1,765	1,712	687	42.4	79.1	118.1	113.1	44.9
Indianapolis, IN	889	744	1,103	1,147	1,033	232.1	192.9	284.9	295.1	265.6
Jacksonville, FL	NR	NR	NR	NR	336	.	.	.	.	98.0
Jersey City, NJ	1	132	4	NR	6	0.9	124.5	3.8	.	5.7
Kansas City, MO	182	171	151	134	149	87.4	82.2	72.5	64.3	71.3
Los Angeles, CA	NR	1,689	1,601	NR	819	.	39.9	37.6	.	19.2
Louisville, KY	106	117	92	108	275	33.6	37.0	29.0	34.0	86.4
Memphis, TN	115	87	97	233	638	28.9	21.7	24.0	57.1	155.0
Miami, FL	NR	NR	NR	NR	485	.	.	.	.	49.8
Milwaukee, WI	1,001	661	672	1,154	1,057	220.6	146.2	149.6	259.3	239.1
Minneapolis, MN	679	712	611	603	480	371.1	387.9	331.2	325.3	258.0
Nashville, TN	21	68	146	168	495	8.6	27.7	58.9	67.0	196.1
New Orleans, LA	27	573	1,182	893	669	11.8	251.8	521.8	396.0	298.4
New York City, NY	1,257	1,207	1,308	2,155	2,086	36.6	35.2	38.0	62.7	60.7
Newark, NJ	10	523	16	8	55	7.2	377.9	11.6	5.8	40.5
Norfolk, VA	60	64	67	42	59	44.5	47.3	50.2	32.5	46.7
Oakland, CA	NR	NR	NR	154	525	.	.	.	26.0	88.5
Oklahoma City, OK	580	384	172	176	163	285.7	186.9	82.8	83.9	77.5
Omaha, NE	247	344	166	349	256	121.5	167.6	80.4	168.1	122.2
Philadelphia, PA	107	601	677	862	633	14.7	83.3	94.6	121.7	90.7
Phoenix, AZ	795	678	887	971	1,083	74.4	62.2	79.3	83.9	90.2
Pittsburgh, PA	145	453	608	620	512	23.2	72.3	97.4	99.9	83.1
Portland, OR	303	267	536	612	501	132.6	115.6	229.3	260.8	212.3

[Continued]

★ 158 ★

Chlamydia: Reported Cases in Men, by Major City

[Continued]

State/Area	Cases					Rates per 100,000 Population				
	1991	1992	1993	1994	1995	1991	1992	1993	1994	1995
Richmond, VA	115	72	107	79	194	125.2	78.7	117.3	87.2	214.0
Rochester, NY	NR	NR	NR	NR	NR	.	.	.	.	.
Sacramento, CA	NR	NR	NR	169	599	.	.	.	31.5	111.1
San Antonio, TX	428	311	491	624	563	73.1	52.0	80.5	100.8	89.4
San Diego, CA	NR	NR	NR	NR	NR	.	.	.	.	.
San Francisco, CA	575	472	517	491	473	158.2	129.4	141.3	134.6	130.0
San Jose, CA	NR	NR	NR	NR	NR	.	.	.	.	.
Seattle, WA	1,124	980	805	823	812	148.6	127.5	103.6	105.4	103.3
St. Louis, MO	204	206	186	203	187	114.3	117.4	108.4	121.0	114.2
St. Paul, MN	253	265	272	295	243	191.3	200.0	205.9	224.1	184.8
St. Petersburg, FL	NR	NR	NR	NR	233	.	.	.	.	57.2
Tampa, FL	NR	NR	NR	NR	417	.	.	.	.	96.7
Toledo, OH	207	159	307	255	160	94.0	72.2	140.0	116.6	73.6
Tucson, AZ	476	262	347	314	370	143.8	77.4	99.8	87.6	100.3
Tulsa, OK	75	51	72	55	82	42.2	28.3	39.7	30.2	45.0
Washington, DC	65	88	111	143	216	23.4	32.2	41.1	54.0	83.4
Wichita, KS	311	306	281	389	288	155.1	150.2	137.0	189.2	139.9
Yonkers, NY	NR	NR	NR	NR	NR	.	.	.	.	.
U.S. CITY TOTAL	17,286	20,832	22,193	23,493	27,380	80.2	78.8	83.4	100.2	89.2
San Juan, PR	44	42	181	215	182	11.2	10.7	46.1	54.8	46.4
TOTAL	17,330	20,874	22,374	23,708	27,562	79.0	77.8	82.9	99.5	88.7

Source: U.S. Department of Health and Human Services. Public Health Service. Centers for Disease Control and Prevention. Division of STD Prevention. *Sexually Transmitted Disease Surveillance, 1995.* U.S. Department of Health and Human Services, Public Health Service, September 1996. *Notes:* NR indicates "no report." 1. Includes cases reported by Washington, D.C.

★ 159 ★

Diseases and Illnesses: Sexually Transmitted Diseases

Chlamydia: Reported Cases in Women, by Major City

This table shows reported cases and rates of chlamydia in women, by selected cities of 200,000 population: United States and outlying areas, 1991-1995.

State/Area	Cases					Rates per 100,000 Population				
	1991	1992	1993	1994	1995	1991	1992	1993	1994	1995
Akron, OH	1,286	1,388	1,523	1,804	1,265	475.4	510.7	557.2	657.0	458.8
Albuquerque, NM	1,608	1,571	1,895	1,876	1,403	642.0	615.4	731.4	711.3	525.6
Atlanta, GA	1,523	3,910	1,035	NR	4,084	444.2	1,126.0	292.8	0	1,116.3
Austin, TX	2,221	1,404	1,816	2,257	2,600	746.8	458.1	575.4	696.8	781.3
Baltimore, MD	3,421	3,894	3,250	3,327	3,693	876.3	1,008.0	853.2	888.6	1,003.2
Birmingham, AL	NR	NR	NR	231	867	0	0	0	66.1	247.7
Boston, MA	2,699	2,406	2,150	1,966	1,696	923.7	836.6	749.0	688.2	587.8
Buffalo, NY	NR	NR	NR	NR	NR	0	0	0	0	0

[Continued]

★ 159 ★

Chlamydia: Reported Cases in Women, by Major City

[Continued]

State/Area	Cases					Rates per 100,000 Population				
	1991	1992	1993	1994	1995	1991	1992	1993	1994	1995
Charlotte, NC	NR	NR	NR	NR	926	0	0	0	0	307.9
Chicago, IL	9,006	11,271	10,152	10,927	9,720	591.0	737.0	663.0	713.8	635.6
Cincinnati, OH	2,405	2,103	2,224	2,370	2,176	525.4	458.8	484.9	518.9	478.8
Cleveland, OH	4,807	4,132	3,186	6,163	5,050	642.6	553.0	427.1	829.6	682.2
Columbus, OH	5,434	4,498	4,144	4,239	2,862	1,074.0	878.6	801.4	814.8	547.3
Corpus Christi, TX	479	326	399	430	978	316.5	212.3	255.6	271.0	613.3
Dallas, TX	2,840	3,092	4,023	3,445	3,950	295.7	318.7	411.0	349.2	397.2
Dayton, OH	1,268	1,266	1,212	1,244	787	423.1	421.6	404.0	417.5	265.2
Denver, CO	2	3	17	NR	NR	0.8	1.2	6.7	0	0
Des Moines, IA	569	829	520	566	571	327.1	469.1	290.2	313.1	312.7
Detroit, MI	NR	39	169	4,138	8,009	0	6.9	30.2	745.1	1,448.3
El Paso, TX	1,032	1,433	1,857	2,011	1,112	325.9	442.9	558.3	586.4	319.3
Fort Worth, TX	1,538	1,034	946	1,905	2,069	253.0	167.8	151.6	299.3	320.1
Honolulu, HI	2,203	2,808	1,936	1,830	1,502	526.9	661.7	452.6	423.1	345.5
Houston, TX	6,432	7,753	7,409	7,665	7,388	440.6	520.3	490.2	500.5	477.6
Indianapolis, IN	4,889	4,352	3,989	3,902	3,629	1,155.5	1,022.3	933.8	910.4	846.5
Jacksonville, FL	NR	NR	NR	NR	1,275	0	0	0	0	355.4
Jersey City, NJ	30	104	33	83	176	26.7	92.5	29.4	74.0	157.4
Kansas City, MO	2,025	2,075	1,524	1,705	1,848	883.7	906.4	665.6	743.8	804.9
Los Angeles, CA	NR	9,094	8,126	NR	3,869	0	213.7	189.5	0	90.2
Louisville, KY	1,270	1,166	1,172	1,022	1,343	360.8	330.1	331.3	288.6	378.8
Memphis, TN	2,560	1,798	1,671	2,256	3,090	585.0	407.4	376.2	502.3	681.4
Miami, FL	NR	NR	NR	NR	1,519	0	0	0	0	143.7
Milwaukee, WI	2,309	856	2,268	4,300	3,275	459.1	171.0	455.9	872.6	669.5
Minneapolis, MN	1,777	1,999	1,767	1,791	1,442	912.2	1,023.9	900.8	909.2	730.3
Nashville, TN	322	767	1,077	1,022	1,431	119.7	282.7	393.2	369.4	514.0
New Orleans, LA	160	1,292	1,962	1,840	2,438	60.9	493.5	752.8	709.4	946.0
New York City, NY	9,705	15,836	14,012	24,317	24,600	250.4	408.8	360.7	626.5	634.8
Newark, NJ	270	515	529	284	1,022	174.8	333.9	343.7	185.9	674.4
Norfolk, VA	1,125	1,011	882	895	768	951.5	853.6	753.7	789.1	690.0
Oakland, CA	NR	NR	NR	825	2,959	0	0	0	134.4	480.2
Oklahoma City, OK	1,498	1,808	1,677	1,350	1,069	682.9	815.4	748.7	596.7	471.6
Omaha, NE	1,062	1,309	726	1,435	1,079	485.7	593.5	327.4	644.0	480.3
Philadelphia, PA	1,044	8,115	9,376	9,095	7,446	124.7	979.5	1,141.0	1,118.7	929.7
Phoenix, AZ	5,734	4,855	4,845	4,247	4,813	521.8	433.0	421.4	356.9	390.6
Pittsburgh, PA	626	2,919	2,587	2,674	2,353	88.4	412.5	367.0	381.9	339.1
Portland, OR	2,531	2,129	1,569	1,460	1,444	1,048.8	873.4	636.3	590.4	581.0
Richmond, VA	1,658	1,143	926	913	1,950	1,517.4	1,051.4	854.3	848.8	1,812.1
Rochester, NY	NR	NR	NR	NR	NR	0	0	0	0	0
Sacramento, CA	NR	NR	NR	767	2,153	0	0	0	136.8	381.7
San Antonio, TX	1,906	3,434	3,956	3,895	3,785	306.2	540.7	610.8	593.1	567.3
San Diego, CA	NR	NR	NR	NR	NR	0	0	0	0	0
San Francisco, CA	1,780	1,695	1,878	1,724	1,535	490.5	464.7	512.1	470.4	418.7
San Jose, CA	NR	NR	NR	NR	NR	0	0	0	0	0
Seattle, WA	3,466	3,086	2,546	2,755	2,474	445.2	390.2	318.3	342.9	305.9
St. Louis, MO	1,744	2,168	2,664	2,810	2,609	818.4	1,035.8	1,301.7	1,405.5	1,338.1

[Continued]

★ 159 ★

Chlamydia: Reported Cases in Women, by Major City

[Continued]

State/Area	Cases					Rates per 100,000 Population				
	1991	1992	1993	1994	1995	1991	1992	1993	1994	1995
St. Paul, MN	827	992	861	824	784	572.4	685.6	597.2	573.8	547.1
St. Petersburg, FL	NR	NR	NR	NR	1,346	0	0	0	0	290.5
Tampa, FL	NR	NR	NR	NR	1,646	0	0	0	0	363.0
Toledo, OH	1,854	1,350	1,460	1,926	805	768.9	560.7	609.1	806.2	339.0
Tucson, AZ	1,645	1,405	1,726	1,533	1,545	476.4	398.0	476.3	410.6	402.8
Tulsa, OK	992	1,083	1,098	774	946	518.9	559.8	564.0	396.3	483.5
Washington, DC	341	588	686	940	1,449	107.6	188.3	222.6	311.0	490.7
Wichita, KS	1,442	1,473	1,081	1,253	1,036	690.8	695.1	506.6	586.6	485.2
Yonkers, NY	NR	NR	NR	NR	NR	0	0	0	0	0
U.S. CITY TOTAL	107,365	135,577	128,537	143,011	159,659	456.9	476.2	448.8	563.8	487.6
San Juan, PR	17	26	196	606	560	3.5	5.4	40.9	126.3	116.7
TOTAL	107,382	135,603	128,733	143,617	160,219	447.8	468.4	442.1	555.6	482.3

Source: U.S. Department of Health and Human Services. Public Health Service. Centers for Disease Control and Prevention. Division of STD Prevention. *Sexually Transmitted Disease Surveillance, 1995.* U.S. Department of Health and Human Services, Public Health Service, September 1996. *Notes:* NR indicates "no report." 1. Includes cases reported by Washington, D.C.

★ 160 ★

Diseases and Illnesses: Sexually Transmitted Diseases

Congenital Syphilis

This table shows reported cases and rates of congenital syphilis in infants less than 1 year of age: United States (excluding outlying areas), 1963-1995.

Year	Cases	Rate per 100,000 live births
1963	367	9.2
1964	336	8.7
1965	335	8.9
1966	333	8.8
1967	156	4.1
1968	274	7.3
1969	264	7.0
1970	323	8.6
1971	422	11.9
1972	360	11.0
1973	295	9.4
1974	250	7.9
1975	169	5.3
1976	160	5.1
1977	134	4.0

[Continued]

★ 160 ★

Congenital Syphilis
[Continued]

Year	Cases	Rate per 100,000 live births
1978	104	3.0
1979	123	3.5
1980	107	3.0
1981	160	4.4
1982	159	4.3
1983	158	4.3
1984	247	6.7
1985	266	7.0
1986	357	9.5
1987	444	11.6
1988	658	16.8
1989	1,807	44.7
1990	3,816	91.0
1991	4,410	107.3
1992	3,850	94.7
1993	3,237	80.7
1994	2,204	55.6
1995	1,548	39.0

Source: U.S. Department of Health and Human Services. Public Health Service. Centers for Disease Control and Prevention. Division of STD Prevention. *Sexually Transmitted Disease Surveillance, 1995.* U.S. Department of Health and Human Services, Public Health Service, September 1996. *Notes:* The surveillance case definition for congenital syphilis changed in 1988 (see Appendix). As of 1995, cases of congenital syphilis in persons <1 year of age per 100,000 live births are obtained using a new reporting form (CDC 73.126). Years 1963-1966 are fiscal years.

★ 161 ★

Diseases and Illnesses: Sexually Transmitted Diseases

Congenital Syphilis, by State

This table shows reported cases and rates of congenital syphilis in infants less than 1 year of age by state/area: United States, 1991-1995.

State/Area	Cases					Rates per 100,000 Population				
	1991	1992	1993	1994	1995	1991	1992	1993	1994	1995
Alabama	21	12	27	18	13	33.4	19.3	42.6	29.6	21.4
Alaska	0	0	0	0	0	0.0	0.0	0.0	0.0	0.0
Arizona	21	18	16	16	10	30.8	26.2	22.6	24.2	15.1
Arkansas	28	34	8	29	27	78.9	97.6	23.4	83.9	78.1
California	719	402	298	194	342	117.9	66.8	50.5	33.3	58.8
Colorado	0	1	8	4	1	0.0	1.8	14.6	7.4	1.8
Connecticut	25	26	10	6	6	51.5	54.7	21.8	14.2	14.2
Delaware	7	4	3	5	1	62.6	37.5	28.4	48.3	9.7
Florida	608	336	235	74	87	313.4	175.3	121.7	38.7	45.5
Georgia	139	178	79	42	44	126.0	160.2	70.3	38.6	40.4

[Continued]

★ 161 ★

Congenital Syphilis, by State
[Continued]

State/Area	Cases					Rates per 100,000 Population				
	1991	1992	1993	1994	1995	1991	1992	1993	1994	1995
Hawaii	0	0	0	0	0	0.0	0.0	0.0	0.0	0.0
Idaho	0	0	0	0	0	0.0	0.0	0.0	0.0	0.0
Illinois	299	396	368	258	182	153.9	206.9	192.6	136.3	96.2
Indiana	0	3	1	11	0	0.0	3.6	1.2	13.2	0.0
Iowa	0	0	1	6	0	0.0	0.0	2.7	16.7	0.0
Kansas	0	4	3	2	1	0.0	10.5	7.9	6.0	3.0
Kentucky	6	8	9	13	9	11.0	14.9	17.2	25.0	17.3
Louisiana	30	1	144	87	31	41.6	1.4	206.2	127.1	45.3
Maine	0	0	0	0	0	0.0	0.0	0.0	0.0	0.0
Maryland	54	43	30	9	23	68.2	55.3	39.7	12.6	32.1
Massachusetts	5	4	6	6	0	5.7	4.6	7.0	7.2	0.0
Michigan	113	73	84	28	27	75.2	50.7	58.5	20.0	19.3
Minnesota	2	6	9	2	2	3.0	9.1	14.1	3.1	3.1
Mississippi	19	26	70	56	63	44.0	60.9	166.0	129.1	145.2
Missouri	15	28	97	72	40	19.1	36.7	125.3	95.5	53.1
Montana	0	0	0	0	0	0.0	0.0	0.0	0.0	0.0
Nebraska	1	4	1	0	0	4.2	17.1	4.4	0.0	0.0
Nevada	14	6	3	3	0	63.6	26.8	14.2	13.9	0.0
New Hampshire	0	0	0	0	0	0.0	0.0	0.0	0.0	0.0
New Jersey	41	104	161	178	93	33.8	86.7	130.9	152.9	79.9
New Mexico	5	0	0	0	0	18.0	0.0	0.0	0.0	0.0
New York	1,077	958	748	388	196	368.0	332.8	268.8	139.0	70.2
North Carolina	53	72	54	44	31	51.8	69.3	53.7	43.2	30.4
North Dakota	0	0	0	0	0	0.0	0.0	0.0	0.0	0.0
Ohio	51	59	71	71	33	30.8	36.4	45.3	43.8	20.4
Oklahoma	12	23	11	15	17	25.1	48.4	23.5	32.8	37.2
Oregon	1	0	4	0	0	2.4	0.0	9.5	0.0	0.0
Pennsylvania	307	274	161	115	64	181.8	166.4	101.1	73.2	40.7
Rhode Island	0	2	1	2	0	0.0	13.8	7.0	14.9	0.0
South Carolina	70	56	82	100	24	121.6	99.7	151.9	196.4	47.1
South Dakota	0	0	0	0	0	0.0	0.0	0.0	0.0	0.0
Tennessee	69	51	52	57	25	92.6	69.3	70.6	75.3	33.0
Texas	262	338	246	224	112	82.5	105.3	74.4	69.5	34.8
Utah	0	0	0	0	0	0.0	0.0	0.0	0.0	0.0
Vermont	0	0	0	0	0	0.0	0.0	0.0	0.0	0.0
Virginia	51	59	23	18	18	52.4	60.7	24.2	18.8	18.8
Washington	9	11	4	3	2	11.3	13.8	5.6	3.8	2.5
West Virginia	1	2	6	2	0	4.4	9.0	27.2	9.3	0.0
Wisconsin	29	10	29	18	11	40.2	14.2	41.9	26.2	16.0
Wyoming	0	1	0	0	0	0.0	14.9	0.0	0.0	0.0
U.S. TOTAL[1]	4,410	3,850	3,237	2,204	1,548	107.3	94.7	80.7	55.6	39.0
Guam	0	0	0	0	0	0.0	0.0	0.0	0.0	0.0
Puerto Rico	28	26	18	20	3	43.8	40.6	28.1	31.3	4.7
Virgin Islands	0	2	1	0	0	0.0	90.3	45.1	0.0	0.0

[Continued]

★ 161 ★

Congenital Syphilis, by State
[Continued]

State/Area	Cases					Rates per 100,000 Population				
	1991	1992	1993	1994	1995	1991	1992	1993	1994	1995
OUTLYING AREAS	28	28	19	20	3	40.2	40.2	27.3	28.7	4.3
TOTAL	4,438	3,878	3,256	2,224	1,551	106.2	93.8	79.7	55.1	38.4

Source: U.S. Department of Health and Human Services. Public Health Service. Centers for Disease Control and Prevention. Division of STD Prevention. *Sexually Transmitted Disease Surveillance, 1995.* U.S. Department of Health and Human Services, Public Health Service, September 1996. *Notes:* The surveillance case definition for congenital syphilis changed in 1988. As of 1995, cases of congenital syphilis in persons <1 year of age per 100,000 live births are obtained using a new reporting form (CDC 73.126). 1. Includes cases reported by Washington, D.C.

★ 162 ★

Diseases and Illnesses: Sexually Transmitted Diseases

Gonorrhea Cases by Age, Gender, and Race/Ethnicity, 1995 - Part 1

This table shows reported cases of gonorrhea by age, gender, and race/ethnicity: United States, 1992-1995.

Age Group	Total			White, Non-Hispanic			Black, Non-Hispanic		
	Total	Male	Female	Total	Male	Female	Total	Male	Female
10-14	6,967	1,074	5,893	1,033	72	961	5,447	929	4,518
15-19	104,758	40,304	64,454	15,664	2,502	13,162	82,897	35,645	47,252
20-24	100,066	52,546	47,520	13,197	4,061	9,136	80,382	45,169	35,213
25-29	51,151	29,775	21,376	7,437	3,211	4,226	40,150	24,523	15,627
30-34	33,731	21,382	12,349	5,624	2,995	2,629	25,852	17,004	8,848
35-39	22,026	15,462	6,564	3,614	2,202	1,412	17,122	12,417	4,705
40-44	11,517	9,153	2,364	1,700	1,190	510	9,204	7,549	1,655
45-54	7,774	6,721	1,053	1,464	1,154	310	5,884	5,243	641
55-64	1,989	1,811	178	355	309	46	1,513	1,399	114
65+	920	754	166	158	127	31	714	599	115
TOTAL	343,010	179,873	163,137	50,520	17,920	32,600	270,867	151,227	119,640

Source: U.S. Department of Health and Human Services. Public Health Service. Centers for Disease Control and Prevention. Division of STD Prevention. *Sexually Transmitted Disease Surveillance, 1995.* U.S. Department of Health and Human Services, Public Health Service, September 1996. *Notes:* In most instances, if age or race/ethnicity was not specified, cases were prorated according to the distribution of cases for which these variables were specified. For the following years, the states/areas listed did not report race/ethnicity for most cases and were excluded: 1992 (New York City and New York state); 1993 (New York City, New York state, and Georgia); 1994 (New York City, New York state, and Georgia); and 1995 (Georgia, New Jersey, New York City, and New York state). Differences between total cases from this table and others in the report are due to different reporting forms and above listed exclusions. Cases in persons aged 0 to 9 years are not shown because some of these may not be due to sexual transmission; however, they are included in the totals.

★ 163 ★

Diseases and Illnesses: Sexually Transmitted Diseases

Gonorrhea Cases by Age, Gender, and Race/Ethnicity, 1995 - Part 2

This table shows reported cases of gonorrhea by age, gender, and race/ethnicity: United States, 1992-1995.

Age Group	Total			Hispanic			Asian/Pacific Islander			American Indian/Alaska Native		
	Total	Male	Female	Total	Male	Female	Total	Male	Female	Total	Male	Female
10-14	6,967	1,074	5,893	415	62	353	35	2	33	37	9	28
15-19	104,758	40,304	64,454	5,289	1,948	3,341	430	94	336	478	115	363
20-24	100,066	52,546	47,520	5,582	2,963	2,619	425	178	247	480	175	305
25-29	51,151	29,775	21,376	3,022	1,767	1,255	281	161	120	261	113	148
30-34	33,731	21,382	12,349	1,886	1,201	685	158	94	64	211	88	123
35-39	22,026	15,462	6,564	1,077	724	353	70	45	25	143	74	69
40-44	11,517	9,153	2,364	507	349	158	46	28	18	60	37	23
45-54	7,774	6,721	1,053	353	277	76	36	23	13	37	24	13
55-64	1,989	1,811	178	108	90	18	9	9	0	4	4	0
65+	920	754	166	31	17	14	11	7	4	6	4	2
TOTAL	343,010	179,873	163,137	18,394	9,438	8,956	1,507	643	864	1,722	645	1,077

Source: U.S. Department of Health and Human Services. Public Health Service. Centers for Disease Control and Prevention. Division of STD Prevention. *Sexually Transmitted Disease Surveillance, 1995.* U.S. Department of Health and Human Services, Public Health Service, September 1996. *Notes:* In most instances, if age or race/ethnicity was not specified, cases were prorated according to the distribution of cases for which these variables were specified. For the following years, the states/areas listed did not report race/ethnicity for most cases and were excluded: 1992 (New York City and New York state); 1993 (New York City, New York state, and Georgia); 1994 (New York City, New York state, and Georgia); and 1995 (Georgia, New Jersey, New York City, and New York state). Differences between total cases from this table and others in the report are due to different reporting forms and above listed exclusions. Cases in persons aged 0 to 9 years are not shown because some of these may not be due to sexual transmission; however, they are included in the totals.

★ 164 ★

Diseases and Illnesses: Sexually Transmitted Diseases

Gonorrhea: Reported Cases and Rates, by State/Area

This table shows reported cases and rates of gonorrhea by state/area: United States and outlying areas, 1991-1995.

State/Area	Cases					Rates per 100,000 Population				
	1991	1992	1993	1994	1995	1991	1992	1993	1994	1995
Alabama	20,878	17,601	15,793	15,881	14,683	510.9	426.1	377.7	376.3	345.2
Alaska	895	653	678	918	660	157.2	111.2	113.4	152.3	109.3
Arizona	4,867	4,187	4,176	3,603	3,844	129.9	109.2	105.9	88.3	91.1
Arkansas	7,262	7,461	7,590	6,892	5,630	306.3	311.5	313.0	280.9	226.7
California	44,883	36,971	29,970	27,593	24,803	147.6	119.6	96.0	87.9	78.5
Colorado	3,900	4,679	3,803	3,632	2,803	115.7	135.0	106.6	99.2	74.8
Connecticut	6,607	5,669	4,658	4,767	4,055	200.8	172.9	142.1	145.6	123.8
Delaware	3,065	1,787	1,586	2,038	2,201	450.6	259.1	226.9	287.9	306.9
Florida	35,400	27,933	23,899	24,367	20,874	266.3	206.7	174.2	174.6	147.4
Georgia	43,075	32,422	31,483	.	21,025	650.3	479.3	456.2	.	292.0
Hawaii	825	686	864	700	563	72.8	59.5	74.1	59.4	47.4
Idaho	173	121	171	98	149	16.7	11.3	15.5	8.6	12.8
Illinois	33,993	29,275	28,412	26,571	21,747	294.9	252.1	243.0	226.0	183.8
Indiana	11,387	9,273	8,656	9,757	8,880	203.2	164.0	151.7	169.5	153.0
Iowa	1,962	1,654	1,915	1,645	1,723	70.3	58.9	67.9	58.1	60.6
Kansas	4,638	4,404	3,771	3,673	2,797	186.2	175.1	148.9	144.0	109.0
Kentucky	5,917	4,671	4,627	5,127	4,751	159.3	124.5	122.0	133.9	123.1

[Continued]

★ 164 ★

Gonorrhea: Reported Cases and Rates, by State/Area
[Continued]

State/Area	Cases					Rates per 100,000 Population				
	1991	1992	1993	1994	1995	1991	1992	1993	1994	1995
Louisiana	14,751	14,153	13,323	11,992	9,292	347.8	331.2	310.7	277.8	214.0
Maine	164	96	80	93	94	13.3	7.8	6.5	7.5	7.6
Maryland	21,831	16,988	13,548	15,137	12,984	449.3	346.0	273.6	302.7	257.5
Massachusetts	6,013	3,587	3,118	3,159	2,658	100.2	59.8	51.8	52.3	43.8
Michigan	26,559	21,467	18,014	18,215	18,220	283.5	227.8	190.5	191.9	190.8
Minnesota	3,097	3,152	2,543	3,346	2,852	69.9	70.5	56.2	73.3	61.9
Mississippi	14,586	12,118	10,468	11,455	9,511	562.7	463.9	396.7	429.0	352.6
Missouri	17,518	14,883	13,148	12,557	11,326	339.7	286.6	251.1	237.8	212.8
Montana	122	110	81	85	65	15.1	13.4	9.6	9.9	7.5
Nebraska	1,777	1,556	714	1,335	1,133	111.7	97.0	44.2	82.2	69.2
Nevada	2,591	2,142	1,869	1,736	1,237	201.6	160.7	135.0	118.7	80.8
New Hampshire	324	145	83	103	118	29.3	13.0	7.4	9.1	10.3
New Jersey	10,576	6,817	6,444	5,269	5,783	136.2	87.3	82.0	66.7	72.8
New Mexico	1,120	921	1,014	1,130	1,054	72.4	58.2	62.7	68.3	62.5
New York	43,800	33,748	30,127	30,997	25,992	242.8	186.5	166.0	170.8	143.3
North Carolina	36,644	26,367	24,187	28,936	23,961	542.8	385.7	347.9	409.3	333.0
North Dakota	83	71	54	35	38	13.1	11.2	8.5	5.5	5.9
Ohio	35,468	27,765	22,286	24,746	23,176	324.5	252.4	201.5	222.9	207.8
Oklahoma	6,924	6,461	4,759	4,888	5,077	218.6	201.5	147.2	150.1	154.9
Oregon	2,172	1,765	1,189	978	854	74.4	59.3	39.2	31.7	27.2
Pennsylvania	24,321	20,135	18,225	13,184	13,038	203.6	167.9	151.5	109.3	108.0
Rhode Island	1,305	669	427	478	545	129.9	66.8	42.7	48.1	55.1
South Carolina	14,232	11,128	10,953	13,067	12,120	400.3	309.6	302.0	358.7	329.9
South Dakota	349	168	270	243	237	49.7	23.7	37.7	33.6	32.5
Tennessee	21,212	15,732	14,285	15,745	13,892	428.6	313.4	280.5	304.2	264.3
Texas	44,181	36,157	30,123	29,757	30,801	254.5	204.4	166.9	161.6	164.5
Utah	335	385	350	303	306	19.0	21.3	18.8	15.9	15.7
Vermont	54	26	25	40	69	9.5	4.5	4.3	6.9	11.8
Virginia	18,171	16,605	12,022	13,414	10,340	289.0	259.9	185.7	204.8	156.2
Washington	4,763	4,169	3,740	2,893	2,765	94.9	81.0	71.2	54.2	50.9
West Virginia	1,245	800	635	805	860	69.2	44.3	34.9	44.1	47.0
Wisconsin	7,113	3,657	6,875	7,776	5,524	143.7	73.2	136.3	153.0	107.8
Wyoming	87	77	85	82	51	19.0	16.6	18.1	17.2	10.6
U.S. TOTAL[1]	623,009	501,777	443,278	418,068	392,848	247.1	196.7	171.9	165.1	149.5
Northeast	93,164	70,892	63,187	58,090	52,352	182.8	138.7	123.2	113.1	101.7
Midwest	143,944	117,325	106,658	109,899	97,653	239.2	193.5	174.7	179.0	158.0
South	319,168	256,694	225,443	206,328	203,689	367.2	291.1	252.1	246.6	221.7
West	66,733	56,866	47,990	43,751	39,154	123.4	103.1	85.6	77.0	68.0
Guam	214	74	83	110	90	151.6	52.4	58.8	77.9	63.8
Puerto Rico	688	422	527	500	618	19.4	11.8	14.6	13.6	16.6
Virgin Islands	311	114	84	60	31	289.3	102.9	75.8	54.2	28.0

[Continued]

★ 164 ★

Gonorrhea: Reported Cases and Rates, by State/Area
[Continued]

State/Area	Cases					Rates per 100,000 Population				
	1991	1992	1993	1994	1995	1991	1992	1993	1994	1995
OUTLYING AREAS	1,213	610	694	670	739	32.0	15.9	17.9	17.0	18.6
TOTAL	624,222	502,387	443,972	418,738	393,587	243.9	194.1	169.7	162.8	147.6

Source: U.S. Department of Health and Human Services. Public Health Service. Centers for Disease Control and Prevention. Division of STD Prevention. *Sexually Transmitted Disease Surveillance, 1995.* U.S. Department of Health and Human Services, Public Health Service, September 1996. *Note:* 1. Includes cases reported by Washington, D.C.

★ 165 ★
Diseases and Illnesses: Sexually Transmitted Diseases

Gonorrhea: Reported Cases and Rates, by State/Area: 1995

This table shows reported cases and rates by state/area, ranked according to rates: United States and outlying areas, 1995.

State/Area	Cases	Rate per 100,000 population	Rank
Mississippi	9,511	352.6	1
Alabama	14,683	345.2	2
North Carolina	23,961	333.0	3
South Carolina	12,120	329.9	4
Delaware	2,201	306.9	5
Georgia	21,025	292.0	6
Tennessee	13,892	264.3	7
Maryland	12,984	257.5	8
Arkansas	5,630	226.7	9
Louisiana	9,292	214.0	10
Missouri	11,326	212.8	11
Ohio	23,176	207.8	12
Michigan	18,220	190.8	13
Illinois	21,747	183.8	14
Texas	30,801	164.5	15
Virginia	10,340	156.2	16
Oklahoma	5,077	154.9	17
Indiana	8,880	153.0	18
U.S. TOTAL[1]	392,848	149.5	
Florida	20,874	147.4	19
New York	25,992	143.3	20
Connecticut	4,055	123.8	21
Kentucky	4,751	123.1	22
Alaska	660	109.3	23
Kansas	2,797	109.0	24

[Continued]

★ 165 ★

Gonorrhea: Reported Cases and Rates, by State/Area: 1995

[Continued]

State/Area	Cases	Rate per 100,000 population	Rank
Pennsylvania	13,038	108.0	25
Wisconsin	5,524	107.8	26
YEAR 2000 Objective[2]		100.0	
Arizona	3,844	91.1	27
Nevada	1,237	80.8	28
California	24,803	78.5	29
Colorado	2,803	74.8	30
New Jersey	5,783	72.8	31
Nebraska	1,133	69.2	32
Guam	90	63.8	33
New Mexico	1,054	62.5	34
Minnesota	2,852	61.9	35
Iowa	1,723	60.6	36
Rhode Island	545	55.1	37
Washington	2,765	50.9	38
Hawaii	563	47.4	39
West Virginia	860	47.0	40
Massachusetts	2,658	43.8	41
South Dakota	237	32.5	42
Virgin Islands	31	28.0	43
Oregon	854	27.2	44
Puerto Rico	618	16.6	45
Utah	306	15.7	46
Idaho	149	12.8	47
Vermont	69	11.8	48
Wyoming	51	10.6	49
New Hampshire	118	10.3	50
Maine	94	7.6	51
Montana	65	7.5	52
North Dakota	38	5.9	53

Source: U.S. Department of Health and Human Services. Public Health Service. Centers for Disease Control and Prevention. Division of STD Prevention. *Sexually Transmitted Disease Surveillance, 1995.* U.S. Department of Health and Human Services, Public Health Service, September 1996. *Notes:* 1. Includes cases reported by Washington, D.C. 2. Revised from 225.0 to 100.0.

★ 166 ★

Diseases and Illnesses: Sexually Transmitted Diseases

Gonorrhea: Reported Cases and Rates in Men, by State/Area: 1991-1995

State/Area	Cases					Rates per 100,000 Population				
	1991	1992	1993	1994	1995	1991	1992	1993	1994	1995
Alabama	11,867	10,018	9,114	8,943	7,698	605.8	505.6	454.4	441.5	377.0
Alaska	475	315	314	487	342	158.5	101.9	99.8	153.9	108.1
Arizona	2,837	2,315	2,291	2,002	2,144	153.3	122.1	117.5	99.3	102.8
Arkansas	4,077	3,581	4,040	3,576	3,031	356.4	309.8	345.2	301.9	252.6
California	27,187	20,927	17,365	15,973	13,127	178.7	135.3	111.2	101.7	83.1
Colorado	2,063	2,426	1,862	1,867	1,402	123.6	141.3	105.3	102.8	75.4
Connecticut	3,682	2,828	2,323	2,328	1,980	230.8	177.8	146.1	146.5	124.5
Delaware	1,695	960	816	964	1,030	513.8	286.9	240.5	280.6	295.8
Florida	21,353	16,418	13,813	13,223	11,435	331.7	250.8	207.7	195.5	166.5
Georgia	25,612	18,836	9,197	.	11,030	797.2	573.3	274.2	.	314.9
Hawaii	498	414	508	331	273	86.6	70.9	86.1	55.6	45.6
Idaho	76	54	69	45	81	14.7	10.2	12.6	8.0	14.0
Illinois	19,533	16,258	17,253	13,371	10,720	348.8	288.0	303.6	233.9	186.3
Indiana	6,168	4,881	4,663	5,272	4,737	226.9	177.9	168.3	188.6	167.9
Iowa	907	736	888	781	773	67.1	54.1	64.9	56.9	56.0
Kansas	2,493	2,282	1,874	1,705	1,269	204.0	184.9	150.7	136.1	100.7
Kentucky	3,198	2,573	2,501	2,898	2,492	177.8	141.5	136.0	156.1	133.0
Louisiana	9,628	8,824	8,201	7,154	5,289	471.3	428.5	396.9	344.0	252.7
Maine	70	43	45	35	38	11.6	7.1	7.5	5.8	6.3
Maryland	12,649	9,826	7,823	7,493	6,661	536.7	412.5	325.5	308.7	272.0
Massachusetts	3,384	2,006	1,692	1,597	1,427	117.4	69.6	58.5	55.0	48.8
Michigan	14,281	11,176	9,027	9,896	10,103	313.8	244.0	196.3	214.4	217.4
Minnesota	1,660	1,660	1,272	1,663	1,364	76.4	75.6	57.3	74.1	60.2
Mississippi	6,859	5,481	4,920	5,452	4,284	552.6	437.8	389.0	425.7	331.1
Missouri	9,730	8,069	7,289	6,681	6,011	391.5	322.2	288.6	262.1	233.8
Montana	60	57	31	41	38	15.0	14.0	7.4	9.6	8.8
Nebraska	876	753	279	619	532	112.9	96.3	35.4	78.1	66.6
Nevada	1,666	1,376	1,217	1,106	789	254.6	202.7	172.6	148.6	101.2
New Hampshire	196	83	40	53	48	36.1	15.2	7.3	9.5	8.5
New Jersey	6,499	4,138	3,646	3,006	3,077	173.1	109.5	95.9	78.6	80.0
New Mexico	596	446	467	484	471	78.3	57.3	58.7	59.3	56.7
New York	23,636	17,713	15,076	14,527	11,993	273.1	204.0	173.0	166.7	137.7
North Carolina	20,967	14,771	13,438	15,897	12,860	641.2	445.6	398.3	463.4	368.2
North Dakota	44	38	22	22	23	13.9	12.0	6.9	6.9	7.2
Ohio	17,737	13,906	11,235	11,972	10,940	336.6	262.0	210.5	223.3	203.1
Oklahoma	3,636	3,492	2,389	2,366	2,313	235.8	223.5	151.7	149.0	144.7
Oregon	1,196	958	624	540	467	83.3	65.5	41.8	35.5	30.2
Pennsylvania	13,243	10,746	9,753	6,732	6,233	231.1	186.7	168.8	116.2	107.4
Rhode Island	750	378	233	237	271	155.5	78.6	48.6	49.6	56.9
South Carolina	9,549	7,096	6,918	8,382	7,388	554.6	407.4	393.6	474.7	414.8
South Dakota	149	66	122	127	120	43.1	18.9	34.6	35.6	33.4
Tennessee	11,392	8,521	7,843	8,965	7,695	477.7	352.1	319.3	358.9	303.2
Texas	26,644	20,054	16,234	16,087	15,793	311.6	230.1	182.5	177.3	171.1
Utah	202	205	185	176	185	23.0	22.8	20.0	18.5	19.1
Vermont	30	16	12	16	26	10.8	5.7	4.3	5.6	9.1
Virginia	10,983	9,697	6,933	7,349	5,414	356.1	309.2	218.1	228.4	166.5
Washington	2,423	2,185	1,985	1,523	1,464	97.4	85.6	76.1	57.5	54.3

[Continued]

★ 166 ★

Gonorrhea: Reported Cases and Rates in Men, by State/Area: 1991-1995
[Continued]

State/Area	Cases					Rates per 100,000 Population				
	1991	1992	1993	1994	1995	1991	1992	1993	1994	1995
West Virginia	653	385	281	376	401	75.5	44.3	32.1	42.8	45.5
Wisconsin	3,369	2,321	3,368	3,884	2,811	139.1	94.8	136.3	155.9	111.9
Wyoming	42	36	34	38	21	18.3	15.5	14.4	15.9	8.7
U.S. TOTAL[1]	355,229	277,657	235,378	222,271	203,563	288.9	223.1	187.1	179.8	158.6
Guam	132	39	43	52	41	181.7	53.7	59.2	71.6	56.4
Puerto Rico	496	302	367	362	413	28.9	17.4	20.9	20.3	22.9
Virgin Islands	207	70	48	33	17	401.2	131.6	90.2	62.0	32.0
OUTLYING AREAS	835	411	458	447	471	45.3	22.1	24.4	23.4	24.4
TOTAL	356,064	278,068	235,836	222,718	204,034	285.3	220.2	184.7	177.4	156.7

Source: U.S. Department of Health and Human Services. Public Health Service. Centers for Disease Control and Prevention. Division of STD Prevention. *Sexually Transmitted Disease Surveillance, 1995.* U.S. Department of Health and Human Services, Public Health Service, September 1996. *Note:* 1. Includes cases reported by Washington, D.C.

★ 167 ★

Diseases and Illnesses: Sexually Transmitted Diseases

Gonorrhea: Reported Cases and Rates in Women, by State/Area: 1991-1995

This table shows reported cases and rates of gonorrhea in women, by state/areas, 1991-1995.

State/Area	Cases					Rates per 100,000 Population				
	1991	1992	1993	1994	1995	1991	1992	1993	1994	1995
Alabama	9,011	7,583	6,679	6,816	6,938	423.5	352.8	307.0	310.6	313.8
Alaska	420	338	364	431	318	155.7	121.4	128.4	150.6	110.7
Arizona	2,030	1,872	1,885	1,601	1,700	107.1	96.5	94.5	77.6	79.8
Arkansas	3,185	3,880	3,550	3,316	2,592	259.5	313.1	283.0	261.3	201.9
California	17,696	16,014	12,605	11,564	11,539	116.4	103.7	80.8	73.7	73.1
Colorado	1,837	2,253	1,941	1,765	1,401	107.9	128.9	107.9	95.6	74.2
Connecticut	2,925	2,841	2,335	2,439	2,075	172.5	168.2	138.3	144.7	123.2
Delaware	1,370	827	770	1,074	1,171	391.0	233.0	214.0	294.8	317.4
Florida	14,047	11,515	10,086	11,144	9,439	204.9	165.3	142.6	154.9	129.3
Georgia	17,463	13,586	6,544	0	9,995	512.0	390.6	184.5	0	270.3
Hawaii	327	272	356	369	290	58.5	47.8	61.8	63.3	49.3
Idaho	97	67	102	53	68	18.6	12.5	18.5	9.3	11.7
Illinois	14,460	13,017	11,159	13,199	11,027	244.1	218.1	185.8	218.5	181.5
Indiana	5,219	4,392	3,993	4,485	4,143	180.9	151.0	136.0	151.6	138.9
Iowa	1,055	918	1,027	864	950	73.3	63.5	70.7	59.3	65.0
Kansas	2,145	2,122	1,897	1,968	1,528	169.0	165.7	147.1	151.6	117.1
Kentucky	2,719	2,098	2,126	2,229	2,259	141.9	108.5	108.8	113.1	113.7
Louisiana	5,123	5,329	5,122	4,838	4,003	233.0	240.7	230.5	216.3	178.0
Maine	94	53	35	58	56	14.8	8.4	5.5	9.1	8.8
Maryland	9,182	7,162	5,725	7,644	6,323	366.9	283.4	224.6	297.1	243.8

[Continued]

★ 167 ★

Gonorrhea: Reported Cases and Rates in Women, by State/Area: 1991-1995
[Continued]

State/Area	Cases					Rates per 100,000 Population				
	1991	1992	1993	1994	1995	1991	1992	1993	1994	1995
Massachusetts	2,629	1,581	1,426	1,562	1,231	84.3	50.7	45.6	49.8	39.1
Michigan	12,278	10,291	8,987	8,319	8,117	254.9	212.5	184.9	170.6	165.6
Minnesota	1,437	1,492	1,271	1,683	1,488	63.7	65.5	55.2	72.4	63.5
Mississippi	7,727	6,637	5,548	6,003	5,218	572.1	487.9	403.8	431.9	371.8
Missouri	7,788	6,814	5,859	5,876	5,315	291.5	253.5	216.2	215.2	193.1
Montana	62	53	50	44	27	15.2	12.8	11.8	10.2	6.2
Nebraska	901	803	434	700	600	110.5	97.8	52.5	84.2	71.6
Nevada	925	766	652	630	448	146.6	117.1	95.9	87.8	59.7
New Hampshire	128	62	43	50	70	22.7	10.9	7.5	8.6	12.0
New Jersey	4,077	2,679	2,798	2,263	2,706	101.6	66.4	68.9	55.5	66.0
New Mexico	524	475	547	646	583	66.7	59.2	66.7	76.9	68.2
New York	20,164	16,035	15,051	16,470	13,999	214.9	170.4	159.4	174.5	148.5
North Carolina	15,677	11,596	10,749	13,039	11,101	450.3	329.2	300.4	358.3	299.8
North Dakota	39	33	32	13	15	12.3	10.4	10.0	4.1	4.7
Ohio	17,731	13,859	11,051	12,774	11,978	313.2	243.4	193.1	222.4	207.8
Oklahoma	3,288	2,947	2,356	2,512	2,764	202.2	179.2	142.2	150.5	164.6
Oregon	976	807	565	438	387	65.8	53.4	36.7	27.9	24.3
Pennsylvania	11,078	9,389	8,472	6,452	6,805	178.2	150.6	135.5	103.0	108.6
Rhode Island	555	291	194	241	274	106.3	55.9	37.4	46.7	53.3
South Carolina	4,683	3,955	3,935	4,486	4,597	255.4	213.5	210.5	239.0	242.9
South Dakota	200	102	148	116	117	56.1	28.3	40.7	31.6	31.6
Tennessee	9,820	7,211	6,442	6,780	6,197	382.9	277.4	244.3	253.1	228.0
Texas	17,537	16,103	13,889	13,670	15,008	199.1	179.5	151.7	146.4	158.1
Utah	133	180	165	127	121	15.0	19.8	17.6	13.2	12.3
Vermont	24	10	13	24	43	8.3	3.4	4.4	8.1	14.4
Virginia	7,188	6,908	5,089	6,025	4,886	224.5	212.4	154.4	180.7	145.1
Washington	2,340	1,984	1,755	1,370	1,301	92.5	76.5	66.3	50.9	47.6
West Virginia	592	415	354	429	459	63.4	44.3	37.5	45.4	48.5
Wisconsin	2,471	1,336	3,507	3,892	2,713	97.8	52.4	136.3	150.2	103.9
Wyoming	45	41	51	44	30	19.7	17.7	21.8	18.5	12.5
U.S. TOTAL[1]	266,507	223,973	192,043	195,353	188,650	206.3	171.5	145.5	150.7	140.3
Guam	82	35	40	58	49	119.7	51.1	58.4	84.7	71.6
Puerto Rico	192	120	160	138	205	10.5	6.5	8.6	7.3	10.7
Virgin Islands	104	44	36	27	14	186.0	76.4	62.5	46.9	24.3
OUTLYING AREAS	378	199	236	223	268	19.3	10.1	11.8	11.0	13.1
TOTAL	266,885	224,172	192,279	195,576	188,918	203.5	169.1	143.5	148.5	138.4

Source: U.S. Department of Health and Human Services. Public Health Service. Centers for Disease Control and Prevention. Division of STD Prevention. *Sexually Transmitted Disease Surveillance, 1995.* U.S. Department of Health and Human Services, Public Health Service, September 1996. *Note:* 1. Includes cases reported by Washington, D.C.

★ 168 ★

Diseases and Illnesses: Sexually Transmitted Diseases

Gonorrhea: Reported Rates, by Age, Gender, and Ethnicity - Part 1

This table shows reported rates of gonorrhea per 100,000 population by age, gender, and race/ethnicity: United States, 1995. Part 1 shows total rates and rates for whites and blacks.

Age Group	Total			White, Non-Hispanic			Black, Non-Hispanic		
	Total	Male	Female	Total	Male	Female	Total	Male	Female
10-14	42.0	12.6	72.8	9.0	1.2	17.2	238.6	80.5	400.4
15-19	664.6	498.4	839.7	142.7	44.5	245.8	3,843.2	3,267.3	4,432.6
20-24	645.9	666.4	624.6	121.1	73.7	169.7	4,238.9	4,880.0	3,627.6
25-29	311.0	360.6	261.0	62.5	53.8	71.3	2,144.5	2,764.3	1,586.4
30-34	177.5	225.4	129.7	39.6	42.1	37.1	1,221.2	1,719.0	784.6
35-39	113.7	160.2	67.6	24.4	29.5	19.1	828.8	1,289.1	426.7
40-44	65.7	105.4	26.7	12.3	17.2	7.4	545.0	961.0	183.2
45-54	28.9	51.0	7.7	6.8	10.8	2.8	239.7	466.7	48.1
55-64	10.9	20.8	1.9	2.4	4.3	0.6	96.2	201.2	13.0
65+	3.1	6.3	1.0	0.6	1.2	0.2	32.7	69.4	8.7
TOTAL	149.9	160.8	139.6	29.1	21.1	36.8	1,086.9	1,279.5	913.1

Source: U.S. Department of Health and Human Services. Public Health Service. Centers for Disease Control and Prevention. Division of STD Prevention. *Sexually Transmitted Disease Surveillance, 1995.* U.S. Department of Health and Human Services, Public Health Service, September 1996. *Notes:* For 1995, the states/areas listed did not report race/ethnicity for most cases: (Georgia, New Jersey, New York City and New York state). Cases and population denominators have been excluded for these states/areas. Rates for the 0 to 9 year age group are not shown; however, these cases are included in the calculation of total rates.

★ 169 ★

Diseases and Illnesses: Sexually Transmitted Diseases

Gonorrhea: Reported Rates by Age, Gender, and Ethnicity - Part 2

This table shows reported rates of gonorrhea per 100,000 population by age, gender, and race/ethnicity: United States, 1995. Part 2 shows total rates and rates for Asians/Pacific Islanders and American Indians/Alaska Natives.

Age Group	Total			Hispanic			Asian/Pacific Islander			American Indian/Alaska Native		
	Total	Male	Female	Total	Male	Female	Total	Male	Female	Total	Male	Female
10-14	42.0	12.6	72.8	21.3	6.2	37.1	5.3	0.6	10.1	16.4	7.9	25.1
15-19	664.6	498.4	839.7	21.3	6.2	37.1	5.3	0.6	10.1	16.4	7.9	25.1
20-24	645.9	666.4	624.6	296.2	285.4	309.5	66.1	55.5	76.6	272.7	194.4	354.5
25-29	311.0	360.6	261.0	167.4	182.0	150.5	40.0	47.4	33.1	152.0	127.6	178.0
30-34	177.5	225.4	129.7	106.1	128.6	81.2	21.5	26.6	16.8	119.3	99.5	139.1
35-39	113.7	160.2	67.6	67.7	88.5	45.7	10.0	13.6	6.8	85.0	89.2	80.9
40-44	65.7	105.4	26.7	40.5	55.4	25.4	7.3	9.7	5.3	40.6	51.7	30.2
45-54	28.9	51.0	7.7	19.9	31.9	8.4	4.1	5.7	2.7	17.8	23.9	12.1
55-64	10.9	20.8	1.9	10.7	18.8	3.4	1.7	3.8	0.0	3.2	6.9	0.0
65+	3.1	6.3	1.0	2.9	3.7	2.3	2.0	3.0	1.3	4.5	7.1	2.6
TOTAL	149.9	160.8	139.6	90.6	90.9	90.3	18.9	16.7	20.9	80.4	60.8	99.5

Source: U.S. Department of Health and Human Services. Public Health Service. Centers for Disease Control and Prevention. Division of STD Prevention. *Sexually Transmitted Disease Surveillance, 1995.* U.S. Department of Health and Human Services, Public Health Service, September 1996. *Notes:* For the year 1995, the states/areas listed did not report race/ethnicity for most cases (Georgia, New Jersey, New York City and New York state). Cases and population denominators have been excluded for these states/areas. Rates for persons in the 0 to 9 year age group are not shown; however, these cases are included in the calculation of total rates.

★ 170 ★

Diseases and Illnesses: Sexually Transmitted Diseases

Gonorrhea: Resistance to Treatment

This table shows results, by selected city, of the Gonococcal Isolate Surveillance Project (GISP): resistance of Neisseria gonorrhoeae to penicillin and tetracycline, 1992-1995.

City	1994					1995				
	Total Isolates	Penicillin Resistance No.	%	Tetracycline Resistance No.	%	Total Isolates	Penicillin Resistance No.	%	Tetracycline Resistance No.	%
Albuquerque, NM	158	19	12.0	34	21.5	167	5	3.0	25	15.0
Anchorage, AK	171	1	0.6	3	1.8	123	5	4.1	7	5.7
Atlanta, GA	229	46	20.1	86	37.6	227	51	22.5	124	54.6
Baltimore, MD	240	41	17.1	63	26.3	240	50	20.8	76	31.7
Birmingham, AL	240	37	15.4	111	46.3	239	53	22.2	60	25.1
Boston, MA	NR	NR	NR	NR	NR	NR	NR	NR	NR	NR
Cincinnati, OH	218	39	17.9	136	62.4	173	23	13.3	98	56.6
Cleveland, OH	240	42	17.5	64	26.7	227	34	15.0	88	38.8
Denver, CO	240	32	13.3	33	13.8	240	14	5.8	21	8.8
Fort Lewis, WA	78	9	11.5	14	17.9	68	12	17.6	6	8.8
Honolulu, HI	74	23	31.1	22	29.7	61	18	29.5	14	23.0
Kansas City, MO	240	24	10.0	13	5.4	240	8	3.3	9	3.8
Long Beach, CA	214	44	20.6	34	15.9	217	44	20.3	46	21.2
Minneapolis, MN	240	22	9.2	25	10.4	240	14	5.8	13	5.4
Nassau County, NY	161	61	37.9	56	34.8	180	54	30.0	30	16.7
New Orleans, LA	210	37	17.6	79	37.6	190	25	13.2	142	74.7
Orange County, CA	201	51	25.4	18	9.0	144	24	16.7	36	25.0
Philadelphia, PA	228	58	25.4	67	29.4	232	52	22.4	32	13.8
Phoenix, AZ	228	18	7.9	18	7.9	240	16	6.7	24	10.0
Portland, OR	240	20	8.3	17	7.1	240	5	2.1	15	6.3
San Diego, CA	240	32	13.3	31	12.9	240	20	8.3	24	10.0
Seattle, WA	206	14	6.8	25	12.1	230	21	9.1	52	22.6
San Francisco, CA	240	26	10.8	36	15.0	240	13	5.4	45	18.8
St Louis, MO	NR	NR	NR	NR	NR	93	16	17.2	29	31.2
San Antonio, TX	221	32	14.5	55	24.9	154	17	11.0	84	54.5
West Palm Beach, FL	239	68	28.5	86	36.0	229	105	45.9	135	59.0
TOTAL	4,996	796	15.9	1,126	22.5	4,874	699	14.3	1,235	25.3

Source: U.S. Department of Health and Human Services. Public Health Service. Centers for Disease Control and Prevention. Division of STD Prevention. *Sexually Transmitted Disease Surveillance, 1995.* U.S. Department of Health and Human Services, Public Health Service, September 1996. *Notes:* NR indicates "no report available." Resistance categories include both plasmid-mediated and chromosomally mediated resistance. Penicillin and tetracycline resistance categories are not mutually exclusive; many isolates are resistant to both antibiotics.

★ 171 ★

Diseases and Illnesses: Sexually Transmitted Diseases

Gonorrhea: Urban Distribution

This table shows reported cases and rates for gonorrhea in selected cities of 200,000+ population: United States and outlying areas, 1991-1995.

State/Area	Cases					Rates per 100,000 Population				
	1991	1992	1993	1994	1995	1991	1992	1993	1994	1995
Akron, OH	1,912	1,488	1,410	1,285	1,043	368.2	285.0	268.5	243.5	196.7
Albuquerque, NM	505	455	560	759	625	103.2	91.2	110.5	147.1	119.7
Atlanta, GA	15,014	10,591	5,002	0	7,330	2,289.8	1,593.7	739.0	0	1,046.1
Austin, TX	1,666	1,312	1,271	1,349	1,600	280.0	214.0	201.4	208.5	240.7
Baltimore, MD	13,007	11,406	8,591	9,099	6,928	1,776.0	1,573.0	1,201.5	1,294.8	1,002.4
Birmingham, AL	8,242	6,101	5,433	5,309	4,321	1,259.3	929.9	827.8	808.1	656.9
Boston, MA	2,867	1,453	1,205	1,199	917	509.5	262.3	217.9	217.9	165.0
Buffalo, NY	2,989	2,519	1,945	1,768	1,691	908.4	764.7	591.2	539.4	518.5
Charlotte, NC	5,375	3,459	2,669	4,137	2,146	1,018.7	645.4	486.4	734.1	370.3
Chicago, IL	21,605	18,454	19,123	16,868	12,586	735.8	626.0	647.9	571.7	426.9
Cincinnati, OH	8,253	5,143	4,355	2,822	2,590	949.5	590.6	499.8	325.1	299.8
Cleveland, OH	8,362	7,349	5,226	6,580	5,746	592.6	521.1	371.1	469.1	411.0
Columbus, OH	5,394	4,070	3,119	4,009	2,887	551.7	411.3	312.1	398.7	285.6
Corpus Christi, TX	516	426	362	344	373	174.0	141.6	118.3	110.6	119.3
Dallas, TX	11,247	7,771	6,820	6,170	8,027	594.6	406.6	353.7	317.5	409.7
Dayton, OH	2,786	2,072	1,518	1,925	1,603	484.1	359.2	263.4	336.2	281.0
Denver, CO	1,839	2,378	2,031	1,735	1,375	388.4	489.8	411.3	351.9	278.1
Des Moines, IA	597	392	482	431	362	179.5	116.0	140.7	124.6	103.6
Detroit, MI	12,647	10,924	9,275	8,637	8,553	1,175.9	1,019.9	871.3	817.4	812.7
El Paso, TX	317	348	279	171	159	51.7	55.4	43.1	25.6	23.4
Fort Worth, TX	2,515	3,337	2,722	2,752	2,442	208.9	273.5	220.4	218.6	191.0
Honolulu, HI	794	657	834	675	543	93.5	76.3	96.2	77.2	61.9
Houston, TX	12,690	10,050	7,732	7,429	6,984	437.3	339.1	257.3	244.0	227.0
Indianapolis, IN	5,952	4,644	4,254	5,430	4,709	738.4	572.3	522.4	664.5	576.0
Jacksonville, FL	4,320	3,096	3,501	3,555	2,476	626.6	442.2	499.7	508.0	352.9
Jersey City, NJ	799	475	324	298	223	366.0	217.4	148.5	136.8	102.6
Kansas City, MO	4,195	4,150	3,160	2,997	3,186	959.3	949.5	722.8	684.6	726.4
Los Angeles, CA	14,699	13,928	11,015	8,774	8,238	175.3	164.0	128.8	102.6	96.3
Louisville, KY	3,166	2,564	2,420	2,637	2,441	474.6	382.8	360.7	392.5	362.7
Memphis, TN	10,974	7,904	6,997	6,973	6,108	1,313.9	938.2	825.3	813.7	706.1
Miami, FL	4,975	3,813	3,204	2,857	2,338	251.6	190.1	160.2	141.3	115.1
Milwaukee, WI	5,517	2,638	3,487	6,284	4,160	576.6	276.9	368.3	670.0	446.7
Minneapolis, MN	1,820	1,840	1,481	1,933	1,689	481.7	485.8	389.1	505.6	440.5
Nashville, TN	2,932	2,348	2,388	3,110	2,622	572.2	454.1	457.5	589.7	494.0
New Orleans, LA	5,368	5,112	5,003	4,056	3,353	1,093.2	1,044.5	1,026.9	836.5	695.8
New York City, NY	29,209	21,813	19,240	19,491	16,499	399.7	298.5	262.6	266.2	225.6
Newark, NJ	2,234	1,451	1,354	1,464	2,222	762.4	495.8	463.7	505.1	772.8
Norfolk, VA	3,391	3,085	2,503	2,519	1,679	1,339.8	1,216.1	998.8	1,038.1	706.7
Oakland, CA	3,034	3,143	1,177	1,185	2,220	256.7	262.8	97.9	98.3	183.5
Oklahoma City, OK	2,212	2,147	1,859	1,763	2,028	523.8	502.6	430.7	404.3	464.0
Omaha, NE	1,045	1,348	566	1,060	880	247.7	316.6	132.2	246.3	202.7
Philadelphia, PA	15,429	12,205	10,580	8,026	6,565	985.0	787.2	688.1	527.6	438.0
Phoenix, AZ	3,689	3,255	3,218	2,797	3,149	170.2	147.1	141.9	119.1	129.5
Pittsburgh, PA	4,396	4,171	3,730	2,602	1,598	329.4	312.6	280.6	197.0	122.0
Portland, OR	1,338	1,127	750	706	543	284.8	237.4	156.1	146.5	112.1

[Continued]

★ 171 ★

Gonorrhea: Urban Distribution
[Continued]

State/Area	Cases					Rates per 100,000 Population				
	1991	1992	1993	1994	1995	1991	1992	1993	1994	1995
Richmond, VA	2,575	3,667	2,029	2,621	2,371	1,280.6	1,831.5	1,016.5	1,322.9	1,195.8
Rochester, NY	3,943	3,445	2,575	2,876	2,210	1,632.3	1,415.0	1,053.7	1,180.1	909.5
Sacramento, CA	1,678	1,171	1,435	1,570	1,684	155.4	107.2	130.8	143.2	152.6
San Antonio, TX	1,902	1,774	1,759	1,738	1,914	157.5	143.9	139.9	136.2	147.6
San Diego, CA	4,297	2,317	3,264	2,837	1,775	168.1	89.1	125.0	107.8	67.1
San Francisco, CA	3,261	2,768	2,224	1,959	1,853	448.9	379.4	303.5	267.9	253.6
San Jose, CA	1,015	887	763	735	475	67.2	58.1	49.4	47.4	30.3
Seattle, WA	2,433	2,026	1,562	1,213	1,295	158.5	129.9	99.0	76.6	81.2
St. Louis, MO	8,189	6,136	5,726	5,228	4,425	2,091.7	1,594.7	1,521.7	1,422.0	1,233.6
St. Paul, MN	606	615	493	656	560	219.0	221.9	178.4	238.3	203.8
St. Petersburg, FL	2,195	1,777	1,280	1,787	1,545	254.7	206.0	148.1	206.2	177.4
Tampa, FL	2,952	2,537	2,395	2,181	1,833	349.2	296.5	276.7	249.6	207.2
Toledo, OH	1,782	1,511	1,556	2,262	944	386.3	327.8	339.0	494.4	207.5
Tucson, AZ	522	438	529	439	359	77.2	63.3	74.5	60.0	47.7
Tulsa, OK	1,703	1,886	1,359	1,444	1,452	461.6	505.0	361.5	382.8	384.0
Washington, DC	9,794	8,310	6,162	6,827	5,687	1,648.0	1,418.6	1,065.9	1,204.0	1,026.1
Wichita, KS	1,460	1,388	1,279	1,078	713	356.8	334.0	305.6	257.2	170.0
Yonkers, NY	199	168	107	131	121	105.5	88.6	56.2	68.6	63.2
U.S. CITY TOTAL	322,339	261,233	220,672	213,552	190,973	478.4	384.5	322.9	314.4	277.2
San Juan, PR	363	197	292	256	349	41.6	22.6	33.5	29.4	40.0
TOTAL	322,702	261,430	220,964	213,808	191,322	472.8	379.9	319.3	310.8	274.3

Source: U.S. Department of Health and Human Services. Public Health Service. Centers for Disease Control and Prevention. Division of STD Prevention. *Sexually Transmitted Disease Surveillance, 1995.* U.S. Department of Health and Human Services, Public Health Service, September 1996.

★ 172 ★

Diseases and Illnesses: Sexually Transmitted Diseases

Gonorrhea: Urban Distribution - Men

This table shows reported cases and rates for gonorrhea in men in selected cities of 200,000+ population: United States and outlying areas, 1991-1995.

State/Area	Cases					Rates per 100,000 Population				
	1991	1992	1993	1994	1995	1991	1992	1993	1994	1995
Akron, OH	971	742	671	524	440	390.2	296.5	266.5	207.0	172.9
Albuquerque, NM	264	211	253	341	301	110.5	86.5	102.2	135.3	117.8
Atlanta, GA	8,607	5,814	2,808	0	3,904	2,751.5	1,832.2	868.5	0	1,165.9
Austin, TX	913	691	672	644	785	306.7	225.3	212.9	199.3	236.4
Baltimore, MD	7,334	6,616	5,015	4,507	3,863	2,144.6	1,952.8	1,501.2	1,372.7	1,195.9
Birmingham, AL	4,913	3,519	3,046	2,801	2,146	1,606.7	1,147.4	992.7	911.6	697.1
Boston, MA	1,659	858	710	614	485	613.4	322.0	267.0	232.1	181.4
Buffalo, NY	1,572	1,310	955	739	707	1,002.8	834.3	608.9	472.8	454.3
Charlotte, NC	3,350	2,201	1,495	2,559	1,323	1,321.1	854.0	566.7	944.4	474.6

[Continued]

★ 172 ★

Gonorrhea: Urban Distribution - Men
[Continued]

State/Area	Cases					Rates per 100,000 Population				
	1991	1992	1993	1994	1995	1991	1992	1993	1994	1995
Chicago, IL	12,614	10,622	12,382	8,438	6,079	893.0	748.8	871.8	594.3	428.3
Cincinnati, OH	4,099	2,628	2,355	1,569	1,308	996.1	637.2	570.6	381.6	319.5
Cleveland, OH	4,440	3,939	2,819	3,257	2,855	669.5	594.0	425.7	493.7	434.0
Columbus, OH	2,483	2,009	1,608	1,924	1,371	526.4	420.7	333.4	396.4	280.9
Corpus Christi, TX	360	275	256	205	181	247.9	186.6	170.9	134.5	118.1
Dallas, TX	7,427	4,823	3,800	3,539	4,269	797.7	512.6	400.4	370.0	442.5
Dayton, OH	1,404	1,012	718	842	726	509.1	365.9	259.8	306.7	265.3
Denver, CO	1,003	1,300	1,022	908	729	435.3	549.9	425.0	378.1	303.3
Des Moines, IA	306	180	248	221	181	193.0	111.6	151.7	133.9	108.4
Detroit, MI	6,701	5,725	4,806	5,347	5,473	1,313.8	1,126.7	951.7	1,066.6	1,095.8
El Paso, TX	195	162	141	78	87	65.6	53.1	44.8	24.1	26.4
Fort Worth, TX	1,598	1,514	1,015	1,381	1,203	268.3	250.7	166.1	221.9	190.3
Honolulu, HI	479	393	487	322	259	111.1	90.0	110.9	72.9	58.5
Houston, TX	7,616	5,975	4,929	4,616	4,008	528.0	405.5	329.9	304.9	262.0
Indianapolis, IN	2,968	2,518	2,182	2,865	2,523	775.0	652.7	563.5	737.2	648.7
Jacksonville, FL	2,695	1,789	2,069	2,156	1,451	799.8	522.5	603.9	630.1	423.1
Jersey City, NJ	513	303	213	190	123	484.5	285.7	201.1	179.8	116.6
Kansas City, MO	2,050	2,067	1,612	1,532	1,630	984.8	993.0	774.3	734.7	779.9
Los Angeles, CA	9,147	8,218	6,006	5,003	4,680	218.7	194.1	140.9	117.4	109.8
Louisville, KY	1,701	1,424	1,349	1,580	1,402	539.8	449.8	425.4	497.3	440.4
Memphis, TN	5,635	4,325	3,808	4,069	3,397	1,417.3	1,078.3	943.6	997.7	825.3
Miami, FL	3,961	3,050	2,499	1,920	1,571	417.7	317.0	260.3	198.0	161.2
Milwaukee, WI	2,727	1,849	1,765	3,018	2,206	600.9	408.9	392.9	678.1	499.0
Minneapolis, MN	1,053	1,070	811	1,056	871	575.4	582.9	439.6	569.7	468.2
Nashville, TN	1,777	1,287	1,430	1,888	1,587	730.0	523.7	576.4	753.1	628.8
New Orleans, LA	4,261	3,917	3,593	2,794	2,265	1,867.0	1,721.0	1,586.0	1,239.0	1,010.2
New York City, NY	15,879	11,537	9,560	9,108	7,707	462.7	336.1	277.7	264.8	224.3
Newark, NJ	1,603	1,063	881	1,006	1,228	1,157.2	768.0	638.1	734.0	903.2
Norfolk, VA	2,396	1,990	1,507	1,501	945	1,776.7	1,471.4	1,128.2	1,161.6	748.4
Oakland, CA	1,710	1,454	565	640	891	294.3	247.4	95.6	108.1	150.2
Oklahoma City, OK	1,154	1,065	846	814	913	568.5	518.4	407.4	388.0	433.9
Omaha, NE	534	649	280	492	417	262.7	316.2	135.6	237.0	199.0
Philadelphia, PA	8,561	6,710	5,994	4,217	3,235	1,174.3	929.5	837.4	595.5	463.4
Phoenix, AZ	2,167	1,857	1,815	1,626	1,824	202.9	170.2	162.3	140.4	152.0
Pittsburgh, PA	2,404	2,180	1,882	1,267	723	383.9	348.0	301.4	204.2	117.4
Portland, OR	758	618	399	395	300	331.7	267.5	170.7	168.3	127.1
Richmond, VA	1,396	1,976	1,180	1,600	1,301	1,520.4	2,159.5	1,293.7	1,766.7	1,435.0
Rochester, NY	2,027	1,774	1,251	1,311	991	1,747.1	1,516.5	1,065.4	1,119.2	848.2
Sacramento, CA	887	564	426	594	769	167.8	105.5	79.4	110.8	142.6
San Antonio, TX	1,096	892	876	872	916	187.2	149.2	143.6	140.9	145.5
San Diego, CA	2,552	1,331	3,051	1,824	0	196.6	100.6	229.7	136.3	0
San Francisco, CA	2,278	1,854	1,557	1,254	1,255	626.6	508.2	425.4	343.8	344.8
San Jose, CA	518	422	363	384	215	67.6	54.5	46.4	48.9	27.1
Seattle, WA	1,294	1,105	889	672	762	171.0	143.8	114.4	86.1	96.9
St. Louis, MO	4,858	3,655	3,473	3,022	2,528	2,723.0	2,083.1	2,023.5	1,801.7	1,544.0
St. Paul, MN	328	295	229	302	262	248.1	222.6	173.3	229.4	199.2

[Continued]

★ 172 ★

Gonorrhea: Urban Distribution - Men
[Continued]

State/Area	Cases					Rates per 100,000 Population				
	1991	1992	1993	1994	1995	1991	1992	1993	1994	1995
St. Petersburg, FL	1,252	1,052	695	912	839	311.0	260.9	172.1	225.0	205.8
Tampa, FL	1,629	1,432	1,347	1,195	1,003	395.4	343.2	319.2	280.6	232.7
Toledo, OH	1,070	767	772	1,191	478	485.9	348.4	352.2	544.7	219.7
Tucson, AZ	300	200	260	210	165	90.6	59.1	74.8	58.6	44.7
Tulsa, OK	962	1,118	764	776	737	541.1	621.0	421.5	426.5	404.0
Washington, DC	6,709	5,313	3,853	4,009	3,449	2,419.5	1,942.3	1,427.1	1,513.9	1,331.9
Wichita, KS	763	726	652	523	319	380.6	356.4	317.9	254.4	155.0
Yonkers, NY	133	104	61	62	59	148.6	115.4	67.4	68.3	64.8
U.S. CITY TOTAL	186,014	148,039	124,976	115,226	100,620	569.5	449.2	377.0	349.7	301.1
San Juan, PR	268	156	215	204	247	68.3	39.8	54.8	52.0	62.9
TOTAL	186,282	148,195	125,191	115,430	100,867	563.6	444.4	373.3	346.2	298.3

Source: U.S. Department of Health and Human Services. Public Health Service. Centers for Disease Control and Prevention. Division of STD Prevention. *Sexually Transmitted Disease Surveillance, 1995.* U.S. Department of Health and Human Services, Public Health Service, September 1996.

★ 173 ★

Diseases and Illnesses: Sexually Transmitted Diseases

Gonorrhea: Urban Distribution - Women

This table shows reported cases and rates for gonorrhea, in women, in selected cities of 200,000+ population: United States and outlying areas, 1991-1995.

State/Area	Cases					Rates per 100,000 Population				
	1991	1992	1993	1994	1995	1991	1992	1993	1994	1995
Akron, OH	941	746	739	761	600	347.8	274.5	270.3	277.1	217.6
Albuquerque, NM	241	244	307	418	324	96.2	95.6	118.5	158.5	121.4
Atlanta, GA	6,407	4,777	2,194	0	3,426	1,868.6	1,375.7	620.6	0	936.4
Austin, TX	753	621	599	705	815	253.2	202.6	189.8	217.6	244.9
Baltimore, MD	5,673	4,790	3,576	4,592	3,065	1,453.1	1,239.9	938.7	1,226.4	832.6
Birmingham, AL	3,329	2,582	2,387	2,423	2,145	954.7	739.1	683.1	692.9	612.9
Boston, MA	1,208	595	495	585	432	413.4	206.9	172.4	204.8	149.7
Buffalo, NY	1,417	1,209	990	1,029	984	822.6	701.3	575.1	600.2	577.1
Charlotte, NC	2,025	1,258	1,174	1,578	823	738.9	452.1	412.1	539.4	273.7
Chicago, IL	8,991	7,832	6,741	8,430	6,507	590.0	512.1	440.2	550.7	425.5
Cincinnati, OH	4,154	2,515	2,000	1,253	1,268	907.5	548.7	436.1	274.3	279.0
Cleveland, OH	3,922	3,410	2,407	3,323	2,856	524.3	456.4	322.7	447.3	385.8
Columbus, OH	2,911	2,061	1,511	2,085	1,498	575.4	402.6	292.2	400.8	286.5
Corpus Christi, TX	156	151	106	139	192	103.1	98.3	67.9	87.6	120.4
Dallas, TX	3,820	2,948	3,020	2,631	3,758	397.7	303.9	308.5	266.7	377.9
Dayton, OH	1,382	1,060	800	1,083	876	461.2	353.0	266.7	363.5	295.2
Denver, CO	836	1,078	1,009	827	646	344.0	432.8	398.3	327.0	254.3
Des Moines, IA	291	212	234	210	181	167.3	120.0	130.6	116.2	99.1
Detroit, MI	5,946	5,199	4,469	3,290	3,080	1,051.4	923.6	798.8	592.4	557.0

[Continued]

★ 173 ★

Gonorrhea: Urban Distribution - Women
[Continued]

State/Area	Cases					Rates per 100,000 Population				
	1991	1992	1993	1994	1995	1991	1992	1993	1994	1995
El Paso, TX	122	186	138	93	72	38.5	57.5	41.5	27.1	20.7
Fort Worth, TX	917	1,823	1,707	1,371	1,239	150.8	295.9	273.6	215.4	191.7
Honolulu, HI	315	264	347	353	284	75.3	62.2	81.1	81.6	65.3
Houston, TX	5,074	4,075	2,803	2,813	2,976	347.6	273.5	185.5	183.7	192.4
Indianapolis, IN	2,984	2,126	2,072	2,565	2,186	705.3	499.4	485.0	598.5	509.9
Jacksonville, FL	1,625	1,307	1,432	1,399	1,025	461.0	365.3	400.0	391.2	285.7
Jersey City, NJ	286	172	111	108	100	254.4	152.9	98.8	96.4	89.4
Kansas City, MO	2,145	2,083	1,548	1,465	1,556	936.1	909.9	676.1	639.1	677.7
Los Angeles, CA	5,552	5,680	5,009	3,771	3,558	132.1	133.5	116.8	87.9	82.9
Louisville, KY	1,465	1,140	1,071	1,057	1,039	416.2	322.8	302.8	298.5	293.1
Memphis, TN	5,339	3,579	3,189	2,904	2,711	1,220.0	810.9	717.9	646.6	597.9
Miami, FL	1,014	763	705	937	767	98.5	73.1	67.7	89.0	72.6
Milwaukee, WI	1,727	789	1,722	3,266	1,954	343.4	157.6	346.1	662.8	399.5
Minneapolis, MN	767	770	670	877	808	393.7	394.4	341.6	445.2	409.2
Nashville, TN	1,155	1,061	958	1,222	1,035	429.3	391.1	349.8	441.6	371.8
New Orleans, LA	1,107	1,195	1,410	1,262	1,088	421.2	456.4	541.0	486.6	422.2
New York City, NY	13,330	10,276	9,680	10,383	8,792	344.0	265.3	249.2	267.5	226.9
Newark, NJ	631	388	473	458	994	408.4	251.5	307.3	299.7	655.9
Norfolk, VA	995	1,095	996	1,004	722	841.6	924.5	851.2	885.2	648.7
Oakland, CA	1,324	1,689	612	494	1,328	220.4	277.8	100.0	80.5	215.5
Oklahoma City, OK	1,058	1,074	1,005	946	1,115	482.3	484.4	448.7	418.1	491.9
Omaha, NE	511	699	285	553	462	233.7	316.9	128.5	248.2	205.7
Philadelphia, PA	6,868	5,495	4,586	3,809	3,330	820.2	663.2	558.1	468.5	415.8
Phoenix, AZ	1,522	1,398	1,403	1,171	1,325	138.5	124.7	122.0	98.4	107.5
Pittsburgh, PA	1,992	1,991	1,848	1,335	875	281.2	281.3	262.1	190.7	126.1
Portland, OR	580	509	351	311	243	240.3	208.8	142.4	125.8	97.8
Richmond, VA	1,179	1,691	848	1,015	1,067	1,079.0	1,555.5	782.4	943.7	991.5
Rochester, NY	1,916	1,671	1,324	1,565	1,219	1,526.3	1,321.1	1,042.9	1,236.4	966.3
Sacramento, CA	791	607	1,009	975	906	143.4	108.8	180.0	173.9	160.6
San Antonio, TX	806	882	883	866	998	129.5	138.9	136.3	131.9	149.6
San Diego, CA	1,745	986	213	291	0	138.7	77.1	16.6	22.5	0
San Francisco, CA	983	914	667	705	598	270.9	250.6	181.9	192.4	163.1
San Jose, CA	497	465	400	351	260	66.7	61.7	52.5	45.8	33.6
Seattle, WA	1,139	921	673	541	533	146.3	116.5	84.1	67.3	65.9
St. Louis, MO	3,331	2,481	2,253	2,206	1,897	1,563.1	1,185.3	1,100.8	1,103.4	972.9
St. Paul, MN	278	320	264	354	298	192.4	221.2	183.1	246.5	207.9
St. Petersburg, FL	943	725	585	875	706	205.3	157.7	127.1	189.7	152.4
Tampa, FL	1,323	1,105	1,048	986	830	305.3	252.0	236.3	220.2	183.0
Toledo, OH	712	744	784	1,071	466	295.3	309.0	327.1	448.3	196.2
Tucson, AZ	222	238	269	229	194	64.3	67.4	74.2	61.3	50.6
Tulsa, OK	741	761	593	668	715	387.6	393.4	304.6	342.0	365.4
Washington, DC	3,085	2,979	2,309	2,818	2,237	973.2	954.0	749.3	932.5	757.5
Wichita, KS	697	662	627	555	394	333.9	312.4	293.8	259.8	184.5
Yonkers, NY	66	64	46	69	62	66.7	64.3	46.0	68.9	61.7
U.S. CITY TOTAL	135,262	113,131	95,684	97,429	88,440	389.6	323.3	271.9	278.5	249.4

[Continued]

★ 173 ★

Gonorrhea: Urban Distribution - Women
[Continued]

State/Area	Cases					Rates per 100,000 Population				
	1991	1992	1993	1994	1995	1991	1992	1993	1994	1995
San Juan, PR	95	41	77	52	102	19.8	8.5	16.1	10.8	21.3
TOTAL	135,357	113,172	95,761	97,481	88,542	384.6	319.0	268.4	274.9	246.3

Source: U.S. Department of Health and Human Services. Public Health Service. Centers for Disease Control and Prevention. Division of STD Prevention. *Sexually Transmitted Disease Surveillance, 1995.* U.S. Department of Health and Human Services, Public Health Service, September 1996.

★ 174 ★

Diseases and Illnesses: Sexually Transmitted Diseases

Gonorrhea: Urban Distribution, Ranked by Rates

This table shows reported cases and rates for gonorrhea in selected cities of 200,000+ population, ranked according to rates: United States and outlying areas, 1995.

City	Number of cases	Rate per 100,000 population	Rank
St. Louis, MO	4,425	1,233.6	1
Richmond, VA	2,371	1,195.8	2
Atlanta, GA	7,330	1,046.1	3
Washington, DC	5,687	1,026.1	4
Baltimore, MD	6,928	1,002.4	5
Rochester, NY	2,210	909.5	6
Detroit, MI	8,553	812.7	7
Newark, NJ	2,222	772.8	8
Kansas City, MO	3,186	726.4	9
Norfolk, VA	1,679	706.7	10
Memphis, TN	6,108	706.1	11
New Orleans, LA	3,353	695.8	12
Birmingham, AL	4,321	656.9	13
Indianapolis, IN	4,709	576.0	14
Buffalo, NY	1,691	518.5	15
Nashville, TN	2,622	494.0	16
Oklahoma City, OK	2,028	464.0	17
Milwaukee, WI	4,160	446.7	18
Minneapolis, MN	1,689	440.5	19
Philadelphia, PA	6,565	438.0	20
Chicago, IL	12,586	426.9	21
Cleveland, OH	5,746	411.0	22
Dallas, TX	8,027	409.7	23
Tulsa, OK	1,452	384.0	24
Charlotte, NC	2,146	370.3	25
Louisville, KY	2,441	362.7	26
Jacksonville, FL	2,476	352.9	27
Cincinnati, OH	2,590	299.8	28

[Continued]

★ 174 ★

Gonorrhea: Urban Distribution, Ranked by Rates
[Continued]

City	Number of cases	Rate per 100,000 population	Rank
Columbus, OH	2,887	285.6	29
Dayton, OH	1,603	281.0	30
Denver, CO	1,375	278.1	31
San Francisco, CA	1,853	253.6	32
Austin, TX	1,600	240.7	33
Houston, TX	6,984	227.0	34
New York City, NY	16,499	225.6	35
Toledo, OH	944	207.5	36
Tampa, FL	1,833	207.2	37
St. Paul, MN	560	203.8	38
Omaha, NE	880	202.7	39
Akron, OH	1,043	196.7	40
Fort Worth, TX	2,442	191.0	41
Oakland, CA	2,220	183.5	42
St. Petersburg, FL	1,545	177.4	43
Wichita, KS	713	170.0	44
Boston, MA	917	165.0	45
Sacramento, CA	1,684	152.6	46
San Antonio, TX	1,914	147.6	47
Phoenix, AZ	3,149	129.5	48
Pittsburgh, PA	1,598	122.0	49
Albuquerque, NM	625	119.7	50
Corpus Christi, TX	373	119.3	51
Miami, FL	2,338	115.1	52
Portland, OR	543	112.1	53
Des Moines, IA	362	103.6	54
Jersey City, NJ	223	102.6	55
YEAR 2000 OBJECTIVE[1]		100.0	
Los Angeles, CA	8,238	96.3	56
Seattle, WA	1,295	81.2	57
San Diego, CA	1,775	67.1	58
Yonkers, NY	121	63.2	59
Honolulu, HI	543	61.9	60
Tucson, AZ	359	47.7	61
San Juan, PR	349	40.0	62
San Jose, CA	475	30.3	63
El Paso, TX	159	23.4	64

Source: U.S. Department of Health and Human Services. Public Health Service. Centers for Disease Control and Prevention. Division of STD Prevention. *Sexually Transmitted Disease Surveillance, 1995.* U.S. Department of Health and Human Services, Public Health Service, September 1996. *Note:* 1. Revised from 225.0 to 100.0.

★ 175 ★

Diseases and Illnesses: Sexually Transmitted Diseases

Leading Sexually Transmitted Diseases: 1995

"According to the Institute of Medicine... STDs and their complications cost America $10 billion per year. In 1995, five of the top ten reported diseases were STDs—syphilis, gonorrhea, AIDS, chlamydia, and hepatitis B."

Source: "The Invisible Worm." *Economist,* 17 May 1997, p. 28. *Note:* STD indicates "sexually transmitted disease."

★ 176 ★

Diseases and Illnesses: Sexually Transmitted Diseases

New Cases of Curable Sexually Transmitted Diseases Worldwide: 1995

[Numbers in millions]

Country/region	Number
Africa	
North/West Africa	10
Sub-Saharan Africa	65
Asia	
Eastern Asia/Pacific	23
Southern/Southeast Asia	150
Australasia	1
Europe	
Eastern Europe/Central Asia	18
Western Europe	16
Latin America/Caribbean	36
North America	14

Source: Ostrovsky, Arkady. "Birthrate Down, Hardship Up." *Financial Times,* 29 May 1997, p. 6. Primary source: World Health Organization, Maternal Health and Safe Motherhood Programme (Geneva), unpublished estimates.

★ 177 ★

Diseases and Illnesses: Sexually Transmitted Diseases

Sexually Transmitted Diseases, by Gender and Reporting Source

Disease	Non-STD Clinic			STD Clinic			Total[1]		
	Male	Female	Total	Male	Female	Total	Male	Female	Total
Total Syphilis	11,650	13,568	25,222	22,966	20,763	43,731	34,616	34,331	68,953
Primary	1,076	445	1,522	3,283	975	4,258	4,359	1,420	5,780
Secondary	1,277	2,278	3,555	3,095	4,070	7,165	4,372	6,348	10,720
Early Latent	3,828	5,210	9,039	8,668	8,896	17,565	12,496	14,106	26,604
Late and Late Latent	4,912	5,103	10,015	7,711	6,628	14,341	12,623	11,731	24,356
Congenital <1 year	NR	NR	NR	NR	NR	NR	679	667	1,406
Total Gonorrhea	67,987	112,465	180,685	135,665	76,185	212,033	203,563	188,650	392,848
Gonococcal PID[2]	NA	2,066	2,066	NA	2,743	2,745	NA	4,809	4,811
Ophthalmia Neonatorum	62	70	132	73	42	115	135	112	247
Other Specified	18,897	28,511	47,468	45,293	24,305	69,713	64,190	52,816	117,181
Not Specified	22,482	35,998	58,480	44,563	24,530	69,093	67,046	60,530	127,576
Chancroid	21	28	49	422	132	554	443	160	606
Granuloma Inguinale	0	0	0	0	0	0	0	0	0
Lymphogranuloma Venereum	35	69	104	67	15	82	102	84	186
Total Chlamydia Trachomatis	28,583	245,087	273,949	30,227	105,434	136,493	65,697	383,956	477,638
Chlamydial PID	NA	1,746	1,765	NA	545	545	NA	2,291	2,310
Ophthalmia Neonatorum	79	93	172	2	6	8	81	99	180
Other Specified	4,457	41,255	45,746	4,768	12,999	18,579	9,225	54,254	64,325
Not Specified	7,061	64,830	71,891	10,429	40,578	51,007	17,499	105,444	122,943
Other and Not Specified PID	NA	2,433	2,433	NA	2,322	2,323	NA	7,065	7,066
Nonspecific Urethritis in Men	5,397	NA	5,397	46,132	NA	46,132	56,667	NA	56,667

Source: U.S. Department of Health and Human Services. Public Health Service. Centers for Disease Control and Prevention. Division of STD Prevention. *Sexually Transmitted Disease Surveillance, 1995.* U.S. Department of Health and Human Services, Public Health Service, September 1996. *Notes:* NA indicates "not applicable." NR indicates "no report." PID indicates "pelvic inflammatory disease. Cases of congenital syphilis in persons <1 year of age are obtained using a new reporting form (CDC 73.126). 1. Totals include unknown gender and reporting source. 2. Pelvic inflammatory disease.

★ 178 ★

Diseases and Illnesses: Sexually Transmitted Diseases

Sexually Transmitted Diseases in the United States

"The U.S. has the highest rate of curable sexually transmitted diseases of any developed country. More than 12 million people—a quarter of them teens — become infected annually."

Source: Cronin, Brian. "Health Report: The Bad News." *Time,* 2 December 1996, p. 25.

★ 179 ★
Diseases and Illnesses: Sexually Transmitted Diseases

Sexually Transmitted Diseases Reported, Excluding Syphilis

This table shows cases of sexually transmitted diseases, excluding syphilis, reported by state health departments, and rates per 100,000 civilian population: United States, 1941-1995.

Year[1]	Chlamydia		Gonorrhea		Chancroid		Granuloma Inguinale		Lympho-granuloma Venereum	
	Cases	Rate	Cases	Rate	Cases	Rate	Cases	Rate	Cases	Rate
1941	NR	-	193,468	146.7	3,384	2.5	639	0.4	1,381	1.0
1942	NR	-	212,403	160.9	5,477	4.1	1,278	0.9	1,888	1.4
1943	NR	-	275,070	213.6	8,354	6.4	1,748	1.3	2,593	2.0
1944	NR	-	300,676	236.5	7,878	6.1	1,759	1.3	2,858	2.2
1945	NR	-	287,181	225.8	5,515	4.3	1,857	1.4	2,631	2.0
1946	NR	-	368,020	275.0	7,091	5.2	2,232	1.6	2,603	1.9
1947	NR	-	380,666	270.0	9,515	6.7	2,330	1.7	2,526	1.8
1948	NR	-	345,501	239.8	7,661	5.3	2,469	1.7	2,429	1.7
1949	NR	-	317,950	217.3	6,707	4.6	2,402	1.6	1,925	1.3
1950	NR	-	286,746	192.5	4,977	3.3	1,783	1.2	1,427	1.0
1951	NR	-	254,470	168.9	4,233	2.8	1,352	0.9	1,300	0.9
1952	NR	-	244,957	160.8	3,738	2.5	951	0.6	1,200	0.8
1953	NR	-	238,340	153.9	3,338	2.2	667	0.4	983	0.6
1954	NR	-	242,050	153.5	3,003	1.9	618	0.4	875	0.6
1955	NR	-	236,197	147.0	2,649	1.7	490	0.3	762	0.5
1956	NR	-	224,346	135.7	2,135	1.3	357	0.2	500	0.3
1957	NR	-	214,496	127.4	1,637	1.0	348	0.2	448	0.3
1958	NR	-	232,386	135.6	1,595	0.9	314	0.2	434	0.3
1959	NR	-	240,254	137.6	1,537	0.9	265	0.2	604	0.3
1960	NR	-	258,933	145.4	1,680	0.9	296	0.2	835	0.5
1961	NR	-	264,158	145.8	1,438	0.8	241	0.1	787	0.4
1962	NR	-	263,714	143.6	1,344	0.7	207	0.1	590	0.3
1963	NR	-	278,289	149.2	1,220	0.7	173	0.1	586	0.3
1964	NR	-	300,666	159.0	1,247	0.7	135	0.1	732	0.4
1965	NR	-	324,925	169.6	982	0.5	155	0.1	878	0.5
1966	NR	-	351,738	181.9	838	0.4	148	0.1	308	0.2
1967	NR	-	404,836	207.3	784	0.4	154	0.1	371	0.2
1968	NR	-	464,543	235.7	845	0.4	156	0.1	485	0.2
1969	NR	-	534,872	268.6	1,104	0.6	154	0.1	520	0.3
1970	NR	-	600,072	297.2	1,416	0.7	124	0.1	612	0.3
1971	NR	-	670,268	327.2	1,320	0.6	89	0.0	692	0.3
1972	NR	-	767,215	369.7	1,414	0.7	81	0.0	756	0.4
1973	NR	-	842,621	402.0	1,165	0.6	62	0.0	408	0.2
1974	NR	-	906,121	428.2	945	0.4	47	0.0	394	0.2
1975	NR	-	999,937	467.7	700	0.3	60	0.0	353	0.2
1976	NR	-	1,001,994	464.1	628	0.3	71	0.0	365	0.2
1977	NR	-	1,002,219	459.5	455	0.2	75	0.0	348	0.2
1978	NR	-	1,013,436	459.7	521	0.2	72	0.0	284	0.1
1979	NR	-	1,004,058	450.3	840	0.4	76	0.0	250	0.1
1980	NR	-	1,004,029	445.1	788	0.3	51	0.0	199	0.1
1981	NR	-	990,864	435.2	850	0.4	66	0.0	263	0.1
1982	NR	-	960,633	417.9	1,392	0.6	17	0.0	235	0.1
1983	NR	-	900,435	387.6	847	0.4	24	0.0	335	0.1

[Continued]

★ 179 ★

Sexually Transmitted Diseases Reported, Excluding Syphilis
[Continued]

Year[1]	Chlamydia		Gonorrhea		Chancroid		Granuloma Inguinale		Lympho-granuloma Venereum	
	Cases	Rate	Cases	Rate	Cases	Rate	Cases	Rate	Cases	Rate
1984	7,594	3.2	878,556	374.8	665	0.3	30	0.0	170	0.1
1985	25,848	10.8	911,419	384.3	2,067	0.9	44	0.0	226	0.1
1986	58,001	24.1	892,229	372.8	3,045	1.3	48	0.0	307	0.1
1987	91,913	47.8	787,532	323.6	4,986	2.0	22	0.0	302	0.1
1988	157,807	81.8	738,160	300.3	4,891	2.0	11	0.0	194	0.1
1989	200,904	96.6	733,294	297.1	4,697	1.9	7	0.0	182	0.1
1990	308,139	145.4	691,368	278.0	4,212	1.7	97	0.0	277	0.1
1991	362,441	163.1	623,009	247.1	3,476	1.4	29	0.0	471	0.2
1992	405,935	173.3	501,777	196.7	1,885	0.7	6	0.0	289	0.1
1993	407,312	172.1	443,278	165.1	1,229	0.5	19	0.0	286	0.1
1994	448,984	184.7	418,068	165.1	773	0.3	3	0.0	235	0.1
1995	477,638	182.2	392,848	149.5	606	0.2	0	0.0	186	0.1

Source: U.S. Department of Health and Human Services. Public Health Service. Centers for Disease Control and Prevention. Division of STD Prevention. *Sexually Transmitted Disease Surveillance, 1995.* U.S. Department of Health and Human Services, Public Health Service, September 1996. *Notes:* NR indicates "no report." Adjustments to the number of cases reported from state health departments were accepted through March 31, 1996. The number of cases and the rates shown here supersede those published in previous reports. Military cases are no longer categorized separately and are included with civilian cases. Georgia has been excluded from gonorrhea numbers for 1994. 1. For 1941-1946, data were reported for the federal fiscal year ending June 30 of the year indicated. From 1947 to the present, data were reported for the calendar year ending December 31. For 1941-1958, data for Alaska and Hawaii were not included.

★ 180 ★

Diseases and Illnesses: Sexually Transmitted Diseases

Syphilis Cases and Rates, 1941-1995[1]

This table shows cases of syphilis reported by state health departments, and rates per 100,000 civilian population, for the United States for the period 1941 to 1995.

Year[1]	Syphilis									
	All Stages		Primary and Secondary		Early Latent		Late and Late Latent		Congenital	
	Cases	Rate	Cases	Rate	Cases	Rate	Cases	Rate	Cases	Rate[2]
1941	485,560	368.2	68,231	51.7	109,018	82.6	202,984	153.9	17,600	13.4
1942	479,601	363.4	75,312	57.0	116,245	88.0	202,064	153.1	16,918	12.8
1943	575,593	447.0	82,204	63.8	149,390	116.0	251,958	195.7	16,164	12.6
1944	467,755	367.9	78,443	61.6	123,038	96.7	202,848	159.6	13,578	10.7
1945	359,114	282.3	77,007	60.5	101,719	79.9	142,187	111.8	12,339	9.7
1946	363,647	271.7	94,957	70.9	107,924	80.6	125,248	93.6	12,106	9.0
1947	355,592	252.3	93,545	66.4	104,124	73.9	122,089	86.6	12,200	8.7
1948	314,313	218.2	68,174	47.3	90,598	62.9	123,312	85.6	13,931	9.7
1949	256,463	175.3	41,942	28.7	75,045	51.3	116,397	79.5	13,952	9.5
1950	217,558	146.0	23,939	16.7	59,256	39.7	113,569	70.2	13,377	9.0
1951	174,924	116.1	14,485	9.6	43,316	28.7	98,311	65.2	11,094	7.4

[Continued]

★ 180 ★

Syphilis Cases and Rates, 1941-1995
[Continued]

| Year[1] | Syphilis | | | | | | | | | |
| | All Stages | | Primary and Secondary | | Early Latent | | Late and Late Latent | | Congenital | |
	Cases	Rate	Cases	Rate	Cases	Rate	Cases	Rate	Cases	Rate[2]
1952	167,762	110.2	10,449	6.9	36,454	24.0	105,238	69.1	8,553	5.6
1953	148,573	95.9	8,637	5.6	28,295	18.3	98,870	63.8	7,675	5.0
1954	130,687	82.9	7,147	4.5	23,861	15.1	89,123	56.5	6,676	4.2
1955	122,392	76.2	6,454	4.0	20,054	12.5	86,526	53.8	5,354	3.3
1956	130,201	78.7	6,392	3.9	19,783	12.0	95,097	57.5	5,491	3.3
1957	123,758	73.5	6,576	3.9	17,796	10.6	91,309	54.2	5,288	3.1
1958	113,884	66.4	7,176	4.2	16,556	9.7	83,027	48.4	4,866	2.8
1959	120,824	69.2	9,799	5.6	17,025	9.8	86,740	49.7	5,130	2.9
1960	122,538	68.8	16,145	9.1	18,017	10.1	81,798	45.9	4,416	2.5
1961	124,658	68.8	19,851	11.0	19,486	10.8	79,304	43.8	4,163	2.3
1962	126,245	68.7	21,067	11.5	19,585	10.7	79,533	43.3	4,070	2.2
1963	124,137	66.6	22,251	11.9	18,235	9.8	78,076	41.9	4,031	2.2
1964	114,325	60.4	22,969	12.1	17,781	9.4	68,629	36.3	3,516	1.9
1965	112,842	58.9	23,338	12.2	17,458	9.1	67,317	35.1	3,564	1.9
1966	105,159	54.4	21,414	11.1	15,950	8.2	63,541	32.9	3,170	1.6
1967	102,581	52.5	21,053	10.8	15,554	8.0	61,975	31.7	2,894	1.5
1968	96,271	48.8	19,019	9.6	15,150	7.7	58,564	29.7	2,381	1.2
1969	92,162	46.3	19,130	9.6	15,402	7.7	54,587	27.4	2,074	1.0
1970	91,382	45.3	21,982	10.9	16,311	8.1	50,348	24.9	1,953	1.0
1971	95,997	46.9	23,783	11.6	19,417	9.5	49,993	24.4	2,052	1.0
1972	91,149	43.9	24,429	11.8	20,784	10.0	43,456	20.9	1,758	0.8
1973	87,469	41.7	24,825	11.8	23,584	11.3	37,054	17.7	1,527	0.7
1974	83,771	39.6	25,385	12.0	25,124	11.9	31,854	15.1	1,138	0.5
1975	80,356	37.6	25,561	12.0	26,569	12.4	27,096	12.7	916	0.4
1976	71,761	33.2	23,731	11.0	25,363	11.7	21,905	10.1	626	0.3
1977	64,621	29.6	20,399	9.4	21,329	9.8	22,313	10.2	463	0.2
1978	64,875	29.4	21,656	9.8	19,628	8.9	23,038	10.4	434	0.2
1979	67,049	30.1	24,874	11.2	20,459	9.2	21,301	9.6	332	0.1
1980	68,832	30.5	27,204	12.1	20,297	9.0	20,979	9.3	277	0.1
1981	72,799	32.0	31,266	13.7	21,033	9.2	20,168	8.9	287	0.1
1982	75,579	32.9	33,613	14.6	21,894	9.5	19,779	8.6	259	0.1
1983	74,637	32.1	32,698	14.1	23,738	10.2	17,896	7.7	239	0.1
1984	69,873	29.8	28,607	12.2	23,132	9.9	17,829	7.6	305	0.1
1985	67,563	28.5	27,131	11.5	21,689	9.2	18,414	7.8	329	0.1
1986	67,771	28.3	27,667	11.6	21,656	9.0	18,046	7.5	410	0.2
1987	87,278	35.9	35,585	14.6	28,233	11.6	22,988	9.4	480	0.2
1988	104,546	42.5	40,474	16.5	35,968	14.6	27,363	11.1	741	0.3
1989	115,067	46.6	45,826	18.6	45,394	18.4	22,032	8.9	1,837	0.7
1990	135,043	54.3	50,578	20.3	55,397	22.3	25,750	10.4	3,865	1.6
1991	128,637	51.0	42,950	17.0	53,855	21.4	27,490	10.9	4,424	1.8
1992	112,816	44.2	33,962	13.3	49,903	19.6	25,084	9.8	3,889	1.5
1993	101,333	39.3	26,496	10.3	41,902	16.3	29,675	11.5	3,260	1.3

[Continued]

★ 180 ★

Syphilis Cases and Rates, 1941-1995
[Continued]

Year[1]	Syphilis									
	All Stages		Primary and Secondary		Early Latent		Late and Late Latent		Congenital	
	Cases	Rate	Cases	Rate	Cases	Rate	Cases	Rate	Cases	Rate[2]
1994	81,696	31.4	20,627	7.9	32,012	12.3	26,840	10.3	2,217	0.9
1995	68,953	26.2	16,500	6.3	26,604	10.1	24,356	9.3	1,548	0.6

Source: U.S. Department of Health and Human Services. Public Health Service. Centers for Disease Control and Prevention. Division of STD Prevention. *Sexually Transmitted Disease Surveillance, 1995.* U.S. Department of Health and Human Services, Public Health Service, September 1996. *Notes:* 1. For 1941-1946, data were reported for the federal fiscal year ending June 30 of the year indicated. From 1947 to the present, data were reported for the calendar year ending December 31. For 1941-1958, data for Alaska and Hawaii were not included. 2. For 1941-1994, rates include all cases of congenitally acquired syphilis per 100,000 population. As of 1995, rates of congenital syphilis in persons <1 year of age per 100,000 population are reported. As of 1995, cases of congenital syphilis in persons <1 year of age per 100,000 live births are obtained using a new reporting form (CDC 73.126). Adjustments to the number of cases reported from state health departments were accepted through March 31, 1996. The number of cases and the rates shown here supersede those published in previous reports. Military cases are no longer categorized separately and are included with civilian cases.

★ 181 ★

Diseases and Illnesses: Sexually Transmitted Diseases

Syphilis: Cases by Age, Gender, Race, and Ethnicity - Part 1

This table shows reported cases of primary and secondary syphilis by age, gender, and race/ethnicity: United States, 1995.

Age Group	Total			White, Non-Hispanic			Black, Non-Hispanic		
	Total	Male	Female	Total	Male	Female	Total	Male	Female
10-14	106	11	95	5	0	5	98	11	87
15-19	1,795	604	1,191	132	28	104	1,601	555	1,046
20-24	3,065	1,476	1,589	241	99	142	2,682	1,303	1,379
25-29	2,852	1,390	1,462	257	121	136	2,433	1,174	1,259
30-34	2,916	1,480	1,436	255	130	125	2,505	1,260	1,245
35-39	2,411	1,368	1,043	253	146	107	2,042	1,147	895
40-44	1,469	977	492	151	98	53	1,264	839	425
45-54	1,272	939	333	140	108	32	1,066	783	283
55-64	384	310	74	51	45	6	317	254	63
65+	186	149	37	29	23	6	139	111	28
TOTAL	16,491	8,722	7,769	1,515	799	716	14,181	7,454	6,727

Source: U.S. Department of Health and Human Services. Public Health Service. Centers for Disease Control and Prevention. Division of STD Prevention. *Sexually Transmitted Disease Surveillance, 1995.* U.S. Department of Health and Human Services, Public Health Service, September 1996. *Notes:* In most instances, if age or race/ethnicity was not specified, cases were prorated according to the distribution of cases for which these variables were specified. Cases from Baltimore, Maryland, were excluded for 1993 because age was not reported for most cases. Differences between total cases from this table and others in the report are due to different reporting forms and above exclusions. Cases in persons age 0 to 9 years are not reported because some of these may not be due to sexual transmission; however, they are included in the totals.

★ 182 ★

Diseases and Illnesses: Sexually Transmitted Diseases

Syphilis: Cases by Age, Gender, Race, and Ethnicity - Part 2

This table shows reported cases of primary and secondary syphilis by age, gender, and race/ethnicity: United States, 1995.

Age Group	Total			Hispanic			Asian/Pacific Islander			American Indian/Alaska Native		
	Total	Male	Female	Total	Male	Female	Total	Male	Female	Total	Male	Female
10-14	106	11	95	3	0	3	0	0	0	0	0	0
15-19	1,795	604	1,191	52	20	32	3	0	3	7	1	6
20-24	3,065	1,476	1,589	126	70	56	12	1	11	4	3	1
25-29	2,852	1,390	1,462	141	86	55	9	3	6	12	6	6
30-34	2,916	1,480	1,436	132	79	53	15	6	9	9	5	4
35-39	2,411	1,368	1,043	108	72	36	5	1	4	3	2	1
40-44	1,469	977	492	46	36	10	4	2	2	4	2	2
45-54	1,272	939	333	58	44	14	3	1	2	5	3	2
55-64	384	310	74	16	11	5	0	0	0	0	0	0
65 +	186	149	37	14	11	3	2	2	0	2	2	0
TOTAL	16,491	8,722	7,769	696	429	267	53	16	37	46	24	22

Source: U.S. Department of Health and Human Services. Public Health Service. Centers for Disease Control and Prevention. Division of STD Prevention. *Sexually Transmitted Disease Surveillance, 1995.* U.S. Department of Health and Human Services, Public Health Service, September 1996. *Notes:* In most instances, if age or race/ethnicity was not specified, cases were prorated according to the distribution of cases for which these variables were specified. Cases from Baltimore, Maryland, were excluded for 1993 because age was not reported for most cases. Differences between total cases from this table and others in the report are due to different reporting forms and above exclusions. Cases in persons age 0 to 9 years are not shown because some of these may not be due to sexual transmission; however, they are included in the totals.

★ 183 ★

Diseases and Illnesses: Sexually Transmitted Diseases

Syphilis, Congenital: Urban Distribution

This table shows reported cases of congenital syphilis in infants less than 1 year of age in selected cities of 200,000+ population: United States and outlying areas, 1986-1995.

City	Cases									
	1986	1987	1988	1989	1990	1991	1992	1993	1994	1995
Akron, OH	0	0	0	0	0	0	0	1	0	0
Albuquerque, NM	0	0	0	0	0	2	0	0	0	0
Atlanta, GA	0	0	1	2	26	48	53	36	11	21
Austin, TX	1	0	0	3	1	5	0	9	3	0
Baltimore, MD	1	1	6	4	8	9	7	5	1	10
Birmingham, AL	0	2	0	0	1	4	0	7	7	8
Boston, MA	1	0	1	5	11	2	4	3	4	0
Buffalo, NY	0	0	0	3	1	5	2	6	1	1
Charlotte, NC	0	0	1	1	6	10	12	10	3	1
Chicago, IL	6	8	14	55	162	245	322	275	177	121
Cincinnati, OH	0	0	0	0	0	3	2	12	15	5
Cleveland, OH	0	0	1	3	12	37	41	47	44	18
Columbus, OH	0	0	0	0	3	1	1	1	1	0
Corpus Christi, TX	1	1	0	0	1	0	0	0	0	0
Dallas, TX	17	15	15	14	25	16	45	22	10	11
Dayton, OH	0	0	1	0	0	1	3	5	5	7
Denver, CO	0	0	0	0	0	0	0	3	3	0

[Continued]

★ 183 ★

Syphilis, Congenital: Urban Distribution

[Continued]

City	Cases									
	1986	1987	1988	1989	1990	1991	1992	1993	1994	1995
Des Moines, IA	0	0	0	0	0	0	0	0	2	0
Detroit, MI	0	3	5	19	61	70	58	72	19	23
El Paso, TX	4	2	0	5	20	15	19	18	10	1
Fort Worth, TX	6	2	3	2	1	20	20	13	7	11
Honolulu, HI	1	0	0	0	0	0	0	0	0	0
Houston, TX	14	12	17	41	106	134	182	119	86	50
Indianapolis, IN	0	0	0	1	0	0	0	0	3	0
Jacksonville, FL	4	7	1	0	0	5	8	8	1	1
Jersey City, NJ	1	0	0	2	16	4	12	7	9	11
Kansas City, MO	0	0	0	0	3	4	14	11	7	2
Los Angeles, CA	30	39	74	41	514	498	343	256	190	155
Louisville, KY	0	0	0	0	2	1	8	7	10	4
Memphis, TN	4	2	20	15	37	59	42	35	35	22
Miami, FL	56	26	81	106	82	255	144	113	14	28
Milwaukee, WI	0	0	0	0	9	28	11	5	15	11
Minneapolis, MN	0	0	0	0	0	0	4	5	1	2
Nashville, TN	0	0	0	1	4	2	2	3	1	1
New Orleans, LA	1	0	0	28	93	27	1	54	23	0
New York City, NY	50	121	133	1,017	1,005	978	898	654	329	0
Newark, NJ	0	0	0	0	23	9	20	73	55	43
Norfolk, VA	0	0	0	0	2	5	9	10	2	8
Oakland, CA	1	7	10	7	35	21	6	7	0	0
Oklahoma City, OK	0	1	0	4	2	7	11	6	12	13
Omaha, NE	0	0	0	1	0	1	4	1	0	0
Philadelphia, PA	10	13	18	23	179	301	266	152	106	64
Phoenix, AZ	0	0	0	0	0	6	17	11	13	6
Pittsburgh, PA	1	1	1	0	2	1	2	2	1	0
Portland, OR	0	3	2	1	0	1	0	2	0	0
Richmond, VA	0	1	0	5	2	7	11	0	0	0
Rochester, NY	0	0	1	4	5	14	12	7	4	4
Sacramento, CA	1	0	1	0	3	6	2	0	0	0
San Antonio, TX	1	5	3	8	3	15	14	9	10	7
San Diego, CA	3	6	12	16	41	35	13	9	0	0
San Francisco, CA	2	0	0	0	26	10	6	7	4	1
San Jose, CA	1	0	1	1	3	3	2	1	0	0
Seattle, WA	0	0	0	1	3	3	6	2	2	0
St. Louis, MO	0	0	0	0	3	5	13	66	49	28
St. Paul, MN	0	0	0	0	0	0	0	2	0	0
St. Petersburg, FL	2	2	5	5	7	29	13	11	0	2
Tampa, FL	3	7	6	12	5	43	14	12	4	9
Toledo, OH	0	0	0	0	0	4	3	3	0	0
Tucson, AZ	0	0	0	1	0	1	0	2	3	1
Tulsa, OK	0	0	0	2	1	1	5	4	1	1
Washington, DC	0	2	5	10	29	246	217	74	28	12
Wichita, KS	0	2	0	0	0	0	1	0	0	0
Yonkers, NY	0	0	2	0	11	13	6	7	8	3

[Continued]

★ 183 ★

Syphilis, Congenital: Urban Distribution

[Continued]

City	Cases									
	1986	1987	1988	1989	1990	1991	1992	1993	1994	1995
U.S. CITY TOTAL	223	291	441	1,469	2,595	3,275	2,931	2,302	1,349	727
San Juan, PR	5	4	4	5	4	15	11	11	10	0
TOTAL	228	295	445	1,474	2,599	3,290	2,942	2,313	1,359	727

Source: U.S. Department of Health and Human Services. Public Health Service. Centers for Disease Control and Prevention. Division of STD Prevention. *Sexually Transmitted Disease Surveillance, 1995.* U.S. Department of Health and Human Services, Public Health Service, September 1996.

★ 184 ★

Diseases and Illnesses: Sexually Transmitted Diseases

Syphilis, Early Latent: Urban Distribution

This table shows reported cases and rates of early latent syphilis in selected cities of 200,000+ population: United States and outlying areas, 1991-1995.

State/Area	Cases					Rates per 100,000 Population				
	1991	1992	1993	1994	1995	1991	1992	1993	1994	1995
Akron, OH	25	28	5	5	6	4.8	5.4	1.0	0.9	1.1
Albuquerque, NM	16	10	10	5	9	3.3	2.0	2.0	1.0	1.7
Atlanta, GA	1,302	1,044	714	515	531	198.6	157.1	105.5	74.5	75.8
Austin, TX	128	113	119	149	79	21.5	18.4	18.9	23.0	11.9
Baltimore, MD	390	276	204	371	369	53.3	38.1	28.5	52.8	53.4
Birmingham, AL	323	364	337	264	289	49.4	55.5	51.3	40.2	43.9
Boston, MA	202	154	111	94	65	35.9	27.8	20.1	17.1	11.7
Buffalo, NY	66	41	38	19	6	20.1	12.4	11.6	5.8	1.8
Charlotte, NC	298	344	245	243	180	56.5	64.2	44.7	43.1	31.1
Chicago, IL	2,154	2,492	1,888	1,307	1,400	73.4	84.5	64.0	44.3	47.5
Cincinnati, OH	42	84	216	260	115	4.8	9.6	24.8	30.0	13.3
Cleveland, OH	262	575	922	599	361	18.6	40.8	65.5	42.7	25.8
Columbus, OH	48	41	34	18	11	4.9	4.1	3.4	1.8	1.1
Corpus Christi, TX	41	44	24	45	29	13.8	14.6	7.8	14.5	9.3
Dallas, TX	815	749	545	520	410	43.1	39.2	28.3	26.8	20.9
Dayton, OH	16	43	43	42	98	2.8	7.5	7.5	7.3	17.2
Denver, CO	23	23	36	34	46	4.9	4.7	7.3	6.9	9.3
Des Moines, IA	32	34	39	60	54	9.6	10.1	11.4	17.3	15.4
Detroit, MI	1,447	957	608	388	364	134.5	89.4	57.1	36.7	34.6
El Paso, TX	85	55	37	42	21	13.9	8.8	5.7	6.3	3.1
Fort Worth, TX	163	233	302	283	280	13.5	19.1	24.5	22.5	21.9
Honolulu, HI	14	9	7	5	0	1.6	1.0	0.8	0.6	0.0
Houston, TX	2,382	2,475	1,622	1,157	892	82.1	83.5	54.0	38.0	29.0
Indianapolis, IN	47	46	128	69	55	5.8	5.7	15.7	8.4	6.7
Jacksonville, FL	197	180	117	128	111	28.6	25.7	16.7	18.3	15.8
Jersey City, NJ	75	74	53	36	30	34.4	33.9	24.3	16.5	13.8
Kansas City, MO	128	150	93	78	29	29.3	34.3	21.3	17.8	6.6

[Continued]

★ 184 ★

Syphilis, Early Latent: Urban Distribution

[Continued]

State/Area	Cases					Rates per 100,000 Population				
	1991	1992	1993	1994	1995	1991	1992	1993	1994	1995
Los Angeles, CA	2,757	2,350	1,755	1,139	997	32.9	27.7	20.5	13.3	11.7
Louisville, KY	22	40	98	109	81	3.3	6.0	14.6	16.2	12.0
Memphis, TN	1,522	1,011	852	717	652	182.2	120.0	100.5	83.7	75.4
Miami, FL	929	880	1,022	686	499	47.0	43.9	51.1	33.9	24.6
Milwaukee, WI	230	264	446	310	229	24.0	27.7	47.1	33.1	24.6
Minneapolis, MN	41	58	56	49	24	10.9	15.3	14.7	12.8	6.3
Nashville, TN	170	147	153	79	97	33.2	28.4	29.3	15.0	18.3
New Orleans, LA	567	573	354	311	215	115.5	117.1	72.7	64.1	44.6
New York City, NY	6,784	5,411	3,769	2,364	1,945	92.8	74.1	51.4	32.3	26.6
Newark, NJ	195	200	170	56	77	66.5	68.3	58.2	19.3	26.8
Norfolk, VA	79	119	98	82	110	31.2	46.9	39.1	33.8	46.3
Oakland, CA	254	241	129	115	60	21.5	20.2	10.7	9.5	5.0
Oklahoma City, OK	79	128	177	142	140	18.7	30.0	41.0	32.6	32.0
Omaha, NE	12	4	4	9	3	2.8	0.9	0.9	2.1	0.7
Philadelphia, PA	3,325	3,348	2,829	1,708	1,100	212.3	215.9	184.0	112.3	73.4
Phoenix, AZ	191	94	81	63	79	8.8	4.2	3.6	2.7	3.2
Pittsburgh, PA	57	45	20	10	13	4.3	3.4	1.5	0.8	1.0
Portland, OR	56	30	15	11	11	11.9	6.3	3.1	2.3	2.3
Richmond, VA	123	115	87	60	70	61.2	57.4	43.6	30.3	35.3
Rochester, NY	101	103	75	59	23	41.8	42.3	30.7	24.2	9.5
Sacramento, CA	104	55	55	33	26	9.6	5.0	5.0	3.0	2.4
San Antonio, TX	291	246	245	240	161	24.1	19.9	19.5	18.8	12.4
San Diego, CA	149	157	94	98	58	5.8	6.0	3.6	3.7	2.2
San Francisco, CA	163	50	29	21	14	22.4	6.9	4.0	2.9	1.9
San Jose, CA	43	45	29	5	4	2.8	2.9	1.9	0.3	0.3
Seattle, WA	17	15	15	7	1	1.1	1.0	1.0	0.4	0.1
St. Louis, MO	50	244	424	391	289	12.8	63.4	112.7	106.3	80.6
St. Paul, MN	9	23	13	14	9	3.3	8.3	4.7	5.1	3.3
St. Petersburg, FL	284	193	161	140	83	32.9	22.4	18.6	16.2	9.5
Tampa, FL	447	385	201	100	79	52.9	45.0	23.2	11.4	8.9
Toledo, OH	87	134	97	28	27	18.9	29.1	21.1	6.1	5.9
Tucson, AZ	10	10	16	22	29	1.5	1.4	2.3	3.0	3.9
Tulsa, OK	36	92	77	27	44	9.8	24.6	20.5	7.2	11.6
Washington, DC	1,224	1,000	837	502	396	206.0	170.7	144.8	88.5	71.4
Wichita, KS	18	19	15	8	12	4.4	4.6	3.6	1.9	2.9
Yonkers, NY	40	60	31	26	16	21.2	31.6	16.3	13.6	8.4
U.S. CITY TOTAL	31,187	28,527	23,026	16,477	13,513	46.3	42.0	33.7	24.0	19.6
San Juan, PR	417	485	558	406	313	47.8	55.6	64.0	46.6	35.9
TOTAL	31,604	29,012	23,584	16,883	13,826	46.3	42.2	34.1	24.3	19.8

Source: U.S. Department of Health and Human Services. Public Health Service. Centers for Disease Control and Prevention. Division of STD Prevention. *Sexually Transmitted Disease Surveillance, 1995.* U.S. Department of Health and Human Services, Public Health Service, September 1996.

★ 185 ★

Diseases and Illnesses: Sexually Transmitted Diseases

Syphilis, Late Latent: Urban Distribution

This table shows reported cases and rates of late latent syphilis in selected cities of 200,000+ population: United States and outlying areas, 1991-1995.

State/Area	Cases					Rates per 100,000 Population				
	1991	1992	1993	1994	1995	1991	1992	1993	1994	1995
Akron, OH	3	1	1	6	1	0.6	0.2	0.2	1.1	0.2
Albuquerque, NM	38	18	60	69	26	7.8	3.6	11.8	13.4	5.0
Atlanta, GA	169	101	141	130	207	25.8	15.2	20.8	18.8	29.5
Austin, TX	41	28	64	48	87	6.9	4.6	10.1	7.4	13.1
Baltimore, MD	124	83	154	109	169	16.9	11.4	21.5	15.5	24.5
Birmingham, AL	151	82	126	132	78	23.1	12.5	19.2	20.1	11.9
Boston, MA	126	126	190	97	88	22.4	22.7	34.4	17.6	15.8
Buffalo, NY	24	23	40	24	23	7.3	7.0	12.2	7.3	7.1
Charlotte, NC	58	62	71	46	41	11.0	11.6	12.9	8.2	7.1
Chicago, IL	180	164	189	203	141	6.1	5.6	6.4	6.9	4.8
Cincinnati, OH	25	18	45	91	26	2.9	2.1	5.2	10.5	3.0
Cleveland, OH	27	68	39	106	108	1.9	4.8	2.8	7.6	7.7
Columbus, OH	52	30	27	44	13	5.3	3.0	2.7	4.4	1.3
Corpus Christi, TX	14	13	8	18	24	4.7	4.3	2.6	5.8	7.7
Dallas, TX	187	225	345	308	334	9.9	11.8	17.9	15.8	17.0
Dayton, OH	11	4	5	62	50	1.9	0.7	0.9	10.8	8.8
Denver, CO	36	37	63	57	65	7.6	7.6	12.8	11.6	13.1
Des Moines, IA	10	2	5	10	11	3.0	0.6	1.5	2.9	3.1
Detroit, MI	176	235	233	211	192	16.4	21.9	21.9	20.0	18.2
El Paso, TX	102	97	150	126	115	16.6	15.4	23.2	18.9	17.0
Fort Worth, TX	100	102	168	112	60	8.3	8.4	13.6	8.9	4.7
Honolulu, HI	15	18	27	32	22	1.8	2.1	3.1	3.7	2.5
Houston, TX	771	614	1,138	1,223	1,283	26.6	20.7	37.9	40.2	41.7
Indianapolis, IN	48	26	35	42	39	6.0	3.2	4.3	5.1	4.8
Jacksonville, FL	52	88	19	51	30	7.5	12.6	2.7	7.3	4.3
Jersey City, NJ	148	112	126	112	70	67.8	51.3	57.7	51.4	32.2
Kansas City, MO	22	22	21	10	13	5.0	5.0	4.8	2.3	3.0
Los Angeles, CA	2,625	2,808	3,075	2,254	1,723	31.3	33.1	36.0	26.4	20.1
Louisville, KY	17	34	54	59	59	2.5	5.1	8.0	8.8	8.8
Memphis, TN	20	285	463	453	442	2.4	33.8	54.6	52.9	51.1
Miami, FL	296	440	640	573	409	15.0	21.9	32.0	28.3	20.1
Milwaukee, WI	47	46	32	81	74	4.9	4.8	3.4	8.6	7.9
Minneapolis, MN	28	34	28	34	36	7.4	9.0	7.4	8.9	9.4
Nashville, TN	11	48	76	54	7	2.1	9.3	14.6	10.2	1.3
New Orleans, LA	289	341	314	307	213	58.9	69.7	64.5	63.3	44.2
New York City, NY	5,012	4,907	4,958	4,678	5,291	68.6	67.2	67.7	63.9	72.4
Newark, NJ	195	133	219	346	232	66.5	45.4	75.0	119.4	80.7
Norfolk, VA	37	26	37	41	31	14.6	10.2	14.8	16.9	13.0
Oakland, CA	187	186	219	170	86	15.8	15.6	18.2	14.1	7.1
Oklahoma City, OK	27	17	31	30	32	6.4	4.0	7.2	6.9	7.3
Omaha, NE	20	19	11	14	11	4.7	4.5	2.6	3.3	2.5
Philadelphia, PA	167	285	255	282	329	10.7	18.4	16.6	18.5	21.9
Phoenix, AZ	167	159	178	133	142	7.7	7.2	7.8	5.7	5.8
Pittsburgh, PA	36	31	25	19	10	2.7	2.3	1.9	1.4	0.8
Portland, OR	50	70	66	34	27	10.6	14.7	13.7	7.1	5.6

[Continued]

★ 185 ★

Syphilis, Late Latent: Urban Distribution
[Continued]

State/Area	Cases					Rates per 100,000 Population				
	1991	1992	1993	1994	1995	1991	1992	1993	1994	1995
Richmond, VA	86	68	61	29	14	42.8	34.0	30.6	14.6	7.1
Rochester, NY	60	87	86	78	59	24.8	35.7	35.2	32.0	24.3
Sacramento, CA	17	13	60	86	41	1.6	1.2	5.5	7.8	3.7
San Antonio, TX	193	128	183	179	174	16.0	10.4	14.6	14.0	13.4
San Diego, CA	138	268	326	296	238	5.4	10.3	12.5	11.3	9.0
San Francisco, CA	302	200	55	19	37	41.6	27.4	7.5	2.6	5.1
San Jose, CA	15	51	74	63	31	1.0	3.3	4.8	4.1	2.0
Seattle, WA	117	121	141	106	87	7.6	7.8	8.9	6.7	5.5
St. Louis, MO	36	30	127	121	60	9.2	7.8	33.8	32.9	16.7
St. Paul, MN	10	5	12	6	12	3.6	1.8	4.3	2.2	4.4
St. Petersburg, FL	80	91	93	103	63	9.3	10.5	10.8	11.9	7.2
Tampa, FL	188	154	286	218	156	22.2	18.0	33.0	25.0	17.6
Toledo, OH	16	12	11	16	3	3.5	2.6	2.4	3.5	0.7
Tucson, AZ	40	49	102	67	47	5.9	7.1	14.4	9.2	6.2
Tulsa, OK	31	17	9	15	13	8.4	4.6	2.4	4.0	3.4
Washington, DC	654	696	450	267	201	110.0	118.8	77.8	47.1	36.3
Wichita, KS	16	21	16	9	14	3.9	5.1	3.8	2.1	3.3
Yonkers, NY	59	34	31	35	43	31.3	17.9	16.3	18.3	22.4
U.S. CITY TOTAL	13,999	14,313	16,294	14,754	13,763	20.8	21.1	23.8	21.5	20.0
San Juan, PR	309	331	540	468	309	35.4	38.0	61.9	53.7	35.4
TOTAL	14,308	14,644	16,834	15,222	14,072	21.0	21.3	24.3	21.9	20.2

Source: U.S. Department of Health and Human Services. Public Health Service. Centers for Disease Control and Prevention. Division of STD Prevention. *Sexually Transmitted Disease Surveillance, 1995.* U.S. Department of Health and Human Services, Public Health Service, September 1996.

★ 186 ★

Diseases and Illnesses: Sexually Transmitted Diseases

Syphilis: Reported Cases and Rates, by State/Area

This table shows reported cases and rates of syphilis by state/area: United States and outlying areas, 1991-1995.

State/Area	Cases					Rates per 100,000 Population				
	1991	1992	1993	1994	1995	1991	1992	1993	1994	1995
Alabama	3,478	2,607	2,333	1,933	1,639	85.1	63.1	55.8	45.8	38.5
Alaska	31	30	51	22	20	5.4	5.1	8.5	3.7	3.3
Arizona	830	540	557	419	415	22.2	14.1	14.1	10.3	9.8
Arkansas	1,929	2,169	1,600	1,328	1,245	81.4	90.6	66.0	54.1	50.1
California	12,856	9,684	9,488	7,321	5,703	42.3	31.3	30.4	23.3	18.1
Colorado	227	207	287	296	304	6.7	6.0	8.0	8.1	8.1
Connecticut	1,345	843	562	337	271	40.9	25.7	17.1	10.3	8.3
Delaware	364	437	274	138	129	53.5	63.4	39.2	19.5	18.0
Florida	10,383	8,319	7,417	5,048	3,470	78.1	61.6	54.1	36.2	24.5

[Continued]

★ 186 ★

Syphilis: Reported Cases and Rates, by State/Area
[Continued]

State/Area	Cases					Rates per 100,000 Population				
	1991	1992	1993	1994	1995	1991	1992	1993	1994	1995
Georgia	8,005	5,950	4,077	3,185	3,678	120.9	88.0	59.1	45.1	51.1
Hawaii	42	41	41	41	25	3.7	3.6	3.5	3.5	2.1
Idaho	36	27	15	10	12	3.5	2.5	1.4	0.9	1.0
Illinois	5,910	6,323	4,881	3,877	3,649	51.3	54.5	41.8	33.0	30.8
Indiana	466	766	1,019	844	880	8.3	13.6	17.9	14.7	15.2
Iowa	161	155	175	235	171	5.8	5.5	6.2	8.3	6.0
Kansas	373	453	293	187	151	15.0	18.0	11.6	7.3	5.9
Kentucky	319	394	651	534	502	8.6	10.5	17.2	14.0	13.0
Louisiana	6,497	6,590	6,854	5,422	3,675	153.2	154.2	159.8	125.6	84.6
Maine	12	12	29	9	4	1.0	1.0	2.3	0.7	0.3
Maryland	3,093	2,207	1,865	1,538	1,471	63.6	45.0	37.7	30.8	29.2
Massachusetts	1,403	1,046	935	622	508	23.4	17.4	15.5	10.3	8.4
Michigan	3,513	2,762	1,952	1,234	1,204	37.5	29.3	20.6	13.0	12.6
Minnesota	208	275	261	201	187	4.7	6.1	5.8	4.4	4.1
Mississippi	2,820	3,447	4,269	4,547	4,549	108.8	132.0	161.8	170.3	168.7
Missouri	952	1,941	2,500	1,985	1,271	18.5	37.4	47.8	37.6	23.9
Montana	13	14	4	9	13	1.6	1.7	0.5	1.1	1.5
Nebraska	62	64	35	46	35	3.9	4.0	2.2	2.8	2.1
Nevada	305	163	139	171	195	23.7	12.2	10.0	11.7	12.7
New Hampshire	38	63	50	18	32	3.4	5.7	4.5	1.6	2.8
New Jersey	3,650	2,736	2,556	2,188	1,490	47.0	35.0	32.5	27.7	18.8
New Mexico	185	138	172	178	138	12.0	8.7	10.6	10.8	8.2
New York	18,379	15,426	12,493	9,376	8,790	101.9	85.3	68.8	51.7	48.5
North Carolina	3,934	5,230	4,448	4,023	3,058	58.3	76.5	64.0	56.9	42.5
North Dakota	2	2	4	1	0	0.3	0.3	0.6	0.2	0.0
Ohio	1,467	2,153	2,889	2,740	1,944	13.4	19.6	26.1	24.7	17.4
Oklahoma	613	812	721	497	585	19.4	25.3	22.3	15.3	17.8
Oregon	277	217	179	100	67	9.5	7.3	5.9	3.2	2.1
Pennsylvania	6,087	5,405	4,257	2,738	1,950	51.0	45.1	35.4	22.7	16.2
Rhode Island	239	182	146	141	90	23.8	18.2	14.6	14.2	9.1
South Carolina	3,296	2,816	2,339	1,945	1,676	92.7	78.4	64.5	53.4	45.6
South Dakota	10	1	3	8	7	1.4	0.1	0.4	1.1	1.0
Tennessee	3,779	3,263	3,241	2,978	2,608	76.4	65.0	63.6	57.5	49.6
Texas	13,356	10,860	9,904	9,028	7,918	76.9	61.4	54.9	49.0	42.3
Utah	82	53	68	51	50	4.6	2.9	3.7	2.7	2.6
Vermont	6	2	1	1	0	1.1	0.3	0.2	0.2	0.0
Virginia	2,751	2,014	1,970	1,919	1,587	43.8	31.5	30.4	29.3	24.0
Washington	570	415	360	281	212	11.4	8.1	6.9	5.3	3.9
West Virginia	366	274	195	179	66	20.3	15.2	10.7	9.8	3.6
Wisconsin	1,015	949	1,112	797	580	20.5	19.0	22.0	15.7	11.3
Wyoming	14	6	9	3	2	3.1	1.3	1.9	0.6	0.4
U.S. TOTAL[1]	128,637	112,816	101,333	81,696	68,953	51.0	44.2	39.3	31.4	26.2
Guam	17	2	5	7	6	12.0	1.4	3.5	5.0	4.3
Puerto Rico	1,940	1,946	2,482	2,018	1,608	54.7	54.4	68.5	54.8	43.2

[Continued]

★ 186 ★

Syphilis: Reported Cases and Rates, by State/Area
[Continued]

State/Area	Cases					Rates per 100,000 Population				
	1991	1992	1993	1994	1995	1991	1992	1993	1994	1995
Virgin Islands	122	51	39	30	19	113.5	46.0	35.2	27.1	17.1
OUTLYING AREAS	2,079	1,999	2,526	2,055	1,633	54.8	52.2	65.2	52.2	41.1
TOTAL	130,716	114,815	103,859	83,751	70,586	51.1	44.4	39.7	31.7	26.5

Source: U.S. Department of Health and Human Services. Public Health Service. Centers for Disease Control and Prevention. Division of STD Prevention. *Sexually Transmitted Disease Surveillance, 1995.* U.S. Department of Health and Human Services, Public Health Service, September 1996. *Note:* 1. Includes cases reported by Washington, D.C.

★ 187 ★

Diseases and Illnesses: Sexually Transmitted Diseases

Syphilis: Reported Cases and Rates, by State/Area

This table shows reported cases and rates of primary and secondary syphilis by state/area: United States and outlying areas, 1991-1995.

State/Area	Cases					Rates per 100,000 Population				
	1991	1992	1993	1994	1995	1991	1992	1993	1994	1995
Alabama	1,594	1,011	869	661	612	39.0	24.5	20.8	15.7	14.4
Alaska	7	5	11	3	2	1.2	0.9	1.8	0.5	0.3
Arizona	334	158	95	50	46	8.9	4.1	2.4	1.2	1.1
Arkansas	895	886	559	446	495	37.7	37.0	23.1	18.2	19.9
California	2,669	1,540	1,073	807	616	8.8	5.0	3.4	2.6	2.0
Colorado	80	62	90	126	100	2.4	1.8	2.5	3.4	2.7
Connecticut	455	257	158	105	86	13.8	7.8	4.8	3.2	2.6
Delaware	194	209	94	27	19	28.5	30.3	13.4	3.8	2.6
Florida	2,723	1,627	1,191	745	383	20.5	12.0	8.7	5.3	2.7
Georgia	2,954	1,811	1,052	820	901	44.6	26.8	15.2	11.6	12.5
Hawaii	10	10	7	4	0	0.9	0.9	0.6	0.3	0.0
Idaho	7	2	2	2	0	0.7	0.2	0.2	0.2	0.0
Illinois	2,446	2,380	1,489	1,099	1,026	21.2	20.5	12.7	9.3	8.7
Indiana	196	294	362	286	321	3.5	5.2	6.3	5.0	5.5
Iowa	68	61	64	75	48	2.4	2.2	2.3	2.6	1.7
Kansas	202	262	130	73	47	8.1	10.4	5.1	2.9	1.8
Kentucky	112	182	331	208	185	3.0	4.9	8.7	5.4	4.8
Louisiana	2,955	2,729	2,598	1,608	1,024	69.7	63.9	60.6	37.3	23.6
Maine	5	8	8	4	2	0.4	0.6	0.6	0.3	0.2
Maryland	1,013	592	359	325	479	20.8	12.1	7.2	6.5	9.5
Massachusetts	492	323	122	90	69	8.2	5.4	2.0	1.5	1.1
Michigan	1,303	951	543	292	304	13.9	10.1	5.7	3.1	3.2
Minnesota	68	90	66	56	45	1.5	2.0	1.5	1.2	1.0
Mississippi	1,234	1,462	1,761	2,084	1,952	47.6	56.0	66.7	78.0	72.4
Missouri	572	1,168	1,354	987	584	11.1	22.5	25.9	18.7	11.0
Montana	6	7	1	3	4	0.7	0.9	0.1	0.4	0.5
Nebraska	18	22	14	10	14	1.1	1.4	0.9	0.6	0.9

[Continued]

★ 187 ★

Syphilis: Reported Cases and Rates, by State/Area

[Continued]

State/Area	Cases					Rates per 100,000 Population				
	1991	1992	1993	1994	1995	1991	1992	1993	1994	1995
Nevada	63	44	20	31	36	4.9	3.3	1.4	2.1	2.4
New Hampshire	20	48	26	4	0	1.8	4.3	2.3	0.4	0.0
New Jersey	1,085	595	328	240	188	14.0	7.6	4.2	3.0	2.4
New Mexico	31	40	34	18	13	2.0	2.5	2.1	1.1	0.8
New York	3,830	2,590	1,390	802	449	21.2	14.3	7.7	4.4	2.5
North Carolina	2,006	2,476	1,937	1,672	1,132	29.7	36.2	27.9	23.7	15.7
North Dakota	0	0	1	0	0	0.0	0.0	0.2	0.0	0.0
Ohio	657	888	1,180	1,187	896	6.0	8.1	10.7	10.7	8.0
Oklahoma	215	346	282	157	197	6.8	10.8	8.7	4.8	6.0
Oregon	89	47	39	22	5	3.0	1.6	1.3	0.7	0.2
Pennsylvania	1,731	1,084	697	404	248	14.5	9.0	5.8	3.3	2.1
Rhode Island	57	30	16	16	4	5.7	3.0	1.6	1.6	0.4
South Carolina	1,526	1,270	921	799	570	42.9	35.3	25.4	21.9	15.5
South Dakota	1	1	2	2	0	0.1	0.1	0.3	0.3	0.0
Tennessee	1,507	1,212	1,156	1,044	906	30.4	24.1	22.7	20.2	17.2
Texas	5,012	3,343	2,530	1,913	1,557	28.9	18.9	14.0	10.4	8.3
Utah	10	9	10	12	4	0.6	0.5	0.5	0.6	0.2
Vermont	2	1	1	0	0	0.4	0.2	0.2	0.0	0.0
Virginia	871	728	660	796	600	13.9	11.4	10.2	12.2	9.1
Washington	185	85	67	36	17	3.7	1.7	1.3	0.7	0.3
West Virginia	29	15	8	8	16	1.6	0.8	0.4	0.4	0.9
Wisconsin	641	579	493	298	185	13.0	11.6	9.8	5.9	3.6
Wyoming	6	2	4	0	1	1.3	0.4	0.9	0.0	0.2
U.S. TOTAL[1]	42,950	33,962	26,496	20,627	16,500	17.0	13.3	10.3	7.9	6.3
Northeast	7,677	4,936	2,746	1,665	1,046	15.1	9.7	5.4	3.2	2.0
Midwest	6,172	6,696	5,698	4,365	3,470	10.3	11.0	9.3	7.1	5.6
South	25,604	20,319	16,599	13,483	11,140	29.5	23.0	18.6	14.9	12.1
West	3,497	2,011	1,453	1,114	844	6.5	3.6	2.6	2.0	1.5
Guam	0	0	0	2	0	0.0	0.0	0.0	1.4	0.0
Puerto Rico	485	437	470	311	285	13.7	12.2	13.0	8.4	7.7
Virgin Islands	65	21	12	7	2	60.5	19.0	10.8	6.3	1.8
OUTLYING AREAS	550	458	482	320	287	14.5	12.0	12.4	8.1	7.2
TOTAL	43,500	34,420	26,978	20,947	16,787	17.0	13.3	10.3	7.9	6.3

Source: U.S. Department of Health and Human Services. Public Health Service. Centers for Disease Control and Prevention. Division of STD Prevention. *Sexually Transmitted Disease Surveillance, 1995.* U.S. Department of Health and Human Services, Public Health Service, September 1996. *Note:* 1. Includes cases reported by Washington, D.C.

★ 188 ★

Diseases and Illnesses: Sexually Transmitted Diseases

Syphilis: Reported Cases and Rates, by State/Area - Men

This table shows reported cases and rates of primary and secondary syphilis in men, by state/area: United States and outlying areas, 1991-1995.

State/Area	Cases					Rates per 100,000 Population				
	1991	1992	1993	1994	1995	1991	1992	1993	1994	1995
Alabama	868	532	480	372	355	44.3	26.9	23.9	18.4	17.4
Alaska	1	2	8	2	1	0.3	0.6	2.5	0.6	0.3
Arizona	194	102	61	37	32	10.5	5.4	3.1	1.8	1.5
Arkansas	432	394	259	217	228	37.8	34.1	22.1	18.3	19.0
California	1,610	953	704	499	373	10.6	6.2	4.5	3.2	2.4
Colorado	49	40	53	78	58	2.9	2.3	3.0	4.3	3.1
Connecticut	244	140	79	51	52	15.3	8.8	5.0	3.2	3.3
Delaware	100	104	37	15	12	30.3	31.1	10.9	4.4	3.4
Florida	1,537	908	691	408	194	23.9	13.9	10.4	6.0	2.8
Georgia	1,633	993	605	470	541	50.8	30.2	18.0	13.7	15.4
Hawaii	8	8	6	4	0	1.4	1.4	1.0	0.7	0.0
Idaho	3	2	2	0	0	0.6	0.4	0.4	0.0	0.0
Illinois	1,336	1,295	787	563	526	23.9	22.9	13.8	9.8	9.1
Indiana	112	167	194	139	169	4.1	6.1	7.0	5.0	6.0
Iowa	39	36	34	34	17	2.9	2.6	2.5	2.5	1.2
Kansas	111	124	70	27	25	9.1	10.0	5.6	2.2	2.0
Kentucky	65	108	184	100	102	3.6	5.9	10.0	5.4	5.4
Louisiana	1,481	1,337	1,241	755	519	72.5	64.9	60.1	36.3	24.8
Maine	2	4	5	1	2	0.3	0.7	0.8	0.2	0.3
Maryland	555	325	217	163	278	23.5	13.6	9.0	6.7	11.4
Massachusetts	289	191	66	51	42	10.0	6.6	2.3	1.8	1.4
Michigan	724	523	274	154	172	15.9	11.4	6.0	3.3	3.7
Minnesota	30	42	38	33	20	1.4	1.9	1.7	1.5	0.9
Mississippi	684	731	818	1,026	952	55.1	58.4	64.7	80.1	73.6
Missouri	309	641	716	537	301	12.4	25.6	28.3	21.1	11.7
Montana	3	4	0	0	2	0.7	1.0	0.0	0.0	0.5
Nebraska	11	11	7	7	10	1.4	1.4	0.9	0.9	1.3
Nevada	29	28	11	22	24	4.4	4.1	1.6	3.0	3.1
New Hampshire	13	36	18	4	0	2.4	6.6	3.3	0.7	0.0
New Jersey	562	303	181	127	116	15.0	8.0	4.8	3.3	3.0
New Mexico	16	27	23	8	10	2.1	3.5	2.9	1.0	1.2
New York	2,140	1,293	810	480	231	24.7	14.9	9.3	5.5	2.7
North Carolina	1,105	1,269	1,006	834	596	33.8	38.3	29.8	24.3	17.1
North Dakota	0	0	1	0	0	0.0	0.0	0.3	0.0	0.0
Ohio	389	507	579	586	479	7.4	9.6	10.8	10.9	8.9
Oklahoma	127	187	149	87	107	8.2	12.0	9.5	5.5	6.7
Oregon	50	28	29	11	3	3.5	1.9	1.9	0.7	0.2
Pennsylvania	1,036	674	417	240	156	18.1	11.7	7.2	4.1	2.7
Rhode Island	35	19	10	9	2	7.3	4.0	2.1	1.9	0.4
South Carolina	817	611	449	396	285	47.4	35.1	25.5	22.4	16.0
South Dakota	0	0	2	2	0	0.0	0.0	0.6	0.6	0.0
Tennessee	747	650	631	534	474	31.3	26.9	25.7	21.4	18.7
Texas	2,751	1,748	1,342	920	787	32.2	20.1	15.1	10.1	8.5
Utah	7	8	6	8	4	0.8	0.9	0.6	0.8	0.4
Vermont	1	0	1	0	0	0.4	0.0	0.4	0.0	0.0

[Continued]

★ 188 ★

Syphilis: Reported Cases and Rates, by State/Area - Men

[Continued]

State/Area	Cases					Rates per 100,000 Population				
	1991	1992	1993	1994	1995	1991	1992	1993	1994	1995
Virginia	481	360	341	396	301	15.6	11.5	10.7	12.3	9.3
Washington	109	51	38	25	11	4.4	2.0	1.5	0.9	0.4
West Virginia	9	5	6	7	5	1.0	0.6	0.7	0.8	0.6
Wisconsin	327	285	218	128	92	13.5	11.6	8.8	5.1	3.7
Wyoming	5	0	2	0	1	2.2	0.0	0.8	0.0	0.4
U.S. TOTAL[1]	23,599	18,026	14,074	10,665	8,731	19.2	14.5	11.2	8.4	6.8
Guam	0	0	0	1	0	0.0	0.0	0.0	1.4	0.0
Puerto Rico	254	225	254	159	144	14.8	13.0	14.5	8.9	8.0
Virgin Islands	38	12	5	3	2	73.6	22.6	9.4	5.6	3.8
OUTLYING AREAS	292	237	259	163	146	15.9	12.7	13.8	8.5	7.6
TOTAL	23,891	18,263	14,333	10,828	8,877	19.1	14.5	11.2	8.4	6.8

Source: U.S. Department of Health and Human Services. Public Health Service. Centers for Disease Control and Prevention. Division of STD Prevention. *Sexually Transmitted Disease Surveillance, 1995.* U.S. Department of Health and Human Services, Public Health Service, September 1996. *Note:* 1. Includes cases reported by Washington, D.C.

★ 189 ★

Diseases and Illnesses: Sexually Transmitted Diseases

Syphilis: Reported Cases and Rates, by State/Area - Women

This table shows reported cases and rates of primary and secondary syphilis, in women, by state/area: United States and outlying areas, 1991-1995.

State/Area	Cases					Rates per 100,000 Population				
	1991	1992	1993	1994	1995	1991	1992	1993	1994	1995
Alabama	726	479	389	289	257	34.1	22.3	17.9	13.2	11.6
Alaska	6	3	3	1	1	2.2	1.1	1.1	0.3	0.3
Arizona	140	56	34	13	14	7.4	2.9	1.7	0.6	0.7
Arkansas	463	492	300	229	267	37.7	39.7	23.9	18.0	20.8
California	1,059	587	369	308	243	7.0	3.8	2.4	2.0	1.5
Colorado	31	22	37	48	42	1.8	1.3	2.1	2.6	2.2
Connecticut	211	117	79	54	34	12.4	6.9	4.7	3.2	2.0
Delaware	94	105	57	12	7	26.8	29.6	15.8	3.3	1.9
Florida	1,186	719	500	337	189	17.3	10.3	7.1	4.7	2.6
Georgia	1,321	818	447	350	360	38.7	23.5	12.6	9.7	9.7
Hawaii	2	2	1	0	0	0.4	0.4	0.2	0.0	0.0
Idaho	4	0	0	2	0	0.8	0.0	0.0	0.4	0.0
Illinois	1,110	1,085	702	536	500	18.7	18.2	11.7	8.9	8.2
Indiana	84	127	168	147	151	2.9	4.4	5.7	5.0	5.1
Iowa	29	25	30	41	31	2.0	1.7	2.1	2.8	2.1
Kansas	91	138	60	46	22	7.2	10.8	4.7	3.5	1.7
Kentucky	47	74	147	108	83	2.5	3.8	7.5	5.5	4.2

[Continued]

★ 189 ★

Syphilis: Reported Cases and Rates, by State/Area - Women
[Continued]

State/Area	Cases					Rates per 100,000 Population				
	1991	1992	1993	1994	1995	1991	1992	1993	1994	1995
Louisiana	1,474	1,392	1,357	853	505	67.1	62.9	61.1	38.1	22.5
Maine	3	4	3	3	0	0.5	0.6	0.5	0.5	0.0
Maryland	458	267	142	129	201	18.3	10.6	5.6	5.0	7.7
Massachusetts	203	132	56	39	27	6.5	4.2	1.8	1.2	0.9
Michigan	579	428	269	138	132	12.0	8.8	5.5	2.8	2.7
Minnesota	38	48	28	23	25	1.7	2.1	1.2	1.0	1.1
Mississippi	550	731	943	1,058	1,000	40.7	53.7	68.6	76.1	71.3
Missouri	263	527	638	450	283	9.8	19.6	23.5	16.5	10.3
Montana	3	3	1	3	2	0.7	0.7	0.2	0.7	0.5
Nebraska	7	11	7	3	4	0.9	1.3	0.8	0.4	0.5
Nevada	34	16	9	9	12	5.4	2.4	1.3	1.3	1.6
New Hampshire	7	12	8	0	0	1.2	2.1	1.4	0.0	0.0
New Jersey	523	292	147	113	72	13.0	7.2	3.6	2.8	1.8
New Mexico	15	13	11	10	3	1.9	1.6	1.3	1.2	0.4
New York	1,690	1,297	580	322	218	18.0	13.8	6.1	3.4	2.3
North Carolina	901	1,207	931	838	536	25.9	34.3	26.0	23.0	14.5
North Dakota	0	0	0	0	0	0.0	0.0	0.0	0.0	0.0
Ohio	268	381	601	601	417	4.7	6.7	10.5	10.5	7.2
Oklahoma	88	159	133	70	90	5.4	9.7	8.0	4.2	5.4
Oregon	39	19	10	11	2	2.6	1.3	0.6	0.7	0.1
Pennsylvania	695	410	280	164	92	11.2	6.6	4.5	2.6	1.5
Rhode Island	22	11	6	7	2	4.2	2.1	1.2	1.4	0.4
South Carolina	709	659	472	403	285	38.7	35.6	25.2	21.5	15.1
South Dakota	1	1	0	0	0	0.3	0.3	0.0	0.0	0.0
Tennessee	760	562	525	510	432	29.6	21.6	19.9	19.0	15.9
Texas	2,261	1,595	1,188	993	770	25.7	17.8	13.0	10.6	8.1
Utah	3	1	4	4	0	0.3	0.1	0.4	0.4	0.0
Vermont	1	1	0	0	0	0.3	0.3	0.0	0.0	0.0
Virginia	390	368	319	400	299	12.2	11.3	9.7	12.0	8.9
Washington	76	34	29	11	6	3.0	1.3	1.1	0.4	0.2
West Virginia	20	10	2	1	11	2.1	1.1	0.2	0.1	1.2
Wisconsin	274	294	275	170	93	10.8	11.5	10.7	6.6	3.6
Wyoming	1	2	2	0	0	0.4	0.9	0.9	0.0	0.0
U.S. TOTAL[1]	19,311	15,936	12,422	9,929	7,768	14.9	12.2	9.4	7.5	5.8
Guam	0	0	0	1	0	0.0	0.0	0.0	1.5	0.0
Puerto Rico	231	212	216	152	141	12.6	11.5	11.6	8.0	7.3
Virgin Islands	27	9	7	4	0	48.3	15.6	12.2	6.9	0.0
OUTLYING AREAS	258	221	223	157	141	13.2	11.2	11.2	7.7	6.9
TOTAL	19,569	16,157	12,645	10,086	7,909	14.9	12.2	9.4	7.5	5.8

Source: U.S. Department of Health and Human Services. Public Health Service. Centers for Disease Control and Prevention. Division of STD Prevention. *Sexually Transmitted Disease Surveillance, 1995.* U.S. Department of Health and Human Services, Public Health Service, September 1996. *Note:* 1. Includes cases reported by Washington, D.C.

★ 190 ★

Diseases and Illnesses: Sexually Transmitted Diseases

Syphilis: Reported Cases and Rates for Late Latent Syphilis, by State/Area

This table shows reported cases and rates of late latent syphilis by state/area: United States and outlying areas, 1991-1995.

State/Area	Cases					Rates per 100,000 Population				
	1991	1992	1993	1994	1995	1991	1992	1993	1994	1995
Alabama	421	303	460	453	334	10.3	7.3	11.0	10.7	7.9
Alaska	22	22	39	18	15	3.9	3.7	6.5	3.0	2.5
Arizona	251	246	330	256	248	6.7	6.4	8.4	6.3	5.9
Arkansas	147	143	154	197	217	6.2	6.0	6.4	8.0	8.7
California	5,244	4,210	5,544	4,493	3,500	17.2	13.6	17.8	14.3	11.1
Colorado	112	92	119	115	134	3.3	2.7	3.3	3.1	3.6
Connecticut	287	220	206	122	86	8.7	6.7	6.3	3.7	2.6
Delaware	49	62	62	47	52	7.2	9.0	8.9	6.6	7.3
Florida	1,962	1,978	2,447	1,909	1,489	14.8	14.6	17.8	13.7	10.5
Georgia	819	656	738	683	1,104	12.4	9.7	10.7	9.7	15.3
Hawaii	18	20	27	32	25	1.6	1.7	2.3	2.7	2.1
Idaho	15	14	12	8	11	1.4	1.3	1.1	0.7	0.9
Illinois	563	545	708	835	728	4.9	4.7	6.1	7.1	6.2
Indiana	91	124	192	209	172	1.6	2.2	3.4	3.6	3.0
Iowa	29	31	28	64	45	1.0	1.1	1.0	2.3	1.6
Kansas	71	77	85	64	62	2.8	3.1	3.4	2.5	2.4
Kentucky	106	107	155	134	143	2.9	2.9	4.1	3.5	3.7
Louisiana	1,251	1,430	1,311	1,409	1,034	29.5	33.5	30.6	32.6	23.8
Maine	1	0	18	0	2	0.1	0.0	1.5	0.0	0.2
Maryland	715	646	842	553	372	14.7	13.2	17.0	11.1	7.4
Massachusetts	358	315	478	326	283	6.0	5.3	7.9	5.4	4.7
Michigan	289	360	348	325	304	3.1	3.8	3.7	3.4	3.2
Minnesota	70	76	90	62	85	1.6	1.7	2.0	1.4	1.8
Mississippi	62	85	380	247	126	2.4	3.3	14.4	9.2	4.7
Missouri	113	125	258	219	135	2.2	2.4	4.9	4.1	2.5
Montana	0	0	0	1	0	0.0	0.0	0.0	0.1	0.0
Nebraska	22	28	12	23	18	1.4	1.7	0.7	1.4	1.1
Nevada	86	45	52	62	89	6.7	3.4	3.8	4.2	5.8
New Hampshire	2	2	7	10	29	0.2	0.2	0.6	0.9	2.5
New Jersey	1,627	1,258	1,482	1,411	893	21.0	16.1	18.9	17.9	11.2
New Mexico	103	58	106	143	100	6.7	3.7	6.6	8.6	5.9
New York	5,796	5,734	6,077	5,503	6,005	32.1	31.7	33.5	30.3	33.1
North Carolina	612	818	779	819	670	9.1	12.0	11.2	11.6	9.3
North Dakota	0	0	0	0	0	0.0	0.0	0.0	0.0	0.0
Ohio	185	185	176	377	281	1.7	1.7	1.6	3.4	2.5
Oklahoma	110	79	85	95	95	3.5	2.5	2.6	2.9	2.9
Oregon	95	113	104	57	45	3.3	3.8	3.4	1.8	1.4
Pennsylvania	460	391	326	322	420	3.9	3.3	2.7	2.7	3.5
Rhode Island	127	127	113	112	72	12.6	12.7	11.3	11.3	7.3
South Carolina	394	360	316	252	266	11.1	10.0	8.7	6.9	7.2
South Dakota	5	0	0	6	6	0.7	0.0	0.0	0.8	0.8
Tennessee	134	426	617	588	540	2.7	8.5	12.1	11.4	10.3
Texas	2,337	1,736	2,740	3,022	3,152	13.5	9.8	15.2	16.4	16.8
Utah	61	34	48	36	39	3.5	1.9	2.6	1.9	2.0
Vermont	3	1	0	1	0	0.5	0.2	0.0	0.2	0.0

[Continued]

★ 190 ★

Syphilis: Reported Cases and Rates for Late Latent Syphilis, by State/Area

[Continued]

State/Area	Cases					Rates per 100,000 Population				
	1991	1992	1993	1994	1995	1991	1992	1993	1994	1995
Virginia	1,016	590	662	492	419	16.2	9.2	10.2	7.5	6.3
Washington	262	255	243	207	181	5.2	5.0	4.6	3.9	3.3
West Virginia	259	224	164	152	38	14.4	12.4	9.0	8.3	2.1
Wisconsin	66	36	81	99	90	1.3	0.7	1.6	1.9	1.8
Wyoming	8	1	4	3	1	1.7	0.2	0.9	0.6	0.2
U.S. TOTAL[1]	27,490	25,084	29,675	26,840	24,356	10.9	9.8	11.5	10.3	9.3
Guam	10	2	3	4	6	7.1	1.4	2.1	2.8	4.3
Puerto Rico	478	527	820	753	582	13.5	14.7	22.6	20.4	15.6
Virgin Islands	2	0	0	0	0	1.9	0.0	0.0	0.0	0.0
OUTLYING AREAS	490	529	823	757	588	12.9	13.8	21.2	19.2	14.8
TOTAL	27,980	25,613	30,498	27,597	24,944	10.9	9.9	11.7	10.4	9.4

Source: U.S. Department of Health and Human Services. Public Health Service. Centers for Disease Control and Prevention. Division of STD Prevention. *Sexually Transmitted Disease Surveillance, 1995.* U.S. Department of Health and Human Services, Public Health Service, September 1996. *Note:* 1. Includes cases reported by Washington, D.C.

★ 191 ★

Diseases and Illnesses: Sexually Transmitted Diseases

Syphilis: Reported Cases and Rates of Early Latent Syphilis, by State/Area

This table shows reported cases and rates of early latent syphilis by state/area: United States and outlying areas, 1991-1995.

State/Area	Cases					Rates per 100,000 Population				
	1991	1992	1993	1994	1995	1991	1992	1993	1994	1995
Alabama	1,441	1,281	978	799	676	35.3	31.0	23.4	18.9	15.9
Alaska	2	3	1	1	3	0.4	0.5	0.2	0.2	0.5
Arizona	224	118	116	97	113	6.0	3.1	2.9	2.4	2.7
Arkansas	859	1,119	879	656	529	36.2	46.7	36.2	26.7	21.3
California	4,278	3,532	2,571	1,825	1,470	14.1	11.4	8.2	5.8	4.7
Colorado	35	52	70	51	68	1.0	1.5	2.0	1.4	1.8
Connecticut	578	340	188	104	92	17.6	10.4	5.7	3.2	2.8
Delaware	114	162	115	59	57	16.8	23.5	16.4	8.3	7.9
Florida	5,090	4,378	3,544	2,320	1,484	38.3	32.4	25.8	16.6	10.5
Georgia	4,093	3,305	2,208	1,639	1,616	61.8	48.9	32.0	23.2	22.4
Hawaii	14	11	7	5	0	1.2	1.0	0.6	0.4	0.0
Idaho	14	11	1	0	1	1.3	1.0	0.1	0.0	0.1
Illinois	2,601	3,002	2,316	1,685	1,774	22.6	25.9	19.8	14.3	15.0
Indiana	178	345	464	338	377	3.2	6.1	8.1	5.9	6.5
Iowa	64	63	82	90	77	2.3	2.2	2.9	3.2	2.7
Kansas	100	110	75	48	40	4.0	4.4	3.0	1.9	1.6
Kentucky	95	97	156	179	166	2.6	2.6	4.1	4.7	4.3

[Continued]

★ 191 ★

Syphilis: Reported Cases and Rates of Early Latent Syphilis, by State/Area
[Continued]

State/Area	Cases					Rates per 100,000 Population				
	1991	1992	1993	1994	1995	1991	1992	1993	1994	1995
Louisiana	2,261	2,430	2,787	2,314	1,598	53.3	56.9	65.0	53.6	36.8
Maine	6	4	3	5	0	0.5	0.3	0.2	0.4	0.0
Maryland	1,311	907	634	651	606	27.0	18.5	12.8	13.0	12.0
Massachusetts	548	404	329	200	154	9.1	6.7	5.5	3.3	2.5
Michigan	1,808	1,378	977	589	567	19.3	14.6	10.3	6.2	5.9
Minnesota	68	103	96	81	55	1.5	2.3	2.1	1.8	1.2
Mississippi	1,505	1,874	2,058	2,160	2,389	58.1	71.7	78.0	80.9	88.6
Missouri	252	620	791	707	506	4.9	11.9	15.1	13.4	9.5
Montana	7	7	3	5	9	0.9	0.9	0.4	0.6	1.0
Nebraska	21	10	8	13	3	1.3	0.6	0.5	0.8	0.2
Nevada	143	78	64	75	68	11.1	5.9	4.6	5.1	4.4
New Hampshire	15	13	17	4	3	1.4	1.2	1.5	0.4	0.3
New Jersey	898	775	579	357	294	11.6	9.9	7.4	4.5	3.7
New Mexico	46	40	32	17	25	3.0	2.5	2.0	1.0	1.5
New York	7,676	6,144	4,278	2,682	2,100	42.6	34.0	23.6	14.8	11.6
North Carolina	1,263	1,864	1,678	1,488	1,231	18.7	27.3	24.1	21.0	17.1
North Dakota	2	2	3	1	0	0.3	0.3	0.5	0.2	0.0
Ohio	574	1,021	1,462	1,105	723	5.3	9.3	13.2	10.0	6.5
Oklahoma	276	362	343	230	280	8.7	11.3	10.6	7.1	8.5
Oregon	92	56	32	21	17	3.2	1.9	1.1	0.7	0.5
Pennsylvania	3,589	3,651	3,072	1,897	1,212	30.0	30.5	25.5	15.7	10.0
Rhode Island	55	23	16	11	14	5.5	2.3	1.6	1.1	1.4
South Carolina	1,305	1,129	1,019	793	791	36.7	31.4	28.1	21.8	21.5
South Dakota	4	0	1	0	1	0.6	0.0	0.1	0.0	0.1
Tennessee	2,069	1,574	1,416	1,289	1,129	41.8	31.4	27.8	24.9	21.5
Texas	5,771	5,443	4,388	3,869	3,015	33.2	30.8	24.3	21.0	16.1
Utah	10	10	10	3	7	0.6	0.6	0.5	0.2	0.4
Vermont	1	0	0	0	0	0.2	0.0	0.0	0.0	0.0
Virginia	811	636	625	613	546	12.9	10.0	9.7	9.4	8.2
Washington	114	64	46	35	12	2.3	1.2	0.9	0.7	0.2
West Virginia	71	27	17	17	11	3.9	1.5	0.9	0.9	0.6
Wisconsin	279	323	509	382	299	5.6	6.5	10.1	7.5	5.8
Wyoming	0	2	1	0	0	0.0	0.4	0.2	0.0	0.0
U.S. TOTAL[1]	53,855	49,903	41,902	32,012	26,604	21.4	19.6	16.3	12.3	10.1
Guam	0	0	2	1	0	0.0	0.0	1.4	0.7	0.0
Puerto Rico	949	956	1,174	934	738	26.8	26.7	32.4	25.3	19.8
Virgin Islands	55	28	26	23	17	51.2	25.3	23.5	20.8	15.3
OUTLYING AREAS	1,004	984	1,202	958	755	26.4	25.7	31.0	24.3	19.0
TOTAL	54,859	50,887	43,104	32,970	27,359	21.4	19.7	16.5	12.5	10.3

Source: U.S. Department of Health and Human Services. Public Health Service. Centers for Disease Control and Prevention. Division of STD Prevention. *Sexually Transmitted Disease Surveillance, 1995.* U.S. Department of Health and Human Services, Public Health Service, September 1996. *Note:* 1. Includes cases reported by Washington, D.C.

★ 192 ★

Diseases and Illnesses: Sexually Transmitted Diseases

Syphilis: State Rankings, 1995

This table shows reported cases and rates for primary and secondary syphilis for states and areas, ranked according to rates. Data are for 1995.

State/Area	Cases	Rate per 100,000 population	Rank
Mississippi	1,952	72.4	1
Louisiana	1,024	23.6	2
Arkansas	495	19.9	3
Tennessee	906	17.2	4
North Carolina	1,132	15.7	5
South Carolina	570	15.5	6
Alabama	612	14.4	7
Georgia	901	12.5	8
Missouri	584	11.0	9
Maryland	479	9.5	10
Virginia	600	9.1	11
Illinois	1,026	8.7	12
Texas	1,557	8.3	13
Ohio	896	8.0	14
Puerto Rico	285	7.7	15
U.S. TOTAL[1]	16,500	6.3	
Oklahoma	197	6.0	16
Indiana	321	5.5	17
Kentucky	185	4.8	18
YEAR 2000 OBJECTIVE[2]		4.0	
Wisconsin	185	3.6	19
Michigan	304	3.2	20
Florida	383	2.7	21
Colorado	100	2.7	22
Delaware	19	2.6	23
Connecticut	86	2.6	24
New York	449	2.5	25
New Jersey	188	2.4	26
Nevada	36	2.4	27
Pennsylvania	248	2.1	28
California	616	2.0	29
Kansas	47	1.8	30
Virgin Islands	2	1.8	31
Iowa	48	1.7	32
Massachusetts	69	1.1	33
Arizona	46	1.1	34
Minnesota	45	1.0	35
West Virginia	16	0.9	36
Nebraska	14	0.9	37
New Mexico	13	0.8	38

[Continued]

★ 192 ★

Syphilis: State Rankings, 1995
[Continued]

State/Area	Cases	Rate per 100,000 population	Rank
Montana	4	0.5	39
Rhode Island	4	0.4	40
Alaska	2	0.3	41
Washington	17	0.3	42
Wyoming	1	0.2	43
Utah	4	0.2	44
Maine	2	0.2	45
Oregon	5	0.2	46
Hawaii	0	0.0	47
Idaho	0	0.0	48
New Hampshire	0	0.0	49
North Dakota	0	0.0	50
South Dakota	0	0.0	51
Vermont	0	0.0	52
Guam	0	0.0	53

Source: U.S. Department of Health and Human Services. Public Health Service. Centers for Disease Control and Prevention. Division of STD Prevention. *Sexually Transmitted Disease Surveillance, 1995.* U.S. Department of Health and Human Services, Public Health Service, September 1996. *Notes:* 1. Includes cases reported by Washington, D.C. 2. Revised from 10.0 to 4.0,

★ 193 ★

Diseases and Illnesses: Sexually Transmitted Diseases

Syphilis: Urban Distribution - Men

This table shows reported cases and rates of primary and secondary stage syphilis in men, in selected cities of 200,000+ population: United States and outlying areas, 1991-1995.

State/Area	Cases					Rates per 100,000 Population				
	1991	1992	1993	1994	1995	1991	1992	1993	1994	1995
Akron, OH	15	7	3	2	1	6.0	2.8	1.2	0.8	0.4
Albuquerque, NM	7	12	10	5	4	2.9	4.9	4.0	2.0	1.6
Atlanta, GA	615	376	221	174	210	196.6	118.5	68.4	52.7	62.7
Austin, TX	59	50	55	31	10	19.8	16.3	17.4	9.6	3.0
Baltimore, MD	128	122	97	87	208	37.4	36.0	29.0	26.5	64.4
Birmingham, AL	193	159	162	154	155	63.1	51.8	52.8	50.1	50.4
Boston, MA	113	46	20	16	25	41.8	17.3	7.5	6.0	9.4
Buffalo, NY	19	11	17	4	1	12.1	7.0	10.8	2.6	0.6
Charlotte, NC	205	173	116	112	64	80.8	67.1	44.0	41.3	23.0
Chicago, IL	1,133	1,031	547	361	328	80.2	72.7	38.5	25.4	23.1
Cincinnati, OH	46	109	206	223	131	11.2	26.4	49.9	54.2	32.0
Cleveland, OH	148	222	235	196	135	22.3	33.5	35.5	29.7	20.5
Columbus, OH	38	7	5	6	2	8.1	1.5	1.0	1.2	0.4
Corpus Christi, TX	19	13	11	10	2	13.1	8.8	7.3	6.6	1.3
Dallas, TX	624	342	212	162	133	67.0	36.3	22.3	16.9	13.8

[Continued]

★ 193 ★

Syphilis: Urban Distribution - Men
[Continued]

State/Area	Cases					Rates per 100,000 Population				
	1991	1992	1993	1994	1995	1991	1992	1993	1994	1995
Dayton, OH	28	46	40	74	144	10.2	16.6	14.5	27.0	52.6
Denver, CO	29	19	29	52	43	12.6	8.0	12.1	21.7	17.9
Des Moines, IA	17	26	18	18	8	10.7	16.1	11.0	10.9	4.8
Detroit, MI	537	309	137	81	76	105.3	60.8	27.1	16.2	15.2
El Paso, TX	20	9	9	5	2	6.7	3.0	2.9	1.5	0.6
Fort Worth, TX	186	172	184	93	67	31.2	28.5	30.1	14.9	10.6
Honolulu, HI	8	7	5	4	0	1.9	1.6	1.1	0.9	0.0
Houston, TX	986	545	327	212	202	68.4	37.0	21.9	14.0	13.2
Indianapolis, IN	19	22	63	32	40	5.0	5.7	16.3	8.2	10.3
Jacksonville, FL	89	52	36	56	28	26.4	15.2	10.5	16.4	8.2
Jersey City, NJ	26	15	10	8	19	24.6	14.1	9.4	7.6	18.0
Kansas City, MO	178	151	96	37	9	85.5	72.5	46.1	17.7	4.3
Los Angeles, CA	687	492	360	206	188	16.4	11.6	8.4	4.8	4.4
Louisville, KY	35	75	154	69	68	11.1	23.7	48.6	21.7	21.4
Memphis, TN	390	310	294	254	239	98.1	77.3	72.8	62.3	58.1
Miami, FL	320	193	178	106	32	33.7	20.1	18.5	10.9	3.3
Milwaukee, WI	311	267	197	121	75	68.5	59.1	43.8	27.2	17.0
Minneapolis, MN	22	27	25	24	10	12.0	14.7	13.6	12.9	5.4
Nashville, TN	151	104	85	51	54	62.0	42.3	34.3	20.3	21.4
New Orleans, LA	392	321	236	105	133	171.8	141.0	104.2	46.6	59.3
New York City, NY	1,767	1,104	666	382	184	51.5	32.2	19.3	11.1	5.4
Newark, NJ	170	90	56	35	29	122.7	65.0	40.6	25.5	21.3
Norfolk, VA	72	80	47	61	68	53.4	59.2	35.2	47.2	53.9
Oakland, CA	99	73	41	27	7	17.0	12.4	6.9	4.6	1.2
Oklahoma City, OK	49	97	89	64	57	24.1	47.2	42.9	30.5	27.1
Omaha, NE	10	11	5	2	5	4.9	5.4	2.4	1.0	2.4
Philadelphia, PA	859	593	313	188	127	117.8	82.1	43.7	26.5	18.2
Phoenix, AZ	170	90	34	21	30	15.9	8.3	3.0	1.8	2.5
Pittsburgh, PA	37	24	8	8	2	5.9	3.8	1.3	1.3	0.3
Portland, OR	31	20	18	9	3	13.6	8.7	7.7	3.8	1.3
Richmond, VA	48	49	30	21	18	52.3	53.5	32.9	23.2	19.9
Rochester, NY	71	49	36	34	8	61.2	41.9	30.7	29.0	6.8
Sacramento, CA	42	19	6	6	3	7.9	3.6	1.1	1.1	0.6
San Antonio, TX	122	62	39	25	23	20.8	10.4	6.4	4.0	3.7
San Diego, CA	172	68	63	66	32	13.2	5.1	4.7	4.9	2.4
San Francisco, CA	121	73	51	32	27	33.3	20.0	13.9	8.8	7.4
San Jose, CA	23	23	18	1	2	3.0	3.0	2.3	0.1	0.3
Seattle, WA	47	33	11	8	4	6.2	4.3	1.4	1.0	0.5
St. Louis, MO	70	336	477	347	196	39.2	191.5	277.9	206.9	119.7
St. Paul, MN	3	10	5	4	3	2.3	7.5	3.8	3.0	2.3
St. Petersburg, FL	129	75	88	43	11	32.0	18.6	21.8	10.6	2.7
Tampa, FL	83	41	16	16	14	20.1	9.8	3.8	3.8	3.2
Toledo, OH	75	86	47	16	13	34.1	39.1	21.4	7.3	6.0
Tucson, AZ	15	5	20	9	1	4.5	1.5	5.8	2.5	0.3
Tulsa, OK	33	39	36	7	25	18.6	21.7	19.9	3.8	13.7
Washington, DC	413	220	168	98	64	148.9	80.4	62.2	37.0	24.7

[Continued]

★ 193 ★

Syphilis: Urban Distribution - Men
[Continued]

State/Area	Cases					Rates per 100,000 Population				
	1991	1992	1993	1994	1995	1991	1992	1993	1994	1995
Wichita, KS	10	2	2	4	8	5.0	1.0	1.0	1.9	3.9
Yonkers, NY	24	16	7	3	1	26.8	17.8	7.7	3.3	1.1
U.S. CITY TOTAL	12,558	9,230	6,797	4,688	3,811	38.4	28.0	20.5	14.1	11.4
San Juan, PR	110	101	95	66	30	28.0	25.7	24.2	16.8	7.6
TOTAL	12,668	9,331	6,892	4,754	3,841	38.3	28.0	20.5	14.1	11.4

Source: U.S. Department of Health and Human Services. Public Health Service. Centers for Disease Control and Prevention. Division of STD Prevention. *Sexually Transmitted Disease Surveillance, 1995.* U.S. Department of Health and Human Services, Public Health Service, September 1996.

★ 194 ★

Diseases and Illnesses: Sexually Transmitted Diseases

Syphilis: Urban Distribution - Women

This table shows reported cases and rates of primary and secondary stage syphilis in women, in selected cities of 200,000+ population: United States and outlying areas, 1991-1995.

State/Area	Cases					Rates per 100,000 Population				
	1991	1992	1993	1994	1995	1991	1992	1993	1994	1995
Akron, OH	14	8	3	0	0	5.2	2.9	1.1	0.0	0.0
Albuquerque, NM	7	10	4	8	2	2.8	3.9	1.5	3.0	0.7
Atlanta, GA	413	231	114	87	110	120.5	66.5	32.2	24.1	30.1
Austin, TX	30	41	45	29	7	10.1	13.4	14.3	9.0	2.1
Baltimore, MD	77	66	47	72	134	19.7	17.1	12.3	19.2	36.4
Birmingham, AL	146	140	133	106	109	41.9	40.1	38.1	30.3	31.1
Boston, MA	95	37	14	8	15	32.5	12.9	4.9	2.8	5.2
Buffalo, NY	18	8	16	4	1	10.4	4.6	9.3	2.3	0.6
Charlotte, NC	160	136	93	102	61	58.4	48.9	32.6	34.9	20.3
Chicago, IL	912	848	469	287	254	59.8	55.5	30.6	18.7	16.6
Cincinnati, OH	28	81	189	250	121	6.1	17.7	41.2	54.7	26.6
Cleveland, OH	107	163	282	215	128	14.3	21.8	37.8	28.9	17.3
Columbus, OH	16	9	3	2	5	3.2	1.8	0.6	0.4	1.0
Corpus Christi, TX	18	11	6	10	6	11.9	7.2	3.8	6.3	3.8
Dallas, TX	591	339	198	130	135	61.5	34.9	20.2	13.2	13.6
Dayton, OH	20	27	36	53	100	6.7	9.0	12.0	17.8	33.7
Denver, CO	22	15	15	31	25	9.1	6.0	5.9	12.3	9.8
Des Moines, IA	13	16	15	19	19	7.5	9.1	8.4	10.5	10.4
Detroit, MI	471	243	140	72	54	83.3	43.2	25.0	13.0	9.8
El Paso, TX	8	4	8	0	0	2.5	1.2	2.4	0.0	0.0
Fort Worth, TX	161	155	167	97	73	26.5	25.2	26.8	15.2	11.3
Honolulu, HI	2	1	1	0	0	0.5	0.2	0.2	0.0	0.0
Houston, TX	696	467	244	231	215	47.7	31.3	16.1	15.1	13.9
Indianapolis, IN	13	33	57	30	34	3.1	7.8	13.3	7.0	7.9

[Continued]

★ 194 ★

Syphilis: Urban Distribution - Women

[Continued]

State/Area	Cases					Rates per 100,000 Population				
	1991	1992	1993	1994	1995	1991	1992	1993	1994	1995
Jacksonville, FL	78	53	37	52	22	22.1	14.8	10.3	14.5	6.1
Jersey City, NJ	36	18	12	6	8	32.0	16.0	10.7	5.4	7.2
Kansas City, MO	137	132	66	36	15	59.8	57.7	28.8	15.7	6.5
Los Angeles, CA	415	291	171	140	119	9.9	6.8	4.0	3.3	2.8
Louisville, KY	20	42	121	78	60	5.7	11.9	34.2	22.0	16.9
Memphis, TN	437	295	255	279	238	99.9	66.8	57.4	62.1	52.5
Miami, FL	189	133	88	69	19	18.4	12.7	8.5	6.6	1.8
Milwaukee, WI	267	280	272	158	75	53.1	55.9	54.7	32.1	15.3
Minneapolis, MN	33	38	18	14	14	16.9	19.5	9.2	7.1	7.1
Nashville, TN	139	120	64	49	43	51.7	44.2	23.4	17.7	15.4
New Orleans, LA	314	259	161	98	88	119.5	98.9	61.8	37.8	34.1
New York City, NY	1,371	1,139	466	247	180	35.4	29.4	12.0	6.4	4.6
Newark, NJ	130	77	44	25	14	84.1	49.9	28.6	16.4	9.2
Norfolk, VA	57	74	42	61	62	48.2	62.5	35.9	53.8	55.7
Oakland, CA	110	50	35	24	8	18.3	8.2	5.7	3.9	1.3
Oklahoma City, OK	33	82	88	51	49	15.0	37.0	39.3	22.5	21.6
Omaha, NE	7	7	3	3	2	3.2	3.2	1.4	1.3	0.9
Philadelphia, PA	552	314	202	110	72	65.9	37.9	24.6	13.5	9.0
Phoenix, AZ	110	53	21	7	13	10.0	4.7	1.8	0.6	1.1
Pittsburgh, PA	57	30	3	1	2	8.0	4.2	0.4	0.1	0.3
Portland, OR	25	14	6	9	1	10.4	5.7	2.4	3.6	0.4
Richmond, VA	48	68	25	18	19	43.9	62.6	23.1	16.7	17.7
Rochester, NY	65	38	35	25	10	51.8	30.0	27.6	19.8	7.9
Sacramento, CA	53	10	2	3	2	9.6	1.8	0.4	0.5	0.4
San Antonio, TX	86	49	42	37	27	13.8	7.7	6.5	5.6	4.0
San Diego, CA	103	42	43	32	20	8.2	3.3	3.4	2.5	1.5
San Francisco, CA	62	24	18	13	5	17.1	6.6	4.9	3.5	1.4
San Jose, CA	13	11	9	3	1	1.7	1.5	1.2	0.4	0.1
Seattle, WA	35	18	11	3	1	4.5	2.3	1.4	0.4	0.1
St. Louis, MO	66	272	431	304	165	31.0	130.0	210.6	152.1	84.6
St. Paul, MN	1	3	5	3	4	0.7	2.1	3.5	2.1	2.8
St. Petersburg, FL	93	57	66	31	9	20.2	12.4	14.3	6.7	1.9
Tampa, FL	55	34	9	15	19	12.7	7.8	2.0	3.3	4.2
Toledo, OH	57	57	50	19	9	23.6	23.7	20.9	8.0	3.8
Tucson, AZ	13	2	12	3	0	3.8	0.6	3.3	0.8	0.0
Tulsa, OK	31	42	25	2	23	16.2	21.7	12.8	1.0	11.8
Washington, DC	351	200	123	72	48	110.7	64.1	39.9	23.8	16.3
Wichita, KS	6	8	4	6	8	2.9	3.8	1.9	2.8	3.7
Yonkers, NY	26	6	4	2	1	26.3	6.0	4.0	2.0	1.0
U.S. CITY TOTAL	9,719	7,531	5,388	3,951	3,083	28.0	21.5	15.3	11.2	8.7

[Continued]

★ 194 ★

Syphilis: Urban Distribution - Women
[Continued]

State/Area	Cases					Rates per 100,000 Population				
	1991	1992	1993	1994	1995	1991	1992	1993	1994	1995
San Juan, PR	89	83	94	65	40	18.6	17.3	19.6	13.6	8.3
TOTAL	9,808	7,614	5,482	4,016	3,123	27.9	21.5	15.4	11.2	8.7

Source: U.S. Department of Health and Human Services. Public Health Service. Centers for Disease Control and Prevention. Division of STD Prevention. *Sexually Transmitted Disease Surveillance, 1995.* U.S. Department of Health and Human Services, Public Health Service, September 1996.

★ 195 ★

Diseases and Illnesses: Sexually Transmitted Diseases

Syphilis: Urban Distribution of All Stages

This table shows reported cases and rates of syphilis, in all its stages, in selected cities of 200,000+ population: United States and outlying areas, 1991-1995.

State/Area	Cases					Rates per 100,000 Population				
	1991	1992	1993	1994	1995	1991	1992	1993	1994	1995
Akron, OH	57	44	13	13	9	11.0	8.4	2.5	2.5	1.7
Albuquerque, NM	70	50	84	87	41	14.3	10.0	16.6	16.9	7.8
Atlanta, GA	2,547	1,805	1,226	917	1,074	388.4	271.6	181.1	132.7	153.3
Austin, TX	263	232	292	260	183	44.2	37.8	46.3	40.2	27.5
Baltimore, MD	728	573	507	673	880	99.4	79.0	70.9	95.8	127.3
Birmingham, AL	817	745	765	664	639	124.8	113.6	116.6	101.1	97.1
Boston, MA	538	367	338	219	193	95.6	66.2	61.1	39.8	34.7
Buffalo, NY	132	85	117	52	31	40.1	25.8	35.6	15.9	9.5
Charlotte, NC	731	727	535	506	347	138.5	135.6	97.5	89.8	59.9
Chicago, IL	4,624	4,857	3,368	2,335	2,244	157.5	164.8	114.1	79.1	76.1
Cincinnati, OH	145	294	668	839	398	16.7	33.8	76.7	96.7	46.1
Cleveland, OH	581	1,069	1,525	1,160	756	41.2	75.8	108.3	82.7	54.1
Columbus, OH	155	88	70	71	31	15.9	8.9	7.0	7.1	3.1
Corpus Christi, TX	92	81	49	83	62	31.0	26.9	16.0	26.7	19.8
Dallas, TX	2,233	1,700	1,322	1,130	1,024	118.1	89.0	68.6	58.1	52.3
Dayton, OH	76	123	129	236	400	13.2	21.3	22.4	41.2	70.1
Denver, CO	110	94	146	177	180	23.2	19.4	29.6	35.9	36.4
Des Moines, IA	72	78	77	110	92	21.7	23.1	22.5	31.8	26.3
Detroit, MI	2,733	1,802	1,190	775	706	254.1	168.2	111.8	73.3	67.1
El Paso, TX	230	184	222	183	142	37.5	29.3	34.3	27.4	20.9
Fort Worth, TX	630	682	834	592	492	52.3	55.9	67.5	47.0	38.5
Honolulu, HI	39	35	40	41	22	4.6	4.1	4.6	4.7	2.5
Houston, TX	4,969	4,283	3,450	2,909	2,680	171.2	144.5	114.8	95.5	87.1
Indianapolis, IN	127	127	283	176	168	15.8	15.7	34.7	21.5	20.5
Jacksonville, FL	421	381	217	289	194	61.1	54.4	31.0	41.3	27.6
Jersey City, NJ	289	232	208	171	138	132.4	106.2	95.3	78.5	63.5
Kansas City, MO	469	469	287	168	69	107.2	107.3	65.7	38.4	15.7
Los Angeles, CA	6,926	6,284	5,619	3,931	3,144	82.6	74.0	65.7	46.0	36.8
Louisville, KY	95	199	434	325	273	14.2	29.7	64.7	48.4	40.6

[Continued]

Syphilis: Urban Distribution of All Stages
[Continued]

State/Area	Cases					Rates per 100,000 Population				
	1991	1992	1993	1994	1995	1991	1992	1993	1994	1995
Memphis, TN	2,428	1,943	1,899	1,738	1,597	290.7	230.6	224.0	202.8	184.6
Miami, FL	1,989	1,790	2,041	1,453	1,014	100.6	89.2	102.0	71.9	49.9
Milwaukee, WI	918	869	952	688	459	95.9	91.2	100.6	73.4	49.3
Minneapolis, MN	125	162	132	122	86	33.1	42.8	34.7	31.9	22.4
Nashville, TN	473	421	381	234	202	92.3	81.4	73.0	44.4	38.1
New Orleans, LA	1,589	1,495	1,120	845	649	323.6	305.5	229.9	174.3	134.7
New York City, NY	15,912	13,459	10,513	8,001	7,791	217.8	184.2	143.5	109.3	106.5
Newark, NJ	699	520	563	518	390	238.5	177.7	192.8	178.7	135.6
Norfolk, VA	250	308	234	247	278	98.8	121.4	93.4	101.8	117.0
Oakland, CA	671	556	431	336	161	56.8	46.5	35.8	27.9	13.3
Oklahoma City, OK	195	337	391	299	288	46.2	78.9	90.6	68.6	65.9
Omaha, NE	50	45	24	28	21	11.9	10.6	5.6	6.5	4.8
Philadelphia, PA	5,204	4,811	3,752	2,394	1,693	332.2	310.3	244.0	157.4	112.9
Phoenix, AZ	657	413	325	237	270	30.3	18.7	14.3	10.1	11.1
Pittsburgh, PA	188	132	58	39	28	14.1	9.9	4.4	3.0	2.1
Portland, OR	163	135	107	63	42	34.7	28.4	22.3	13.1	8.7
Richmond, VA	313	311	203	128	121	155.7	155.3	101.7	64.6	61.0
Rochester, NY	311	289	239	200	104	128.7	118.7	97.8	82.1	42.8
Sacramento, CA	222	99	123	128	72	20.6	9.1	11.2	11.7	6.5
San Antonio, TX	707	499	518	491	395	58.5	40.5	41.2	38.5	30.5
San Diego, CA	597	548	535	492	348	23.4	21.1	20.5	18.7	13.2
San Francisco, CA	658	353	160	89	83	90.6	48.4	21.8	12.2	11.4
San Jose, CA	97	132	131	72	38	6.4	8.6	8.5	4.6	2.4
Seattle, WA	219	193	180	126	93	14.3	12.4	11.4	8.0	5.8
St. Louis, MO	227	895	1,525	1,212	736	58.0	232.6	405.3	329.7	205.2
St. Paul, MN	23	41	37	27	28	8.3	14.8	13.4	9.8	10.2
St. Petersburg, FL	615	429	419	317	170	71.4	49.7	48.5	36.6	19.5
Tampa, FL	816	628	524	355	277	96.5	73.4	60.5	40.6	31.3
Toledo, OH	239	292	208	79	52	51.8	63.4	45.3	17.3	11.4
Tucson, AZ	79	66	152	104	78	11.7	9.5	21.4	14.2	10.4
Tulsa, OK	132	198	151	52	105	35.8	53.0	40.2	13.8	27.8
Washington, DC	2,888	2,333	1,652	967	727	485.9	398.3	285.8	170.5	131.2
Wichita, KS	50	51	37	27	42	12.2	12.3	8.8	6.4	10.0
Yonkers, NY	162	122	80	74	63	85.9	64.3	42.0	38.8	32.9
U.S. CITY TOTAL	70,765	62,565	53,812	41,274	35,113	105.0	92.1	78.7	60.1	51.0
San Juan, PR	940	1,013	1,298	1,015	693	107.8	116.2	148.8	116.4	79.5
TOTAL	71,705	63,578	55,110	42,289	35,806	105.1	92.4	79.6	60.9	51.3

Source: U.S. Department of Health and Human Services. Public Health Service. Centers for Disease Control and Prevention. Division of STD Prevention. *Sexually Transmitted Disease Surveillance, 1995.* U.S. Department of Health and Human Services, Public Health Service, September 1996.

Diseases and Illnesses: Sexually Transmitted Diseases

Syphilis: Urban Distribution of Primary and Secondary Stages

This table shows reported cases and rates of syphilis in primary and secondary stages in selected cities of 200,000+ population: United States and outlying areas, 1991-1995.

State/Area	Cases					Rates per 100,000 Population				
	1991	1992	1993	1994	1995	1991	1992	1993	1994	1995
Akron, OH	29	15	6	2	1	5.6	2.9	1.1	0.4	0.2
Albuquerque, NM	14	22	14	13	6	2.9	4.4	2.8	2.5	1.1
Atlanta, GA	1,028	607	335	261	320	156.8	91.3	49.5	37.8	45.7
Austin, TX	89	91	100	60	17	15.0	14.8	15.8	9.3	2.6
Baltimore, MD	205	188	144	192	342	28.0	25.9	20.1	27.3	49.5
Birmingham, AL	339	299	295	260	264	51.8	45.6	44.9	39.6	40.1
Boston, MA	208	83	34	24	40	37.0	15.0	6.1	4.4	7.2
Buffalo, NY	37	19	33	8	2	11.2	5.8	10.0	2.4	0.6
Charlotte, NC	365	309	209	214	125	69.2	57.7	38.1	38.0	21.6
Chicago, IL	2,045	1,879	1,016	648	582	69.6	63.7	34.4	22.0	19.7
Cincinnati, OH	74	190	395	473	252	8.5	21.8	45.3	54.5	29.2
Cleveland, OH	255	385	517	411	263	18.1	27.3	36.7	29.3	18.8
Columbus, OH	54	16	8	8	7	5.5	1.6	0.8	0.8	0.7
Corpus Christi, TX	37	24	17	20	8	12.5	8.0	5.6	6.4	2.6
Dallas, TX	1,215	681	410	292	268	64.2	35.6	21.3	15.0	13.7
Dayton, OH	48	73	76	127	244	8.3	12.7	13.2	22.2	42.8
Denver, CO	51	34	44	83	68	10.8	7.0	8.9	16.8	13.8
Des Moines, IA	30	42	33	37	27	9.0	12.4	9.6	10.7	7.7
Detroit, MI	1,008	552	277	153	130	93.7	51.5	26.0	14.5	12.4
El Paso, TX	28	13	17	5	2	4.6	2.1	2.6	0.7	0.3
Fort Worth, TX	347	327	351	190	140	28.8	26.8	28.4	15.1	10.9
Honolulu, HI	10	8	6	4	0	1.2	0.9	0.7	0.5	0.0
Houston, TX	1,682	1,012	571	443	417	58.0	34.1	19.0	14.5	13.6
Indianapolis, IN	32	55	120	62	74	4.0	6.8	14.7	7.6	9.1
Jacksonville, FL	167	105	73	108	50	24.2	15.0	10.4	15.4	7.1
Jersey City, NJ	62	33	22	14	27	28.4	15.1	10.1	6.4	12.4
Kansas City, MO	315	283	162	73	24	72.0	64.7	37.1	16.7	5.5
Los Angeles, CA	1,102	783	531	346	307	13.1	9.2	6.2	4.0	3.6
Louisville, KY	55	117	275	147	128	8.2	17.5	41.0	21.9	19.0
Memphis, TN	827	605	549	533	477	99.0	71.8	64.8	62.2	55.1
Miami, FL	509	326	266	175	51	25.7	16.3	13.3	8.7	2.5
Milwaukee, WI	613	547	469	279	150	64.1	57.4	49.5	29.7	16.1
Minneapolis, MN	55	65	43	38	24	14.6	17.2	11.3	9.9	6.3
Nashville, TN	290	224	149	100	97	56.6	43.3	28.5	19.0	18.3
New Orleans, LA	706	580	397	203	221	143.8	118.5	81.5	41.9	45.9
New York City, NY	3,138	2,243	1,132	629	364	42.9	30.7	15.4	8.6	5.0
Newark, NJ	300	167	100	60	43	102.4	57.1	34.2	20.7	15.0
Norfolk, VA	129	154	89	122	130	51.0	60.7	35.5	50.3	54.7
Oakland, CA	209	123	76	51	15	17.7	10.3	6.3	4.2	1.2
Oklahoma City, OK	82	179	177	115	106	19.4	41.9	41.0	26.4	24.3
Omaha, NE	17	18	8	5	7	4.0	4.2	1.9	1.2	1.6
Philadelphia, PA	1,411	907	515	298	199	90.1	58.5	33.5	19.6	13.3
Phoenix, AZ	280	143	55	28	43	12.9	6.5	2.4	1.2	1.8
Pittsburgh, PA	94	54	11	9	4	7.0	4.0	0.8	0.7	0.3
Portland, OR	56	34	24	18	4	11.9	7.2	5.0	3.7	0.8

[Continued]

★ 196 ★

Syphilis: Urban Distribution of Primary and Secondary Stages
[Continued]

State/Area	Cases					Rates per 100,000 Population				
	1991	1992	1993	1994	1995	1991	1992	1993	1994	1995
Richmond, VA	96	117	55	39	37	47.7	58.4	27.6	19.7	18.7
Rochester, NY	136	87	71	59	18	56.3	35.7	29.1	24.2	7.4
Sacramento, CA	95	29	8	9	5	8.8	2.7	0.7	0.8	0.5
San Antonio, TX	208	111	81	62	50	17.2	9.0	6.4	4.9	3.9
San Diego, CA	275	110	106	98	52	10.8	4.2	4.1	3.7	2.0
San Francisco, CA	183	97	69	45	32	25.2	13.3	9.4	6.2	4.4
San Jose, CA	36	34	27	4	3	2.4	2.2	1.7	0.3	0.2
Seattle, WA	82	51	22	11	5	5.3	3.3	1.4	0.7	0.3
St. Louis, MO	136	608	908	651	361	34.7	158.0	241.3	177.1	100.6
St. Paul, MN	4	13	10	7	7	1.4	4.7	3.6	2.5	2.5
St. Petersburg, FL	222	132	154	74	20	25.8	15.3	17.8	8.5	2.3
Tampa, FL	138	75	25	31	33	16.3	8.8	2.9	3.5	3.7
Toledo, OH	132	143	97	35	22	28.6	31.0	21.1	7.6	4.8
Tucson, AZ	28	7	32	12	1	4.1	1.0	4.5	1.6	0.1
Tulsa, OK	64	81	61	9	48	17.3	21.7	16.2	2.4	12.7
Washington, DC	764	420	291	170	112	128.6	71.7	50.3	30.0	20.2
Wichita, KS	16	10	6	10	16	3.9	2.4	1.4	2.4	3.8
Yonkers, NY	50	22	11	5	2	26.5	11.6	5.8	2.6	1.0
U.S. CITY TOTAL	22,312	16,761	12,185	8,672	6,894	33.1	24.7	17.8	12.6	10.0
San Juan, PR	199	184	189	131	70	22.8	21.1	21.7	15.0	8.0
TOTAL	22,511	16,945	12,374	8,803	6,964	33.0	24.6	17.9	12.7	10.0

Source: U.S. Department of Health and Human Services. Public Health Service. Centers for Disease Control and Prevention. Division of STD Prevention. *Sexually Transmitted Disease Surveillance, 1995.* U.S. Department of Health and Human Services, Public Health Service, September 1996.

★ 197 ★

Diseases and Illnesses: Sexually Transmitted Diseases

Syphilis: Urban Distribution, Ranked by Rate: 1995

This table shows reported cases and rates of syphilis, in all its stages, in selected cities of 200,000+ population: United States and outlying areas, 1995.

City	Cases	Rate per 100,000 population	Rank
St. Louis, MO	361	100.6	1
Memphis, TN	477	55.1	2
Norfolk, VA	130	54.7	3
Baltimore, MD	342	49.5	4
New Orleans, LA	221	45.9	5
Atlanta, GA	320	45.7	6

[Continued]

★ 197 ★

Syphilis: Urban Distribution, Ranked by Rate: 1995
[Continued]

City	Cases	Rate per 100,000 population	Rank
Dayton, OH	244	42.8	7
Birmingham, AL	264	40.1	8
Cincinnati, OH	252	29.2	9
Oklahoma City, OK	106	24.3	10
Charlotte, NC	125	21.6	11
Washington, DC	112	20.2	12
Chicago, IL	582	19.7	13
Louisville, KY	128	19.0	14
Cleveland, OH	263	18.8	15
Richmond, VA	37	18.7	16
Nashville, TN	97	18.3	17
Milwaukee, WI	150	16.1	18
Newark, NJ	43	15.0	19
Denver, CO	68	13.8	20
Dallas, TX	268	13.7	21
Houston, TX	417	13.6	22
Philadelphia, PA	199	13.3	23
Tulsa, OK	48	12.7	24
Jersey City, NJ	27	12.4	25
Detroit, MI	130	12.4	26
Fort Worth, TX	140	10.9	27
Indianapolis, IN	74	9.1	28
San Juan, PR	70	8.0	29
Des Moines, IA	27	7.7	30
Rochester, NY	18	7.4	31
Boston, MA	40	7.2	32
Jacksonville, FL	50	7.1	33
Minneapolis, MN	24	6.3	34
Kansas City, MO	24	5.5	35
New York City, NY	364	5.0	36
Toledo, OH	22	4.8	37
San Francisco, CA	32	4.4	38
YEAR 2000 OBJECTIVE[1]		4.0	
San Antonio, TX	50	3.9	39
Wichita, KS	16	3.8	40
Tampa, FL	33	3.7	41
Los Angeles, CA	307	3.6	42
Corpus Christi, TX	8	2.6	43
Austin, TX	17	2.6	44
St. Paul, MN	7	2.5	45
Miami, FL	51	2.5	46
St. Petersburg, FL	20	2.3	47
San Diego, CA	52	2.0	48

[Continued]

★ 197 ★

Syphilis: Urban Distribution, Ranked by Rate: 1995
[Continued]

City	Cases	Rate per 100,000 population	Rank
Phoenix, AZ	43	1.8	49
Omaha, NE	7	1.6	50
Oakland, CA	15	1.2	51
Albuquerque, NM	6	1.1	52
Yonkers, NY	2	1.0	53
Portland, OR	4	0.8	54
Columbus, OH	7	0.7	55
Buffalo, NY	2	0.6	56
Sacramento, CA	5	0.5	57
Seattle, WA	5	0.3	58
Pittsburgh, PA	4	0.3	59
El Paso, TX	2	0.3	60
San Jose, CA	3	0.2	61
Akron, OH	1	0.2	62
Tucson, AZ	1	0.1	63
Honolulu, HI	0	0.0	64

Source: U.S. Department of Health and Human Services. Public Health Service. Centers for Disease Control and Prevention. Division of STD Prevention. *Sexually Transmitted Disease Surveillance, 1995.* U.S. Department of Health and Human Services, Public Health Service, September 1996. *Note:* 1. Revised from 10.0 to 4.0.

Diseases and Illnesses: Tuberculosis

★ 198 ★

Tuberculosis Deaths Worldwide: 1995

"More people died from tuberculosis (TB) in 1995 than in any other year in history, according to a report by the World Health Organization (WHO). According to WHO, nearly three million people died from TB in 1995, surpassing the worst years of the epidemic around 1900, when an estimated 2.1 million people died annually."

Source: "Public Health News & Notes: TB Deaths Reach Historic Levels." *Public Health Reports,* vol. III, no. 4 (July/August 1996), p. 292.

★ 199 ★

Diseases and Illnesses: Tuberculosis

Tuberculosis: Highest Rates

Total U.S. tuberculosis cases declined by 6.7% in 1996.

[Rate is number of cases per 100,000 people]

State	Rate
District of Columbia	25.6
Hawaii	16.9
Alaska	15.8
New York	14.2
California	13.5
Texas	11.0

Source: "TB Cases Decline in U.S." *USA TODAY,* 12 May 1997, p. 1A. Primary source: Centers for Disease Control and Prevention.

★ 200 ★

Diseases and Illnesses: Tuberculosis

Tuberculosis Rates, by State: 1996

[In number of cases per 100,000 people]

State	Case rate per 100,000
District of Columbia	25.6
Hawaii	16.9
Alaska	15.8
New York	14.2
California	13.5
Texas	11.0
Georgia	10.7
New Jersey	10.3
Alabama	9.9
Florida	9.8
Louisiana	9.7
Tennessee	9.5
South Carolina	9.4
Mississippi	9.2
Arkansas	9.0
Illinois	8.9
Nevada	8.5
North Carolina	7.6
Kentucky	6.7
Arizona	6.4
Maryland	6.3
Oklahoma	6.1

[Continued]

★ 200 ★

Tuberculosis Rates, by State: 1996
[Continued]

State	Case rate per 100,000
Delaware	5.9
Oregon	5.9
Virginia	5.3
New Mexico	5.2
Washington	5.2
Pennsylvania	4.8
Michigan	4.6
Massachusetts	4.3
Connecticut	4.2
Missouri	4.2
Indiana	3.5
Rhode Island	3.5
West Virginia	3.1
Kansas	2.9
Utah	2.9
Minnesota	2.8
Colorado	2.7
Ohio	2.7
South Dakota	2.6
Iowa	2.5
Montana	2.2
Wisconsin	2.2
New Hampshire	1.8
Maine	1.7
Wyoming	1.5
Nebraska	1.3
North Dakota	1.2
Idaho	0.9
Vermont	0.7

Source: Manning, Anita. "TB Cases in USA Continue to Drop." *USA TODAY,* 24 March 1997, p. 8D. Primary source: U.S. Centers for Disease Control and Prevention.

Environmental Health

★ 201 ★

Cryptosporidiosis Cases: 1984-1995

Cryptosporidium, a parasite, has been linked to 11 waterborne illness outbreaks since 1984. Table shows where the outbreaks occurred, the number of persons affected and the number of confirmed cases of cryptosporidiosis (shown in parentheses).

Location	Number affected (confirmed cases)
Bexar County, TX	2,000 (47)
Bernalillo County, NM	NA (78)
Carroll County, GA	13,000
Berks County, PA	551
Jackson County, OR	15,000
Milwaukee County, WI	403,000
Yakima County, WA	7 (3)
Cook County, MN	27 (5)
Clark County, NV	(78)
Walla Walla County, WA	86 (15)
Alachua County, FL	(72)

Source: Wright, Andrew G. "Battling A Bad Bug." *ENR,* 2 June 1997, p. 24. Primary source: Helena Solo-Gabriele, American Water Works Association 1996.

★ 202 ★

Environmental Health

Pollution-Related Death Rates

City	Number of deaths
Los Angeles, CA	5,873
New York, NY	4,024
Chicago, IL	3,479
Philadelphia, PA	2,599
Detroit, MI	2,123

Source: Thompson, Dick. "America's Deadliest Cities." *Time,* 9 December 1996, p. 71. Primary source: Natural Resources Defense Council.

★ 203 ★

Environmental Health

Proposed Stricter Air Quality Standards

The Environmental Protection Agency proposes to expand regulation of particulate matter to cover particles as small as 2.5 microns in diameter (currently, the standard is 10 microns), and to lower the acceptable level of ozone from 0.12 parts per million cubic feet of air to 0.08 parts per million. In addition, the agency proposes to expand monitoring time of ozone from one hour to eight hours.

By EPA's calculation, if fully adopted the new rule annually would cut premature deaths by 20,000, cases of aggravated asthma by 250,000, cases of acute childhood respiratory problems by 250,000, bronchitis cases by 60,000, hospital admissions by 9,000, and cases of significant breathing problems by 1.5 million. The dollar benefits, says EPA, would reach $115 billion.

Source: Miller, William H. "Clean-Air Contention: EPA's proposed stricter air-quality standards stir heated controversy—and vehement industry opposition." *Industry Week,* 5 May 1997, p. 14.

Health Status

★ 204 ★

Health Prognoses for Men and Women After Myocardial Infarction, by Event

Data refer to problems occurring within 6 years of the first MI (myocardial infarction).

[In percentages]

Within 6 years after an MI	Men	Women
Will have another MI	23	31
Will develop angina	41	34
Will be disabled with heart failure	20	20
Will have a stroke	9	18
Will experience sudden death	13	6

Source: "News Pulse: Affairs of the Heart." *Nursing95* (March 1995), p. 8.

★ 205 ★

Health Status

Respondent-Assessed Health Status, by Selected Characteristics: 1994

[Data are based on household interviews of a sample of the civilian noninstitutionalized population].

Characteristic	Percent with poor or fair health
Total[1,2]	9.6
Age	
Under 15 years	2.9
Under 5 years	2.9
5-14 years	2.9
15-44 years	6.4
45-64 years	16.6
65 years and over	28.0
65-74 years	25.6
75 years and over	31.3
Sex and age	
Male[1]	9.0
Under 15 years	3.1
15-44 years	5.4
45-64 years	15.3
65-74 years	26.6
75 years and over	31.9
Female[1]	
Under 15 years	10.1
15-44 years	2.7
45-64 years	7.4
65-74 years	17.7
75 years and over	24.9
	30.8
Race and age	
White[1]	8.6
Under 15 years	2.5
15-44 years	5.6
45-64 years	14.9
65-74 years	24.2
75 years and over	29.8
Black[1]	16.1
Under 15 years	4.9
15-44 years	10.6
45-64 years	30.2
65-74 years	40.3
75 years and over	46.8

[Continued]

★ 205 ★

Respondent-Assessed Health Status, by Selected Characteristics: 1994

[Continued]

Characteristic	Percent with poor or fair health
Family income[1,3]	
Less than $14,000	20.4
$14,000-$24,999	12.3
$25,000-$34,999	7.9
$35,000-$49,999	6.2
$50,000 or more	3.9
Geographic region[1]	
Northeast	8.1
Midwest	8.6
South	11.2
West	9.4
Location of residence[1]	
Within MSA	9.2
Outside MSA	10.8

Source: U.S. Department of Health and Human Services. Public Health Service. Centers for Disease Control and Prevention. National Center for Health Statistics. *Health, United States, 1995.* Hyattsville, MD: Public Health Service, 1996, p. 172. Primary source: Centers for Disease Control and Prevention, National Center for Health Statistics, Division of Health Interview Statistics. Data from the National Health Interview Survey. *Notes:* 1. Age adjusted. 2. Includes all other races not shown separately and unknown family income. 3. Family income categories for 1989-94.

Hearing Loss

★ 206 ★

Causes of Hearing Loss: 1996

Cause	Decibels	Hours before hearing damage can occur
Jet takeoff	120+	.25
Rock concert	90-120	.25
Subway train	100+	2.0
Stereo headphones	100+	2.0
Lawn mower	90	8.0

[Continued]

★ 206 ★

Causes of Hearing Loss: 1996
[Continued]

Cause	Decibels	Hours before hearing damage can occur
Motorcycle	90	8.0
Busy city street	70	N/A
Normal talking	40-60	N/A
Quiet home	20-40	N/A

Source: "The Human Condition: Hearing Loss." *Time* (Fall 1996), p. 86. Primary source: Deafness Research Foundation; National Institute on Deafness and Other Communication Disorders. *Note:* NA indicates "not available."

Home Health Care

★ 207 ★

Caregivers, by Sex and Family Role

Family role	Percentage
Daughters	29.0
Wives	23.0
Females (Other)	20.0
Husbands	13.0
Sons	8.0
Males (Other)	7.0

Source: Marosy, John Paul. "Elder Caregiving in the 21st Century." *CARING Magazine* (May 1997), p. 15.

★ 208 ★

Home Health Care

Elderly Home Health Patients: 1994

Covers the civilian noninstitutionalized population 65 years old and over who are home health care patients. Home health care is provided to individuals and families in their place of residence. Based on the 1994 National Home and Hospice Care Survey.

ITEM	CURRENT PATIENTS[1]		DIS-CHARGES[2]	
	Number (1,000)	Per-cent	Number (1,000)	Per-cent
Total 65 years old and over	1,379.8	100.0	3,826.5	100.0
Received help with –				
Bathing or showering	746.6	54.1	1,580.1	41.3
Dressing	632.4	45.8	1,307.7	34.2
Eating	127.1	9.2	223.3	5.8
Transferring in/out of a bed or chair	436.3	31.6	1,048.0	27.4
Using the toilet	336.6	24.4	759.7	19.9
Doing light housework	564.4	40.9	918.4	24.0
Managing money	27.4	2.0	40.4	1.1
Shopping for groceries or clothes	252.5	18.3	454.1	11.9
Using the telephone	47.0	3.4	40.6	1.1
Preparing meals	351.4	25.5	728.8	19.0
Taking medications	340.4	24.7	755.6	19.7
Primary source of payment of last billing:				
Private insurance	26.2	1.9	315.5	8.2
Own income	63.1	4.6	116.1	3.0
Medicare	1,004.6	72.8	3,068.5	80.2
Medicaid	120.5	8.7	108.9	2.8
Services rendered last billing period:				
Skilled nursing	1,122.4	81.3	3,302.8	86.3
Personal care	585.5	42.4	1,176.7	30.8
Social services	124.6	9.0	368.4	9.6
Counseling	48.3	3.5	165.7	4.3
Medications	74.3	5.4	190.2	5.0
Physical therapy	232.3	16.8	933.9	24.4
Homemaker/companion services	322.2	23.4	612.4	16.0
Referral services	20.8	1.5	66.4	1.7
Dietary and nutrition services	44.1	3.2	76.0	2.0
Physician services	16.2	1.2	48.9	1.3
High tech care	13.9	1.0	39.8	1.0

[Continued]

★ 208 ★

Elderly Home Health Patients: 1994
[Continued]

ITEM	CURRENT PATIENTS[1]		DIS-CHARGES[2]	
	Number (1,000)	Per-cent	Number (1,000)	Per-cent
Occupational/vocational therapy	39.0	2.8	164.2	4.3
Speech therapy/audiology	17.0	1.2	46.9	1.2

Source: 1996 Statistical Abstract of the United States on CD-ROM [machine-readable datafiles]. CD-8A-97. Washington, DC: U.S. Department of Commerce, Economics and Statistics Administration, Bureau of the Census, Data User Services Division, January 1997. Primary source: U.S. National Center for Health Statistics, unpublished data. Notes: 1. Patients on the rolls of the agency as of midnight the day prior to the survey. 2. Patients removed from the rolls of the agency during the 12 months prior to the day of the survey. A patient could be included more than once if the individual had more than one episode of care during the year.

★ 209 ★

Home Health Care

Home Health and Hospice Care Patients, by Selected Characteristic: 1994

ITEM	CURRENT PATIENTS[1]			DISCHARGES[2]		
	Total	Home health agency	Hospice	Total	Home health agency	Hospice
Total (1,000)	1,950.3	1,889.4	61.0	5,600.2	5,272.2	328.0
PERCENT DISTRIBUTION Age:						
Under 45 years old	12.6	12.7	9.0	14.3	14.9	6.2
45-54 years old	4.4	4.4	6.3	5.3	5.2	6.9
55-64 years old	10.1	9.9	15.6	7.8	7.4	13.9
65 years old and over	72.8	73.0	69.1	72.6	72.5	73.0
65-69 years old	9.3	9.3	9.5	9.4	9.2	11.6
70-74 years old	12.6	12.6	13.8	14.6	14.5	16.2
75-79 years old	14.9	15.0	12.3	16.4	16.5	15.5
80-84 years old	15.9	15.9	16.5	18.1	18.5	12.4
85 years old and over	20.1	20.2	16.9	14.1	13.9	17.4
Sex:						
Male	32.8	32.5	44.7	41.0	40.3	52.3
Female	67.2	67.5	55.3	59.0	59.7	47.7
Race:						
White	63.8	63.3	80.8	66.8	66.0	79.4
Black	15.6	15.9	7.2	8.6	8.6	7.3
Other or unknown	20.6	20.8	12.0	24.7	25.4	13.3

[Continued]

★ 209 ★

Home Health and Hospice Care Patients, by Selected Characteristic: 1994

[Continued]

ITEM	CURRENT PATIENTS[1]			DISCHARGES[2]		
	Total	Home health agency	Hospice	Total	Home health agency	Hospice
Marital status:[3]						
Married	31.2	30.6	48.4	38.3	37.7	48.9
Widowed	36.0	36.2	30.6	30.6	30.7	29.7
Divorced or separated	4.8	4.7	6.0	4.7	4.6	5.5
Never married	16.5	16.7	11.4	14.9	15.2	9.2
Unknown	11.5	11.7	3.7	11.5	11.8	6.8

Source: 1996 Statistical Abstract of the United States on CD-ROM [machine-readable datafiles]. CD-8A-97. Washington, DC: U.S. Department of Commerce, Economics and Statistics Administration, Bureau of the Census, Data User Services Division, January 1997. Primary source: National Center for Health Statistics, Advance Data, no. 274, 24 April, 1996. Notes: 1. Patients on the rolls of the agency as of midnight the day prior to the survey. 2. Patients removed from the rolls of the agency during the 12 months prior to the day of the survey. A patient could be included more than once if the individual had more than one episode of care during the year. 3. For current patients, marital status at admission; for discharged patients, status at time of discharge.

★ 210 ★

Home Health Care

Home Health Care Patients Age 45 Years and Older, by Sex and Age: 1994

Sex	45-64 years	65-74 years	75-84 years	85 years and over
Women	3.5	20.1	53.5	132.2
Men	3.0	14.8	35.6	80.0

Source: U.S. Department of Health and Human Services. Public Health Service. Centers for Disease Control and Prevention. National Center for Health Statistics. Health, United States, 1995. Hyattsville, MD: Public Health Service, 1996, p. 69. Primary source: Substance Abuse and Mental Health Services Administration, Office of Applied Studies, National Household Survey on Drug Abuse.

Immunization and Vaccinations

★ 211 ★

Children Immunized Against Specified Diseases: 1991 to 1994

In percent. Covers civilian noninstitutionalized population ages 19 months to 35 months. Based on estimates from the National Health Interview Survey. Excludes respondents with unknown or missing information.

VACCINATION	1991, total	1992, total	1993, total	1994			
				Total	White	Black	Other
Diphtheria-tetanus-pertussis (DPT)/ diphtheria-tetanus:							
3+ doses	68.8	83.0	88.2	89.5	90.5	84.7	88.2
4+ doses	43.3	59.0	72.1	70.0	70.7	64.2	77.4
Polio: 3+ doses	53.2	72.4	78.9	79.1	80.1	72.9	82.1
Hib 3+ doses[1]:	1.7	28.2	55.0	75.2	76.7	67.8	72.6
Hepatitis B: 3+ doses	(NA)	(NA)	16.3	34.8	34.1	36.9	39.9
Measles containing	82.0	82.5	84.1	90.2	91.6	85.8	81.1
3 DPT/3 polio/1 MMR[2]	50.0	68.7	74.5	77.1	78.5	69.9	76.5
4 DPT/3 polio/1 MMR [2, 3]	37.0	55.3	67.1	67.3	68.3	60.5	72.2

Source: 1996 Statistical Abstract of the United States on CD-ROM [machine-readable datafiles]. CD-8A-97. Washington, DC: U.S. Department of Commerce, Economics and Statistics Administration, Bureau of the Census, Data User Services Division, January 1997. Primary source: U.S. Centers for Disease Control and Prevention, Atlanta, GA, the National Health Interview Survey. Notes: NA Not available. 1. Haemophilus B. 2. Measles, measles/rubella, measles/mumps, and measles/mumps/ rubella. 3. Up-to-date for age.

★ 212 ★

Immunization and Vaccinations

Medicare-Paid Influenza Vaccination Rates, by Race and State: 1993

[In percentages]

State	Race		
	White	Black	Total[1]
Alabama	39	19	35
Alaska	19	18	16
Arizona[2]	44	22	42
Arkansas	46	24	44
California[2]	28	15	26
Colorado	47	21	46
Connecticut	35	22	35
Delaware	32	17	30
District of Columbia	32	14	20
Florida	41	18	40
Georgia	38	16	33

[Continued]

★ 212 ★

Medicare-Paid Influenza Vaccination Rates, by Race and State: 1993
[Continued]

State	Race		
	White	Black	Total[1]
Hawaii	34	24	36
Idaho	47	31	46
Illinois	31	11	29
Indiana	42	19	41
Iowa	49	27	49
Kansas	46	21	45
Kentucky	35	21	34
Louisiana	29	14	26
Maine	42	31	42
Maryland	37	17	34
Massachusetts	18	9	17
Michigan	33	18	32
Minnesota	43	26	43
Mississippi	27	15	24
Missouri	36	16	34
Montana	48	35	48
Nebraska	46	22	45
Nevada	23	15	23
New Hampshire	35	28	34
New Jersey[2]	27	16	26
New Mexico	28	14	27
New York	34	13	31
North Carolina	41	18	37
North Dakota	41	28	41
Ohio	36	21	35
Oklahoma	39	18	38
Oregon	46	25	45
Pennsylvania	40	22	38
Rhode Island	41	27	40
South Carolina[2]	36	18	32
South Dakota	41	32	40
Tennessee	46	21	43
Texas	34	15	32
Utah	34	20	34
Vermont	34	33	33
Virginia	45	24	41
Washington	42	24	42
West Virginia	29	19	29
Wisconsin	45	27	45

[Continued]

★ 212 ★

Medicare-Paid Influenza Vaccination Rates, by Race and State: 1993

[Continued]

State	Race		
	White	Black	Total[1]
Wyoming	29	24	29
Total	37	17	35

Source: U.S. Department of Health and Human Services. Public Health Service. Centers for Disease Control and Prevention. National Center for Health Statistics. "International Notes: Dengue Type 3 Infection—Nicaragua and Panama, October-November 1994." *CDC Surveillance Summaries. Morbidity and Mortality Weekly Report* vol. 44, no. 2, 20 January 1995, p. 26. *Notes:* 1. Includes persons in all racial groups and persons of unknown race. 2. After the mailing of the original estimates from the Medicare claims data to the 63 federal vaccination grant programs, California and South Carolina reported 473,062 and 23,322 influenza vaccinations administered to persons aged >65 years, respectively, which were not billed to Medicare in 1993. Arizona estimated that an additional 40,000 persons received vaccine that was not billed to Medicare, and New Jersey estimated 80,000-100,000 doses were not billed. This additional information is not reflected in the table.

★ 213 ★

Immunization and Vaccinations

Vaccinations, 4:3:1 Series, by Selected Urban Area: 1994-1995

Coverage level/ Area	4:3:1 Series coverage percentage
>85%	
Boston, MA	87
Santa Clara County, CA	85
75%-84%	
Baltimore, MD	80
Cuyahoga County, OH	84
Dade County, FL	77
El Paso County, TX	82
Fulton-DeKalb Counties, GA	77
Jefferson County, AL	78
Kings County, WA	78
Maricopa County, AZ	77
Marion County, IN	81
Milwaukee County, WI	80
New York, NY	76
65%-74%	
Bexar County, TX	67
Dallas County, TX	71
Davidson County, TN	69
Washington, DC	72

[Continued]

★ 213 ★

Vaccinations, 4:3:1 Series, by Selected Urban Area: 1994-1995

[Continued]

Coverage level/ Area	4:3:1 Series coverage percentage
Duval County, FL	74
Franklin County, OH	71
Los Angeles County, CA	73
Orleans Parish, LA	67
Philadelphia County, PA	71
San Diego County, CA	74
Shelby County, TN	73
<65%	
Chicago, IL	61
Detroit, MI	52
Houston, TX	62
Newark, NJ	62

Source: U.S. Department of Health and Human Services. Public Health Service. Centers for Disease Control and Prevention. National Center for Health Statistics. "Vaccination Coverage Levels." *Morbidity and Mortality Weekly Report,* vol. 45, no. 7, 23 February 1996, p. 148. Primary source: National Immunization Survey, United States, April 1994 - March 1995.

★ 214 ★

Immunization and Vaccinations

Vaccinations, 4:3:1 Series, by State: 1994-1995

Coverage level/ State	4:3:1 Series coverage percentage
>85%	
Connecticut	86
Massachusetts	85
Vermont	87
75%-84%	
Arizona	77
Colorado	76
Delaware	81
Florida	79
Georgia	76
Hawaii	84
Iowa	83
Kansas	82
Kentucky	81
Maine	83
Maryland	79

[Continued]

★ 214 ★

Vaccinations, 4:3:1 Series, by State: 1994-1995
[Continued]

Coverage level/ State	4:3:1 Series coverage percentage
Minnesota	78
Mississippi	80
New Hampshire	84
New York	76
North Carolina	83
North Dakota	82
Pennsylvania	78
Rhode Island	83
South Carolina	81
South Dakota	76
Virginia	78
Washington	75
Wisconsin	76
Wyoming	79
65%-74%	
Alabama	74
Alaska	72
Arkansas	69
California	73
Idaho	66
Illinois	69
Indiana	72
Louisiana	74
Missouri	67
Montana	72
Nebraska	72
Nevada	68
New Jersey	70
New Mexico	73
Ohio	74
Oklahoma	73
Oregon	67
Tennessee	73
Texas	71
Utah	70
West Virginia	69

[Continued]

★ 214 ★

Vaccinations, 4:3:1 Series, by State: 1994-1995
[Continued]

Coverage level/ State	4:3:1 Series coverage percentage
<65%	
Michigan	63
Total	75

Source: U.S. Department of Health and Human Services. Public Health Service. Centers for Disease Control and Prevention. "Vaccination Coverage Levels." *Morbidity and Mortality Weekly Report,* vol. 45, no. 7, 23 February 1996, p. 148. Primary source: National Immunization Survey, United States, April 1994 - March 1995.

★ 215 ★

Immunization and Vaccinations

Vaccinations, 4:3:1:3 Series, by Selected Urban Area: 1994-1995

Coverage level/ Area	4:3:1:3 Series coverage percentage
>85%	
Boston, MA	87
75%-84%	
Baltimore, MD	77
Cuyahoga County, OH	82
El Paso County, TX	79
Fulton/DeKalb Counties, GA	75
Jefferson County, AL	75
Marion County, IN	78
Milwaukee County, WI	77
New York, NY	75
Santa Clara County, CA	80
65%-74%	
Dade County, FL	74
Dallas County, TX	66
Davidson County, TN	67
Washington, DC	67
Duval County, FL	71
Franklin County, OH	70
Kings County, WA	74
Los Angeles County, CA	68
Maricopa County, AZ	74
Orleans Parish, LA	66
Philadelphia County, PA	69

[Continued]

★ 215 ★

Vaccinations, 4:3:1:3 Series, by Selected Urban Area: 1994-1995

[Continued]

Coverage level/ Area	4:3:1:3 Series coverage percentage
San Diego County, CA	72
Shelby County, TN	71
<65%	
Bexar County, TX	64
Chicago, IL	61
Detroit, MI	46
Houston, TX	58
Newark, NJ	55

Source: U.S. Department of Health and Human Services. Public Health Service. Centers for Disease Control and Prevention. National Center for Health Statistics. "Vaccination Coverage Levels." *Morbidity and Mortality Weekly Report,* vol. 45, no. 7, 23 February 1996, p. 148 Primary source: National Immunization Survey, United States, April 1994 - March 1995.

★ 216 ★

Immunization and Vaccinations

Vaccinations, 4:3:1:3 Series, by State: 1994-1995

Coverage level/ State	4:3:1:3 Series coverage percentage
>85%	
Vermont	86
75%-84%	
Connecticut	84
Delaware	79
Florida	78
Georgia	75
Hawaii	80
Iowa	82
Kansas	79
Kentucky	80
Maine	80
Maryland	77
Massachusetts	83
Minnesota	77
Mississippi	80
New Hampshire	82
New York	75
North Carolina	79
North Dakota	80

[Continued]

★ 216 ★

Vaccinations, 4:3:1:3 Series, by State: 1994-1995
[Continued]

Coverage level/ State	4:3:1:3 Series coverage percentage
Pennsylvania	76
Rhode Island	81
South Carolina	79
Virginia	77
Wyoming	76
65%-74%	
Alabama	73
Alaska	68
Arizona	74
Arkansas	66
California	70
Colorado	73
Idaho	65
Indiana	70
Louisiana	72
Missouri	66
Montana	71
Nebraska	67
Nevada	65
New Jersey	69
New Mexico	70
Ohio	73
Oklahoma	70
Oregon	65
South Dakota	74
Tennessee	70
Texas	68
Utah	67
Washington	73
West Virginia	68
Wisconsin	74
<65%	
Illinois	64
Michigan	59
Total	72

Source: U.S. Department of Health and Human Services. Public Health Service. Centers for Disease Control and Prevention. National Center for Health Statistics. "Vaccination Coverage Levels." *Morbidity and Mortality Weekly Report,* vol. 45, no. 7, 23 February 1996, p. 148 Primary source: National Immunization Survey, United States, April 1994 - March 1995.

Injuries and Accidents

★ 217 ★

Accidental Deaths From Police Pursuits, 1995: Top 10 States

State	Total fatalities
California	57
Texas	25
Florida	23
Georgia	23
Illinois	19
Michigan	16
Ohio	14
Indiana	13
Pennsylvania	12
North Carolina	11

Source: Heinlein, Gary. "No Pursuit Without Risks, Police Driving School Teaches." *Detroit News,* 16 January 1997, p. 1E.

★ 218 ★

Injuries and Accidents

Accidental Deaths From Snowmobiles: 1996-97

Data refer to deaths in the states with the most snowmobiles.

State	1996-97	Average
Michigan	31	26
Wisconsin	29	24.8
Minnesota	28	21
New York	9	14.8
New Hampshire	8	4.6
Maine	7	6.4
Idaho	4	0.4
Illinois	2	5
Pennsylvania	1	3.8
Vermont	1	0.2

Source: Nasser, Haya Ed. "Snowmobiles Skid Into Danger." *USA TODAY,* 28 February 1997, p. 3A.

★ 219 ★

Injuries and Accidents

Accidents Associated with Car Phones

"According to a study published last week in the *New England Journal of Medicine*, drivers using car phones are four times as likely to be involved in an accident as those minding only the road—about the same rate found among motorists driving at the legal blood-alcohol limit."

Source: Kluger, Jeffrey. "Distress Calls: A New Study Links Car Phones with Accidents." *Time,* 24 February 1997, p. 52.

★ 220 ★

Injuries and Accidents

Boating Accident Fatalities, by Cause: 1994

Type of accident	Percentage
Falls overboard	26
Collision with object	9
Collision with another vessel	12
Struck by boat/propeller	2
Capsizing	28
Flooding/sinking	11
Groundings	2
Other	10

Source: Squires, Sally. "High Seas: The Hazards of Drunk Boating." *Washington Post,* 2 July 1996, p. 10.

★ 221 ★

Injuries and Accidents

Dog Bites That Required Medical Attention: 1986 and 1994

Year	Dog bites
1986	585,000
1994	800,000

Source: Wulf, Steve. "Man's Best Friend?" *Time,* 23 June 1997, p. 58.

★ 222 ★

Injuries and Accidents

Fatalities Resulting from Motor Vehicle Crashes, by Vehicle Size and Type: 1991-1994

[In number of fatalities per million registered vehicles]

Vehicle	Number of crashes
Small pickup	217
Small car	200
Average	169
Sport-utility	163
Medium car	159
Standard pickup	134
Large car	130
Minivan	114
Standard van	86

Source: "Rollover Fatality Rates." *Automotive News,* 10 June 1996, p. 47. Primary source: National Highway Traffic Safety Administration.

★ 223 ★

Injuries and Accidents

Fatalities Resulting From Unintentional Injuries, by Type: 1995

Class	1995
Total	93,000
Motor vehicle	42,300
Public (excluding motor vehicle)	22,000
Home	26,000
Work	4,800

Source: "The National Unintentional-Injury Fatality Toll." *Safety & Health* (May 1996), p. 69.

★ 224 ★

Injuries and Accidents

Fatalities Resulting From Vehicle Rollovers, by Vehicle Type: 1991-1994

[In number of fatalities per million registered vehicles]

Vehicle	Number of fatalities
Sport-utility	98
Small pickup	93
Standard pickup	59
Average	47
Small car	47
Minivan	40
Standard van	34
Medium car	28
Large car	19

Source: "Rollover Fatality Rates." *Automotive News,* 10 June 1996, p. 47. Primary source: National Highway Traffic Safety Administration.

★ 225 ★

Injuries and Accidents

Head Injuries Resulting from Car Crashes: A Comparison of Air Bag and Seat Belt Use

[In percentages]

Injury	Air bag only	Belt only	Air bag and belt
Brain injuries	25.0	4.0	0.6
Facial lacerations	30.8	10.0	6.6
Facial abrasions	2.4	7.1	11.7
Facial contusions	19.0	14.7	3.2
Facial fractures	2.3	3.0	0.0

Source: "Stats on Bags & Belts." *Current Health* (April 1996), p. 2.

★ 226 ★

Injuries and Accidents

Number of Sports Injuries in 1995, by Sport

Sport	Number of injuries
Basketball	694,000
Cycling	600,000
Football	390,000
Snow skiing	330,000
Skating	322,000
Baseball	219,000
Soccer	157,000
Softball	156,000
Volleyball	87,000
Field and ice hockey	77,000

Source: Montague, Jim. "Currents: The Most Dangerous Games." *Hospitals & Health Networks,* 5 September 1996, p. 10. Primary source: American Academy of Orthopedic Surgeons, 1996.

★ 227 ★

Injuries and Accidents

Sports Injuries, by Sport: 1995

[Rate is number of injuries and accidents per 1,000 participants]

Sport	Rate
Basketball	14.9
Baseball	13.5
Football[1]	12.0
Ice Hockey	9.6
Soccer	9.3
Volleyball[2]	2.0

Source: "Notebook: Blood Sports." *Time,* 17 June 1996, p. 22. Primary source: U.S. Consumer Product Safety Commission; Sporting Goods Manufacturers Association. *Notes:* 1. Touch and tackle. 2. Hard surface and sand.

★ 228 ★
Injuries and Accidents

Sports-Related Injuries to Children, by Sport: 1996

Data refer to annual sports injuries sustained by children ages 5 to 14.

Sport	Organized	Unorganized and informal
Football	61,000	117,000
Basketball	56,000	165,500
Baseball	53,000	116,000
Soccer	28,000	41,000
Hockey[1]	21,000	NA
Gymnastics	13,500	21,000
Volleyball	7,500	15,000

Source: Bates, Karl Leif. "Most Doctors Don't Know When to Bench a Player." *Detroit News,* 28 May 1997, p. 1C. Primary source: U.S. Consumer Product Safety Commission. *Notes:* NA indicates "not applicable." 1. All kinds.

★ 229 ★
Injuries and Accidents

Sports With the Most Expensive Injuries Treated in Emergency Rooms: 1995

Sport	Number of injuries	Cost (billions)
Cycling	599,874	4.29
Basketball	693,933	3.60
Snow skiing	330,289	2.40
Football	390,180	2.20
Skating, all types	322,311	1.96

Source: "Big-Ticket Sports Injuries." *USA TODAY,* 8 August 1996, p. 1C. Primary source: Consumer Product Safety Commission; American Academy of Orthopedic Surgeons.

★ 230 ★

Injuries and Accidents

States with the Highest Bicycle Fatality Rates: 1996

[Rate is in deaths per 1,000,000 persons]

State	Rate
Florida	8.8
Arizona	7.0
Louisiana	5.9
South Carolina	5.4
North Carolina	4.5

Source: "Road Sign." *Time,* 2 June 1997, p. 24. Primary source: Environmental Working Group.

★ 231 ★

Injuries and Accidents

States with the Lowest Bicycle Fatality Rates: 1996

[Rate is in deaths per 1,000,000 persons]

State	Rate
North Dakota	1.7
Oklahoma	1.6
New Hampshire	1.4
West Virginia	1.2
Rhode Island	1.1

Source: "Road Sign." *Time,* 2 June 1997, p. 24. Primary source: Environmental Working Group.

★ 232 ★

Injuries and Accidents

United States Deaths and Death Rates, 1994: All Injuries

[Rate is number of deaths per 100,000 persons]

Age Group	Total		Male		Female	
	Deaths	Rate	Deaths	Rate	Deaths	Rate
00-04	4,286	21.72	2,512	24.88	1,774	18.41
05-09	1,777	9.42	1,100	11.38	677	7.35
10-14	2,696	14.38	1,847	19.23	849	9.28
15-19	12,257	69.57	9,643	106.71	2,614	30.46
20-24	15,136	82.49	12,456	133.60	2,680	29.69
25-29	13,212	68.79	10,545	109.45	2,667	27.87
30-34	14,301	64.53	11,228	101.60	3,073	27.65

[Continued]

★ 232 ★

United States Deaths and Death Rates, 1994: All Injuries
[Continued]

Age Group	Total Deaths	Total Rate	Male Deaths	Male Rate	Female Deaths	Female Rate
35-39	13,829	63.04	10,565	96.85	3,264	29.59
40-44	11,698	59.42	9,056	93.14	2,642	26.51
45-49	8,867	53.18	6,639	81.18	2,228	26.23
50-54	6,589	49.95	4,808	75.01	1,781	26.27
55-59	5,241	47.94	3,802	72.53	1,439	25.28
60-64	5,113	50.71	3,626	76.48	1,487	27.83
65-69	5,564	55.78	3,694	82.04	1,870	34.17
70-74	6,340	72.56	4,056	107.04	2,284	46.15
75-79	6,881	104.71	4,166	156.86	2,715	69.33
80-84	6,897	158.63	3,752	242.07	3,145	112.41
85+	10,067	286.14	4,262	435.08	5,805	228.67
Unknown	189		157		32	
Total	150,940	57.98	107,914	84.91	43,026	32.29

Source: National Center for Injury Prevention and Control, Centers for Disease Control and Prevention, State Injury Mortality Statistics, downloaded from http://www.cdc.gov.ncip/ncipchm.htm on March 10, 1995.

★ 233 ★

Injuries and Accidents

United States Deaths and Death Rates, 1994: Firearm Homicide/Legal Intervention
[Rate is number of deaths per 100,000 persons]

Age Group	Total Deaths	Total Rate	Male Deaths	Male Rate	Female Deaths	Female Rate
00-04	71	0.36	38	0.38	33	0.34
05-09	73	0.39	36	0.37	37	0.40
10-14	325	1.73	241	2.51	84	0.92
15-19	3,150	17.88	2,826	31.27	324	3.78
20-24	3,833	20.89	3,415	36.63	418	4.63
25-29	2,799	14.57	2,414	25.06	385	4.02
30-34	2,384	10.76	1,973	17.85	411	3.70
35-39	1,808	8.24	1,461	13.39	347	3.15
40-44	1,217	6.18	1,007	10.36	210	2.11
45-49	760	4.56	609	7.45	151	1.78
50-54	473	3.59	371	5.79	102	1.50
55-59	302	2.76	241	4.60	61	1.07
60-64	229	2.27	170	3.59	59	1.10
65-69	156	1.56	117	2.60	39	0.71
70-74	126	1.44	82	2.16	44	0.89
75-79	79	1.20	48	1.81	31	0.79
80-84	40	0.92	17	1.10	23	0.82
85+	19	0.54	8	0.82	11	0.43

[Continued]

★ 233 ★

United States Deaths and Death Rates, 1994: Firearm Homicide/Legal Intervention

[Continued]

Age Group	Total Deaths	Total Rate	Male Deaths	Male Rate	Female Deaths	Female Rate
Unknown	22		19		3	
Total	17,866	6.86	15,093	11.88	2,773	2.08

Source: National Center for Injury Prevention and Control, Centers for Disease Control and Prevention, State Injury Mortality Statistics, downloaded from http://www.cdc.gov.ncip/ ncipchm.htm on March 10, 1995.

★ 234 ★

Injuries and Accidents

United States Deaths and Death Rates, 1994: Firearm-Related

[Rate is number of deaths per 100,000 persons]

Age Group	Total Deaths	Total Rate	Male Deaths	Male Rate	Female Deaths	Female Rate
00-04	107	0.54	62	0.61	45	0.47
05-09	105	0.56	57	0.59	48	0.52
10-14	660	3.52	517	5.38	143	1.56
15-19	4,961	28.16	4,442	49.16	519	6.05
20-24	6,095	33.22	5,467	58.64	628	6.96
25-29	4,725	24.60	4,096	42.51	629	6.57
30-34	4,349	19.62	3,632	32.87	717	6.45
35-39	3,670	16.73	2,991	27.42	679	6.16
40-44	2,849	14.47	2,369	24.37	480	4.82
45-49	2,192	13.15	1,801	22.02	391	4.60
50-54	1,624	12.31	1,307	20.39	317	4.67
55-59	1,243	11.37	1,067	20.35	176	3.09
60-64	1,161	11.51	978	20.63	183	3.43
65-69	1,144	11.47	984	21.85	160	2.92
70-74	1,209	13.84	1,059	27.95	150	3.03
75-79	1,100	16.74	996	37.50	104	2.66
80-84	749	17.23	682	44.00	67	2.39
85+	532	15.12	487	49.71	45	1.77
Unknown	30		27		3	
Total	38,505	14.79	33,021	25.98	5,484	4.12

Source: National Center for Injury Prevention and Control, Centers for Disease Control and Prevention, State Injury Mortality Statistics, downloaded from http://www.cdc.gov.ncip/ ncipchm.htm on March 10, 1995.

★ 235 ★

Injuries and Accidents

United States Deaths and Death Rates, 1994: Firearm Suicide

[Rate is number per 100,000 persons]

Age Group	Total Deaths	Total Rate	Male Deaths	Male Rate	Female Deaths	Female Rate
00-04	0	0.00	0	0.00	0	0.00
05-09	1	0.01	1	0.01	0	0.00
10-14	187	1.00	139	1.45	48	0.52
15-19	1,377	7.82	1,204	13.32	173	2.02
20-24	1,967	10.72	1,784	19.14	183	2.03
25-29	1,750	9.11	1,531	15.89	219	2.29
30-34	1,782	8.04	1,506	13.63	276	2.48
35-39	1,733	7.90	1,424	13.05	309	2.80
40-44	1,531	7.78	1,275	13.11	256	2.57
45-49	1,351	8.10	1,124	13.74	227	2.67
50-54	1,092	8.28	894	13.95	198	2.92
55-59	902	8.25	794	15.15	108	1.90
60-64	895	8.88	776	16.37	119	2.23
65-69	958	9.60	841	18.68	117	2.14
70-74	1,052	12.04	950	25.07	102	2.06
75-79	991	15.08	920	34.64	71	1.81
80-84	693	15.94	649	41.87	44	1.57
85+	497	14.13	469	47.88	28	1.10
Unknown	6		6			
Total	18,765	7.21	16,287	12.82	2,478	1.86

Source: National Center for Injury Prevention and Control, Centers for Disease Control and Prevention, State Injury Mortality Statistics, downloaded from http://www.cdc.gov/ncip/ncipchm.htm on March 10, 1995.

★ 236 ★

Injuries and Accidents

United States Deaths and Death Rates, 1994: Homicide

[Rate is number per 100,000 persons]

Age Group	Total Deaths	Total Rate	Male Deaths	Male Rate	Female Deaths	Female Rate
00-04	786	3.98	444	4.40	342	3.55
05-09	156	0.83	75	0.78	81	0.88
10-14	413	2.20	279	2.91	134	1.46
15-19	3,532	20.05	3,082	34.11	450	5.24
20-24	4,481	24.42	3,841	41.20	640	7.09
25-29	3,548	18.47	2,869	29.78	679	7.09
30-34	3,206	14.47	2,487	22.51	719	6.47
35-39	2,641	12.04	1,990	18.24	651	5.90

[Continued]

★ 236 ★

United States Deaths and Death Rates, 1994:
Homicide

[Continued]

Age Group	Total Deaths	Total Rate	Male Deaths	Male Rate	Female Deaths	Female Rate
40-44	1,806	9.17	1,431	14.72	375	3.76
45-49	1,139	6.83	880	10.76	259	3.05
50-54	751	5.69	579	9.03	172	2.54
55-59	500	4.57	384	7.33	116	2.04
60-64	398	3.95	295	6.22	103	1.93
65-69	346	3.47	243	5.40	103	1.88
70-74	285	3.26	169	4.46	116	2.34
75-79	222	3.38	127	4.78	95	2.43
80-84	165	3.80	78	5.03	87	3.11
85+	120	3.41	54	5.51	66	2.60
Unknown	52		35		17	
Total	24,547	9.43	19,342	15.22	5,205	3.91

Source: National Center for Injury Prevention and Control, Centers for Disease Control and Prevention, State Injury Mortality Statistics, downloaded from http://www.cdc.gov.ncip/ncipchm.htm on March 10, 1995.

★ 237 ★

Injuries and Accidents

United States Deaths and Death Rates, 1994:
Homicide/Legal Intervention

[Rate is number per 100,000 persons]

Age Group	Total Deaths	Total Rate	Male Deaths	Male Rate	Female Deaths	Female Rate
00-04	786	3.98	444	4.40	342	3.55
05-09	156	0.83	75	0.78	81	0.88
10-14	416	2.22	282	2.94	134	1.46
15-19	3,569	20.26	3,118	34.51	451	5.26
20-24	4,547	24.78	3,906	41.90	641	7.10
25-29	3,607	18.78	2,926	30.37	681	7.12
30-34	3,281	14.80	2,559	23.16	722	6.50
35-39	2,698	12.30	2,044	18.74	654	5.93
40-44	1,833	9.31	1,458	15.00	375	3.76
45-49	1,162	6.97	903	11.04	259	3.05
50-54	767	5.81	593	9.25	174	2.57
55-59	502	4.59	386	7.36	116	2.04
60-64	402	3.99	299	6.31	103	1.93
65-69	348	3.49	245	5.44	103	1.88
70-74	288	3.30	172	4.54	116	2.34
75-79	225	3.42	129	4.86	96	2.45
80-84	165	3.80	78	5.03	87	3.11
85+	122	3.47	55	5.61	67	2.64

[Continued]

★ 237 ★

United States Deaths and Death Rates, 1994: Homicide/Legal Intervention

[Continued]

Age Group	Total		Male		Female	
	Deaths	Rate	Deaths	Rate	Deaths	Rate
Unknown	52		35		17	
Total	24,926	9.57	19,707	15.51	5,219	3.92

Source: National Center for Injury Prevention and Control, Centers for Disease Control and Prevention, State Injury Mortality Statistics, downloaded from http://www.cdc.gov.ncip/ncipchm.htm on March 10, 1995.

★ 238 ★

Injuries and Accidents

United States Deaths and Death Rates, 1994: Motor Vehicle Occupant, Traffic-Related

[Rate is number per 100,000 persons]

Age Group	Total		Male		Female	
	Deaths	Rate	Deaths	Rate	Deaths	Rate
00-04	564	2.86	282	2.79	282	2.93
05-09	365	1.93	203	2.10	162	1.76
10-14	535	2.85	281	2.93	254	2.78
15-19	3,506	19.90	2,314	25.61	1,192	13.89
20-24	3,427	18.68	2,500	26.81	927	10.27
25-29	2,340	12.18	1,656	17.19	684	7.15
30-34	2,181	9.84	1,526	13.81	655	5.89
35-39	1,906	8.69	1,286	11.79	620	5.62
40-44	1,503	7.63	1,003	10.32	500	5.02
45-49	1,272	7.63	832	10.17	440	5.18
50-54	1,037	7.86	666	10.39	371	5.47
55-59	853	7.80	537	10.24	316	5.55
60-64	848	8.41	508	10.72	340	6.36
65-69	961	9.63	527	11.70	434	7.93
70-74	1,083	12.39	576	15.20	507	10.24
75-79	1,007	15.32	512	19.28	495	12.64
80-84	836	19.23	415	26.78	421	15.05
85+	585	16.63	332	33.89	253	9.97
Unknown	9		6		3	
Total	24,818	9.53	15,962	12.56	8,856	6.65

Source: National Center for Injury Prevention and Control, Centers for Disease Control and Prevention, State Injury Mortality Statistics, downloaded from http://www.cdc.gov.ncip/ncipchm.htm on March 10, 1995.

★ 239 ★

Injuries and Accidents

United States Deaths and Death Rates, 1994: Motor Vehicle-Pedestrian, Traffic-Related

[Rate is number per 100,000 persons]

Age Group	Total Deaths	Total Rate	Male Deaths	Male Rate	Female Deaths	Female Rate
00-04	280	1.42	179	1.77	101	1.05
05-09	315	1.67	220	2.28	95	1.03
10-14	259	1.38	169	1.76	90	0.98
15-19	273	1.55	191	2.11	82	0.96
20-24	352	1.92	270	2.90	82	0.91
25-29	372	1.94	285	2.96	87	0.91
30-34	487	2.20	372	3.37	115	1.03
35-39	510	2.32	375	3.44	135	1.22
40-44	436	2.21	338	3.48	98	0.98
45-49	339	2.03	239	2.92	100	1.18
50-54	307	2.33	213	3.32	94	1.39
55-59	260	2.38	180	3.43	80	1.41
60-64	238	2.36	159	3.35	79	1.48
65-69	258	2.59	157	3.49	101	1.85
70-74	255	2.92	143	3.77	112	2.26
75-79	311	4.73	174	6.55	137	3.50
80-84	296	6.81	161	10.39	135	4.83
85+	218	6.20	114	11.64	104	4.10
Unknown	20		19		1	
Total	5,786	2.22	3,958	3.11	1,828	1.37

Source: National Center for Injury Prevention and Control, Centers for Disease Control and Prevention, State Injury Mortality Statistics, downloaded from http://www.cdc.gov.ncip/ncipchm.htm on March 10, 1995.

★ 240 ★

Injuries and Accidents

United States Deaths and Death Rates, 1994: Motor Vehicle Related, Overall

[Rate is number per 100,000 persons]

Age Group	Total Deaths	Total Rate	Male Deaths	Male Rate	Female Deaths	Female Rate
00-04	1,140	5.78	628	6.22	512	5.31
05-09	893	4.73	558	5.78	335	3.64
10-14	1,134	6.05	703	7.32	431	4.71
15-19	5,172	29.36	3,527	39.03	1,645	19.17
20-24	5,512	30.04	4,157	44.59	1,355	15.01
25-29	3,955	20.59	2,929	30.40	1,026	10.72
30-34	3,858	17.41	2,829	25.60	1,029	9.26
35-39	3,416	15.57	2,441	22.38	975	8.84

[Continued]

★ 240 ★

United States Deaths and Death Rates, 1994: Motor Vehicle Related, Overall

[Continued]

Age Group	Total Deaths	Total Rate	Male Deaths	Male Rate	Female Deaths	Female Rate
40-44	2,796	14.20	1,988	20.45	808	8.11
45-49	2,328	13.96	1,599	19.55	729	8.58
50-54	1,859	14.09	1,237	19.30	622	9.17
55-59	1,494	13.66	978	18.66	516	9.07
60-64	1,436	14.24	911	19.22	525	9.83
65-69	1,651	16.55	965	21.43	686	12.54
70-74	1,743	19.95	953	25.15	790	15.96
75-79	1,738	26.45	937	35.28	801	20.45
80-84	1,460	33.58	773	49.87	687	24.55
85+	1,027	29.19	585	59.72	442	17.41
Unknown	34		30		4	
Total	42,646	16.38	28,728	22.60	13,918	10.44

Source: National Center for Injury Prevention and Control, Centers for Disease Control and Prevention, State Injury Mortality Statistics, downloaded from http://www.cdc.gov.ncip/ncipchm.htm on March 10, 1995.

★ 241 ★

Injuries and Accidents

United States Deaths and Death Rates, 1994: Motor Vehicle, Traffic-Related

[Rate is number per 100,000 persons]

Age Group	Total Deaths	Total Rate	Male Deaths	Male Rate	Female Deaths	Female Rate
00-04	979	4.96	533	5.28	446	4.63
05-09	857	4.54	532	5.51	325	3.53
10-14	1,096	5.84	670	6.98	426	4.66
15-19	5,108	28.99	3,475	38.46	1,633	19.03
20-24	5,437	29.63	4,094	43.91	1,343	14.88
25-29	3,882	20.21	2,873	29.82	1,009	10.54
30-34	3,773	17.02	2,756	24.94	1,017	9.15
35-39	3,335	15.20	2,374	21.76	961	8.71
40-44	2,740	13.92	1,943	19.98	797	8.00
45-49	2,287	13.72	1,564	19.12	723	8.51
50-54	1,825	13.84	1,212	18.91	613	9.04
55-59	1,467	13.42	956	18.24	511	8.98
60-64	1,397	13.85	880	18.56	517	9.68
65-69	1,606	16.10	931	20.68	675	12.33
70-74	1,697	19.42	923	24.36	774	15.64
75-79	1,688	25.69	907	34.15	781	19.94
80-84	1,424	32.75	756	48.78	668	23.88
85+	998	28.37	567	57.88	431	16.98

[Continued]

★ 241 ★

United States Deaths and Death Rates, 1994: Motor Vehicle, Traffic-Related

[Continued]

Age Group	Total Deaths	Total Rate	Male Deaths	Male Rate	Female Deaths	Female Rate
Unknown	33		29		4	
Total	41,629	15.99	27,975	22.01	13,654	10.25

Source: National Center for Injury Prevention and Control, Centers for Disease Control and Prevention, State Injury Mortality Statistics, downloaded from http://www.cdc.gov.ncip/ncipchm.htm on March 10, 1995.

★ 242 ★

Injuries and Accidents

United States Deaths and Death Rates, 1994: Motor Vehicle, Unintentional

[Rate is number per 100,000 persons]

Age Group	Total Deaths	Total Rate	Male Deaths	Male Rate	Female Deaths	Female Rate
00-04	1,139	5.77	628	6.22	511	5.30
05-09	893	4.73	558	5.78	335	3.64
10-14	1,133	6.04	702	7.31	431	4.71
15-19	5,160	29.29	3,517	38.92	1,643	19.15
20-24	5,500	29.97	4,147	44.48	1,353	14.99
25-29	3,937	20.50	2,915	30.26	1,022	10.68
30-34	3,843	17.34	2,817	25.49	1,026	9.23
35-39	3,404	15.52	2,431	22.28	973	8.82
40-44	2,782	14.13	1,978	20.34	804	8.07
45-49	2,321	13.92	1,593	19.48	728	8.57
50-54	1,853	14.05	1,232	19.22	621	9.16
55-59	1,491	13.64	977	18.64	514	9.03
60-64	1,432	14.20	908	19.15	524	9.81
65-69	1,648	16.52	964	21.41	684	12.50
70-74	1,737	19.88	950	25.07	787	15.90
75-79	1,734	26.39	933	35.13	801	20.45
80-84	1,457	33.51	771	49.74	686	24.52
85+	1,026	29.16	584	59.62	442	17.41
Unknown	34		30		4	
Total	42,524	16.33	28,635	22.53	13,889	10.42

Source: National Center for Injury Prevention and Control, Centers for Disease Control and Prevention, State Injury Mortality Statistics, downloaded from http://www.cdc.gov.ncip/ncipchm.htm on March 10, 1995.

★ 243 ★

Injuries and Accidents

United States Deaths and Death Rates, 1994:
Suffocation

[Rate is number per 100,000 persons]

Age Group	Total Deaths	Total Rate	Male Deaths	Male Rate	Female Deaths	Female Rate
05-09	77	0.41	42	0.43	35	0.38
10-14	209	1.11	149	1.55	60	0.66
15-19	454	2.58	368	4.07	86	1.00
20-24	731	3.98	594	6.37	137	1.52
25-29	855	4.45	670	6.95	185	1.93
30-34	889	4.01	719	6.51	170	1.53
35-39	834	3.80	658	6.03	176	1.60
40-44	658	3.34	521	5.36	137	1.37
45-49	440	2.64	316	3.86	124	1.46
50-54	370	2.81	265	4.13	105	1.55
55-59	278	2.54	195	3.72	83	1.46
60-64	312	3.09	216	4.56	96	1.80
65-69	362	3.63	236	5.24	126	2.30
70-74	472	5.40	294	7.76	178	3.60
75-79	559	8.51	309	11.63	250	6.38
80-84	607	13.96	326	21.03	281	10.04
85+	1,075	30.56	401	40.94	674	26.55
Unknown	17		14		3	
Total	9,835	3.78	6,676	5.25	3,159	2.37

Source: National Center for Injury Prevention and Control, Centers for Disease Control and Prevention, State Injury Mortality Statistics, downloaded from http://www.cdc.gov.ncip/ncipchm.htm on March 10, 1995.

★ 244 ★

Injuries and Accidents

United States Deaths and Death Rates, 1994:
Suffocation, Unintentional

[Rate is number per 100,000 persons]

Age Group	Total Deaths	Total Rate	Male Deaths	Male Rate	Female Deaths	Female Rate
00-04	566	2.87	342	3.39	224	2.32
05-09	53	0.28	31	0.32	22	0.24
10-14	72	0.38	59	0.61	13	0.14
15-19	54	0.31	47	0.52	7	0.08
20-24	74	0.40	62	0.67	12	0.13
25-29	88	0.46	73	0.76	15	0.16
30-34	122	0.55	99	0.90	23	0.21
35-39	137	0.62	101	0.93	36	0.33
40-44	160	0.81	117	1.20	43	0.43

[Continued]

★ 244 ★

United States Deaths and Death Rates, 1994:
Suffocation, Unintentional
[Continued]

Age Group	Total Deaths	Total Rate	Male Deaths	Male Rate	Female Deaths	Female Rate
45-49	128	0.77	87	1.06	41	0.48
50-54	126	0.96	87	1.36	39	0.58
55-59	115	1.05	77	1.47	38	0.67
60-64	152	1.51	96	2.02	56	1.05
65-69	220	2.21	135	3.00	85	1.55
70-74	296	3.39	180	4.75	116	2.34
75-79	382	5.81	204	7.68	178	4.55
80-84	475	10.93	242	15.61	233	8.33
85+	918	26.09	317	32.36	601	23.67
Unknown	5		5			
Total	4,143	1.59	2,361	1.86	1,782	1.34

Source: National Center for Injury Prevention and Control, Centers for Disease Control and Prevention, State Injury Mortality Statistics, downloaded from http://www.cdc.gov.ncip/ncipchm.htm on March 10, 1995.

★ 245 ★

Injuries and Accidents

United States Deaths and Death Rates, 1994: Suicide
[Rate is number per 100,000]

Age Group	Total Deaths	Total Rate	Male Deaths	Male Rate	Female Deaths	Female Rate
00-04	0	0.00	0	0.00	0	0.00
05-09	4	0.02	4	0.04	0	0.00
10-14	318	1.70	230	2.40	88	0.96
15-19	1,948	11.06	1,649	18.25	299	3.48
20-24	3,008	16.39	2,653	28.46	355	3.93
25-29	3,026	15.76	2,555	26.52	471	4.92
30-34	3,328	15.02	2,740	24.79	588	5.29
35-39	3,397	15.48	2,662	24.40	735	6.66
40-44	2,978	15.13	2,308	23.74	670	6.72
45-49	2,407	14.44	1,825	22.31	582	6.85
50-54	1,889	14.32	1,404	21.90	485	7.15
55-59	1,462	13.37	1,128	21.52	334	5.87
60-64	1,350	13.39	1,070	22.57	280	5.24
65-69	1,384	13.87	1,091	24.23	293	5.35
70-74	1,481	16.95	1,209	31.91	272	5.50
75-79	1,351	20.56	1,148	43.23	203	5.18
80-84	981	22.56	828	53.42	153	5.47
85+	811	23.05	653	66.66	158	6.22

[Continued]

★ 245 ★

United States Deaths and Death Rates, 1994: Suicide
[Continued]

Age Group	Total Deaths	Total Rate	Male Deaths	Male Rate	Female Deaths	Female Rate
Unknown	19		17		2	
Total	31,142	11.96	25,174	19.81	5,968	4.48

Source: National Center for Injury Prevention and Control, Centers for Disease Control and Prevention, State Injury Mortality Statistics, downloaded from http://www.cdc.gov.ncip/ncipchm.htm on March 10, 1995.

★ 246 ★

Injuries and Accidents

United States Deaths and Death Rates, 1994: Unintentional Drowning

[Rate is number per 100,000 persons]

Age Group	Total Deaths	Total Rate	Male Deaths	Male Rate	Female Deaths	Female Rate
00-04	548	2.78	340	3.37	208	2.16
05-09	189	1.00	141	1.46	48	0.52
10-14	221	1.18	180	1.87	41	0.45
15-19	358	2.03	323	3.57	35	0.41
20-24	313	1.71	293	3.14	20	0.22
25-29	304	1.58	276	2.86	28	0.29
30-34	358	1.62	322	2.91	36	0.32
35-39	330	1.50	283	2.59	47	0.43
40-44	265	1.35	218	2.24	47	0.47
45-49	207	1.24	173	2.12	34	0.40
50-54	142	1.08	120	1.87	22	0.32
55-59	128	1.17	107	2.04	21	0.37
60-64	105	1.04	86	1.81	19	0.36
65-69	91	0.91	71	1.58	20	0.37
70-74	85	0.97	57	1.50	28	0.57
75-79	111	1.69	74	2.79	37	0.94
80-84	94	2.16	53	3.42	41	1.47
85 +	66	1.88	37	3.78	29	1.14
Unknown	27		25		2	
Total	3,942	1.51	3,179	2.50	763	0.57

Source: National Center for Injury Prevention and Control, Centers for Disease Control and Prevention, State Injury Mortality Statistics, downloaded from http://www.cdc.gov.ncip/ncipchm.htm on March 10, 1995.

★ 247 ★

Injuries and Accidents

United States Deaths and Death Rates, 1994: Unintentional Fall

[Rate is number per 100,000 persons]

Age Group	Total Deaths	Total Rate	Male Deaths	Male Rate	Female Deaths	Female Rate
00-04	78	0.40	56	0.55	22	0.23
05-09	26	0.14	21	0.22	5	0.05
10-14	30	0.16	21	0.22	9	0.10
15-19	94	0.53	83	0.92	11	0.13
20-24	125	0.68	116	1.24	9	0.10
25-29	173	0.90	150	1.56	23	0.24
30-34	204	0.92	177	1.60	27	0.24
35-39	272	1.24	231	2.12	41	0.37
40-44	364	1.85	301	3.10	63	0.63
45-49	300	1.80	240	2.93	60	0.71
50-54	283	2.15	231	3.60	52	0.77
55-59	331	3.03	250	4.77	81	1.42
60-64	434	4.30	323	6.81	111	2.08
65-69	527	5.28	337	7.48	190	3.47
70-74	795	9.10	490	12.93	305	6.16
75-79	1,170	17.80	647	24.36	523	13.36
80-84	1,655	38.07	806	52.00	849	30.34
85+	3,223	91.61	1,209	123.42	2,014	79.34
Unknown	4		3		1	
Total	10,088	3.87	5,692	4.48	4,396	3.30

Source: National Center for Injury Prevention and Control, Centers for Disease Control and Prevention, State Injury Mortality Statistics, downloaded from http://www.cdc.gov.ncip/ncipchm.htm on March 10, 1995.

★ 248 ★

Injuries and Accidents

United States Deaths and Death Rates, 1994: Unintentional Fire/Flame

[Rate is number per 100,000 persons]

Age Group	Total Deaths	Total Rate	Male Deaths	Male Rate	Female Deaths	Female Rate
00-04	694	3.52	428	4.24	266	2.76
05-09	246	1.30	139	1.44	107	1.16
10-14	99	0.53	56	0.58	43	0.47
15-19	87	0.49	55	0.61	32	0.37
20-24	161	0.88	101	1.08	60	0.66
25-29	185	0.96	123	1.28	62	0.65
30-34	214	0.97	154	1.39	60	0.54
35-39	200	0.91	137	1.26	63	0.57

[Continued]

★ 248 ★

United States Deaths and Death Rates, 1994:
Unintentional Fire/Flame
[Continued]

Age Group	Total		Male		Female	
	Deaths	Rate	Deaths	Rate	Deaths	Rate
40-44	221	1.12	177	1.82	44	0.44
45-49	203	1.22	135	1.65	68	0.80
50-54	149	1.13	108	1.68	41	0.60
55-59	150	1.37	90	1.72	60	1.05
60-64	208	2.06	131	2.76	77	1.44
65-69	200	2.00	112	2.49	88	1.61
70-74	227	2.60	114	3.01	113	2.28
75-79	240	3.65	133	5.01	107	2.73
80-84	250	5.75	135	8.71	115	4.11
85+	249	7.08	112	11.43	137	5.40
Unknown	3		3			
Total	3,986	1.53	2,443	1.92	1,543	1.16

Source: National Center for Injury Prevention and Control, Centers for Disease Control and Prevention, State Injury Mortality Statistics, downloaded from http://www.cdc.gov.ncip/ncipchm.htm on March 10, 1995.

★ 249 ★

Injuries and Accidents

United States Deaths and Death Rates, 1994:
Unintentional Injury

Age Group	Total		Male		Female	
	Deaths	Rate	Deaths	Rate	Deaths	Rate
00-04	3,406	17.26	2,023	20.03	1,383	14.35
05-09	1,595	8.45	1,009	10.44	586	6.37
10-14	1,913	10.20	1,296	13.50	617	6.74
15-19	6,565	37.26	4,721	52.24	1,844	21.49
20-24	7,333	39.96	5,696	61.10	1,637	18.13
25-29	6,252	32.55	4,822	50.05	1,430	14.94
30-34	7,200	32.49	5,570	50.40	1,630	14.67
35-39	7,155	32.61	5,421	49.69	1,734	15.72
40-44	6,405	32.53	4,916	50.56	1,489	14.94
45-49	4,997	29.97	3,679	44.98	1,318	15.52
50-54	3,771	28.59	2,699	42.11	1,072	15.81
55-59	3,154	28.85	2,207	42.10	947	16.64
60-64	3,278	32.51	2,209	46.59	1,069	20.01
65-69	3,772	37.81	2,324	51.61	1,448	26.46
70-74	4,507	51.58	2,631	69.43	1,876	37.91
75-79	5,249	79.87	2,851	107.35	2,398	61.24
80-84	5,708	131.29	2,821	182.01	2,887	103.19
85+	9,078	258.03	3,525	359.84	5,553	218.75

[Continued]

★ 249 ★

United States Deaths and Death Rates, 1994:
Unintentional Injury
[Continued]

Age Group	Total		Male		Female	
	Deaths	Rate	Deaths	Rate	Deaths	Rate
Unknown	99		89		10	
Total	91,437	35.12	60,509	47.61	30,928	23.21

Source: National Center for Injury Prevention and Control, Centers for Disease Control and Prevention, State Injury Mortality Statistics, downloaded from http://www.cdc.gov.ncip/ncipchm.htm on March 10, 1995.

★ 250 ★

Injuries and Accidents

United States Deaths and Death Rates, 1994:
Unintentional Poisoning
[Rate is number per 100,000 persons]

Age Group	Total		Male		Female	
	Deaths	Rate	Deaths	Rate	Deaths	Rate
00-04	52	0.26	26	0.26	26	0.27
05-09	20	0.11	10	0.10	10	0.11
10-14	35	0.19	21	0.22	14	0.15
15-19	148	0.84	115	1.27	33	0.38
20-24	414	2.26	321	3.44	93	1.03
25-29	813	4.23	652	6.77	161	1.68
30-34	1,504	6.79	1,196	10.82	308	2.77
35-39	1,809	8.25	1,406	12.89	403	3.65
40-44	1,664	8.45	1,346	13.84	318	3.19
45-49	925	5.55	723	8.84	202	2.38
50-54	437	3.31	304	4.74	133	1.96
55-59	239	2.19	164	3.13	75	1.32
60-64	183	1.81	114	2.40	69	1.29
65-69	154	1.54	90	2.00	64	1.17
70-74	163	1.87	86	2.27	77	1.56
75-79	144	2.19	78	2.94	66	1.69
80-84	112	2.58	45	2.90	67	2.39
85+	171	4.86	56	5.72	115	4.53
Unknown	7		6		1	
Total	8,994	3.45	6,759	5.32	2,235	1.68

Source: National Center for Injury Prevention and Control, Centers for Disease Control and Prevention, State Injury Mortality Statistics, downloaded from http://www.cdc.gov.ncip/ncipchm.htm on March 10, 1995.

Life Expectancy

★ 251 ★

Expectation of Life at Birth, 1970 to 1994, and Projections, 1995 to 2010

In years. Beginning 1970, excludes deaths of nonresidents of the United States.

YEAR	TOTAL			WHITE			BLACK AND OTHER			BLACK		
	Total	Male	Female	Total	Male	Female	Total	Male	Female	Total	Male	Female
1970	70.8	67.1	74.7	71.7	68.0	75.6	65.3	61.3	69.4	64.1	60.0	68.3
1975	72.6	68.8	76.6	73.4	69.5	77.3	68.0	63.7	72.4	66.8	62.4	71.3
1980	73.7	70.0	77.4	74.4	70.7	78.1	69.5	65.3	73.6	68.1	63.8	72.5
1982	74.5	70.8	78.1	75.1	71.5	78.7	70.9	66.8	74.9	69.4	65.1	73.6
1983	74.6	71.0	78.1	75.2	71.6	78.7	70.9	67.0	74.7	69.4	65.2	73.5
1984	74.7	71.1	78.2	75.3	71.8	78.7	71.1	67.2	74.9	69.5	65.3	73.6
1985	74.7	71.1	78.2	75.3	71.8	78.7	71.0	67.0	74.8	69.3	65.0	73.4
1986	74.7	71.2	78.2	75.4	71.9	78.8	70.9	66.8	74.9	69.1	64.8	73.4
1987	74.9	71.4	78.3	75.6	72.1	78.9	71.0	66.9	75.0	69.1	64.7	73.4
1988	74.9	71.4	78.3	75.6	72.2	78.9	70.8	66.7	74.8	68.9	64.4	73.2
1989	75.1	71.7	78.5	75.9	72.5	79.2	70.9	66.7	74.9	68.8	64.3	73.3
1990	75.4	71.8	78.8	76.1	72.7	79.4	71.2	67.0	75.2	69.1	64.5	73.6
1991	75.5	72.0	78.9	76.3	72.9	79.6	71.5	67.3	75.5	69.3	64.6	73.8
1992	75.8	72.3	79.1	76.5	73.2	79.8	71.8	67.7	75.7	69.6	65.0	73.9
1993	75.5	72.2	78.8	76.3	73.1	79.5	71.5	67.3	75.5	69.2	64.6	73.7
1994	75.7	72.3	79.0	76.4	73.2	79.6	71.7	67.5	75.8	69.6	64.9	74.1
Projections:[1]												
1995	76.3	72.5	79.3	77.0	73.6	80.1	72.5	68.2	76.8	70.3	64.8	74.5
2000	76.7	73.0	79.7	77.6	74.2	80.5	72.9	68.3	77.5	70.2	64.6	74.7
2005	77.3	73.5	80.2	78.2	74.7	81.0	73.6	69.1	78.1	70.7	64.5	75.0
2010	77.9	74.1	80.6	78.8	75.5	81.6	74.3	69.9	78.7	71.3	65.1	75.5

Source: 1996 Statistical Abstract of the United States on CD-ROM [machine-readable datafiles]. CD-8A-97. Washington, DC: U.S. Department of Commerce, Economics and Statistics Administration, Bureau of the Census, Data User Services Division, January 1997. Primary source: Except as noted, U.S. National Center for Health Statistics, *Vital Statistics of the United States*, annual, and *Monthly Vital Statistics Reports. Notes:* NA Not available. 1. Based on middle mortality assumptions; for details, see source: U.S. Bureau of the Census, Current Population Reports, P25-1104.

★ 252 ★

Life Expectancy

Life Expectancy at Birth, Age 65, and Age 75, by Race and Sex: 1994

[Data are based on the National Vital Statistics System]

Specified age and year	All races			White			Black		
	Both sexes	Male	Female	Both sexes	Male	Female	Both sexes	Male	Female
At birth	75.7	72.3	79.0	76.4	73.2	79.6	69.6	64.9	74.1
At 65 years	17.4	15.5	18.9	---	---	---	---	---	---
At 75 years	11.0	9.6	11.9	---	---	---	---	---	---

Source: U.S. Department of Health and Human Services. Public Health Service. Centers for Disease Control and Prevention. National Center for Health Statistics. *Health, United States, 1995.* Hyattsville, MD: Public Health Service, 1996, p. 109.

Men's Health

★ 253 ★

Death from Prostate Cancer

"In patients whose prostate cancer hasn't spread, the odds of dying from the disease within 10 years drops to less than 5% if the entire gland is surgically removed."

Source: Cronin, Brian. "Health Report: The Good News." *Time,* 14 July 1997, p. 19. Primary source: *J.A.M.A.*

★ 254 ★
Men's Health

Diagnostic/Nonsurgical Procedures for Males Discharged From Non-Federal Short Stay Hospitals, by Age and Procedure: 1993

[Data are based on a sample of hospital records]

Sex, age, and surgical category	Procedures in thousands 1993[1,2]	Procedures per 1,000 population 1993[1,2]
All ages[3,4,5]	7,787	60.5
Angiocardiography using contrast material	832	6.5
Computerized axial tomography (CAT scan)	565	4.3
Diagnostic ultrasound	572	4.4
Cystoscopy	195	1.5
Endoscopy of small intestine without biopsy	223	1.7
Radioisotope scan	173	1.3
Arteriography using contrast material	192	1.5
Endoscopy of large intestine without biopsy	146	1.1
Under 15 years[3,5]	582	20.0
Spinal tap	76	2.6
Computerized axial tomography (CAT scan)	32	1.1
Diagnostic ultrasound	31	1.1
Electroencephalogram	11	0.4
Application of cast or splint	6[6]	0.2[6]
Radioisotope scan	7[6]	0.2[6]
Cystoscopy	[6]	[6]
15-44 years[3,5]	1,741	29.8
Computerized axial tomography (CAT scan)	160	2.7
Diagnostic ultrasound	95	1.6
Angiocardiography using contrast material	101	1.7
Endoscopy of small intestine without biopsy	46	0.8
Spinal tap	44	0.8
Arthroscopy of knee	41	0.7
Contrast myelogram	21	0.4
Cystoscopy	22	0.4
Endoscopy of large intestine without biopsy	25	0.4
Application of cast or splint	13	0.2
45-64 years[3,5]	2,182	91.3
Angiocardiography using contrast material	383	16.0
Diagnostic ultrasound	163	6.8
Computerized axial tomography (CAT scan)	128	5.3
Endoscopy of small intestine without biopsy	65	2.7
Cystoscopy	47	2.0
Radioisotope scan	51	2.1

[Continued]

★ 254 ★

Diagnostic/Nonsurgical Procedures for Males Discharged From Non-Federal Short Stay Hospitals, by Age and Procedure: 1993
[Continued]

Sex, age, and surgical category	Procedures in thousands 1993[1,2]	Procedures per 1,000 population 1993[1,2]
Arteriography using contrast material	71	3.0
Endoscopy of large intestine without biopsy	44	1.8
65-74 years[3,5]	1,675	203.4
Angiocardiography using contrast material	239	29.0
Diagnostic ultrasound	139	16.8
Computerized axial tomography (CAT scan)	116	14.1
Cystoscopy	58	7.1
Endoscopy of small intestine without biopsy	46	5.6
Arteriography using contrast material	53	6.4
Radioisotope scan	44	5.4
Endoscopy of large intestine without biopsy	27	3.2
75 years and over[3,5]	1,606	317.6
Diagnostic ultrasound	145	28.7
Computerized axial tomography (CAT scan)	130	25.6
Cystoscopy	65	12.8
Angiocardiography using contrast material	103	20.3
Endoscopy of small intestine without biopsy	65	12.8
Endoscopy of large intestine without biopsy	50	9.9
Radioisotope scan	39	7.6
Arteriography using contrast material	38	7.6

Source: U.S. Department of Health and Human Services. Public Health Service. Centers for Disease Control and Prevention. National Center for Health Statistics. *Health, United States, 1995.* Hyattsville, MD: Public Health Service, 1996. p. 207. Primary source: Centers for Disease Control and Prevention, National Center for Health Statistics, Division of Health Interview Statistics. Data from National Hospital Discharge Survey. *Notes:* Excludes newborn infants. Data do not reflect total use; procedures for outpatients are not included in the National Hospital Discharge Survey. For example, CAT scans have been performed 1. Comparisons of data from 1983-93 with data from earlier years should be made with caution as estimates of change may reflect improvements in the design (see Appendix I) rather than true changes in hospital use. 2. In 1993 children's hospitals had a high rate of nonresponse which may have resulted in underestimates of hospital utilization by children. 3. Beginning in 1989 the definition of some surgical and diagnostic and other nonsurgical procedures was revised, thus causing a discontinuity in the totals. 4. Rates are age adjusted. 5. Includes nonsurgical procedures not shown. 6. Statistics based on fewer than 5,000 estimated discharges are not shown; those based on 5,000-9,000 estimated discharges are to be used with caution.

★ 255 ★

Men's Health

Operations for Men Discharged from Non-Federal Short-Stay Hospitals, by Age and Surgical Category: 1993

[Data are based on a sample of hospital records]

Sex, age, and surgical category	Operations in thousands 1993[1,2]	Operations per 1,000 population 1993[1,2]
All ages[3,4,5]	8,355	64.7
Cardiac catheterization	613	4.8
Prostatectomy	317	2.4
Reduction of fracture (excluding skull, nose, and jaw)	294	2.3
Direct heart revascularization (coronary bypass)	353	2.8
Excision or destruction of intervertebral disc and spinal fusion	272	2.0
Operations on muscles, tendons, fascia, and bursa	158	1.2
Repair of inguinal hernia	96	0.8
Under 15 years [3,5]	459	15.8
Reduction of fracture (excluding skull, nose, and jaw)	37	1.3
Appendectomy, excluding incidental[6]	27	0.9
Tonsillectomy, with or without adenoidectomy	16	0.6
Myringotomy	16	0.5
Repair of inguinal hernia	9[7]	0.3[7]
Circumcision	18	0.6
15-44 years[3,5]	2,133	36.6
Reduction of fracture (excluding skull, nose, and jaw)	148	2.5
Excision or destruction of intervertebral disc and spinal fusion	160	2.7
Appendectomy, excluding incidental[6]	82	1.4
Operations on muscles, tendons, fascia, and bursa	74	1.3
Debridement of wound, infection, or burn	77	1.3
Excision of semilunar cartilage of knee	28	0.5
Repair of inguinal hernia	17	0.3
45-64 years[3,5]	2,458	102.8
Cardiac catheterization	282	11.8
Direct heart revascularization (coronary bypass)	162	6.8
Excision or destruction of intervertebral disc and spinal fusion	86	3.6
Prostatectomy	66	2.8
Reduction of fracture (excluding skull, nose, and jaw)	50	2.1
Operations on muscles, tendons, fascia, and bursa	42	1.8
Repair of inguinal hernia	23	1.0
65-74 years[3,5]	1,870	227.1
Cardiac catheterization	180	21.9
Prostatectomy	139	16.9

[Continued]

★ 255 ★

Operations for Men Discharged from Non-Federal Short-Stay Hospitals, by Age and Surgical Category: 1993
[Continued]

Sex, age, and surgical category	Operations in thousands 1993[1,2]	Operations per 1,000 population 1993[1,2]
Direct heart revascularization (coronary bypass)	129	15.7
Biopsies on the digestive system	30	3.6
Pacemaker insertion or replacement	35	4.3
Repair of inguinal hernia	28	3.4
Extraction of lens	6[7]	0.7[7]
75 years and over[3,5]	1,435	283.7
Prostatectomy	110	21.8
Pacemaker insertion or replacement	78	15.5
Cardiac catheterization	78	15.5
Biopsies on the digestive system	37	7.2
Direct heart revascularization (coronary bypass)	44	8.7
Repair of inguinal hernia	19	3.8
Extraction of lens	10	2.1
Insertion of prosthetic lens (pseudophakos)	10	2.0

Source: U.S. Department of Health and Human Services. Public Health Service. Centers for Disease Control and Prevention. National Center for Health Statistics. *Health, United States, 1995.* Hyattsville, MD: Public Health Service, 1996. p. 205. Primary source: Centers for Disease Control and Prevention, National Center for Health Statistics, Division of Health Interview Statistics. Data from National Hospital Discharge Survey. *Notes:* Excludes newborn infants. Data do not reflect total use of operations because operations for outpatients are not included in the National Hospital Discharge Survey. In recent years, for example, lens extractions and myringotomies have been performed on outpatients as well as inpatients. Rates are based on the civilian population as of July 1. In each sex and age group, data are shown for the five most common operations in 1980 and 1991. Surgical categories are based on the International Classification of Diseases, 9th Revision, Clinical Modification. For a listing of the code numbers, see Appendix II, table VII. 1. Comparisons of data from 1983-93 with data from earlier years should be made with caution as estimates of change may reflect improvements in the design (see Appendix I) rather than true changes in hospital use. 2. In 1993 children's hospitals had a high rate of nonresponse which may have resulted in underestimates of hospital utilization by children. 3. Beginning in 1989 the definition of some surgical and diagnostic and other nonsurgical procedures was revised, thus causing a discontinuity in the trends for the totals and selected surgical procedures. 4. Rates are age adjusted. 5. Includes operations not listed in table. 6. Limited to estimated number of appendectomies, excluding those performed incidental to other abdominal surgery. 7. Statistics based on fewer than 5,000 estimated discharges are not shown; those based on 5,000-9,000 estimated discharges are to be used with caution.

★ 256 ★

Men's Health

Prostate Cancer Rates, by Race: 1990-1992
[Rate is number of cases per 100,000 men ages 50-74]

Race/ethnicity	Rate
White	405.5
Black	477.2

Source: Merrill, PhD, Ray M. "Trends in Prostate Cancer Incidence and Surgery." *Primary Care & Cancer* (June 1996), p. 33. Primary source: Surveillance, Epidemiology, and End Results (SEER) Program.

★ 257 ★

Men's Health

Radical Prostatectomy Rates, by Race: 1990-1992

[Rate is number of cases per 100,000 men ages 50-74]

Race/ethnicity	Rate
White	201.1
Black	153.1

Source: Merrill, PhD, Ray M. "Trends in Prostate Cancer Incidence and Surgery." *Primary Care & Cancer* (June 1996), p. 33. Primary source: Surveillance, Epidemiology, and End Results (SEER) Program.

Mental Health

★ 258 ★

Depression and Stroke

"...A 29-year study finds that clinically depressed adults may face a 50% increased risk of dying from stroke. Depression—which is treatable—may somehow alter blood-platelet activity, which in turn may trigger clot formation."

Source: Cronin, Brian. "Health Report: The Bad News." *Time,* 28 April 1997, p. 26. Primary source: *Epidemiology;* Society of Behavioral Medicine meeting; Centers for Disease Control and Prevention.

★ 259 ★
Mental Health

Fees Paid to Mental Health Professionals

Table shows out-of-pocket costs for patients who do not have or use insurance for a typical 45-minute session. Insurers pay fees that are $10-$15 less.

Provider	Hourly Fee ($)
Psychiatrists	110
Psychologists	90
Marriage/family therapists	75
Social workers	75
Professional counselors	70

Source: "Mental Disorders: The Toll." *USA TODAY,* 28 May 1996. Primary sources: National Institute of Mental Health; Dorothy Rice, University of California, San Francisco; *Psychotherapy Finances.*

★ 260 ★
Mental Health

Mental Health Treatment, by Provider: 1995

Provider	Percentage
Family doctors	
Drugs & counseling	48
Drugs	37
Counseling	15
Mental-health specialists	
Drugs & therapy	17
Drugs	3
Therapy	80

Source: "Mental Health: Does Therapy Help?" Consumer Reports (November 1995), p. 738. Primary source: Based on a survey of 4,000 readers of *Consumer Reports.*

★ 261 ★

Mental Health

Mental Illness in the U.S.

"Research conducted by National Institute of Mental Health (NIMH) shows that anxiety disorders are the most common of all mental illnesses in America: more than 23 million people are affected each year. Fear, worry, or anxiety in situations when most people would not experience them could indicate an anxiety disorder."

Source: "Public Health News & Notes: Anxiety Disorders Lead Mental Ills in United States." *Public Health Records,* vol. III, no. 4 (July/August 1996), p. 293.

★ 262 ★

Mental Health

Population Affected by Mental Disorders

Data refer to the number of adults who suffer from any mental disorder, and particular disorders, at some point during any 1-year period.

Disorder	Sufferers (millions)	% of pop.
Any mental disorder[1]	40.7	22.1
Schizophrenia	2.0	1.1
Depressive disorders	17.5	9.5
Anxiety disorders	23.2	12.6
Other	8.2	4.4

Source: "Mental Disorders: The Toll." *USA TODAY,* 28 May 1996. Primary sources: National Institute of Mental Health; Dorothy Rice, University of California, San Francisco; *Psychotherapy Finances. Notes:* 1. Data are based on 1990 Census count of 184 million people 18 years old and older. Data do not include statistics on substance abuse. Some people have more than one mental disorder.

★ 263 ★

Mental Health

Psychiatric Care Coverage, by Type

Payer	Percentage
Commercial insurance	20
Blue Cross/Blue Shield	11
Medicare	7
Medicaid	5
HMO/PPO	4

[Continued]

★ 263 ★

Psychiatric Care Coverage, by Type
[Continued]

Payer	Percentage
Self-pay	47
Other	6

Source: "Paying for Psychiatric Care." *American Medical News,* 27 May 1996, p. 2. Primary source: U.S. Department of Health and Human Services, National Center for Health Statistics (December 1993).

Pregnancy and Childbirth

★ 264 ★

Hospital Births Attended by Midwives

The table shows the number of hospital births attended by certified nurse-midwives, i.e., registered nurses with either a master's degree or a certificate in midwifery.

Year	Number of births
1975	19,686
1981	55,537
1987	98,425
1989	122,892
1990	139,229
1991	158,068
1992	176,117

Source: "Going Natural." *American Health* (November 1995), p. 26. Primary source: National Center for Health Statistics.

★ 265 ★

Pregnancy and Childbirth

Leading Pregnancy Drug Prescriptions: 1995

[In number of prescriptions written per 1,000 deliveries]

Drug	Rate of prescriptions
Amoxicillin	230
Acetominophen products	139
Terconazole	130
Ampicillin	118
Erythromycin	114
Codeine	108
Nitrofurantoin	97
Docusate Sodium	96
Metronidazole	87
Cephalexin	81

Source: "News You Can Use: The Top 10 Pregnancy Drugs." *U.S. News & World Report,* 27 March 1995, p. 60.

★ 266 ★

Pregnancy and Childbirth

Live Births, by Method of Delivery, 1992-1994: Cesarean

Year and race of mother	Cesarean		
	Total	Primary	Repeat
All races[1]			
1994	830,517	520,647	309,870
1993	861,987	539,251	322,736
1992	888,622	554,662	333,960
White			
1994	656,400	407,946	248,454
1993	682,355	423,540	258,815
1992	705,841	437,398	268,443
Black			
1994	138,067	88,636	49,431
1993	143,452	91,677	51,775
1992	146,480	93,165	53,315

Source: Ventura, S.J., J.A. Martin, T.J. Mathews, and S.C. Clarke. "Advance Report of Final Natality Statistics, 1994." Monthly Vital Statistics Report vol. 44, no. 11, supp., p. 71. Hyattsville, Maryland: National Center for Health Statistics, 1996. *Note:* 1. Includes races other than white and black.

★ 267 ★

Pregnancy and Childbirth

Live Births, by Method of Delivery, 1992-1994: Vaginal

Year and race of mother	Vaginal	
	Total	After pervious cesarean
All races[1]		
1994	3,087,576	110,341
1993	3,098,796	103,581
1992	3,100,710	97,549
White		
1994	2,435,965	88,471
1993	2,435,229	82,995
1992	2,434,959	77,977
Black		
1994	493,879	16,970
1993	509,816	16,179
1992	514,929	15,382

Source: Ventura, S.J., J.A. Martin, T.J. Mathews, and S.C. Clarke. "Advance Report of Final Natality Statistics, 1994." Monthly Vital Statistics Report, vol. 44, no. 11, supp., p. 71. Hyattsville, Maryland: National Center for Health Statistics, 1996. *Note:* 1. Includes races other than white and black.

★ 268 ★

Pregnancy and Childbirth

Live Births, by Race: 1992-1994

Year and race of mother	All births
All races[1]	
1994	3,952,767
1993	4,000,240
1992	4,065,014
White	
1994	3,121,004
1993	3,149,833
1992	3,201,678
Black	
1994	636,391

[Continued]

★ 268 ★

Live Births, by Race: 1992-1994
[Continued]

Year and race of mother	All births
1993	658,875
1992	673,633

Source: Ventura, S.J., J.A. Martin, T.J. Mathews, and S.C. Clarke. "Advance Report of Final Natality Statistics, 1994." Monthly Vital Statistics Report, vol. 44, no. 11, supp., p. 71. Hyattsville, Maryland: National Center for Health Statistics, 1996. *Note:* 1. Includes races other than white and black.

★ 269 ★

Pregnancy and Childbirth

Live Births, by Race, Ethnicity, and Prenatal Care Begun in First Trimester: 1992 and 1993
[In percent of live births]

Characteristic	1992	1993
Percent of live births[1]		
All mothers	77.7	78.9
White	80.8	81.8
Black	63.9	66.0
American Indian or Alaska Native	62.1	63.4
Asian or Pacific Islander	76.6	77.6
Chinese	83.8	84.6
Japanese	88.2	87.2
Filipino	78.7	79.3
Hawaiian and part Hawaiian	69.9	70.6
Other Asian or Pacific Islander	72.8	74.4
Hispanic origin (selected States)[2,3]	64.2	66.6
Mexican American	62.1	64.8
Puerto Rican	67.8	70.0
Cuban	86.8	88.9
Central and South American	66.8	68.7
Other and unknown Hispanic	68.0	70.0
White, non-Hispanic (selected States)[2]	84.9	85.6
Black, non-Hispanic (selected States)[2]	64.0	66.1

Source: U.S. Department of Health and Human Services. Public Health Service. Centers for Disease Control and Prevention. National Center for Health Statistics. *Health, United States, 1995.* Hyattsville, MD: Public Health Service, 1996. *Notes:* Data for 1970 and 1975 exclude births that occurred in States not reporting prenatal care (see Appendix I). The race groups, white and black, include persons of Hispanic and non-Hispanic origin. Conversely, persons of Hispanic origin may be of any race. 1. Excludes live births for whom trimester prenatal care began is unknown. 2. Trend data for Hispanics and non-Hispanics are affected by expansion of the reporting area for an Hispanic-origin item on the birth certificate and by immigration. These two factors affect numbers of events, composition of the Hispanic population, and maternal and infant health characteristics. The number of States in the reporting area increased from 22 in 1980, to 23 and the District of Columbia (DC) in 1983-87, 30 and DC in 1988, 47 and DC in 1989, 48 and DC in 1990, 49 and DC in 1991-92, and 50 and DC in 1993 (see Appendix I, National Vital Statistics System). 3. Includes mothers of all races.

★ 270 ★

Pregnancy and Childbirth

Live Births, by Race, Ethnicity, and Prenatal Care Begun in First Trimester or Not At All: 1992 and 1993

[In percent of live births]

Characteristic	1992	1993
All mothers	5.2	4.8
White	4.2	3.9
Black	9.9	9.0
American Indian or Alaska Native	11.0	10.3
Asian or Pacific Islander	4.9	4.6
Chinese	2.9	2.9
Japanese	2.4	2.8
Filipino	4.3	4.0
Hawaiian and part Hawaiian	7.0	6.7
Other Asian or Pacific Islander	5.9	5.4
Hispanic origin (selected States)[1,2]	9.5	8.8
Mexican American	10.5	9.7
Puerto Rican	8.0	7.1
Cuban	2.1	1.8
Central and South American	7.9	7.3
Other and unknown	7.5	7.0
White, non-Hispanic (selected States)[1]	2.8	2.7
Black, non-Hispanic (selected States)[1]	9.8	9.0

Source: U.S. Department of Health and Human Services. Public Health Service. Centers for Disease Control and Prevention. National Center for Health Statistics. *Health, United States, 1995.* Hyattsville, MD: Public Health Service, 1996. *Notes:* Data for 1970 and 1975 exclude births that occurred in States not reporting prenatal care (see Appendix I). The race groups, white and black, include persons of Hispanic and non-Hispanic origin. Conversely, persons of Hispanic origin may be of any race. 1. Trend data for Hispanics and non-Hispanics are affected by expansion of the reporting area for an Hispanic-origin item on the birth certificate and by immigration. These two factors affect numbers of events, composition of the Hispanic population, and maternal and infant health characteristics. The number of States in the reporting area increased from 22 in 1980, to 23 and the District of Columbia (DC) in 1983-87, 30 and DC in 1988, 47 and DC in 1989, 48 and DC in 1990, 49 and DC in 1991-92, and 50 and DC in 1993 (see Appendix I, National Vital Statistics System). 2. Includes mothers of all races.

★ 271 ★

Pregnancy and Childbirth

Live Births Rates, by Method of Delivery, 1992-1994: Cesarean and Vaginal Cesarean

Year and race of mother	Cesarean delivery rate		Rate of vaginal cesarean birth after previous cesarean[3]
	Total[1]	Primary[2]	
All races[4]			
1994	21.2	14.9	26.3
1993	21.8	15.3	24.3
1992	22.3	15.6	22.6
White			
1994	21.2	14.8	26.3
1993	21.9	15.3	24.3
1992	22.5	15.7	22.5
Black			
1994	21.8	15.7	25.6
1993	22.0	15.7	23.8
1992	22.1	15.7	22.4

Source: Ventura, S.J., J.A. Martin, T.J. Mathews, and S.C. Clarke. "Advance Report of Final Natality Statistics, 1994." Monthly Vital Statistics Report, vol. 44, no. 11, supp., p. 71. Hyattsville, Maryland: National Center for Health Statistics, 1996. *Notes:* 1. Percent of all live births by cesarean delivery. 2. Number of primary cesarean per 100 live births women who have not had a previous cesarean. 3. Number of vaginal births after previous cesarean delivery per 100 births to women with previous cesarean delivery. 4. Includes races other than white and black.

Religion and Medicine

★ 272 ★

Effect of Religious Faith on Blood Pressure

"A survey of 30 years of research on blood pressure showed that churchgoers have lower blood pressure than non-churchgoers—5mm lower, according to [Dr. David] Larson, even when adjusted to account for smoking and other risk factors."

Source: Wallis, Claudia. "Healing." *Time,* 24 June 1996, p. 59.

★ 273 ★

Religion and Medicine

Effect of Religious Faith on Heart Surgery Patients

"A 1995 study at Dartmouth-Hitchcock Medical Center found that one of the best predictors of survival among 232 heart-surgery patients was the degree to which the patients said they drew comfort and strength from religious faith. Those who did not had more than three times the death rate of those who did."

Source: Wallis, Claudia. "Healing." *Time,* 24 June 1996, p. 59.

Women's Health

★ 274 ★

Annual Deaths From Unsafe Abortions Worldwide

Data are estimated.

	Annual deaths from unsafe abortions
North America	-
Latin America	6,000
Caribbean	6,000
Europe	100
Africa	23,000
Former USSR	500
Asia	40,000
Oceania	500

Source: Ostrovsky, Arkady. "Birthrate Down, Hardship Up." *Financial Times,* 29 May 1997, p. 6. Primary source: World Health Organization, Maternal Health and Safe Motherhood Programme (Geneva), unpublished estimates. *Note:* "-" indicates "negligible."

★ 275 ★

Women's Health

Breast Cancer Surgery by City, 1995: Highest Percentages

Data refer to women over age 65 who have had either a lumpectomy or a partial mastectomy.

City	Percentage
Elyria, OH	48
Paterson, NJ	38
Boston, MA	32
Philadelphia, PA	31
New York, NY	29
Los Angeles, CA	22

Source: Chang, Trina. "Health Care Compared: Breast Cancer Surgery." *American Health* (May 1996), p. 25.

★ 276 ★

Women's Health

Breast Cancer Surgery by City, 1995: Lowest Percentages

Data refer to women over age 65 who have had either a lumpectomy or a partial mastectomy.

City	Percentage
Rapid City, SD	1
Ogden, UT	2
Fort Smith, AR	4
Yakima, WA	4
Fort Collins, CO	5
Houston, TX	13

Source: Chang, Trina. "Health Care Compared: Breast Cancer Surgery." *American Health* (May 1996), p. 25.

★ 277 ★

Women's Health

Cervical Cancer Screening, by Age Group

The table shows the percentage of women in each age group who reported having had a pap test within the preceding 36 months.

Age group	Percentage
18-29 years	73.0
30-39 years	76.0
40-49 years	71.0
50-59 years	64.0
70 years and older	43.0

Source: "Cervical Cancer Screening by Age, 1987 and 1992." *Primary Care & Cancer* (April 1996), p. 17. Primary source: *MMWR Morbidity & Mortality Weekly Report* 45:57-61, 1996.

★ 278 ★

Women's Health

Diagnostic/Nonsurgical Procedures for Females Discharged From Non-Federal Short-Stay Hospitals, by Age and Procedure: 1993

[Data are based on a sample of hospital records]

Age and procedure category	Procedures in thousands 1993[1,2]	Procedures per 1,000 population 1993[1,2]
All ages[3,4,5]	11,055	71.9
Diagnostic ultrasound	848	5.3
Computerized axial tomography (CAT scan)	594	3.7
Angiocardiography using contrast material	561	3.5
Radioisotope scan	239	1.4
Laparoscopy (excluding that for ligation and division of fallopian tubes)	152	1.1
Endoscopy of large intestine without biopsy	201	1.2
Cystoscopy	105	0.7
Under 5 years[3,5]	474	17.1
Spinal tap	64	2.3
Diagnostic ultrasound	30	1.1
Computerized axial tomography (CAT scan)	27	1.0
Electroencephalogram	9[6]	0.3[6]
Radioisotope scan	5[6]	0.2[6]
Application of cast or splint	5[6]	0.2[6]
Cystoscopy	[6]	[6]

[Continued]

★ 278 ★

Diagnostic/Nonsurgical Procedures for Females Discharged From Non-Federal Short-Stay Hospitals, by Age and Procedure: 1993

[Continued]

Age and procedure category	Procedures in thousands 1993[1,2]	Procedures per 1,000 population 1993[1,2]
15-44 years[3,5]	4,442	75.3
Diagnostic ultrasound	259	4.4
Laparoscopy (excluding that for ligation and division of fallopian tubes)	111	1.9
Computerized axial tomography (CAT scan)	113	1.9
Biliary tract x-ray	50	0.8
Radioisotope scan	37	0.6
Endoscopy of large intestine without biopsy	21	0.4
Cystoscopy	36	0.6
Contrast myelogram	15	0.3
45-64 years[3,5]	1,914	74.6
Angiocardiography using contrast material	203	7.9
Diagnostic ultrasound	155	6.0
Computerized axial tomography (CAT scan)	123	4.8
Radioisotope scan	58	2.2
Laparoscopy (excluding that for ligation and division of fallopian tubes)	30	1.2
Endoscopy of small intestine without biopsy	62	2.4
Endoscopy of large intestine without biopsy	46	1.8
Cystoscopy	28	1.1
65-74 years[3,5]	1,744	167.4
Angiocardiography using contrast material	192	18.4
Diagnostic ultrasound	157	15.1
Computerized axial tomography (CAT scan)	121	11.6
Radioisotope scan	60	5.8
Endoscopy of small intestine without biopsy	62	6.0
Endoscopy of large intestine without biopsy	44	4.2
Arteriography using contrast material	44	4.2
Cystoscopy	18	1.8
75 years and over[3,5]	2,482	273.3
Computerized axial tomography (CAT scan)	210	23.1
Diagnostic ultrasound	247	27.2
Angiocardiography using contrast material	120	13.2
Endoscopy of large intestine without biopsy	89	9.8
Endoscopy of small intestine without biopsy	106	11.6

[Continued]

★ 278 ★

Diagnostic/Nonsurgical Procedures for Females Discharged From Non-Federal Short-Stay Hospitals, by Age and Procedure: 1993

[Continued]

Age and procedure category	Procedures in thousands 1993[1,2]	Procedures per 1,000 population 1993[1,2]
Radioisotope scan	79	8.6
Cystoscopy	21	2.4

Source: U.S. Department of Health and Human Services. Public Health Service. Centers for Disease Control and Prevention. National Center for Health Statistics. *Health, United States, 1995.* Hyattsville, MD: Public Health Service, 1996. p. 208. Primary source: Centers for Disease Control and Prevention, National Center for Health Statistics, Division of Health Interview Statistics. Data from National Hospital Discharge Survey. *Notes:* Excludes newborn infants. Data do not reflect total use of procedures for outpatients are not included in the National Hospital Discharge Survey. For example, CAT scans have been performed on outpatients as well as inpatients. Rates are based on the civilian population as of July 1. In each sex and age group, data are shown for the five most common in 1980 and 1991. Procedure categories are based on the International Classification of Diseases, 9th Revision, Clinical Modification. For a listing of the code numbers. 1. Comparisons of data from 1983-93 with data from earlier years should be made with caution as estimates of change may reflect improvements in the design (see Appendix I) rather than true changes in hospital use. 2. In 1993 children's hospitals had a high rate of nonresponse which may have resulted in underestimates of hospital utilization by children. 3. Beginning in 1989 the definition of some surgical and diagnostic and other nonsurgical procedures was revised, thus causing a discontinuity in the totals. 4. Rates are age adjusted. 5. Includes nonsurgical procedures not shown. 6. Statistics based on fewer than 5,000 estimated discharges are not shown; those based on 5,000-9,000 estimated discharges are to be used with caution.

★ 279 ★

Women's Health

Menopause and Emotional Health

"Though menopause may seem like a cheerless event, it may actually alleviate emotional distress. The rate of women who suffer from anxiety or depression drops from 10.8% in women under 55 to 5.3% in those 55 and older."

Source: Cronin, Brian. "Health Report: The Good News." *Time,* 14 July 1997, p. 19. Primary source: Royal College of Psychiatrists meeting.

★ 280 ★

Women's Health

Miscarriage Risk, by Age: 1996

Age	Percentage
20	0.0-10.0
25	0.0-10.0
30	10.0
35	10.0-20.0
40	10.0-20.0
45	30.0-40.0
45+	50.0-60.0

Source: "The Risks of Racing the Reproductive Clock." *Business Week,* 5 May 1997, p. 96. Primary source: *Reproductive Potential in the Older Woman.*

★ 281 ★

Women's Health

New Mothers, by Age Group: 1980 and 1995

Age	1980	1995
35-39	18,200	82,700
40-44	2,000	13,700

Source: "The Risks of Racing the Reproductive Clock." *Business Week,* 5 May 1997, p. 96. Primary source: *Reproductive Potential in the Older Woman.*

★ 282 ★

Women's Health

Operations for Women Discharged from Non-Federal Short-Stay Hospitals, by Age and Surgical Category: 1993

[Data are based on a sample of hospital records]

Age and surgical category	Operations in thousands 1993[1,2]	Operations per 1,000 population 1993[1,2]
All ages[3,4,5]	14,411	96.4
Procedures to assist delivery[3]	2,428	16.8
Cesarean section[7]	917	6.3
Repair of current obstetrical laceration	860	5.9
Hysterectomy	562	3.9

[Continued]

★ 282 ★

Operations for Women Discharged from Non-Federal Short-Stay Hospitals, by Age and Surgical Category: 1993
[Continued]

Age and surgical category	Operations in thousands 1993[1,2]	Operations per 1,000 population 1993[1,2]
Oophorectomy and salpingo-oophorectomy	443	3.1
Bilateral destruction or occlusion of fallopian tubes	384	2.6
Diagnostic dilation and curettage of uterus	64	0.4
Under 15 years[3,5]	349	12.6
Tonsillectomy, with or without adenoidectomy	15	0.5
Reduction of fracture (excluding skull, nose, and jaw)	24	0.9
Appendectomy, excluding incidental[6]	23	0.8
Myringotomy	14	0.5
Operations on muscles, tendons, fascia, and bursa	6[8]	0.2[8]
Adenoidectomy without tonsillectomy	[8]	[8]
15-44 years[3,5]	7,706	130.6
Procedures to assist delivery[3]	2,418	41.0
Cesarean section[7]	915	15.5
Repair of current obstetrical laceration	857	14.5
Bilateral destruction or occlusion of fallopian tubes	383	6.5
Hysterectomy	326	5.5
Diagnostic dilation and curettage of uterus	36	0.6
45-64 years[3,5]	2,623	102.3
Hysterectomy	172	6.7
Cardiac catheterization	138	5.4
Oophorectomy and salpingo-oophorectomy	164	6.4
Cholecystectomy	104	4.0
Excision or destruction of intervertebral disc and spinal fusion	89	3.5
Diagnostic dilation and curettage of uterus	19	0.7
Biopsies on the integumentary system (breast, skin, and subcutaneous tissue)	14	0.5
65-74 years[3,5]	1,799	172.7
Cardiac catheterization	141	13.6
Cholecystectomy	59	5.7
Biopsies on the digestive system	46	4.4
Arthroplasty and replacement of hip	44	4.2
Reduction of fracture (excluding skull, nose, and jaw)	55	5.3
Extraction of lens	12	1.2
Insertion of prosthetic lens (pseudophakos)	11	1.0

[Continued]

★ 282 ★

Operations for Women Discharged from Non-Federal Short-Stay Hospitals, by Age and Surgical Category: 1993

[Continued]

Age and surgical category	Operations in thousands 1993[1,2]	Operations per 1,000 population 1993[1,2]
75 years and over[3,5]	1,935	213.1
Reduction of fracture (excluding skull, nose, and jaw)	139	15.3
Pacemaker insertion or replacement	80	8.9
Cardiac catheterization	85	9.4
Arthroplasty and replacement of hip	85	9.4
Biopsies on the digestive system	57	6.2
Extraction of lens	22	2.5
Insertion of prosthetic lens (pseudophakos)	20	2.2

Source: U.S. Department of Health and Human Services. Public Health Service. Centers for Disease Control and Prevention. National Center for Health Statistics. *Health, United States, 1995.* Hyattsville, MD: Public Health Service, 1996. p. 206. Primary source: Centers for Disease Control and Prevention, National Center for Health Statistics, Division of Health Interview Statistics. Data from National Hospital Discharge Survey. *Notes:* Excludes newborn infants. Data do not reflect total use of operations because operations for outpatients are not included in the National Hospital Discharge Survey. In recent years, for example, lens extractions and myringotomies have been performed on outpatients as well as inpatients. Rates are based on the civilian population as of July 1. In each sex and age group, data are shown for the five most common operations in 1980 and 1991. Surgical categories are based on the International Classification of Diseases, 9th Revision, Clinical Modification. For a listing of the code numbers, see Appendix II, table VII. 1. Comparisons of data from 1983-93 with data from earlier years should be made with caution as estimates of change may reflect improvements in the design (see Appendix I) rather than true changes in hospital use. 2. In 1993 children's hospitals had a high rate of nonresponse which may have resulted in underestimates of hospital utilization by children. 3. Beginning in 1989 the definition of some surgical and diagnostic and other nonsurgical procedures was revised, thus causing a discontinuity in the trends for the totals and selected surgical procedures. 4. Rates are age adjusted. 5. Includes operations not listed in table. 6. Limited to estimated number of appendectomies, excluding those performed incidental to other abdominal surgery. 7. Cesarean sections accounted for 16.5 percent of all deliveries in 1980, 22.7 percent in 1985, 23.5 percent in 1991, and 22.8 percent in 1993. 8. Statistics based on fewer than 5,000 estimated discharges are not shown; those based on 5,000-9,000 estimated discharges are to be used with caution.

★ 283 ★

Women's Health

Projected Fertility Rates, by Race and Age Group: 1995 and 2010

The total fertility rate is the number of births that 1,000 women would have in their lifetime if, at each year of age, they experienced the birth rates occurring in the specified year. Birth rates represent live births per 1,000 women in age group indicated. Projections are based on middle fertility assumptions.

AGE GROUP	ALL RACES[1]		WHITE		BLACK		AMERICAN INDIAN, ESKIMO, ALEUT		ASIAN AND PACIFIC ISLANDER		HISPANIC	
	1995	2010	1995	2010	1995	2010	1995	2010	1995	2010	1995	2010
Total fertility rate	2,055	2,108	1,984	2,046	4.8	2,438	2,151	2,159	1,953	1,954	2,977	
Birth rates:												
10 to 14 years old	1.4	1.6	0.8	0.9	109.6	4.8	1.7	1.7	0.8	0.8	2.6	2.3
15 to 19 years old	59.4	63.6	50.7	56.0	157.4	111.5	78.7	81.8	28.5	28.7	103.7	95.8
20 to 24 years old	115.4	118.2	108.9	112.6	112.0	158.7	143.3	143.7	80.3	79.5	184.1	172.6
25 to 29 years old	117.8	119.5	118.7	120.7	66.6	113.1	108.3	109.0	121.6	121.7	152.4	143.7

[Continued]

★ 283 ★

Projected Fertility Rates, by Race and Age Group: 1995 and 2010

[Continued]

AGE GROUP	ALL RACES[1]		WHITE		BLACK		AMERICAN INDIAN, ESKIMO, ALEUT		ASIAN AND PACIFIC ISLANDER		HISPANIC	
	1995	2010	1995	2010	1995	2010	1995	2010	1995	2010	1995	2010
30 to 34 years old	78.9	81.0	80.0	82.0	27.8	67.8	61.7	62.9	100.9	101.1	96.7	91.5
35 to 39 years old	31.6	32.1	31.5	31.7	5.4	27.7	27.4	27.4	47.9	47.3	45.3	40.5
40 to 44 years old	5.6	5.9	5.4	5.6	0.3	5.3	6.0	6.0	10.4	10.3	10.8	8.5
45 to 49 years old	0.3	0.3	0.2	0.2	0.3	0.2	0.3	0.3	1.0	1.0	0.6	0.5

Source: 1996 Statistical Abstract of the United States on CD-ROM [machine-readable datafiles]. CD-8A-97. Washington, DC: U.S. Department of Commerce, Economics and Statistics Administration, Bureau of the Census, Data User Services Division, January 1997. Primary source: U.S. Bureau of the Census, *Current Population Reports*, P25-1130. *Note:* 1. Persons of Hispanic origin may be of any race.

★ 284 ★

Women's Health

Women Age 40 and Older Who Have Had a Mammogram Within the Past Two Years, by Selected Characteristics: 1993

[Data are based on household interviews of a sample of the civilian noninstitutionalized population].

Characteristic	Percentage
Age	
40 years and over	59.7
50 years and over	59.7
40-49 years	59.9
50-64 years	65.1
65 years and over	54.2
Age, race, and Hispanic origin	
40 years and over:	
White, non-Hispanic	60.6
Black, non-Hispanic	59.2
Hispanic	50.9
40-49 years:	
White, non-Hispanic	61.6
Black, non-Hispanic	55.6
Hispanic	52.6
50 years and over:	
White, non-Hispanic	60.2
Black, non-Hispanic	61.4
Hispanic	49.7

[Continued]

★ 284 ★

Women Age 40 and Older Who Have Had a Mammogram Within the Past Two Years, by Selected Characteristics: 1993
[Continued]

Characteristic	Percentage
50-64 years:	
White, non-Hispanic	66.2
Black, non-Hispanic	65.5
Hispanic	59.2
65 years and over:	
White, non-Hispanic	54.7
Black, non-Hispanic	56.3
Hispanic	35.7
Age and poverty status[2]	
40 years and over:	
Below poverty	41.6
At or above poverty	62.8
40-49 years:	
Below poverty	37.3
At or above poverty	62.7
50 years and over:	
Below poverty	43.4
At or above poverty	62.8
50-64 years:	
Below poverty	46.8
At or above poverty	67.6
65 years and over:	
Below poverty	41.0
At or above poverty	57.5
Age and education	
40 years of age and over:	
Less than 12 years	46.4
12 years	59.0
13 years or more	69.5
40-49 years of age:	
Less than 12 years	43.6
12 years	56.5
13 years or more	66.1

[Continued]

★ 284 ★

Women Age 40 and Older Who Have Had a Mammogram Within the Past Two Years, by Selected Characteristics: 1993

[Continued]

Characteristic	Percentage
50 years of age and over:	
Less than 12 years	46.9
12 years	60.1
13 years or more	72.5
50-64 years of age:	
Less than 12 years	51.4
12 years	62.4
13 years or more	78.5
65 years of age and over:	
Less than 12 years	44.2
12 years	57.4
13 years or more	64.8

Source: U.S. Department of Health and Human Services. Public Health Service. Centers for Disease Control and Prevention. National Center for Health Statistics. *Health, United States, 1995.* Hyattsville, MD: Public Health Service, 1996. p. 191. Primary source: Centers for Disease Control and Prevention, National Center for Health Statistics, Division of Health Interview Statistics. Data from National Health Interview Survey. *Notes:* 1. Questions concerning use of mammography differed slightly on the National Health Interview Survey across the years for which data are shown. In 1987 and 1990 women were asked to report when they had their last mammogram. In 1991 women were asked whether they had a mammogram in the past 2 years. In 1993 women were asked whether they had a mammogram within the past year, between 1 and 2 years ago, or over 2 years ago. 2. Poverty status is based on family income and family size using Bureau of the Census poverty thresholds.

★ 285 ★

Women's Health

Breast Implants, by Women's Lifestyles: 1996

The table presents a profile of women who are more likely to have breast implants, based on lifestyles. Data are in percentages.

Characteristic	With implants	Without implants
Have at least a year of college	70	59
Have 7 or more drinks a week	30	17
Have 14 or more sexual partners	39	5
Use hair dye	85	59

Source: "Notebook: Implant Insights." *Time,* 9 June 1997, p. 18. Primary source: *Journal of the American Medical Association.*

Chapter 3
HEALTH CARE ESTABLISHMENT

The tables in this chapter present a comprehensive view of the Health Care Establishment, i.e., the institutional view of health care. Statistical profiles of health care establishments (hospitals, clinics, doctors' offices, etc) are provided for the national, state, and metropolitan level. Additionally, tables are included profiling HMOs, hospitals, nursing homes, and specialized centers. Data on drugs and medicines, including pharmaceutical producers, on insurance carriers, and on merger and acquisition activity in this field round out the chapter's coverage. Tables presenting data on the financial aspects of this "establishment" are in Chapter 6 - Health Expenditures and Funding. Data on health care insurance programs are in Chapter 7 - Health Care Programs. Related material can be found in Chapter 8 - Medical Professions, Chapter 9 - Medical Practices and Producedures, and in Chapter 11 - International Comparisons.

Centers

★ 286 ★

Growth of Diagnostic Centers in the U.S., 1984-1994

This table shows the number of freestanding imaging centers. The most frequently performed procedures are ultrasound, mammography, and x-ray.

Year	Number of centers
1984	698
1985	911
1986	1,095
1987	1,278
1988	1,464
1989	1,647
1990	1,822
1991	1,962
1992	2,055

[Continued]

★ 286 ★

Growth of Diagnostic Centers in the U.S., 1984-1994

[Continued]

Year	Number of centers
1993	2,118
1994	2,151

Source: "Imaging News: Diagnostic Imaging Centers in the U.S., 1984-1994." *Diagnostic Imaging* (February 1996), p. 21.

★ 287 ★

Centers

Leading Cancer Centers, by Amount of Federal Research Grant: 1995

Center (city)	Amount ($ mil.)
Fred Hutchinson Cancer Research Center (Seattle, WA)	47.4
Johns Hopkins University Oncology Center (Baltimore, MD)	36.7
University of Texas M.D. Anderson Cancer Center (Houston, TX)	34.7
University of Pittsburgh Cancer Institute (Pittsburgh, PA)	33.9
Memorial Sloan-Kettering Institute for Cancer Research (New York, NY)	32.4

Source: "Top Centers." *Detroit News,* 8 July 1996, p. A4.

Characteristics

★ 288 ★

Health Service Establishments: Employment, Hours, and Earnings

This table shows employment, hours, and earnings in private sector[1] health service establishments, by selected type of establishment, 1992-1996.

Item	Calendar year				1996	
	1992	1993	1994	1995	Q1	Q2
Total Employment (in 1,000's)						
Nonfarm Private Sector	89,959	91,889	95,044	97,892	97,489	100,024
Health Services	8,490	8,756	8,992	9,257	9,441	9,540
Offices and Clinics of Physicians	1,463	1,506	1,545	1,606	1,639	1,665

[Continued]

★ 288 ★

Health Service Establishments: Employment, Hours, and Earnings
[Continued]

Item	Calendar year				1996	
	1992	1993	1994	1995	Q1	Q2
Offices and Clinics of Dentists	541	556	574	597	614	622
Nursing Homes	1,533	1,585	1,649	1,693	1,717	1,735
Private Hospitals	3,750	3,779	3,763	3,784	3,828	3,846
Home Health Care Services	398	469	559	626	647	658
Non-Supervisory Employment (in 1,000's)						
Nonfarm Private Sector	72,930	74,777	77,610	80,123	79,615	81,962
Health Services	7,546	7,770	7,966	8,200	8,366	8,455
Offices and Clinics of Physicians	1,202	1,231	1,261	1,311	1,340	1,363
Offices and Clinics of Dentists	473	487	501	521	539	546
Nursing Homes	1,385	1,431	1,487	1,527	1,546	1,562
Private Hospitals	3,442	3,464	3,441	3,460	3,503	3,520
Home Health Care Services	369	435	518	579	599	608
Average Weekly Hours						
Nonfarm Private Sector	34.4	34.5	34.7	34.5	33.9	34.4
Health Services	32.8	32.8	32.8	32.8	32.5	32.5
Offices and Clinics of Physicians	32.2	32.2	32.4	32.5	32.6	32.7
Offices and Clinics of Dentists	28.4	28.3	28.1	28.0	27.9	28.1
Nursing Homes	32.3	32.2	32.3	32.5	32.2	32.3
Private Hospitals	34.4	34.6	34.7	34.5	34.4	34.3
Home Health Care Services	27.4	27.8	28.2	28.6	27.7	27.8
Average Hourly Earnings						
Nonfarm Private Sector	10.57	10.83	11.12	11.44	11.70	11.75
Health Services	11.39	11.78	12.10	12.45	12.73	12.76
Offices and Clinics of Physicians	11.42	11.89	12.26	12.52	12.88	13.01
Offices and Clinics of Dentists	11.02	11.44	11.97	12.40	12.68	12.76
Nursing Homes	7.86	8.17	8.50	8.76	8.92	8.93
Private Hospitals	13.03	13.46	13.83	14.30	14.62	14.62
Home Health Care Services	10.00	10.41	10.67	10.91	11.11	11.12
Addenda: Hospital Employment (in 1,000's)						
Total	5,068	5,100	5,077	5,092	5,135	5,151
Private	3,750	3,779	3,763	3,784	3,828	3,846
Federal	235	234	234	232	231	229
State	419	414	407	397	390	385
Local	665	673	673	679	685	689

Source: U.S. Department of Labor. Bureau of Labor Statistics. *Employment and Earnings.* Washington, DC: U.S. Government Printing Office. Monthly reports for January 1992-June 1996. Data presented here conform to the 1987 Standard Industrial Classification. Q designates quarter of year. Quarterly data are not seasonally adjusted. *Notes:* 1. Excludes hospitals, clinics, and other health-related establishments run by all governments.

Drugs and Medicine

★ 289 ★

AIDS Drug-Treatment Funding, 1995: Leading States

[In millions of dollars]

State	Cost
California	8.4
New York	8.3
Florida	5.6
Puerto Rico	2.5
New Jersey	2.1
Texas	1.4
Illinois	1.3
Georgia	1

Source: Georges, Christopher. "Costly New AIDS Drug Therapy Finds Support in Congress, Due to Efforts of Unlikely Alliance." *Wall Street Journal,* 11 July 1996, p. A18. Primary source: National Association of State and Territorial AIDS Directors.

★ 290 ★

Drugs and Medicine

AIDS-Infected Children and Drugs

"The first major study of AIDS-infected kids concludes that the AIDS drug DDI, taken alone with AZT, is vastly superior to AZT alone in halting the progress of the disease."

Source: Cronin, Brian. "Health Report: The Good News." *Time,* 23 June 1997, p. 23. Primary source: *New England Journal of Medicine.*

★ 291 ★

Drugs and Medicine

AIDS Patients Receiving Treatment, 1995: Leading States

[In thousands of patients]

State	Total patients served
New York	17
California	9
Florida	6
Texas	5
Puerto Rico	5
Illinois	2
New Jersey	2
Georgia	2

Source: Georges, Christopher. "Costly New AIDS Drug Therapy Finds Support in Congress, Due to Efforts of Unlikely Alliance." *Wall Street Journal,* 11 July 1996, p. A18. Primary source: National Association of State and Territorial AIDS Directors.

★ 292 ★

Drugs and Medicine

Balloon Angioplasty and Drugs

"Balloon-angioplasty patients given a 'super-aspirin' called ReoPro had their risk of postoperative heart attack or death cut by half."

Source: Cronin, Brian. "Health Report: The Good News." *Time,* 23 June 1997, p. 23. Primary source: *New England Journal of Medicine.*

★ 293 ★

Drugs and Medicine

Blood-Pressure Drug Prescriptions Written: 1994-95

According to the source, the blood-pressure drug market is estimated at $20 billion.

Drug	1995 prescriptions (millions)	Percent change from 1994
Calcium channel blockers	90.5	3.6
ACE inhibitors	66.4	11.0
Beta blockers	54.7	6.8

Source: McGinley, Laurie, and Elyse Tanouye. "FDA to Assess Drugs to Treat Hypertension." *Wall Street Journal,* 25 January 1996, p. B1. Primary source: IMS America.

★ 294 ★

Drugs and Medicine

Bypass Surgery Drugs

"In a major study, an experimental drug called Acadesine cut in half the risk of a patient's dying during or soon after the heart operation. It also reduced by at least 25% the chance of a heart attack or stroke from surgery."

Source: Cronin, Brian. "Health Report: The Good News." *Time,* 3 February 1997, p. 14. Primary source: *New England Journal of Medicine; Journal of the American Medical Association;* Food and Drug Administration.

★ 295 ★

Drugs and Medicine

Cancer Drug Research, by Cancer Type: 1995

Data refer to the number of drugs currently in development for each type of cancer.

Type of cancer	Number
Bladder cancer	8
Brain cancer	14
Breast cancer	48
Colon cancer	30
Esophageal cancer	2
Head/neck cancer	9
Kidney cancer	12
Leukemia	26

[Continued]

★ 295 ★

Cancer Drug Research, by Cancer Type: 1995
[Continued]

Type of cancer	Number
Liver cancer	5
Lung cancer	37
Lymphoma	26
Multiple myeloma	5
Neuroblastoma	3
Ovarian cancer	23
Pancreatic cancer	10
Prostate cancer	25
Skin cancer	31
Solid tumors	24
Stomach cancer	5
Uterine cancer	6
Others	49

Source: "More Than 200 Cancer Medicines Now in Development." *Medical Marketing & Media* (July 1995), p. 16. Primary source: Pharmaceutical Research and Manufacturers of America.

★ 296 ★

Drugs and Medicine

Cost of Adverse Reactions to Drugs

"Hospital patients pay as much as $4 billion a year for treatment of adverse reactions to drugs they're prescribed. Up to half the problems could be avoided with simple measures—like better tracking of patients' allergies."

Source: Cronin, Brian. "Health Report: The Bad News." *Time,* 3 February 1997, p. 14. Primary source: *Journal of the American Medical Association;* National Institutes of Health.

★ 297 ★

Drugs and Medicine

Drugs Being Tested for Treatment of Mental Illness, by Disorder: 1996

According to the source, in addition to the drugs listed in the table, pharmaceutical companies are developing one drug for post-traumatic stress and one for attention-deficit hyperactivity disorder.

Disorder	Number
Anxiety disorder	12
Dementias	19
Eating disorder	3
Mood disorder	13
Anxiety disorder	17
Substance abuse/ dependence disorder	8
Other disorders	2

Source: "Spotlight: Medicines in Testing for Mental Illness." *Medical Tribune,* (Family Physician Edition), 23 May 1996, p. 1. Primary source: Pharmaceutical Research Manufacturers of America.

★ 298 ★

Drugs and Medicine

Drugs for Treatment of AIDS and Hepatitis B

"...sold by Glaxo Wellcome PLC as Epivir, the drug is part of the combination therapy revolutionizing AIDS treatment. In 1996, the first full year since its launch, Epivir produced $315 million in revenues. Analysts say sales could reach $840 million by 2000."

"Now, the same chemical compound, renamed lamivudine, could be the most effective treatment yet for hepatitis B, which affects 350 million people worldwide—killing 2 million annually. On April 10, data from a trial involving 358 patients in Hong Kong, Taiwan, and Singapore were presented at a meeting of the European Association for the Study of the Liver. Ninety-six percent of patients receiving a 100-milligram dose of the drug experienced dramatic suppression of the hepatitis B virus (HBV) with few side effects. What's more, 67% also had reduced liver inflammation—a sign of healthier tissue."

Source: Flynn, Julia. "A Hepatitis Drug That May Cure Glaxo." *Business Week,* 12 May 1997, p. 104.

★ 299 ★

Drugs and Medicine

Leading Brand-Name Prescription Drugs, by Number of Prescriptions Written: 1996

Manufacturers' names are shown in parentheses in the table. According to the source, in 1996, the number of prescriptions dispensed in drugstores expanded 5.5%, to 2.3 billion.

Brand	Total Rxs (000s)
Pondimin (Robins)	7,330
Sporanox (Janssen)	1,509
Neurontin (Warner-Lambert)	1,498
Zithromax (Pfizer)	12,459
Imdur (Schering)	3,508
Ionamin (Fisons)	1,747
Adipex-P (Gate)	1,095
Demadex (Boehringer-Mannheim)	1,313
Flonase (Glaxo Wellcome)	4,325
Zocor (Merck)	11,786

Source: "Special Report: Annual Rx Survey." *Drug Topics,* 7 April 1997, p. 48. Primary source: Scott-Levin Associates, Newtown, Pennsylvania.

★ 300 ★

Drugs and Medicine

Leading Brands in the Cholesterol-Reducer Market

Brand (Company)	Market share ($ mil.)
Zocor (Merck)	1,000.0
Mevacor (Merck)	791.9
Pravachol (Bristol-Myers)	564.7

Source: Wilke, Michael. "3 Agencies Vie for Colestid OTC Biz." *Advertising Age,* 7 July 1997, p. 3.

★ 301 ★

Drugs and Medicine

Protease Inhibitors for HIV Patients: 1997

The table shows the percentage of all protease inhibitor prescriptions accounted for by each drug. Pharmaceutical manufacturers' names are shown in parentheses.

Drug	Percentage
Crixivan (Merck)	52
Invirase (Roche)	23
Norvir (Abbott)	14
Viracept (Agouron)	11

Source: Armstrong, Larry. "Besting AIDS—and the Drug Giants." *Business Week,* 9 June 1997, p. 79. Primary source: Bloomberg Financial Markets.

★ 302 ★

Drugs and Medicine

Prozac Prescription Growth in the United States: 1988-1996

According to the source, 24 million people use Prozac throughout the world. Eighteen million Prozac users live in the United States.

[Number of prescriptions is in millions]

Year	Number
1988	2.469
1989	6.133
1990	10.655
1991	10.028
1992	11.443
1993	12.163
1994	16.427
1995	18.838
1996	20.705

Source: "Prozac Prescription Growth." *USA TODAY,* 9 July 1997, p. 1A. Primary source: IMS America; Eli Lilly & Company.

★ 303 ★

Drugs and Medicine

States With the Most Pharmaceutical Companies: 1995

State	Number
North Carolina	44
Florida	23
Texas	16
New York	15
Michigan	14
Ohio	12
Missouri	12
California	12
New Jersey	11
Indiana	11

Source: "Recent Locations: Top U.S. States." *Site Selection* (February 1996), p. 95. Primary source: Conway Data New Plant Database.

★ 304 ★

Drugs and Medicine

Top Ten Drugs Dispensed in Retail Pharmacies: Covered by All Insurers

Drug	Total Rxs (000s)
Premarin	19,175
Trimox	16,523
Amoxil	16,414
Hydrocodone W/APAP	14,236
Cephalexin	12,813
Zantac	12,711
Synthroid	12,533
Amoxicillin	12,249
Acetaminophen w/codeine	10,878
Lanoxin	10,552

Source: "News & Trends: Brands on Top, No Matter Who Pays." *Business & Health* (November 1995), p. 14.

★ 305 ★

Drugs and Medicine

Top Ten Drugs Dispensed in Retail Pharmacies: Covered by Medicaid Program

Drug	Total Rxs (000s)
Amoxil	3.040
Acetaminophen w/codeine	1,993
Furosemide	1,835
Zantac	1,820
Albuterol Sulfate	1,654
Amoxicillin	1,651
Trimox	1,628
Proventil	1,484
Procardia	1,413
Lanoxin	1,291

Source: "News & Trends: Brands on Top, No Matter Who Pays." *Business & Health* (November 1995), p. 14.

★ 306 ★

Drugs and Medicine

Zantac Sales: 1996

"After years of litigation, Glaxo Wellcome looks certain to lose patent protection in America for Zantac, its anti-ulcer pill, on July 26th. Last year this drug probably provided around half the firm's operating profits of $4.7 billion. The company's patent on Zovirax which treats herpes and chicken-pox, expired last week. Henceforth other drug firms will be able to make cheap copies of Glaxo's best-selling medicines."

Source: "Coping with Unwellcome News." *Economist,* 26 April 1997, p. 59.

Establishment Data

★ 307 ★

Private Health Service Establishments

This table shows the percent change in employment, hours, and earnings in private health service establishments, by selected type of establishment, for the 1992-1996 period.

Item	Calendar year				1996	
	1992	1993	1994	1995	Q1	Q2
Total Employment (in 1,000s)						
Nonfarm Private Sector	0.1	2.1	3.4	3.0	1.9	2.2
Health Services	3.8	3.1	2.7	2.9	3.5	3.6
Offices and Clinics	4.2	2.9	2.6	3.9	3.9	4.3
Offices and Clinics	2.5	2.9	3.1	4.1	5.2	4.8
Nursing Homes	2.7	3.4	4.0	2.7	2.8	3.1
Private Hospitals	2.6	0.8	-0.4	0.6	1.8	1.9
Home Health Care Service	15.5	17.9	19.3	11.9	7.3	6.2
Non-Supervisory Employment (in 1,000s)						
Nonfarm Private Sector	0.4	2.5	3.8	3.2	2.0	2.3
Health Services	3.7	3.0	2.5	2.9	3.6	3.6
Offices and Clinic	4.0	2.4	2.5	4.0	4.2	4.6
Offices and Clinic	2.1	2.8	3.0	4.0	5.6	5.6
Nursing Homes	2.8	3.3	3.9	2.7	2.7	2.9
Private Hospitals	2.7	0.6	-0.7	0.6	2.0	2.0
Home Health Care Service	15.6	17.9	19.1	11.9	7.3	6.1
Average Weekly Hours						
Nonfarm Private Sector	0.2	0.3	0.5	-0.6	-1.1	0.2
Health Services	0.7	0.1	0.1	-0.2	-0.8	-0.5
Offices and Clinic	0.8	0.2	0.5	0.2	0.4	1.0
Offices and Clinic	0.2	-0.3	-0.5	-0.6	-0.6	0.6
Nursing Homes	0.5	-0.3	0.3	0.5	-0.3	0.0
Private Hospitals	0.6	0.5	0.2	-0.3	-0.9	-0.9
Home Health Care Service	4.8	1.4	1.7	1.2	-3.4	-3.2
Average Hourly Earnings						
Nonfarm Private Sector	2.4	2.5	2.7	2.8	3.1	3.4
Health Services	3.9	3.4	2.7	2.9	3.0	3.2
Offices and Clinic	2.5	4.2	3.1	2.1	3.4	4.6
Offices and Clinic	3.8	3.8	4.6	3.6	3.5	3.3
Nursing Homes	3.9	4.0	4.0	3.1	2.4	2.3
Private Hospitals	4.2	3.3	2.7	3.4	3.1	3.3
Home Health Care Service	6.6	4.1	2.5	2.3	2.4	2.6
Addenda: Hospital Employment (in 000s)						
Total	2.2	0.6	-0.5	0.3	1.4	1.4
Private	2.6	0.8	-0.4	0.6	1.8	1.9

[Continued]

★ 307 ★

Private Health Service Establishments
[Continued]

Item	Calendar year				1996	
	1992	1993	1994	1995	Q1	Q2
Federal	0.5	-0.4	0.0	-0.7	0.2	-1.3
State	0.5	-1.2	-1.6	-2.5	-3.3	-3.2
Local	1.8	1.3	0.0	0.8	1.7	1.9

Source: U.S. Department of Labor. Bureau of labor Statistics. *Employment and Earnings.* Washington. U.S. Government Printing Office. Monthly reports for January 1992-June 1996. *Notes:* Data presented here conform to the 1987 Standard Industrial Classification. Q designates quarter of year. Quarterly data are not seasonally adjusted.

★ 308 ★

Establishment Data

Private Health Services Establishments: Change in Characteristics

This table shows percent change in implied non-supervisory payrolls, employment, average weekly hours, and average hourly earnings in private[1] health service establishments by selected type of establishment for the period 1992-1996.

Item	Calendar year				1996	
	1992	1993	1994	1995	Q1	Q2
Percent change from the same period the year before						
Health Services						
Payrolls	8.5	6.6	5.4	5.5	5.6	6.5
Employment	3.7	3.0	2.5	2.9	3.6	3.6
Average Weekly Hours	0.7	0.1	0.1	-0.2	-0.8	-0.5
Average Hourly Earnings	3.9	3.4	2.7	2.9	3.0	3.2
Offices and Clinics of Physicians						
Payrolls	7.5	6.9	6.2	6.4	8.2	10.6
Employment	4.0	2.4	2.5	4.0	4.2	4.6
Average Weekly Hours	0.8	0.2	0.5	0.2	0.4	1.0
Average Hourly Earnings	2.5	4.2	3.1	2.1	3.4	4.6
Offices and Clinics of Dentists						
Payrolls	6.1	6.5	7.3	7.1	8.7	9.8
Employment	2.1	2.8	3.0	4.0	5.6	5.6
Average Weekly Hours	0.2	-0.3	-0.5	-0.6	-0.6	0.6
Average Hourly Earnings	3.8	3.8	4.6	3.6	3.5	3.3
Nursing Homes						
Payrolls	7.4	7.1	8.3	6.5	4.8	5.3
Employment	2.8	3.3	3.9	2.7	2.7	2.9
Average Weekly Hours	0.5	-0.3	0.3	0.5	-0.3	0.0
Average Hourly Earnings	3.9	4.0	4.0	3.1	2.4	2.3

[Continued]

★ 308 ★

Private Health Services Establishments: Change in Characteristics

[Continued]

Item	Calendar year				1996	
	1992	1993	1994	1995	Q1	Q2
Private Hospitals						
Payrolls	7.6	4.5	2.2	3.6	4.2	4.4
Employment	2.7	0.6	-0.7	0.6	2.0	2.0
Average Weekly Hours	0.6	0.5	0.2	-0.3	-0.9	-0.9
Average Hourly Earnings	4.2	3.3	2.7	3.4	3.1	3.3
Home Health Care Services						
Payrolls	29.1	24.4	24.1	15.7	6.2	5.3
Employment	15.6	17.9	19.1	11.9	7.3	6.1
Average Weekly Hours	4.8	1.4	1.7	1.2	-3.4	-3.2
Average Hourly Earnings	6.6	4.1	2.5	2.3	2.4	2.6
Nonfarm Private Sector						
Payrolls	3.1	5.4	7.1	5.6	4.0	6.0
Employment	0.4	2.5	3.8	3.2	2.0	2.3
Average Weekly Hours	0.2	0.3	0.5	-0.6	-1.1	0.2
Average Hourly Earnings	2.4	2.5	2.7	2.8	3.1	3.4

Source: U.S. Department of Labor. Bureau of Labor Statistics. *Employment and Earnings.* Washington, DC: U.S. Government Printing Office. Monthly reports for January 1992-June 1996. *Notes:* Data presented here conform to the 1987 Standard Industrial Classification Q. designates quarter of year. Quarterly data are not seasonally adjusted. 1. Excludes hospitals, clinics, and other health-related establishments run by all governments.

★ 309 ★

Establishment Data

Home Health Care Agency Growth: 1989-1994

According to the National Association for Home Care (NAHC), between 1989 and 1994, the total number of home health care agencies has grown by 26%.

Year	Number
1989	5676
1990	5695
1991	5780
1992	6004
1993	6497
1994	7521

Source: "Home Health Care Update 95." *Nursing95* (July 1995), p. 57.

★ 310 ★

Establishment Data

Clinics of Doctors of Medicine and Dentists by Major Metro Area, Non-Taxed Establishments: 1992

Area	Establish-ments	Revenues in $1,000	Employ-ment	Payroll in $1,000	Payroll per employee
United States	3,302	16,621,893	157,758	5,295,773	33,569
Albany – Schenectady – Troy, NY MSA	18	-	-	-	-
Albuquerque, NM MSA	12	12,863	294	5,557	18,901
Allentown – Bethlehem – Easton, PA MSA	4	-	-	-	-
Atlanta, GA MSA	25	55,129	1,091	26,242	24,053
Austin – San Marcos, TX MSA	5	4,121	67	1,453	21,687
Baton Rouge, LA MSA	2	-	-	-	-
Birmingham, AL MSA	19	-	-	-	-
Boston – Worcester – Lawrence, MA – NH – ME – CT CMSA	100	-	-	-	-
Buffalo – Niagara Falls, NY MSA	16	-	-	-	-
Charlotte – Gastonia – Rock Hill, NC – SC MSA	5	-	-	-	-
Chicago – Gary – Kenosha, IL – IN – WI CMSA	75	337,209	3,051	101,263	33,190
Cincinnati – Hamilton, OH – KY – IN CMSA	41	-	-	-	-
Cleveland – Akron, OH CMSA	49	478,665	3,473	79,461	22,880
Columbus, OH MSA	18	26,310	326	11,307	34,684
Dallas – Fort Worth, TX CMSA	31	-	-	-	-
Dayton – Springfield, OH MSA	6	-	-	-	-
Denver – Boulder – Greeley, CO CMSA	38	-	-	-	-
Des Moines, IA MSA	4	-	-	-	-
Detroit – Ann Arbor – Flint, MI CMSA	94	-	-	-	-
Fresno, CA MSA	13	47,939	320	8,089	25,278
Grand Rapids – Muskegon – Holland, MI MSA	12	8,934	141	3,523	24,986
Greensboro – Winston-Salem – High Point, NC MSA	2	-	-	-	-
Greenville – Spartanburg – Anderson, SC MSA	7	-	-	-	-
Harrisburg – Lebanon – Carlisle, PA MSA	14	22,701	545	12,617	23,150
Hartford, CT MSA	13	31,134	488	14,236	29,172
Honolulu, HI MSA	19	-	-	-	-
Houston – Galveston – Brazoria, TX CMSA	10	5,980	114	2,272	19,930
Indianapolis, IN MSA	23	-	-	-	-
Jacksonville, FL MSA	10	28,483	486	17,841	36,710
Kalamazoo – Battle Creek, MI MSA	10	23,113	371	13,710	36,954
Kansas City, MO – KS MSA	31	115,538	1,322	41,907	31,700
Knoxville, TN MSA	2	-	-	-	-
Lansing – East Lansing, MI MSA	7	-	-	-	-

[Continued]

★ 310 ★

Clinics of Doctors of Medicine and Dentists by Major Metro Area, Non-Taxed Establishments: 1992
[Continued]

Area	Establish-ments	Revenues in $1,000	Employ-ment	Payroll in $1,000	Payroll per employee
Lexington, KY MSA	2	-	-	-	-
Little Rock – North Little Rock, AR MSA	1	-	-	-	-
Los Angeles – Riverside – Orange County, CA CMSA	157	-	-	-	-
Louisville, KY – IN MSA	9	-	-	-	-
Madison, WI MSA	7	-	-	-	-
Memphis, TN – AR – MS MSA	8	8,984	164	3,901	23,787
Miami – Fort Lauderdale, FL CMSA	18	-	-	-	-
Milwaukee – Racine, WI CMSA	19	-	-	-	-
Minneapolis – St. Paul, MN – WI MSA	71	575,917	7,033	247,441	35,183
Nashville, TN MSA	3	-	-	-	-
New Orleans, LA MSA	9	-	-	-	-
New York – Northern New Jersey – Long Island, NY – NJ – CT CMSA	137	-	-	-	-
Norfolk – Virginia Beach – Newport News, VA – NC MSA	18	-	-	-	-
Oklahoma City, OK MSA	12	13,121	350	6,067	17,334
Omaha, NE – IA MSA	6	-	-	-	-
Orlando, FL MSA	12	12,964	217	7,026	32,378
Philadelphia – Wilmington – Atlantic City, PA – NJ – DE – MD CMSA	63	-	-	-	-
Phoenix – Mesa, AZ MSA	26	43,911	676	16,897	24,996
Pittsburgh, PA MSA	43	154,284	1,064	37,097	34,866
Portland – Salem, OR – WA CMSA	44	-	-	-	-
Providence – Fall River – Warwick, RI – MA MSA	25	79,726	785	27,585	35,140
Raleigh – Durham – Chapel Hill, NC MSA	10	-	-	-	-
Richmond – Petersburg, VA MSA	5	1,031	27	466	17,259
Rochester, NY MSA	14	52,646	701	16,553	23,613
Sacramento – Yolo, CA CMSA	24	-	-	-	-
St. Louis, MO – IL MSA	21	68,894	707	26,096	36,911
Salt Lake City – Ogden, UT MSA	14	-	-	-	-
San Antonio, TX MSA	18	18,160	423	8,914	21,073
San Diego, CA MSA	65	832,029	5,262	156,545	29,750
San Francisco – Oakland – San Jose, CA CMSA	90	-	-	-	-
Santa Barbara – Santa Maria – Lompoc, CA MSA	15	-	-	-	-
Scranton – Wilkes-Barre – Hazleton, PA MSA	30	63,320	730	34,379	47,095
Seattle – Tacoma – Bremerton, WA CMSA	79	-	-	-	-
Springfield, MA MSA	10	-	-	-	-

[Continued]

★ 310 ★

Clinics of Doctors of Medicine and Dentists by Major Metro Area, Non-Taxed Establishments: 1992

[Continued]

Area	Establish-ments	Revenues in $1,000	Employ-ment	Payroll in $1,000	Payroll per employee
Syracuse, NY MSA	15	-	-	-	-
Tampa – St. Petersburg – Clearwater, FL MSA	11	9,831	149	2,745	18,423
Toledo, OH MSA	3	-	-	-	-
Tucson, AZ MSA	13	-	-	-	-
Tulsa, OK MSA	3	-	-	-	-
Washington – Baltimore, DC – MD – VA – WV CMSA	84	744,433	6,877	264,645	38,483
West Palm Beach – Boca Raton, FL MSA	4	989	16	456	28,500
Wichita, KS MSA	6	-	-	-	-
Youngstown – Warren, OH MSA	2	-	-	-	-

Source: U.S. Department of Commerce. Bureau of the Census. *1992 Economic Census Report Series,* CD-ROM 1i, Washington, DC, October 1996. *Notes:* - means no data reported. 1. HS stands for total health service establishments, revenues, employment, or payroll.

★ 311 ★

Establishment Data

Clinics of Doctors of Medicine and Dentists by State, Non-Taxed Establishments: 1992

Area	Establish-ments	Revenues in $1,000	Employ-ment	Payroll in $1,000	Payroll per employee
United States	3,302	16,621,893	157,758	5,295,773	33,569
Alabama	80	246,816	3,085	99,777	32,343
Alaska	11	12,517	268	6,435	24,011
Arizona	55	142,289	1,582	40,735	25,749
Arkansas	21	13,527	264	5,842	22,129
California	447	4,651,722	19,573	610,301	31,181
Colorado	63	348,485	2,691	71,732	26,656
Connecticut	34	156,530	1,527	48,650	31,860
Delaware	4	2,721	59	1,632	27,661
District of Columbia	18	230,619	1,574	93,680	59,517
Florida	118	266,357	3,455	111,281	32,209
Georgia	46	118,801	1,621	39,206	24,186
Hawaii	25	-	-	-	-
Idaho	19	12,277	271	6,059	22,358
Illinois	88	355,690	3,352	107,401	32,041
Indiana	70	140,657	1,489	43,331	29,101
Iowa	19	38,246	630	12,451	19,763
Kansas	20	45,974	588	12,746	21,677
Kentucky	38	49,429	748	17,361	23,210

[Continued]

★ 311 ★

Clinics of Doctors of Medicine and Dentists by State, Non-Taxed Establishments: 1992
[Continued]

Area	Establish-ments	Revenues in $1,000	Employ-ment	Payroll in $1,000	Payroll per employee
Louisiana	17	23,212	382	9,258	24,236
Maine	41	31,621	662	16,493	24,914
Maryland	52	385,700	3,800	129,181	33,995
Massachusetts	120	1,058,223	11,844	516,052	43,571
Michigan	153	757,513	7,668	265,002	34,559
Minnesota	97	1,447,679	19,642	797,918	40,623
Mississippi	45	43,767	811	17,579	21,676
Missouri	51	157,278	1,832	63,255	34,528
Montana	13	6,167	202	2,840	14,059
Nebraska	18	35,134	628	20,499	32,642
Nevada	3	-	-	-	-
New Hampshire	15	-	-	-	-
New Jersey	35	93,495	1,143	32,532	28,462
New Mexico	46	33,896	842	15,343	18,222
New York	230	1,189,276	15,148	522,425	34,488
North Carolina	79	238,662	2,121	41,966	19,786
North Dakota	9	5,045	91	2,691	29,571
Ohio	150	652,713	5,719	144,381	25,246
Oklahoma	17	35,849	694	18,688	26,928
Oregon	53	-	-	-	-
Pennsylvania	237	559,657	6,518	261,861	40,175
Rhode Island	23	-	-	-	-
South Carolina	42	40,777	782	19,217	24,574
South Dakota	13	9,620	241	5,607	23,266
Tennessee	31	21,304	420	11,654	27,748
Texas	121	204,278	3,299	65,612	19,888
Utah	24	10,074	166	3,580	21,566
Vermont	30	59,651	613	21,225	34,625
Virginia	76	318,295	3,134	92,669	29,569
Washington	117	971,587	11,007	375,716	34,134
West Virginia	78	82,431	1,564	36,684	23,455
Wisconsin	85	638,823	6,383	252,453	39,551
Wyoming	5	-	-	-	-

Source: U.S. Department of Commerce. Bureau of the Census. *1992 Economic Census Report Series,* CD-ROM 1i, Washington, DC, October 1996. *Notes:* - means no data reported. 1. HS stands for total health service establishments, revenues, employment, or payroll.

★ 312 ★

Establishment Data

Commercial Economic, Sociological, and Educational Research Establishments by Major Metro Area: 1992

Area	Establishments		Revenues		Employment		Payroll		
	Number	% of HS[1] in area	Total ($000)	% of HS[1] in area	Number	% of HS[1] in area	Total ($000)	% of HS[1] in area	Payroll per employee
United States	5,165	1.17	6,138,318	2.05	100,729	2.26	2,238,657	1.73	22,225
Albany – Schenectady – Troy, NY MSA	12	0.92	3,107	0.38	175	1.33	1,485	0.41	8,486
Albuquerque, NM MSA	15	1.41	-	-	-	-	-	-	-
Allentown – Bethlehem – Easton, PA MSA	9	0.73	-	-	-	-	-	-	-
Anchorage, AK MSA	10	2.06	5,092	1.39	56	1.55	1,902	1.33	33,964
Appleton – Oshkosh – Neenah, WI MSA	6	1.15	3,331	0.92	199	3.47	1,448	0.80	7,276
Atlanta, GA MSA	101	1.66	93,750	1.95	2,092	3.50	30,353	1.50	14,509
Augusta – Aiken, GA – SC MSA	3	0.42	-	-	-	-	-	-	-
Austin – San Marcos, TX MSA	30	1.91	27,129	2.27	598	3.22	13,037	2.69	21,801
Bakersfield, CA MSA	2	0.26	-	-	-	-	-	-	-
Baton Rouge, LA MSA	3	0.34	-	-	-	-	-	-	-
Beaumont – Port Arthur, TX MSA	0	0.00	0	0.00	0	0.00	0	0.00	0
Birmingham, AL MSA	15	1.09	5,418	0.36	203	1.01	1,788	0.28	8,808
Boise City, ID MSA	8	1.34	3,751	0.99	78	1.34	831	0.49	10,654
Boston – Worcester – Lawrence, MA – NH – ME – CT CMSA	173	1.77	329,730	4.66	4,030	3.50	127,940	3.93	31,747
Buffalo – Niagara Falls, NY MSA	22	1.10	6,380	0.58	285	1.32	2,286	0.46	8,021
Canton – Massillon, OH MSA	0	0.00	0	0.00	0	0.00	0	0.00	0
Charleston – North Charleston, SC MSA	7	0.86	-	-	-	-	-	-	-
Charlotte – Gastonia – Rock Hill, NC – SC MSA	19	1.19	5,791	0.41	175	0.86	1,984	0.30	11,337
Chattanooga, TN – GA MSA	4	0.53	-	-	-	-	-	-	-
Chicago – Gary – Kenosha, IL – IN – WI CMSA	311	2.14	-	-	-	-	-	-	-
Cincinnati – Hamilton, OH – KY – IN CMSA	68	2.17	-	-	-	-	-	-	-
Cleveland – Akron, OH CMSA	40	0.74	-	-	-	-	-	-	-
Colorado Springs, CO MSA	13	1.46	2,441	0.55	49	0.74	1,248	0.62	25,469
Columbia, SC MSA	9	1.21	-	-	-	-	-	-	-
Columbus, OH MSA	28	1.15	-	-	-	-	-	-	-
Corpus Christi, TX MSA	5	0.67	-	-	-	-	-	-	-
Dallas – Fort Worth, TX CMSA	106	1.27	110,488	1.69	1,925	2.24	39,415	1.49	20,475
Davenport – Moline – Rock Island, IA – IL MSA	5	0.74	-	-	-	-	-	-	-
Dayton – Springfield, OH MSA	9	0.55	2,593	0.23	101	0.57	1,178	0.21	11,663
Daytona Beach, FL MSA	7	0.95	10,314	1.93	106	1.27	6,010	2.73	56,698
Denver – Boulder – Greeley, CO CMSA	100	2.29	97,829	3.85	1,675	4.69	34,241	3.06	20,442
Des Moines, IA MSA	12	1.63	4,849	0.95	152	2.14	2,008	0.76	13,211
Detroit – Ann Arbor – Flint, MI CMSA	85	0.90	-	-	-	-	-	-	-
El Paso, TX MSA	6	0.75	-	-	-	-	-	-	-
Eugene – Springfield, OR MSA	7	1.20	2,933	0.87	22	0.41	596	0.38	27,091
Fort Myers – Cape Coral, FL MSA	4	0.56	-	-	-	-	-	-	-
Fort Pierce – Port St. Lucie, FL MSA	3	0.58	851	0.19	11	0.18	374	0.20	34,000
Fort Wayne, IN MSA	4	0.57	5,724	1.03	406	4.30	2,542	0.99	6,261
Fresno, CA MSA	9	0.61	2,524	0.29	139	1.13	1,142	0.31	8,216
Grand Rapids – Muskegon – Holland, MI MSA	16	1.05	7,394	0.82	313	2.18	3,432	0.79	10,965
Greensboro – Winston-Salem – High Point, NC MSA	21	1.39	33,343	2.81	575	3.36	8,412	1.59	14,630
Greenville – Spartanburg – Anderson, SC MSA	7	0.60	4,106	0.53	100	0.83	1,543	0.41	15,430
Harrisburg – Lebanon – Carlisle, PA MSA	8	0.81	-	-	-	-	-	-	-
Hartford, CT MSA	21	0.93	-	-	-	-	-	-	-

[Continued]

269

Commercial Economic, Sociological, and Educational Research Establishments by Major Metro Area: 1992

[Continued]

Area	Establishments		Revenues		Employment		Payroll		
	Number	% of HS[1] in area	Total ($000)	% of HS[1] in area	Number	% of HS[1] in area	Total ($000)	% of HS[1] in area	Payroll per employee
Honolulu, HI MSA	10	0.59	-	-	-	-	-	-	-
Houston – Galveston – Brazoria, TX CMSA	70	0.99	-	-	-	-	-	-	-
Huntsville, AL MSA	4	0.75	-	-	-	-	-	-	-
Indianapolis, IN MSA	27	1.06	42,373	2.11	557	1.73	14,829	1.58	26,623
Jackson, MS MSA	5	0.78	-	-	-	-	-	-	-
Jacksonville, FL MSA	18	1.02	6,559	0.50	185	1.08	2,498	0.45	13,503
Johnson City – Kingsport – Bristol, TN – VA MSA	1	0.14	-	-	-	-	-	-	-
Kalamazoo – Battle Creek, MI MSA	2	0.27	-	-	-	-	-	-	-
Kansas City, MO – KS MSA	43	1.51	24,298	1.11	1,154	3.42	10,462	1.06	9,066
Knoxville, TN MSA	10	0.84	-	-	-	-	-	-	-
Lafayette, LA MSA	3	0.47	-	-	-	-	-	-	-
Lakeland – Winter Haven, FL MSA	2	0.41	-	-	-	-	-	-	-
Lancaster, PA MSA	2	0.33	-	-	-	-	-	-	-
Lansing – East Lansing, MI MSA	9	1.23	5,256	1.31	87	1.38	2,413	1.27	27,736
Las Vegas, NV – AZ MSA	7	0.45	3,765	0.22	71	0.38	1,872	0.27	26,366
Lexington, KY MSA	3	0.37	552	0.09	45	0.50	376	0.14	8,356
Little Rock – North Little Rock, AR MSA	12	1.15	5,521	0.71	225	2.01	1,764	0.48	7,840
Los Angeles – Riverside – Orange County, CA CMSA	346	1.13	350,353	1.49	5,439	1.96	126,196	1.38	23,202
Louisville, KY – IN MSA	19	1.10	7,404	0.44	356	1.38	2,772	0.39	7,787
Macon, GA MSA	1	0.18	-	-	-	-	-	-	-
Madison, WI MSA	19	3.67	-	-	-	-	-	-	-
Melbourne – Titusville – Palm Bay, FL MSA	5	0.62	787	0.15	31	0.43	211	0.08	6,806
Memphis, TN – AR – MS MSA	21	1.28	11,257	0.91	299	1.83	6,244	1.16	20,883
Miami – Fort Lauderdale, FL CMSA	78	0.85	45,039	0.66	739	0.85	18,462	0.66	24,982
Milwaukee – Racine, WI CMSA	29	0.96	-	-	-	-	-	-	-
Minneapolis – St. Paul, MN – WI MSA	101	2.71	92,730	3.20	1,755	3.52	33,505	2.23	19,091
Mobile, AL MSA	0	0.00	0	0.00	0	0.00	0	0.00	0
Modesto, CA MSA	1	0.15	-	-	-	-	-	-	-
Montgomery, AL MSA	3	0.61	-	-	-	-	-	-	-
Nashville, TN MSA	17	0.87	-	-	-	-	-	-	-
New Orleans, LA MSA	13	0.54	4,103	0.19	275	0.93	1,748	0.21	6,356
New York – Northern New Jersey – Long Island, NY – NJ – CT- CMSA	882	2.17	1,539,253	5.89	15,543	4.66	506,028	4.63	32,557
Norfolk – Virginia Beach – Newport News, VA – NC MSA	15	0.66	21,811	1.61	1,335	6.10	7,990	1.23	5,985
Oklahoma City, OK MSA	12	0.61	-	-	-	-	-	-	-
Omaha, NE – IA MSA	17	1.68	34,934	4.26	840	6.75	10,946	2.93	13,031
Orlando, FL MSA	35	1.38	10,853	0.57	350	1.39	4,213	0.51	12,037
Pensacola, FL MSA	4	0.76	-	-	-	-	-	-	-
Peoria – Pekin, IL MSA	7	1.38	-	-	-	-	-	-	-
Philadelphia – Wilmington – Atlantic City, PA – NJ – DE – MD CMSA	168	1.45	304,405	4.17	5,492	5.50	135,184	4.15	24,615
Phoenix – Mesa, AZ MSA	62	1.29	75,746	2.41	1,709	4.43	29,981	2.18	17,543
Pittsburgh, PA MSA	52	1.09	-	-	-	-	-	-	-
Portland, ME MSA	9	1.66	2,232	0.58	71	1.21	875	0.49	12,324
Portland – Salem, OR – WA CMSA	51	1.44	-	-	-	-	-	-	-
Providence – Fall River – Warwick, RI – MA MSA	14	0.68	-	-	-	-	-	-	-
Raleigh – Durham – Chapel Hill, NC MSA	30	2.09	22,856	1.88	328	1.91	9,135	1.81	27,851

[Continued]

★ 312 ★

Commercial Economic, Sociological, and Educational Research Establishments by Major Metro Area: 1992

[Continued]

Area	Establishments		Revenues		Employment		Payroll		
	Number	% of HS[1] in area	Total ($000)	% of HS[1] in area	Number	% of HS[1] in area	Total ($000)	% of HS[1] in area	Payroll per employee
Reno, NV MSA	3	0.45	-	-	-	-	-	-	-
Richmond – Petersburg, VA MSA	21	1.31	13,310	0.85	322	1.45	5,412	0.82	16,807
Rochester, NY MSA	23	1.50	29,886	3.61	491	3.52	11,467	3.27	23,354
Rockford, IL MSA	8	1.68	-	-	-	-	-	-	-
Sacramento – Yolo, CA CMSA	28	0.97	-	-	-	-	-	-	-
Saginaw – Bay City – Midland, MI MSA	1	0.15	-	-	-	-	-	-	-
St. Louis, MO – IL MSA	57	1.28	48,465	1.69	1,173	2.69	17,670	1.42	15,064
Salinas, CA MSA	9	1.48	-	-	-	-	-	-	-
Salt Lake City – Ogden, UT MSA	19	0.92	5,068	0.37	437	1.98	2,527	0.44	5,783
San Antonio, TX MSA	26	0.99	-	-	-	-	-	-	-
San Diego, CA MSA	74	1.50	40,988	1.26	755	1.81	16,606	1.23	21,995
San Francisco – Oakland – San Jose, CA CMSA	245	1.74	-	-	-	-	-	-	-
Santa Barbara – Santa Maria – Lompoc, CA MSA	10	1.20	8,385	1.96	90	1.71	3,469	1.95	38,544
Sarasota – Bradenton, FL MSA	13	1.06	18,553	1.89	375	2.60	5,122	1.26	13,659
Scranton – Wilkes-Barre – Hazleton, PA MSA	4	0.35	-	-	-	-	-	-	-
Seattle – Tacoma – Bremerton, WA CMSA	90	1.49	48,731	1.37	1,001	1.85	17,980	1.16	17,962
Shreveport – Bossier City, LA MSA	4	0.62	-	-	-	-	-	-	-
Spokane, WA MSA	4	0.54	834	0.16	55	0.70	390	0.17	7,091
Springfield, MO MSA	3	0.65	672	0.17	17	0.25	193	0.10	11,353
Springfield, MA MSA	9	0.99	26,099	3.91	403	3.34	10,765	3.35	26,712
Stockton – Lodi, CA MSA	2	0.24	-	-	-	-	-	-	-
Syracuse, NY MSA	13	1.19	8,702	1.26	347	3.54	4,258	1.35	12,271
Tallahassee, FL MSA	16	4.03	8,144	2.36	256	5.43	3,222	2.11	12,586
Tampa – St. Petersburg – Clearwater, FL MSA	41	0.83	161,050	3.70	2,360	3.86	38,701	2.24	16,399
Toledo, OH MSA	18	1.60	50,499	6.49	1,313	10.45	21,918	5.52	16,693
Tucson, AZ MSA	12	0.95	-	-	-	-	-	-	-
Tulsa, OK MSA	17	1.24	-	-	-	-	-	-	-
Washington – Baltimore, DC – MD – VA – WV CMSA	349	2.70	-	-	-	-	-	-	-
West Palm Beach – Boca Raton, FL MSA	22	0.82	8,703	0.44	147	0.60	3,299	0.39	22,442
Wichita, KS MSA	13	1.70	-	-	-	-	-	-	-
Youngstown – Warren, OH MSA	1	0.08	-	-	-	-	-	-	-

Source: U.S. Department of Commerce. Bureau of the Census. *1992 Economic Census Report Series,* CD-ROM 1i, Washington, DC, October 1996. *Notes:* - means no data reported. 1. HS stands for total health service establishments, revenues, employment, or payroll.

★ 313 ★

Establishment Data

Commercial Economic, Sociological, and Educational Research Establishments by Major Metro Area, Non-Taxed: 1992

Area	Establish-ments	Revenues in $1,000	Employ-ment	Payroll in $1,000	Payroll per employee
United States	536	352,374	4,712	134,236	28,488
Albany – Schenectady – Troy, NY MSA	3	336	3	91	30,333
Atlanta, GA MSA	3	1,121	16	386	24,125
Boston – Worcester – Lawrence, MA – NH – ME – CT CMSA	30	-	-	-	-
Buffalo – Niagara Falls, NY MSA	0	0	0	0	0
Chicago – Gary – Kenosha, IL – IN – WI CMSA	23	-	-	-	-
Cincinnati – Hamilton, OH – KY – IN CMSA	3	331	7	168	24,000
Cleveland – Akron, OH CMSA	4	-	-	-	-
Columbus, OH MSA	3	-	-	-	-
Dallas – Fort Worth, TX CMSA	6	-	-	-	-
Denver – Boulder – Greeley, CO CMSA	10	-	-	-	-
Detroit – Ann Arbor – Flint, MI CMSA	4	692	12	386	32,167
Hartford, CT MSA	4	-	-	-	-
Houston – Galveston – Brazoria, TX CMSA	3	-	-	-	-
Indianapolis, IN MSA	4	-	-	-	-
Kansas City, MO – KS MSA	2	-	-	-	-
Los Angeles – Riverside – Orange County, CA CMSA	27	14,102	125	3,795	30,360
Miami – Fort Lauderdale, FL CMSA	3	-	-	-	-
Milwaukee – Racine, WI CMSA	6	1,269	20	536	26,800
Minneapolis – St. Paul, MN – WI MSA	5	-	-	-	-
New York – Northern New Jersey – Long Island, NY – NJ – CT- CMSA	52	-	-	-	-
Philadelphia – Wilmington – Atlantic City, PA – NJ – DE – MD CMSA	6	-	-	-	-
Phoenix – Mesa, AZ MSA	3	-	-	-	-
Pittsburgh, PA MSA	7	-	-	-	-
Portland – Salem, OR – WA CMSA	9	-	-	-	-
Providence – Fall River – Warwick, RI – MA MSA	3	-	-	-	-
Sacramento – Yolo, CA CMSA	7	-	-	-	-
St. Louis, MO – IL MSA	6	1,792	73	829	11,356
San Diego, CA MSA	5	-	-	-	-
San Francisco – Oakland – San Jose, CA CMSA	35	22,018	334	7,963	23,841
Seattle – Tacoma – Bremerton, WA CMSA	6	-	-	-	-
Tampa – St. Petersburg – Clearwater, FL MSA	2	-	-	-	-

[Continued]

★ 313 ★

Commercial Economic, Sociological, and Educational Research Establishments by Major Metro Area, Non-Taxed: 1992

[Continued]

Area	Establish-ments	Revenues in $1,000	Employ-ment	Payroll in $1,000	Payroll per employee
Washington – Baltimore, DC – MD – VA – WV CMSA	70	-	-	-	-

Source: U.S. Department of Commerce. Bureau of the Census. *1992 Economic Census Report Series,* CD-ROM 1i, Washington, DC, October 1996. *Notes:* - means no data reported. 1. HS stands for total health service establishments, revenues, employment, or payroll.

★ 314 ★

Establishment Data

Commercial Economic, Sociological, and Educational Research Establishments by State: 1992

Area	Establishments		Revenues		Employment		Payroll		
	Number	% of HS[1] in area	Total ($000)	% of HS[1] in area	Number	% of HS[1] in area	Total ($000)	% of HS[1] in area	Payroll per employee
United States	5,165	1.17	6,138,318	2.05	100,729	2.26	2,238,657	1.73	22,225
Alabama	27	0.49	12,910	0.26	295	0.38	5,156	0.24	17,478
Alaska	15	1.75	6,613	1.22	88	1.56	2,590	1.19	29,432
Arizona	77	1.08	83,534	1.83	1,926	3.28	33,161	1.70	17,218
Arkansas	17	0.48	6,239	0.26	278	0.65	2,000	0.19	7,194
California	738	1.20	698,608	1.62	10,261	1.91	247,300	1.43	24,101
Colorado	124	1.77	104,434	2.79	1,800	3.26	37,177	2.27	20,654
Connecticut	140	2.12	244,562	4.98	1,733	2.40	72,348	3.08	41,747
Delaware	11	0.92	-	-	-	-	-	-	-
District of Columbia	108	7.83	155,961	19.54	1,654	17.05	64,300	18.54	38,875
Florida	263	0.89	277,906	1.19	4,655	1.48	84,231	0.87	18,095
Georgia	119	1.07	98,857	1.15	2,278	1.88	32,246	0.88	14,155
Hawaii	11	0.49	-	-	-	-	-	-	-
Idaho	11	0.63	-	-	-	-	-	-	-
Illinois	339	1.81	530,373	4.29	8,294	4.42	210,465	3.76	25,376
Indiana	57	0.65	70,888	1.16	1,356	1.27	29,297	1.07	21,605
Iowa	38	0.91	48,765	2.09	1,165	2.59	20,091	1.81	17,245
Kansas	44	1.14	26,134	0.86	1,769	3.31	11,761	0.89	6,648
Kentucky	31	0.56	27,962	0.68	669	1.00	11,221	0.63	16,773
Louisiana	27	0.40	6,680	0.12	350	0.41	2,647	0.12	7,563
Maine	20	0.93	4,703	0.40	122	0.55	1,574	0.30	12,902
Maryland	144	1.57	336,585	5.97	4,956	6.20	117,479	4.71	23,704
Massachusetts	177	1.67	356,383	4.67	4,400	3.46	138,742	3.91	31,532
Michigan	118	0.75	177,612	2.04	4,952	3.51	67,191	1.63	13,568
Minnesota	108	1.83	92,948	2.26	1,771	2.34	33,753	1.62	19,059
Mississippi	11	0.36	4,500	0.22	106	0.29	2,481	0.28	23,406

[Continued]

★314★

Commercial Economic, Sociological, and Educational Research Establishments by State: 1992

[Continued]

Area	Establishments		Revenues		Employment		Payroll		
	Number	% of HS[1] in area	Total ($000)	% of HS[1] in area	Number	% of HS[1] in area	Total ($000)	% of HS[1] in area	Payroll per employee
Missouri	84	1.00	54,286	0.99	1,396	1.47	19,881	0.81	14,241
Montana	11	0.74	-	-	-	-	-	-	-
Nebraska	33	1.40	-	-	-	-	-	-	-
Nevada	10	0.43	-	-	-	-	-	-	-
New Hampshire	21	1.14	7,587	0.64	109	0.57	2,711	0.50	24,872
New Jersey	268	1.62	554,141	5.33	5,758	4.51	168,327	3.81	29,234
New Mexico	23	0.96	7,214	0.49	291	1.23	2,773	0.45	9,529
New York	606	1.87	843,744	4.25	10,248	3.68	303,625	3.68	29,628
North Carolina	87	0.98	66,009	0.99	1,189	1.11	21,522	0.72	18,101
North Dakota	3	0.39	-	-	-	-	-	-	-
Ohio	164	0.88	232,597	2.00	4,332	2.17	81,812	1.47	18,886
Oklahoma	31	0.58	11,890	0.36	460	0.78	4,236	0.30	9,209
Oregon	54	0.96	24,730	0.84	717	1.49	9,588	0.74	13,372
Pennsylvania	231	1.06	317,761	2.52	6,337	3.44	143,073	2.53	22,577
Rhode Island	15	0.79	-	-	-	-	-	-	-
South Carolina	28	0.60	8,165	0.26	244	0.49	2,912	0.21	11,934
South Dakota	7	0.72	-	-	-	-	-	-	-
Tennessee	53	0.64	-	-	-	-	-	-	-
Texas	271	0.90	229,168	1.00	4,410	1.27	90,370	0.98	20,492
Utah	28	0.92	10,655	0.58	927	3.00	5,630	0.75	6,073
Vermont	10	1.08	4,133	1.02	78	1.03	2,012	1.22	25,795
Virginia	157	1.61	158,361	2.37	3,130	3.06	61,191	2.02	19,550
Washington	109	1.18	54,135	1.00	1,133	1.30	20,111	0.84	17,750
West Virginia	11	0.41	6,598	0.37	263	0.91	2,429	0.34	9,236
Wisconsin	67	0.93	32,687	0.69	1,317	1.55	13,572	0.58	10,305
Wyoming	8	1.12	1,252	0.39	13	0.23	506	0.37	38,923

Source: U.S. Department of Commerce. Bureau of the Census. *1992 Economic Census Report Series,* CD-ROM 1i, Washington, DC, October 1996. *Notes:* - means no data reported. 1. HS stands for total health service establishments, revenues, employment, or payroll.

★ 315 ★

Establishment Data

Commercial Economic, Sociological, and Educational Research Establishments by State, Non-Taxed: 1992

Area	Establish-ments	Revenues in $1,000	Employ-ment	Payroll in $1,000	Payroll per employee
United States	536	352,374	4,712	134,236	28,488
Alabama	4	251	4	69	17,250
Alaska	3	-	-	-	-
Arizona	10	2,289	34	663	19,500
Arkansas	3	-	-	-	-
California	79	-	-	-	-
Colorado	15	-	-	-	-
Connecticut	6	2,162	41	725	17,683
Delaware	0	0	0	0	0
District of Columbia	39	39,630	308	11,781	38,250
Florida	6	-	-	-	-
Georgia	3	1,121	16	386	24,125
Hawaii	4	-	-	-	-
Idaho	1	-	-	-	-
Illinois	28	46,838	942	19,827	21,048
Indiana	13	-	-	-	-
Iowa	5	1,452	25	362	14,480
Kansas	3	-	-	-	-
Kentucky	6	-	-	-	-
Louisiana	3	267	8	124	15,500
Maine	1	-	-	-	-
Maryland	14	-	-	-	-
Massachusetts	33	-	-	-	-
Michigan	15	-	-	-	-
Minnesota	5	-	-	-	-
Mississippi	3	-	-	-	-
Missouri	8	2,234	98	1,281	13,071
Montana	7	3,070	57	1,246	21,860
Nebraska	4	-	-	-	-
Nevada	1	-	-	-	-
New Hampshire	2	-	-	-	-
New Jersey	11	3,934	65	1,468	22,585
New Mexico	6	-	-	-	-
New York	50	-	-	-	-
North Carolina	9	1,874	37	650	17,568
North Dakota	1	-	-	-	-
Ohio	11	2,389	47	1,001	21,298
Oklahoma	3	-	-	-	-
Oregon	13	14,041	158	5,776	36,557
Pennsylvania	22	-	-	-	-
Rhode Island	3	-	-	-	-
South Carolina	3	-	-	-	-
South Dakota	1	-	-	-	-
Tennessee	5	-	-	-	-

[Continued]

★ 315 ★

Commercial Economic, Sociological, and Educational Research Establishments by State, Non-Taxed: 1992

[Continued]

Area	Establish- ments	Revenues in $1,000	Employ- ment	Payroll in $1,000	Payroll per employee
Texas	17	-	-	-	-
Utah	6	1,386	19	552	29,053
Vermont	2	-	-	-	-
Virginia	24	-	-	-	-
Washington	9	-	-	-	-
West Virginia	1	-	-	-	-
Wisconsin	14	-	-	-	-
Wyoming	1	-	-	-	-

Source: U.S. Department of Commerce. Bureau of the Census. *1992 Economic Census Report Series,* CD-ROM 1i, Washington, DC, October 1996. *Notes:* - means no data reported. 1. HS stands for total health service establishments, revenues, employment, or payroll.

★ 316 ★

Establishment Data

Commercial Medical and Biological Research Establishments by Major Metro Area: 1992

Area	Establishments		Revenues		Employment		Payroll		
	Number	% of HS[1] in area	Total ($000)	% of HS[1] in area	Number	% of HS[1] in area	Total ($000)	% of HS[1] in area	Payroll per employee
United States	1,458	0.33	2,875,397	0.96	28,264	0.63	1,204,507	0.93	42,616
Atlanta, GA MSA	10	0.16	-	-	-	-	-	-	-
Boston – Worcester – Lawrence, MA – NH – ME – CT CMSA	112	1.15	455,046	6.44	3,063	2.66	156,770	4.82	51,182
Chicago – Gary – Kenosha, IL – IN – WI CMSA	28	0.19	-	-	-	-	-	-	-
Cincinnati – Hamilton, OH – KY – IN CMSA	6	0.19	-	-	-	-	-	-	-
Cleveland – Akron, OH CMSA	7	0.13	-	-	-	-	-	-	-
Dallas – Fort Worth, TX CMSA	10	0.12	-	-	-	-	-	-	-
Denver – Boulder – Greeley, CO CMSA	30	0.69	91,308	3.59	863	2.42	49,863	4.45	57,779
Detroit – Ann Arbor – Flint, MI CMSA	20	0.21	-	-	-	-	-	-	-
Houston – Galveston – Brazoria, TX CMSA	25	0.35	-	-	-	-	-	-	-
Indianapolis, IN MSA	7	0.28	2,408	0.12	30	0.09	781	0.08	26,033
Kansas City, MO – KS MSA	11	0.39	11,137	0.51	151	0.45	5,464	0.55	36,185
Los Angeles – Riverside – Orange County, CA CMSA	75	0.25	105,785	0.45	923	0.33	45,022	0.49	48,778
Miami – Fort Lauderdale, FL CMSA	18	0.20	14,346	0.21	135	0.16	5,026	0.18	37,230
Milwaukee – Racine, WI CMSA	2	0.07	-	-	-	-	-	-	-
Minneapolis – St. Paul, MN – WI MSA	34	0.91	34,798	1.20	341	0.68	14,296	0.95	41,924
New York – Northern New Jersey – Long Island, NY – NJ – CT- CMSA	137	0.34	-	-	-	-	-	-	-
Orlando, FL MSA	11	0.43	-	-	-	-	-	-	-
Philadelphia – Wilmington – Atlantic City, PA – NJ – DE – MD CMSA	41	0.35	263,720	3.61	1,964	1.97	105,433	3.24	53,683
Phoenix – Mesa, AZ MSA	12	0.25	-	-	-	-	-	-	-

[Continued]

★ 316 ★

Commercial Medical and Biological Research Establishments by Major Metro Area: 1992

[Continued]

Area	Establishments		Revenues		Employment		Payroll		
	Number	% of HS[1] in area	Total ($000)	% of HS[1] in area	Number	% of HS[1] in area	Total ($000)	% of HS[1] in area	Payroll per employee
Pittsburgh, PA MSA	1	0.02	-	-	-	-	-	-	-
Portland – Salem, OR – WA CMSA	13	0.37	-	-	-	-	-	-	-
Sacramento – Yolo, CA CMSA	9	0.31	-	-	-	-	-	-	-
St. Louis, MO – IL MSA	10	0.22	-	-	-	-	-	-	-
San Diego, CA MSA	53	1.08	128,413	3.93	1,442	3.46	68,913	5.12	47,790
San Francisco – Oakland – San Jose, CA CMSA	123	0.88	-	-	-	-	-	-	-
Seattle – Tacoma – Bremerton, WA CMSA	34	0.56	-	-	-	-	-	-	-
Tampa – St. Petersburg – Clearwater, FL MSA	12	0.24	-	-	-	-	-	-	-
Washington – Baltimore, DC – MD – VA – WV CMSA	95	0.73	-	-	-	-	-	-	-
West Palm Beach – Boca Raton, FL MSA	3	0.11	-	-	-	-	-	-	-

Source: U.S. Department of Commerce. Bureau of the Census. *1992 Economic Census Report Series,* CD-ROM 1i, Washington, DC, October 1996. *Notes:* - means no data reported. 1. HS stands for total health service establishments, revenues, employment, or payroll.

★ 317 ★

Establishment Data

Commercial Medical and Biological Research Establishments by State: 1992

Area	Establishments		Revenues		Employment		Payroll		
	Number	% of HS[1] in area	Total ($000)	% of HS[1] in area	Number	% of HS[1] in area	Total ($000)	% of HS[1] in area	Payroll per employee
United States	1,458	0.33	2,875,397	0.96	28,264	0.63	1,204,507	0.93	42,616
Alabama	17	0.31	9,547	0.19	115	0.15	3,594	0.17	31,252
Alaska	6	0.70	3,558	0.66	37	0.65	1,278	0.59	34,541
Arizona	22	0.31	10,639	0.23	127	0.22	5,088	0.26	40,063
Arkansas	9	0.25	3,946	0.16	94	0.22	2,381	0.22	25,330
California	290	0.47	611,251	1.42	5,421	1.01	270,253	1.57	49,853
Colorado	39	0.56	96,810	2.59	963	1.74	53,112	3.24	55,153
Connecticut	16	0.24	32,609	0.66	237	0.33	11,327	0.48	47,793
Delaware	2	0.17	-	-	-	-	-	-	-
District of Columbia	5	0.36	-	-	-	-	-	-	-
Florida	63	0.21	93,342	0.40	1,760	0.56	49,457	0.51	28,101
Georgia	16	0.14	12,010	0.14	120	0.10	4,230	0.12	35,250
Hawaii	1	0.04	-	-	-	-	-	-	-
Idaho	2	0.12	-	-	-	-	-	-	-
Illinois	35	0.19	18,334	0.15	215	0.11	6,639	0.12	30,879
Indiana	17	0.20	13,023	0.21	200	0.19	5,458	0.20	27,290
Iowa	9	0.22	-	-	-	-	-	-	-
Kansas	13	0.34	18,822	0.62	246	0.46	9,052	0.68	36,797
Kentucky	10	0.18	6,865	0.17	118	0.18	3,619	0.20	30,669
Louisiana	17	0.25	7,803	0.14	96	0.11	3,717	0.17	38,719

[Continued]

★ 317 ★

Commercial Medical and Biological Research Establishments by State: 1992
[Continued]

Area	Establishments		Revenues		Employment		Payroll		
	Number	% of HS[1] in area	Total ($000)	% of HS[1] in area	Number	% of HS[1] in area	Total ($000)	% of HS[1] in area	Payroll per employee
Maine	6	0.28	2,062	0.18	32	0.15	605	0.11	18,906
Maryland	75	0.82	255,106	4.52	3,072	3.85	107,778	4.32	35,084
Massachusetts	115	1.08	465,604	6.11	3,288	2.58	161,369	4.55	49,078
Michigan	30	0.19	44,020	0.51	572	0.41	16,087	0.39	28,124
Minnesota	40	0.68	37,250	0.91	372	0.49	14,952	0.72	40,194
Mississippi	5	0.16	782	0.04	6	0.02	144	0.02	24,000
Missouri	22	0.26	15,221	0.28	133	0.14	4,472	0.18	33,624
Montana	6	0.40	-	-	-	-	-	-	-
Nebraska	6	0.25	-	-	-	-	-	-	-
Nevada	6	0.26	2,046	0.09	13	0.05	402	0.04	30,923
New Hampshire	7	0.38	4,831	0.41	44	0.23	1,924	0.35	43,727
New Jersey	65	0.39	163,350	1.57	1,444	1.13	68,025	1.54	47,109
New Mexico	8	0.33	6,927	0.47	121	0.51	2,967	0.48	24,521
New York	84	0.26	142,672	0.72	1,664	0.60	72,406	0.88	43,513
North Carolina	37	0.42	78,225	1.18	869	0.81	31,657	1.06	36,429
North Dakota	2	0.26	-	-	-	-	-	-	-
Ohio	41	0.22	49,641	0.43	664	0.33	22,562	0.40	33,979
Oklahoma	7	0.13	1,493	0.05	37	0.06	749	0.05	20,243
Oregon	23	0.41	7,710	0.26	108	0.22	3,023	0.23	27,991
Pennsylvania	52	0.24	269,630	2.13	2,036	1.10	109,656	1.94	53,859
Rhode Island	6	0.32	6,926	0.65	68	0.37	4,654	1.00	68,441
South Carolina	6	0.13	1,610	0.05	15	0.03	558	0.04	37,200
South Dakota	0	0.00	0	0.00	0	0.00	0	0.00	0
Tennessee	21	0.26	-	-	-	-	-	-	-
Texas	80	0.27	139,924	0.61	1,570	0.45	54,019	0.59	34,407
Utah	25	0.82	23,916	1.30	329	1.06	13,140	1.74	39,939
Vermont	3	0.32	1,171	0.29	14	0.19	519	0.31	37,071
Virginia	30	0.31	42,398	0.63	344	0.34	14,945	0.49	43,445
Washington	42	0.46	-	-	-	-	-	-	-
West Virginia	2	0.07	-	-	-	-	-	-	-
Wisconsin	15	0.21	-	-	-	-	-	-	-
Wyoming	2	0.28	-	-	-	-	-	-	-

Source: U.S. Department of Commerce. Bureau of the Census. *1992 Economic Census Report Series,* CD-ROM 1i, Washington, DC, October 1996. *Notes:* - means no data reported. 1. HS stands for total health service establishments, revenues, employment, or payroll.

★ 318 ★

Establishment Data

Commercial Physical and Biological Research Establishments by Major Metro Area: 1992

Area	Establishments		Revenues		Employment		Payroll		
	Number	% of HS[1] in area	Total ($000)	% of HS[1] in area	Number	% of HS[1] in area	Total ($000)	% of HS[1] in area	Payroll per employee
United States	3,826	0.87	11,788,343	3.94	111,124	2.50	4,989,952	3.87	44,904
Albany – Schenectady – Troy, NY MSA	12	0.92	-	-	-	-	-	-	-
Albuquerque, NM MSA	40	3.75	89,552	10.73	1,332	10.53	50,271	13.34	37,741
Allentown – Bethlehem – Easton, PA MSA	10	0.81	-	-	-	-	-	-	-
Anchorage, AK MSA	6	1.23	4,160	1.14	46	1.27	1,580	1.11	34,348
Appleton – Oshkosh – Neenah, WI MSA	0	0.00	0	0.00	0	0.00	0	0.00	0
Atlanta, GA MSA	33	0.54	30,462	0.63	290	0.48	12,225	0.61	42,155
Augusta – Aiken, GA – SC MSA	4	0.56	-	-	-	-	-	-	-
Austin – San Marcos, TX MSA	42	2.67	112,729	9.42	1,104	5.94	44,356	9.14	40,178
Bakersfield, CA MSA	8	1.05	-	-	-	-	-	-	-
Baton Rouge, LA MSA	6	0.68	-	-	-	-	-	-	-
Beaumont – Port Arthur, TX MSA	0	0.00	0	0.00	0	0.00	0	0.00	0
Birmingham, AL MSA	10	0.73	8,671	0.57	105	0.52	3,677	0.57	35,019
Boise City, ID MSA	4	0.67	-	-	-	-	-	-	-
Boston – Worcester – Lawrence, MA – NH – ME – CT CMSA	257	2.63	776,350	10.98	5,972	5.19	312,656	9.60	52,354
Buffalo – Niagara Falls, NY MSA	18	0.90	-	-	-	-	-	-	-
Canton – Massillon, OH MSA	5	0.72	-	-	-	-	-	-	-
Charleston – North Charleston, SC MSA	7	0.86	1,096	0.19	19	0.21	406	0.17	21,368
Charlotte – Gastonia – Rock Hill, NC – SC MSA	6	0.37	2,492	0.18	19	0.09	659	0.10	34,684
Chattanooga, TN – GA MSA	4	0.53	-	-	-	-	-	-	-
Chicago – Gary – Kenosha, IL – IN – WI CMSA	70	0.48	-	-	-	-	-	-	-
Cincinnati – Hamilton, OH – KY – IN CMSA	16	0.51	-	-	-	-	-	-	-
Cleveland – Akron, OH CMSA	28	0.52	-	-	-	-	-	-	-
Colorado Springs, CO MSA	15	1.69	65,792	14.81	642	9.72	30,603	15.20	47,668
Columbia, SC MSA	1	0.13	-	-	-	-	-	-	-
Columbus, OH MSA	19	0.78	-	-	-	-	-	-	-
Corpus Christi, TX MSA	3	0.40	-	-	-	-	-	-	-
Dallas – Fort Worth, TX CMSA	37	0.44	176,332	2.70	2,194	2.55	103,462	3.91	47,157
Davenport – Moline – Rock Island, IA – IL MSA	1	0.15	-	-	-	-	-	-	-
Dayton – Springfield, OH MSA	37	2.25	132,598	11.59	1,364	7.70	52,154	9.25	38,236
Daytona Beach, FL MSA	2	0.27	-	-	-	-	-	-	-
Denver – Boulder – Greeley, CO CMSA	88	2.01	-	-	-	-	-	-	-
Des Moines, IA MSA	4	0.54	-	-	-	-	-	-	-
Detroit – Ann Arbor – Flint, MI CMSA	72	0.76	-	-	-	-	-	-	-
El Paso, TX MSA	8	1.01	5,534	0.71	86	0.80	2,699	0.92	31,384
Eugene – Springfield, OR MSA	7	1.20	1,813	0.54	37	0.68	895	0.58	24,189
Fort Myers – Cape Coral, FL MSA	2	0.28	-	-	-	-	-	-	-
Fort Pierce – Port St. Lucie, FL MSA	2	0.39	-	-	-	-	-	-	-
Fort Wayne, IN MSA	2	0.29	-	-	-	-	-	-	-
Fresno, CA MSA	7	0.47	8,509	0.98	102	0.83	4,189	1.13	41,069
Grand Rapids – Muskegon – Holland, MI MSA	5	0.33	1,180	0.13	9	0.06	376	0.09	41,778
Greensboro – Winston-Salem – High Point, NC MSA	11	0.73	5,905	0.50	55	0.32	2,403	0.46	43,691
Greenville – Spartanburg – Anderson, SC MSA	6	0.51	1,952	0.25	8	0.07	735	0.20	91,875
Harrisburg – Lebanon – Carlisle, PA MSA	6	0.61	-	-	-	-	-	-	-
Hartford, CT MSA	12	0.53	-	-	-	-	-	-	-

[Continued]

★318★

Commercial Physical and Biological Research Establishments by Major Metro Area: 1992
[Continued]

Area	Establishments		Revenues		Employment		Payroll		
	Number	% of HS[1] in area	Total ($000)	% of HS[1] in area	Number	% of HS[1] in area	Total ($000)	% of HS[1] in area	Payroll per employee
Honolulu, HI MSA	10	0.59	-	-	-	-	-	-	-
Houston – Galveston – Brazoria, TX CMSA	62	0.88	142,022	2.42	1,306	1.75	56,528	2.41	43,283
Huntsville, AL MSA	31	5.82	128,983	28.22	1,451	22.18	62,499	32.70	43,073
Indianapolis, IN MSA	17	0.67	15,096	0.75	253	0.79	5,975	0.63	23,617
Jackson, MS MSA	2	0.31	-	-	-	-	-	-	-
Jacksonville, FL MSA	4	0.23	7,397	0.57	93	0.54	3,519	0.63	37,839
Johnson City – Kingsport – Bristol, TN – VA MSA	3	0.43	-	-	-	-	-	-	-
Kalamazoo – Battle Creek, MI MSA	3	0.41	-	-	-	-	-	-	-
Kansas City, MO – KS MSA	21	0.74	15,679	0.72	240	0.71	7,297	0.74	30,404
Knoxville, TN MSA	17	1.42	-	-	-	-	-	-	-
Lafayette, LA MSA	4	0.63	-	-	-	-	-	-	-
Lakeland – Winter Haven, FL MSA	2	0.41	-	-	-	-	-	-	-
Lancaster, PA MSA	2	0.33	-	-	-	-	-	-	-
Lansing – East Lansing, MI MSA	1	0.14	-	-	-	-	-	-	-
Las Vegas, NV – AZ MSA	15	0.96	314,909	18.65	3,074	16.66	129,339	18.99	42,075
Lexington, KY MSA	3	0.37	585	0.10	9	0.10	396	0.14	44,000
Little Rock – North Little Rock, AR MSA	3	0.29	-	-	-	-	-	-	-
Los Angeles – Riverside – Orange County, CA CMSA	242	0.79	719,402	3.06	6,766	2.44	358,929	3.93	53,049
Louisville, KY – IN MSA	8	0.47	1,932	0.12	30	0.12	395	0.06	13,167
Macon, GA MSA	1	0.18	-	-	-	-	-	-	-
Madison, WI MSA	13	2.51	16,540	3.19	254	3.53	8,916	3.80	35,102
Melbourne – Titusville – Palm Bay, FL MSA	16	1.97	16,884	3.11	250	3.44	9,122	3.64	36,488
Memphis, TN – AR – MS MSA	6	0.36	1,122	0.09	20	0.12	576	0.11	28,800
Miami – Fort Lauderdale, FL CMSA	30	0.33	21,880	0.32	239	0.27	8,452	0.30	35,364
Milwaukee – Racine, WI CMSA	9	0.30	-	-	-	-	-	-	-
Minneapolis – St. Paul, MN – WI MSA	59	1.58	55,110	1.90	513	1.03	22,565	1.50	43,986
Mobile, AL MSA	2	0.31	-	-	-	-	-	-	-
Modesto, CA MSA	4	0.59	-	-	-	-	-	-	-
Montgomery, AL MSA	8	1.63	2,163	0.43	30	0.40	437	0.21	14,567
Nashville, TN MSA	9	0.46	13,544	0.73	98	0.39	4,158	0.54	42,429
New Orleans, LA MSA	10	0.41	7,079	0.32	86	0.29	3,387	0.40	39,384
New York – Northern New Jersey – Long Island, NY – NJ – CT- CMSA	323	0.80	-	-	-	-	-	-	-
Norfolk – Virginia Beach – Newport News, VA – NC MSA	22	0.98	38,333	2.83	630	2.88	24,178	3.74	38,378
Oklahoma City, OK MSA	8	0.41	-	-	-	-	-	-	-
Omaha, NE – IA MSA	4	0.40	-	-	-	-	-	-	-
Orlando, FL MSA	25	0.99	78,125	4.11	1,540	6.11	41,415	5.06	26,893
Pensacola, FL MSA	2	0.38	-	-	-	-	-	-	-
Peoria – Pekin, IL MSA	2	0.39	-	-	-	-	-	-	-
Philadelphia – Wilmington – Atlantic City, PA – NJ – DE – MD CMSA	89	0.77	-	-	-	-	-	-	-
Phoenix – Mesa, AZ MSA	23	0.48	-	-	-	-	-	-	-
Pittsburgh, PA MSA	25	0.52	-	-	-	-	-	-	-
Portland, ME MSA	8	1.48	3,950	1.03	71	1.21	1,357	0.76	19,113
Portland – Salem, OR – WA CMSA	31	0.87	-	-	-	-	-	-	-
Providence – Fall River – Warwick, RI – MA MSA	15	0.72	-	-	-	-	-	-	-
Raleigh – Durham – Chapel Hill, NC MSA	39	2.71	52,625	4.33	523	3.04	22,096	4.38	42,249

[Continued]

★318★

Commercial Physical and Biological Research Establishments by Major Metro Area: 1992

[Continued]

Area	Establishments		Revenues		Employment		Payroll		
	Number	% of HS[1] in area	Total ($000)	% of HS[1] in area	Number	% of HS[1] in area	Total ($000)	% of HS[1] in area	Payroll per employee
Reno, NV MSA	4	0.60	-	-	-	-	-	-	-
Richmond – Petersburg, VA MSA	7	0.44	-	-	-	-	-	-	-
Rochester, NY MSA	10	0.65	6,278	0.76	76	0.55	3,004	0.86	39,526
Rockford, IL MSA	1	0.21	-	-	-	-	-	-	-
Sacramento – Yolo, CA CMSA	21	0.73	-	-	-	-	-	-	-
Saginaw – Bay City – Midland, MI MSA	4	0.59	-	-	-	-	-	-	-
St. Louis, MO – IL MSA	27	0.61	58,186	2.03	337	0.77	17,113	1.38	50,780
Salinas, CA MSA	13	2.14	4,660	1.56	47	1.07	2,132	1.74	45,362
Salt Lake City – Ogden, UT MSA	26	1.26	35,346	2.56	468	2.12	16,980	2.96	36,282
San Antonio, TX MSA	21	0.80	-	-	-	-	-	-	-
San Diego, CA MSA	136	2.76	604,106	18.50	6,027	14.47	267,235	19.85	44,340
San Francisco – Oakland – San Jose, CA CMSA	319	2.27	-	-	-	-	-	-	-
Santa Barbara – Santa Maria – Lompoc, CA MSA	33	3.95	99,752	23.36	855	16.21	42,156	23.69	49,305
Sarasota – Bradenton, FL MSA	6	0.49	1,399	0.14	11	0.08	640	0.16	58,182
Scranton – Wilkes-Barre – Hazleton, PA MSA	4	0.35	-	-	-	-	-	-	-
Seattle – Tacoma – Bremerton, WA CMSA	68	1.12	-	-	-	-	-	-	-
Shreveport – Bossier City, LA MSA	2	0.31	-	-	-	-	-	-	-
Spokane, WA MSA	6	0.82	1,481	0.29	22	0.28	585	0.25	26,591
Springfield, MO MSA	1	0.22	-	-	-	-	-	-	-
Springfield, MA MSA	8	0.88	15,066	2.25	242	2.00	6,051	1.89	25,004
Stockton – Lodi, CA MSA	4	0.48	-	-	-	-	-	-	-
Syracuse, NY MSA	6	0.55	10,218	1.48	107	1.09	3,961	1.26	37,019
Tallahassee, FL MSA	3	0.76	-	-	-	-	-	-	-
Tampa – St. Petersburg – Clearwater, FL MSA	27	0.55	-	-	-	-	-	-	-
Toledo, OH MSA	10	0.89	16,335	2.10	213	1.70	6,387	1.61	29,986
Tucson, AZ MSA	20	1.59	72,050	7.29	266	1.95	11,357	2.82	42,695
Tulsa, OK MSA	4	0.29	-	-	-	-	-	-	-
Washington – Baltimore, DC – MD – VA – WV CMSA	296	2.29	-	-	-	-	-	-	-
West Palm Beach – Boca Raton, FL MSA	16	0.60	9,181	0.46	130	0.53	4,412	0.52	33,938
Wichita, KS MSA	2	0.26	-	-	-	-	-	-	-
Youngstown – Warren, OH MSA	0	0.00	0	0.00	0	0.00	0	0.00	0

Source: U.S. Department of Commerce. Bureau of the Census. *1992 Economic Census Report Series,* CD-ROM 1i, Washington, DC, October 1996. *Notes:* - means no data reported. 1. HS stands for total health service establishments, revenues, employment, or payroll.

★319★

Establishment Data

Commercial Physical and Biological Research Establishments by Major Metro Area, Non-Taxed: 1992

Area	Establish-ments	Revenues in $1,000	Employ-ment	Payroll in $1,000	Payroll per employee
United States	344	4,978,474	47,973	2,091,951	43,607
Albany – Schenectady – Troy, NY MSA	0	0	0	0	0
Atlanta, GA MSA	2	-	-	-	-
Boston – Worcester – Lawrence, MA – NH – ME – CT CMSA	20	-	-	-	-
Buffalo – Niagara Falls, NY MSA	2	-	-	-	-
Chicago – Gary – Kenosha, IL – IN – WI CMSA	9	670,039	8,549	322,669	37,743
Cincinnati – Hamilton, OH – KY – IN CMSA	2	-	-	-	-
Cleveland – Akron, OH CMSA	1	-	-	-	-
Columbus, OH MSA	2	-	-	-	-
Dallas – Fort Worth, TX CMSA	4	-	-	-	-
Denver – Boulder – Greeley, CO CMSA	4	-	-	-	-
Detroit – Ann Arbor – Flint, MI CMSA	5	-	-	-	-
Hartford, CT MSA	0	0	0	0	0
Houston – Galveston – Brazoria, TX CMSA	6	-	-	-	-
Indianapolis, IN MSA	1	-	-	-	-
Kansas City, MO – KS MSA	4	-	-	-	-
Los Angeles – Riverside – Orange County, CA CMSA	24	-	-	-	-
Miami – Fort Lauderdale, FL CMSA	2	-	-	-	-
Milwaukee – Racine, WI CMSA	1	-	-	-	-
Minneapolis – St. Paul, MN – WI MSA	4	1,270	15	526	35,067
New York – Northern New Jersey – Long Island, NY – NJ – CT- CMSA	30	337,097	4,037	183,749	45,516
Philadelphia – Wilmington – Atlantic City, PA – NJ – DE – MD CMSA	11	25,257	330	9,666	29,291
Phoenix – Mesa, AZ MSA	2	-	-	-	-
Pittsburgh, PA MSA	9	17,073	198	4,991	25,207
Portland – Salem, OR – WA CMSA	4	-	-	-	-
Providence – Fall River – Warwick, RI – MA MSA	4	1,942	35	915	26,143
Sacramento – Yolo, CA CMSA	2	-	-	-	-
St. Louis, MO – IL MSA	2	-	-	-	-
San Diego, CA MSA	9	-	-	-	-
San Francisco – Oakland – San Jose, CA CMSA	18	-	-	-	-
Seattle – Tacoma – Bremerton, WA CMSA	6	-	-	-	-
Tampa – St. Petersburg – Clearwater, FL MSA	2	-	-	-	-

[Continued]

★ 319 ★

Commercial Physical and Biological Research Establishments by Major Metro Area, Non-Taxed: 1992

[Continued]

Area	Establish-ments	Revenues in $1,000	Employ-ment	Payroll in $1,000	Payroll per employee
Washington – Baltimore, DC – MD – VA – WV CMSA	50	-	-	-	-

Source: U.S. Department of Commerce. Bureau of the Census. *1992 Economic Census Report Series,* CD-ROM 1i, Washington, DC, October 1996. *Notes:* - means no data reported. 1. HS stands for total health service establishments, revenues, employment, or payroll.

★ 320 ★

Establishment Data

Commercial Physical and Biological Research Establishments by State: 1992

Area	Establishments		Revenues		Employment		Payroll		
	Number	% of HS[1] in area	Total ($000)	% of HS[1] in area	Number	% of HS[1] in area	Total ($000)	% of HS[1] in area	Payroll per employee
United States	3,826	0.87	11,788,343	3.94	111,124	2.50	4,989,952	3.87	44,904
Alabama	56	1.01	141,692	2.88	1,605	2.08	67,208	3.18	41,874
Alaska	12	1.40	6,831	1.26	81	1.43	2,799	1.29	34,556
Arizona	52	0.73	124,409	2.72	651	1.11	26,929	1.38	41,366
Arkansas	13	0.36	6,683	0.27	179	0.42	4,459	0.42	24,911
California	802	1.30	2,289,107	5.32	20,616	3.85	1,040,305	6.03	50,461
Colorado	117	1.67	214,388	5.74	2,245	4.06	108,017	6.58	48,114
Connecticut	58	0.88	109,385	2.23	839	1.16	42,104	1.79	50,184
Delaware	4	0.33	-	-	-	-	-	-	-
District of Columbia	21	1.52	-	-	-	-	-	-	-
Florida	166	0.56	184,727	0.79	2,840	0.90	90,153	0.94	31,744
Georgia	49	0.44	38,604	0.45	426	0.35	16,695	0.45	39,190
Hawaii	12	0.54	-	-	-	-	-	-	-
Idaho	14	0.81	-	-	-	-	-	-	-
Illinois	88	0.47	216,870	1.75	2,287	1.22	100,889	1.80	44,114
Indiana	35	0.40	33,018	0.54	518	0.49	13,051	0.48	25,195
Iowa	13	0.31	5,316	0.23	72	0.16	1,772	0.16	24,611
Kansas	26	0.67	23,976	0.79	355	0.66	11,253	0.85	31,699
Kentucky	23	0.42	13,004	0.32	190	0.28	5,908	0.33	31,095
Louisiana	26	0.38	10,830	0.20	129	0.15	4,721	0.22	36,597
Maine	13	0.60	4,468	0.38	79	0.36	1,569	0.29	19,861
Maryland	160	1.75	581,171	10.30	6,119	7.66	243,453	9.75	39,786
Massachusetts	257	2.42	782,740	10.26	6,178	4.86	314,451	8.87	50,899
Michigan	95	0.60	288,805	3.32	2,740	1.94	114,947	2.79	41,951
Minnesota	74	1.25	60,375	1.47	593	0.78	24,169	1.16	40,757
Mississippi	21	0.68	10,074	0.48	119	0.32	4,103	0.47	34,479
Missouri	42	0.50	68,665	1.25	496	0.52	23,069	0.94	46,510
Montana	10	0.67	-	-	-	-	-	-	-

[Continued]

★ 320 ★

Commercial Physical and Biological Research Establishments by State: 1992

[Continued]

Area	Establishments Number	Establishments % of HS[1] in area	Revenues Total ($000)	Revenues % of HS[1] in area	Employment Number	Employment % of HS[1] in area	Payroll Total ($000)	Payroll % of HS[1] in area	Payroll per employee
Nebraska	13	0.55	-	-	-	-	-	-	-
Nevada	25	1.08	318,848	14.17	3,113	12.33	130,699	14.27	41,985
New Hampshire	28	1.52	21,947	1.85	200	1.04	10,213	1.88	51,065
New Jersey	163	0.99	809,528	7.78	6,254	4.90	374,035	8.46	59,807
New Mexico	58	2.42	115,057	7.78	1,678	7.10	62,669	10.13	37,347
New York	196	0.60	691,027	3.48	5,844	2.10	273,030	3.31	46,720
North Carolina	73	0.82	102,940	1.55	1,095	1.02	41,566	1.39	37,960
North Dakota	7	0.90	-	-	-	-	-	-	-
Ohio	127	0.68	564,924	4.85	5,638	2.82	231,323	4.15	41,029
Oklahoma	19	0.36	4,179	0.13	77	0.13	1,623	0.11	21,078
Oregon	59	1.05	32,114	1.09	400	0.83	14,376	1.11	35,940
Pennsylvania	138	0.63	701,136	5.55	5,909	3.20	283,845	5.01	48,036
Rhode Island	15	0.79	13,370	1.26	174	0.96	7,804	1.67	44,851
South Carolina	18	0.39	4,793	0.15	45	0.09	1,829	0.13	40,644
South Dakota	1	0.10	-	-	-	-	-	-	-
Tennessee	50	0.61	-	-	-	-	-	-	-
Texas	211	0.70	481,209	2.10	5,215	1.51	227,235	2.46	43,573
Utah	40	1.31	43,021	2.33	593	1.92	20,128	2.67	33,943
Vermont	9	0.97	4,462	1.10	39	0.52	1,647	1.00	42,231
Virginia	173	1.77	399,928	5.99	4,145	4.06	172,399	5.69	41,592
Washington	93	1.01	611,777	11.33	5,458	6.24	228,867	9.61	41,932
West Virginia	13	0.48	10,479	0.59	99	0.34	3,401	0.48	34,354
Wisconsin	33	0.46	79,706	1.68	759	0.89	28,172	1.20	37,117
Wyoming	5	0.70	633	0.20	4	0.07	206	0.15	51,500

Source: U.S. Department of Commerce. Bureau of the Census. *1992 Economic Census Report Series,* CD-ROM 1i, Washington, DC, October 1996. *Notes:* - means no data reported. 1. HS stands for total health service establishments, revenues, employment, or payroll.

★ 321 ★

Establishment Data

Commercial Physical and Biological Research Establishments by State, Non-Taxed: 1992

Area	Establish-ments	Revenues in $1,000	Employ-ment	Payroll in $1,000	Payroll per employee
United States	344	4,978,474	47,973	2,091,951	43,607
Alabama	4	-	-	-	-
Alaska	0	0	0	0	0
Arizona	6	-	-	-	-
Arkansas	0	0	0	0	0
California	55	331,917	3,530	161,062	45,627

[Continued]

★ 321 ★

Commercial Physical and Biological Research Establishments by State, Non-Taxed: 1992
[Continued]

Area	Establish-ments	Revenues in $1,000	Employ-ment	Payroll in $1,000	Payroll per employee
Colorado	5	-	-	-	-
Connecticut	3	-	-	-	-
Delaware	0	0	0	0	0
District of Columbia	14	35,544	342	13,384	39,135
Florida	7	12,568	157	6,867	43,739
Georgia	3	-	-	-	-
Hawaii	2	-	-	-	-
Idaho	5	-	-	-	-
Illinois	9	670,039	8,549	322,669	37,743
Indiana	2	-	-	-	-
Iowa	1	-	-	-	-
Kansas	2	-	-	-	-
Kentucky	1	-	-	-	-
Louisiana	4	-	-	-	-
Maine	0	0	0	0	0
Maryland	25	590,779	4,666	217,760	46,670
Massachusetts	24	872,070	8,661	436,116	50,354
Michigan	13	-	-	-	-
Minnesota	4	1,270	15	526	35,067
Mississippi	4	9,937	188	5,269	28,027
Missouri	6	-	-	-	-
Montana	0	0	0	0	0
Nebraska	1	-	-	-	-
Nevada	0	0	0	0	0
New Hampshire	2	-	-	-	-
New Jersey	6	-	-	-	-
New Mexico	5	14,865	312	11,545	37,003
New York	28	332,561	4,066	184,027	45,260
North Carolina	7	-	-	-	-
North Dakota	0	0	0	0	0
Ohio	6	-	-	-	-
Oklahoma	1	-	-	-	-
Oregon	4	-	-	-	-
Pennsylvania	26	72,829	782	25,298	32,350
Rhode Island	4	1,942	35	915	26,143
South Carolina	1	-	-	-	-
South Dakota	0	0	0	0	0
Tennessee	8	-	-	-	-
Texas	15	-	-	-	-
Utah	4	3,895	93	1,835	19,731
Vermont	0	0	0	0	0
Virginia	16	551,106	4,794	248,866	51,912
Washington	7	13,110	150	4,732	31,547
West Virginia	1	-	-	-	-

[Continued]

★ 321 ★

Commercial Physical and Biological Research Establishments by State, Non-Taxed: 1992

[Continued]

Area	Establish-ments	Revenues in $1,000	Employ-ment	Payroll in $1,000	Payroll per employee
Wisconsin	2	-	-	-	-
Wyoming	1	-	-	-	-

Source: U.S. Department of Commerce. Bureau of the Census. *1992 Economic Census Report Series,* CD-ROM 1i, Washington, DC, October 1996. *Notes:* - means no data reported. 1. HS stands for total health service establishments, revenues, employment, or payroll.

★ 322 ★

Establishment Data

Commercial Physical Research Establishments by Major Metro Area: 1992

Area	Establishments		Revenues		Employment		Payroll		
	Number	% of HS[1] in area	Total ($000)	% of HS[1] in area	Number	% of HS[1] in area	Total ($000)	% of HS[1] in area	Payroll per employee
United States	2,368	0.54	8,912,946	2.98	82,860	1.86	3,785,445	2.93	45,685
Atlanta, GA MSA	23	0.38	-	-	-	-	-	-	-
Boston – Worcester – Lawrence, MA – NH – ME – CT CMSA	145	1.48	321,304	4.54	2,909	2.53	155,886	4.79	53,587
Chicago – Gary – Kenosha, IL – IN – WI CMSA	42	0.29	184,187	1.89	1,965	1.44	91,078	2.07	46,350
Cincinnati – Hamilton, OH – KY – IN CMSA	10	0.32	9,694	0.48	36	0.10	2,274	0.22	63,167
Cleveland – Akron, OH CMSA	21	0.39	-	-	-	-	-	-	-
Dallas – Fort Worth, TX CMSA	27	0.32	-	-	-	-	-	-	-
Denver – Boulder – Greeley, CO CMSA	58	1.33	-	-	-	-	-	-	-
Detroit – Ann Arbor – Flint, MI CMSA	52	0.55	-	-	-	-	-	-	-
Houston – Galveston – Brazoria, TX CMSA	37	0.52	-	-	-	-	-	-	-
Indianapolis, IN MSA	10	0.39	12,688	0.63	223	0.69	5,194	0.55	23,291
Kansas City, MO – KS MSA	10	0.35	4,542	0.21	89	0.26	1,833	0.19	20,596
Los Angeles – Riverside – Orange County, CA CMSA	167	0.55	613,617	2.61	5,843	2.10	313,907	3.43	53,724
Miami – Fort Lauderdale, FL CMSA	12	0.13	7,534	0.11	104	0.12	3,426	0.12	32,942
Milwaukee – Racine, WI CMSA	7	0.23	-	-	-	-	-	-	-
Minneapolis – St. Paul, MN – WI MSA	25	0.67	20,312	0.70	172	0.34	8,269	0.55	48,076
New York – Northern New Jersey – Long Island, NY – NJ – CT- CMSA	186	0.46	746,369	2.86	5,513	1.65	344,077	3.15	62,412
Orlando, FL MSA	14	0.55	-	-	-	-	-	-	-
Philadelphia – Wilmington – Atlantic City, PA – NJ – DE – MD CMSA	48	0.41	-	-	-	-	-	-	-
Phoenix – Mesa, AZ MSA	11	0.23	-	-	-	-	-	-	-
Pittsburgh, PA MSA	24	0.50	-	-	-	-	-	-	-
Portland – Salem, OR – WA CMSA	18	0.51	-	-	-	-	-	-	-
Sacramento – Yolo, CA CMSA	12	0.42	-	-	-	-	-	-	-
St. Louis, MO – IL MSA	17	0.38	-	-	-	-	-	-	-
San Diego, CA MSA	83	1.68	475,693	14.57	4,585	11.01	198,322	14.73	43,255
San Francisco – Oakland – San Jose, CA CMSA	196	1.40	460,719	5.11	3,618	3.18	202,529	5.36	55,978
Seattle – Tacoma – Bremerton, WA CMSA	34	0.56	-	-	-	-	-	-	-

[Continued]

★ 322 ★

Commercial Physical Research Establishments by Major Metro Area: 1992

[Continued]

Area	Establishments		Revenues		Employment		Payroll		
	Number	% of HS[1] in area	Total ($000)	% of HS[1] in area	Number	% of HS[1] in area	Total ($000)	% of HS[1] in area	Payroll per employee
Tampa – St. Petersburg – Clearwater, FL MSA	15	0.30	13,662	0.31	148	0.24	5,458	0.32	36,878
Washington – Baltimore, DC – MD – VA – WV CMSA	201	1.55	671,783	8.31	6,407	5.82	279,141	7.78	43,568
West Palm Beach – Boca Raton, FL MSA	13	0.48	-	-	-	-	-	-	-

Source: U.S. Department of Commerce. Bureau of the Census. *1992 Economic Census Report Series,* CD-ROM 1i, Washington, DC, October 1996. *Notes: -* means no data reported. 1. HS stands for total health service establishments, revenues, employment, or payroll.

★ 323 ★

Establishment Data

Commercial Physical Research Establishments by State: 1992

Area	Establishments		Revenues		Employment		Payroll		
	Number	% of HS[1] in area	Total ($000)	% of HS[1] in area	Number	% of HS[1] in area	Total ($000)	% of HS[1] in area	Payroll per employee
United States	2,368	0.54	8,912,946	2.98	82,860	1.86	3,785,445	2.93	45,685
Alabama	39	0.71	132,145	2.68	1,490	1.93	63,614	3.01	42,694
Alaska	6	0.70	3,273	0.60	44	0.78	1,521	0.70	34,568
Arizona	30	0.42	113,770	2.49	524	0.89	21,841	1.12	41,681
Arkansas	4	0.11	2,737	0.11	85	0.20	2,078	0.20	24,447
California	512	0.83	1,677,856	3.90	15,195	2.84	770,052	4.47	50,678
Colorado	78	1.11	117,578	3.15	1,282	2.32	54,905	3.35	42,828
Connecticut	42	0.64	76,776	1.56	602	0.83	30,777	1.31	51,125
Delaware	2	0.17	-	-	-	-	-	-	-
District of Columbia	16	1.16	-	-	-	-	-	-	-
Florida	103	0.35	91,385	0.39	1,080	0.34	40,696	0.42	37,681
Georgia	33	0.30	26,594	0.31	306	0.25	12,465	0.34	40,735
Hawaii	11	0.49	-	-	-	-	-	-	-
Idaho	12	0.69	-	-	-	-	-	-	-
Illinois	53	0.28	198,536	1.60	2,072	1.10	94,250	1.68	45,487
Indiana	18	0.21	19,995	0.33	318	0.30	7,593	0.28	23,877
Iowa	4	0.10	-	-	-	-	-	-	-
Kansas	13	0.34	5,154	0.17	109	0.20	2,201	0.17	20,193
Kentucky	13	0.24	6,139	0.15	72	0.11	2,289	0.13	31,792
Louisiana	9	0.13	3,027	0.05	33	0.04	1,004	0.05	30,424
Maine	7	0.32	2,406	0.20	47	0.21	964	0.18	20,511
Maryland	85	0.93	326,065	5.78	3,047	3.81	135,675	5.44	44,527
Massachusetts	142	1.34	317,136	4.16	2,890	2.27	153,082	4.32	52,970
Michigan	65	0.41	244,785	2.81	2,168	1.54	98,860	2.40	45,600
Minnesota	34	0.58	23,125	0.56	221	0.29	9,217	0.44	41,706
Mississippi	16	0.52	9,292	0.45	113	0.31	3,959	0.45	35,035
Missouri	20	0.24	53,444	0.97	363	0.38	18,597	0.76	51,231

[Continued]

★ 323 ★

Commercial Physical Research Establishments by State: 1992
[Continued]

Area	Establishments		Revenues		Employment		Payroll		
	Number	% of HS[1] in area	Total ($000)	% of HS[1] in area	Number	% of HS[1] in area	Total ($000)	% of HS[1] in area	Payroll per employee
Montana	4	0.27	-	-	-	-	-	-	-
Nebraska	7	0.30	-	-	-	-	-	-	-
Nevada	19	0.82	316,802	14.08	3,100	12.27	130,297	14.22	42,031
New Hampshire	21	1.14	17,116	1.44	156	0.81	8,289	1.53	53,135
New Jersey	98	0.59	646,178	6.21	4,810	3.77	306,010	6.93	63,620
New Mexico	50	2.08	108,130	7.32	1,557	6.58	59,702	9.65	38,344
New York	112	0.35	548,355	2.76	4,180	1.50	200,624	2.43	47,996
North Carolina	36	0.41	24,715	0.37	226	0.21	9,909	0.33	43,845
North Dakota	5	0.65	-	-	-	-	-	-	-
Ohio	86	0.46	515,283	4.43	4,974	2.49	208,761	3.75	41,970
Oklahoma	12	0.22	2,686	0.08	40	0.07	874	0.06	21,850
Oregon	36	0.64	24,404	0.82	292	0.61	11,353	0.88	38,880
Pennsylvania	86	0.40	431,506	3.42	3,873	2.10	174,189	3.08	44,975
Rhode Island	9	0.47	6,444	0.61	106	0.58	3,150	0.67	29,717
South Carolina	12	0.26	3,183	0.10	30	0.06	1,271	0.09	42,367
South Dakota	1	0.10	-	-	-	-	-	-	-
Tennessee	29	0.35	-	-	-	-	-	-	-
Texas	131	0.44	341,285	1.49	3,645	1.05	173,216	1.88	47,522
Utah	15	0.49	19,105	1.03	264	0.85	6,988	0.93	26,470
Vermont	6	0.65	3,291	0.81	25	0.33	1,128	0.68	45,120
Virginia	143	1.47	357,530	5.35	3,801	3.72	157,454	5.20	41,424
Washington	51	0.55	-	-	-	-	-	-	-
West Virginia	11	0.41	-	-	-	-	-	-	-
Wisconsin	18	0.25	-	-	-	-	-	-	-
Wyoming	3	0.42	-	-	-	-	-	-	-

Source: U.S. Department of Commerce. Bureau of the Census. *1992 Economic Census Report Series,* CD-ROM 1i, Washington, DC, October 1996. *Notes:* - means no data reported. 1. HS stands for total health service establishments, revenues, employment, or payroll.

★ 324 ★

Establishment Data

Dental Clinics by Major Metro Area: 1992

Area	Establishments		Revenues		Employment		Payroll		
	Number	% of HS[1] in area	Total ($000)	% of HS[1] in area	Number	% of HS[1] in area	Total ($000)	% of HS[1] in area	Payroll per employee
United States	604	0.14	351,169	0.12	5,232	0.12	138,169	0.11	26,408
Atlanta, GA MSA	7	0.11	16,164	0.34	271	0.45	9,724	0.48	35,882
Boston – Worcester – Lawrence, MA – NH – ME – CT CMSA	10	0.10	-	-	-	-	-	-	-
Chicago – Gary – Kenosha, IL – IN – WI CMSA	23	0.16	-	-	-	-	-	-	-

[Continued]

★ 324 ★

Dental Clinics by Major Metro Area: 1992
[Continued]

Area	Establishments		Revenues		Employment		Payroll		
	Number	% of HS[1] in area	Total ($000)	% of HS[1] in area	Number	% of HS[1] in area	Total ($000)	% of HS[1] in area	Payroll per employee
Cincinnati – Hamilton, OH – KY – IN CMSA	1	0.03	-	-	-	-	-	-	-
Cleveland – Akron, OH CMSA	2	0.04	-	-	-	-	-	-	-
Dallas – Fort Worth, TX CMSA	9	0.11	2,614	0.04	29	0.03	816	0.03	28,138
Denver – Boulder – Greeley, CO CMSA	7	0.16	-	-	-	-	-	-	-
Detroit – Ann Arbor – Flint, MI CMSA	21	0.22	-	-	-	-	-	-	-
Houston – Galveston – Brazoria, TX CMSA	9	0.13	-	-	-	-	-	-	-
Indianapolis, IN MSA	2	0.08	-	-	-	-	-	-	-
Kansas City, MO – KS MSA	2	0.07	-	-	-	-	-	-	-
Los Angeles – Riverside – Orange County, CA CMSA	56	0.18	51,126	0.22	740	0.27	14,811	0.16	20,015
Miami – Fort Lauderdale, FL CMSA	7	0.08	-	-	-	-	-	-	-
Milwaukee – Racine, WI CMSA	12	0.40	-	-	-	-	-	-	-
Minneapolis – St. Paul, MN – WI MSA	10	0.27	-	-	-	-	-	-	-
New York – Northern New Jersey – Long Island, NY – NJ – CT- CMSA	35	0.09	18,805	0.07	286	0.09	6,585	0.06	23,024
Orlando, FL MSA	5	0.20	1,265	0.07	19	0.08	425	0.05	22,368
Philadelphia – Wilmington – Atlantic City, PA – NJ – DE – MD CMSA	12	0.10	-	-	-	-	-	-	-
Phoenix – Mesa, AZ MSA	8	0.17	2,757	0.09	44	0.11	1,106	0.08	25,136
Pittsburgh, PA MSA	5	0.10	-	-	-	-	-	-	-
Portland – Salem, OR – WA CMSA	30	0.85	-	-	-	-	-	-	-
Sacramento – Yolo, CA CMSA	8	0.28	3,830	0.20	60	0.24	1,565	0.19	26,083
St. Louis, MO – IL MSA	1	0.02	-	-	-	-	-	-	-
San Diego, CA MSA	5	0.10	2,735	0.08	46	0.11	1,300	0.10	28,261
San Francisco – Oakland – San Jose, CA CMSA	24	0.17	16,755	0.19	158	0.14	4,450	0.12	28,165
Seattle – Tacoma – Bremerton, WA CMSA	25	0.41	12,026	0.34	168	0.31	5,384	0.35	32,048
Tampa – St. Petersburg – Clearwater, FL MSA	5	0.10	2,144	0.05	43	0.07	853	0.05	19,837
Washington – Baltimore, DC – MD – VA – WV CMSA	14	0.11	-	-	-	-	-	-	-
West Palm Beach – Boca Raton, FL MSA	4	0.15	1,285	0.07	25	0.10	450	0.05	18,000

Source: U.S. Department of Commerce. Bureau of the Census. *1992 Economic Census Report Series,* CD-ROM 1i, Washington, DC, October 1996. *Notes:* - means no data reported. 1. HS stands for total health service establishments, revenues, employment, or payroll.

★ 325 ★

Establishment Data

Dental Clinics by Major Metro Area, Non-Taxed: 1992

Area	Establish-ments	Revenues in $1,000	Employ-ment	Payroll in $1,000	Payroll per employee
United States	115	73,640	1,422	31,107	21,876
Albany–Schenectady–Troy, NY MSA	0	0	0	0	0
Atlanta, GA MSA	0	0	0	0	0
Boston–Worcester–Lawrence, MA–NH–ME–CT CMSA	0	0	0	0	0
Buffalo–Niagara Falls, NY MSA	0	0	0	0	0
Chicago–Gary–Kenosha, IL–IN–WI CMSA	0	0	0	0	0
Cincinnati–Hamilton, OH–KY–IN CMSA	1	-	-	-	-
Cleveland–Akron, OH CMSA	1	-	-	-	-
Columbus, OH MSA	0	0	0	0	0
Dallas–Fort Worth, TX CMSA	5	-	-	-	-
Denver–Boulder–Greeley, CO CMSA	3	-	-	-	-
Detroit–Ann Arbor–Flint, MI CMSA	1	-	-	-	-
Hartford, CT MSA	0	0	0	0	0
Houston–Galveston–Brazoria, TX CMSA	0	0	0	0	0
Indianapolis, IN MSA	1	-	-	-	-
Kansas City, MO–KS MSA	1	-	-	-	-
Los Angeles–Riverside–Orange County, CA CMSA	11	-	-	-	-
Miami–Fort Lauderdale, FL CMSA	0	0	0	0	0
Milwaukee–Racine, WI CMSA	0	0	0	0	0
Minneapolis–St. Paul, MN–WI MSA	4	-	-	-	-
New York–Northern New Jersey–Long Island, NY–NJ–CT- CMSA	5	1,803	44	1,303	29,614
Philadelphia–Wilmington–Atlantic City, PA–NJ–DE–MD CMSA	3	-	-	-	-
Phoenix–Mesa, AZ MSA	0	0	0	0	0
Pittsburgh, PA MSA	0	0	0	0	0
Portland–Salem, OR–WA CMSA	10	-	-	-	-
Providence–Fall River–Warwick, RI–MA MSA	0	0	0	0	0
Sacramento–Yolo, CA CMSA	0	0	0	0	0
St. Louis, MO–IL MSA	0	0	0	0	0
San Diego, CA MSA	0	0	0	0	0
San Francisco–Oakland–San Jose, CA CMSA	3	-	-	-	-
Seattle–Tacoma–Bremerton, WA CMSA	5	-	-	-	-
Tampa–St. Petersburg–Clearwater, FL MSA	1	-	-	-	-

[Continued]

★ 325 ★

Dental Clinics by Major Metro Area, Non-Taxed: 1992

[Continued]

Area	Establish-ments	Revenues in $1,000	Employ-ment	Payroll in $1,000	Payroll per employee
Washington – Baltimore, DC – MD – VA – WV CMSA	1	-	-	-	-

Source: U.S. Department of Commerce. Bureau of the Census. *1992 Economic Census Report Series,* CD-ROM 1i, Washington, DC, October 1996. *Notes:* - means no data reported. 1. HS stands for total health service establishments, revenues, employment, or payroll.

★ 326 ★

Establishment Data

Dental Clinics by State: 1992

Area	Establishments		Revenues		Employment		Payroll		
	Number	% of HS[1] in area	Total ($000)	% of HS[1] in area	Number	% of HS[1] in area	Total ($000)	% of HS[1] in area	Payroll per employee
United States	604	0.14	351,169	0.12	5,232	0.12	138,169	0.11	26,408
Alabama	6	0.11	1,453	0.03	25	0.03	579	0.03	23,160
Alaska	4	0.47	-	-	-	-	-	-	-
Arizona	16	0.23	6,788	0.15	119	0.20	3,262	0.17	27,412
Arkansas	5	0.14	1,463	0.06	26	0.06	571	0.05	21,962
California	104	0.17	84,026	0.20	1,142	0.21	24,223	0.14	21,211
Colorado	8	0.11	-	-	-	-	-	-	-
Connecticut	5	0.08	2,961	0.06	43	0.06	1,525	0.07	35,465
Delaware	0	0.00	0	0.00	0	0.00	0	0.00	0
District of Columbia	2	0.15	-	-	-	-	-	-	-
Florida	34	0.11	10,986	0.05	218	0.07	3,925	0.04	18,005
Georgia	11	0.10	19,032	0.22	310	0.26	10,962	0.30	35,361
Hawaii	14	0.63	9,414	0.72	108	0.69	3,307	0.56	30,620
Idaho	1	0.06	-	-	-	-	-	-	-
Illinois	26	0.14	9,689	0.08	144	0.08	4,079	0.07	28,326
Indiana	10	0.11	4,520	0.07	61	0.06	1,997	0.07	32,738
Iowa	3	0.07	785	0.03	13	0.03	257	0.02	19,769
Kansas	6	0.16	1,474	0.05	24	0.04	534	0.04	22,250
Kentucky	4	0.07	141	0.00	11	0.02	63	0.00	5,727
Louisiana	7	0.10	6,257	0.11	62	0.07	1,071	0.05	17,274
Maine	1	0.05	-	-	-	-	-	-	-
Maryland	11	0.12	4,760	0.08	71	0.09	1,975	0.08	27,817
Massachusetts	11	0.10	3,483	0.05	69	0.05	1,575	0.04	22,826
Michigan	30	0.19	14,265	0.16	242	0.17	6,988	0.17	28,876
Minnesota	12	0.20	-	-	-	-	-	-	-
Mississippi	6	0.19	1,375	0.07	25	0.07	456	0.05	18,240
Missouri	2	0.02	-	-	-	-	-	-	-
Montana	2	0.13	-	-	-	-	-	-	-
Nebraska	2	0.08	-	-	-	-	-	-	-

[Continued]

★ 326 ★

Dental Clinics by State: 1992

[Continued]

Area	Establishments		Revenues		Employment		Payroll		
	Number	% of HS[1] in area	Total ($000)	% of HS[1] in area	Number	% of HS[1] in area	Total ($000)	% of HS[1] in area	Payroll per employee
Nevada	1	0.04	-	-	-	-	-	-	-
New Hampshire	0	0.00	0	0.00	0	0.00	0	0.00	0
New Jersey	10	0.06	4,805	0.05	70	0.05	2,218	0.05	31,686
New Mexico	4	0.17	1,344	0.09	28	0.12	566	0.09	20,214
New York	38	0.12	21,194	0.11	328	0.12	6,995	0.08	21,326
North Carolina	12	0.14	13,738	0.21	231	0.22	6,362	0.21	27,541
North Dakota	2	0.26	-	-	-	-	-	-	-
Ohio	8	0.04	3,603	0.03	38	0.02	1,021	0.02	26,868
Oklahoma	9	0.17	2,297	0.07	35	0.06	1,168	0.08	33,371
Oregon	39	0.69	19,213	0.65	292	0.61	10,610	0.82	36,336
Pennsylvania	21	0.10	5,765	0.05	103	0.06	2,380	0.04	23,107
Rhode Island	3	0.16	-	-	-	-	-	-	-
South Carolina	3	0.06	-	-	-	-	-	-	-
South Dakota	3	0.31	830	0.15	14	0.15	155	0.06	11,071
Tennessee	0	0.00	0	0.00	0	0.00	0	0.00	0
Texas	32	0.11	15,825	0.07	203	0.06	4,902	0.05	24,148
Utah	5	0.16	1,387	0.08	21	0.07	568	0.08	27,048
Vermont	1	0.11	-	-	-	-	-	-	-
Virginia	7	0.07	1,819	0.03	34	0.03	963	0.03	28,324
Washington	38	0.41	18,017	0.33	263	0.30	8,402	0.35	31,947
West Virginia	2	0.07	-	-	-	-	-	-	-
Wisconsin	23	0.32	25,281	0.53	346	0.41	10,552	0.45	30,497
Wyoming	0	0.00	0	0.00	0	0.00	0	0.00	0

Source: U.S. Department of Commerce. Bureau of the Census. *1992 Economic Census Report Series,* CD-ROM 1i, Washington, DC, October 1996.
Notes: - means no data reported. 1. HS stands for total health service establishments, revenues, employment, or payroll.

★ 327 ★

Establishment Data

Dental Clinics by State, Non-Taxed: 1992

Area	Establish-ments	Revenues in $1,000	Employ-ment	Payroll in $1,000	Payroll per employee
United States	115	73,640	1,422	31,107	21,876
Alabama	1	-	-	-	-
Alaska	0	0	0	0	0
Arizona	1	-	-	-	-
Arkansas	1	-	-	-	-
California	20	9,955	231	5,068	21,939
Colorado	4	2,760	62	1,556	25,097
Connecticut	0	0	0	0	0

[Continued]

★ 327 ★

Dental Clinics by State, Non-Taxed: 1992
[Continued]

Area	Establish-ments	Revenues in $1,000	Employ-ment	Payroll in $1,000	Payroll per employee
Delaware	0	0	0	0	0
District of Columbia	1	-	-	-	-
Florida	3	-	-	-	-
Georgia	1	-	-	-	-
Hawaii	1	-	-	-	-
Idaho	0	0	0	0	0
Illinois	0	0	0	0	0
Indiana	2	-	-	-	-
Iowa	1	-	-	-	-
Kansas	1	-	-	-	-
Kentucky	2	-	-	-	-
Louisiana	0	0	0	0	0
Maine	1	-	-	-	-
Maryland	0	0	0	0	0
Massachusetts	0	0	0	0	0
Michigan	4	2,030	20	417	20,850
Minnesota	4	-	-	-	-
Mississippi	0	0	0	0	0
Missouri	0	0	0	0	0
Montana	0	0	0	0	0
Nebraska	0	0	0	0	0
Nevada	0	0	0	0	0
New Hampshire	0	0	0	0	0
New Jersey	3	-	-	-	-
New Mexico	6	1,536	31	596	19,226
New York	5	1,780	47	1,328	28,255
North Carolina	3	-	-	-	-
North Dakota	0	0	0	0	0
Ohio	7	-	-	-	-
Oklahoma	1	-	-	-	-
Oregon	9	-	-	-	-
Pennsylvania	3	-	-	-	-
Rhode Island	0	0	0	0	0
South Carolina	3	-	-	-	-
South Dakota	0	0	0	0	0
Tennessee	0	0	0	0	0
Texas	6	-	-	-	-
Utah	2	-	-	-	-
Vermont	4	-	-	-	-
Virginia	2	-	-	-	-
Washington	7	-	-	-	-
West Virginia	4	-	-	-	-

[Continued]

★ 327 ★

Dental Clinics by State, Non-Taxed: 1992

[Continued]

Area	Establish-ments	Revenues in $1,000	Employ-ment	Payroll in $1,000	Payroll per employee
Wisconsin	2	-	-	-	-
Wyoming	0	0	0	0	0

Source: U.S. Department of Commerce. Bureau of the Census. *1992 Economic Census Report Series,* CD-ROM 1i, Washington, DC, October 1996. *Notes:* - means no data reported. 1. HS stands for total health service establishments, revenues, employment, or payroll.

★ 328 ★

Establishment Data

Dental Laboratories by Major Metro Area: 1992

Area	Establishments		Revenues		Employment		Payroll		
	Number	% of HS[1] in area	Total ($000)	% of HS[1] in area	Number	% of HS[1] in area	Total ($000)	% of HS[1] in area	Payroll per employee
United States	7,527	1.70	1,948,464	0.65	39,106	0.88	824,312	0.64	21,079
Albany – Schenectady – Troy, NY MSA	15	1.15	4,702	0.58	146	1.11	2,374	0.65	16,260
Albuquerque, NM MSA	35	3.28	6,462	0.77	137	1.08	2,352	0.62	17,168
Allentown – Bethlehem – Easton, PA MSA	14	1.13	2,430	0.35	46	0.49	831	0.27	18,065
Anchorage, AK MSA	9	1.85	3,100	0.85	54	1.49	1,249	0.87	23,130
Appleton – Oshkosh – Neenah, WI MSA	8	1.54	3,879	1.07	88	1.53	2,252	1.24	25,591
Atlanta, GA MSA	132	2.17	37,834	0.79	850	1.42	17,814	0.88	20,958
Augusta – Aiken, GA – SC MSA	9	1.27	1,107	0.17	33	0.36	407	0.14	12,333
Austin – San Marcos, TX MSA	27	1.72	4,646	0.39	103	0.55	1,742	0.36	16,913
Bakersfield, CA MSA	11	1.45	1,961	0.36	32	0.39	448	0.20	14,000
Baton Rouge, LA MSA	15	1.69	3,661	0.49	77	0.70	1,592	0.52	20,675
Beaumont – Port Arthur, TX MSA	12	1.66	1,647	0.29	38	0.37	715	0.30	18,816
Birmingham, AL MSA	32	2.32	8,417	0.56	191	0.95	3,838	0.60	20,094
Boise City, ID MSA	22	3.67	-	-	-	-	-	-	-
Boston – Worcester – Lawrence, MA – NH – ME – CT CMSA	137	1.40	35,657	0.50	694	0.60	15,527	0.48	22,373
Buffalo – Niagara Falls, NY MSA	32	1.61	14,747	1.33	274	1.27	5,363	1.07	19,573
Canton – Massillon, OH MSA	8	1.15	1,813	0.44	36	0.50	653	0.31	18,139
Charleston – North Charleston, SC MSA	13	1.59	2,174	0.37	41	0.45	910	0.39	22,195
Charlotte – Gastonia – Rock Hill, NC – SC MSA	32	2.00	12,221	0.87	260	1.28	6,518	0.99	25,069
Chattanooga, TN – GA MSA	14	1.84	3,249	0.45	75	0.75	1,451	0.47	19,347
Chicago – Gary – Kenosha, IL – IN – WI CMSA	258	1.77	-	-	-	-	-	-	-
Cincinnati – Hamilton, OH – KY – IN CMSA	46	1.47	-	-	-	-	-	-	-
Cleveland – Akron, OH CMSA	78	1.45	20,223	0.62	517	1.01	9,812	0.64	18,979
Colorado Springs, CO MSA	12	1.35	3,334	0.75	75	1.14	2,060	1.02	27,467
Columbia, SC MSA	6	0.81	636	0.13	16	0.22	200	0.08	12,500
Columbus, OH MSA	39	1.60	9,912	0.56	242	0.86	4,704	0.58	19,438
Corpus Christi, TX MSA	8	1.07	1,424	0.25	37	0.44	547	0.24	14,784
Dallas – Fort Worth, TX CMSA	128	1.54	28,936	0.44	583	0.68	11,460	0.43	19,657
Davenport – Moline – Rock Island, IA – IL MSA	16	2.36	4,608	1.28	126	2.10	2,309	1.46	18,325
Dayton – Springfield, OH MSA	34	2.06	8,237	0.72	185	1.04	3,670	0.65	19,838

[Continued]

★ 328 ★

Dental Laboratories by Major Metro Area: 1992

[Continued]

Area	Establishments		Revenues		Employment		Payroll		
	Number	% of HS[1] in area	Total ($000)	% of HS[1] in area	Number	% of HS[1] in area	Total ($000)	% of HS[1] in area	Payroll per employee
Daytona Beach, FL MSA	14	1.89	2,037	0.38	34	0.41	495	0.22	14,559
Denver – Boulder – Greeley, CO CMSA	93	2.13	21,358	0.84	429	1.20	8,794	0.79	20,499
Des Moines, IA MSA	18	2.44	4,752	0.93	109	1.53	2,276	0.86	20,881
Detroit – Ann Arbor – Flint, MI CMSA	181	1.92	51,739	0.95	1,038	1.23	23,132	0.91	22,285
El Paso, TX MSA	10	1.26	1,681	0.22	63	0.59	760	0.26	12,063
Eugene – Springfield, OR MSA	18	3.08	-	-	-	-	-	-	-
Fort Myers – Cape Coral, FL MSA	14	1.96	2,766	0.42	66	0.80	1,271	0.41	19,258
Fort Pierce – Port St. Lucie, FL MSA	9	1.73	1,606	0.36	33	0.53	600	0.32	18,182
Fort Wayne, IN MSA	14	2.00	4,201	0.76	103	1.09	2,146	0.84	20,835
Fresno, CA MSA	28	1.89	6,236	0.72	126	1.02	2,101	0.57	16,675
Grand Rapids – Muskegon – Holland, MI MSA	29	1.90	9,145	1.02	189	1.32	4,091	0.95	21,646
Greensboro – Winston-Salem – High Point, NC MSA	42	2.78	8,128	0.68	157	0.92	3,444	0.65	21,936
Greenville – Spartanburg – Anderson, SC MSA	27	2.30	3,685	0.47	89	0.74	1,560	0.41	17,528
Harrisburg – Lebanon – Carlisle, PA MSA	19	1.93	8,977	1.38	266	2.79	4,610	1.49	17,331
Hartford, CT MSA	33	1.45	8,941	0.51	178	0.65	4,063	0.48	22,826
Honolulu, HI MSA	30	1.78	8,702	0.84	171	1.42	4,129	0.87	24,146
Houston – Galveston – Brazoria, TX CMSA	86	1.22	25,718	0.44	476	0.64	10,506	0.45	22,071
Huntsville, AL MSA	19	3.56	9,196	2.01	190	2.90	4,103	2.15	21,595
Indianapolis, IN MSA	39	1.53	16,020	0.80	390	1.21	8,004	0.85	20,523
Jackson, MS MSA	17	2.67	4,725	0.93	101	1.40	1,990	0.95	19,703
Jacksonville, FL MSA	31	1.75	7,513	0.57	175	1.02	3,289	0.59	18,794
Johnson City – Kingsport – Bristol, TN – VA MSA	15	2.17	4,342	0.71	99	1.01	1,822	0.67	18,404
Kalamazoo – Battle Creek, MI MSA	13	1.76	2,931	0.67	62	0.87	1,259	0.59	20,306
Kansas City, MO – KS MSA	47	1.65	29,825	1.36	576	1.71	12,640	1.28	21,944
Knoxville, TN MSA	24	2.01	4,082	0.50	84	0.79	1,420	0.36	16,905
Lafayette, LA MSA	5	0.78	669	0.15	19	0.27	252	0.14	13,263
Lakeland – Winter Haven, FL MSA	13	2.67	3,048	0.76	72	1.13	1,495	0.89	20,764
Lancaster, PA MSA	9	1.49	1,853	0.49	51	0.81	830	0.43	16,275
Lansing – East Lansing, MI MSA	12	1.64	5,975	1.49	125	1.99	3,126	1.64	25,008
Las Vegas, NV – AZ MSA	25	1.61	6,386	0.38	110	0.60	2,802	0.41	25,473
Lexington, KY MSA	17	2.10	2,064	0.35	28	0.31	736	0.27	26,286
Little Rock – North Little Rock, AR MSA	10	0.96	1,525	0.20	42	0.38	536	0.15	12,762
Los Angeles – Riverside – Orange County, CA CMSA	484	1.58	124,697	0.53	2,196	0.79	47,139	0.52	21,466
Louisville, KY – IN MSA	28	1.63	7,528	0.45	177	0.69	3,239	0.45	18,299
Macon, GA MSA	9	1.65	3,184	0.56	57	0.76	1,562	0.69	27,404
Madison, WI MSA	14	2.70	6,817	1.32	159	2.21	3,936	1.68	24,755
Melbourne – Titusville – Palm Bay, FL MSA	16	1.97	2,940	0.54	61	0.84	1,231	0.49	20,180
Memphis, TN – AR – MS MSA	30	1.82	11,667	0.94	167	1.02	3,553	0.66	21,275
Miami – Fort Lauderdale, FL CMSA	152	1.66	24,525	0.36	512	0.59	9,923	0.35	19,381
Milwaukee – Racine, WI CMSA	50	1.65	16,633	0.81	399	1.17	7,836	0.75	19,639
Minneapolis – St. Paul, MN – WI MSA	102	2.74	45,114	1.56	955	1.91	21,688	1.45	22,710
Mobile, AL MSA	20	3.12	2,503	0.45	66	0.69	1,024	0.39	15,515
Modesto, CA MSA	17	2.52	-	-	-	-	-	-	-
Montgomery, AL MSA	11	2.24	2,283	0.46	43	0.58	899	0.43	20,907
Nashville, TN MSA	42	2.16	8,072	0.44	173	0.68	3,822	0.49	22,092
New Orleans, LA MSA	32	1.32	8,935	0.41	225	0.76	4,082	0.49	18,142
New York – Northern New Jersey – Long Island, NY – NJ – CT- CMSA	662	1.63	-	-	-	-	-	-	-

[Continued]

★ 328 ★

Dental Laboratories by Major Metro Area: 1992
[Continued]

Area	Establishments		Revenues		Employment		Payroll		
	Number	% of HS[1] in area	Total ($000)	% of HS[1] in area	Number	% of HS[1] in area	Total ($000)	% of HS[1] in area	Payroll per employee
Norfolk – Virginia Beach – Newport News, VA – NC MSA	28	1.24	8,925	0.66	194	0.89	4,491	0.69	23,149
Oklahoma City, OK MSA	27	1.37	4,886	0.38	112	0.57	1,935	0.35	17,277
Omaha, NE – IA MSA	17	1.68	5,340	0.65	138	1.11	2,608	0.70	18,899
Orlando, FL MSA	49	1.93	10,650	0.56	259	1.03	4,950	0.60	19,112
Pensacola, FL MSA	14	2.66	-	-	-	-	-	-	-
Peoria – Pekin, IL MSA	7	1.38	-	-	-	-	-	-	-
Philadelphia – Wilmington – Atlantic City, PA – NJ – DE – MD CMSA	159	1.37	-	-	-	-	-	-	-
Phoenix – Mesa, AZ MSA	100	2.08	22,850	0.73	432	1.12	9,418	0.69	21,801
Pittsburgh, PA MSA	39	0.82	7,458	0.27	179	0.47	2,674	0.21	14,939
Portland, ME MSA	6	1.11	2,827	0.74	73	1.24	1,465	0.82	20,068
Portland – Salem, OR – WA CMSA	79	2.23	-	-	-	-	-	-	-
Providence – Fall River – Warwick, RI – MA MSA	31	1.49	7,614	0.65	119	0.60	3,577	0.68	30,059
Raleigh – Durham – Chapel Hill, NC MSA	44	3.06	-	-	-	-	-	-	-
Reno, NV MSA	17	2.55	3,082	0.59	51	0.86	1,033	0.47	20,255
Richmond – Petersburg, VA MSA	23	1.44	4,980	0.32	116	0.52	2,427	0.37	20,922
Rochester, NY MSA	27	1.76	8,552	1.03	197	1.41	3,636	1.04	18,457
Rockford, IL MSA	6	1.26	2,169	0.60	46	0.85	1,118	0.68	24,304
Sacramento – Yolo, CA CMSA	66	2.28	-	-	-	-	-	-	-
Saginaw – Bay City – Midland, MI MSA	11	1.61	2,474	0.65	43	0.67	1,019	0.52	23,698
St. Louis, MO – IL MSA	106	2.38	27,891	0.97	603	1.38	12,535	1.01	20,788
Salinas, CA MSA	13	2.14	2,796	0.93	40	0.91	946	0.77	23,650
Salt Lake City – Ogden, UT MSA	58	2.82	-	-	-	-	-	-	-
San Antonio, TX MSA	40	1.52	12,664	0.70	291	1.01	6,049	0.81	20,787
San Diego, CA MSA	91	1.85	17,615	0.54	325	0.78	6,301	0.47	19,388
San Francisco – Oakland – San Jose, CA CMSA	340	2.42	86,788	0.96	1,528	1.34	32,586	0.86	21,326
Santa Barbara – Santa Maria – Lompoc, CA MSA	21	2.51	9,502	2.22	120	2.28	2,829	1.59	23,575
Sarasota – Bradenton, FL MSA	19	1.55	3,164	0.32	53	0.37	1,131	0.28	21,340
Scranton – Wilkes-Barre – Hazleton, PA MSA	13	1.14	2,759	0.44	57	0.54	1,048	0.40	18,386
Seattle – Tacoma – Bremerton, WA CMSA	149	2.46	37,202	1.05	676	1.25	15,313	0.99	22,652
Shreveport – Bossier City, LA MSA	15	2.34	2,855	0.50	53	0.62	844	0.36	15,925
Spokane, WA MSA	21	2.86	4,514	0.88	84	1.07	1,612	0.69	19,190
Springfield, MO MSA	10	2.17	2,703	0.70	59	0.86	1,080	0.55	18,305
Springfield, MA MSA	19	2.10	4,514	0.68	104	0.86	2,180	0.68	20,962
Stockton – Lodi, CA MSA	15	1.80	3,134	0.61	49	0.61	903	0.40	18,429
Syracuse, NY MSA	21	1.92	6,547	0.95	108	1.10	2,221	0.71	20,565
Tallahassee, FL MSA	9	2.27	1,695	0.49	45	0.95	918	0.60	20,400
Tampa – St. Petersburg – Clearwater, FL MSA	91	1.84	26,126	0.60	568	0.93	11,661	0.68	20,530
Toledo, OH MSA	17	1.51	7,139	0.92	169	1.35	3,093	0.78	18,302
Tucson, AZ MSA	33	2.62	5,708	0.58	148	1.09	2,801	0.70	18,926
Tulsa, OK MSA	25	1.83	7,853	0.83	161	1.13	3,472	0.82	21,565
Washington – Baltimore, DC – MD – VA – WV CMSA	160	1.24	-	-	-	-	-	-	-
West Palm Beach – Boca Raton, FL MSA	46	1.71	9,010	0.46	187	0.76	4,105	0.49	21,952
Wichita, KS MSA	20	2.61	8,832	0.91	208	1.54	4,215	1.02	20,264
Youngstown – Warren, OH MSA	16	1.33	1,644	0.24	45	0.37	534	0.17	11,867

Source: U.S. Department of Commerce. Bureau of the Census. *1992 Economic Census Report Series,* CD-ROM 1i, Washington, DC, October 1996. *Notes:* - means no data reported. 1. HS stands for total health service establishments, revenues, employment, or payroll.

★ 329 ★

Establishment Data

Dental Laboratories by State: 1992

Area	Establishments		Revenues		Employment		Payroll		
	Number	% of HS[1] in area	Total ($000)	% of HS[1] in area	Number	% of HS[1] in area	Total ($000)	% of HS[1] in area	Payroll per employee
United States	7,527	1.70	1,948,464	0.65	39,106	0.88	824,312	0.64	21,079
Alabama	126	2.28	31,649	0.64	690	0.89	13,858	0.66	20,084
Alaska	12	1.40	3,455	0.64	61	1.08	1,411	0.65	23,131
Arizona	150	2.11	33,077	0.72	632	1.08	13,647	0.70	21,593
Arkansas	43	1.21	13,733	0.56	275	0.64	5,170	0.49	18,800
California	1,167	1.90	288,269	0.67	5,033	0.94	104,936	0.61	20,850
Colorado	143	2.04	30,135	0.81	618	1.12	12,715	0.77	20,574
Connecticut	87	1.32	27,239	0.55	459	0.63	11,825	0.50	25,763
Delaware	11	0.92	4,979	0.63	128	1.10	2,661	0.73	20,789
District of Columbia	11	0.80	1,617	0.20	23	0.24	664	0.19	28,870
Florida	526	1.78	106,564	0.46	2,314	0.73	45,785	0.48	19,786
Georgia	213	1.92	65,952	0.76	1,406	1.16	30,443	0.83	21,652
Hawaii	38	1.71	10,524	0.80	196	1.25	4,631	0.79	23,628
Idaho	47	2.71	9,553	0.97	156	0.92	3,289	0.79	21,083
Illinois	328	1.75	89,085	0.72	1,817	0.97	41,680	0.74	22,939
Indiana	146	1.68	43,180	0.71	1,043	0.98	19,325	0.70	18,528
Iowa	71	1.70	19,648	0.84	462	1.03	9,097	0.82	19,690
Kansas	56	1.45	34,213	1.12	675	1.26	14,429	1.09	21,376
Kentucky	77	1.40	15,076	0.37	292	0.44	6,068	0.34	20,781
Louisiana	86	1.26	18,912	0.34	429	0.50	7,715	0.35	17,984
Maine	17	0.79	4,890	0.42	121	0.55	2,264	0.42	18,711
Maryland	113	1.24	28,669	0.51	655	0.82	13,926	0.56	21,261
Massachusetts	142	1.34	34,697	0.45	688	0.54	15,282	0.43	22,212
Michigan	289	1.84	79,880	0.92	1,604	1.14	35,312	0.86	22,015
Minnesota	148	2.51	58,256	1.42	1,230	1.62	27,882	1.34	22,668
Mississippi	51	1.65	10,555	0.51	237	0.64	4,138	0.47	17,460
Missouri	146	1.73	43,120	0.78	968	1.02	20,018	0.82	20,680
Montana	30	2.01	4,346	0.67	59	0.55	1,359	0.52	23,034
Nebraska	46	1.95	12,811	0.82	297	1.10	5,744	0.80	19,340
Nevada	44	1.90	8,542	0.38	147	0.58	3,279	0.36	22,306
New Hampshire	33	1.80	8,621	0.73	167	0.87	3,487	0.64	20,880
New Jersey	254	1.54	76,518	0.74	1,279	1.00	34,515	0.78	26,986
New Mexico	46	1.92	8,625	0.58	165	0.70	2,839	0.46	17,206
New York	546	1.69	182,700	0.92	3,411	1.23	77,208	0.94	22,635
North Carolina	234	2.64	44,672	0.67	995	0.93	19,932	0.67	20,032
North Dakota	12	1.55	5,638	0.90	139	1.52	3,107	1.02	22,353
Ohio	264	1.42	61,802	0.53	1,487	0.74	27,760	0.50	18,668
Oklahoma	71	1.33	14,821	0.45	310	0.52	5,921	0.42	19,100
Oregon	131	2.32	29,926	1.01	539	1.12	11,426	0.88	21,199
Pennsylvania	256	1.18	67,210	0.53	1,477	0.80	28,995	0.51	19,631
Rhode Island	31	1.63	7,601	0.72	120	0.66	3,626	0.78	30,217
South Carolina	68	1.46	13,282	0.42	294	0.59	5,978	0.43	20,333
South Dakota	25	2.58	4,911	0.87	109	1.20	1,507	0.58	13,826
Tennessee	155	1.88	37,314	0.55	715	0.71	14,282	0.50	19,975
Texas	407	1.36	93,256	0.41	1,908	0.55	37,575	0.41	19,693

[Continued]

297

★ 329 ★

Dental Laboratories by State: 1992
[Continued]

Area	Establishments		Revenues		Employment		Payroll		
	Number	% of HS[1] in area	Total ($000)	% of HS[1] in area	Number	% of HS[1] in area	Total ($000)	% of HS[1] in area	Payroll per employee
Utah	83	2.72	21,715	1.18	450	1.46	7,556	1.00	16,791
Vermont	15	1.61	2,538	0.63	51	0.68	947	0.57	18,569
Virginia	136	1.39	29,067	0.44	623	0.61	13,456	0.44	21,599
Washington	235	2.55	53,369	0.99	955	1.09	20,526	0.86	21,493
West Virginia	27	1.00	8,830	0.49	187	0.65	4,041	0.57	21,610
Wisconsin	120	1.66	42,146	0.89	980	1.15	20,736	0.88	21,159
Wyoming	14	1.96	1,276	0.39	30	0.53	339	0.25	11,300

Source: U.S. Department of Commerce. Bureau of the Census. *1992 Economic Census Report Series,* CD-ROM 1i, Washington, DC, October 1996. *Notes:* - means no data reported. 1. HS stands for total health service establishments, revenues, employment, or payroll.

★ 330 ★

Establishment Data

Diet and Weight Reducing Services by Major Metro Area: 1992

	Establishments	Revenues ($ 000)	Employment	Payroll ($ 000)	Payroll per employee
United States	3,795	1,512,047	39,522	373,901	9,461
Atlanta, GA MSA	51	25,311	729	6,428	8,818
Boston – Worcester – Lawrence, MA – NH – ME – CT CMSA	181	57,072	1,901	16,989	8,937
Chicago – Gary – Kenosha, IL – IN – WI CMSA	110	75,765	1,658	21,819	13,160
Cincinnati – Hamilton, OH – KY – IN CMSA	23	-	-	-	-
Cleveland – Akron, OH CMSA	54	15,566	284	4,693	16,525
Dallas – Fort Worth, TX CMSA	70	32,937	874	8,599	9,839
Denver – Boulder – Greeley, CO CMSA	33	-	-	-	-
Detroit – Ann Arbor – Flint, MI CMSA	71	15,074	339	3,945	11,637
Houston – Galveston – Brazoria, TX CMSA	16	-	-	-	-
Indianapolis, IN MSA	34	16,636	759	4,490	5,916
Kansas City, MO – KS MSA	42	15,943	492	4,312	8,764
Los Angeles – Riverside – Orange County, CA CMSA	216	-	-	-	-
Miami – Fort Lauderdale, FL CMSA	55	27,919	674	8,055	11,951
Milwaukee – Racine, WI CMSA	34	-	-	-	-
Minneapolis – St. Paul, MN – WI MSA	32	20,393	1,094	4,356	3,982
New York – Northern New Jersey – Long Island, NY – NJ – CT- CMSA	258	-	-	-	-
Orlando, FL MSA	28	13,558	670	3,565	5,321

[Continued]

★ 330 ★

Diet and Weight Reducing Services by Major Metro Area: 1992

[Continued]

	Establish ments	Revenues ($ 000)	Employ- ment	Payroll ($ 000)	Payroll per employee
Philadelphia – Wilmington – Atlantic City, PA – NJ – DE – MD CMSA	82	-	-	-	-
Phoenix – Mesa, AZ MSA	24	20,197	379	5,728	15,113
Pittsburgh, PA MSA	37	26,073	262	4,202	16,038
Portland – Salem, OR – WA CMSA	28	-	-	-	-
Sacramento – Yolo, CA CMSA	35	-	-	-	-
St. Louis, MO – IL MSA	42	26,069	803	5,902	7,350
San Diego, CA MSA	52	23,520	412	5,524	13,408
San Francisco – Oakland – San Jose, CA CMSA	131	45,130	801	10,349	12,920
Seattle – Tacoma – Bremerton, WA CMSA	51	-	-	-	-
Tampa – St. Petersburg – Clearwater, FL MSA	29	9,086	148	1,428	9,649
Washington – Baltimore, DC – MD – VA – WV CMSA	121	-	-	-	-
West Palm Beach – Boca Raton, FL MSA	20	12,012	431	3,068	7,118

Source: U.S. Department of Commerce. Bureau of the Census. *1992 Economic Census Report Series,* CD-ROM 1i, Washington, DC, October 1996. *Note:* - means no data reported.

★ 331 ★

Establishment Data

Diet and Weight Reducing Services by State: 1992

	Establish ments	Revenues ($ 000)	Employ- ment	Payroll ($ 000)	Payroll per employee
United States	3,795	1,512,047	39,522	373,901	9,461
Alabama	66	13,748	286	2,617	9,150
Alaska	9	1,411	39	386	9,897
Arizona	30	22,028	421	6,098	14,485
Arkansas	24	5,107	301	1,491	4,953
California	505	213,595	3,821	49,230	12,884
Colorado	44	12,627	228	2,240	9,825
Connecticut	40	13,779	309	3,824	12,375
Delaware	17	6,641	169	1,724	10,201
District of Columbia	4	-	-	-	-
Florida	217	88,239	2,623	20,612	7,858
Georgia	82	33,139	900	7,935	8,817
Hawaii	5	-	-	-	-
Idaho	39	4,046	144	868	6,028
Illinois	154	85,813	2,066	23,922	11,579
Indiana	98	31,603	1,180	8,047	6,819

[Continued]

★ 331 ★

Diet and Weight Reducing Services by State: 1992
[Continued]

	Establish ments	Revenues ($ 000)	Employ- ment	Payroll ($ 000)	Payroll per employee
Iowa	45	9,374	390	2,223	5,700
Kansas	47	16,985	692	4,015	5,802
Kentucky	49	13,181	484	4,056	8,380
Louisiana	39	14,676	375	3,770	10,053
Maine	15	13,551	519	3,813	7,347
Maryland	79	38,756	1,146	9,058	7,904
Massachusetts	192	59,940	1,962	18,077	9,214
Michigan	119	24,839	658	5,954	9,049
Minnesota	57	23,547	1,202	4,853	4,037
Mississippi	20	5,990	254	1,554	6,118
Missouri	85	37,095	1,185	9,082	7,664
Montana	11	1,239	27	229	8,481
Nebraska	31	7,875	335	1,922	5,737
Nevada	20	6,876	252	2,098	8,325
New Hampshire	19	4,680	204	1,733	8,495
New Jersey	119	77,473	1,807	18,936	10,479
New Mexico	12	4,952	179	1,278	7,140
New York	217	157,121	2,536	34,859	13,746
North Carolina	110	22,107	579	5,907	10,202
North Dakota	16	2,880	96	696	7,250
Ohio	282	61,275	1,655	17,195	10,390
Oklahoma	37	11,413	391	3,381	8,647
Oregon	43	18,297	523	4,228	8,084
Pennsylvania	148	83,749	1,807	19,336	10,701
Rhode Island	36	15,233	640	6,169	9,639
South Carolina	35	9,442	351	2,992	8,524
South Dakota	6	1,102	28	282	10,071
Tennessee	64	22,663	587	6,064	10,330
Texas	146	67,106	2,297	18,198	7,923
Utah	52	9,440	389	2,451	6,301
Vermont	7	2,056	175	929	5,309
Virginia	126	46,290	1,034	9,554	9,240
Washington	73	50,124	961	10,660	11,093
West Virginia	17	4,674	344	1,013	2,945
Wisconsin	72	31,030	884	7,720	8,733
Wyoming	15	-	-	-	-

Source: U.S. Department of Commerce. Bureau of the Census. *1992 Economic Census Report Series,* CD-ROM 1i, Washington, DC, October 1996. *Note:* - means no data reported.

★ 332 ★

Establishment Data

General Medical and Surgical Hospitals by Major Metro Area: 1992

Area	Establishments		Revenues		Employment		Payroll		
	Number	% of HS[1] in area	Total ($000)	% of HS[1] in area	Number	% of HS[1] in area	Total ($000)	% of HS[1] in area	Payroll per employee
United States	704	0.16	24,162,290	8.08	323,141	7.26	8,012,918	6.21	24,797
Albany – Schenectady – Troy, NY MSA	0	0.00	0	0.00	0	0.00	0	0.00	0
Albuquerque, NM MSA	1	0.09	-	-	-	-	-	-	-
Allentown – Bethlehem – Easton, PA MSA	0	0.00	0	0.00	0	0.00	0	0.00	0
Anchorage, AK MSA	1	0.21	-	-	-	-	-	-	-
Appleton – Oshkosh – Neenah, WI MSA	0	0.00	0	0.00	0	0.00	0	0.00	0
Atlanta, GA MSA	15	0.25	533,489	11.07	6,380	10.66	150,822	7.47	23,640
Augusta – Aiken, GA – SC MSA	2	0.28	-	-	-	-	-	-	-
Austin – San Marcos, TX MSA	3	0.19	-	-	-	-	-	-	-
Bakersfield, CA MSA	2	0.26	-	-	-	-	-	-	-
Baton Rouge, LA MSA	2	0.23	-	-	-	-	-	-	-
Beaumont – Port Arthur, TX MSA	4	0.55	-	-	-	-	-	-	-
Birmingham, AL MSA	4	0.29	-	-	-	-	-	-	-
Boise City, ID MSA	1	0.17	-	-	-	-	-	-	-
Boston – Worcester – Lawrence, MA – NH – ME – CT CMSA	4	0.04	105,703	1.49	1,677	1.46	38,176	1.17	22,764
Buffalo – Niagara Falls, NY MSA	0	0.00	0	0.00	0	0.00	0	0.00	0
Canton – Massillon, OH MSA	0	0.00	0	0.00	0	0.00	0	0.00	0
Charleston – North Charleston, SC MSA	2	0.25	-	-	-	-	-	-	-
Charlotte – Gastonia – Rock Hill, NC – SC MSA	1	0.06	-	-	-	-	-	-	-
Chattanooga, TN – GA MSA	5	0.66	144,960	20.21	1,902	19.07	45,582	14.91	23,965
Chicago – Gary – Kenosha, IL – IN – WI CMSA	7	0.05	-	-	-	-	-	-	-
Cincinnati – Hamilton, OH – KY – IN CMSA	1	0.03	-	-	-	-	-	-	-
Cleveland – Akron, OH CMSA	0	0.00	0	0.00	0	0.00	0	0.00	0
Colorado Springs, CO MSA	0	0.00	0	0.00	0	0.00	0	0.00	0
Columbia, SC MSA	0	0.00	0	0.00	0	0.00	0	0.00	0
Columbus, OH MSA	2	0.08	-	-	-	-	-	-	-
Corpus Christi, TX MSA	4	0.53	-	-	-	-	-	-	-
Dallas – Fort Worth, TX CMSA	26	0.31	-	-	-	-	-	-	-
Davenport – Moline – Rock Island, IA – IL MSA	1	0.15	-	-	-	-	-	-	-
Dayton – Springfield, OH MSA	0	0.00	0	0.00	0	0.00	0	0.00	0
Daytona Beach, FL MSA	2	0.27	-	-	-	-	-	-	-
Denver – Boulder – Greeley, CO CMSA	2	0.05	-	-	-	-	-	-	-
Des Moines, IA MSA	1	0.14	-	-	-	-	-	-	-
Detroit – Ann Arbor – Flint, MI CMSA	0	0.00	0	0.00	0	0.00	0	0.00	0
El Paso, TX MSA	6	0.75	-	-	-	-	-	-	-
Eugene – Springfield, OR MSA	0	0.00	0	0.00	0	0.00	0	0.00	0
Fort Myers – Cape Coral, FL MSA	3	0.42	-	-	-	-	-	-	-
Fort Pierce – Port St. Lucie, FL MSA	2	0.39	-	-	-	-	-	-	-
Fort Wayne, IN MSA	0	0.00	0	0.00	0	0.00	0	0.00	0
Fresno, CA MSA	1	0.07	-	-	-	-	-	-	-
Grand Rapids – Muskegon – Holland, MI MSA	0	0.00	0	0.00	0	0.00	0	0.00	0
Greensboro – Winston-Salem – High Point, NC MSA	0	0.00	0	0.00	0	0.00	0	0.00	0
Greenville – Spartanburg – Anderson, SC MSA	3	0.26	-	-	-	-	-	-	-
Harrisburg – Lebanon – Carlisle, PA MSA	0	0.00	0	0.00	0	0.00	0	0.00	0
Hartford, CT MSA	0	0.00	0	0.00	0	0.00	0	0.00	0
Honolulu, HI MSA	1	0.06	-	-	-	-	-	-	-

[Continued]

★ 332 ★

General Medical and Surgical Hospitals by Major Metro Area: 1992
[Continued]

Area	Establishments		Revenues		Employment		Payroll		
	Number	% of HS[1] in area	Total ($000)	% of HS[1] in area	Number	% of HS[1] in area	Total ($000)	% of HS[1] in area	Payroll per employee
Houston – Galveston – Brazoria, TX CMSA	36	0.51	-	-	-	-	-	-	-
Huntsville, AL MSA	3	0.56	-	-	-	-	-	-	-
Indianapolis, IN MSA	2	0.08	-	-	-	-	-	-	-
Jackson, MS MSA	1	0.16	-	-	-	-	-	-	-
Jacksonville, FL MSA	1	0.06	-	-	-	-	-	-	-
Johnson City – Kingsport – Bristol, TN – VA MSA	4	0.58	-	-	-	-	-	-	-
Kalamazoo – Battle Creek, MI MSA	0	0.00	0	0.00	0	0.00	0	0.00	0
Kansas City, MO – KS MSA	1	0.04	-	-	-	-	-	-	-
Knoxville, TN MSA	1	0.08	-	-	-	-	-	-	-
Lafayette, LA MSA	3	0.47	-	-	-	-	-	-	-
Lakeland – Winter Haven, FL MSA	1	0.21	-	-	-	-	-	-	-
Lancaster, PA MSA	0	0.00	0	0.00	0	0.00	0	0.00	0
Lansing – East Lansing, MI MSA	0	0.00	0	0.00	0	0.00	0	0.00	0
Las Vegas, NV – AZ MSA	6	0.39	478,660	28.35	4,762	25.81	140,440	20.62	29,492
Lexington, KY MSA	3	0.37	-	-	-	-	-	-	-
Little Rock – North Little Rock, AR MSA	1	0.10	-	-	-	-	-	-	-
Los Angeles – Riverside – Orange County, CA CMSA	86	0.28	-	-	-	-	-	-	-
Louisville, KY – IN MSA	5	0.29	-	-	-	-	-	-	-
Macon, GA MSA	3	0.55	-	-	-	-	-	-	-
Madison, WI MSA	0	0.00	0	0.00	0	0.00	0	0.00	0
Melbourne – Titusville – Palm Bay, FL MSA	0	0.00	0	0.00	0	0.00	0	0.00	0
Memphis, TN – AR – MS MSA	2	0.12	-	-	-	-	-	-	-
Miami – Fort Lauderdale, FL CMSA	26	0.28	1,323,659	19.35	17,155	19.73	451,873	16.11	26,341
Milwaukee – Racine, WI CMSA	0	0.00	0	0.00	0	0.00	0	0.00	0
Minneapolis – St. Paul, MN – WI MSA	0	0.00	0	0.00	0	0.00	0	0.00	0
Mobile, AL MSA	1	0.16	-	-	-	-	-	-	-
Modesto, CA MSA	1	0.15	-	-	-	-	-	-	-
Montgomery, AL MSA	3	0.61	-	-	-	-	-	-	-
Nashville, TN MSA	6	0.31	-	-	-	-	-	-	-
New Orleans, LA MSA	16	0.66	524,631	23.98	6,243	21.08	171,911	20.44	27,537
New York – Northern New Jersey – Long Island, NY – NJ – CT- CMSA	13	0.03	615,304	2.36	9,126	2.74	298,345	2.73	32,692
Norfolk – Virginia Beach – Newport News, VA – NC MSA	0	0.00	0	0.00	0	0.00	0	0.00	0
Oklahoma City, OK MSA	2	0.10	-	-	-	-	-	-	-
Omaha, NE – IA MSA	1	0.10	-	-	-	-	-	-	-
Orlando, FL MSA	6	0.24	244,694	12.86	3,017	11.96	77,466	9.47	25,676
Pensacola, FL MSA	2	0.38	-	-	-	-	-	-	-
Peoria – Pekin, IL MSA	0	0.00	0	0.00	0	0.00	0	0.00	0
Philadelphia – Wilmington – Atlantic City, PA – NJ – DE – MD CMSA	0	0.00	0	0.00	0	0.00	0	0.00	0
Phoenix – Mesa, AZ MSA	4	0.08	-	-	-	-	-	-	-
Pittsburgh, PA MSA	0	0.00	0	0.00	0	0.00	0	0.00	0
Portland, ME MSA	0	0.00	0	0.00	0	0.00	0	0.00	0
Portland – Salem, OR – WA CMSA	4	0.11	-	-	-	-	-	-	-
Providence – Fall River – Warwick, RI – MA MSA	0	0.00	0	0.00	0	0.00	0	0.00	0
Raleigh – Durham – Chapel Hill, NC MSA	2	0.14	-	-	-	-	-	-	-
Reno, NV MSA	1	0.15	-	-	-	-	-	-	-
Richmond – Petersburg, VA MSA	6	0.38	509,773	32.57	6,012	27.06	156,593	23.67	26,047
Rochester, NY MSA	0	0.00	0	0.00	0	0.00	0	0.00	0

[Continued]

★ 332 ★

General Medical and Surgical Hospitals by Major Metro Area: 1992
[Continued]

Area	Establishments		Revenues		Employment		Payroll		
	Number	% of HS[1] in area	Total ($000)	% of HS[1] in area	Number	% of HS[1] in area	Total ($000)	% of HS[1] in area	Payroll per employee
Rockford, IL MSA	0	0.00	0	0.00	0	0.00	0	0.00	0
Sacramento – Yolo, CA CMSA	0	0.00	0	0.00	0	0.00	0	0.00	0
Saginaw – Bay City – Midland, MI MSA	0	0.00	0	0.00	0	0.00	0	0.00	0
St. Louis, MO – IL MSA	2	0.04	-	-	-	-	-	-	-
Salinas, CA MSA	0	0.00	0	0.00	0	0.00	0	0.00	0
Salt Lake City – Ogden, UT MSA	4	0.19	-	-	-	-	-	-	-
San Antonio, TX MSA	6	0.23	240,944	13.38	3,557	12.37	90,522	12.13	25,449
San Diego, CA MSA	5	0.10	219,145	6.71	2,485	5.97	69,108	5.13	27,810
San Francisco – Oakland – San Jose, CA CMSA	9	0.06	-	-	-	-	-	-	-
Santa Barbara – Santa Maria – Lompoc, CA MSA	1	0.12	-	-	-	-	-	-	-
Sarasota – Bradenton, FL MSA	3	0.24	-	-	-	-	-	-	-
Scranton – Wilkes-Barre – Hazleton, PA MSA	0	0.00	0	0.00	0	0.00	0	0.00	0
Seattle – Tacoma – Bremerton, WA CMSA	4	0.07	-	-	-	-	-	-	-
Shreveport – Bossier City, LA MSA	5	0.78	96,907	16.95	1,535	18.06	31,547	13.62	20,552
Spokane, WA MSA	1	0.14	-	-	-	-	-	-	-
Springfield, MO MSA	2	0.43	-	-	-	-	-	-	-
Springfield, MA MSA	0	0.00	0	0.00	0	0.00	0	0.00	0
Stockton – Lodi, CA MSA	1	0.12	-	-	-	-	-	-	-
Syracuse, NY MSA	0	0.00	0	0.00	0	0.00	0	0.00	0
Tallahassee, FL MSA	2	0.50	-	-	-	-	-	-	-
Tampa – St. Petersburg – Clearwater, FL MSA	20	0.41	864,673	19.84	11,241	18.37	260,888	15.12	23,209
Toledo, OH MSA	0	0.00	0	0.00	0	0.00	0	0.00	0
Tucson, AZ MSA	3	0.24	-	-	-	-	-	-	-
Tulsa, OK MSA	3	0.22	-	-	-	-	-	-	-
Washington – Baltimore, DC – MD – VA – WV CMSA	3	0.02	-	-	-	-	-	-	-
West Palm Beach – Boca Raton, FL MSA	7	0.26	352,702	17.84	4,180	17.01	123,785	14.68	29,614
Wichita, KS MSA	1	0.13	-	-	-	-	-	-	-
Youngstown – Warren, OH MSA	1	0.08	-	-	-	-	-	-	-

Source: U.S. Department of Commerce. Bureau of the Census. *1992 Economic Census Report Series,* CD-ROM 1i, Washington, DC, October 1996. *Notes:* - means no data reported. 1. HS stands for total health service establishments, revenues, employment, or payroll. 2. MSA stands for Metropolitan Statistical Area. 3. CMSA stands for Consolidated Metropolitan Statistical Area.

★ 333 ★

Establishment Data

General Medical and Surgical Hospitals by Major Metro Area, Non-Taxed: 1992

Area	Establish-ments	Revenues in $1,000	Employ-ment	Payroll in $1,000	Payroll per employee
United States	4,920	254,391,214	4,087,892	112,136,788	27,431
Albany – Schenectady – Troy, NY MSA[2]	14	-	-	-	-
Albuquerque, NM MSA	10	-	-	-	-
Allentown – Bethlehem – Easton, PA MSA	9	-	-	-	-
Atlanta, GA MSA	27	2,535,871	38,101	1,011,086	26,537

[Continued]

★ 333 ★

General Medical and Surgical Hospitals by Major Metro Area, Non-Taxed: 1992
[Continued]

Area	Establish-ments	Revenues in $1,000	Employ-ment	Payroll in $1,000	Payroll per employee
Austin–San Marcos, TX MSA	9	-	-	-	-
Baton Rouge, LA MSA	6	376,776	6,789	143,103	21,079
Birmingham, AL MSA	13	-	-	-	-
Boston–Worcester–Lawrence, MA–NH–ME–CT CMSA[3]	81	-	-	-	-
Buffalo–Niagara Falls, NY MSA	21	-	-	-	-
Charlotte–Gastonia–Rock Hill, NC–SC MSA	11	1,073,629	16,647	446,528	26,823
Chicago–Gary–Kenosha, IL–IN–WI CMSA	99	-	-	-	-
Cincinnati–Hamilton, OH–KY–IN CMSA	24	-	-	-	-
Cleveland–Akron, OH CMSA	45	-	-	-	-
Columbus, OH MSA	14	-	-	-	-
Dallas–Fort Worth, TX CMSA	37	-	-	-	-
Dayton–Springfield, OH MSA	13	1,385,709	22,124	607,745	27,470
Denver–Boulder–Greeley, CO CMSA	22	-	-	-	-
Des Moines, IA MSA	7	-	-	-	-
Detroit–Ann Arbor–Flint, MI CMSA	69	6,737,678	105,386	3,038,485	28,832
Fresno, CA MSA	12	-	-	-	-
Grand Rapids–Muskegon–Holland, MI MSA	13	815,035	14,797	353,152	23,866
Greensboro–Winston-Salem–High Point, NC MSA	17	1,088,018	18,446	489,646	26,545
Greenville–Spartanburg–Anderson, SC MSA	11	-	-	-	-
Harrisburg–Lebanon–Carlisle, PA MSA	10	-	-	-	-
Hartford, CT MSA	16	-	-	-	-
Honolulu, HI MSA	10	-	-	-	-
Houston–Galveston–Brazoria, TX CMSA	28	-	-	-	-
Indianapolis, IN MSA	22	2,130,720	33,234	898,624	27,039
Jacksonville, FL MSA	13	-	-	-	-
Kalamazoo–Battle Creek, MI MSA	8	423,482	7,398	190,152	25,703
Kansas City, MO–KS MSA	36	1,957,117	35,137	857,191	24,396
Knoxville, TN MSA	9	-	-	-	-
Lansing–East Lansing, MI MSA	7	465,205	7,882	197,599	25,070
Lexington, KY MSA	9	-	-	-	-
Little Rock–North Little Rock, AR MSA	10	-	-	-	-
Los Angeles–Riverside–Orange County, CA CMSA	127	-	-	-	-
Louisville, KY–IN MSA	12	907,207	15,497	379,468	24,487
Madison, WI MSA	6	-	-	-	-

[Continued]

★ 333 ★

General Medical and Surgical Hospitals by Major Metro Area, Non-Taxed: 1992
[Continued]

Area	Establish-ments	Revenues in $1,000	Employ-ment	Payroll in $1,000	Payroll per employee
Memphis, TN–AR–MS MSA	15	-	-	-	-
Miami–Fort Lauderdale, FL CMSA	22	2,734,982	36,639	1,197,780	32,691
Milwaukee–Racine, WI CMSA	24	-	-	-	-
Minneapolis–St. Paul, MN–WI MSA	35	-	-	-	-
Nashville, TN MSA	17	-	-	-	-
New Orleans, LA MSA	15	1,509,262	23,956	666,677	27,829
New York–Northern New Jersey–Long Island, NY–NJ–CT- CMSA	210	27,449,248	400,654	13,745,244	34,307
Norfolk–Virginia Beach–Newport News, VA–NC MSA	20	-	-	-	-
Oklahoma City, OK MSA	19	1,089,266	19,472	466,758	23,971
Omaha, NE–IA MSA	11	842,306	14,552	386,682	26,572
Orlando, FL MSA	13	-	-	-	-
Philadelphia–Wilmington–Atlantic City, PA–NJ–DE–MD CMSA	99	-	-	-	-
Phoenix–Mesa, AZ MSA	29	-	-	-	-
Pittsburgh, PA MSA	41	-	-	-	-
Portland–Salem, OR–WA CMSA	22	-	-	-	-
Providence–Fall River–Warwick, RI–MA MSA	16	-	-	-	-
Raleigh–Durham–Chapel Hill, NC MSA	13	1,434,345	21,857	641,040	29,329
Richmond–Petersburg, VA MSA	10	-	-	-	-
Rochester, NY MSA	17	1,078,425	21,411	524,713	24,507
Sacramento–Yolo, CA CMSA	17	-	-	-	-
St. Louis, MO–IL MSA	42	-	-	-	-
Salt Lake City–Ogden, UT MSA	10	-	-	-	-
San Antonio, TX MSA	15	1,471,275	22,796	726,810	31,883
San Diego, CA MSA	23	2,176,663	29,487	914,153	31,002
San Francisco–Oakland–San Jose, CA CMSA	78	7,498,002	91,883	3,466,068	37,723
Santa Barbara–Santa Maria–Lompoc, CA MSA	7	-	-	-	-
Scranton–Wilkes-Barre–Hazleton, PA MSA	16	738,361	13,608	331,294	24,346
Seattle–Tacoma–Bremerton, WA CMSA	37	3,118,620	46,039	1,392,998	30,257
Springfield, MA MSA	10	594,155	10,627	283,941	26,719
Syracuse, NY MSA	10	-	-	-	-
Tampa–St. Petersburg–Clearwater, FL MSA	18	1,692,690	25,092	715,636	28,520
Toledo, OH MSA	11	-	-	-	-
Tucson, AZ MSA	7	-	-	-	-
Tulsa, OK MSA	11	-	-	-	-
Washington–Baltimore, DC–MD–VA–WV CMSA	71	-	-	-	-

[Continued]

★ 333 ★

General Medical and Surgical Hospitals by Major Metro Area, Non-Taxed: 1992
[Continued]

Area	Establish-ments	Revenues in $1,000	Employ-ment	Payroll in $1,000	Payroll per employee
West Palm Beach – Boca Raton, FL MSA	8	-	-	-	-
Wichita, KS MSA	9	-	-	-	-
Youngstown – Warren, OH MSA	9	-	-	-	-

Source: U.S. Department of Commerce. Bureau of the Census. *1992 Economic Census Report Series,* CD-ROM 1i, Washington, DC, October 1996. *Notes:* - means no data reported. 1. HS stands for total health service establishments, revenues, employment, or payroll. 2. MSA stands for Metropolitan Statistical Area. 3. CMSA stands for Consolidated Metropolitan Statistical Area.

★ 334 ★

Establishment Data

General Medical and Surgical Hospitals by State: 1992

Area	Establishments		Revenues		Employment		Payroll		
	Number	% of HS[1] in area	Total ($000)	% of HS[1] in area	Number	% of HS[1] in area	Total ($000)	% of HS[1] in area	Payroll per employee
United States	704	0.16	24,162,290	8.08	323,141	7.26	8,012,918	6.21	24,797
Alabama	31	0.56	970,042	19.70	13,370	17.29	287,129	13.61	21,476
Alaska	1	0.12	-	-	-	-	-	-	-
Arizona	8	0.11	318,040	6.96	4,548	7.74	99,887	5.12	21,963
Arkansas	13	0.36	278,132	11.42	4,056	9.50	79,632	7.48	19,633
California	114	0.19	3,874,600	9.01	49,541	9.24	1,453,439	8.43	29,338
Colorado	3	0.04	-	-	-	-	-	-	-
Connecticut	0	0.00	0	0.00	0	0.00	0	0.00	0
Delaware	0	0.00	0	0.00	0	0.00	0	0.00	0
District of Columbia	0	0.00	0	0.00	0	0.00	0	0.00	0
Florida	95	0.32	4,123,939	17.69	53,968	17.12	1,336,507	13.87	24,765
Georgia	36	0.32	1,107,715	12.84	14,056	11.62	313,454	8.54	22,300
Hawaii	1	0.04	-	-	-	-	-	-	-
Idaho	3	0.17	-	-	-	-	-	-	-
Illinois	10	0.05	475,784	3.85	7,218	3.85	189,905	3.39	26,310
Indiana	5	0.06	169,002	2.78	2,747	2.57	57,542	2.10	20,947
Iowa	2	0.05	-	-	-	-	-	-	-
Kansas	5	0.13	-	-	-	-	-	-	-
Kentucky	23	0.42	730,738	17.74	10,670	15.91	248,204	13.96	23,262
Louisiana	40	0.59	940,812	17.02	12,637	14.64	309,054	14.20	24,456
Maine	0	0.00	0	0.00	0	0.00	0	0.00	0
Maryland	2	0.02	-	-	-	-	-	-	-
Massachusetts	2	0.02	-	-	-	-	-	-	-
Michigan	0	0.00	0	0.00	0	0.00	0	0.00	0
Minnesota	0	0.00	0	0.00	0	0.00	0	0.00	0
Mississippi	14	0.45	218,563	10.49	3,668	9.96	73,078	8.31	19,923
Missouri	11	0.13	373,586	6.80	5,565	5.87	121,773	4.98	21,882
Montana	1	0.07	-	-	-	-	-	-	-

[Continued]

★ 334 ★

General Medical and Surgical Hospitals by State: 1992

[Continued]

Area	Establishments		Revenues		Employment		Payroll		
	Number	% of HS[1] in area	Total ($000)	% of HS[1] in area	Number	% of HS[1] in area	Total ($000)	% of HS[1] in area	Payroll per employee
Nebraska	1	0.04	-	-	-	-	-	-	-
Nevada	6	0.26	-	-	-	-	-	-	-
New Hampshire	2	0.11	-	-	-	-	-	-	-
New Jersey	0	0.00	0	0.00	0	0.00	0	0.00	0
New Mexico	5	0.21	-	-	-	-	-	-	-
New York	13	0.04	615,304	3.10	9,126	3.28	298,345	3.62	32,692
North Carolina	12	0.14	353,765	5.31	5,095	4.75	111,857	3.75	21,954
North Dakota	1	0.13	-	-	-	-	-	-	-
Ohio	3	0.02	-	-	-	-	-	-	-
Oklahoma	11	0.21	313,020	9.56	4,694	7.95	100,090	7.08	21,323
Oregon	7	0.12	-	-	-	-	-	-	-
Pennsylvania	1	0.00	-	-	-	-	-	-	-
Rhode Island	0	0.00	0	0.00	0	0.00	0	0.00	0
South Carolina	12	0.26	449,969	14.36	6,326	12.64	135,337	9.70	21,394
South Dakota	0	0.00	0	0.00	0	0.00	0	0.00	0
Tennessee	48	0.58	1,005,997	14.91	14,445	14.40	325,505	11.34	22,534
Texas	123	0.41	4,327,310	18.88	53,894	15.56	1,327,291	14.40	24,628
Utah	8	0.26	255,420	13.83	3,847	12.45	77,023	10.20	20,022
Vermont	0	0.00	0	0.00	0	0.00	0	0.00	0
Virginia	13	0.13	820,513	12.28	10,274	10.05	239,897	7.92	23,350
Washington	5	0.05	112,746	2.09	1,537	1.76	38,193	1.60	24,849
West Virginia	10	0.37	180,031	10.07	2,770	9.59	59,449	8.44	21,462
Wisconsin	1	0.01	-	-	-	-	-	-	-
Wyoming	2	0.28	-	-	-	-	-	-	-

Source: U.S. Department of Commerce. Bureau of the Census. *1992 Economic Census Report Series,* CD-ROM 1i, Washington, DC, October 1996. *Notes:* - means no data reported. 1. HS stands for total health service establishments, revenues, employment, or payroll.

★ 335 ★

Establishment Data

General Medical and Surgical Hospitals by State, Non-Taxed: 1992

Area	Establish-ments	Revenues in $1,000	Employ-ment	Payroll in $1,000	Payroll per employee
United States	4,920	254,391,214	4,087,892	112,136,788	27,431
Alabama	89	3,726,237	60,658	1,497,509	24,688
Alaska	25	-	-	-	-
Arizona	67	3,439,245	50,768	1,394,134	27,461
Arkansas	73	2,044,575	37,366	845,857	22,637
California	359	27,901,348	364,300	11,748,855	32,250

[Continued]

★ 335 ★

General Medical and Surgical Hospitals by State, Non-Taxed: 1992

[Continued]

Area	Establish-ments	Revenues in $1,000	Employ-ment	Payroll in $1,000	Payroll per employee
Colorado	73	3,219,257	50,331	1,366,451	27,149
Connecticut	39	3,786,612	58,247	1,872,180	32,142
Delaware	11	-	-	-	-
District of Columbia	12	2,186,445	29,842	1,015,935	34,044
Florida	139	10,919,750	160,327	4,595,643	28,664
Georgia	127	5,828,956	97,389	2,472,231	25,385
Hawaii	19	1,032,395	15,676	498,279	31,786
Idaho	39	683,596	11,842	273,175	23,068
Illinois	205	13,186,555	218,065	5,700,581	26,142
Indiana	116	5,933,791	101,129	2,461,754	24,343
Iowa	123	2,846,264	58,593	1,234,789	21,074
Kansas	134	2,159,512	43,823	991,725	22,630
Kentucky	86	3,228,323	58,079	1,338,764	23,051
Louisiana	99	4,123,581	71,142	1,784,082	25,078
Maine	40	1,206,565	22,536	569,767	25,283
Maryland	53	4,627,686	78,427	2,118,750	27,016
Massachusetts	95	7,779,679	125,266	3,545,140	28,301
Michigan	179	10,395,142	170,870	4,633,596	27,118
Minnesota	150	4,162,651	76,885	1,931,371	25,120
Mississippi	94	2,239,209	41,388	934,333	22,575
Missouri	129	6,109,390	108,767	2,657,307	24,431
Montana	59	-	-	-	-
Nebraska	91	1,527,541	29,349	684,488	23,322
Nevada	19	-	-	-	-
New Hampshire	26	-	-	-	-
New Jersey	101	8,834,956	136,496	4,113,650	30,138
New Mexico	42	1,105,057	19,076	499,883	26,205
New York	244	23,851,395	374,942	12,174,406	32,470
North Carolina	124	6,436,550	106,292	2,803,250	26,373
North Dakota	52	800,852	16,199	357,528	22,071
Ohio	193	12,688,956	210,784	5,431,308	25,767
Oklahoma	113	2,650,428	50,015	1,140,240	22,798
Oregon	60	2,602,828	41,550	1,142,428	27,495
Pennsylvania	229	15,485,156	253,828	6,873,855	27,081
Rhode Island	16	1,071,723	19,162	564,723	29,471
South Carolina	62	3,194,874	49,207	1,296,697	26,352
South Dakota	62	-	-	-	-
Tennessee	97	5,185,221	84,446	2,129,066	25,212
Texas	311	12,876,951	197,134	5,404,542	27,416
Utah	33	-	-	-	-
Vermont	16	-	-	-	-
Virginia	89	5,352,328	87,453	2,301,323	26,315
Washington	99	4,649,823	71,148	2,080,876	29,247
West Virginia	51	1,916,620	32,415	807,972	24,926

[Continued]

★ 335 ★

General Medical and Surgical Hospitals by State, Non-Taxed: 1992
[Continued]

Area	Establish-ments	Revenues in $1,000	Employ-ment	Payroll in $1,000	Payroll per employee
Wisconsin	129	4,709,713	84,779	1,957,097	23,085
Wyoming	27	-	-	-	

Source: U.S. Department of Commerce. Bureau of the Census. *1992 Economic Census Report Series,* CD-ROM 1i, Washington, DC, October 1996. *Notes:* - means no data reported. 1. HS stands for total health service establishments, revenues, employment, or payroll.

★ 336 ★

Establishment Data

General Medical and Surgical Hospitals (Government), by Major Metro Area, Non-Taxed: 1992

Area	Establish-ments	Revenues in $1,000	Employ-ment	Payroll in $1,000	Payroll per employee
United States	1,739	64,213,954	1,044,580	31,076,135	29,750
Albany – Schenectady – Troy, NY MSA	1	-	-	-	-
Atlanta, GA MSA	13	961,683	16,248	411,140	25,304
Boston – Worcester – Lawrence, MA – NH – ME – CT CMSA	12	-	-	-	-
Buffalo – Niagara Falls, NY MSA	2	-	-	-	-
Chicago – Gary – Kenosha, IL – IN – WI CMSA	9	-	-	-	-
Cincinnati – Hamilton, OH – KY – IN CMSA	4	-	-	-	-
Cleveland – Akron, OH CMSA	3	-	-	-	-
Columbus, OH MSA	3	-	-	-	-
Dallas – Fort Worth, TX CMSA	10	-	-	-	-
Denver – Boulder – Greeley, CO CMSA	4	-	-	-	-
Detroit – Ann Arbor – Flint, MI CMSA	10	1,219,639	16,930	547,473	32,337
Hartford, CT MSA	2	-	-	-	-
Houston – Galveston – Brazoria, TX CMSA	13	-	-	-	-
Indianapolis, IN MSA	11	803,873	12,274	343,251	27,966
Kansas City, MO – KS MSA	11	530,676	11,283	272,832	24,181
Los Angeles – Riverside – Orange County, CA CMSA	30	-	-	-	-
Miami – Fort Lauderdale, FL CMSA	8	1,406,229	17,524	677,994	38,689
Milwaukee – Racine, WI CMSA	2	-	-	-	-
Minneapolis – St. Paul, MN – WI MSA	7	-	-	-	-
New York – Northern New Jersey – Long Island, NY – NJ – CT- CMSA	30	5,350,613	78,147	2,951,536	37,769

[Continued]

★ 336 ★

General Medical and Surgical Hospitals (Government), by Major Metro Area, Non-Taxed: 1992

[Continued]

Area	Establish-ments	Revenues in $1,000	Employ-ment	Payroll in $1,000	Payroll per employee
Philadelphia – Wilmington – Atlantic City, PA – NJ – DE – MD CMSA	6	-	-	-	-
Phoenix – Mesa, AZ MSA	6	-	-	-	-
Pittsburgh, PA MSA	2	-	-	-	-
Portland – Salem, OR – WA CMSA	3	-	-	-	-
Providence – Fall River – Warwick, RI – MA MSA	2	-	-	-	-
Sacramento – Yolo, CA CMSA	2	-	-	-	-
St. Louis, MO – IL MSA	6	-	-	-	-
San Diego, CA MSA	8	927,388	12,133	393,430	32,426
San Francisco – Oakland – San Jose, CA CMSA	25	3,164,751	39,535	1,667,762	42,184
Seattle – Tacoma – Bremerton, WA CMSA	13	1,150,171	18,121	588,964	32,502
Tampa – St. Petersburg – Clearwater, FL MSA	4	643,546	8,900	306,936	34,487
Washington – Baltimore, DC – MD – VA – WV CMSA	9	-	-	-	-

Source: U.S. Department of Commerce. Bureau of the Census. *1992 Economic Census Report Series,* CD-ROM 1i, Washington, DC, October 1996. *Notes:* - means no data reported. 1. HS stands for total health service establishments, revenues, employment, or payroll.

★ 337 ★

Establishment Data

General Medical and Surgical Hospitals (Government), by State, Non-Taxed: 1992

Area	Establish-ments	Revenues in $1,000	Employ-ment	Payroll in $1,000	Payroll per employee
United States	1,739	64,213,954	1,044,580	31,076,135	29,750
Alabama	59	2,269,898	36,203	938,676	25,928
Alaska	18	-	-	-	-
Arizona	19	686,066	12,585	392,709	31,205
Arkansas	31	628,486	12,584	311,768	24,775
California	125	10,004,432	130,766	4,584,382	35,058
Colorado	35	1,113,817	16,572	517,738	31,242
Connecticut	4	261,267	3,620	129,383	35,741
Delaware	2	-	-	-	-
District of Columbia	3	640,122	8,392	309,577	36,890
Florida	42	3,614,321	49,235	1,709,771	34,727
Georgia	84	2,828,685	51,071	1,293,055	25,319
Hawaii	8	312,940	5,216	188,428	36,125

[Continued]

★ 337 ★

General Medical and Surgical Hospitals (Government), by State, Non-Taxed: 1992
[Continued]

Area	Establish-ments	Revenues in $1,000	Employ-ment	Payroll in $1,000	Payroll per employee
Idaho	29	303,848	5,761	126,590	21,974
Illinois	45	1,746,178	32,378	990,296	30,585
Indiana	53	1,631,768	29,203	714,654	24,472
Iowa	66	928,737	20,049	423,639	21,130
Kansas	73	718,625	17,778	379,026	21,320
Kentucky	18	664,358	13,193	328,868	24,927
Louisiana	69	1,900,900	36,639	915,525	24,988
Maine	5	113,753	2,295	68,306	29,763
Maryland	6	428,084	6,031	252,787	41,915
Massachusetts	12	805,696	13,299	403,218	30,319
Michigan	42	1,795,175	27,569	815,704	29,588
Minnesota	67	1,177,421	23,209	595,226	25,646
Mississippi	66	1,354,029	25,723	608,265	23,647
Missouri	47	1,078,468	20,876	557,875	26,723
Montana	16	-	-	-	-
Nebraska	46	492,042	9,746	247,557	25,401
Nevada	13	-	-	-	-
New Hampshire	1	-	-	-	-
New Jersey	7	630,122	9,280	387,306	41,736
New Mexico	20	545,952	9,787	276,725	28,275
New York	40	5,475,042	82,431	2,979,777	36,149
North Carolina	38	2,037,926	33,032	920,102	27,855
North Dakota	5	106,037	1,812	65,263	36,017
Ohio	26	1,905,328	30,510	899,403	29,479
Oklahoma	72	1,078,824	21,617	516,409	23,889
Oregon	19	542,212	8,892	308,437	34,687
Pennsylvania	12	533,900	8,959	315,580	35,225
Rhode Island	3	128,862	2,155	69,001	32,019
South Carolina	36	1,493,972	23,636	654,258	27,681
South Dakota	18	-	-	-	-
Tennessee	38	1,573,466	27,843	700,552	25,161
Texas	183	4,854,545	80,798	2,348,264	29,063
Utah	11	-	-	-	-
Vermont	1	-	-	-	-
Virginia	14	1,633,902	25,643	802,548	31,297
Washington	50	1,550,742	25,401	793,220	31,228
West Virginia	15	327,890	5,931	176,624	29,780
Wisconsin	9	703,357	9,914	287,263	28,975
Wyoming	18	-	-	-	-

Source: U.S. Department of Commerce. Bureau of the Census. *1992 Economic Census Report Series,* CD-ROM 1i, Washington, DC, October 1996. *Notes:* - means no data reported. 1. HS stands for total health service establishments, revenues, employment, or payroll.

★ 338 ★

Establishment Data

General Medical and Surgical Hospitals (Nongovernment), by Major Metro Area, Non-Taxed: 1992

Area	Establish-ments	Revenues in $1,000	Employ-ment	Payroll in $1,000	Payroll per employee
United States	3,181	190,177,260	3,043,312	81,060,653	26,636
Albany – Schenectady – Troy, NY MSA	13	808,843	16,493	389,411	23,611
Atlanta, GA MSA	14	1,574,188	21,853	599,946	27,454
Boston – Worcester – Lawrence, MA – NH – ME – CT CMSA	69	6,278,245	99,198	2,794,463	28,171
Buffalo – Niagara Falls, NY MSA	19	919,430	19,426	455,131	23,429
Chicago – Gary – Kenosha, IL – IN – WI CMSA	90	-	-	-	-
Cincinnati – Hamilton, OH – KY – IN CMSA	20	-	-	-	-
Cleveland – Akron, OH CMSA	42	-	-	-	-
Columbus, OH MSA	11	1,087,590	15,901	424,669	26,707
Dallas – Fort Worth, TX CMSA	27	2,080,733	27,906	760,798	27,263
Denver – Boulder – Greeley, CO CMSA	18	1,464,604	21,957	582,443	26,527
Detroit – Ann Arbor – Flint, MI CMSA	59	5,518,039	88,456	2,491,012	28,161
Hartford, CT MSA	14	1,236,680	19,447	609,801	31,357
Houston – Galveston – Brazoria, TX CMSA	15	-	-	-	-
Indianapolis, IN MSA	11	1,326,847	20,960	555,373	26,497
Kansas City, MO – KS MSA	25	1,426,441	23,854	584,359	24,497
Los Angeles – Riverside – Orange County, CA CMSA	97	-	-	-	-
Miami – Fort Lauderdale, FL CMSA	14	1,328,753	19,115	519,786	27,193
Milwaukee – Racine, WI CMSA	22	-	-	-	-
Minneapolis – St. Paul, MN – WI MSA	28	1,895,695	31,026	832,565	26,834
New York – Northern New Jersey – Long Island, NY – NJ – CT- CMSA	180	22,098,635	322,507	10,793,708	33,468
Philadelphia – Wilmington – Atlantic City, PA – NJ – DE – MD CMSA	93	7,888,173	119,607	3,505,420	29,308
Phoenix – Mesa, AZ MSA	23	1,892,655	25,089	651,540	25,969
Pittsburgh, PA MSA	39	3,613,737	56,920	1,521,767	26,735
Portland – Salem, OR – WA CMSA	19	-	-	-	-
Providence – Fall River – Warwick, RI – MA MSA	14	1,060,627	18,660	539,946	28,936
Sacramento – Yolo, CA CMSA	15	-	-	-	-
St. Louis, MO – IL MSA	36	3,054,100	53,111	1,293,482	24,354
San Diego, CA MSA	15	1,249,275	17,354	520,723	30,006
San Francisco – Oakland – San Jose, CA CMSA	53	4,333,251	52,348	1,798,306	34,353
Seattle – Tacoma – Bremerton, WA CMSA	24	1,968,449	27,918	804,034	28,800
Tampa – St. Petersburg – Clearwater, FL MSA	14	1,049,144	16,192	408,700	25,241

[Continued]

★ 338 ★

General Medical and Surgical Hospitals (Nongovernment), by Major Metro Area, Non-Taxed: 1992

[Continued]

Area	Establish-ments	Revenues in $1,000	Employ-ment	Payroll in $1,000	Payroll per employee
Washington–Baltimore, DC–MD–VA–WV CMSA	62	6,429,564	103,452	2,849,393	27,543

Source: U.S. Department of Commerce. Bureau of the Census. *1992 Economic Census Report Series,* CD-ROM 1i, Washington, DC, October 1996. *Notes:* - means no data reported. 1. HS stands for total health service establishments, revenues, employment, or payroll.

★ 339 ★

Establishment Data

General Medical and Surgical Hospitals (Nongovernment), by State, Non-Taxed: 1992

Area	Establish-ments	Revenues in $1,000	Employ-ment	Payroll in $1,000	Payroll per employee
United States	3,181	190,177,260	3,043,312	81,060,653	26,636
Alabama	30	1,456,339	24,455	558,833	22,851
Alaska	7	308,928	3,705	132,154	35,669
Arizona	48	2,753,179	38,183	1,001,425	26,227
Arkansas	42	1,416,089	24,782	534,089	21,551
California	234	17,896,916	233,534	7,164,473	30,679
Colorado	38	2,105,440	33,759	848,713	25,140
Connecticut	35	3,525,345	54,627	1,742,797	31,904
Delaware	9	684,690	11,072	306,428	27,676
District of Columbia	9	1,546,323	21,450	706,358	32,930
Florida	97	7,305,429	111,092	2,885,872	25,977
Georgia	43	3,000,271	46,318	1,179,176	25,458
Hawaii	11	719,455	10,460	309,851	29,622
Idaho	10	379,748	6,081	146,585	24,105
Illinois	160	11,440,377	185,687	4,710,285	25,367
Indiana	63	4,302,023	71,926	1,747,100	24,290
Iowa	57	1,917,527	38,544	811,150	21,045
Kansas	61	1,440,887	26,045	612,699	23,525
Kentucky	68	2,563,965	44,886	1,009,896	22,499
Louisiana	30	2,222,681	34,503	868,557	25,173
Maine	35	1,092,812	20,241	501,461	24,775
Maryland	47	4,199,602	72,396	1,865,963	25,774
Massachusetts	83	6,973,983	111,967	3,141,922	28,061
Michigan	137	8,599,967	143,301	3,817,892	26,642
Minnesota	83	2,985,230	53,676	1,336,145	24,893
Mississippi	28	885,180	15,665	326,068	20,815
Missouri	82	5,030,922	87,891	2,099,432	23,887
Montana	43	711,784	12,704	290,471	22,865

[Continued]

★ 339 ★

General Medical and Surgical Hospitals (Nongovernment), by State, Non-Taxed: 1992

[Continued]

Area	Establish-ments	Revenues in $1,000	Employ-ment	Payroll in $1,000	Payroll per employee
Nebraska	45	1,035,499	19,603	436,931	22,289
Nevada	6	366,906	4,513	130,049	28,817
New Hampshire	25	981,655	15,494	411,577	26,564
New Jersey	94	8,204,834	127,216	3,726,344	29,291
New Mexico	22	559,105	9,289	223,158	24,024
New York	204	18,376,353	292,511	9,194,629	31,433
North Carolina	86	4,398,624	73,260	1,883,148	25,705
North Dakota	47	694,815	14,387	292,265	20,315
Ohio	167	10,783,628	180,274	4,531,905	25,139
Oklahoma	41	1,571,604	28,398	623,831	21,967
Oregon	41	2,060,616	32,658	833,991	25,537
Pennsylvania	217	14,951,256	244,869	6,558,275	26,783
Rhode Island	13	942,861	17,007	495,722	29,148
South Carolina	26	1,700,902	25,571	642,439	25,124
South Dakota	44	654,551	13,298	272,444	20,488
Tennessee	59	3,611,755	56,603	1,428,514	25,237
Texas	128	8,022,406	116,336	3,056,278	26,271
Utah	22	-	-	-	-
Vermont	15	460,064	8,478	205,394	24,227
Virginia	75	3,718,426	61,810	1,498,775	24,248
Washington	49	3,099,081	45,747	1,287,656	28,147
West Virginia	36	1,588,730	26,484	631,348	23,839
Wisconsin	120	4,006,356	74,865	1,669,834	22,305
Wyoming	9	-	-	-	-

Source: U.S. Department of Commerce. Bureau of the Census. *1992 Economic Census Report Series,* CD-ROM 1i, Washington, DC, October 1996. *Notes:* - means no data reported. 1. HS stands for total health service establishments, revenues, employment, or payroll.

★ 340 ★

Establishment Data

General Medical Clinics by Major Metro Area: 1992

Area	Establishments		Revenues		Employment		Payroll		
	Number	% of HS[1] in area	Total ($000)	% of HS[1] in area	Number	% of HS[1] in area	Total ($000)	% of HS[1] in area	Payroll per employee
United States	4,736	1.07	12,590,420	4.21	125,343	2.82	5,072,094	3.93	40,466
Albany – Schenectady – Troy, NY MSA	10	0.76	13,760	1.70	210	1.59	9,597	2.64	45,700
Albuquerque, NM MSA	21	1.97	-	-	-	-	-	-	-
Allentown – Bethlehem – Easton, PA MSA	7	0.57	12,427	1.81	96	1.03	4,487	1.47	46,740
Anchorage, AK MSA	2	0.41	-	-	-	-	-	-	-
Appleton – Oshkosh – Neenah, WI MSA	7	1.34	12,945	3.58	90	1.57	9,171	5.05	101,900
Atlanta, GA MSA	72	1.18	107,463	2.23	1,390	2.32	37,258	1.85	26,804

[Continued]

★ 340 ★

General Medical Clinics by Major Metro Area: 1992
[Continued]

Area	Establishments		Revenues		Employment		Payroll		
	Number	% of HS[1] in area	Total ($000)	% of HS[1] in area	Number	% of HS[1] in area	Total ($000)	% of HS[1] in area	Payroll per employee
Augusta – Aiken, GA – SC MSA	7	0.98	14,054	2.19	258	2.79	7,948	2.82	30,806
Austin – San Marcos, TX MSA	55	3.50	80,646	6.74	915	4.93	31,390	6.47	34,306
Bakersfield, CA MSA	16	2.11	26,598	4.88	354	4.34	12,069	5.51	34,093
Baton Rouge, LA MSA	15	1.69	14,671	1.98	185	1.68	6,091	2.01	32,924
Beaumont – Port Arthur, TX MSA	7	0.97	9,469	1.65	60	0.59	3,547	1.47	59,117
Birmingham, AL MSA	26	1.89	23,904	1.58	458	2.27	7,134	1.11	15,576
Boise City, ID MSA	4	0.67	-	-	-	-	-	-	-
Boston – Worcester – Lawrence, MA – NH – ME – CT CMSA	90	0.92	84,205	1.19	853	0.74	43,192	1.33	50,635
Buffalo – Niagara Falls, NY MSA	15	0.75	7,310	0.66	72	0.33	3,279	0.66	45,542
Canton – Massillon, OH MSA	5	0.72	1,880	0.46	15	0.21	1,167	0.55	77,800
Charleston – North Charleston, SC MSA	12	1.47	13,647	2.31	230	2.52	4,422	1.89	19,226
Charlotte – Gastonia – Rock Hill, NC – SC MSA	39	2.43	81,577	5.83	809	3.97	24,440	3.72	30,210
Chattanooga, TN – GA MSA	10	1.31	11,953	1.67	148	1.48	5,621	1.84	37,980
Chicago – Gary – Kenosha, IL – IN – WI CMSA	151	1.04	-	-	-	-	-	-	-
Cincinnati – Hamilton, OH – KY – IN CMSA	20	0.64	-	-	-	-	-	-	-
Cleveland – Akron, OH CMSA	72	1.34	87,766	2.70	1,003	1.95	27,451	1.79	27,369
Colorado Springs, CO MSA	12	1.35	14,268	3.21	191	2.89	5,717	2.84	29,932
Columbia, SC MSA	16	2.15	10,974	2.27	127	1.77	4,948	2.06	38,961
Columbus, OH MSA	22	0.90	30,888	1.76	342	1.22	13,675	1.68	39,985
Corpus Christi, TX MSA	6	0.80	8,818	1.53	84	0.99	2,274	1.01	27,071
Dallas – Fort Worth, TX CMSA	82	0.99	186,269	2.85	1,579	1.83	73,066	2.76	46,274
Davenport – Moline – Rock Island, IA – IL MSA	5	0.74	4,350	1.20	34	0.57	1,636	1.03	48,118
Dayton – Springfield, OH MSA	31	1.88	28,942	2.53	340	1.92	11,986	2.13	35,253
Daytona Beach, FL MSA	11	1.49	-	-	-	-	-	-	-
Denver – Boulder – Greeley, CO CMSA	47	1.08	-	-	-	-	-	-	-
Des Moines, IA MSA	5	0.68	4,064	0.80	48	0.67	1,463	0.55	30,479
Detroit – Ann Arbor – Flint, MI CMSA	89	0.94	-	-	-	-	-	-	-
El Paso, TX MSA	12	1.51	23,723	3.05	223	2.08	6,775	2.32	30,381
Eugene – Springfield, OR MSA	8	1.37	14,927	4.45	102	1.89	3,234	2.08	31,706
Fort Myers – Cape Coral, FL MSA	9	1.26	7,290	1.10	116	1.41	4,036	1.30	34,793
Fort Pierce – Port St. Lucie, FL MSA	4	0.77	1,910	0.43	32	0.52	979	0.52	30,594
Fort Wayne, IN MSA	18	2.57	31,546	5.70	496	5.26	15,349	6.00	30,946
Fresno, CA MSA	22	1.49	80,718	9.29	782	6.35	36,250	9.77	46,355
Grand Rapids – Muskegon – Holland, MI MSA	20	1.31	25,338	2.82	275	1.92	6,349	1.47	23,087
Greensboro – Winston-Salem – High Point, NC MSA	12	0.80	80,240	6.76	566	3.31	22,066	4.18	38,986
Greenville – Spartanburg – Anderson, SC MSA	12	1.02	15,255	1.96	120	1.00	7,263	1.93	60,525
Harrisburg – Lebanon – Carlisle, PA MSA	11	1.11	18,940	2.90	197	2.07	9,048	2.93	45,929
Hartford, CT MSA	22	0.97	-	-	-	-	-	-	-
Honolulu, HI MSA	31	1.84	68,320	6.58	514	4.27	49,748	10.42	96,786
Houston – Galveston – Brazoria, TX CMSA	73	1.03	-	-	-	-	-	-	-
Huntsville, AL MSA	3	0.56	-	-	-	-	-	-	-
Indianapolis, IN MSA	23	0.90	37,260	1.86	254	0.79	15,484	1.65	60,961
Jackson, MS MSA	9	1.41	13,002	2.57	152	2.11	3,913	1.87	25,743
Jacksonville, FL MSA	44	2.48	125,068	9.57	1,728	10.09	67,222	12.08	38,902
Johnson City – Kingsport – Bristol, TN – VA MSA	6	0.87	6,538	1.07	56	0.57	3,653	1.34	65,232

[Continued]

315

★ 340 ★

General Medical Clinics by Major Metro Area: 1992
[Continued]

Area	Establishments		Revenues		Employment		Payroll		
	Number	% of HS[1] in area	Total ($000)	% of HS[1] in area	Number	% of HS[1] in area	Total ($000)	% of HS[1] in area	Payroll per employee
Kalamazoo – Battle Creek, MI MSA	2	0.27	-	-	-	-	-	-	-
Kansas City, MO – KS MSA	70	2.45	87,643	4.01	983	2.91	41,262	4.17	41,976
Knoxville, TN MSA	9	0.75	10,763	1.33	166	1.56	3,603	0.92	21,705
Lafayette, LA MSA	7	1.10	8,720	1.94	52	0.74	2,536	1.38	48,769
Lakeland – Winter Haven, FL MSA	9	1.85	27,556	6.86	326	5.13	6,387	3.81	19,592
Lancaster, PA MSA	4	0.66	3,590	0.94	86	1.36	2,792	1.46	32,465
Lansing – East Lansing, MI MSA	5	0.68	11,080	2.77	335	5.32	5,384	2.83	16,072
Las Vegas, NV – AZ MSA	31	1.99	92,747	5.49	961	5.21	33,033	4.85	34,374
Lexington, KY MSA	8	0.99	7,223	1.22	129	1.43	3,673	1.33	28,473
Little Rock – North Little Rock, AR MSA	13	1.25	11,317	1.46	98	0.88	3,517	0.96	35,888
Los Angeles – Riverside – Orange County, CA CMSA	518	1.69	2,608,691	11.11	25,599	9.22	982,969	10.75	38,399
Louisville, KY – IN MSA	13	0.76	18,897	1.13	199	0.77	8,546	1.20	42,945
Macon, GA MSA	4	0.74	-	-	-	-	-	-	-
Madison, WI MSA	3	0.58	3,847	0.74	30	0.42	2,010	0.86	67,000
Melbourne – Titusville – Palm Bay, FL MSA	10	1.23	11,178	2.06	110	1.51	3,546	1.42	32,236
Memphis, TN – AR – MS MSA	27	1.64	27,162	2.19	331	2.03	9,119	1.70	27,550
Miami – Fort Lauderdale, FL CMSA	145	1.59	344,285	5.03	2,883	3.32	93,749	3.34	32,518
Milwaukee – Racine, WI CMSA	33	1.09	38,721	1.90	433	1.27	20,902	2.01	48,273
Minneapolis – St. Paul, MN – WI MSA	28	0.75	53,340	1.84	765	1.53	27,180	1.81	35,529
Mobile, AL MSA	3	0.47	7,820	1.39	211	2.21	3,154	1.20	14,948
Modesto, CA MSA	8	1.19	12,878	2.13	83	1.04	3,015	1.22	36,325
Montgomery, AL MSA	2	0.41	-	-	-	-	-	-	-
Nashville, TN MSA	31	1.60	70,816	3.82	705	2.79	23,501	3.03	33,335
New Orleans, LA MSA	33	1.36	30,179	1.38	419	1.41	10,097	1.20	24,098
New York – Northern New Jersey – Long Island, NY – NJ – CT- CMSA	224	0.55	-	-	-	-	-	-	-
Norfolk – Virginia Beach – Newport News, VA – NC MSA	14	0.62	23,002	1.70	389	1.78	10,563	1.63	27,154
Oklahoma City, OK MSA	15	0.76	27,378	2.11	436	2.23	13,555	2.42	31,089
Omaha, NE – IA MSA	10	0.99	22,655	2.76	273	2.19	9,552	2.56	34,989
Orlando, FL MSA	47	1.86	115,891	6.09	929	3.68	37,632	4.60	40,508
Pensacola, FL MSA	4	0.76	-	-	-	-	-	-	-
Peoria – Pekin, IL MSA	5	0.98	-	-	-	-	-	-	-
Philadelphia – Wilmington – Atlantic City, PA – NJ – DE – MD CMSA	80	0.69	183,076	2.51	1,965	1.97	77,461	2.38	39,420
Phoenix – Mesa, AZ MSA	70	1.46	332,822	10.58	2,700	7.01	115,655	8.42	42,835
Pittsburgh, PA MSA	24	0.50	31,242	1.15	266	0.70	11,697	0.94	43,974
Portland, ME MSA	6	1.11	2,853	0.74	42	0.71	1,538	0.86	36,619
Portland – Salem, OR – WA CMSA	34	0.96	-	-	-	-	-	-	-
Providence – Fall River – Warwick, RI – MA MSA	12	0.58	15,064	1.28	234	1.18	5,434	1.03	23,222
Raleigh – Durham – Chapel Hill, NC MSA	23	1.60	60,120	4.95	368	2.14	20,085	3.98	54,579
Reno, NV MSA	12	1.80	12,955	2.49	121	2.03	3,921	1.80	32,405
Richmond – Petersburg, VA MSA	12	0.75	31,600	2.02	469	2.11	7,794	1.18	16,618
Rochester, NY MSA	2	0.13	-	-	-	-	-	-	-
Rockford, IL MSA	5	1.05	-	-	-	-	-	-	-
Sacramento – Yolo, CA CMSA	19	0.66	-	-	-	-	-	-	-
Saginaw – Bay City – Midland, MI MSA	6	0.88	6,418	1.68	93	1.45	3,582	1.81	38,516
St. Louis, MO – IL MSA	67	1.51	265,016	9.26	1,857	4.26	51,189	4.12	27,565
Salinas, CA MSA	2	0.33	-	-	-	-	-	-	-
Salt Lake City – Ogden, UT MSA	21	1.02	-	-	-	-	-	-	-
San Antonio, TX MSA	19	0.72	27,211	1.51	310	1.08	8,292	1.11	26,748
San Diego, CA MSA	87	1.77	372,707	11.42	3,714	8.92	181,196	13.46	48,787

[Continued]

★ 340 ★

General Medical Clinics by Major Metro Area: 1992

[Continued]

Area	Establishments		Revenues		Employment		Payroll		
	Number	% of HS[1] in area	Total ($000)	% of HS[1] in area	Number	% of HS[1] in area	Total ($000)	% of HS[1] in area	Payroll per employee
San Francisco – Oakland – San Jose, CA CMSA	129	0.92	-	-	-	-	-	-	-
Santa Barbara – Santa Maria – Lompoc, CA MSA	13	1.56	-	-	-	-	-	-	-
Sarasota – Bradenton, FL MSA	10	0.81	8,798	0.90	113	0.78	2,058	0.50	18,212
Scranton – Wilkes-Barre – Hazleton, PA MSA	7	0.61	3,703	0.59	73	0.69	1,380	0.53	18,904
Seattle – Tacoma – Bremerton, WA CMSA	75	1.24	102,998	2.89	695	1.28	27,074	1.74	38,955
Shreveport – Bossier City, LA MSA	6	0.93	5,157	0.90	79	0.93	1,546	0.67	19,570
Spokane, WA MSA	3	0.41	2,791	0.55	26	0.33	1,668	0.71	64,154
Springfield, MO MSA	8	1.74	-	-	-	-	-	-	-
Springfield, MA MSA	8	0.88	17,972	2.69	127	1.05	7,612	2.37	59,937
Stockton – Lodi, CA MSA	6	0.72	-	-	-	-	-	-	-
Syracuse, NY MSA	6	0.55	9,643	1.40	95	0.97	3,388	1.08	35,663
Tallahassee, FL MSA	2	0.50	-	-	-	-	-	-	-
Tampa – St. Petersburg – Clearwater, FL MSA	64	1.30	132,775	3.05	1,598	2.61	38,450	2.23	24,061
Toledo, OH MSA	22	1.95	60,253	7.74	667	5.31	36,207	9.13	54,283
Tucson, AZ MSA	16	1.27	44,730	4.53	468	3.44	17,946	4.46	38,346
Tulsa, OK MSA	21	1.54	26,490	2.79	393	2.75	14,797	3.48	37,651
Washington – Baltimore, DC – MD – VA – WV CMSA	143	1.11	-	-	-	-	-	-	-
West Palm Beach – Boca Raton, FL MSA	21	0.78	58,388	2.95	454	1.85	13,856	1.64	30,520
Wichita, KS MSA	6	0.78	14,554	1.50	104	0.77	3,421	0.82	32,894
Youngstown – Warren, OH MSA	3	0.25	5,242	0.75	75	0.61	1,445	0.45	19,267

Source: U.S. Department of Commerce. Bureau of the Census. *1992 Economic Census Report Series,* CD-ROM 1i, Washington, DC, October 1996. *Notes:* - means no data reported. 1. HS stands for total health service establishments, revenues, employment, or payroll.

★ 341 ★

Establishment Data

General Medical Clinics by Major Metro Area, Non-Taxed: 1992

Area	Establish-ments	Revenues in $1,000	Employ-ment	Payroll in $1,000	Payroll per employee
United States	3,187	16,548,253	156,336	5,264,666	33,675
Albany – Schenectady – Troy, NY MSA	18	-	-	-	-
Atlanta, GA MSA	25	55,129	1,091	26,242	24,053
Boston – Worcester – Lawrence, MA – NH – ME – CT CMSA	100	-	-	-	-
Buffalo – Niagara Falls, NY MSA	16	-	-	-	-
Chicago – Gary – Kenosha, IL – IN – WI CMSA	75	337,209	3,051	101,263	33,190
Cincinnati – Hamilton, OH – KY – IN CMSA	40	-	-	-	-
Cleveland – Akron, OH CMSA	48	-	-	-	-
Columbus, OH MSA	18	26,310	326	11,307	34,684

[Continued]

★ 341 ★

General Medical Clinics by Major Metro Area, Non-Taxed: 1992
[Continued]

Area	Establish-ments	Revenues in $1,000	Employ-ment	Payroll in $1,000	Payroll per employee
Dallas–Fort Worth, TX CMSA	26	-	-	-	-
Denver–Boulder–Greeley, CO CMSA	35	-	-	-	-
Detroit–Ann Arbor–Flint, MI CMSA	93	-	-	-	-
Hartford, CT MSA	13	31,134	488	14,236	29,172
Houston–Galveston–Brazoria, TX CMSA	10	5,980	114	2,272	19,930
Indianapolis, IN MSA	22	-	-	-	-
Kansas City, MO–KS MSA	30	-	-	-	-
Los Angeles–Riverside–Orange County, CA CMSA	146	-	-	-	-
Miami–Fort Lauderdale, FL CMSA	18	-	-	-	-
Milwaukee–Racine, WI CMSA	19	-	-	-	-
Minneapolis–St. Paul, MN–WI MSA	67	-	-	-	-
New York–Northern New Jersey–Long Island, NY–NJ–CT- CMSA	132	-	-	-	-
Philadelphia–Wilmington–Atlantic City, PA–NJ–DE–MD CMSA	60	-	-	-	-
Phoenix–Mesa, AZ MSA	26	43,911	676	16,897	24,996
Pittsburgh, PA MSA	43	154,284	1,064	37,097	34,866
Portland–Salem, OR–WA CMSA	34	-	-	-	-
Providence–Fall River–Warwick, RI–MA MSA	25	79,726	785	27,585	35,140
Sacramento–Yolo, CA CMSA	24	-	-	-	-
St. Louis, MO–IL MSA	21	68,894	707	26,096	36,911
San Diego, CA MSA	65	832,029	5,262	156,545	29,750
San Francisco–Oakland–San Jose, CA CMSA	87	-	-	-	-
Seattle–Tacoma–Bremerton, WA CMSA	74	-	-	-	-
Tampa–St. Petersburg–Clearwater, FL MSA	10	-	-	-	-
Washington–Baltimore, DC–MD–VA–WV CMSA	83	-	-	-	-

Source: U.S. Department of Commerce. Bureau of the Census. *1992 Economic Census Report Series,* CD-ROM 1i, Washington, DC, October 1996. *Notes:* - means no data reported. 1. HS stands for total health service establishments, revenues, employment, or payroll.

★ 342 ★

Establishment Data

General Medical Clinics by State: 1992

Area	Establishments		Revenues		Employment		Payroll		
	Number	% of HS[1] in area	Total ($000)	% of HS[1] in area	Number	% of HS[1] in area	Total ($000)	% of HS[1] in area	Payroll per employee
United States	4,736	1.07	12,590,420	4.21	125,343	2.82	5,072,094	3.93	40,466
Alabama	57	1.03	68,005	1.38	1,150	1.49	19,457	0.92	16,919
Alaska	6	0.70	11,074	2.04	115	2.03	3,176	1.46	27,617
Arizona	102	1.44	387,401	8.48	3,368	5.73	137,960	7.07	40,962
Arkansas	46	1.29	114,221	4.69	1,292	3.03	44,305	4.16	34,292
California	849	1.38	5,527,687	12.86	51,561	9.62	2,399,928	13.92	46,545
Colorado	75	1.07	107,263	2.87	1,210	2.19	38,670	2.36	31,959
Connecticut	43	0.65	68,242	1.39	858	1.19	26,862	1.14	31,308
Delaware	15	1.25	36,233	4.59	444	3.82	14,292	3.93	32,189
District of Columbia	10	0.73	6,863	0.86	46	0.47	3,280	0.95	71,304
Florida	412	1.39	940,627	4.04	9,393	2.98	301,436	3.13	32,092
Georgia	115	1.04	165,753	1.92	2,285	1.89	58,228	1.59	25,483
Hawaii	47	2.11	82,083	6.26	676	4.32	59,582	10.11	88,139
Idaho	12	0.69	10,752	1.09	157	0.93	2,922	0.70	18,611
Illinois	189	1.01	324,790	2.63	3,907	2.08	117,635	2.10	30,109
Indiana	88	1.01	109,231	1.79	1,147	1.08	46,593	1.70	40,622
Iowa	64	1.53	62,933	2.69	777	1.73	29,326	2.64	37,743
Kansas	68	1.76	97,394	3.20	1,219	2.28	37,150	2.81	30,476
Kentucky	39	0.71	44,107	1.07	539	0.80	21,036	1.18	39,028
Louisiana	80	1.17	103,070	1.86	1,136	1.32	37,867	1.74	33,334
Maine	12	0.56	8,519	0.72	114	0.52	4,364	0.82	38,281
Maryland	108	1.18	221,621	3.93	2,894	3.62	94,628	3.79	32,698
Massachusetts	90	0.85	84,872	1.11	812	0.64	36,794	1.04	45,313
Michigan	137	0.87	280,526	3.22	2,235	1.59	70,724	1.72	31,644
Minnesota	46	0.78	67,920	1.65	1,025	1.35	33,709	1.62	32,887
Mississippi	39	1.26	33,610	1.61	359	0.97	11,574	1.32	32,240
Missouri	140	1.66	357,556	6.51	3,085	3.25	111,022	4.54	35,988
Montana	11	0.74	8,338	1.28	111	1.03	2,341	0.90	21,090
Nebraska	23	0.98	30,534	1.96	430	1.59	13,195	1.84	30,686
Nevada	44	1.90	105,793	4.70	1,092	4.32	37,044	4.04	33,923
New Hampshire	30	1.63	70,825	5.96	558	2.91	51,177	9.43	91,715
New Jersey	118	0.72	266,094	2.56	2,513	1.97	109,527	2.48	43,584
New Mexico	30	1.25	-	-	-	-	-	-	-
New York	178	0.55	283,635	1.43	3,119	1.12	124,337	1.51	39,864
North Carolina	103	1.16	252,045	3.79	2,049	1.91	77,750	2.61	37,945
North Dakota	5	0.65	7,037	1.12	69	0.75	1,385	0.46	20,072
Ohio	194	1.05	270,266	2.32	3,083	1.54	115,321	2.07	37,405
Oklahoma	49	0.92	60,284	1.84	911	1.54	31,025	2.20	34,056
Oregon	61	1.08	83,132	2.81	1,110	2.31	34,950	2.69	31,486
Pennsylvania	136	0.63	190,956	1.51	1,835	1.00	80,221	1.42	43,717
Rhode Island	12	0.63	13,055	1.23	210	1.16	4,992	1.07	23,771
South Carolina	65	1.40	57,630	1.84	728	1.45	24,631	1.77	33,834
South Dakota	14	1.45	12,141	2.15	136	1.49	3,275	1.26	24,081
Tennessee	93	1.13	134,079	1.99	1,549	1.54	47,300	1.65	30,536
Texas	341	1.14	715,142	3.12	5,808	1.68	267,014	2.90	45,973

[Continued]

★ 342 ★

General Medical Clinics by State: 1992
[Continued]

Area	Establishments		Revenues		Employment		Payroll		
	Number	% of HS[1] in area	Total ($000)	% of HS[1] in area	Number	% of HS[1] in area	Total ($000)	% of HS[1] in area	Payroll per employee
Utah	29	0.95	153,170	8.29	1,900	6.15	45,450	6.02	23,921
Vermont	7	0.75	4,147	1.02	68	0.90	2,732	1.66	40,176
Virginia	75	0.77	119,967	1.80	1,668	1.63	37,956	1.25	22,755
Washington	104	1.13	140,932	2.61	1,071	1.22	44,992	1.89	42,009
West Virginia	32	1.19	40,110	2.24	730	2.53	16,609	2.36	22,752
Wisconsin	88	1.22	118,253	2.50	1,416	1.67	67,030	2.86	47,338
Wyoming	5	0.70	-	-	-	-	-	-	-

Source: U.S. Department of Commerce. Bureau of the Census. *1992 Economic Census Report Series,* CD-ROM 1i, Washington, DC, October 1996. *Notes:* - means no data reported. 1. HS stands for total health service establishments, revenues, employment, or payroll.

★ 343 ★

Establishment Data

General Medical Clinics by State, Non-Taxed: 1992

Area	Establish- ments	Revenues in $1,000	Employ- ment	Payroll in $1,000	Payroll per employee
United States	3,187	16,548,253	156,336	5,264,666	33,675
Alabama	79	-	-	-	-
Alaska	11	12,517	268	6,435	24,011
Arizona	54	-	-	-	-
Arkansas	20	-	-	-	-
California	427	4,641,767	19,342	605,233	31,291
Colorado	59	345,725	2,629	70,176	26,693
Connecticut	34	156,530	1,527	48,650	31,860
Delaware	4	2,721	59	1,632	27,661
District of Columbia	17	-	-	-	-
Florida	115	-	-	-	-
Georgia	45	-	-	-	-
Hawaii	24	-	-	-	-
Idaho	19	12,277	271	6,059	22,358
Illinois	88	355,690	3,352	107,401	32,041
Indiana	68	-	-	-	-
Iowa	18	-	-	-	-
Kansas	19	-	-	-	-
Kentucky	36	-	-	-	-
Louisiana	17	23,212	382	9,258	24,236
Maine	40	-	-	-	-
Maryland	52	385,700	3,800	129,181	33,995
Massachusetts	120	1,058,223	11,844	516,052	43,571
Michigan	149	755,483	7,648	264,585	34,595

[Continued]

★ 343 ★

General Medical Clinics by State, Non-Taxed: 1992

[Continued]

Area	Establish-ments	Revenues in $1,000	Employ-ment	Payroll in $1,000	Payroll per employee
Minnesota	93	-	-	-	-
Mississippi	45	43,767	811	17,579	21,676
Missouri	51	157,278	1,832	63,255	34,528
Montana	13	6,167	202	2,840	14,059
Nebraska	18	35,134	628	20,499	32,642
Nevada	3	-	-	-	-
New Hampshire	15	-	-	-	-
New Jersey	32	-	-	-	-
New Mexico	40	32,360	811	14,747	18,184
New York	225	1,187,496	15,101	521,097	34,507
North Carolina	76	-	-	-	-
North Dakota	9	5,045	91	2,691	29,571
Ohio	143	-	-	-	-
Oklahoma	16	-	-	-	-
Oregon	44	-	-	-	-
Pennsylvania	234	-	-	-	-
Rhode Island	23	-	-	-	-
South Carolina	39	-	-	-	-
South Dakota	13	9,620	241	5,607	23,266
Tennessee	31	21,304	420	11,654	27,748
Texas	115	-	-	-	-
Utah	22	-	-	-	-
Vermont	26	-	-	-	-
Virginia	74	-	-	-	-
Washington	110	-	-	-	-
West Virginia	74	-	-	-	-
Wisconsin	83	-	-	-	-
Wyoming	5	-	-	-	-

Source: U.S. Department of Commerce. Bureau of the Census. *1992 Economic Census Report Series,* CD-ROM 1i, Washington, DC, October 1996. *Notes:* - means no data reported. 1. HS stands for total health service establishments, revenues, employment, or payroll.

★ 344 ★

Establishment Data

Home Health Care Services Establishments by Major Metro Area: 1992

Area	Establishments		Revenues		Employment		Payroll		
	Number	% of HS[1] in area	Total ($000)	% of HS[1] in area	Number	% of HS[1] in area	Total ($000)	% of HS[1] in area	Payroll per employee
United States	8,045	1.82	10,413,844	3.48	341,889	7.68	4,853,090	3.76	14,195
Albany – Schenectady – Troy, NY MSA	36	2.75	54,893	6.80	2,132	16.14	26,899	7.40	12,617
Albuquerque, NM MSA	18	1.69	13,442	1.61	444	3.51	5,352	1.42	12,054
Allentown – Bethlehem – Easton, PA MSA	18	1.45	16,191	2.35	756	8.09	9,617	3.14	12,721

[Continued]

★ 344 ★

Home Health Care Services Establishments by Major Metro Area: 1992

[Continued]

Area	Establishments		Revenues		Employment		Payroll		
	Number	% of HS[1] in area	Total ($000)	% of HS[1] in area	Number	% of HS[1] in area	Total ($000)	% of HS[1] in area	Payroll per employee
Anchorage, AK MSA	3	0.62	-	-	-	-	-	-	-
Appleton – Oshkosh – Neenah, WI MSA	11	2.11	7,035	1.94	350	6.11	3,965	2.18	11,329
Atlanta, GA MSA	152	2.49	233,609	4.85	4,246	7.09	95,217	4.72	22,425
Augusta – Aiken, GA – SC MSA	20	2.81	24,291	3.78	907	9.80	12,966	4.60	14,295
Austin – San Marcos, TX MSA	40	2.55	43,413	3.63	1,446	7.78	20,453	4.21	14,145
Bakersfield, CA MSA	11	1.45	16,678	3.06	442	5.41	8,423	3.84	19,057
Baton Rouge, LA MSA	39	4.41	41,181	5.55	1,178	10.68	21,272	7.01	18,058
Beaumont – Port Arthur, TX MSA	27	3.73	50,323	8.74	2,659	26.01	29,816	12.38	11,213
Birmingham, AL MSA	37	2.69	55,852	3.70	2,076	10.28	26,215	4.09	12,628
Boise City, ID MSA	4	0.67	3,435	0.91	234	4.01	2,342	1.38	10,009
Boston – Worcester – Lawrence, MA – NH – ME – CT CMSA	159	1.63	268,282	3.79	9,008	7.82	120,840	3.71	13,415
Buffalo – Niagara Falls, NY MSA	40	2.01	113,048	10.22	5,247	24.23	62,887	12.60	11,985
Canton – Massillon, OH MSA	9	1.30	4,742	1.15	193	2.71	2,660	1.26	13,782
Charleston – North Charleston, SC MSA	9	1.10	7,886	1.33	220	2.41	3,929	1.68	17,859
Charlotte – Gastonia – Rock Hill, NC – SC MSA	43	2.68	72,125	5.16	2,247	11.04	37,837	5.75	16,839
Chattanooga, TN – GA MSA	28	3.68	59,089	8.24	1,233	12.36	24,556	8.03	19,916
Chicago – Gary – Kenosha, IL – IN – WI CMSA	215	1.48	-	-	-	-	-	-	-
Cincinnati – Hamilton, OH – KY – IN CMSA	66	2.10	-	-	-	-	-	-	-
Cleveland – Akron, OH CMSA	96	1.79	120,194	3.69	3,591	7.00	52,515	3.42	14,624
Colorado Springs, CO MSA	12	1.35	13,870	3.12	468	7.08	6,219	3.09	13,288
Columbia, SC MSA	14	1.88	20,670	4.28	648	9.03	8,308	3.46	12,821
Columbus, OH MSA	46	1.89	58,419	3.32	1,991	7.07	22,328	2.75	11,214
Corpus Christi, TX MSA	13	1.73	14,838	2.57	757	8.95	5,592	2.48	7,387
Dallas – Fort Worth, TX CMSA	151	1.82	264,028	4.05	7,504	8.72	103,668	3.91	13,815
Davenport – Moline – Rock Island, IA – IL MSA	11	1.62	10,651	2.95	399	6.65	5,088	3.22	12,752
Dayton – Springfield, OH MSA	23	1.40	25,427	2.22	1,265	7.14	13,845	2.46	10,945
Daytona Beach, FL MSA	18	2.43	29,742	5.56	705	8.42	10,804	4.91	15,325
Denver – Boulder – Greeley, CO CMSA	72	1.65	-	-	-	-	-	-	-
Des Moines, IA MSA	11	1.49	9,675	1.90	478	6.72	5,649	2.13	11,818
Detroit – Ann Arbor – Flint, MI CMSA	134	1.42	132,890	2.44	4,631	5.51	66,476	2.61	14,355
El Paso, TX MSA	26	3.27	23,891	3.08	1,590	14.84	13,110	4.49	8,245
Eugene – Springfield, OR MSA	10	1.71	4,251	1.27	196	3.62	2,131	1.37	10,872
Fort Myers – Cape Coral, FL MSA	14	1.96	15,295	2.30	460	5.59	7,871	2.54	17,111
Fort Pierce – Port St. Lucie, FL MSA	14	2.70	-	-	-	-	-	-	-
Fort Wayne, IN MSA	14	2.00	18,656	3.37	587	6.22	9,902	3.87	16,869
Fresno, CA MSA	20	1.35	18,015	2.07	526	4.27	7,992	2.15	15,194
Grand Rapids – Muskegon – Holland, MI MSA	28	1.84	20,367	2.27	756	5.27	9,559	2.21	12,644
Greensboro – Winston-Salem – High Point, NC MSA	33	2.19	30,467	2.57	1,088	6.37	16,056	3.04	14,757
Greenville – Spartanburg – Anderson, SC MSA	15	1.28	13,395	1.72	475	3.96	8,093	2.15	17,038
Harrisburg – Lebanon – Carlisle, PA MSA	21	2.13	14,972	2.29	426	4.47	5,969	1.93	14,012
Hartford, CT MSA	30	1.32	49,484	2.81	1,908	6.99	27,136	3.19	14,222
Honolulu, HI MSA	2	0.12	-	-	-	-	-	-	-
Houston – Galveston – Brazoria, TX CMSA	108	1.53	-	-	-	-	-	-	-
Huntsville, AL MSA	16	3.00	13,261	2.90	458	7.00	7,110	3.72	15,524
Indianapolis, IN MSA	45	1.77	77,276	3.85	2,028	6.30	32,699	3.47	16,124
Jackson, MS MSA	17	2.67	27,745	5.48	781	10.83	13,414	6.41	17,175

[Continued]

★ 344 ★

Home Health Care Services Establishments by Major Metro Area: 1992

[Continued]

Area	Establishments		Revenues		Employment		Payroll		
	Number	% of HS[1] in area	Total ($000)	% of HS[1] in area	Number	% of HS[1] in area	Total ($000)	% of HS[1] in area	Payroll per employee
Jacksonville, FL MSA	31	1.75	24,229	1.85	744	4.35	11,227	2.02	15,090
Johnson City – Kingsport – Bristol, TN – VA MSA	23	3.33	34,648	5.67	795	8.07	14,833	5.45	18,658
Kalamazoo – Battle Creek, MI MSA	16	2.17	15,332	3.52	773	10.81	8,246	3.84	10,668
Kansas City, MO – KS MSA	59	2.07	81,112	3.71	2,344	6.94	32,814	3.31	13,999
Knoxville, TN MSA	39	3.26	53,983	6.65	962	9.02	22,815	5.84	23,716
Lafayette, LA MSA	22	3.45	15,559	3.46	309	4.38	6,725	3.66	21,764
Lakeland – Winter Haven, FL MSA	12	2.46	10,203	2.54	486	7.65	6,200	3.70	12,757
Lancaster, PA MSA	7	1.16	7,666	2.02	397	6.27	3,972	2.08	10,005
Lansing – East Lansing, MI MSA	20	2.74	11,889	2.97	560	8.90	6,792	3.57	12,129
Las Vegas, NV – AZ MSA	36	2.31	56,018	3.32	1,241	6.73	24,590	3.61	19,815
Lexington, KY MSA	9	1.11	10,746	1.81	436	4.83	5,110	1.85	11,720
Little Rock – North Little Rock, AR MSA	16	1.54	23,273	2.99	421	3.76	7,146	1.94	16,974
Los Angeles – Riverside – Orange County, CA CMSA	329	1.08	542,042	2.31	9,377	3.38	196,802	2.15	20,988
Louisville, KY – IN MSA	20	1.16	56,435	3.36	1,819	7.04	23,709	3.32	13,034
Macon, GA MSA	24	4.41	19,357	3.43	546	7.24	8,824	3.90	16,161
Madison, WI MSA	14	2.70	16,754	3.24	497	6.90	9,494	4.05	19,103
Melbourne – Titusville – Palm Bay, FL MSA	15	1.85	14,369	2.65	520	7.15	9,569	3.82	18,402
Memphis, TN – AR – MS MSA	42	2.55	106,791	8.60	1,859	11.38	38,321	7.13	20,614
Miami – Fort Lauderdale, FL CMSA	329	3.60	440,314	6.44	9,586	11.03	170,041	6.06	17,738
Milwaukee – Racine, WI CMSA	37	1.22	-	-	-	-	-	-	-
Minneapolis – St. Paul, MN – WI MSA	69	1.85	118,390	4.09	4,508	9.03	62,104	4.14	13,776
Mobile, AL MSA	18	2.80	43,801	7.80	1,897	19.85	24,253	9.24	12,785
Modesto, CA MSA	5	0.74	-	-	-	-	-	-	-
Montgomery, AL MSA	14	2.85	13,004	2.59	712	9.59	7,245	3.44	10,176
Nashville, TN MSA	66	3.40	95,447	5.15	2,423	9.57	45,934	5.92	18,957
New Orleans, LA MSA	90	3.71	88,650	4.05	2,275	7.68	42,456	5.05	18,662
New York – Northern New Jersey – Long Island, NY – NJ – CT- CMSA	596	1.47	1,301,206	4.98	49,515	14.84	727,120	6.66	14,685
Norfolk – Virginia Beach – Newport News, VA – NC MSA	42	1.86	42,963	3.17	2,468	11.28	24,900	3.85	10,089
Oklahoma City, OK MSA	34	1.73	45,634	3.51	841	4.29	16,752	2.99	19,919
Omaha, NE – IA MSA	21	2.08	39,708	4.84	1,159	9.32	14,604	3.91	12,601
Orlando, FL MSA	66	2.61	83,340	4.38	2,895	11.48	34,203	4.18	11,815
Pensacola, FL MSA	15	2.85	22,989	4.40	520	6.51	9,883	4.17	19,006
Peoria – Pekin, IL MSA	10	1.97	16,117	4.45	545	9.32	5,510	2.93	10,110
Philadelphia – Wilmington – Atlantic City, PA – NJ – DE – MD CMSA	181	1.56	-	-	-	-	-	-	-
Phoenix – Mesa, AZ MSA	64	1.33	89,241	2.84	2,082	5.40	35,737	2.60	17,165
Pittsburgh, PA MSA	86	1.81	115,889	4.26	3,419	8.96	45,799	3.67	13,395
Portland, ME MSA	14	2.59	22,216	5.80	717	12.19	8,564	4.78	11,944
Portland – Salem, OR – WA CMSA	50	1.41	-	-	-	-	-	-	-
Providence – Fall River – Warwick, RI – MA MSA	30	1.45	22,939	1.94	848	4.27	10,509	1.98	12,393
Raleigh – Durham – Chapel Hill, NC MSA	39	2.71	36,231	2.98	1,164	6.77	16,492	3.27	14,168
Reno, NV MSA	9	1.35	-	-	-	-	-	-	-
Richmond – Petersburg, VA MSA	44	2.75	39,706	2.54	1,949	8.77	22,270	3.37	11,426
Rochester, NY MSA	26	1.70	48,334	5.84	2,078	14.91	29,269	8.35	14,085
Rockford, IL MSA	10	2.10	6,262	1.73	284	5.23	3,012	1.83	10,606
Sacramento – Yolo, CA CMSA	34	1.18	-	-	-	-	-	-	-
Saginaw – Bay City – Midland, MI MSA	13	1.91	16,910	4.42	672	10.46	10,237	5.18	15,234
St. Louis, MO – IL MSA	84	1.89	118,430	4.14	3,026	6.94	44,084	3.55	14,568
Salinas, CA MSA	12	1.97	20,901	6.99	469	10.66	10,453	8.54	22,288

[Continued]

★ 344 ★

Home Health Care Services Establishments by Major Metro Area: 1992

[Continued]

Area	Establishments		Revenues		Employment		Payroll		
	Number	% of HS[1] in area	Total ($000)	% of HS[1] in area	Number	% of HS[1] in area	Total ($000)	% of HS[1] in area	Payroll per employee
Salt Lake City – Ogden, UT MSA	30	1.46	39,887	2.89	1,424	6.45	18,364	3.20	12,896
San Antonio, TX MSA	56	2.13	95,320	5.29	5,057	17.59	41,784	5.60	8,263
San Diego, CA MSA	61	1.24	65,020	1.99	1,792	4.30	29,219	2.17	16,305
San Francisco – Oakland – San Jose, CA CMSA	152	1.08	-	-	-	-	-	-	-
Santa Barbara – Santa Maria – Lompoc, CA MSA	9	1.08	7,331	1.72	120	2.28	2,628	1.48	21,900
Sarasota – Bradenton, FL MSA	31	2.53	39,751	4.05	1,373	9.51	17,697	4.34	12,889
Scranton – Wilkes-Barre – Hazleton, PA MSA	43	3.76	35,481	5.62	1,376	12.96	19,164	7.31	13,927
Seattle – Tacoma – Bremerton, WA CMSA	66	1.09	98,060	2.75	2,904	5.36	42,437	2.73	14,613
Shreveport – Bossier City, LA MSA	13	2.02	16,269	2.85	493	5.80	7,160	3.09	14,523
Spokane, WA MSA	14	1.90	15,673	3.07	613	7.82	6,280	2.69	10,245
Springfield, MO MSA	16	3.48	12,727	3.31	619	9.01	6,413	3.24	10,360
Springfield, MA MSA	14	1.55	26,423	3.95	1,152	9.54	12,861	4.01	11,164
Stockton – Lodi, CA MSA	8	0.96	7,620	1.47	391	4.87	5,169	2.27	13,220
Syracuse, NY MSA	18	1.65	29,404	4.26	1,145	11.68	13,239	4.21	11,562
Tallahassee, FL MSA	10	2.52	7,878	2.28	414	8.78	4,611	3.02	11,138
Tampa – St. Petersburg – Clearwater, FL MSA	135	2.73	247,595	5.68	6,845	11.19	101,738	5.90	14,863
Toledo, OH MSA	19	1.69	13,725	1.76	675	5.37	6,383	1.61	9,456
Tucson, AZ MSA	21	1.67	31,137	3.15	804	5.90	11,812	2.94	14,692
Tulsa, OK MSA	24	1.75	-	-	-	-	-	-	-
Washington – Baltimore, DC – MD – VA – WV CMSA	169	1.31	-	-	-	-	-	-	-
West Palm Beach – Boca Raton, FL MSA	67	2.49	81,556	4.13	2,558	10.41	41,309	4.90	16,149
Wichita, KS MSA	16	2.09	-	-	-	-	-	-	-
Youngstown – Warren, OH MSA	14	1.16	18,250	2.63	551	4.48	8,784	2.74	15,942

Source: U.S. Department of Commerce. Bureau of the Census. *1992 Economic Census Report Series*, CD-ROM 1i, Washington, DC, October 1996. *Notes:* - means no data reported. 1. HS stands for total health service establishments, revenues, employment, or payroll.

★ 345 ★

Establishment Data

Home Health Care Services Establishments by Major Metro Area, Non-Taxed: 1992

Area	Establish-ments	Revenues in $1,000	Employ-ment	Payroll in $1,000	Payroll per employee
United States	2,215	5,713,903	193,424	3,236,612	16,733
Albany – Schenectady – Troy, NY MSA	9	33,417	1,027	19,320	18,812
Atlanta, GA MSA	17	45,656	805	21,467	26,667
Boston – Worcester – Lawrence, MA – NH – ME – CT CMSA	118	319,515	8,746	168,965	19,319
Buffalo – Niagara Falls, NY MSA	9	25,463	793	11,369	14,337
Chicago – Gary – Kenosha, IL – IN – WI CMSA	63	-	-	-	-

[Continued]

★ 345 ★

Home Health Care Services Establishments by Major Metro Area, Non-Taxed: 1992

[Continued]

Area	Establish-ments	Revenues in $1,000	Employ-ment	Payroll in $1,000	Payroll per employee
Cincinnati – Hamilton, OH – KY – IN CMSA	11	-	-	-	-
Cleveland – Akron, OH CMSA	22	-	-	-	-
Columbus, OH MSA	8	13,972	511	6,837	13,380
Dallas – Fort Worth, TX CMSA	18	76,183	3,974	40,223	10,122
Denver – Boulder – Greeley, CO CMSA	25	-	-	-	-
Detroit – Ann Arbor – Flint, MI CMSA	57	-	-	-	-
Hartford, CT MSA	21	55,590	1,740	34,802	20,001
Houston – Galveston – Brazoria, TX CMSA	23	-	-	-	-
Indianapolis, IN MSA	9	-	-	-	-
Kansas City, MO – KS MSA	15	27,516	842	15,300	18,171
Los Angeles – Riverside – Orange County, CA CMSA	56	-	-	-	-
Miami – Fort Lauderdale, FL CMSA	20	98,982	1,068	28,325	26,522
Milwaukee – Racine, WI CMSA	15	-	-	-	-
Minneapolis – St. Paul, MN – WI MSA	21	58,917	1,964	33,481	17,047
New York – Northern New Jersey – Long Island, NY – NJ – CT- CMSA	190	-	-	-	-
Philadelphia – Wilmington – Atlantic City, PA – NJ – DE – MD CMSA	52	-	-	-	-
Phoenix – Mesa, AZ MSA	7	-	-	-	-
Pittsburgh, PA MSA	21	-	-	-	-
Portland – Salem, OR – WA CMSA	11	-	-	-	-
Providence – Fall River – Warwick, RI – MA MSA	22	67,332	1,749	37,379	21,372
Sacramento – Yolo, CA CMSA	5	-	-	-	-
St. Louis, MO – IL MSA	18	-	-	-	-
San Diego, CA MSA	8	41,733	1,220	22,887	18,760
San Francisco – Oakland – San Jose, CA CMSA	31	-	-	-	-
Seattle – Tacoma – Bremerton, WA CMSA	23	71,948	2,533	42,030	16,593
Tampa – St. Petersburg – Clearwater, FL MSA	6	-	-	-	-
Washington – Baltimore, DC – MD – VA – WV CMSA	34	-	-	-	-

Source: U.S. Department of Commerce. Bureau of the Census. *1992 Economic Census Report Series,* CD-ROM 1i, Washington, DC, October 1996. *Notes:* - means no data reported. 1. HS stands for total health service establishments, revenues, employment, or payroll.

★ 346 ★
Establishment Data

Home Health Care Services Establishments by State: 1992

Area	Establishments		Revenues		Employment		Payroll		
	Number	% of HS[1] in area	Total ($000)	% of HS[1] in area	Number	% of HS[1] in area	Total ($000)	% of HS[1] in area	Payroll per employee
United States	8,045	1.82	10,413,844	3.48	341,889	7.68	4,853,090	3.76	14,195
Alabama	142	2.57	180,748	3.67	6,432	8.32	88,070	4.17	13,692
Alaska	8	0.93	-	-	-	-	-	-	-
Arizona	102	1.44	127,209	2.78	3,043	5.18	50,222	2.57	16,504
Arkansas	48	1.35	46,366	1.90	1,342	3.14	16,610	1.56	12,377
California	694	1.13	939,952	2.19	20,995	3.92	383,504	2.22	18,266
Colorado	109	1.55	90,071	2.41	3,148	5.70	40,273	2.45	12,793
Connecticut	103	1.56	157,899	3.22	5,655	7.82	81,588	3.48	14,428
Delaware	14	1.17	9,844	1.25	471	4.05	5,351	1.47	11,361
District of Columbia	16	1.16	-	-	-	-	-	-	-
Florida	852	2.88	1,141,072	4.90	30,852	9.79	485,872	5.04	15,748
Georgia	359	3.24	455,758	5.28	9,797	8.10	196,429	5.35	20,050
Hawaii	5	0.22	-	-	-	-	-	-	-
Idaho	30	1.73	18,231	1.85	906	5.35	10,484	2.52	11,572
Illinois	292	1.56	507,002	4.10	14,648	7.81	220,316	3.94	15,041
Indiana	152	1.75	173,804	2.85	6,579	6.17	87,468	3.19	13,295
Iowa	58	1.39	37,084	1.59	1,621	3.60	17,028	1.53	10,505
Kansas	82	2.12	84,345	2.77	2,450	4.58	33,508	2.53	13,677
Kentucky	85	1.54	121,810	2.96	3,887	5.80	54,589	3.07	14,044
Louisiana	263	3.86	257,721	4.66	6,635	7.69	123,995	5.70	18,688
Maine	41	1.90	40,030	3.40	1,406	6.39	16,414	3.08	11,674
Maryland	129	1.41	188,344	3.34	3,696	4.63	74,770	3.00	20,230
Massachusetts	178	1.68	300,928	3.95	10,876	8.55	139,254	3.93	12,804
Michigan	270	1.72	227,965	2.62	8,948	6.35	118,822	2.89	13,279
Minnesota	108	1.83	141,816	3.45	6,286	8.29	76,824	3.69	12,221
Mississippi	92	2.98	108,658	5.21	2,874	7.80	50,324	5.72	17,510
Missouri	165	1.96	181,958	3.31	6,112	6.45	75,621	3.09	12,373
Montana	18	1.21	8,958	1.38	235	2.18	3,795	1.46	16,149
Nebraska	35	1.48	48,085	3.09	1,623	6.02	19,157	2.67	11,803
Nevada	44	1.90	69,163	3.07	1,605	6.35	30,264	3.30	18,856
New Hampshire	36	1.96	21,453	1.81	739	3.85	10,581	1.95	14,318
New Jersey	220	1.33	320,155	3.08	8,208	6.43	144,831	3.28	17,645
New Mexico	46	1.92	29,702	2.01	1,364	5.77	14,007	2.26	10,269
New York	532	1.64	1,231,855	6.20	52,324	18.80	715,048	8.67	13,666
North Carolina	205	2.31	213,085	3.20	7,796	7.27	110,291	3.70	14,147
North Dakota	15	1.94	8,612	1.37	409	4.47	4,263	1.40	10,423
Ohio	313	1.69	324,480	2.79	12,150	6.09	148,930	2.67	12,258
Oklahoma	108	2.02	132,577	4.05	3,127	5.29	55,369	3.92	17,707
Oregon	73	1.29	44,981	1.52	1,715	3.56	21,934	1.69	12,790
Pennsylvania	364	1.67	385,688	3.05	13,555	7.35	174,954	3.09	12,907
Rhode Island	25	1.32	19,907	1.88	843	4.64	9,444	2.02	11,203
South Carolina	72	1.55	60,143	1.92	2,098	4.19	29,410	2.11	14,018
South Dakota	7	0.72	1,528	0.27	211	2.32	813	0.31	3,853
Tennessee	335	4.07	514,425	7.62	10,860	10.83	216,786	7.55	19,962
Texas	667	2.23	883,368	3.85	41,638	12.02	418,039	4.53	10,040

[Continued]

★ 346 ★

Home Health Care Services Establishments by State: 1992

[Continued]

Area	Establishments		Revenues		Employment		Payroll		
	Number	% of HS[1] in area	Total ($000)	% of HS[1] in area	Number	% of HS[1] in area	Total ($000)	% of HS[1] in area	Payroll per employee
Utah	43	1.41	47,867	2.59	1,737	5.62	22,651	3.00	13,040
Vermont	11	1.18	5,722	1.41	269	3.56	3,334	2.02	12,394
Virginia	185	1.90	175,874	2.63	7,623	7.46	88,541	2.92	11,615
Washington	105	1.14	128,443	2.38	4,347	4.97	58,282	2.45	13,407
West Virginia	48	1.78	39,908	2.23	1,417	4.91	17,345	2.46	12,241
Wisconsin	124	1.72	128,281	2.71	6,147	7.23	74,237	3.17	12,077
Wyoming	17	2.38	4,706	1.45	285	5.06	2,561	1.89	8,986

Source: U.S. Department of Commerce. Bureau of the Census. *1992 Economic Census Report Series,* CD-ROM 1i, Washington, DC, October 1996. *Notes:* - means no data reported. 1. HS stands for total health service establishments, revenues, employment, or payroll.

★ 347 ★

Establishment Data

Home Health Care Services Establishments by State, Non-Taxed: 1992

Area	Establish-ments	Revenues in $1,000	Employ-ment	Payroll in $1,000	Payroll per employee
United States	2,215	5,713,903	193,424	3,236,612	16,733
Alabama	33	57,489	1,989	31,970	16,073
Alaska	2	-	-	-	-
Arizona	12	29,720	951	16,039	16,865
Arkansas	24	31,812	1,432	15,711	10,971
California	128	348,026	8,300	200,712	24,182
Colorado	41	51,412	1,794	27,275	15,203
Connecticut	64	161,528	4,852	92,111	18,984
Delaware	12	32,288	1,060	19,239	18,150
District of Columbia	6	-	-	-	-
Florida	95	292,163	5,813	120,608	20,748
Georgia	55	87,686	1,809	41,614	23,004
Hawaii	10	11,366	370	7,762	20,978
Idaho	2	-	-	-	-
Illinois	95	158,194	5,132	88,093	17,165
Indiana	48	72,773	2,436	42,575	17,477
Iowa	44	39,437	1,397	20,686	14,807
Kansas	22	22,134	659	11,114	16,865
Kentucky	45	60,270	1,387	27,670	19,950
Louisiana	4	3,632	77	1,814	23,558
Maine	38	46,776	1,572	27,502	17,495
Maryland	26	42,914	1,137	25,405	22,344
Massachusetts	127	361,658	9,892	193,688	19,580

[Continued]

★ 347 ★

Home Health Care Services Establishments by State, Non-Taxed: 1992

[Continued]

Area	Establish-ments	Revenues in $1,000	Employ-ment	Payroll in $1,000	Payroll per employee
Michigan	120	266,911	6,582	132,893	20,190
Minnesota	31	63,213	2,190	36,055	16,463
Mississippi	12	44,129	1,135	24,894	21,933
Missouri	38	62,327	2,064	33,941	16,444
Montana	8	15,586	1,745	11,026	6,319
Nebraska	5	-	-	-	-
Nevada	12	-	-	-	-
New Hampshire	43	40,363	1,739	24,390	14,025
New Jersey	59	217,932	6,508	118,166	18,157
New Mexico	22	23,009	1,267	14,231	11,232
New York	180	1,609,720	54,809	1,038,793	18,953
North Carolina	56	127,534	4,059	67,748	16,691
North Dakota	8	-	-	-	-
Ohio	93	160,560	4,806	82,343	17,133
Oklahoma	19	-	-	-	-
Oregon	15	48,824	1,248	19,326	15,486
Pennsylvania	165	292,663	8,338	152,999	18,350
Rhode Island	20	61,593	1,501	33,839	22,544
South Carolina	9	16,393	416	8,662	20,822
South Dakota	8	-	-	-	-
Tennessee	39	78,301	1,997	37,178	18,617
Texas	129	280,617	26,175	168,395	6,433
Utah	3	-	-	-	-
Vermont	23	-	-	-	-
Virginia	31	58,651	1,828	31,087	17,006
Washington	51	113,873	4,530	68,338	15,086
West Virginia	16	26,938	772	12,230	15,842
Wisconsin	56	84,983	3,801	48,794	12,837
Wyoming	11	-	-	-	-

Source: U.S. Department of Commerce. Bureau of the Census. *1992 Economic Census Report Series,* CD-ROM 1i, Washington, DC, October 1996. *Notes:* - means no data reported. 1. HS stands for total health service establishments, revenues, employment, or payroll.

★ 348 ★

Establishment Data

Hospitals by Major Metro Area: 1992

Area	Establishments		Revenues		Employment		Payroll		
	Number	% of HS[1] in area	Total ($000)	% of HS[1] in area	Number	% of HS[1] in area	Total ($000)	% of HS[1] in area	Payroll per employee
United States	1,403	0.32	31,082,975	10.39	428,150	9.62	10,556,433	8.18	24,656
Abilene, TX MSA	2	0.75	-	-	-	-	-	-	-
Albany, GA MSA	1	0.53							
Albany – Schenectady – Troy, NY MSA	3	0.23	54,368	6.73	944	7.15	25,843	7.11	27,376
Albuquerque, NM MSA	6	0.56	190,589	22.84	3,377	26.70	80,106	21.25	23,721
Alexandria, LA MSA	2	0.74	-	-	-	-	-	-	-
Allentown – Bethlehem – Easton, PA MSA	0	0.00	0	0.00	0	0.00	0	0.00	0
Altoona, PA MSA	2	0.83	-	-	-	-	-	-	-
Amarillo, TX MSA	1	0.24	-	-	-	-	-	-	-
Anchorage, AK MSA	3	0.62	-	-	-	-	-	-	-
Anniston, AL MSA	0	0.00	0	0.00	0	0.00	0	0.00	0
Appleton – Oshkosh – Neenah, WI MSA	0	0.00	0	0.00	0	0.00	0	0.00	0
Asheville, NC MSA	2	0.46	-	-	-	-	-	-	-
Athens, GA MSA	1	0.42	-	-	-	-	-	-	-
Atlanta, GA MSA	25	0.41	663,802	13.77	8,186	13.68	190,855	9.46	23,315
Augusta – Aiken, GA – SC MSA	5	0.70	-	-	-	-	-	-	-
Austin – San Marcos, TX MSA	15	0.95	236,834	19.79	3,455	18.60	79,409	16.36	22,984
Bakersfield, CA MSA	4	0.53	59,738	10.95	946	11.59	20,572	9.39	21,746
Bangor, ME MSA	0	0.00	0	0.00	0	0.00	0	0.00	0
Barnstable – Yarmouth, MA MSA	0	0.00	0	0.00	0	0.00	0	0.00	0
Baton Rouge, LA MSA	6	0.68	105,184	14.18	1,551	14.06	37,494	12.36	24,174
Beaumont – Port Arthur, TX MSA	6	0.83	165,921	28.83	2,293	22.43	50,020	20.77	21,814
Bellingham, WA MSA	0	0.00	0	0.00	0	0.00	0	0.00	0
Benton Harbor, MI MSA	1	0.42	-	-	-	-	-	-	-
Billings, MT MSA	1	0.39	-	-	-	-	-	-	-
Biloxi – Gulfport – Pascagoula, MS MSA	5	1.06	86,529	28.42	1,405	27.79	28,866	23.64	20,545
Binghamton, NY MSA	0	0.00	0	0.00	0	0.00	0	0.00	0
Birmingham, AL MSA	8	0.58	-	-	-	-	-	-	-
Bismarck, ND MSA	0	0.00	0	0.00	0	0.00	0	0.00	0
Bloomington, IN MSA	1	0.55	-	-	-	-	-	-	-
Bloomington – Normal, IL MSA	0	0.00	0	0.00	0	0.00	0	0.00	0
Boise City, ID MSA	4	0.67	-	-	-	-	-	-	-
Boston – Worcester – Lawrence, MA – NH – ME – CT CMSA	25	0.26	415,499	5.88	7,220	6.27	192,059	5.90	26,601
Brownsville – Harlingen – San Benito, TX MSA	3	1.02	-	-	-	-	-	-	-
Bryan – College Station, TX MSA	3	1.55	-	-	-	-	-	-	-
Buffalo – Niagara Falls, NY MSA	1	0.05	-	-	-	-	-	-	-
Burlington, VT MSA	0	0.00	0	0.00	0	0.00	0	0.00	0
Canton – Massillon, OH MSA	0	0.00	0	0.00	0	0.00	0	0.00	0
Casper, WY MSA	1	0.79	-	-	-	-	-	-	-
Cedar Rapids, IA MSA	0	0.00	0	0.00	0	0.00	0	0.00	0
Champaign – Urbana, IL MSA	0	0.00	0	0.00	0	0.00	0	0.00	0
Charleston – North Charleston, SC MSA	5	0.61	147,981	25.00	2,274	24.96	45,741	19.57	20,115
Charleston, WV MSA	2	0.40	-	-	-	-	-	-	-
Charlotte – Gastonia – Rock Hill, NC – SC MSA	4	0.25	144,521	10.34	1,644	8.08	40,761	6.20	24,794
Charlottesville, VA MSA	2	0.81	-	-	-	-	-	-	-
Chattanooga, TN – GA MSA	9	1.18	176,972	24.67	2,423	24.30	57,693	18.88	23,811
Cheyenne, WY MSA	0	0.00	0	0.00	0	0.00	0	0.00	0
Chicago – Gary – Kenosha, IL – IN – WI CMSA	25	0.17	-	-	-	-	-	-	-
Chico – Paradise, CA MSA	2	0.41	-	-	-	-	-	-	-

[Continued]

★ 348 ★

Hospitals by Major Metro Area: 1992
[Continued]

Area	Establishments		Revenues		Employment		Payroll		
	Number	% of HS[1] in area	Total ($000)	% of HS[1] in area	Number	% of HS[1] in area	Total ($000)	% of HS[1] in area	Payroll per employee
Cincinnati – Hamilton, OH – KY – IN CMSA	3	0.10	14,318	0.71	263	0.76	4,763	0.47	18,110
Clarksville – Hopkinsville, TN – KY MSA	1	0.53	-	-	-	-	-	-	-
Cleveland – Akron, OH CMSA	3	0.06	-	-	-	-	-	-	-
Colorado Springs, CO MSA	3	0.34	-	-	-	-	-	-	-
Columbia, MO MSA	2	0.81	-	-	-	-	-	-	-
Columbia, SC MSA	2	0.27	-	-	-	-	-	-	-
Columbus, GA – AL MSA	2	0.61	-	-	-	-	-	-	-
Columbus, OH MSA	2	0.08	-	-	-	-	-	-	-
Corpus Christi, TX MSA	8	1.07	161,717	28.00	2,192	25.93	51,424	22.77	23,460
Cumberland, MD – WV MSA	2	1.03	-	-	-	-	-	-	-
Dallas – Fort Worth, TX CMSA	64	0.77	1,413,007	21.66	17,511	20.34	449,727	16.97	25,683
Danville, VA MSA	0	0.00	0	0.00	0	0.00	0	0.00	0
Davenport – Moline – Rock Island, IA – IL MSA	1	0.15	-	-	-	-	-	-	-
Dayton – Springfield, OH MSA	2	0.12	-	-	-	-	-	-	-
Daytona Beach, FL MSA	3	0.41	-	-	-	-	-	-	-
Decatur, AL MSA	3	1.48	-	-	-	-	-	-	-
Decatur, IL MSA	0	0.00	0	0.00	0	0.00	0	0.00	0
Denver – Boulder – Greeley, CO CMSA	9	0.21	-	-	-	-	-	-	-
Des Moines, IA MSA	1	0.14	-	-	-	-	-	-	-
Detroit – Ann Arbor – Flint, MI CMSA	7	0.07	53,879	0.99	1,031	1.23	21,438	0.84	20,793
Dothan, AL MSA	2	0.91	-	-	-	-	-	-	-
Dover, DE MSA	0	0.00	0	0.00	0	0.00	0	0.00	0
Dubuque, IA MSA	0	0.00	0	0.00	0	0.00	0	0.00	0
Duluth – Superior, MN – WI MSA	0	0.00	0	0.00	0	0.00	0	0.00	0
Eau Claire, WI MSA	0	0.00	0	0.00	0	0.00	0	0.00	0
El Paso, TX MSA	8	1.01	-	-	-	-	-	-	-
Elkhart – Goshen, IN MSA	0	0.00	0	0.00	0	0.00	0	0.00	0
Elmira, NY MSA	0	0.00	0	0.00	0	0.00	0	0.00	0
Enid, OK MSA	3	2.54	-	-	-	-	-	-	-
Erie, PA MSA	2	0.41	-	-	-	-	-	-	-
Eugene – Springfield, OR MSA	0	0.00	0	0.00	0	0.00	0	0.00	0
Evansville – Henderson, IN – KY MSA	2	0.41	-	-	-	-	-	-	-
Fargo – Moorhead, ND – MN MSA	1	0.46	-	-	-	-	-	-	-
Fayetteville, NC MSA	2	0.73	-	-	-	-	-	-	-
Fayetteville – Springdale – Rogers, AR MSA	2	0.58	-	-	-	-	-	-	-
Florence, AL MSA	2	0.82	-	-	-	-	-	-	-
Florence, SC MSA	0	0.00	0	0.00	0	0.00	0	0.00	0
Fort Collins – Loveland, CO MSA	0	0.00	0	0.00	0	0.00	0	0.00	0
Fort Myers – Cape Coral, FL MSA	5	0.70	-	-	-	-	-	-	-
Fort Pierce – Port St. Lucie, FL MSA	4	0.77	-	-	-	-	-	-	-
Fort Smith, AR – OK MSA	2	0.70	-	-	-	-	-	-	-
Fort Walton Beach, FL MSA	5	2.01	96,505	42.74	1,465	40.21	31,159	35.90	21,269
Fort Wayne, IN MSA	1	0.14	-	-	-	-	-	-	-
Fresno, CA MSA	4	0.27	28,295	3.26	493	4.00	13,021	3.51	26,412
Gadsden, AL MSA	2	1.12	-	-	-	-	-	-	-
Gainesville, FL MSA	1	0.22	-	-	-	-	-	-	-
Glens Falls, NY MSA	0	0.00	0	0.00	0	0.00	0	0.00	0
Goldsboro, NC MSA	0	0.00	0	0.00	0	0.00	0	0.00	0
Grand Forks, ND – MN MSA	0	0.00	0	0.00	0	0.00	0	0.00	0
Grand Rapids – Muskegon – Holland, MI MSA	1	0.07	-	-	-	-	-	-	-
Great Falls, MT MSA	0	0.00	0	0.00	0	0.00	0	0.00	0
Green Bay, WI MSA	1	0.34	-	-	-	-	-	-	-

[Continued]

★ 348 ★

Hospitals by Major Metro Area: 1992

[Continued]

Area	Establishments		Revenues		Employment		Payroll		
	Number	% of HS[1] in area	Total ($000)	% of HS[1] in area	Number	% of HS[1] in area	Total ($000)	% of HS[1] in area	Payroll per employee
Greensboro – Winston-Salem – High Point, NC MSA	2	0.13	-	-	-	-	-	-	-
Greenville, NC MSA	0	0.00	0	0.00	0	0.00	0	0.00	0
Greenville – Spartanburg – Anderson, SC MSA	4	0.34	51,299	6.58	724	6.04	16,778	4.45	23,174
Harrisburg – Lebanon – Carlisle, PA MSA	1	0.10	-	-	-	-	-	-	-
Hartford, CT MSA	1	0.04	-	-	-	-	-	-	-
Hickory – Morganton, NC MSA	2	0.55	-	-	-	-	-	-	-
Honolulu, HI MSA	2	0.12	-	-	-	-	-	-	-
Houma, LA MSA	1	0.38	-	-	-	-	-	-	-
Houston – Galveston – Brazoria, TX CMSA	62	0.88	-	-	-	-	-	-	-
Huntington – Ashland, WV – KY – OH MSA	2	0.41	-	-	-	-	-	-	-
Huntsville, AL MSA	5	0.94	123,641	27.05	1,785	27.28	38,664	20.23	21,661
Indianapolis, IN MSA	9	0.35	142,466	7.11	2,207	6.86	51,755	5.50	23,450
Iowa City, IA MSA	0	0.00	0	0.00	0	0.00	0	0.00	0
Jackson, MI MSA	0	0.00	0	0.00	0	0.00	0	0.00	0
Jackson, MS MSA	4	0.63	-	-	-	-	-	-	-
Jackson, TN MSA	1	0.65	-	-	-	-	-	-	-
Jacksonville, FL MSA	5	0.28	82,095	6.28	1,157	6.76	27,861	5.01	24,080
Jacksonville, NC MSA	1	0.93	-	-	-	-	-	-	-
Jamestown, NY MSA	0	0.00	0	0.00	0	0.00	0	0.00	0
Janesville – Beloit, WI MSA	0	0.00	0	0.00	0	0.00	0	0.00	0
Johnson City – Kingsport – Bristol, TN – VA MSA	7	1.01	146,533	23.99	2,079	21.11	47,180	17.33	22,694
Johnstown, PA MSA	0	0.00	0	0.00	0	0.00	0	0.00	0
Joplin, MO MSA	1	0.33	-	-	-	-	-	-	-
Kalamazoo – Battle Creek, MI MSA	0	0.00	0	0.00	0	0.00	0	0.00	0
Kansas City, MO – KS MSA	12	0.42	176,809	8.09	2,437	7.22	61,828	6.24	25,371
Killeen – Temple, TX MSA	1	0.46	-	-	-	-	-	-	-
Knoxville, TN MSA	2	0.17	-	-	-	-	-	-	-
Kokomo, IN MSA	1	0.56	-	-	-	-	-	-	-
La Crosse, WI – MN MSA	0	0.00	0	0.00	0	0.00	0	0.00	0
Lafayette, LA MSA	5	0.78	83,419	18.55	1,245	17.66	24,981	13.61	20,065
Lafayette, IN MSA	1	0.53	-	-	-	-	-	-	-
Lake Charles, LA MSA	2	0.67	-	-	-	-	-	-	-
Lakeland – Winter Haven, FL MSA	2	0.41	-	-	-	-	-	-	-
Lancaster, PA MSA	0	0.00	0	0.00	0	0.00	0	0.00	0
Lansing – East Lansing, MI MSA	1	0.14	-	-	-	-	-	-	-
Laredo, TX MSA	2	1.39	-	-	-	-	-	-	-
Las Cruces, NM MSA	2	0.91	-	-	-	-	-	-	-
Las Vegas, NV – AZ MSA	10	0.64	528,663	31.31	5,339	28.94	152,788	22.43	28,617
Lawrence, KS MSA	0	0.00	0	0.00	0	0.00	0	0.00	0
Lawton, OK MSA	2	1.29	-	-	-	-	-	-	-
Lewiston – Auburn, ME MSA	0	0.00	0	0.00	0	0.00	0	0.00	0
Lexington, KY MSA	4	0.49	75,494	12.74	1,189	13.16	26,192	9.50	22,029
Lima, OH MSA	0	0.00	0	0.00	0	0.00	0	0.00	0
Lincoln, NE MSA	0	0.00	0	0.00	0	0.00	0	0.00	0
Little Rock – North Little Rock, AR MSA	6	0.58	117,540	15.12	1,518	13.57	37,886	10.31	24,958
Longview – Marshall, TX MSA	2	0.62	-	-	-	-	-	-	-
Los Angeles – Riverside – Orange County, CA CMSA	127	0.42	3,165,574	13.48	41,403	14.91	1,192,006	13.04	28,790
Louisville, KY – IN MSA	8	0.47	-	-	-	-	-	-	-
Lubbock, TX MSA	3	0.55	50,322	13.20	666	12.21	13,888	9.21	20,853
Lynchburg, VA MSA	0	0.00	0	0.00	0	0.00	0	0.00	0

[Continued]

★ 348 ★

Hospitals by Major Metro Area: 1992
[Continued]

Area	Establishments		Revenues		Employment		Payroll		
	Number	% of HS[1] in area	Total ($000)	% of HS[1] in area	Number	% of HS[1] in area	Total ($000)	% of HS[1] in area	Payroll per employee
Macon, GA MSA	6	1.10	-	-	-	-	-	-	-
Madison, WI MSA	1	0.19	-	-	-	-	-	-	-
Mansfield, OH MSA	1	0.35	-	-	-	-	-	-	-
McAllen – Edinburg – Mission, TX MSA	3	0.75	-	-	-	-	-	-	-
Medford – Ashland, OR MSA	0	0.00	0	0.00	0	0.00	0	0.00	0
Melbourne – Titusville – Palm Bay, FL MSA	2	0.25	-	-	-	-	-	-	-
Memphis, TN – AR – MS MSA	5	0.30	104,716	8.43	1,678	10.27	37,421	6.96	22,301
Merced, CA MSA	1	0.41	-	-	-	-	-	-	-
Miami – Fort Lauderdale, FL CMSA	41	0.45	1,491,583	21.80	19,781	22.75	515,005	18.36	26,035
Milwaukee – Racine, WI CMSA	4	0.13	-	-	-	-	-	-	-
Minneapolis – St. Paul, MN – WI MSA	1	0.03	-	-	-	-	-	-	-
Mobile, AL MSA	2	0.31	-	-	-	-	-	-	-
Modesto, CA MSA	2	0.30	-	-	-	-	-	-	-
Monroe, LA MSA	4	1.43	-	-	-	-	-	-	-
Montgomery, AL MSA	4	0.81	130,374	25.99	1,793	24.16	42,228	20.04	23,552
Muncie, IN MSA	0	0.00	0	0.00	0	0.00	0	0.00	0
Myrtle Beach, SC MSA	2	0.87	-	-	-	-	-	-	-
Naples, FL MSA	1	0.26	-	-	-	-	-	-	-
Nashville, TN MSA	13	0.67	408,255	22.02	5,515	21.79	133,029	17.14	24,121
New London – Norwich, CT – RI MSA	0	0.00	0	0.00	0	0.00	0	0.00	0
New Orleans, LA MSA	30	1.24	624,063	28.52	8,056	27.21	206,244	24.52	25,601
New York – Northern New Jersey – Long Island, NY – NJ – CT- CMSA	28	0.07	912,509	3.49	13,493	4.05	420,510	3.85	31,165
Norfolk – Virginia Beach – Newport News, VA – NC MSA	7	0.31	65,949	4.86	1,441	6.58	25,987	4.02	18,034
Ocala, FL MSA	3	0.89	-	-	-	-	-	-	-
Odessa – Midland, TX MSA	3	0.77	-	-	-	-	-	-	-
Oklahoma City, OK MSA	6	0.30	190,221	14.65	2,488	12.71	57,259	10.21	23,014
Omaha, NE – IA MSA	2	0.20	-	-	-	-	-	-	-
Orlando, FL MSA	10	0.39	275,349	14.48	3,458	13.71	87,477	10.69	25,297
Owensboro, KY MSA	0	0.00	0	0.00	0	0.00	0	0.00	0
Panama City, FL MSA	2	0.81	-	-	-	-	-	-	-
Parkersburg – Marietta, WV – OH MSA	1	0.40	-	-	-	-	-	-	-
Pensacola, FL MSA	4	0.76	-	-	-	-	-	-	-
Peoria – Pekin, IL MSA	0	0.00	0	0.00	0	0.00	0	0.00	0
Philadelphia – Wilmington – Atlantic City, PA – NJ – DE – MD CMSA	15	0.13	-	-	-	-	-	-	-
Phoenix – Mesa, AZ MSA	11	0.23	251,564	8.00	3,433	8.91	85,215	6.20	24,822
Pine Bluff, AR MSA	0	0.00	0	0.00	0	0.00	0	0.00	0
Pittsburgh, PA MSA	3	0.06	-	-	-	-	-	-	-
Pittsfield, MA MSA	0	0.00	0	0.00	0	0.00	0	0.00	0
Portland, ME MSA	2	0.37	-	-	-	-	-	-	-
Portland – Salem, OR – WA CMSA	8	0.23	-	-	-	-	-	-	-
Providence – Fall River – Warwick, RI – MA MSA	0	0.00	0	0.00	0	0.00	0	0.00	0
Provo – Orem, UT MSA	2	0.44	-	-	-	-	-	-	-
Pueblo, CO MSA	0	0.00	0	0.00	0	0.00	0	0.00	0
Punta Gorda, FL MSA	1	0.42	-	-	-	-	-	-	-
Raleigh – Durham – Chapel Hill, NC MSA	5	0.35	99,516	8.19	1,431	8.32	38,064	7.54	26,600
Rapid City, SD MSA	0	0.00	0	0.00	0	0.00	0	0.00	0
Reading, PA MSA	0	0.00	0	0.00	0	0.00	0	0.00	0
Redding, CA MSA	2	0.54	-	-	-	-	-	-	-
Reno, NV MSA	3	0.45	-	-	-	-	-	-	-
Richland – Kennewick – Pasco, WA MSA	0	0.00	0	0.00	0	0.00	0	0.00	0
Richmond – Petersburg, VA MSA	11	0.69	570,326	36.44	6,896	31.03	175,432	26.52	25,440

[Continued]

★ 348 ★

Hospitals by Major Metro Area: 1992
[Continued]

Area	Establishments		Revenues		Employment		Payroll		
	Number	% of HS[1] in area	Total ($000)	% of HS[1] in area	Number	% of HS[1] in area	Total ($000)	% of HS[1] in area	Payroll per employee
Roanoke, VA MSA	3	0.78	-	-	-	-	-	-	-
Rochester, MN MSA	0	0.00	0	0.00	0	0.00	0	0.00	0
Rochester, NY MSA	0	0.00	0	0.00	0	0.00	0	0.00	0
Rockford, IL MSA	1	0.21	-	-	-	-	-	-	-
Rocky Mount, NC MSA	4	2.52	44,044	24.80	755	25.63	13,875	20.28	18,377
Sacramento – Yolo, CA CMSA	5	0.17	33,155	1.72	468	1.88	12,325	1.49	26,335
Saginaw – Bay City – Midland, MI MSA	0	0.00	0	0.00	0	0.00	0	0.00	0
St. Cloud, MN MSA	0	0.00	0	0.00	0	0.00	0	0.00	0
St. Joseph, MO MSA	0	0.00	0	0.00	0	0.00	0	0.00	0
St. Louis, MO – IL MSA	5	0.11	125,662	4.39	1,311	3.01	37,830	3.05	28,856
Salinas, CA MSA	0	0.00	0	0.00	0	0.00	0	0.00	0
Salt Lake City – Ogden, UT MSA	11	0.53	-	-	-	-	-	-	-
San Angelo, TX MSA	2	1.32	-	-	-	-	-	-	-
San Antonio, TX MSA	17	0.65	339,874	18.87	5,087	17.69	124,990	16.75	24,570
San Diego, CA MSA	13	0.26	300,734	9.21	3,773	9.06	102,543	7.62	27,178
San Francisco – Oakland – San Jose, CA CMSA	27	0.19	-	-	-	-	-	-	-
San Luis Obispo – Atascadero – Paso Robles, CA MSA	3	0.62	115,221	34.73	1,450	30.50	36,785	29.56	25,369
Santa Barbara – Santa Maria – Lompoc, CA MSA	2	0.24	-	-	-	-	-	-	-
Santa Fe, NM MSA	1	0.33	-	-	-	-	-	-	-
Sarasota – Bradenton, FL MSA	7	0.57	222,599	22.67	3,160	21.88	68,457	16.80	21,664
Savannah, GA MSA	1	0.23	-	-	-	-	-	-	-
Scranton – Wilkes-Barre – Hazleton, PA MSA	1	0.09	-	-	-	-	-	-	-
Seattle – Tacoma – Bremerton, WA CMSA	7	0.12	-	-	-	-	-	-	-
Sharon, PA MSA	0	0.00	0	0.00	0	0.00	0	0.00	0
Sheboygan, WI MSA	0	0.00	0	0.00	0	0.00	0	0.00	0
Sherman – Denison, TX MSA	2	0.90	-	-	-	-	-	-	-
Shreveport – Bossier City, LA MSA	9	1.40	142,511	24.93	1,950	22.94	43,173	18.64	22,140
Sioux City, IA – NE MSA	0	0.00	0	0.00	0	0.00	0	0.00	0
Sioux Falls, SD MSA	2	0.85	-	-	-	-	-	-	-
South Bend, IN MSA	1	0.20	-	-	-	-	-	-	-
Spokane, WA MSA	2	0.27	-	-	-	-	-	-	-
Springfield, IL MSA	1	0.32	-	-	-	-	-	-	-
Springfield, MO MSA	3	0.65	49,223	12.80	956	13.92	18,718	9.45	19,579
Springfield, MA MSA	2	0.22	-	-	-	-	-	-	-
State College, PA MSA	2	1.22	-	-	-	-	-	-	-
Steubenville – Weirton, OH – WV MSA	0	0.00	0	0.00	0	0.00	0	0.00	0
Stockton – Lodi, CA MSA	1	0.12	-	-	-	-	-	-	-
Sumter, SC MSA	0	0.00	0	0.00	0	0.00	0	0.00	0
Syracuse, NY MSA	1	0.09	-	-	-	-	-	-	-
Tallahassee, FL MSA	3	0.76	-	-	-	-	-	-	-
Tampa – St. Petersburg – Clearwater, FL MSA	32	0.65	1,029,857	23.63	13,556	22.15	318,691	18.47	23,509
Terre Haute, IN MSA	3	1.20	-	-	-	-	-	-	-
Texarkana, TX – Texarkana, AR MSA	4	1.90	37,927	20.06	485	17.19	12,639	15.19	26,060
Toledo, OH MSA	1	0.09	-	-	-	-	-	-	-
Topeka, KS MSA	2	0.71	-	-	-	-	-	-	-
Tucson, AZ MSA	10	0.79	200,696	20.32	3,014	22.13	66,762	16.60	22,151
Tulsa, OK MSA	7	0.51	101,453	10.68	1,598	11.20	36,220	8.52	22,666
Tuscaloosa, AL MSA	1	0.52	-	-	-	-	-	-	-
Tyler, TX MSA	0	0.00	0	0.00	0	0.00	0	0.00	0
Utica – Rome, NY MSA	0	0.00	0	0.00	0	0.00	0	0.00	0
Victoria, TX MSA	2	1.05	-	-	-	-	-	-	-

[Continued]

★ 348 ★

Hospitals by Major Metro Area: 1992

[Continued]

Area	Establishments		Revenues		Employment		Payroll		
	Number	% of HS[1] in area	Total ($000)	% of HS[1] in area	Number	% of HS[1] in area	Total ($000)	% of HS[1] in area	Payroll per employee
Visalia – Tulare – Porterville, CA MSA	2	0.44	-	-	-	-	-	-	-
Waco, TX MSA	1	0.34	-	-	-	-	-	-	-
Washington – Baltimore, DC – MD – VA – WV CMSA	15	0.12	-	-	-	-	-	-	-
Waterloo – Cedar Falls, IA MSA	0	0.00	0	0.00	0	0.00	0	0.00	0
Wausau, WI MSA	0	0.00	0	0.00	0	0.00	0	0.00	0
West Palm Beach – Boca Raton, FL MSA	13	0.48	413,674	20.93	5,000	20.35	143,735	17.05	28,747
Wheeling, WV – OH MSA	1	0.33	-	-	-	-	-	-	-
Wichita, KS MSA	5	0.65	-	-	-	-	-	-	-
Wichita Falls, TX MSA	2	0.90	-	-	-	-	-	-	-
Williamsport, PA MSA	0	0.00	0	0.00	0	0.00	0	0.00	0
Wilmington, NC MSA	2	0.63	-	-	-	-	-	-	-
Yakima, WA MSA	0	0.00	0	0.00	0	0.00	0	0.00	0
York, PA MSA	1	0.20	-	-	-	-	-	-	-
Youngstown – Warren, OH MSA	2	0.17	-	-	-	-	-	-	-
Yuba City, CA MSA	1	0.51	-	-	-	-	-	-	-
Yuma, AZ MSA	0	0.00	0	0.00	0	0.00	0	0.00	0

Source: U.S. Department of Commerce. Bureau of the Census. *1992 Economic Census Report Series*, CD-ROM 1i, Washington, DC, October 1996. *Notes:* - means no data reported. 1. HS stands for total health service establishments, revenues, employment, or payroll.

★ 349 ★

Establishment Data

Hospitals by Major Metro Area, Non-Taxed: 1992

Area	Establish- ments	Revenues in $1,000	Employ- ment	Payroll in $1,000	Payroll per employee
United States	5,717	279,735,236	4,566,323	126,202,009	27,638
Albany – Schenectady – Troy, NY MSA	16	956,602	19,225	484,294	25,191
Albuquerque, NM MSA	16	647,265	11,733	304,356	25,940
Allentown – Bethlehem – Easton, PA MSA	11	738,343	13,425	364,047	27,117
Atlanta, GA MSA	39	3,112,662	47,000	1,250,853	26,614
Austin – San Marcos, TX MSA	10	508,656	8,780	228,418	26,016
Baton Rouge, LA MSA	9	476,662	8,381	186,854	22,295
Birmingham, AL MSA	15	1,531,843	21,620	592,801	27,419
Boston – Worcester – Lawrence, MA – NH – ME – CT CMSA	117	-	-	-	-
Buffalo – Niagara Falls, NY MSA	26	1,494,748	30,378	785,761	25,866
Charlotte – Gastonia – Rock Hill, NC – SC MSA	15	1,190,956	18,761	517,141	27,565
Chicago – Gary – Kenosha, IL – IN – WI CMSA	116	-	-	-	-
Cincinnati – Hamilton, OH – KY – IN CMSA	32	-	-	-	-

[Continued]

★ 349 ★

Hospitals by Major Metro Area, Non-Taxed: 1992
[Continued]

Area	Establish-ments	Revenues in $1,000	Employ-ment	Payroll in $1,000	Payroll per employee
Cleveland – Akron, OH CMSA	55	4,534,031	72,307	2,066,030	28,573
Columbus, OH MSA	20	1,720,110	26,281	696,647	26,508
Dallas – Fort Worth, TX CMSA	44	3,266,607	48,273	1,336,571	27,688
Dayton – Springfield, OH MSA	17	1,509,343	24,515	670,963	27,369
Denver – Boulder – Greeley, CO CMSA	32	2,392,081	35,323	1,016,688	28,783
Des Moines, IA MSA	8	665,998	12,304	294,838	23,963
Detroit – Ann Arbor – Flint, MI CMSA	87	-	-	-	-
Fresno, CA MSA	13	727,017	11,232	329,423	29,329
Grand Rapids – Muskegon – Holland, MI MSA	16	885,723	16,442	391,920	23,837
Greensboro – Winston-Salem – High Point, NC MSA	23	1,142,878	19,737	523,618	26,530
Greenville – Spartanburg – Anderson, SC MSA	15	822,171	12,950	328,032	25,331
Harrisburg – Lebanon – Carlisle, PA MSA	13	822,613	14,389	415,516	28,877
Hartford, CT MSA	26	1,613,795	25,286	831,691	32,891
Honolulu, HI MSA	15	1,054,109	16,339	514,413	31,484
Houston – Galveston – Brazoria, TX CMSA	34	3,912,487	52,594	1,634,451	31,077
Indianapolis, IN MSA	28	2,225,573	35,239	959,775	27,236
Jacksonville, FL MSA	15	1,058,331	15,296	418,485	27,359
Kalamazoo – Battle Creek, MI MSA	13	570,054	10,255	294,707	28,738
Kansas City, MO – KS MSA	42	2,128,436	39,134	958,036	24,481
Knoxville, TN MSA	12	954,879	14,578	355,620	24,394
Lansing – East Lansing, MI MSA	7	465,205	7,882	197,599	25,070
Lexington, KY MSA	12	688,111	12,035	306,546	25,471
Little Rock – North Little Rock, AR MSA	13	1,060,225	17,888	461,736	25,813
Los Angeles – Riverside – Orange County, CA CMSA	148	13,930,521	179,971	5,729,868	31,838
Louisville, KY – IN MSA	15	971,241	16,915	411,010	24,299
Madison, WI MSA	8	643,693	10,849	298,270	27,493
Memphis, TN – AR – MS MSA	18	1,552,320	25,973	662,839	25,520
Miami – Fort Lauderdale, FL CMSA	26	2,958,457	39,951	1,294,429	32,400
Milwaukee – Racine, WI CMSA	35	-	-	-	-
Minneapolis – St. Paul, MN – WI MSA	43	2,906,955	47,803	1,354,193	28,329
Nashville, TN MSA	19	1,428,334	22,238	620,547	27,905
New Orleans, LA MSA	19	1,641,496	26,153	720,281	27,541
New York – Northern New Jersey – Long Island, NY – NJ – CT- CMSA	282	-	-	-	-
Norfolk – Virginia Beach – Newport News, VA – NC MSA	23	1,671,628	27,353	768,052	28,079
Oklahoma City, OK MSA	24	1,155,427	20,917	504,556	24,122
Omaha, NE – IA MSA	15	948,144	16,341	438,131	26,812

[Continued]

★ 349 ★

Hospitals by Major Metro Area, Non-Taxed: 1992
[Continued]

Area	Establish-ments	Revenues in $1,000	Employ-ment	Payroll in $1,000	Payroll per employee
Orlando, FL MSA	17	1,134,669	18,628	510,954	27,429
Philadelphia – Wilmington – Atlantic City, PA – NJ – DE – MD CMSA	131	9,645,343	147,379	4,382,943	29,739
Phoenix – Mesa, AZ MSA	35	2,405,240	33,907	922,330	27,202
Pittsburgh, PA MSA	55	4,508,713	71,503	1,983,241	27,736
Portland – Salem, OR – WA CMSA	26	-	-	-	-
Providence – Fall River – Warwick, RI – MA MSA	23	1,377,996	24,555	714,950	29,116
Raleigh – Durham – Chapel Hill, NC MSA	17	1,505,817	23,455	684,338	29,177
Richmond – Petersburg, VA MSA	15	952,190	16,341	430,774	26,362
Rochester, NY MSA	20	1,219,609	24,655	622,027	25,229
Sacramento – Yolo, CA CMSA	18	-	-	-	-
St. Louis, MO – IL MSA	53	3,723,087	64,358	1,615,793	25,106
Salt Lake City – Ogden, UT MSA	14	971,027	16,248	414,689	25,522
San Antonio, TX MSA	22	1,627,484	26,169	808,637	30,901
San Diego, CA MSA	30	2,374,624	33,205	1,009,564	30,404
San Francisco – Oakland – San Jose, CA CMSA	88	8,112,614	102,116	3,830,518	37,511
Santa Barbara – Santa Maria – Lompoc, CA MSA	8	294,466	4,369	122,828	28,114
Scranton – Wilkes-Barre – Hazleton, PA MSA	22	809,089	15,133	365,849	24,176
Seattle – Tacoma – Bremerton, WA CMSA	44	3,475,208	50,657	1,546,119	30,521
Springfield, MA MSA	15	702,790	12,738	350,827	27,542
Syracuse, NY MSA	11	764,683	14,871	390,364	26,250
Tampa – St. Petersburg – Clearwater, FL MSA	23	1,903,760	28,303	800,216	28,273
Toledo, OH MSA	12	1,049,372	18,492	458,410	24,790
Tucson, AZ MSA	10	659,060	10,419	311,055	29,855
Tulsa, OK MSA	14	737,680	13,450	312,129	23,207
Washington – Baltimore, DC – MD – VA – WV CMSA	95	-	-	-	-
West Palm Beach – Boca Raton, FL MSA	10	653,843	9,696	276,462	28,513
Wichita, KS MSA	10	565,618	8,510	253,493	29,788
Youngstown – Warren, OH MSA	11	751,121	12,540	330,702	26,372

Source: U.S. Department of Commerce. Bureau of the Census. *1992 Economic Census Report Series,* CD-ROM 1i, Washington, DC, October 1996. *Notes:* - means no data reported. 1. HS stands for total health service establishments, revenues, employment, or payroll.

★ 350 ★

Establishment Data

Hospitals by State: 1992

Area	Establishments		Revenues		Employment		Payroll		
	Number	% of HS[1] in area	Total ($000)	% of HS[1] in area	Number	% of HS[1] in area	Total ($000)	% of HS[1] in area	Payroll per employee
United States	1,403	0.32	31,082,975	10.39	428,150	9.62	10,556,433	8.18	24,656
Alabama	42	0.76	1,090,520	22.14	14,759	19.08	324,254	15.37	21,970
Alaska	3	0.35	-	-	-	-	-	-	-
Arizona	24	0.34	463,969	10.16	6,659	11.34	155,693	7.98	23,381
Arkansas	24	0.67	386,849	15.88	5,626	13.18	117,815	11.07	20,941
California	199	0.32	4,589,732	10.68	60,181	11.23	1,725,177	10.00	28,666
Colorado	13	0.19	223,987	5.99	2,850	5.16	74,762	4.55	26,232
Connecticut	3	0.05	-	-	-	-	-	-	-
Delaware	3	0.25	23,651	2.99	396	3.41	9,317	2.56	23,528
District of Columbia	1	0.07	-	-	-	-	-	-	-
Florida	160	0.54	4,795,458	20.58	63,442	20.13	1,564,118	16.24	24,654
Georgia	58	0.52	1,348,157	15.63	17,260	14.26	385,680	10.51	22,345
Hawaii	2	0.09	-	-	-	-	-	-	-
Idaho	10	0.58	150,377	15.24	2,347	13.87	49,490	11.90	21,086
Illinois	28	0.15	766,083	6.19	11,116	5.92	298,170	5.33	26,823
Indiana	26	0.30	362,531	5.95	5,274	4.94	115,594	4.21	21,918
Iowa	2	0.05	-	-	-	-	-	-	-
Kansas	17	0.44	473,814	15.54	6,492	12.15	160,426	12.13	24,711
Kentucky	32	0.58	813,909	19.76	11,949	17.82	276,976	15.58	23,180
Louisiana	72	1.06	1,208,855	21.87	16,962	19.65	398,347	18.30	23,485
Maine	2	0.09	-	-	-	-	-	-	-
Maryland	12	0.13	149,373	2.65	2,757	3.45	62,396	2.50	22,632
Massachusetts	19	0.18	272,389	3.57	4,916	3.86	141,334	3.99	28,750
Michigan	10	0.06	79,682	0.92	1,428	1.01	30,033	0.73	21,032
Minnesota	1	0.02	-	-	-	-	-	-	-
Mississippi	21	0.68	284,208	13.64	4,638	12.59	94,735	10.77	20,426
Missouri	24	0.28	470,019	8.55	7,128	7.52	159,473	6.52	22,373
Montana	4	0.27	19,772	3.04	320	2.97	7,997	3.08	24,991
Nebraska	3	0.13	-	-	-	-	-	-	-
Nevada	12	0.52	563,642	25.05	5,955	23.58	167,069	18.24	28,055
New Hampshire	12	0.65	170,668	14.37	3,037	15.81	67,084	12.36	22,089
New Jersey	5	0.03	113,124	1.09	1,582	1.24	35,195	0.80	22,247
New Mexico	16	0.67	315,596	21.35	5,184	21.92	116,829	18.88	22,536
New York	29	0.09	899,620	4.53	13,884	4.99	431,443	5.23	31,075
North Carolina	27	0.30	524,762	7.88	7,520	7.01	170,038	5.70	22,611
North Dakota	1	0.13	-	-	-	-	-	-	-
Ohio	13	0.07	145,695	1.25	2,641	1.32	56,432	1.01	21,368
Oklahoma	24	0.45	422,724	12.91	6,431	10.89	138,898	9.83	21,598
Oregon	11	0.20	143,744	4.86	2,322	4.82	51,611	3.98	22,227
Pennsylvania	25	0.11	319,412	2.53	5,127	2.78	126,847	2.24	24,741
Rhode Island	0	0.00	0	0.00	0	0.00	0	0.00	0
South Carolina	21	0.45	518,511	16.55	7,275	14.54	160,290	11.49	22,033
South Dakota	2	0.21	-	-	-	-	-	-	-
Tennessee	64	0.78	1,176,450	17.43	17,187	17.14	387,565	13.50	22,550
Texas	237	0.79	5,418,834	23.64	70,011	20.21	1,709,808	18.54	24,422

[Continued]

★ 350 ★

Hospitals by State: 1992
[Continued]

| Area | Establishments | | Revenues | | Employment | | Payroll | | |
	Number	% of HS[1] in area	Total ($000)	% of HS[1] in area	Number	% of HS[1] in area	Total ($000)	% of HS[1] in area	Payroll per employee
Utah	17	0.56	321,988	17.44	4,913	15.89	101,068	13.39	20,572
Vermont	0	0.00	0	0.00	0	0.00	0	0.00	0
Virginia	34	0.35	1,007,493	15.08	13,627	13.34	307,496	10.16	22,565
Washington	9	0.10	135,372	2.51	1,965	2.25	47,556	2.00	24,202
West Virginia	17	0.63	250,432	14.01	3,845	13.32	83,550	11.87	21,730
Wisconsin	8	0.11	57,052	1.20	1,031	1.21	18,826	0.80	18,260
Wyoming	4	0.56	-	-	-	-	-	-	-

Source: U.S. Department of Commerce. Bureau of the Census. *1992 Economic Census Report Series,* CD-ROM 1i, Washington, DC, October 1996. *Notes:* - means no data reported. 1. HS stands for total health service establishments, revenues, employment, or payroll.

★ 351 ★
Establishment Data

Hospitals by State, Non-Taxed: 1992

Area	Establish-ments	Revenues in $1,000	Employ-ment	Payroll in $1,000	Payroll per employee
United States	5,717	279,735,236	4,566,323	126,202,009	27,638
Alabama	98	4,024,178	67,084	1,664,686	24,815
Alaska	26	596,703	7,640	274,339	35,908
Arizona	76	3,600,559	53,483	1,464,695	27,386
Arkansas	78	2,215,046	40,922	926,252	22,635
California	405	29,962,335	397,857	12,923,725	32,483
Colorado	87	3,652,021	58,174	1,600,044	27,504
Connecticut	63	4,255,354	66,254	2,165,200	32,680
Delaware	13	879,404	14,114	409,987	29,048
District of Columbia	17	2,704,309	38,375	1,275,270	33,232
Florida	169	11,732,751	175,737	5,004,644	28,478
Georgia	152	6,731,196	114,970	2,919,328	25,392
Hawaii	27	1,241,615	19,482	603,959	31,001
Idaho	44	730,153	13,079	303,173	23,180
Illinois	229	13,949,196	233,937	6,169,021	26,370
Indiana	137	6,228,340	108,347	2,669,868	24,642
Iowa	131	3,017,768	62,893	1,372,258	21,819
Kansas	145	2,382,443	49,908	1,147,948	23,001
Kentucky	96	3,371,748	61,570	1,414,340	22,971
Louisiana	114	4,451,802	77,389	1,943,972	25,119
Maine	45	1,292,158	24,588	631,158	25,669
Maryland	73	5,291,084	89,932	2,468,416	27,448
Massachusetts	141	9,442,398	154,068	4,455,037	28,916
Michigan	209	11,364,639	187,209	5,157,089	27,547

[Continued]

★ 351 ★

Hospitals by State, Non-Taxed: 1992

[Continued]

Area	Establish- ments	Revenues in $1,000	Employ- ment	Payroll in $1,000	Payroll per employee
Minnesota	166	4,669,274	86,423	2,238,538	25,902
Mississippi	97	2,343,484	44,958	998,245	22,204
Missouri	151	6,747,443	122,050	2,962,873	24,276
Montana	61	845,040	15,490	367,804	23,745
Nebraska	101	1,711,480	33,452	788,134	23,560
Nevada	20	733,300	9,815	287,590	29,301
New Hampshire	29	1,080,201	17,747	471,640	26,576
New Jersey	130	9,729,684	154,585	4,675,221	30,244
New Mexico	51	1,242,439	22,672	580,914	25,623
New York	297	26,822,860	429,785	14,037,207	32,661
North Carolina	147	6,884,202	115,902	3,070,419	26,492
North Dakota	56	843,084	17,409	387,804	22,276
Ohio	230	13,853,145	232,413	6,076,133	26,144
Oklahoma	126	2,809,388	53,691	1,231,793	22,942
Oregon	68	2,691,841	43,529	1,212,826	27,862
Pennsylvania	289	17,700,037	290,397	7,981,360	27,484
Rhode Island	21	1,257,773	22,678	664,173	29,287
South Carolina	72	3,315,243	52,072	1,363,573	26,186
South Dakota	63	838,177	17,234	380,006	22,050
Tennessee	111	5,594,181	92,596	2,328,776	25,150
Texas	348	14,662,414	229,740	6,268,975	27,287
Utah	39	1,304,884	22,591	560,674	24,818
Vermont	18	545,676	9,782	252,795	25,843
Virginia	108	5,786,108	99,034	2,557,534	25,825
Washington	110	5,058,466	76,902	2,266,845	29,477
West Virginia	55	1,992,715	34,281	849,790	24,789
Wisconsin	149	5,205,751	94,916	2,209,839	23,282
Wyoming	29	349,746	7,167	166,119	23,178

Source: U.S. Department of Commerce. Bureau of the Census. *1992 Economic Census Report Series,* CD-ROM 1i, Washington, DC, October 1996. *Notes:* - means no data reported. 1. HS stands for total health service establishments, revenues, employment, or payroll.

★ 352 ★

Establishment Data

Intermediate Care Facilities by Major Metro Area: 1992

Area	Establishments		Revenues		Employment		Payroll		
	Number	% of HS[1] in area	Total ($000)	% of HS[1] in area	Number	% of HS[1] in area	Total ($000)	% of HS[1] in area	Payroll per employee
United States	3,375	0.76	4,207,093	1.41	164,704	3.70	2,007,501	1.56	12,189
Albany – Schenectady – Troy, NY MSA	0	0.00	0	0.00	0	0.00	0	0.00	0
Albuquerque, NM MSA	3	0.28	-	-	-	-	-	-	-
Allentown – Bethlehem – Easton, PA MSA	1	0.08	-	-	-	-	-	-	-

[Continued]

★ 352 ★

Intermediate Care Facilities by Major Metro Area: 1992
[Continued]

Area	Establishments		Revenues		Employment		Payroll		
	Number	% of HS[1] in area	Total ($000)	% of HS[1] in area	Number	% of HS[1] in area	Total ($000)	% of HS[1] in area	Payroll per employee
Anchorage, AK MSA	0	0.00	0	0.00	0	0.00	0	0.00	0
Appleton – Oshkosh – Neenah, WI MSA	0	0.00	0	0.00	0	0.00	0	0.00	0
Atlanta, GA MSA	8	0.13	5,648	0.12	176	0.29	2,247	0.11	12,767
Augusta – Aiken, GA – SC MSA	1	0.14	-	-	-	-	-	-	-
Austin – San Marcos, TX MSA	26	1.65	-	-	-	-	-	-	-
Bakersfield, CA MSA	1	0.13	-	-	-	-	-	-	-
Baton Rouge, LA MSA	6	0.68	-	-	-	-	-	-	-
Beaumont – Port Arthur, TX MSA	5	0.69	-	-	-	-	-	-	-
Birmingham, AL MSA	1	0.07	-	-	-	-	-	-	-
Boise City, ID MSA	7	1.17	7,905	2.10	324	5.55	4,067	2.40	12,552
Boston – Worcester – Lawrence, MA – NH – ME – CT CMSA	118	1.21	186,776	2.64	6,251	5.43	102,485	3.15	16,395
Buffalo – Niagara Falls, NY MSA	1	0.05	-	-	-	-	-	-	-
Canton – Massillon, OH MSA	18	2.60	-	-	-	-	-	-	-
Charleston – North Charleston, SC MSA	0	0.00	0	0.00	0	0.00	0	0.00	0
Charlotte – Gastonia – Rock Hill, NC – SC MSA	15	0.94	11,694	0.84	426	2.09	5,411	0.82	12,702
Chattanooga, TN – GA MSA	2	0.26	-	-	-	-	-	-	-
Chicago – Gary – Kenosha, IL – IN – WI CMSA	65	0.45	-	-	-	-	-	-	-
Cincinnati – Hamilton, OH – KY – IN CMSA	37	1.18	-	-	-	-	-	-	-
Cleveland – Akron, OH CMSA	53	0.99	-	-	-	-	-	-	-
Colorado Springs, CO MSA	8	0.90	1,317	0.30	64	0.97	563	0.28	8,797
Columbia, SC MSA	0	0.00	0	0.00	0	0.00	0	0.00	0
Columbus, OH MSA	32	1.32	29,383	1.67	1,026	3.65	12,471	1.54	12,155
Corpus Christi, TX MSA	8	1.07	-	-	-	-	-	-	-
Dallas – Fort Worth, TX CMSA	44	0.53	47,535	0.73	1,923	2.23	22,377	0.84	11,637
Davenport – Moline – Rock Island, IA – IL MSA	8	1.18	-	-	-	-	-	-	-
Dayton – Springfield, OH MSA	11	0.67	-	-	-	-	-	-	-
Daytona Beach, FL MSA	2	0.27	-	-	-	-	-	-	-
Denver – Boulder – Greeley, CO CMSA	14	0.32	-	-	-	-	-	-	-
Des Moines, IA MSA	17	2.30	25,061	4.93	968	13.60	12,051	4.54	12,449
Detroit – Ann Arbor – Flint, MI CMSA	40	0.42	-	-	-	-	-	-	-
El Paso, TX MSA	2	0.25	-	-	-	-	-	-	-
Eugene – Springfield, OR MSA	3	0.51	-	-	-	-	-	-	-
Fort Myers – Cape Coral, FL MSA	1	0.14	-	-	-	-	-	-	-
Fort Pierce – Port St. Lucie, FL MSA	1	0.19	-	-	-	-	-	-	-
Fort Wayne, IN MSA	17	2.43	-	-	-	-	-	-	-
Fresno, CA MSA	8	0.54	-	-	-	-	-	-	-
Grand Rapids – Muskegon – Holland, MI MSA	6	0.39	5,840	0.65	232	1.62	2,590	0.60	11,164
Greensboro – Winston-Salem – High Point, NC MSA	9	0.60	9,947	0.84	378	2.21	5,384	1.02	14,243
Greenville – Spartanburg – Anderson, SC MSA	1	0.09	-	-	-	-	-	-	-
Harrisburg – Lebanon – Carlisle, PA MSA	6	0.61	5,643	0.86	236	2.48	2,165	0.70	9,174
Hartford, CT MSA	8	0.35	-	-	-	-	-	-	-
Honolulu, HI MSA	4	0.24	-	-	-	-	-	-	-
Houston – Galveston – Brazoria, TX CMSA	36	0.51	35,002	0.60	1,233	1.65	15,199	0.65	12,327
Huntsville, AL MSA	2	0.38	-	-	-	-	-	-	-
Indianapolis, IN MSA	68	2.68	61,527	3.07	2,277	7.08	30,784	3.27	13,520
Jackson, MS MSA	3	0.47	-	-	-	-	-	-	-

[Continued]

★ 352 ★

Intermediate Care Facilities by Major Metro Area: 1992

[Continued]

Area	Establishments		Revenues		Employment		Payroll		
	Number	% of HS[1] in area	Total ($000)	% of HS[1] in area	Number	% of HS[1] in area	Total ($000)	% of HS[1] in area	Payroll per employee
Jacksonville, FL MSA	8	0.45	-	-	-	-	-	-	-
Johnson City – Kingsport – Bristol, TN – VA MSA	8	1.16	-	-	-	-	-	-	-
Kalamazoo – Battle Creek, MI MSA	4	0.54	-	-	-	-	-	-	-
Kansas City, MO – KS MSA	23	0.81	17,007	0.78	938	2.78	8,245	0.83	8,790
Knoxville, TN MSA	2	0.17	-	-	-	-	-	-	-
Lafayette, LA MSA	2	0.31	-	-	-	-	-	-	-
Lakeland – Winter Haven, FL MSA	4	0.82	-	-	-	-	-	-	-
Lancaster, PA MSA	3	0.50	-	-	-	-	-	-	-
Lansing – East Lansing, MI MSA	6	0.82	-	-	-	-	-	-	-
Las Vegas, NV – AZ MSA	4	0.26	-	-	-	-	-	-	-
Lexington, KY MSA	5	0.62	-	-	-	-	-	-	-
Little Rock – North Little Rock, AR MSA	2	0.19	-	-	-	-	-	-	-
Los Angeles – Riverside – Orange County, CA CMSA	89	0.29							
Louisville, KY – IN MSA	15	0.87	-	-	-	-	-	-	-
Macon, GA MSA	2	0.37	-	-	-	-	-	-	-
Madison, WI MSA	22	4.25							
Melbourne – Titusville – Palm Bay, FL MSA	3	0.37	-	-	-	-	-	-	-
Memphis, TN – AR – MS MSA	8	0.49	-	-	-	-	-	-	-
Miami – Fort Lauderdale, FL CMSA	21	0.23	-	-	-	-	-	-	-
Milwaukee – Racine, WI CMSA	10	0.33	-	-	-	-	-	-	-
Minneapolis – St. Paul, MN – WI MSA	110	2.95	46,371	1.60	2,117	4.24	26,516	1.77	12,525
Mobile, AL MSA	3	0.47	-	-	-	-	-	-	-
Modesto, CA MSA	0	0.00	0	0.00	0	0.00	0	0.00	0
Montgomery, AL MSA	2	0.41	-	-	-	-	-	-	-
Nashville, TN MSA	16	0.82	36,241	1.95	1,586	6.27	17,739	2.29	11,185
New Orleans, LA MSA	15	0.62	32,972	1.51	1,079	3.64	11,892	1.41	11,021
New York – Northern New Jersey – Long Island, NY – NJ – CT- CMSA	59	0.15	94,389	0.36	2,675	0.80	45,207	0.41	16,900
Norfolk – Virginia Beach – Newport News, VA – NC MSA	16	0.71	50,837	3.75	1,877	8.58	26,697	4.13	14,223
Oklahoma City, OK MSA	38	1.93	49,433	3.81	2,413	12.32	22,963	4.10	9,516
Omaha, NE – IA MSA	6	0.59	-	-	-	-	-	-	-
Orlando, FL MSA	11	0.43	-	-	-	-	-	-	-
Pensacola, FL MSA	2	0.38	-	-	-	-	-	-	-
Peoria – Pekin, IL MSA	7	1.38	-	-	-	-	-	-	-
Philadelphia – Wilmington – Atlantic City, PA – NJ – DE – MD CMSA	39	0.34	-	-	-	-	-	-	-
Phoenix – Mesa, AZ MSA	6	0.12	-	-	-	-	-	-	-
Pittsburgh, PA MSA	8	0.17	12,540	0.46	287	0.75	5,313	0.43	18,512
Portland, ME MSA	12	2.22	33,772	8.81	1,147	19.50	17,949	10.01	15,649
Portland – Salem, OR – WA CMSA	41	1.16	-	-	-	-	-	-	-
Providence – Fall River – Warwick, RI – MA MSA	13	0.63	-	-	-	-	-	-	-
Raleigh – Durham – Chapel Hill, NC MSA	18	1.25	8,681	0.71	246	1.43	4,017	0.80	16,329
Reno, NV MSA	3	0.45	-	-	-	-	-	-	-
Richmond – Petersburg, VA MSA	8	0.50	15,293	0.98	565	2.54	7,060	1.07	12,496
Rochester, NY MSA	0	0.00	0	0.00	0	0.00	0	0.00	0
Rockford, IL MSA	11	2.31	13,121	3.62	480	8.84	5,703	3.47	11,881
Sacramento – Yolo, CA CMSA	8	0.28	6,812	0.35	269	1.08	3,472	0.42	12,907
Saginaw – Bay City – Midland, MI MSA	4	0.59	-	-	-	-	-	-	-
St. Louis, MO – IL MSA	37	0.83	49,815	1.74	2,115	4.85	21,876	1.76	10,343
Salinas, CA MSA	0	0.00	0	0.00	0	0.00	0	0.00	0

[Continued]

★ 352 ★

Intermediate Care Facilities by Major Metro Area: 1992

[Continued]

Area	Establishments		Revenues		Employment		Payroll		
	Number	% of HS[1] in area	Total ($000)	% of HS[1] in area	Number	% of HS[1] in area	Total ($000)	% of HS[1] in area	Payroll per employee
Salt Lake City – Ogden, UT MSA	26	1.26	-	-	-	-	-	-	-
San Antonio, TX MSA	14	0.53	-	-	-	-	-	-	-
San Diego, CA MSA	9	0.18	8,161	0.25	364	0.87	3,364	0.25	9,242
San Francisco – Oakland – San Jose, CA CMSA	21	0.15	12,809	0.14	466	0.41	6,661	0.18	14,294
Santa Barbara – Santa Maria – Lompoc, CA MSA	0	0.00	0	0.00	0	0.00	0	0.00	0
Sarasota – Bradenton, FL MSA	2	0.16	-	-	-	-	-	-	-
Scranton – Wilkes-Barre – Hazleton, PA MSA	8	0.70	15,866	2.51	605	5.70	8,221	3.14	13,588
Seattle – Tacoma – Bremerton, WA CMSA	14	0.23	14,532	0.41	462	0.85	7,628	0.49	16,511
Shreveport – Bossier City, LA MSA	5	0.78	7,096	1.24	241	2.83	2,741	1.18	11,373
Spokane, WA MSA	2	0.27	-	-	-	-	-	-	-
Springfield, MO MSA	5	1.09	-	-	-	-	-	-	-
Springfield, MA MSA	3	0.33	3,238	0.48	129	1.07	1,889	0.59	14,643
Stockton – Lodi, CA MSA	1	0.12	-	-	-	-	-	-	-
Syracuse, NY MSA	1	0.09	-	-	-	-	-	-	-
Tallahassee, FL MSA	0	0.00	0	0.00	0	0.00	0	0.00	0
Tampa – St. Petersburg – Clearwater, FL MSA	8	0.16	17,544	0.40	565	0.92	7,501	0.43	13,276
Toledo, OH MSA	12	1.07	-	-	-	-	-	-	-
Tucson, AZ MSA	4	0.32	-	-	-	-	-	-	-
Tulsa, OK MSA	31	2.27	44,982	4.73	1,971	13.81	20,322	4.78	10,311
Washington – Baltimore, DC – MD – VA – WV CMSA	84	0.65	128,615	1.59	4,169	3.79	63,285	1.76	15,180
West Palm Beach – Boca Raton, FL MSA	9	0.33	-	-	-	-	-	-	-
Wichita, KS MSA	12	1.57	-	-	-	-	-	-	-
Youngstown – Warren, OH MSA	8	0.67	-	-	-	-	-	-	-

Source: U.S. Department of Commerce. Bureau of the Census. *1992 Economic Census Report Series,* CD-ROM 1i, Washington, DC, October 1996. *Notes:* - means no data reported. 1. HS stands for total health service establishments, revenues, employment, or payroll.

★ 353 ★

Establishment Data

Intermediate Care Facilities by Major Metro Area, Non-Taxed: 1992

Area	Establish- ments	Revenues in $1,000	Employ- ment	Payroll in $1,000	Payroll per employee
United States	2,791	2,949,580	113,526	1,515,629	13,351
Albany – Schenectady – Troy, NY MSA	30	31,981	1,288	17,399	13,509
Atlanta, GA MSA	10	-	-	-	-
Boston – Worcester – Lawrence, MA – NH – ME – CT CMSA	72	-	-	-	-
Buffalo – Niagara Falls, NY MSA	22	-	-	-	-
Chicago – Gary – Kenosha, IL – IN – WI CMSA	49	-	-	-	-
Cincinnati – Hamilton, OH – KY – IN CMSA	32	31,917	1,097	16,762	15,280

[Continued]

★ 353 ★

Intermediate Care Facilities by Major Metro Area, Non-Taxed: 1992

[Continued]

Area	Establish- ments	Revenues in $1,000	Employ- ment	Payroll in $1,000	Payroll per employee
Cleveland – Akron, OH CMSA	61	-	-	-	-
Columbus, OH MSA	44	-	-	-	-
Dallas – Fort Worth, TX CMSA	6	-	-	-	-
Denver – Boulder – Greeley, CO CMSA	6	13,844	354	5,797	16,376
Detroit – Ann Arbor – Flint, MI CMSA	97	41,551	1,753	23,491	13,400
Hartford, CT MSA	11	-	-	-	-
Houston – Galveston – Brazoria, TX CMSA	10	-	-	-	-
Indianapolis, IN MSA	9	-	-	-	-
Kansas City, MO – KS MSA	14	-	-	-	-
Los Angeles – Riverside – Orange County, CA CMSA	24	-	-	-	-
Miami – Fort Lauderdale, FL CMSA	6	17,129	367	9,624	26,223
Milwaukee – Racine, WI CMSA	32	-	-	-	-
Minneapolis – St. Paul, MN – WI MSA	51	35,964	1,462	20,626	14,108
New York – Northern New Jersey – Long Island, NY – NJ – CT- CMSA	304	340,987	10,779	182,425	16,924
Philadelphia – Wilmington – Atlantic City, PA – NJ – DE – MD CMSA	108	-	-	-	-
Phoenix – Mesa, AZ MSA	21	-	-	-	-
Pittsburgh, PA MSA	39	29,402	912	15,232	16,702
Portland – Salem, OR – WA CMSA	8	-	-	-	-
Providence – Fall River – Warwick, RI – MA MSA	35	-	-	-	-
Sacramento – Yolo, CA CMSA	2	-	-	-	-
St. Louis, MO – IL MSA	48	71,508	2,774	33,486	12,071
San Diego, CA MSA	24	-	-	-	-
San Francisco – Oakland – San Jose, CA CMSA	16	-	-	-	-
Seattle – Tacoma – Bremerton, WA CMSA	2	-	-	-	-
Tampa – St. Petersburg – Clearwater, FL MSA	8	-	-	-	-
Washington – Baltimore, DC – MD – VA – WV CMSA	88	78,284	2,734	38,133	13,948

Source: U.S. Department of Commerce. Bureau of the Census. *1992 Economic Census Report Series,* CD-ROM 1i, Washington, DC, October 1996. *Notes:* - means no data reported. 1. HS stands for total health service establishments, revenues, employment, or payroll.

★ 354 ★

Establishment Data

Intermediate Care Facilities by State: 1992

Area	Establishments		Revenues		Employment		Payroll		
	Number	% of HS[1] in area	Total ($000)	% of HS[1] in area	Number	% of HS[1] in area	Total ($000)	% of HS[1] in area	Payroll per employee
United States	3,375	0.76	4,207,093	1.41	164,704	3.70	2,007,501	1.56	12,189
Alabama	11	0.20	12,170	0.25	486	0.63	4,869	0.23	10,019
Alaska	0	0.00	0	0.00	0	0.00	0	0.00	0
Arizona	10	0.14	9,369	0.21	211	0.36	3,454	0.18	16,370
Arkansas	14	0.39	20,895	0.86	972	2.28	10,270	0.97	10,566
California	147	0.24	99,235	0.23	3,743	0.70	52,041	0.30	13,904
Colorado	27	0.39	14,363	0.38	558	1.01	6,945	0.42	12,446
Connecticut	39	0.59	77,843	1.59	1,868	2.58	36,430	1.55	19,502
Delaware	2	0.17	-	-	-	-	-	-	-
District of Columbia	33	2.39	-	-	-	-	-	-	-
Florida	81	0.27	134,299	0.58	4,316	1.37	59,914	0.62	13,882
Georgia	24	0.22	25,031	0.29	948	0.78	11,807	0.32	12,455
Hawaii	7	0.31	24,275	1.85	628	4.01	11,005	1.87	17,524
Idaho	15	0.87	-	-	-	-	-	-	-
Illinois	218	1.17	327,927	2.65	11,795	6.29	130,487	2.33	11,063
Indiana	215	2.47	277,537	4.56	10,074	9.44	125,114	4.56	12,419
Iowa	137	3.27	160,814	6.88	7,878	17.52	84,400	7.59	10,713
Kansas	105	2.72	116,010	3.81	5,754	10.76	60,788	4.60	10,564
Kentucky	69	1.25	136,496	3.31	5,303	7.91	63,324	3.56	11,941
Louisiana	72	1.06	127,718	2.31	5,116	5.93	52,097	2.39	10,183
Maine	70	3.24	144,779	12.30	5,467	24.85	76,896	14.43	14,065
Maryland	44	0.48	64,760	1.15	2,356	2.95	32,286	1.29	13,704
Massachusetts	109	1.03	156,816	2.06	5,327	4.19	89,817	2.53	16,861
Michigan	94	0.60	77,045	0.88	3,266	2.32	40,935	0.99	12,534
Minnesota	173	2.93	76,452	1.86	3,697	4.88	43,094	2.07	11,656
Mississippi	17	0.55	45,509	2.18	1,766	4.79	18,395	2.09	10,416
Missouri	125	1.48	95,592	1.74	4,673	4.93	43,430	1.78	9,294
Montana	2	0.13	-	-	-	-	-	-	-
Nebraska	37	1.57	-	-	-	-	-	-	-
Nevada	7	0.30	5,321	0.24	207	0.82	2,281	0.25	11,019
New Hampshire	30	1.63	-	-	-	-	-	-	-
New Jersey	16	0.10	25,584	0.25	716	0.56	11,938	0.27	16,673
New Mexico	6	0.25	12,872	0.87	454	1.92	5,888	0.95	12,969
New York	29	0.09	45,552	0.23	1,484	0.53	21,997	0.27	14,823
North Carolina	83	0.94	73,342	1.10	2,959	2.76	35,832	1.20	12,109
North Dakota	16	2.06	-	-	-	-	-	-	-
Ohio	265	1.43	368,401	3.16	13,742	6.88	180,330	3.24	13,123
Oklahoma	209	3.92	245,634	7.50	11,939	20.21	116,743	8.26	9,778
Oregon	50	0.89	68,903	2.33	3,075	6.39	40,702	3.14	13,236
Pennsylvania	78	0.36	94,577	0.75	2,982	1.62	44,454	0.79	14,907
Rhode Island	17	0.90	-	-	-	-	-	-	-
South Carolina	9	0.19	7,789	0.25	262	0.52	3,380	0.24	12,901
South Dakota	6	0.62	-	-	-	-	-	-	-
Tennessee	85	1.03	176,049	2.61	7,084	7.06	75,282	2.62	10,627
Texas	292	0.98	283,039	1.23	11,867	3.43	129,621	1.41	10,923

[Continued]

★ 354 ★

Intermediate Care Facilities by State: 1992

[Continued]

Area	Establishments		Revenues		Employment		Payroll		
	Number	% of HS[1] in area	Total ($000)	% of HS[1] in area	Number	% of HS[1] in area	Total ($000)	% of HS[1] in area	Payroll per employee
Utah	48	1.57	-	-	-	-	-	-	-
Vermont	13	1.40	13,896	3.43	609	8.07	7,206	4.37	11,833
Virginia	74	0.76	184,828	2.77	6,916	6.77	94,405	3.12	13,650
Washington	21	0.23	26,458	0.49	910	1.04	13,191	0.55	14,496
West Virginia	69	2.56	105,795	5.92	3,944	13.66	45,797	6.50	11,612
Wisconsin	54	0.75	36,121	0.76	1,346	1.58	19,883	0.85	14,772
Wyoming	1	0.14	-	-	-	-	-	-	-

Source: U.S. Department of Commerce. Bureau of the Census. *1992 Economic Census Report Series,* CD-ROM 1i, Washington, DC, October 1996. *Notes:* - means no data reported. 1. HS stands for total health service establishments, revenues, employment, or payroll.

★ 355 ★

Establishment Data

Intermediate Care Facilities by State, Non-Taxed: 1992

Area	Establish-ments	Revenues in $1,000	Employ-ment	Payroll in $1,000	Payroll per employee
United States	2,791	2,949,580	113,526	1,515,629	13,351
Alabama	15	-	-	-	-
Alaska	7	-	-	-	-
Arizona	27	-	-	-	-
Arkansas	26	-	-	-	-
California	82	58,249	2,276	29,838	13,110
Colorado	8	-	-	-	-
Connecticut	33	27,002	721	13,970	19,376
Delaware	6	-	-	-	-
District of Columbia	11	19,412	511	8,819	17,258
Florida	45	88,909	3,209	42,839	13,350
Georgia	15	-	-	-	-
Hawaii	4	-	-	-	-
Idaho	13	-	-	-	-
Illinois	166	257,716	8,861	121,828	13,749
Indiana	77	120,140	4,788	59,489	12,425
Iowa	115	202,876	9,834	108,949	11,079
Kansas	62	-	-	-	-
Kentucky	11	16,092	762	9,247	12,135
Louisiana	105	93,336	3,857	38,489	9,979
Maine	38	48,648	1,901	27,641	14,540
Maryland	75	51,783	1,829	26,099	14,270
Massachusetts	73	51,511	1,673	26,805	16,022
Michigan	180	84,727	3,528	46,926	13,301

[Continued]

★ 355 ★

Intermediate Care Facilities by State, Non-Taxed: 1992
[Continued]

Area	Establish-ments	Revenues in $1,000	Employ-ment	Payroll in $1,000	Payroll per employee
Minnesota	135	80,992	3,927	46,307	11,792
Mississippi	2	-	-	-	-
Missouri	41	66,230	3,144	36,670	11,663
Montana	12	-	-	-	-
Nebraska	18	-	-	-	-
Nevada	3	-	-	-	-
New Hampshire	14	-	-	-	-
New Jersey	34	26,216	773	13,067	16,904
New Mexico	8	-	-	-	-
New York	427	459,941	15,305	247,291	16,158
North Carolina	60	63,796	2,474	34,041	13,759
North Dakota	34	15,709	869	7,489	8,618
Ohio	237	241,686	9,660	131,083	13,570
Oklahoma	22	26,997	1,224	14,024	11,458
Oregon	17	-	-	-	-
Pennsylvania	197	186,373	7,356	95,949	13,044
Rhode Island	48	-	-	-	-
South Carolina	44	-	-	-	-
South Dakota	9	11,788	593	6,274	10,580
Tennessee	32	38,405	1,636	18,513	11,316
Texas	87	71,670	2,921	33,513	11,473
Utah	2	-	-	-	-
Vermont	12	15,839	568	8,797	15,488
Virginia	32	84,839	3,100	43,270	13,958
Washington	6	8,681	233	4,017	17,240
West Virginia	10	-	-	-	-
Wisconsin	52	46,040	1,641	23,196	14,135
Wyoming	2	-	-	-	-

Source: U.S. Department of Commerce. Bureau of the Census. *1992 Economic Census Report Series,* CD-ROM 1i, Washington, DC, October 1996. *Notes:* - means no data reported. 1. HS stands for total health service establishments, revenues, employment, or payroll.

★ 356 ★

Establishment Data

Kidney Dialysis Centers by Major Metro Area: 1992

Area	Establishments		Revenues		Employment		Payroll		
	Number	% of HS[1] in area	Total ($000)	% of HS[1] in area	Number	% of HS[1] in area	Total ($000)	% of HS[1] in area	Payroll per employee
United States	1,119	0.25	2,060,263	0.69	21,195	0.48	558,112	0.43	26,332
Albany – Schenectady – Troy, NY MSA	3	0.23	-	-	-	-	-	-	-
Albuquerque, NM MSA	3	0.28	-	-	-	-	-	-	-
Allentown – Bethlehem – Easton, PA MSA	3	0.24	-	-	-	-	-	-	-

[Continued]

★ 356 ★

Kidney Dialysis Centers by Major Metro Area: 1992
[Continued]

Area	Establishments		Revenues		Employment		Payroll		
	Number	% of HS[1] in area	Total ($000)	% of HS[1] in area	Number	% of HS[1] in area	Total ($000)	% of HS[1] in area	Payroll per employee
Anchorage, AK MSA	0	0.00	0	0.00	0	0.00	0	0.00	0
Appleton – Oshkosh – Neenah, WI MSA	1	0.19	-	-	-	-	-	-	-
Atlanta, GA MSA	20	0.33	31,236	0.65	244	0.41	6,129	0.30	25,119
Augusta – Aiken, GA – SC MSA	8	1.13	-	-	-	-	-	-	-
Austin – San Marcos, TX MSA	2	0.13	-	-	-	-	-	-	-
Bakersfield, CA MSA	3	0.40	-	-	-	-	-	-	-
Baton Rouge, LA MSA	5	0.56	-	-	-	-	-	-	-
Beaumont – Port Arthur, TX MSA	3	0.41	4,766	0.83	38	0.37	822	0.34	21,632
Birmingham, AL MSA	3	0.22	-	-	-	-	-	-	-
Boise City, ID MSA	0	0.00	0	0.00	0	0.00	0	0.00	0
Boston – Worcester – Lawrence, MA – NH – ME – CT CMSA	16	0.16	-	-	-	-	-	-	-
Buffalo – Niagara Falls, NY MSA	2	0.10	-	-	-	-	-	-	-
Canton – Massillon, OH MSA	1	0.14	-	-	-	-	-	-	-
Charleston – North Charleston, SC MSA	2	0.25	-	-	-	-	-	-	-
Charlotte – Gastonia – Rock Hill, NC – SC MSA	9	0.56	-	-	-	-	-	-	-
Chattanooga, TN – GA MSA	0	0.00	0	0.00	0	0.00	0	0.00	0
Chicago – Gary – Kenosha, IL – IN – WI CMSA	30	0.21	53,270	0.55	636	0.47	16,132	0.37	25,365
Cincinnati – Hamilton, OH – KY – IN CMSA	0	0.00	0	0.00	0	0.00	0	0.00	0
Cleveland – Akron, OH CMSA	1	0.02	-	-	-	-	-	-	-
Colorado Springs, CO MSA	2	0.23	-	-	-	-	-	-	-
Columbia, SC MSA	4	0.54	-	-	-	-	-	-	-
Columbus, OH MSA	3	0.12	-	-	-	-	-	-	-
Corpus Christi, TX MSA	4	0.53	10,073	1.74	108	1.28	2,162	0.96	20,019
Dallas – Fort Worth, TX CMSA	40	0.48	-	-	-	-	-	-	-
Davenport – Moline – Rock Island, IA – IL MSA	1	0.15	-	-	-	-	-	-	-
Dayton – Springfield, OH MSA	4	0.24	-	-	-	-	-	-	-
Daytona Beach, FL MSA	5	0.68	5,099	0.95	49	0.59	1,128	0.51	23,020
Denver – Boulder – Greeley, CO CMSA	8	0.18	-	-	-	-	-	-	-
Des Moines, IA MSA	1	0.14	-	-	-	-	-	-	-
Detroit – Ann Arbor – Flint, MI CMSA	12	0.13	-	-	-	-	-	-	-
El Paso, TX MSA	6	0.75	-	-	-	-	-	-	-
Eugene – Springfield, OR MSA	1	0.17	-	-	-	-	-	-	-
Fort Myers – Cape Coral, FL MSA	1	0.14	-	-	-	-	-	-	-
Fort Pierce – Port St. Lucie, FL MSA	4	0.77	-	-	-	-	-	-	-
Fort Wayne, IN MSA	3	0.43	-	-	-	-	-	-	-
Fresno, CA MSA	4	0.27	3,350	0.39	53	0.43	873	0.24	16,472
Grand Rapids – Muskegon – Holland, MI MSA	0	0.00	0	0.00	0	0.00	0	0.00	0
Greensboro – Winston-Salem – High Point, NC MSA	7	0.46	21,200	1.79	148	0.87	4,557	0.86	30,791
Greenville – Spartanburg – Anderson, SC MSA	5	0.43	10,176	1.30	111	0.93	2,789	0.74	25,126
Harrisburg – Lebanon – Carlisle, PA MSA	1	0.10	-	-	-	-	-	-	-
Hartford, CT MSA	2	0.09	-	-	-	-	-	-	-
Honolulu, HI MSA	0	0.00	0	0.00	0	0.00	0	0.00	0
Houston – Galveston – Brazoria, TX CMSA	21	0.30	-	-	-	-	-	-	-
Huntsville, AL MSA	3	0.56	-	-	-	-	-	-	-
Indianapolis, IN MSA	4	0.16	-	-	-	-	-	-	-
Jackson, MS MSA	5	0.78	-	-	-	-	-	-	-

[Continued]

★ 356 ★

Kidney Dialysis Centers by Major Metro Area: 1992

[Continued]

Area	Establishments		Revenues		Employment		Payroll		
	Number	% of HS[1] in area	Total ($000)	% of HS[1] in area	Number	% of HS[1] in area	Total ($000)	% of HS[1] in area	Payroll per employee
Jacksonville, FL MSA	4	0.23	-	-	-	-	-	-	-
Johnson City – Kingsport – Bristol, TN – VA MSA	3	0.43	-	-	-	-	-	-	-
Kalamazoo – Battle Creek, MI MSA	0	0.00	0	0.00	0	0.00	0	0.00	0
Kansas City, MO – KS MSA	6	0.21	15,687	0.72	150	0.44	3,746	0.38	24,973
Knoxville, TN MSA	2	0.17	-	-	-	-	-	-	-
Lafayette, LA MSA	3	0.47	-	-	-	-	-	-	-
Lakeland – Winter Haven, FL MSA	3	0.62	-	-	-	-	-	-	-
Lancaster, PA MSA	0	0.00	0	0.00	0	0.00	0	0.00	0
Lansing – East Lansing, MI MSA	0	0.00	0	0.00	0	0.00	0	0.00	0
Las Vegas, NV – AZ MSA	3	0.19	-	-	-	-	-	-	-
Lexington, KY MSA	1	0.12	-	-	-	-	-	-	-
Little Rock – North Little Rock, AR MSA	6	0.58	-	-	-	-	-	-	-
Los Angeles – Riverside – Orange County, CA CMSA	101	0.33	198,578	0.85	2,062	0.74	58,281	0.64	28,264
Louisville, KY – IN MSA	5	0.29	-	-	-	-	-	-	-
Macon, GA MSA	7	1.29	-	-	-	-	-	-	-
Madison, WI MSA	0	0.00	0	0.00	0	0.00	0	0.00	0
Melbourne – Titusville – Palm Bay, FL MSA	1	0.12	-	-	-	-	-	-	-
Memphis, TN – AR – MS MSA	2	0.12	-	-	-	-	-	-	-
Miami – Fort Lauderdale, FL CMSA	33	0.36	47,826	0.70	639	0.74	14,844	0.53	23,230
Milwaukee – Racine, WI CMSA	2	0.07	-	-	-	-	-	-	-
Minneapolis – St. Paul, MN – WI MSA	1	0.03	-	-	-	-	-	-	-
Mobile, AL MSA	4	0.62	-	-	-	-	-	-	-
Modesto, CA MSA	0	0.00	0	0.00	0	0.00	0	0.00	0
Montgomery, AL MSA	3	0.61	-	-	-	-	-	-	-
Nashville, TN MSA	9	0.46	-	-	-	-	-	-	-
New Orleans, LA MSA	20	0.83	22,892	1.05	319	1.08	6,479	0.77	20,310
New York – Northern New Jersey – Long Island, NY – NJ – CT- CMSA	39	0.10	126,309	0.48	1,331	0.40	42,213	0.39	31,715
Norfolk – Virginia Beach – Newport News, VA – NC MSA	5	0.22	11,142	0.82	130	0.59	3,033	0.47	23,331
Oklahoma City, OK MSA	3	0.15	-	-	-	-	-	-	-
Omaha, NE – IA MSA	0	0.00	0	0.00	0	0.00	0	0.00	0
Orlando, FL MSA	9	0.36	10,796	0.57	100	0.40	2,123	0.26	21,230
Pensacola, FL MSA	0	0.00	0	0.00	0	0.00	0	0.00	0
Peoria – Pekin, IL MSA	0	0.00	0	0.00	0	0.00	0	0.00	0
Philadelphia – Wilmington – Atlantic City, PA – NJ – DE – MD CMSA	37	0.32	-	-	-	-	-	-	-
Phoenix – Mesa, AZ MSA	15	0.31	-	-	-	-	-	-	-
Pittsburgh, PA MSA	11	0.23	-	-	-	-	-	-	-
Portland, ME MSA	3	0.55	-	-	-	-	-	-	-
Portland – Salem, OR – WA CMSA	3	0.08	-	-	-	-	-	-	-
Providence – Fall River – Warwick, RI – MA MSA	3	0.14	-	-	-	-	-	-	-
Raleigh – Durham – Chapel Hill, NC MSA	5	0.35	-	-	-	-	-	-	-
Reno, NV MSA	0	0.00	0	0.00	0	0.00	0	0.00	0
Richmond – Petersburg, VA MSA	6	0.38	-	-	-	-	-	-	-
Rochester, NY MSA	0	0.00	0	0.00	0	0.00	0	0.00	0
Rockford, IL MSA	0	0.00	0	0.00	0	0.00	0	0.00	0
Sacramento – Yolo, CA CMSA	11	0.38	-	-	-	-	-	-	-
Saginaw – Bay City – Midland, MI MSA	0	0.00	0	0.00	0	0.00	0	0.00	0
St. Louis, MO – IL MSA	13	0.29	14,642	0.51	162	0.37	4,328	0.35	26,716
Salinas, CA MSA	1	0.16	-	-	-	-	-	-	-

[Continued]

★ 356 ★

Kidney Dialysis Centers by Major Metro Area: 1992

[Continued]

Area	Establishments		Revenues		Employment		Payroll		
	Number	% of HS[1] in area	Total ($000)	% of HS[1] in area	Number	% of HS[1] in area	Total ($000)	% of HS[1] in area	Payroll per employee
Salt Lake City – Ogden, UT MSA	0	0.00	0	0.00	0	0.00	0	0.00	0
San Antonio, TX MSA	16	0.61	34,510	1.92	363	1.26	7,917	1.06	21,810
San Diego, CA MSA	13	0.26	23,959	0.73	273	0.66	7,408	0.55	27,136
San Francisco – Oakland – San Jose, CA CMSA	28	0.20	-	-	-	-	-	-	-
Santa Barbara – Santa Maria – Lompoc, CA MSA	1	0.12	-	-	-	-	-	-	-
Sarasota – Bradenton, FL MSA	6	0.49	7,824	0.80	86	0.60	1,923	0.47	22,360
Scranton – Wilkes-Barre – Hazleton, PA MSA	2	0.17	-	-	-	-	-	-	-
Seattle – Tacoma – Bremerton, WA CMSA	1	0.02	-	-	-	-	-	-	-
Shreveport – Bossier City, LA MSA	5	0.78	-	-	-	-	-	-	-
Spokane, WA MSA	0	0.00	0	0.00	0	0.00	0	0.00	0
Springfield, MO MSA	0	0.00	0	0.00	0	0.00	0	0.00	0
Springfield, MA MSA	2	0.22	-	-	-	-	-	-	-
Stockton – Lodi, CA MSA	3	0.36	-	-	-	-	-	-	-
Syracuse, NY MSA	0	0.00	0	0.00	0	0.00	0	0.00	0
Tallahassee, FL MSA	2	0.50	-	-	-	-	-	-	-
Tampa – St. Petersburg – Clearwater, FL MSA	21	0.43	28,553	0.66	259	0.42	6,627	0.38	25,587
Toledo, OH MSA	1	0.09	-	-	-	-	-	-	-
Tucson, AZ MSA	0	0.00	0	0.00	0	0.00	0	0.00	0
Tulsa, OK MSA	1	0.07	-	-	-	-	-	-	-
Washington – Baltimore, DC – MD – VA – WV CMSA	58	0.45	95,079	1.18	987	0.90	26,152	0.73	26,496
West Palm Beach – Boca Raton, FL MSA	12	0.45	12,534	0.63	141	0.57	3,111	0.37	22,064
Wichita, KS MSA	1	0.13	-	-	-	-	-	-	-
Youngstown – Warren, OH MSA	2	0.17	-	-	-	-	-	-	-

Source: U.S. Department of Commerce. Bureau of the Census. *1992 Economic Census Report Series,* CD-ROM 1i, Washington, DC, October 1996. *Notes:* - means no data reported. 1. HS stands for total health service establishments, revenues, employment, or payroll.

★ 357 ★

Establishment Data

Kidney Dialysis Centers by Major Metro Area, Non-Taxed: 1992

Area	Establish- ments	Revenues in $1,000	Employ- ment	Payroll in $1,000	Payroll per employee
United States	196	400,191	5,309	133,404	25,128
Albany – Schenectady – Troy, NY MSA	0	0	0	0	0
Atlanta, GA MSA	3	-	-	-	-
Boston – Worcester – Lawrence, MA – NH – ME – CT CMSA	1	-	-	-	-
Buffalo – Niagara Falls, NY MSA	0	0	0	0	0
Chicago – Gary – Kenosha, IL – IN – WI CMSA	0	0	0	0	0
Cincinnati – Hamilton, OH – KY – IN CMSA	5	-	-	-	-

[Continued]

★ 357 ★

Kidney Dialysis Centers by Major Metro Area, Non-Taxed: 1992
[Continued]

Area	Establish-ments	Revenues in $1,000	Employ-ment	Payroll in $1,000	Payroll per employee
Cleveland – Akron, OH CMSA	4	-	-	-	-
Columbus, OH MSA	0	0	0	0	0
Dallas – Fort Worth, TX CMSA	1	-	-	-	-
Denver – Boulder – Greeley, CO CMSA	1	-	-	-	-
Detroit – Ann Arbor – Flint, MI CMSA	7	-	-	-	-
Hartford, CT MSA	0	0	0	0	0
Houston – Galveston – Brazoria, TX CMSA	0	0	0	0	0
Indianapolis, IN MSA	0	0	0	0	0
Kansas City, MO – KS MSA	1	-	-	-	-
Los Angeles – Riverside – Orange County, CA CMSA	1	-	-	-	-
Miami – Fort Lauderdale, FL CMSA	2	-	-	-	-
Milwaukee – Racine, WI CMSA	0	0	0	0	0
Minneapolis – St. Paul, MN – WI MSA	8	-	-	-	-
New York – Northern New Jersey – Long Island, NY – NJ – CT- CMSA	8	-	-	-	-
Philadelphia – Wilmington – Atlantic City, PA – NJ – DE – MD CMSA	4	-	-	-	-
Phoenix – Mesa, AZ MSA	0	0	0	0	0
Pittsburgh, PA MSA	5	-	-	-	-
Portland – Salem, OR – WA CMSA	0	0	0	0	0
Providence – Fall River – Warwick, RI – MA MSA	1	-	-	-	-
Sacramento – Yolo, CA CMSA	2	-	-	-	-
St. Louis, MO – IL MSA	1	-	-	-	-
San Diego, CA MSA	0	0	0	0	0
San Francisco – Oakland – San Jose, CA CMSA	7	-	-	-	-
Seattle – Tacoma – Bremerton, WA CMSA	8	-	-	-	-
Tampa – St. Petersburg – Clearwater, FL MSA	0	0	0	0	0
Washington – Baltimore, DC – MD – VA – WV CMSA	5	-	-	-	-

Source: U.S. Department of Commerce. Bureau of the Census. *1992 Economic Census Report Series,* CD-ROM 1i, Washington, DC, October 1996. *Notes:* - means no data reported. 1. HS stands for total health service establishments, revenues, employment, or payroll.

★ 358 ★

Establishment Data

Kidney Dialysis Centers by State: 1992

Area	Establishments		Revenues		Employment		Payroll		
	Number	% of HS[1] in area	Total ($000)	% of HS[1] in area	Number	% of HS[1] in area	Total ($000)	% of HS[1] in area	Payroll per employee
United States	1,119	0.25	2,060,263	0.69	21,195	0.48	558,112	0.43	26,332
Alabama	32	0.58	62,374	1.27	597	0.77	13,135	0.62	22,002
Alaska	0	0.00	0	0.00	0	0.00	0	0.00	0
Arizona	19	0.27	25,134	0.55	315	0.54	6,660	0.34	21,143
Arkansas	17	0.48	13,841	0.57	158	0.37	3,911	0.37	24,753
California	178	0.29	319,426	0.74	3,492	0.65	99,651	0.58	28,537
Colorado	12	0.17	22,910	0.61	275	0.50	9,175	0.56	33,364
Connecticut	5	0.08	12,978	0.26	129	0.18	4,174	0.18	32,357
Delaware	4	0.33	-	-	-	-	-	-	-
District of Columbia	11	0.80	23,057	2.89	248	2.56	6,592	1.90	26,581
Florida	117	0.40	155,668	0.67	1,747	0.55	40,206	0.42	23,014
Georgia	60	0.54	82,707	0.96	813	0.67	18,036	0.49	22,185
Hawaii	0	0.00	0	0.00	0	0.00	0	0.00	0
Idaho	0	0.00	0	0.00	0	0.00	0	0.00	0
Illinois	38	0.20	62,963	0.51	781	0.42	19,618	0.35	25,119
Indiana	13	0.15	32,984	0.54	218	0.20	5,814	0.21	26,670
Iowa	1	0.02	-	-	-	-	-	-	-
Kansas	7	0.18	16,166	0.53	169	0.32	4,094	0.31	24,225
Kentucky	11	0.20	19,330	0.47	206	0.31	4,439	0.25	21,549
Louisiana	56	0.82	77,428	1.40	769	0.89	18,494	0.85	24,049
Maine	4	0.19	11,848	1.01	104	0.47	2,452	0.46	23,577
Maryland	33	0.36	54,753	0.97	597	0.75	15,663	0.63	26,236
Massachusetts	18	0.17	-	-	-	-	-	-	-
Michigan	14	0.09	35,884	0.41	363	0.26	9,029	0.22	24,873
Minnesota	1	0.02	-	-	-	-	-	-	-
Mississippi	13	0.42	15,700	0.75	192	0.52	4,856	0.55	25,292
Missouri	16	0.19	24,697	0.45	229	0.24	6,221	0.25	27,166
Montana	0	0.00	0	0.00	0	0.00	0	0.00	0
Nebraska	0	0.00	0	0.00	0	0.00	0	0.00	0
Nevada	3	0.13	-	-	-	-	-	-	-
New Hampshire	4	0.22	-	-	-	-	-	-	-
New Jersey	11	0.07	-	-	-	-	-	-	-
New Mexico	9	0.38	12,710	0.86	125	0.53	3,626	0.59	29,008
New York	31	0.10	97,380	0.49	1,107	0.40	34,195	0.41	30,890
North Carolina	47	0.53	94,152	1.41	855	0.80	21,127	0.71	24,710
North Dakota	0	0.00	0	0.00	0	0.00	0	0.00	0
Ohio	15	0.08	34,203	0.29	313	0.16	8,240	0.15	26,326
Oklahoma	7	0.13	6,772	0.21	59	0.10	1,755	0.12	29,746
Oregon	6	0.11	11,273	0.38	103	0.21	3,082	0.24	29,922
Pennsylvania	62	0.29	124,492	0.99	1,400	0.76	35,372	0.62	25,266
Rhode Island	2	0.11	-	-	-	-	-	-	-
South Carolina	29	0.62	42,330	1.35	484	0.97	10,737	0.77	22,184
South Dakota	0	0.00	0	0.00	0	0.00	0	0.00	0
Tennessee	25	0.30	97,775	1.45	1,074	1.07	29,474	1.03	27,443
Texas	125	0.42	280,242	1.22	2,311	0.67	65,076	0.71	28,159

[Continued]

★ 358 ★

Kidney Dialysis Centers by State: 1992

[Continued]

Area	Establishments		Revenues		Employment		Payroll		
	Number	% of HS[1] in area	Total ($000)	% of HS[1] in area	Number	% of HS[1] in area	Total ($000)	% of HS[1] in area	Payroll per employee
Utah	1	0.03	-	-	-	-	-	-	-
Vermont	0	0.00	0	0.00	0	0.00	0	0.00	0
Virginia	44	0.45	59,056	0.88	597	0.58	14,769	0.49	24,739
Washington	2	0.02	-	-	-	-	-	-	-
West Virginia	9	0.33	-	-	-	-	-	-	-
Wisconsin	5	0.07	10,294	0.22	93	0.11	2,983	0.13	32,075
Wyoming	2	0.28	-	-	-	-	-	-	-

Source: U.S. Department of Commerce. Bureau of the Census. *1992 Economic Census Report Series,* CD-ROM 1i, Washington, DC, October 1996. *Notes:* - means no data reported. 1. HS stands for total health service establishments, revenues, employment, or payroll.

★ 359 ★

Establishment Data

Kidney Dialysis Centers by State, Non-Taxed: 1992

Area	Establish-ments	Revenues in $1,000	Employ-ment	Payroll in $1,000	Payroll per employee
United States	196	400,191	5,309	133,404	25,128
Alabama	3	-	-	-	-
Alaska	2	-	-	-	-
Arizona	5	-	-	-	-
Arkansas	2	-	-	-	-
California	15	28,638	416	10,793	25,945
Colorado	1	-	-	-	-
Connecticut	0	0	0	0	0
Delaware	0	0	0	0	0
District of Columbia	0	0	0	0	0
Florida	10	12,627	197	4,060	20,609
Georgia	8	-	-	-	-
Hawaii	5	-	-	-	-
Idaho	0	0	0	0	0
Illinois	0	0	0	0	0
Indiana	1	-	-	-	-
Iowa	0	0	0	0	0
Kansas	0	0	0	0	0
Kentucky	5	-	-	-	-
Louisiana	1	-	-	-	-
Maine	0	0	0	0	0
Maryland	5	-	-	-	-
Massachusetts	1	-	-	-	-
Michigan	8	-	-	-	-

[Continued]

★ 359 ★

Kidney Dialysis Centers by State, Non-Taxed: 1992
[Continued]

Area	Establish-ments	Revenues in $1,000	Employ-ment	Payroll in $1,000	Payroll per employee
Minnesota	15	-	-	-	-
Mississippi	21	-	-	-	-
Missouri	9	-	-	-	-
Montana	0	0	0	0	0
Nebraska	1	-	-	-	-
Nevada	0	0	0	0	0
New Hampshire	0	0	0	0	0
New Jersey	2	-	-	-	-
New Mexico	5	-	-	-	-
New York	9	28,815	433	11,953	27,605
North Carolina	1	-	-	-	-
North Dakota	0	0	0	0	0
Ohio	10	35,406	476	12,651	26,578
Oklahoma	0	0	0	0	0
Oregon	0	0	0	0	0
Pennsylvania	8	-	-	-	-
Rhode Island	2	-	-	-	-
South Carolina	7	-	-	-	-
South Dakota	0	0	0	0	0
Tennessee	22	-	-	-	-
Texas	2	-	-	-	-
Utah	0	0	0	0	0
Vermont	0	0	0	0	0
Virginia	0	0	0	0	0
Washington	9	-	-	-	-
West Virginia	0	0	0	0	0
Wisconsin	1	-	-	-	-
Wyoming	0	0	0	0	0

Source: U.S. Department of Commerce. Bureau of the Census. *1992 Economic Census Report Series,* CD-ROM 1i, Washington, DC, October 1996. *Notes:* - means no data reported. 1. HS stands for total health service establishments, revenues, employment, or payroll.

★ 360 ★

Establishment Data

Medical Equipment Rental and Leasing Establishments by Major Metro Area: 1992

	Establish ments	Revenues ($ 000)	Employ- ment	Payroll ($ 000)	Payroll per employee
United States	3,276	3,109,843	31,062	766,734	24,684
Albany – Schenectady – Troy, NY MSA	11	9,194	169	3,733	22,089
Albuquerque, NM MSA	8	9,553	63	1,543	24,492
Allentown – Bethlehem – Easton, PA MSA	11	11,480	131	3,787	28,908
Anchorage, AK MSA	1	-	-	-	-
Appleton – Oshkosh – Neenah, WI MSA	4	-	-	-	-
Atlanta, GA MSA	38	29,284	366	9,761	26,669
Augusta – Aiken, GA – SC MSA	7	7,537	104	1,967	18,913
Austin – San Marcos, TX MSA	8	4,589	53	851	16,057
Bakersfield, CA MSA	15	12,328	88	3,127	35,534
Baton Rouge, LA MSA	4	1,651	19	258	13,579
Beaumont – Port Arthur, TX MSA	6	3,701	56	977	17,446
Birmingham, AL MSA	8	8,432	72	1,379	19,153
Boise City, ID MSA	4	-	-	-	-
Boston – Worcester – Lawrence, MA – NH – ME – CT CMSA	54	72,550	434	12,977	29,901
Buffalo – Niagara Falls, NY MSA	13	15,375	193	5,545	28,731
Canton – Massillon, OH MSA	1	-	-	-	-
Charleston – North Charleston, SC MSA	4	3,083	37	866	23,405
Charlotte – Gastonia – Rock Hill, NC – SC MSA	13	8,521	91	1,864	20,484
Chattanooga, TN – GA MSA	8	-	-	-	-
Chicago – Gary – Kenosha, IL – IN – WI CMSA	71	-	-	-	-
Cincinnati – Hamilton, OH – KY – IN CMSA	23	26,876	327	6,831	20,890
Cleveland – Akron, OH CMSA	35	43,579	404	10,735	26,572
Colorado Springs, CO MSA	6	6,149	41	1,029	25,098
Columbia, SC MSA	5	5,802	44	770	17,500
Columbus, OH MSA	19	21,556	162	3,966	24,481
Corpus Christi, TX MSA	5	-	-	-	-
Dallas – Fort Worth, TX CMSA	56	57,167	672	13,894	20,676
Davenport – Moline – Rock Island, IA – IL MSA	4	3,757	36	709	19,694
Dayton – Springfield, OH MSA	9	8,427	44	1,313	29,841
Daytona Beach, FL MSA	9	6,103	66	1,271	19,258
Denver – Boulder – Greeley, CO CMSA	31	52,533	513	12,803	24,957
Des Moines, IA MSA	7	6,556	68	2,029	29,838
Detroit – Ann Arbor – Flint, MI CMSA	67	-	-	-	-
El Paso, TX MSA	7	8,905	88	2,090	23,750
Eugene – Springfield, OR MSA	5	2,082	27	522	19,333
Fort Myers – Cape Coral, FL MSA	4	4,323	39	1,228	31,487

[Continued]

★ 360 ★

Medical Equipment Rental and Leasing Establishments by Major Metro Area: 1992

[Continued]

	Establish ments	Revenues ($ 000)	Employ- ment	Payroll ($ 000)	Payroll per employee
Fort Pierce – Port St. Lucie, FL MSA	4	-	-	-	-
Fort Wayne, IN MSA	6	4,554	68	940	13,824
Fresno, CA MSA	9	7,574	84	1,765	21,012
Grand Rapids – Muskegon – Holland, MI MSA	10	10,762	122	3,282	26,902
Greensboro – Winston-Salem – High Point, NC MSA	8	10,091	118	2,614	22,153
Greenville – Spartanburg – Anderson, SC MSA	10	-	-	-	-
Harrisburg – Lebanon – Carlisle, PA MSA	11	7,802	83	1,565	18,855
Hartford, CT MSA	9	18,574	228	4,999	21,925
Honolulu, HI MSA	3	10,236	76	1,894	24,921
Houston – Galveston – Brazoria, TX CMSA	41	42,961	541	12,295	22,726
Huntsville, AL MSA	4	2,027	32	459	14,344
Indianapolis, IN MSA	15	39,935	360	8,088	22,467
Jackson, MS MSA	5	-	-	-	-
Jacksonville, FL MSA	17	15,957	192	4,259	22,182
Johnson City – Kingsport – Bristol, TN – VA MSA	14	-	-	-	-
Kalamazoo – Battle Creek, MI MSA	3	-	-	-	-
Kansas City, MO – KS MSA	21	34,419	273	6,256	22,916
Knoxville, TN MSA	13	11,951	129	3,086	23,922
Lafayette, LA MSA	6	2,745	42	1,086	25,857
Lakeland – Winter Haven, FL MSA	7	3,061	32	635	19,844
Lancaster, PA MSA	6	-	-	-	-
Lansing – East Lansing, MI MSA	8	-	-	-	-
Las Vegas, NV – AZ MSA	14	12,538	98	2,299	23,459
Lexington, KY MSA	8	4,432	58	1,201	20,707
Little Rock – North Little Rock, AR MSA	11	10,160	53	1,430	26,981
Los Angeles – Riverside – Orange County, CA CMSA	144	218,513	1,716	48,496	28,261
Louisville, KY – IN MSA	21	17,813	204	4,481	21,966
Macon, GA MSA	4	1,608	28	402	14,357
Madison, WI MSA	6	-	-	-	-
Melbourne – Titusville – Palm Bay, FL MSA	6	-	-	-	-
Memphis, TN – AR – MS MSA	13	8,020	98	1,894	19,327
Miami – Fort Lauderdale, FL CMSA	127	59,501	624	14,804	23,724
Milwaukee – Racine, WI CMSA	11	-	-	-	-
Minneapolis – St. Paul, MN – WI MSA	21	39,214	401	8,449	21,070
Mobile, AL MSA	11	4,598	63	1,030	16,349

[Continued]

★ 360 ★

Medical Equipment Rental and Leasing Establishments by Major Metro Area: 1992
[Continued]

	Establish ments	Revenues ($ 000)	Employ- ment	Payroll ($ 000)	Payroll per employee
Modesto, CA MSA	4	-	-	-	-
Montgomery, AL MSA	6	3,899	46	804	17,478
Nashville, TN MSA	17	13,460	132	3,052	23,121
New Orleans, LA MSA	16	15,533	173	3,600	20,809
New York – Northern New Jersey – Long Island, NY – NJ – CT- CMSA	160	173,490	1,563	47,431	30,346
Norfolk – Virginia Beach – Newport News, VA – NC MSA	11	9,944	92	2,565	27,880
Oklahoma City, OK MSA	15	8,997	99	1,763	17,808
Omaha, NE – IA MSA	11	11,613	96	2,319	24,156
Orlando, FL MSA	29	26,889	232	6,486	27,957
Pensacola, FL MSA	9	3,776	51	833	16,333
Peoria – Pekin, IL MSA	8	-	-	-	-
Philadelphia – Wilmington – Atlantic City, PA – NJ – DE – MD CMSA	69	198,969	2,002	69,882	34,906
Phoenix – Mesa, AZ MSA	30	28,551	240	6,372	26,550
Pittsburgh, PA MSA	47	72,498	776	16,644	21,448
Portland, ME MSA	4	-	-	-	-
Portland – Salem, OR – WA CMSA	9	-	-	-	-
Providence – Fall River – Warwick, RI – MA MSA	10	6,310	84	1,739	20,702
Raleigh – Durham – Chapel Hill, NC MSA	8	19,057	190	5,922	31,168
Reno, NV MSA	7	7,579	79	1,836	23,241
Richmond – Petersburg, VA MSA	12	5,776	94	1,663	17,691
Rochester, NY MSA	8	5,148	53	1,474	27,811
Rockford, IL MSA	3	-	-	-	-
Sacramento – Yolo, CA CMSA	10	-	-	-	-
Saginaw – Bay City – Midland, MI MSA	5	3,425	36	644	17,889
St. Louis, MO – IL MSA	34	47,079	484	11,203	23,147
Salinas, CA MSA	2	-	-	-	-
Salt Lake City – Ogden, UT MSA	15	-	-	-	-
San Antonio, TX MSA	24	17,480	183	4,226	23,093
San Diego, CA MSA	21	52,048	451	15,165	33,625
San Francisco – Oakland – San Jose, CA CMSA	48	-	-	-	-
Santa Barbara – Santa Maria – Lompoc, CA MSA	4	3,445	30	770	25,667
Sarasota – Bradenton, FL MSA	10	3,711	48	963	20,062
Scranton – Wilkes-Barre – Hazleton, PA MSA	16	9,465	114	2,730	23,947
Seattle – Tacoma – Bremerton, WA CMSA	21	-	-	-	-
Shreveport – Bossier City, LA MSA	5	-	-	-	-
Spokane, WA MSA	5	-	-	-	-

[Continued]

★ 360 ★

Medical Equipment Rental and Leasing Establishments by Major Metro Area: 1992

[Continued]

	Establish ments	Revenues ($ 000)	Employ- ment	Payroll ($ 000)	Payroll per employee
Springfield, MO MSA	5	-	-	-	-
Springfield, MA MSA	9	-	-	-	-
Stockton–Lodi, CA MSA	4	-	-	-	-
Syracuse, NY MSA	7	4,370	62	1,031	16,629
Tallahassee, FL MSA	5	2,779	23	504	21,913
Tampa–St. Petersburg–Clearwater, FL MSA	43	33,100	324	8,060	24,877
Toledo, OH MSA	6	12,714	159	4,169	26,220
Tucson, AZ MSA	10	12,541	125	4,324	34,592
Tulsa, OK MSA	12	11,276	107	2,243	20,963
Washington–Baltimore, DC–MD–VA–WV CMSA	50	-	-	-	-
West Palm Beach–Boca Raton, FL MSA	11	4,483	54	1,208	22,370
Wichita, KS MSA	8	6,540	72	1,581	21,958
Youngstown–Warren, OH MSA	8	-	-	-	-

Source: U.S. Department of Commerce. Bureau of the Census. *1992 Economic Census Report Series,* CD-ROM 1i, Washington, DC, October 1996. *Note:* - means no data reported.

★ 361 ★

Establishment Data

Medical Equipment Rental and Leasing Establishments by State: 1992

	Establish ments	Revenues ($ 000)	Employ- ment	Payroll ($ 000)	Payroll per employee
United States	3,276	3,109,843	31,062	766,734	24,684
Alabama	62	28,052	362	5,829	16,102
Alaska	3	-	-	-	-
Arizona	49	45,180	425	11,820	27,812
Arkansas	66	33,845	360	7,149	19,858
California	296	409,248	3,467	97,189	28,033
Colorado	56	68,558	695	16,521	23,771
Connecticut	32	39,418	409	9,916	24,244
Delaware	6	5,622	41	1,021	24,902
Florida	322	187,923	1,953	45,942	23,524
Georgia	94	62,925	719	17,087	23,765
Hawaii	6	11,144	84	2,078	24,738
Idaho	8	3,460	40	930	23,250
Illinois	125	145,203	1,239	34,238	27,634
Indiana	66	100,612	981	20,496	20,893

[Continued]

★ 361 ★

Medical Equipment Rental and Leasing Establishments by State: 1992
[Continued]

	Establish ments	Revenues ($ 000)	Employ- ment	Payroll ($ 000)	Payroll per employee
Iowa	42	28,306	263	5,729	21,783
Kansas	31	32,055	317	6,441	20,319
Kentucky	91	48,361	595	12,070	20,286
Louisiana	52	31,988	371	7,027	18,941
Maine	20	13,718	164	3,947	24,067
Maryland	45	67,813	593	17,818	30,047
Massachusetts	63	81,733	537	14,655	27,291
Michigan	129	129,853	1,295	34,442	26,596
Minnesota	33	47,837	483	10,520	21,781
Mississippi	28	13,794	154	2,804	18,208
Missouri	68	74,612	790	17,531	22,191
Montana	17	5,727	89	1,664	18,697
Nebraska	29	20,780	234	4,784	20,444
Nevada	25	21,737	199	4,971	24,980
New Hampshire	19	11,977	105	2,672	25,448
New Jersey	76	202,611	1,792	65,967	36,812
New Mexico	23	14,366	122	2,528	20,721
New York	161	151,387	1,613	44,251	27,434
North Carolina	80	64,490	668	16,098	24,099
North Dakota	9	7,357	99	1,729	17,465
Ohio	113	127,805	1,348	30,691	22,768
Oklahoma	48	26,268	306	5,501	17,977
Oregon	26	23,528	254	5,345	21,043
Pennsylvania	188	207,879	2,398	56,907	23,731
Rhode Island	5	-	-	-	-
South Carolina	31	20,720	225	4,933	21,924
South Dakota	12	-	-	-	-
Tennessee	102	66,969	747	16,604	22,228
Texas	258	194,236	2,188	48,253	22,053
Utah	21	22,128	155	3,402	21,948
Vermont	5	2,574	35	650	18,571
Virginia	86	54,083	696	14,909	21,421
Washington	35	45,349	500	10,905	21,810
West Virginia	45	42,970	376	8,340	22,181
Wisconsin	50	41,768	338	7,577	22,417
Wyoming	19	7,564	100	1,742	17,420

Source: U.S. Department of Commerce. Bureau of the Census. *1992 Economic Census Report Series*, CD-ROM 1i, Washington, DC, October 1996. *Note:* - means no data reported.

★ 362 ★

Establishment Data

Medical Laboratories by Major Metro Area: 1992

Area	Establishments		Revenues		Employment		Payroll		
	Number	% of HS[1] in area	Total ($000)	% of HS[1] in area	Number	% of HS[1] in area	Total ($000)	% of HS[1] in area	Payroll per employee
United States	8,434	1.91	12,511,336	4.18	138,760	3.12	3,979,942	3.08	28,682
Albany – Schenectady – Troy, NY MSA	23	1.76	35,900	4.44	467	3.54	11,284	3.11	24,163
Albuquerque, NM MSA	35	3.28	45,814	5.49	471	3.72	12,600	3.34	26,752
Allentown – Bethlehem – Easton, PA MSA	29	2.34	23,700	3.45	185	1.98	4,445	1.45	24,027
Anchorage, AK MSA	11	2.26	8,805	2.41	91	2.51	2,550	1.78	28,022
Appleton – Oshkosh – Neenah, WI MSA	10	1.92	6,956	1.92	92	1.60	2,203	1.21	23,946
Atlanta, GA MSA	124	2.04	195,034	4.05	1,916	3.20	59,421	2.94	31,013
Augusta – Aiken, GA – SC MSA	10	1.41	13,727	2.13	143	1.55	4,308	1.53	30,126
Austin – San Marcos, TX MSA	27	1.72	49,800	4.16	547	2.94	11,864	2.44	21,689
Bakersfield, CA MSA	19	2.50	15,973	2.93	257	3.15	7,023	3.20	27,327
Baton Rouge, LA MSA	18	2.03	42,930	5.79	572	5.19	12,651	4.17	22,117
Beaumont – Port Arthur, TX MSA	13	1.80	7,224	1.26	101	0.99	3,222	1.34	31,901
Birmingham, AL MSA	34	2.47	63,433	4.20	899	4.45	18,314	2.86	20,372
Boise City, ID MSA	4	0.67	-	-	-	-	-	-	-
Boston – Worcester – Lawrence, MA – NH – ME – CT CMSA	217	2.22	431,594	6.10	4,717	4.10	141,833	4.36	30,068
Buffalo – Niagara Falls, NY MSA	28	1.40	39,698	3.59	505	2.33	14,666	2.94	29,042
Canton – Massillon, OH MSA	13	1.88	10,172	2.46	121	1.70	5,512	2.61	45,554
Charleston – North Charleston, SC MSA	8	0.98	7,404	1.25	39	0.43	1,244	0.53	31,897
Charlotte – Gastonia – Rock Hill, NC – SC MSA	19	1.19	14,058	1.01	163	0.80	4,429	0.67	27,172
Chattanooga, TN – GA MSA	8	1.05	50,203	7.00	653	6.55	12,890	4.22	19,740
Chicago – Gary – Kenosha, IL – IN – WI CMSA	260	1.79	329,588	3.39	3,781	2.77	102,348	2.33	27,069
Cincinnati – Hamilton, OH – KY – IN CMSA	53	1.69	-	-	-	-	-	-	-
Cleveland – Akron, OH CMSA	107	1.99	97,951	3.01	1,154	2.25	33,755	2.20	29,250
Colorado Springs, CO MSA	16	1.80	9,798	2.21	93	1.41	2,962	1.47	31,849
Columbia, SC MSA	10	1.34	15,097	3.13	186	2.59	4,265	1.78	22,930
Columbus, OH MSA	41	1.69	175,168	9.95	2,481	8.81	48,952	6.03	19,731
Corpus Christi, TX MSA	6	0.80	4,539	0.79	82	0.97	1,582	0.70	19,293
Dallas – Fort Worth, TX CMSA	165	1.98	240,736	3.69	2,723	3.16	71,727	2.71	26,341
Davenport – Moline – Rock Island, IA – IL MSA	12	1.77	23,866	6.61	322	5.37	6,866	4.34	21,323
Dayton – Springfield, OH MSA	34	2.06	50,510	4.41	743	4.19	14,915	2.65	20,074
Daytona Beach, FL MSA	23	3.11	11,025	2.06	143	1.71	2,459	1.12	17,196
Denver – Boulder – Greeley, CO CMSA	69	1.58	88,476	3.48	1,082	3.03	28,187	2.52	26,051
Des Moines, IA MSA	6	0.81	8,611	1.69	117	1.64	3,085	1.16	26,368
Detroit – Ann Arbor – Flint, MI CMSA	149	1.58	320,558	5.88	4,040	4.81	104,009	4.08	25,745
El Paso, TX MSA	19	2.39	22,882	2.95	277	2.59	6,681	2.29	24,119
Eugene – Springfield, OR MSA	9	1.54	-	-	-	-	-	-	-
Fort Myers – Cape Coral, FL MSA	12	1.68	5,465	0.82	61	0.74	1,296	0.42	21,246
Fort Pierce – Port St. Lucie, FL MSA	17	3.28	11,694	2.61	101	1.63	2,772	1.49	27,446
Fort Wayne, IN MSA	15	2.14	15,584	2.82	160	1.70	5,423	2.12	33,894
Fresno, CA MSA	30	2.03	30,935	3.56	394	3.20	10,194	2.75	25,873
Grand Rapids – Muskegon – Holland, MI MSA	25	1.64	63,490	7.07	935	6.51	22,446	5.19	24,006
Greensboro – Winston-Salem – High Point, NC MSA	34	2.25	103,107	8.69	1,077	6.30	30,175	5.72	28,018
Greenville – Spartanburg – Anderson, SC MSA	14	1.19	11,664	1.50	148	1.23	3,871	1.03	26,155
Harrisburg – Lebanon – Carlisle, PA MSA	21	2.13	24,732	3.79	199	2.09	4,547	1.47	22,849
Hartford, CT MSA	74	3.26	91,714	5.21	1,045	3.83	30,710	3.61	29,388
Honolulu, HI MSA	23	1.37	-	-	-	-	-	-	-

[Continued]

359

★ 362 ★

Medical Laboratories by Major Metro Area: 1992
[Continued]

Area	Establishments		Revenues		Employment		Payroll		
	Number	% of HS[1] in area	Total ($000)	% of HS[1] in area	Number	% of HS[1] in area	Total ($000)	% of HS[1] in area	Payroll per employee
Houston – Galveston – Brazoria, TX CMSA	142	2.01	183,892	3.13	1,968	2.63	53,589	2.29	27,230
Huntsville, AL MSA	17	3.19	31,904	6.98	285	4.36	10,577	5.53	37,112
Indianapolis, IN MSA	69	2.71	121,655	6.07	1,152	3.58	44,011	4.68	38,204
Jackson, MS MSA	12	1.88	15,416	3.04	209	2.90	5,437	2.60	26,014
Jacksonville, FL MSA	28	1.58	34,979	2.68	272	1.59	6,150	1.11	22,610
Johnson City – Kingsport – Bristol, TN – VA MSA	9	1.30	12,798	2.09	120	1.22	5,680	2.09	47,333
Kalamazoo – Battle Creek, MI MSA	12	1.63	16,475	3.78	295	4.12	6,273	2.92	21,264
Kansas City, MO – KS MSA	57	2.00	201,534	9.22	1,793	5.31	56,227	5.68	31,359
Knoxville, TN MSA	23	1.92	35,468	4.37	390	3.66	14,144	3.62	36,267
Lafayette, LA MSA	16	2.51	9,756	2.17	128	1.82	2,398	1.31	18,734
Lakeland – Winter Haven, FL MSA	7	1.44	2,747	0.68	39	0.61	716	0.43	18,359
Lancaster, PA MSA	11	1.82	9,069	2.38	103	1.63	1,963	1.03	19,058
Lansing – East Lansing, MI MSA	21	2.87	32,236	8.05	392	6.23	12,222	6.42	31,179
Las Vegas, NV – AZ MSA	25	1.61	64,445	3.82	731	3.96	23,615	3.47	32,305
Lexington, KY MSA	21	2.59	41,977	7.09	427	4.73	10,608	3.85	24,843
Little Rock – North Little Rock, AR MSA	17	1.63	13,369	1.72	129	1.15	2,542	0.69	19,705
Los Angeles – Riverside – Orange County, CA CMSA	658	2.15	1,269,794	5.41	11,762	4.24	379,779	4.15	32,289
Louisville, KY – IN MSA	15	0.87	73,349	4.37	921	3.56	23,114	3.24	25,097
Macon, GA MSA	16	2.94	23,885	4.23	127	1.68	4,873	2.15	38,370
Madison, WI MSA	9	1.74	15,252	2.95	149	2.07	4,975	2.12	33,389
Melbourne – Titusville – Palm Bay, FL MSA	24	2.95	12,163	2.24	127	1.75	2,319	0.93	18,260
Memphis, TN – AR – MS MSA	28	1.70	63,838	5.14	622	3.81	17,109	3.18	27,506
Miami – Fort Lauderdale, FL CMSA	302	3.30	281,270	4.11	3,081	3.54	78,201	2.79	25,382
Milwaukee – Racine, WI CMSA	42	1.39	101,549	4.97	1,590	4.66	39,288	3.78	24,709
Minneapolis – St. Paul, MN – WI MSA	46	1.24	70,436	2.43	622	1.25	23,188	1.55	37,280
Mobile, AL MSA	10	1.56	8,055	1.44	126	1.32	2,994	1.14	23,762
Modesto, CA MSA	15	2.22	26,403	4.37	333	4.15	9,708	3.92	29,153
Montgomery, AL MSA	12	2.44	24,038	4.79	290	3.91	10,734	5.09	37,014
Nashville, TN MSA	49	2.52	136,889	7.38	1,419	5.61	50,675	6.53	35,712
New Orleans, LA MSA	47	1.94	59,687	2.73	812	2.74	17,743	2.11	21,851
New York – Northern New Jersey – Long Island, NY – NJ – CT- CMSA	829	2.04	1,611,800	6.17	15,625	4.68	522,565	4.78	33,444
Norfolk – Virginia Beach – Newport News, VA – NC MSA	31	1.37	23,316	1.72	238	1.09	6,887	1.06	28,937
Oklahoma City, OK MSA	46	2.34	53,609	4.13	645	3.29	21,333	3.81	33,074
Omaha, NE – IA MSA	15	1.49	25,996	3.17	360	2.89	12,413	3.32	34,481
Orlando, FL MSA	61	2.41	60,001	3.15	784	3.11	20,108	2.46	25,648
Pensacola, FL MSA	10	1.90	-	-	-	-	-	-	-
Peoria – Pekin, IL MSA	6	1.18	-	-	-	-	-	-	-
Philadelphia – Wilmington – Atlantic City, PA – NJ – DE – MD CMSA	296	2.55	-	-	-	-	-	-	-
Phoenix – Mesa, AZ MSA	89	1.85	129,237	4.11	1,185	3.08	47,042	3.42	39,698
Pittsburgh, PA MSA	124	2.60	169,984	6.25	2,318	6.08	51,716	4.14	22,311
Portland, ME MSA	12	2.22	17,432	4.55	148	2.52	3,154	1.76	21,311
Portland – Salem, OR – WA CMSA	40	1.13	-	-	-	-	-	-	-
Providence – Fall River – Warwick, RI – MA MSA	95	4.58	62,242	5.28	841	4.24	25,673	4.85	30,527
Raleigh – Durham – Chapel Hill, NC MSA	19	1.32	-	-	-	-	-	-	-
Reno, NV MSA	25	3.75	54,442	10.44	452	7.59	12,241	5.62	27,082
Richmond – Petersburg, VA MSA	25	1.56	33,381	2.13	547	2.46	9,788	1.48	17,894
Rochester, NY MSA	35	2.29	37,487	4.53	419	3.01	10,583	3.02	25,258

[Continued]

★ 362 ★

Medical Laboratories by Major Metro Area: 1992
[Continued]

Area	Establishments		Revenues		Employment		Payroll		
	Number	% of HS[1] in area	Total ($000)	% of HS[1] in area	Number	% of HS[1] in area	Total ($000)	% of HS[1] in area	Payroll per employee
Rockford, IL MSA	3	0.63	587	0.16	5	0.09	165	0.10	33,000
Sacramento–Yolo, CA CMSA	75	2.59	-	-	-	-	-	-	-
Saginaw–Bay City–Midland, MI MSA	16	2.35	20,372	5.33	352	5.48	9,346	4.73	26,551
St. Louis, MO–IL MSA	71	1.60	71,747	2.51	774	1.78	24,049	1.94	31,071
Salinas, CA MSA	10	1.64	3,783	1.26	27	0.61	1,975	1.61	73,148
Salt Lake City–Ogden, UT MSA	33	1.60	-	-	-	-	-	-	-
San Antonio, TX MSA	75	2.86	108,707	6.04	1,165	4.05	41,789	5.60	35,870
San Diego, CA MSA	106	2.15	181,145	5.55	2,282	5.48	69,665	5.18	30,528
San Francisco–Oakland–San Jose, CA CMSA	285	2.03	341,819	3.79	3,595	3.16	118,516	3.14	32,967
Santa Barbara–Santa Maria–Lompoc, CA MSA	13	1.56	13,502	3.16	224	4.25	5,040	2.83	22,500
Sarasota–Bradenton, FL MSA	30	2.44	24,507	2.50	266	1.84	6,543	1.61	24,598
Scranton–Wilkes-Barre–Hazleton, PA MSA	33	2.88	36,482	5.78	420	3.95	9,445	3.60	22,488
Seattle–Tacoma–Bremerton, WA CMSA	130	2.15	199,726	5.61	2,325	4.29	71,471	4.60	30,740
Shreveport–Bossier City, LA MSA	12	1.87	15,101	2.64	95	1.12	5,867	2.53	61,758
Spokane, WA MSA	20	2.72	29,950	5.87	468	5.97	9,696	4.15	20,718
Springfield, MO MSA	6	1.30	8,817	2.29	51	0.74	2,952	1.49	57,882
Springfield, MA MSA	20	2.21	33,557	5.02	180	1.49	11,620	3.62	64,556
Stockton–Lodi, CA MSA	16	1.92	14,791	2.86	117	1.46	3,243	1.43	27,718
Syracuse, NY MSA	22	2.01	29,923	4.33	239	2.44	5,843	1.86	24,448
Tallahassee, FL MSA	8	2.02	11,032	3.19	130	2.76	3,007	1.97	23,131
Tampa–St. Petersburg–Clearwater, FL MSA	123	2.49	214,603	4.92	2,595	4.24	61,297	3.55	23,621
Toledo, OH MSA	27	2.40	18,876	2.42	247	1.97	6,235	1.57	25,243
Tucson, AZ MSA	31	2.46	32,572	3.30	407	2.99	8,502	2.11	20,889
Tulsa, OK MSA	26	1.90	42,548	4.48	504	3.53	17,815	4.19	35,347
Washington–Baltimore, DC–MD–VA–WV CMSA	249	1.93	-	-	-	-	-	-	-
West Palm Beach–Boca Raton, FL MSA	61	2.27	44,441	2.25	391	1.59	9,289	1.10	23,757
Wichita, KS MSA	16	2.09	23,921	2.47	191	1.41	6,307	1.52	33,021
Youngstown–Warren, OH MSA	20	1.66	19,499	2.81	219	1.78	4,591	1.43	20,963

Source: U.S. Department of Commerce. Bureau of the Census. *1992 Economic Census Report Series,* CD-ROM 1i, Washington, DC, October 1996. *Notes:* - means no data reported. 1. HS stands for total health service establishments, revenues, employment, or payroll.

★ 363 ★

Establishment Data

Medical Laboratories by State: 1992

Area	Establishments		Revenues		Employment		Payroll		
	Number	% of HS[1] in area	Total ($000)	% of HS[1] in area	Number	% of HS[1] in area	Total ($000)	% of HS[1] in area	Payroll per employee
United States	8,434	1.91	12,511,336	4.18	138,760	3.12	3,979,942	3.08	28,682
Alabama	116	2.10	168,931	3.43	2,100	2.72	54,196	2.57	25,808
Alaska	15	1.75	11,042	2.04	103	1.82	3,690	1.70	35,825
Arizona	137	1.93	169,550	3.71	1,685	2.87	57,847	2.97	34,331
Arkansas	44	1.23	44,102	1.81	504	1.18	13,575	1.28	26,935

[Continued]

★ 363 ★

Medical Laboratories by State: 1992
[Continued]

Area	Establishments		Revenues		Employment		Payroll		
	Number	% of HS[1] in area	Total ($000)	% of HS[1] in area	Number	% of HS[1] in area	Total ($000)	% of HS[1] in area	Payroll per employee
California	1,296	2.11	2,068,574	4.81	20,758	3.87	660,793	3.83	31,833
Colorado	98	1.40	105,691	2.83	1,248	2.26	33,457	2.04	26,808
Connecticut	195	2.96	235,653	4.80	2,698	3.73	82,670	3.52	30,641
Delaware	58	4.84	50,682	6.42	594	5.11	16,661	4.58	28,049
District of Columbia	11	0.80	11,352	1.42	64	0.66	5,396	1.56	84,312
Florida	768	2.59	768,179	3.30	8,562	2.72	207,367	2.15	24,219
Georgia	204	1.84	291,822	3.38	2,924	2.42	88,451	2.41	30,250
Hawaii	33	1.48	69,169	5.28	802	5.13	23,994	4.07	29,918
Idaho	25	1.44	22,889	2.32	264	1.56	6,460	1.55	24,470
Illinois	310	1.66	376,662	3.04	4,356	2.32	116,293	2.08	26,697
Indiana	172	1.98	239,552	3.93	2,778	2.60	89,394	3.26	32,179
Iowa	49	1.17	60,220	2.57	764	1.70	20,954	1.88	27,427
Kansas	56	1.45	180,898	5.93	1,707	3.19	51,977	3.93	30,449
Kentucky	94	1.71	153,232	3.72	1,763	2.63	44,610	2.51	25,303
Louisiana	136	1.99	154,851	2.80	1,933	2.24	47,507	2.18	24,577
Maine	28	1.30	39,893	3.39	369	1.68	8,666	1.63	23,485
Maryland	189	2.07	300,026	5.32	4,004	5.01	109,977	4.41	27,467
Massachusetts	225	2.12	449,633	5.90	4,616	3.63	147,762	4.17	32,011
Michigan	247	1.57	464,351	5.33	6,126	4.35	159,061	3.86	25,965
Minnesota	61	1.03	95,899	2.34	917	1.21	29,970	1.44	32,683
Mississippi	55	1.78	65,122	3.13	886	2.41	18,619	2.12	21,015
Missouri	137	1.63	173,179	3.15	1,586	1.67	52,485	2.15	33,093
Montana	21	1.41	12,375	1.90	146	1.35	4,505	1.74	30,856
Nebraska	45	1.91	61,745	3.97	840	3.11	25,642	3.58	30,526
Nevada	50	2.16	119,121	5.29	1,180	4.67	35,916	3.92	30,437
New Hampshire	39	2.12	37,127	3.13	574	2.99	13,333	2.46	23,228
New Jersey	346	2.10	889,888	8.55	7,682	6.02	268,482	6.08	34,949
New Mexico	62	2.58	74,898	5.07	874	3.70	21,226	3.43	24,286
New York	601	1.85	860,102	4.33	9,588	3.45	282,863	3.43	29,502
North Carolina	103	1.16	398,248	5.98	4,351	4.06	95,537	3.20	21,957
North Dakota	16	2.06	22,157	3.53	170	1.86	7,190	2.37	42,294
Ohio	324	1.75	449,887	3.86	6,126	3.07	141,866	2.55	23,158
Oklahoma	97	1.82	107,695	3.29	1,320	2.23	44,096	3.12	33,406
Oregon	70	1.24	85,114	2.88	1,234	2.56	37,778	2.91	30,614
Pennsylvania	498	2.29	653,541	5.17	7,322	3.97	187,562	3.31	25,616
Rhode Island	92	4.85	61,561	5.81	873	4.81	26,084	5.58	29,879
South Carolina	45	0.97	49,563	1.58	551	1.10	14,178	1.02	25,731
South Dakota	11	1.14	36,487	6.47	319	3.50	18,886	7.25	59,204
Tennessee	130	1.58	306,430	4.54	3,298	3.29	102,923	3.58	31,208
Texas	581	1.94	719,179	3.14	7,864	2.27	222,185	2.41	28,253
Utah	44	1.44	78,641	4.26	1,080	3.49	27,157	3.60	25,145
Vermont	8	0.86	4,375	1.08	61	0.81	1,215	0.74	19,918
Virginia	153	1.57	237,257	3.55	3,262	3.19	85,572	2.83	26,233
Washington	190	2.06	267,350	4.95	3,276	3.74	96,445	4.05	29,440

[Continued]

★ 363 ★

Medical Laboratories by State: 1992

[Continued]

Area	Establishments		Revenues		Employment		Payroll		
	Number	% of HS[1] in area	Total ($000)	% of HS[1] in area	Number	% of HS[1] in area	Total ($000)	% of HS[1] in area	Payroll per employee
West Virginia	55	2.04	57,383	3.21	515	1.78	12,476	1.77	24,225
Wisconsin	84	1.16	145,760	3.08	2,097	2.47	54,026	2.31	25,763
Wyoming	10	1.40	4,298	1.33	46	0.82	967	0.71	21,022

Source: U.S. Department of Commerce. Bureau of the Census. *1992 Economic Census Report Series,* CD-ROM 1i, Washington, DC, October 1996. *Notes:* - means no data reported. 1. HS stands for total health service establishments, revenues, employment, or payroll.

★ 364 ★

Establishment Data

Nursing and Personal Care Facilities by Major Metro Area, Non-Taxed: 1992

Area	Establish-ments	Revenues in $1,000	Employ-ment	Payroll in $1,000	Payroll per employee
United States	5,925	15,220,487	497,895	7,590,981	15,246
Albany – Schenectady – Troy, NY MSA	47	126,093	4,326	66,111	15,282
Albuquerque, NM MSA	6	26,683	853	14,035	16,454
Allentown – Bethlehem – Easton, PA MSA	25	84,139	2,162	36,898	17,067
Atlanta, GA MSA	24	50,668	1,716	25,827	15,051
Austin – San Marcos, TX MSA	10	22,911	883	11,744	13,300
Baton Rouge, LA MSA	16	26,977	940	11,183	11,897
Birmingham, AL MSA	8	-	-	-	-
Boston – Worcester – Lawrence, MA – NH – ME – CT CMSA	144	-	-	-	-
Buffalo – Niagara Falls, NY MSA	46	157,935	5,234	82,026	15,672
Charlotte – Gastonia – Rock Hill, NC – SC MSA	21	43,965	1,424	21,534	15,122
Chicago – Gary – Kenosha, IL – IN – WI CMSA	145	-	-	-	-
Cincinnati – Hamilton, OH – KY – IN CMSA	66	-	-	-	-
Cleveland – Akron, OH CMSA	92	206,175	6,921	108,626	15,695
Columbus, OH MSA	64	116,776	4,037	59,147	14,651
Dallas – Fort Worth, TX CMSA	25	-	-	-	-
Dayton – Springfield, OH MSA	47	135,426	3,871	56,074	14,486
Denver – Boulder – Greeley, CO CMSA	20	-	-	-	-
Des Moines, IA MSA	15	41,322	1,512	21,004	13,892
Detroit – Ann Arbor – Flint, MI CMSA	172	-	-	-	-
Fresno, CA MSA	9	21,327	744	10,334	13,890
Grand Rapids – Muskegon – Holland, MI MSA	39	93,120	3,578	46,954	13,123

[Continued]

★ 364 ★

Nursing and Personal Care Facilities by Major Metro Area, Non-Taxed: 1992

[Continued]

Area	Establish-ments	Revenues in $1,000	Employ-ment	Payroll in $1,000	Payroll per employee
Greensboro – Winston-Salem – High Point, NC MSA	26	65,614	2,901	32,904	11,342
Greenville – Spartanburg – Anderson, SC MSA	11	-	-	-	-
Harrisburg – Lebanon – Carlisle, PA MSA	54	101,362	3,553	49,931	14,053
Hartford, CT MSA	30	123,491	2,931	66,688	22,753
Honolulu, HI MSA	8	-	-	-	-
Houston – Galveston – Brazoria, TX CMSA	18	-	-	-	-
Indianapolis, IN MSA	23	-	-	-	-
Jacksonville, FL MSA	16	67,463	1,978	27,611	13,959
Kalamazoo – Battle Creek, MI MSA	12	42,055	1,545	18,099	11,715
Kansas City, MO – KS MSA	31	84,909	3,184	43,382	13,625
Knoxville, TN MSA	9	-	-	-	-
Lansing – East Lansing, MI MSA	6	-	-	-	-
Lexington, KY MSA	10	-	-	-	-
Little Rock – North Little Rock, AR MSA	10	-	-	-	-
Los Angeles – Riverside – Orange County, CA CMSA	93	-	-	-	-
Louisville, KY – IN MSA	27	-	-	-	-
Madison, WI MSA	8	26,914	1,046	15,378	14,702
Memphis, TN – AR – MS MSA	11	31,017	1,062	12,866	12,115
Miami – Fort Lauderdale, FL CMSA	21	-	-	-	-
Milwaukee – Racine, WI CMSA	66	-	-	-	-
Minneapolis – St. Paul, MN – WI MSA	124	377,696	13,249	194,964	14,715
Nashville, TN MSA	10	-	-	-	-
New Orleans, LA MSA	31	46,781	1,807	20,813	11,518
New York – Northern New Jersey – Long Island, NY – NJ – CT- CMSA	533	-	-	-	-
Norfolk – Virginia Beach – Newport News, VA – NC MSA	19	69,841	2,396	33,635	14,038
Oklahoma City, OK MSA	12	23,638	979	12,485	12,753
Omaha, NE – IA MSA	13	40,358	1,646	22,232	13,507
Orlando, FL MSA	19	88,005	2,295	33,498	14,596
Philadelphia – Wilmington – Atlantic City, PA – NJ – DE – MD CMSA	224	-	-	-	-
Phoenix – Mesa, AZ MSA	53	137,649	3,898	59,014	15,140
Pittsburgh, PA MSA	76	226,298	6,515	95,682	14,686
Portland – Salem, OR – WA CMSA	28	-	-	-	-
Providence – Fall River – Warwick, RI – MA MSA	63	130,214	4,049	68,372	16,886
Raleigh – Durham – Chapel Hill, NC MSA	7	-	-	-	-

[Continued]

★ 364 ★

Nursing and Personal Care Facilities by Major Metro Area, Non-Taxed: 1992

[Continued]

Area	Establish-ments	Revenues in $1,000	Employ-ment	Payroll in $1,000	Payroll per employee
Richmond – Petersburg, VA MSA	9	21,961	816	11,500	14,093
Rochester, NY MSA	57	140,167	4,802	76,823	15,998
Sacramento – Yolo, CA CMSA	19	-	-	-	-
St. Louis, MO – IL MSA	81	194,304	6,403	83,963	13,113
Salt Lake City – Ogden, UT MSA	10	25,565	860	12,516	14,553
San Antonio, TX MSA	15	49,095	1,731	22,756	13,146
San Diego, CA MSA	36	70,770	2,103	30,714	14,605
San Francisco – Oakland – San Jose, CA CMSA	53	-	-	-	-
Santa Barbara – Santa Maria – Lompoc, CA MSA	4	-	-	-	-
Scranton – Wilkes-Barre – Hazleton, PA MSA	31	115,561	4,290	62,674	14,609
Seattle – Tacoma – Bremerton, WA CMSA	31	-	-	-	-
Springfield, MA MSA	15	-	-	-	-
Syracuse, NY MSA	15	97,773	2,923	50,052	17,124
Tampa – St. Petersburg – Clearwater, FL MSA	28	98,547	2,875	41,157	14,315
Toledo, OH MSA	15	49,679	1,993	27,588	13,842
Tucson, AZ MSA	5	-	-	-	-
Tulsa, OK MSA	5	-	-	-	-
Washington – Baltimore, DC – MD – VA – WV CMSA	153	-	-	-	-
West Palm Beach – Boca Raton, FL MSA	15	85,107	2,169	34,859	16,071
Wichita, KS MSA	16	36,647	1,389	17,964	12,933
Youngstown – Warren, OH MSA	24	32,557	1,282	15,205	11,860

Source: U.S. Department of Commerce. Bureau of the Census. *1992 Economic Census Report Series*, CD-ROM 1i, Washington, DC, October 1996. Notes: - means no data reported. 1. HS stands for total health service establishments, revenues, employment, or payroll.

★ 365 ★

Establishment Data

Nursing and Personal Care Facilities by State, Non-Taxed: 1992

Area	Establish-ments	Revenues in $1,000	Employ-ment	Payroll in $1,000	Payroll per employee
United States	5,925	15,220,487	497,895	7,590,981	15,246
Alabama	33	53,669	2,620	25,943	9,902
Alaska	15	42,843	991	20,842	21,031
Arizona	70	163,427	4,884	73,498	15,049
Arkansas	45	46,658	1,776	19,682	11,082

[Continued]

★ 365 ★

Nursing and Personal Care Facilities by State, Non-Taxed: 1992
[Continued]

Area	Establish-ments	Revenues in $1,000	Employ-ment	Payroll in $1,000	Payroll per employee
California	244	567,874	16,386	272,343	16,620
Colorado	41	113,704	3,987	54,181	13,589
Connecticut	83	353,534	8,920	190,102	21,312
Delaware	16	53,006	1,726	25,836	14,969
District of Columbia	15	49,586	1,172	25,378	21,654
Florida	161	669,095	18,634	279,117	14,979
Georgia	56	125,996	4,711	61,462	13,046
Hawaii	12	-	-	-	-
Idaho	24	34,039	1,298	16,485	12,700
Illinois	351	814,109	27,992	389,309	13,908
Indiana	135	288,527	10,347	140,565	13,585
Iowa	186	354,147	16,479	189,775	11,516
Kansas	124	209,479	8,884	105,288	11,851
Kentucky	65	173,141	6,601	85,490	12,951
Louisiana	128	150,631	6,257	66,348	10,604
Maine	54	86,493	3,169	46,355	14,628
Maryland	133	385,700	11,309	183,009	16,183
Massachusetts	168	511,225	14,613	277,697	19,003
Michigan	319	533,404	18,097	253,567	14,012
Minnesota	321	724,217	28,650	383,608	13,389
Mississippi	16	33,649	1,255	17,529	13,967
Missouri	119	292,266	11,670	142,401	12,202
Montana	31	40,269	1,776	21,994	12,384
Nebraska	67	142,729	6,270	79,117	12,618
Nevada	3	-	-	-	-
New Hampshire	21	-	-	-	-
New Jersey	126	472,038	12,572	240,111	19,099
New Mexico	26	70,394	2,629	36,023	13,702
New York	679	2,765,134	69,139	1,438,261	20,802
North Carolina	108	228,559	8,840	115,514	13,067
North Dakota	99	165,980	7,723	90,893	11,769
Ohio	384	837,962	29,161	421,255	14,446
Oklahoma	39	57,291	2,403	28,676	11,933
Oregon	50	124,304	4,581	64,752	14,135
Pennsylvania	515	1,497,270	46,370	688,647	14,851
Rhode Island	72	118,615	3,665	60,205	16,427
South Carolina	62	66,449	2,256	32,520	14,415
South Dakota	59	100,637	5,074	55,342	10,907
Tennessee	67	152,648	5,812	67,240	11,569
Texas	186	352,001	12,621	166,910	13,225
Utah	15	33,514	1,474	17,006	11,537
Vermont	24	30,207	1,134	16,802	14,817
Virginia	73	233,049	8,020	113,218	14,117
Washington	63	230,745	7,656	122,390	15,986

[Continued]

★ 365 ★

Nursing and Personal Care Facilities by State, Non-Taxed: 1992

[Continued]

Area	Establish-ments	Revenues in $1,000	Employ-ment	Payroll in $1,000	Payroll per employee
West Virginia	24	60,612	2,422	30,219	12,477
Wisconsin	190	504,970	20,453	284,024	13,887
Wyoming	8	19,244	950	11,156	11,743

Source: U.S. Department of Commerce. Bureau of the Census. *1992 Economic Census Report Series,* CD-ROM 1i, Washington, DC, October 1996. *Notes:* - means no data reported. 1. HS stands for total health service establishments, revenues, employment, or payroll.

★ 366 ★

Establishment Data

Offices and Clinics of Chiropractors by Major Metro Area: 1992

Area	Establishments		Revenues		Employment		Payroll		
	Number	% of HS[1] in area	Total ($000)	% of HS[1] in area	Number	% of HS[1] in area	Total ($000)	% of HS[1] in area	Payroll per employee
United States	27,329	6.19	5,917,909	1.98	84,730	1.90	1,652,165	1.28	19,499
Albany – Schenectady – Troy, NY MSA	75	5.73	14,690	1.82	248	1.88	3,860	1.06	15,565
Albuquerque, NM MSA	78	7.31	17,469	2.09	285	2.25	4,863	1.29	17,063
Allentown – Bethlehem – Easton, PA MSA	72	5.82	15,126	2.20	213	2.28	3,373	1.10	15,836
Anchorage, AK MSA	34	7.00	12,932	3.54	124	3.43	4,609	3.23	37,169
Appleton – Oshkosh – Neenah, WI MSA	49	9.40	12,856	3.55	199	3.47	4,551	2.51	22,869
Atlanta, GA MSA	510	8.37	105,866	2.20	1,539	2.57	29,590	1.47	19,227
Augusta – Aiken, GA – SC MSA	28	3.94	6,110	0.95	105	1.13	2,104	0.75	20,038
Austin – San Marcos, TX MSA	111	7.07	29,399	2.46	529	2.85	8,806	1.81	16,647
Bakersfield, CA MSA	67	8.83	18,114	3.32	242	2.96	4,408	2.01	18,215
Baton Rouge, LA MSA	50	5.65	9,056	1.22	179	1.62	2,825	0.93	15,782
Beaumont – Port Arthur, TX MSA	19	2.63	4,560	0.79	56	0.55	1,111	0.46	19,839
Birmingham, AL MSA	48	3.49	8,467	0.56	129	0.64	2,279	0.36	17,667
Boise City, ID MSA	49	8.18	9,176	2.43	112	1.92	1,627	0.96	14,527
Boston – Worcester – Lawrence, MA – NH – ME – CT CMSA	517	5.29	145,061	2.05	1,774	1.54	42,629	1.31	24,030
Buffalo – Niagara Falls, NY MSA	75	3.76	13,009	1.18	234	1.08	2,880	0.58	12,308
Canton – Massillon, OH MSA	47	6.78	14,110	3.42	252	3.53	5,469	2.59	21,702
Charleston – North Charleston, SC MSA	52	6.37	10,836	1.83	114	1.25	3,748	1.60	32,877
Charlotte – Gastonia – Rock Hill, NC – SC MSA	96	5.99	28,614	2.05	375	1.84	11,110	1.69	29,627
Chattanooga, TN – GA MSA	40	5.26	8,677	1.21	135	1.35	2,470	0.81	18,296
Chicago – Gary – Kenosha, IL – IN – WI CMSA	629	4.32	137,345	1.41	2,054	1.51	39,659	0.90	19,308
Cincinnati – Hamilton, OH – KY – IN CMSA	174	5.55	54,782	2.70	788	2.26	16,146	1.59	20,490
Cleveland – Akron, OH CMSA	151	2.81	42,552	1.31	657	1.28	16,179	1.05	24,626
Colorado Springs, CO MSA	87	9.80	14,128	3.18	261	3.95	4,453	2.21	17,061
Columbia, SC MSA	48	6.44	8,596	1.78	120	1.67	2,151	0.90	17,925
Columbus, OH MSA	103	4.24	28,266	1.61	376	1.34	8,523	1.05	22,668
Corpus Christi, TX MSA	29	3.86	5,678	0.98	71	0.84	1,836	0.81	25,859
Dallas – Fort Worth, TX CMSA	397	4.77	93,144	1.43	1,461	1.70	28,777	1.09	19,697

[Continued]

★ 366 ★

Offices and Clinics of Chiropractors by Major Metro Area: 1992
[Continued]

Area	Establishments		Revenues		Employment		Payroll		
	Number	% of HS[1] in area	Total ($000)	% of HS[1] in area	Number	% of HS[1] in area	Total ($000)	% of HS[1] in area	Payroll per employee
Davenport – Moline – Rock Island, IA – IL MSA	85	12.54	12,412	3.44	227	3.78	4,055	2.57	17,863
Dayton – Springfield, OH MSA	68	4.13	22,022	1.92	294	1.66	5,939	1.05	20,201
Daytona Beach, FL MSA	57	7.70	12,791	2.39	168	2.01	3,709	1.69	22,077
Denver – Boulder – Greeley, CO CMSA	341	7.80	63,279	2.49	914	2.56	17,836	1.59	19,514
Des Moines, IA MSA	41	5.56	6,173	1.21	109	1.53	1,331	0.50	12,211
Detroit – Ann Arbor – Flint, MI CMSA	525	5.57	92,919	1.70	1,526	1.82	28,264	1.11	18,522
El Paso, TX MSA	37	4.65	10,512	1.35	163	1.52	3,437	1.18	21,086
Eugene – Springfield, OR MSA	41	7.02	6,049	1.80	89	1.65	1,576	1.01	17,708
Fort Myers – Cape Coral, FL MSA	64	8.96	13,057	1.96	174	2.11	4,442	1.43	25,529
Fort Pierce – Port St. Lucie, FL MSA	43	8.29	9,676	2.16	136	2.20	2,513	1.35	18,478
Fort Wayne, IN MSA	36	5.14	8,085	1.46	113	1.20	2,510	0.98	22,212
Fresno, CA MSA	123	8.31	25,927	2.99	375	3.05	6,766	1.82	18,043
Grand Rapids – Muskegon – Holland, MI MSA	101	6.62	16,009	1.78	242	1.69	3,511	0.81	14,508
Greensboro – Winston-Salem – High Point, NC MSA	70	4.64	15,995	1.35	235	1.37	4,129	0.78	17,570
Greenville – Spartanburg – Anderson, SC MSA	82	6.97	14,636	1.88	231	1.93	3,900	1.03	16,883
Harrisburg – Lebanon – Carlisle, PA MSA	71	7.19	17,079	2.62	253	2.66	4,952	1.60	19,573
Hartford, CT MSA	103	4.54	29,933	1.70	327	1.20	7,093	0.83	21,691
Honolulu, HI MSA	76	4.52	24,916	2.40	260	2.16	8,462	1.77	32,546
Houston – Galveston – Brazoria, TX CMSA	354	5.01	85,084	1.45	1,228	1.64	26,135	1.11	21,283
Huntsville, AL MSA	33	6.19	8,539	1.87	112	1.71	1,904	1.00	17,000
Indianapolis, IN MSA	101	3.97	25,931	1.29	362	1.13	8,372	0.89	23,127
Jackson, MS MSA	16	2.51	2,933	0.58	44	0.61	544	0.26	12,364
Jacksonville, FL MSA	88	4.96	22,041	1.69	358	2.09	7,350	1.32	20,531
Johnson City – Kingsport – Bristol, TN – VA MSA	36	5.22	6,546	1.07	96	0.97	1,765	0.65	18,385
Kalamazoo – Battle Creek, MI MSA	37	5.01	6,345	1.46	96	1.34	1,223	0.57	12,740
Kansas City, MO – KS MSA	188	6.58	28,185	1.29	505	1.50	8,254	0.83	16,345
Knoxville, TN MSA	60	5.02	14,986	1.85	251	2.35	5,622	1.44	22,398
Lafayette, LA MSA	24	3.76	4,527	1.01	83	1.18	1,250	0.68	15,060
Lakeland – Winter Haven, FL MSA	33	6.78	10,321	2.57	178	2.80	4,599	2.75	25,837
Lancaster, PA MSA	54	8.94	9,186	2.41	139	2.20	1,733	0.91	12,468
Lansing – East Lansing, MI MSA	37	5.06	6,087	1.52	107	1.70	1,513	0.80	14,140
Las Vegas, NV – AZ MSA	118	7.58	35,600	2.11	410	2.22	12,127	1.78	29,578
Lexington, KY MSA	31	3.82	5,869	0.99	94	1.04	1,775	0.64	18,883
Little Rock – North Little Rock, AR MSA	54	5.19	10,844	1.39	171	1.53	3,740	1.02	21,871
Los Angeles – Riverside – Orange County, CA CMSA	1,873	6.12	450,985	1.92	5,603	2.02	118,847	1.30	21,211
Louisville, KY – IN MSA	80	4.65	15,378	0.92	229	0.89	3,643	0.51	15,908
Macon, GA MSA	23	4.23	6,446	1.14	92	1.22	2,248	0.99	24,435
Madison, WI MSA	44	8.49	13,855	2.68	191	2.65	5,389	2.30	28,215
Melbourne – Titusville – Palm Bay, FL MSA	71	8.73	14,312	2.64	236	3.25	4,657	1.86	19,733
Memphis, TN – AR – MS MSA	37	2.25	8,618	0.69	118	0.72	2,148	0.40	18,203
Miami – Fort Lauderdale, FL CMSA	465	5.09	109,138	1.60	1,582	1.82	36,608	1.30	23,140
Milwaukee – Racine, WI CMSA	186	6.14	40,136	1.96	590	1.73	11,918	1.15	20,200
Minneapolis – St. Paul, MN – WI MSA	493	13.24	104,079	3.59	1,626	3.26	30,232	2.02	18,593
Mobile, AL MSA	38	5.92	6,137	1.09	143	1.50	1,855	0.71	12,972
Modesto, CA MSA	78	11.56	17,570	2.91	240	2.99	4,765	1.92	19,854
Montgomery, AL MSA	19	3.87	2,179	0.43	35	0.47	512	0.24	14,629
Nashville, TN MSA	104	5.35	20,632	1.11	250	0.99	4,392	0.57	17,568

[Continued]

Offices and Clinics of Chiropractors by Major Metro Area: 1992

[Continued]

Area	Establishments		Revenues		Employment		Payroll		
	Number	% of HS[1] in area	Total ($000)	% of HS[1] in area	Number	% of HS[1] in area	Total ($000)	% of HS[1] in area	Payroll per employee
New Orleans, LA MSA	90	3.71	19,399	0.89	307	1.04	5,904	0.70	19,231
New York – Northern New Jersey – Long Island, NY – NJ – CT- CMSA	2,555	6.29	649,378	2.49	7,807	2.34	161,866	1.48	20,733
Norfolk – Virginia Beach – Newport News, VA – NC MSA	88	3.90	21,468	1.58	304	1.39	7,335	1.13	24,128
Oklahoma City, OK MSA	87	4.42	20,879	1.61	299	1.53	7,129	1.27	23,843
Omaha, NE – IA MSA	61	6.05	11,178	1.36	166	1.33	2,725	0.73	16,416
Orlando, FL MSA	165	6.51	43,713	2.30	518	2.05	14,043	1.72	27,110
Pensacola, FL MSA	33	6.26	8,621	1.65	141	1.76	3,415	1.44	24,220
Peoria – Pekin, IL MSA	47	9.25	8,875	2.45	141	2.41	3,048	1.62	21,617
Philadelphia – Wilmington – Atlantic City, PA – NJ – DE – MD CMSA	584	5.04	137,535	1.88	2,021	2.02	41,398	1.27	20,484
Phoenix – Mesa, AZ MSA	444	9.23	91,436	2.91	1,303	3.38	28,402	2.07	21,797
Pittsburgh, PA MSA	333	6.99	88,040	3.24	1,187	3.11	25,099	2.01	21,145
Portland, ME MSA	30	5.55	4,627	1.21	70	1.19	931	0.52	13,300
Portland – Salem, OR – WA CMSA	274	7.73	41,292	2.07	632	2.03	9,829	1.11	15,552
Providence – Fall River – Warwick, RI – MA MSA	86	4.15	20,980	1.78	244	1.23	5,856	1.11	24,000
Raleigh – Durham – Chapel Hill, NC MSA	73	5.08	15,416	1.27	186	1.08	4,055	0.80	21,801
Reno, NV MSA	41	6.15	10,941	2.10	110	1.85	2,573	1.18	23,391
Richmond – Petersburg, VA MSA	37	2.31	7,382	0.47	96	0.43	1,802	0.27	18,771
Rochester, NY MSA	68	4.44	10,788	1.30	189	1.36	2,101	0.60	11,116
Rockford, IL MSA	44	9.22	10,389	2.87	149	2.74	3,376	2.05	22,658
Sacramento – Yolo, CA CMSA	278	9.62	-	-	-	-	-	-	-
Saginaw – Bay City – Midland, MI MSA	28	4.11	4,275	1.12	73	1.14	1,052	0.53	14,411
St. Louis, MO – IL MSA	320	7.19	56,212	1.96	904	2.07	16,805	1.35	18,590
Salinas, CA MSA	51	8.39	13,554	4.53	200	4.55	3,351	2.74	16,755
Salt Lake City – Ogden, UT MSA	85	4.13	17,754	1.29	327	1.48	4,331	0.75	13,245
San Antonio, TX MSA	90	3.43	22,785	1.26	262	0.91	6,098	0.82	23,275
San Diego, CA MSA	387	7.85	81,038	2.48	965	2.32	18,384	1.37	19,051
San Francisco – Oakland – San Jose, CA CMSA	1,036	7.38	213,106	2.36	2,944	2.59	52,353	1.39	17,783
Santa Barbara – Santa Maria – Lompoc, CA MSA	80	9.57	16,887	3.95	209	3.96	3,632	2.04	17,378
Sarasota – Bradenton, FL MSA	85	6.93	18,465	1.88	264	1.83	6,273	1.54	23,761
Scranton – Wilkes-Barre – Hazleton, PA MSA	72	6.29	14,609	2.31	223	2.10	3,590	1.37	16,099
Seattle – Tacoma – Bremerton, WA CMSA	507	8.37	98,220	2.76	1,304	2.41	22,892	1.47	17,555
Shreveport – Bossier City, LA MSA	24	3.74	6,787	1.19	85	1.00	1,767	0.76	20,788
Spokane, WA MSA	54	7.35	8,477	1.66	127	1.62	2,087	0.89	16,433
Springfield, MO MSA	35	7.61	4,856	1.26	68	0.99	909	0.46	13,368
Springfield, MA MSA	57	6.30	17,616	2.64	225	1.86	6,076	1.89	27,004
Stockton – Lodi, CA MSA	68	8.14	18,752	3.62	234	2.91	6,127	2.69	26,184
Syracuse, NY MSA	48	4.40	9,903	1.43	139	1.42	2,502	0.79	18,000
Tallahassee, FL MSA	23	5.79	5,541	1.60	69	1.46	1,702	1.12	24,667
Tampa – St. Petersburg – Clearwater, FL MSA	325	6.58	80,557	1.85	1,147	1.87	27,649	1.60	24,105
Toledo, OH MSA	56	4.97	11,613	1.49	173	1.38	3,734	0.94	21,584
Tucson, AZ MSA	86	6.82	17,373	1.76	238	1.75	3,892	0.97	16,353
Tulsa, OK MSA	100	7.31	23,808	2.51	261	1.83	5,663	1.33	21,697
Washington – Baltimore, DC – MD – VA – WV CMSA	343	2.65	108,488	1.34	1,459	1.33	34,840	0.97	23,879
West Palm Beach – Boca Raton, FL MSA	195	7.25	50,883	2.57	686	2.79	18,692	2.22	27,248

[Continued]

★ 366 ★

Offices and Clinics of Chiropractors by Major Metro Area: 1992

[Continued]

Area	Establishments		Revenues		Employment		Payroll		
	Number	% of HS[1] in area	Total ($000)	% of HS[1] in area	Number	% of HS[1] in area	Total ($000)	% of HS[1] in area	Payroll per employee
Wichita, KS MSA	60	7.84	16,660	1.72	271	2.00	5,246	1.26	19,358
Youngstown – Warren, OH MSA	47	3.91	12,633	1.82	187	1.52	3,595	1.12	19,225

Source: U.S. Department of Commerce. Bureau of the Census. *1992 Economic Census Report Series,* CD-ROM 1i, Washington, DC, October 1996. *Notes:* - means no data reported. 1. HS stands for total health service establishments, revenues, employment, or payroll.

★ 367 ★

Establishment Data

Offices and Clinics of Chiropractors by State: 1992

Area	Establishments		Revenues		Employment		Payroll		
	Number	% of HS[1] in area	Total ($000)	% of HS[1] in area	Number	% of HS[1] in area	Total ($000)	% of HS[1] in area	Payroll per employee
United States	27,329	6.19	5,917,909	1.98	84,730	1.90	1,652,165	1.28	19,499
Alabama	282	5.11	50,995	1.04	859	1.11	14,243	0.67	16,581
Alaska	71	8.28	21,901	4.04	227	4.01	6,719	3.09	29,599
Arizona	622	8.75	123,169	2.70	1,760	3.00	36,023	1.85	20,468
Arkansas	237	6.65	39,365	1.62	641	1.50	10,847	1.02	16,922
California	4,364	7.10	972,152	2.26	12,604	2.35	244,193	1.42	19,374
Colorado	589	8.40	100,648	2.69	1,529	2.77	27,504	1.68	17,988
Connecticut	347	5.26	101,975	2.08	1,207	1.67	27,507	1.17	22,790
Delaware	50	4.17	13,666	1.73	205	1.76	6,155	1.69	30,024
District of Columbia	13	0.94	4,109	0.51	50	0.52	1,100	0.32	22,000
Florida	1,847	6.24	444,248	1.91	6,337	2.01	147,465	1.53	23,270
Georgia	760	6.85	154,081	1.79	2,334	1.93	45,004	1.23	19,282
Hawaii	119	5.35	38,828	2.96	408	2.61	12,898	2.19	31,613
Idaho	134	7.73	22,470	2.28	326	1.93	4,224	1.02	12,957
Illinois	1,068	5.71	216,560	1.75	3,447	1.84	63,264	1.13	18,353
Indiana	436	5.01	98,161	1.61	1,422	1.33	28,856	1.05	20,293
Iowa	446	10.66	68,192	2.92	1,353	3.01	17,276	1.55	12,769
Kansas	321	8.30	58,992	1.94	994	1.86	18,238	1.38	18,348
Kentucky	269	4.88	51,115	1.24	855	1.28	15,304	0.86	17,899
Louisiana	284	4.16	58,506	1.06	933	1.08	16,581	0.76	17,772
Maine	126	5.84	26,779	2.27	428	1.95	7,584	1.42	17,720
Maryland	231	2.53	76,300	1.35	1,053	1.32	24,578	0.98	23,341
Massachusetts	575	5.42	163,870	2.15	1,986	1.56	48,870	1.38	24,607
Michigan	938	5.96	155,693	1.79	2,572	1.83	42,977	1.04	16,710
Minnesota	824	13.95	160,994	3.92	2,668	3.52	47,335	2.27	17,742
Mississippi	113	3.66	19,203	0.92	354	0.96	5,165	0.59	14,590
Missouri	598	7.10	89,333	1.63	1,542	1.63	23,687	0.97	15,361
Montana	117	7.85	16,310	2.50	260	2.41	3,017	1.16	11,604
Nebraska	163	6.92	30,074	1.93	464	1.72	8,002	1.12	17,246
Nevada	166	7.16	47,657	2.12	521	2.06	14,776	1.61	28,361

[Continued]

★ 367 ★

Offices and Clinics of Chiropractors by State: 1992
[Continued]

Area	Establishments		Revenues		Employment		Payroll		
	Number	% of HS[1] in area	Total ($000)	% of HS[1] in area	Number	% of HS[1] in area	Total ($000)	% of HS[1] in area	Payroll per employee
New Hampshire	108	5.88	21,688	1.83	321	1.67	5,836	1.08	18,181
New Jersey	1,245	7.54	326,710	3.14	3,936	3.08	87,611	1.98	22,259
New Mexico	185	7.71	34,298	2.32	549	2.32	8,638	1.40	15,734
New York	1,741	5.37	388,348	1.95	5,122	1.84	88,721	1.08	17,322
North Carolina	439	4.95	99,116	1.49	1,385	1.29	31,073	1.04	22,435
North Dakota	90	11.61	14,992	2.39	230	2.52	4,163	1.37	18,100
Ohio	871	4.69	237,979	2.04	3,463	1.73	75,464	1.35	21,792
Oklahoma	316	5.92	66,456	2.03	895	1.52	17,924	1.27	20,027
Oregon	428	7.59	60,225	2.04	990	2.06	15,097	1.16	15,249
Pennsylvania	1,310	6.03	293,051	2.32	4,293	2.33	78,006	1.38	18,171
Rhode Island	79	4.16	17,967	1.69	220	1.21	5,322	1.14	24,191
South Carolina	319	6.87	60,285	1.92	848	1.69	17,420	1.25	20,542
South Dakota	118	12.19	20,907	3.71	321	3.53	4,165	1.60	12,975
Tennessee	356	4.33	74,113	1.10	1,065	1.06	19,705	0.69	18,502
Texas	1,426	4.76	331,418	1.45	5,025	1.45	97,305	1.06	19,364
Utah	153	5.01	27,714	1.50	502	1.62	6,474	0.86	12,896
Vermont	65	6.99	10,566	2.61	173	2.29	2,045	1.24	11,821
Virginia	355	3.64	85,384	1.28	1,184	1.16	27,519	0.91	23,242
Washington	804	8.72	147,177	2.72	2,079	2.38	34,526	1.45	16,607
West Virginia	105	3.90	24,442	1.37	392	1.36	7,390	1.05	18,852
Wisconsin	665	9.21	142,761	3.01	2,295	2.70	46,829	2.00	20,405
Wyoming	41	5.75	6,966	2.15	103	1.83	1,540	1.14	14,951

Source: U.S. Department of Commerce. Bureau of the Census. *1992 Economic Census Report Series,* CD-ROM 1i, Washington, DC, October 1996. *Notes:* - means no data reported. 1. HS stands for total health service establishments, revenues, employment, or payroll.

★ 368 ★

Establishment Data

Offices and Clinics of Optometrists by Major Metro Area: 1992

Area	Establishments		Revenues		Employment		Payroll		
	Number	% of HS[1] in area	Total ($000)	% of HS[1] in area	Number	% of HS[1] in area	Total ($000)	% of HS[1] in area	Payroll per employee
United States	17,135	3.88	4,939,521	1.65	68,596	1.54	1,300,969	1.01	18,966
Albany – Schenectady – Troy, NY MSA	32	2.44	7,939	0.98	118	0.89	1,800	0.50	15,254
Albuquerque, NM MSA	37	3.47	10,925	1.31	158	1.25	2,593	0.69	16,411
Allentown – Bethlehem – Easton, PA MSA	50	4.04	13,991	2.03	196	2.10	3,708	1.21	18,918
Anchorage, AK MSA	21	4.32	8,873	2.43	90	2.49	2,710	1.90	30,111
Appleton – Oshkosh – Neenah, WI MSA	24	4.61	6,627	1.83	85	1.48	1,996	1.10	23,482
Atlanta, GA MSA	180	2.95	49,376	1.02	677	1.13	16,075	0.80	23,744
Augusta – Aiken, GA – SC MSA	25	3.52	8,828	1.37	118	1.28	3,025	1.07	25,636
Austin – San Marcos, TX MSA	60	3.82	18,803	1.57	257	1.38	5,205	1.07	20,253
Bakersfield, CA MSA	33	4.35	10,669	1.96	145	1.78	2,116	0.97	14,593
Baton Rouge, LA MSA	19	2.15	6,448	0.87	76	0.69	2,063	0.68	27,145

[Continued]

★ 368 ★

Offices and Clinics of Optometrists by Major Metro Area: 1992

[Continued]

Area	Establishments		Revenues		Employment		Payroll		
	Number	% of HS[1] in area	Total ($000)	% of HS[1] in area	Number	% of HS[1] in area	Total ($000)	% of HS[1] in area	Payroll per employee
Beaumont – Port Arthur, TX MSA	17	2.35	6,051	1.05	89	0.87	1,780	0.74	20,000
Birmingham, AL MSA	44	3.20	16,425	1.09	203	1.01	4,876	0.76	24,020
Boise City, ID MSA	28	4.67	8,084	2.14	131	2.24	1,732	1.02	13,221
Boston – Worcester – Lawrence, MA – NH – ME – CT CMSA	325	3.33	89,236	1.26	1,214	1.05	25,131	0.77	20,701
Buffalo – Niagara Falls, NY MSA	48	2.41	16,069	1.45	234	1.08	4,430	0.89	18,932
Canton – Massillon, OH MSA	34	4.91	6,515	1.58	100	1.40	1,806	0.86	18,060
Charleston – North Charleston, SC MSA	26	3.19	5,445	0.92	103	1.13	1,478	0.63	14,350
Charlotte – Gastonia – Rock Hill, NC – SC MSA	96	5.99	25,770	1.84	327	1.61	5,991	0.91	18,321
Chattanooga, TN – GA MSA	29	3.81	6,307	0.88	93	0.93	1,590	0.52	17,097
Chicago – Gary – Kenosha, IL – IN – WI CMSA	487	3.35	-	-	-	-	-	-	-
Cincinnati – Hamilton, OH – KY – IN CMSA	115	3.67	31,522	1.55	466	1.34	9,541	0.94	20,474
Cleveland – Akron, OH CMSA	180	3.35	47,315	1.45	726	1.41	13,408	0.87	18,468
Colorado Springs, CO MSA	21	2.36	7,152	1.61	114	1.73	2,491	1.24	21,851
Columbia, SC MSA	28	3.76	7,749	1.60	116	1.62	2,661	1.11	22,940
Columbus, OH MSA	120	4.94	28,295	1.61	466	1.66	7,518	0.93	16,133
Corpus Christi, TX MSA	16	2.13	3,460	0.60	53	0.63	621	0.28	11,717
Dallas – Fort Worth, TX CMSA	280	3.37	82,321	1.26	1,029	1.20	19,138	0.72	18,599
Davenport – Moline – Rock Island, IA – IL MSA	24	3.54	6,989	1.93	103	1.72	1,501	0.95	14,573
Dayton – Springfield, OH MSA	83	5.04	25,354	2.22	373	2.10	7,383	1.31	19,794
Daytona Beach, FL MSA	26	3.51	9,120	1.71	111	1.33	4,091	1.86	36,856
Denver – Boulder – Greeley, CO CMSA	147	3.36	43,132	1.70	680	1.90	14,187	1.27	20,863
Des Moines, IA MSA	28	3.79	8,527	1.68	143	2.01	2,950	1.11	20,629
Detroit – Ann Arbor – Flint, MI CMSA	293	3.11	114,396	2.10	1,499	1.78	34,926	1.37	23,300
El Paso, TX MSA	24	3.02	6,919	0.89	89	0.83	1,836	0.63	20,629
Eugene – Springfield, OR MSA	23	3.94	4,589	1.37	74	1.37	1,109	0.71	14,986
Fort Myers – Cape Coral, FL MSA	26	3.64	8,508	1.28	126	1.53	2,460	0.79	19,524
Fort Pierce – Port St. Lucie, FL MSA	18	3.47	6,916	1.54	99	1.60	2,026	1.09	20,465
Fort Wayne, IN MSA	40	5.71	10,353	1.87	155	1.64	2,802	1.09	18,077
Fresno, CA MSA	61	4.12	22,960	2.64	329	2.67	6,351	1.71	19,304
Grand Rapids – Muskegon – Holland, MI MSA	73	4.79	19,321	2.15	250	1.74	4,394	1.02	17,576
Greensboro – Winston-Salem – High Point, NC MSA	80	5.30	30,093	2.54	388	2.27	10,890	2.06	28,067
Greenville – Spartanburg – Anderson, SC MSA	52	4.42	18,058	2.32	232	1.93	5,748	1.52	24,776
Harrisburg – Lebanon – Carlisle, PA MSA	55	5.57	19,361	2.97	267	2.80	5,308	1.72	19,880
Hartford, CT MSA	78	3.44	24,434	1.39	286	1.05	5,156	0.61	18,028
Honolulu, HI MSA	77	4.58	21,635	2.09	262	2.18	5,095	1.07	19,447
Houston – Galveston – Brazoria, TX CMSA	238	3.37	81,700	1.39	1,067	1.43	23,715	1.01	22,226
Huntsville, AL MSA	16	3.00	5,053	1.11	61	0.93	1,199	0.63	19,656
Indianapolis, IN MSA	102	4.01	28,807	1.44	394	1.22	8,158	0.87	20,706
Jackson, MS MSA	16	2.51	5,160	1.02	66	0.92	1,217	0.58	18,439
Jacksonville, FL MSA	61	3.44	18,450	1.41	275	1.61	6,734	1.21	24,487
Johnson City – Kingsport – Bristol, TN – VA MSA	35	5.07	9,041	1.48	131	1.33	2,041	0.75	15,580
Kalamazoo – Battle Creek, MI MSA	31	4.20	8,211	1.89	117	1.64	2,263	1.05	19,342
Kansas City, MO – KS MSA	76	2.66	19,298	0.88	257	0.76	5,005	0.51	19,475
Knoxville, TN MSA	39	3.26	11,631	1.43	118	1.11	2,369	0.61	20,076
Lafayette, LA MSA	19	2.98	3,897	0.87	73	1.04	1,241	0.68	17,000

[Continued]

★ 368 ★

Offices and Clinics of Optometrists by Major Metro Area: 1992
[Continued]

Area	Establishments		Revenues		Employment		Payroll		
	Number	% of HS[1] in area	Total ($000)	% of HS[1] in area	Number	% of HS[1] in area	Total ($000)	% of HS[1] in area	Payroll per employee
Lakeland – Winter Haven, FL MSA	19	3.90	6,443	1.60	85	1.34	2,032	1.21	23,906
Lancaster, PA MSA	26	4.30	7,422	1.95	105	1.66	1,478	0.77	14,076
Lansing – East Lansing, MI MSA	32	4.38	11,526	2.88	173	2.75	4,089	2.15	23,636
Las Vegas, NV – AZ MSA	69	4.43	22,953	1.36	341	1.85	7,781	1.14	22,818
Lexington, KY MSA	34	4.19	9,102	1.54	142	1.57	2,586	0.94	18,211
Little Rock – North Little Rock, AR MSA	41	3.94	12,543	1.61	202	1.81	3,467	0.94	17,163
Los Angeles – Riverside – Orange County, CA CMSA	1,117	3.65	374,294	1.59	4,519	1.63	93,152	1.02	20,613
Louisville, KY – IN MSA	40	2.33	10,444	0.62	165	0.64	3,231	0.45	19,582
Macon, GA MSA	14	2.57	3,682	0.65	60	0.80	1,389	0.61	23,150
Madison, WI MSA	25	4.83	6,114	1.18	95	1.32	1,636	0.70	17,221
Melbourne – Titusville – Palm Bay, FL MSA	26	3.20	6,182	1.14	74	1.02	1,673	0.67	22,608
Memphis, TN – AR – MS MSA	70	4.25	21,488	1.73	297	1.82	5,202	0.97	17,515
Miami – Fort Lauderdale, FL CMSA	239	2.61	51,160	0.75	666	0.77	15,713	0.56	23,593
Milwaukee – Racine, WI CMSA	85	2.81	25,392	1.24	408	1.19	7,139	0.69	17,498
Minneapolis – St. Paul, MN – WI MSA	129	3.46	31,673	1.09	509	1.02	9,048	0.60	17,776
Mobile, AL MSA	18	2.80	2,604	0.46	43	0.45	638	0.24	14,837
Modesto, CA MSA	37	5.48	14,150	2.34	225	2.81	4,022	1.62	17,876
Montgomery, AL MSA	15	3.05	3,476	0.69	54	0.73	986	0.47	18,259
Nashville, TN MSA	75	3.86	18,991	1.02	283	1.12	4,746	0.61	16,770
New Orleans, LA MSA	46	1.90	12,766	0.58	187	0.63	3,851	0.46	20,594
New York – Northern New Jersey – Long Island, NY – NJ – CT- CMSA	1,047	2.58	-	-	-	-	-	-	-
Norfolk – Virginia Beach – Newport News, VA – NC MSA	98	4.34	23,906	1.76	350	1.60	6,179	0.96	17,654
Oklahoma City, OK MSA	89	4.52	23,612	1.82	333	1.70	6,526	1.16	19,598
Omaha, NE – IA MSA	29	2.87	8,176	1.00	104	0.84	2,333	0.62	22,433
Orlando, FL MSA	86	3.40	23,980	1.26	305	1.21	7,239	0.88	23,734
Pensacola, FL MSA	17	3.23	3,843	0.74	62	0.78	1,034	0.44	16,677
Peoria – Pekin, IL MSA	18	3.54	4,934	1.36	77	1.32	1,202	0.64	15,610
Philadelphia – Wilmington – Atlantic City, PA – NJ – DE – MD CMSA	387	3.34	102,529	1.40	1,444	1.45	28,585	0.88	19,796
Phoenix – Mesa, AZ MSA	101	2.10	25,030	0.80	323	0.84	6,400	0.47	19,814
Pittsburgh, PA MSA	185	3.88	47,895	1.76	720	1.89	10,515	0.84	14,604
Portland, ME MSA	26	4.81	7,530	1.96	105	1.78	1,766	0.99	16,819
Portland – Salem, OR – WA CMSA	119	3.36	27,645	1.39	419	1.35	6,300	0.71	15,036
Providence – Fall River – Warwick, RI – MA MSA	88	4.24	23,634	2.00	327	1.65	5,228	0.99	15,988
Raleigh – Durham – Chapel Hill, NC MSA	75	5.22	23,316	1.92	318	1.85	7,197	1.43	22,632
Reno, NV MSA	31	4.65	11,563	2.22	119	2.00	2,853	1.31	23,975
Richmond – Petersburg, VA MSA	64	4.00	17,006	1.09	270	1.22	4,527	0.68	16,767
Rochester, NY MSA	48	3.14	12,471	1.51	174	1.25	2,915	0.83	16,753
Rockford, IL MSA	19	3.98	5,643	1.56	84	1.55	1,153	0.70	13,726
Sacramento – Yolo, CA CMSA	136	4.70	-	-	-	-	-	-	-
Saginaw – Bay City – Midland, MI MSA	26	3.81	9,636	2.52	148	2.30	3,525	1.78	23,818
St. Louis, MO – IL MSA	132	2.97	43,166	1.51	690	1.58	13,510	1.09	19,580
Salinas, CA MSA	25	4.11	7,471	2.50	99	2.25	2,060	1.68	20,808
Salt Lake City – Ogden, UT MSA	48	2.33	13,087	0.95	210	0.95	3,348	0.58	15,943
San Antonio, TX MSA	89	3.39	22,388	1.24	328	1.14	6,373	0.85	19,430
San Diego, CA MSA	180	3.65	61,845	1.89	719	1.73	14,294	1.06	19,880
San Francisco – Oakland – San Jose, CA CMSA	512	3.65	150,309	1.67	1,908	1.68	32,594	0.86	17,083
Santa Barbara – Santa Maria – Lompoc, CA MSA	36	4.31	7,519	1.76	103	1.95	1,710	0.96	16,602

[Continued]

★ 368 ★

Offices and Clinics of Optometrists by Major Metro Area: 1992

[Continued]

Area	Establishments		Revenues		Employment		Payroll		
	Number	% of HS[1] in area	Total ($000)	% of HS[1] in area	Number	% of HS[1] in area	Total ($000)	% of HS[1] in area	Payroll per employee
Sarasota – Bradenton, FL MSA	36	2.93	9,214	0.94	104	0.72	2,568	0.63	24,692
Scranton – Wilkes-Barre – Hazleton, PA MSA	50	4.37	19,429	3.08	220	2.07	5,563	2.12	25,286
Seattle – Tacoma – Bremerton, WA CMSA	187	3.09	50,537	1.42	719	1.33	12,274	0.79	17,071
Shreveport – Bossier City, LA MSA	20	3.12	3,232	0.57	52	0.61	659	0.28	12,673
Spokane, WA MSA	20	2.72	7,226	1.42	84	1.07	1,393	0.60	16,583
Springfield, MO MSA	7	1.52	3,010	0.78	46	0.67	1,140	0.58	24,783
Springfield, MA MSA	34	3.76	7,853	1.18	105	0.87	2,086	0.65	19,867
Stockton – Lodi, CA MSA	43	5.15	15,591	3.01	188	2.34	4,389	1.93	23,346
Syracuse, NY MSA	28	2.56	6,902	1.00	99	1.01	1,782	0.57	18,000
Tallahassee, FL MSA	15	3.78	4,294	1.24	67	1.42	1,652	1.08	24,657
Tampa – St. Petersburg – Clearwater, FL MSA	111	2.25	24,296	0.56	309	0.51	7,104	0.41	22,990
Toledo, OH MSA	41	3.64	15,824	2.03	188	1.50	4,755	1.20	25,293
Tucson, AZ MSA	37	2.93	12,778	1.29	179	1.31	3,178	0.79	17,754
Tulsa, OK MSA	69	5.04	15,510	1.63	224	1.57	3,088	0.73	13,786
Washington – Baltimore, DC – MD – VA – WV CMSA	356	2.75	-	-	-	-	-	-	-
West Palm Beach – Boca Raton, FL MSA	72	2.68	20,137	1.02	227	0.92	6,530	0.77	28,767
Wichita, KS MSA	48	6.27	20,054	2.07	271	2.00	5,971	1.44	22,033
Youngstown – Warren, OH MSA	50	4.16	10,426	1.50	138	1.12	2,348	0.73	17,014

Source: U.S. Department of Commerce. Bureau of the Census. *1992 Economic Census Report Series,* CD-ROM 1i, Washington, DC, October 1996. *Notes:* - means no data reported. 1. HS stands for total health service establishments, revenues, employment, or payroll.

★ 369 ★

Establishment Data

Offices and Clinics of Optometrists by State: 1992

Area	Establishments		Revenues		Employment		Payroll		
	Number	% of HS[1] in area	Total ($000)	% of HS[1] in area	Number	% of HS[1] in area	Total ($000)	% of HS[1] in area	Payroll per employee
United States	17,135	3.88	4,939,521	1.65	68,596	1.54	1,300,969	1.01	18,966
Alabama	229	4.15	65,608	1.33	900	1.16	16,647	0.79	18,497
Alaska	44	5.13	17,112	3.16	177	3.13	4,975	2.29	28,107
Arizona	189	2.66	49,165	1.08	672	1.14	12,392	0.64	18,440
Arkansas	202	5.67	56,672	2.33	916	2.15	14,930	1.40	16,299
California	2,382	3.88	754,317	1.75	9,465	1.77	180,920	1.05	19,115
Colorado	257	3.67	73,235	1.96	1,134	2.05	22,381	1.36	19,736
Connecticut	228	3.46	73,960	1.51	907	1.25	18,355	0.78	20,237
Delaware	40	3.34	12,873	1.63	203	1.75	4,150	1.14	20,443
District of Columbia	24	1.74	9,216	1.15	112	1.15	2,773	0.80	24,759
Florida	854	2.89	221,280	0.95	2,943	0.93	70,085	0.73	23,814
Georgia	373	3.36	102,345	1.19	1,472	1.22	31,969	0.87	21,718
Hawaii	99	4.45	27,647	2.11	330	2.11	6,542	1.11	19,824
Idaho	94	5.42	24,607	2.49	357	2.11	4,963	1.19	13,902
Illinois	698	3.73	213,734	1.73	3,177	1.69	59,910	1.07	18,857

[Continued]

★ 369 ★

Offices and Clinics of Optometrists by State: 1992
[Continued]

Area	Establishments		Revenues		Employment		Payroll		
	Number	% of HS[1] in area	Total ($000)	% of HS[1] in area	Number	% of HS[1] in area	Total ($000)	% of HS[1] in area	Payroll per employee
Indiana	463	5.32	133,059	2.18	1,924	1.80	35,972	1.31	18,696
Iowa	270	6.45	79,034	3.38	1,202	2.67	21,633	1.95	17,998
Kansas	247	6.39	78,371	2.57	1,103	2.06	19,769	1.49	17,923
Kentucky	248	4.50	72,650	1.76	1,015	1.51	18,574	1.04	18,300
Louisiana	196	2.87	48,393	0.88	743	0.86	13,470	0.62	18,129
Maine	123	5.70	35,347	3.00	448	2.04	7,856	1.47	17,536
Maryland	235	2.57	78,104	1.38	1,184	1.48	24,496	0.98	20,689
Massachusetts	370	3.49	97,781	1.28	1,326	1.04	27,119	0.77	20,452
Michigan	607	3.86	203,832	2.34	2,754	1.95	59,857	1.45	21,735
Minnesota	281	4.76	71,690	1.75	1,073	1.42	18,669	0.90	17,399
Mississippi	148	4.80	37,655	1.81	545	1.48	8,758	1.00	16,070
Missouri	301	3.57	88,489	1.61	1,325	1.40	25,130	1.03	18,966
Montana	103	6.91	24,435	3.75	360	3.34	5,830	2.25	16,194
Nebraska	121	5.13	38,725	2.49	604	2.24	11,207	1.56	18,555
Nevada	110	4.74	36,924	1.64	503	1.99	11,163	1.22	22,193
New Hampshire	74	4.03	20,073	1.69	272	1.42	4,834	0.89	17,772
New Jersey	550	3.33	147,976	1.42	1,928	1.51	35,814	0.81	18,576
New Mexico	104	4.34	30,091	2.04	420	1.78	6,623	1.07	15,769
New York	791	2.44	226,940	1.14	2,959	1.06	58,592	0.71	19,801
North Carolina	498	5.61	146,551	2.20	2,024	1.89	42,591	1.43	21,043
North Dakota	64	8.26	21,635	3.45	333	3.64	6,177	2.03	18,550
Ohio	836	4.50	218,608	1.88	3,293	1.65	58,464	1.05	17,754
Oklahoma	317	5.94	76,308	2.33	1,086	1.84	17,892	1.27	16,475
Oregon	222	3.94	51,605	1.74	765	1.59	11,225	0.87	14,673
Pennsylvania	869	4.00	246,226	1.95	3,521	1.91	62,361	1.10	17,711
Rhode Island	72	3.79	21,103	1.99	285	1.57	4,638	0.99	16,274
South Carolina	198	4.26	58,093	1.85	810	1.62	16,886	1.21	20,847
South Dakota	80	8.26	19,165	3.40	285	3.13	4,860	1.86	17,053
Tennessee	364	4.42	101,398	1.50	1,379	1.37	22,892	0.80	16,600
Texas	1,100	3.67	329,294	1.44	4,476	1.29	86,299	0.94	19,280
Utah	81	2.65	21,944	1.19	341	1.10	5,782	0.77	16,956
Vermont	50	5.38	11,768	2.90	136	1.80	1,992	1.21	14,647
Virginia	436	4.47	115,755	1.73	1,720	1.68	32,780	1.08	19,058
Washington	341	3.70	95,398	1.77	1,353	1.55	22,321	0.94	16,497
West Virginia	151	5.61	43,184	2.42	579	2.01	8,617	1.22	14,883
Wisconsin	347	4.81	94,432	1.99	1,536	1.81	24,995	1.07	16,273
Wyoming	54	7.57	15,714	4.84	221	3.93	3,839	2.84	17,371

Source: U.S. Department of Commerce. Bureau of the Census. *1992 Economic Census Report Series,* CD-ROM 1i, Washington, DC, October 1996. *Notes:* - means no data reported. 1. HS stands for total health service establishments, revenues, employment, or payroll.

★ 370 ★
Establishment Data

Offices and Clinics of Podiatrists by Major Metro Areas: 1992

Area	Establishments		Revenues		Employment		Payroll		
	Number	% of HS[1] in area	Total ($000)	% of HS[1] in area	Number	% of HS[1] in area	Total ($000)	% of HS[1] in area	Payroll per employee
United States	7,948	1.80	1,920,076	0.64	26,429	0.59	624,211	0.48	23,618
Albany – Schenectady – Troy, NY MSA	33	2.52	6,677	0.83	89	0.67	1,559	0.43	17,517
Albuquerque, NM MSA	17	1.59	4,744	0.57	78	0.62	1,347	0.36	17,269
Allentown – Bethlehem – Easton, PA MSA	37	2.99	6,611	0.96	113	1.21	1,954	0.64	17,292
Anchorage, AK MSA	4	0.82	-	-	-	-	-	-	-
Appleton – Oshkosh – Neenah, WI MSA	6	1.15	1,311	0.36	17	0.30	292	0.16	17,176
Atlanta, GA MSA	87	1.43	29,803	0.62	328	0.55	13,347	0.66	40,692
Augusta – Aiken, GA – SC MSA	7	0.98	2,549	0.40	34	0.37	844	0.30	24,824
Austin – San Marcos, TX MSA	16	1.02	2,748	0.23	40	0.22	851	0.18	21,275
Bakersfield, CA MSA	10	1.32	2,285	0.42	30	0.37	676	0.31	22,533
Baton Rouge, LA MSA	7	0.79	1,735	0.23	27	0.24	850	0.28	31,481
Beaumont – Port Arthur, TX MSA	4	0.55	2,968	0.52	33	0.32	1,429	0.59	43,303
Birmingham, AL MSA	11	0.80	4,157	0.28	56	0.28	1,996	0.31	35,643
Boise City, ID MSA	7	1.17	2,716	0.72	34	0.58	977	0.58	28,735
Boston – Worcester – Lawrence, MA – NH – ME – CT CMSA	186	1.90	40,066	0.57	549	0.48	11,959	0.37	21,783
Buffalo – Niagara Falls, NY MSA	63	3.16	11,396	1.03	233	1.08	3,165	0.63	13,584
Canton – Massillon, OH MSA	14	2.02	3,138	0.76	47	0.66	1,137	0.54	24,191
Charleston – North Charleston, SC MSA	4	0.49	719	0.12	12	0.13	168	0.07	14,000
Charlotte – Gastonia – Rock Hill, NC – SC MSA	33	2.06	8,279	0.59	120	0.59	3,003	0.46	25,025
Chattanooga, TN – GA MSA	9	1.18	2,636	0.37	42	0.42	844	0.28	20,095
Chicago – Gary – Kenosha, IL – IN – WI CMSA	344	2.36	-	-	-	-	-	-	-
Cincinnati – Hamilton, OH – KY – IN CMSA	66	2.10	14,935	0.74	230	0.66	6,111	0.60	26,570
Cleveland – Akron, OH CMSA	183	3.41	34,137	1.05	570	1.11	10,306	0.67	18,081
Colorado Springs, CO MSA	14	1.58	3,730	0.84	56	0.85	1,445	0.72	25,804
Columbia, SC MSA	13	1.74	2,367	0.49	35	0.49	736	0.31	21,029
Columbus, OH MSA	61	2.51	17,336	0.99	232	0.82	6,851	0.84	29,530
Corpus Christi, TX MSA	8	1.07	2,519	0.44	36	0.43	1,083	0.48	30,083
Dallas – Fort Worth, TX CMSA	120	1.44	30,657	0.47	356	0.41	9,830	0.37	27,612
Davenport – Moline – Rock Island, IA – IL MSA	12	1.77	1,882	0.52	20	0.33	265	0.17	13,250
Dayton – Springfield, OH MSA	29	1.76	6,686	0.58	93	0.52	2,060	0.37	22,151
Daytona Beach, FL MSA	18	2.43	2,958	0.55	49	0.59	943	0.43	19,245
Denver – Boulder – Greeley, CO CMSA	62	1.42	-	-	-	-	-	-	-
Des Moines, IA MSA	16	2.17	2,812	0.55	57	0.80	918	0.35	16,105
Detroit – Ann Arbor – Flint, MI CMSA	305	3.24	88,458	1.62	1,334	1.59	37,138	1.46	27,840
El Paso, TX MSA	13	1.63	3,627	0.47	52	0.49	1,178	0.40	22,654
Eugene – Springfield, OR MSA	4	0.68	654	0.19	7	0.13	149	0.10	21,286
Fort Myers – Cape Coral, FL MSA	23	3.22	7,610	1.14	87	1.06	2,175	0.70	25,000
Fort Pierce – Port St. Lucie, FL MSA	14	2.70	4,272	0.95	49	0.79	1,195	0.64	24,388
Fort Wayne, IN MSA	14	2.00	2,977	0.54	45	0.48	1,422	0.56	31,600
Fresno, CA MSA	21	1.42	3,852	0.44	58	0.47	1,149	0.31	19,810
Grand Rapids – Muskegon – Holland, MI MSA	28	1.84	5,953	0.66	95	0.66	2,483	0.57	26,137
Greensboro – Winston-Salem – High Point, NC MSA	25	1.66	6,830	0.58	96	0.56	2,848	0.54	29,667
Greenville – Spartanburg – Anderson, SC MSA	9	0.77	2,963	0.38	34	0.28	1,580	0.42	46,471
Harrisburg – Lebanon – Carlisle, PA MSA	21	2.13	3,830	0.59	44	0.46	1,094	0.35	24,864
Hartford, CT MSA	54	2.38	15,213	0.86	193	0.71	6,804	0.80	35,254
Honolulu, HI MSA	11	0.65	2,218	0.21	22	0.18	343	0.07	15,591

[Continued]

★ 370 ★

Offices and Clinics of Podiatrists by Major Metro Areas: 1992

[Continued]

Area	Establishments		Revenues		Employment		Payroll		
	Number	% of HS[1] in area	Total ($000)	% of HS[1] in area	Number	% of HS[1] in area	Total ($000)	% of HS[1] in area	Payroll per employee
Houston – Galveston – Brazoria, TX CMSA	114	1.61	34,328	0.58	353	0.47	10,218	0.44	28,946
Huntsville, AL MSA	5	0.94	2,910	0.64	50	0.76	1,304	0.68	26,080
Indianapolis, IN MSA	52	2.05	15,663	0.78	250	0.78	7,653	0.81	30,612
Jackson, MS MSA	5	0.78	1,015	0.20	14	0.19	155	0.07	11,071
Jacksonville, FL MSA	30	1.69	10,229	0.78	133	0.78	3,276	0.59	24,632
Johnson City – Kingsport – Bristol, TN – VA MSA	7	1.01	1,316	0.22	22	0.22	504	0.19	22,909
Kalamazoo – Battle Creek, MI MSA	8	1.08	3,088	0.71	46	0.64	1,625	0.76	35,326
Kansas City, MO – KS MSA	35	1.23	10,200	0.47	139	0.41	4,369	0.44	31,432
Knoxville, TN MSA	19	1.59	5,420	0.67	92	0.86	2,301	0.59	25,011
Lafayette, LA MSA	4	0.63	1,636	0.36	17	0.24	172	0.09	10,118
Lakeland – Winter Haven, FL MSA	7	1.44	2,589	0.64	34	0.54	849	0.51	24,971
Lancaster, PA MSA	13	2.15	2,763	0.73	48	0.76	806	0.42	16,792
Lansing – East Lansing, MI MSA	10	1.37	2,923	0.73	33	0.52	861	0.45	26,091
Las Vegas, NV – AZ MSA	17	1.09	4,653	0.28	53	0.29	1,077	0.16	20,321
Lexington, KY MSA	4	0.49	837	0.14	8	0.09	144	0.05	18,000
Little Rock – North Little Rock, AR MSA	7	0.67	1,458	0.19	22	0.20	437	0.12	19,864
Los Angeles – Riverside – Orange County, CA CMSA	445	1.45	113,569	0.48	1,286	0.46	34,667	0.38	26,957
Louisville, KY – IN MSA	21	1.22	5,141	0.31	79	0.31	1,373	0.19	17,380
Macon, GA MSA	5	0.92	1,331	0.24	19	0.25	473	0.21	24,895
Madison, WI MSA	5	0.97	1,511	0.29	23	0.32	262	0.11	11,391
Melbourne – Titusville – Palm Bay, FL MSA	12	1.48	3,948	0.73	57	0.78	1,627	0.65	28,544
Memphis, TN – AR – MS MSA	18	1.09	6,281	0.51	75	0.46	2,154	0.40	28,720
Miami – Fort Lauderdale, FL CMSA	178	1.95	40,075	0.59	607	0.70	14,995	0.53	24,703
Milwaukee – Racine, WI CMSA	61	2.01	13,221	0.65	206	0.60	4,934	0.47	23,951
Minneapolis – St. Paul, MN – WI MSA	34	0.91	6,638	0.23	106	0.21	2,437	0.16	22,991
Mobile, AL MSA	9	1.40	1,856	0.33	28	0.29	456	0.17	16,286
Modesto, CA MSA	8	1.19	1,399	0.23	17	0.21	208	0.08	12,235
Montgomery, AL MSA	3	0.61	880	0.18	10	0.13	247	0.12	24,700
Nashville, TN MSA	21	1.08	4,883	0.26	53	0.21	876	0.11	16,528
New Orleans, LA MSA	21	0.87	5,775	0.26	59	0.20	1,808	0.21	30,644
New York – Northern New Jersey – Long Island, NY – NJ – CT- CMSA	1,159	2.85	275,619	1.06	3,228	0.97	70,445	0.64	21,823
Norfolk – Virginia Beach – Newport News, VA – NC MSA	36	1.60	9,532	0.70	148	0.68	4,352	0.67	29,405
Oklahoma City, OK MSA	24	1.22	9,252	0.71	126	0.64	3,398	0.61	26,968
Omaha, NE – IA MSA	15	1.49	3,216	0.39	66	0.53	1,226	0.33	18,576
Orlando, FL MSA	45	1.78	15,089	0.79	187	0.74	5,619	0.69	30,048
Pensacola, FL MSA	5	0.95	2,353	0.45	29	0.36	605	0.26	20,862
Peoria – Pekin, IL MSA	11	2.17	2,419	0.67	58	0.99	972	0.52	16,759
Philadelphia – Wilmington – Atlantic City, PA – NJ – DE – MD CMSA	351	3.03	72,263	0.99	1,169	1.17	21,055	0.65	18,011
Phoenix – Mesa, AZ MSA	82	1.71	20,862	0.66	291	0.76	8,470	0.62	29,107
Pittsburgh, PA MSA	114	2.39	25,284	0.93	377	0.99	7,500	0.60	19,894
Portland, ME MSA	9	1.66	1,646	0.43	21	0.36	472	0.26	22,476
Portland – Salem, OR – WA CMSA	40	1.13	-	-	-	-	-	-	-
Providence – Fall River – Warwick, RI – MA MSA	52	2.51	11,916	1.01	181	0.91	3,583	0.68	19,796
Raleigh – Durham – Chapel Hill, NC MSA	16	1.11	6,232	0.51	70	0.41	2,723	0.54	38,900
Reno, NV MSA	9	1.35	2,725	0.52	33	0.55	994	0.46	30,121
Richmond – Petersburg, VA MSA	28	1.75	6,341	0.41	94	0.42	2,288	0.35	24,340
Rochester, NY MSA	33	2.16	9,021	1.09	121	0.87	1,784	0.51	14,744

[Continued]

★ 370 ★

Offices and Clinics of Podiatrists by Major Metro Areas: 1992

[Continued]

Area	Establishments		Revenues		Employment		Payroll		
	Number	% of HS[1] in area	Total ($000)	% of HS[1] in area	Number	% of HS[1] in area	Total ($000)	% of HS[1] in area	Payroll per employee
Rockford, IL MSA	11	2.31	2,580	0.71	33	0.61	1,119	0.68	33,909
Sacramento – Yolo, CA CMSA	47	1.63	-	-	-	-	-	-	-
Saginaw – Bay City – Midland, MI MSA	10	1.47	4,003	1.05	53	0.83	1,444	0.73	27,245
St. Louis, MO – IL MSA	73	1.64	18,980	0.66	278	0.64	6,550	0.53	23,561
Salinas, CA MSA	11	1.81	2,759	0.92	32	0.73	826	0.67	25,812
Salt Lake City – Ogden, UT MSA	33	1.60	6,901	0.50	128	0.58	2,168	0.38	16,938
San Antonio, TX MSA	40	1.52	10,390	0.58	142	0.49	3,781	0.51	26,627
San Diego, CA MSA	72	1.46	12,626	0.39	172	0.41	2,880	0.21	16,744
San Francisco – Oakland – San Jose, CA CMSA	246	1.75	53,764	0.60	653	0.57	15,069	0.40	23,077
Santa Barbara – Santa Maria – Lompoc, CA MSA	8	0.96	2,187	0.51	31	0.59	1,180	0.66	38,065
Sarasota – Bradenton, FL MSA	24	1.96	7,093	0.72	88	0.61	2,636	0.65	29,955
Scranton – Wilkes-Barre – Hazleton, PA MSA	36	3.15	5,954	0.94	116	1.09	1,517	0.58	13,078
Seattle – Tacoma – Bremerton, WA CMSA	97	1.60	20,902	0.59	280	0.52	5,533	0.36	19,761
Shreveport – Bossier City, LA MSA	7	1.09	2,411	0.42	35	0.41	637	0.27	18,200
Spokane, WA MSA	20	2.72	4,420	0.87	56	0.71	1,447	0.62	25,839
Springfield, MO MSA	9	1.96	1,192	0.31	15	0.22	207	0.10	13,800
Springfield, MA MSA	22	2.43	4,028	0.60	57	0.47	1,122	0.35	19,684
Stockton – Lodi, CA MSA	12	1.44	2,882	0.56	47	0.59	985	0.43	20,957
Syracuse, NY MSA	24	2.20	5,069	0.73	90	0.92	1,741	0.55	19,344
Tallahassee, FL MSA	3	0.76	-	-	-	-	-	-	-
Tampa – St. Petersburg – Clearwater, FL MSA	92	1.86	21,737	0.50	313	0.51	8,174	0.47	26,115
Toledo, OH MSA	30	2.66	8,775	1.13	126	1.00	3,459	0.87	27,452
Tucson, AZ MSA	27	2.14	4,503	0.46	65	0.48	1,215	0.30	18,692
Tulsa, OK MSA	14	1.02	2,652	0.28	36	0.25	570	0.13	15,833
Washington – Baltimore, DC – MD – VA – WV CMSA	296	2.29	79,177	0.98	1,075	0.98	31,024	0.86	28,860
West Palm Beach – Boca Raton, FL MSA	74	2.75	17,534	0.89	261	1.06	5,346	0.63	20,483
Wichita, KS MSA	7	0.92	2,338	0.24	29	0.21	682	0.16	23,517
Youngstown – Warren, OH MSA	39	3.24	10,125	1.46	122	0.99	3,474	1.08	28,475

Source: U.S. Department of Commerce. Bureau of the Census. *1992 Economic Census Report Series*, CD-ROM 1i, Washington, DC, October 1996. *Notes:* - means no data reported. 1. HS stands for total health service establishments, revenues, employment, or payroll.

★ 371 ★

Establishment Data

Offices and Clinics of Podiatrists by State: 1992

Area	Establishments		Revenues		Employment		Payroll		
	Number	% of HS[1] in area	Total ($000)	% of HS[1] in area	Number	% of HS[1] in area	Total ($000)	% of HS[1] in area	Payroll per employee
United States	7,948	1.80	1,920,076	0.64	26,429	0.59	624,211	0.48	23,618
Alabama	49	0.89	15,910	0.32	229	0.30	6,751	0.32	29,480
Alaska	5	0.58	2,222	0.41	21	0.37	277	0.13	13,190
Arizona	121	1.70	27,962	0.61	404	0.69	10,532	0.54	26,069
Arkansas	20	0.56	5,017	0.21	71	0.17	1,868	0.18	26,310

[Continued]

★ 371 ★

Offices and Clinics of Podiatrists by State: 1992
[Continued]

Area	Establishments		Revenues		Employment		Payroll		
	Number	% of HS[1] in area	Total ($000)	% of HS[1] in area	Number	% of HS[1] in area	Total ($000)	% of HS[1] in area	Payroll per employee
California	930	1.51	217,602	0.51	2,665	0.50	65,253	0.38	24,485
Colorado	88	1.25	18,980	0.51	295	0.53	6,355	0.39	21,542
Connecticut	152	2.30	48,830	0.99	561	0.78	17,606	0.75	31,383
Delaware	25	2.09	6,801	0.86	92	0.79	2,999	0.82	32,598
District of Columbia	32	2.32	8,181	1.02	111	1.14	2,965	0.85	26,712
Florida	564	1.91	147,168	0.63	2,082	0.66	52,398	0.54	25,167
Georgia	139	1.25	47,600	0.55	573	0.47	18,570	0.51	32,408
Hawaii	16	0.72	3,871	0.30	43	0.27	970	0.16	22,558
Idaho	17	0.98	5,283	0.54	78	0.46	1,655	0.40	21,218
Illinois	419	2.24	105,745	0.85	1,370	0.73	35,880	0.64	26,190
Indiana	166	1.91	41,792	0.69	633	0.59	16,546	0.60	26,139
Iowa	75	1.79	14,998	0.64	270	0.60	5,046	0.45	18,689
Kansas	55	1.42	12,107	0.40	196	0.37	4,122	0.31	21,031
Kentucky	46	0.83	10,299	0.25	165	0.25	2,944	0.17	17,842
Louisiana	48	0.70	13,876	0.25	176	0.20	4,081	0.19	23,188
Maine	36	1.67	6,464	0.55	94	0.43	1,682	0.32	17,894
Maryland	211	2.31	56,379	1.00	780	0.98	22,521	0.90	28,873
Massachusetts	208	1.96	43,366	0.57	594	0.47	12,618	0.36	21,242
Michigan	400	2.54	112,871	1.30	1,680	1.19	46,109	1.12	27,446
Minnesota	60	1.02	12,440	0.30	188	0.25	4,336	0.21	23,064
Mississippi	18	0.58	3,801	0.18	68	0.18	891	0.10	13,103
Missouri	98	1.16	24,462	0.45	353	0.37	8,739	0.36	24,756
Montana	16	1.07	3,441	0.53	38	0.35	768	0.30	20,211
Nebraska	34	1.44	7,020	0.45	110	0.41	2,678	0.37	24,345
Nevada	28	1.21	7,995	0.36	88	0.35	2,388	0.26	27,136
New Hampshire	24	1.31	5,180	0.44	69	0.36	1,857	0.34	26,913
New Jersey	449	2.72	103,924	1.00	1,299	1.02	26,066	0.59	20,066
New Mexico	33	1.38	8,215	0.56	145	0.61	2,549	0.41	17,579
New York	938	2.89	209,057	1.05	2,702	0.97	52,675	0.64	19,495
North Carolina	140	1.58	35,032	0.53	528	0.49	12,469	0.42	23,616
North Dakota	7	0.90	1,382	0.22	26	0.28	424	0.14	16,308
Ohio	490	2.64	109,704	0.94	1,682	0.84	38,259	0.69	22,746
Oklahoma	52	0.97	14,850	0.45	209	0.35	5,106	0.36	24,431
Oregon	61	1.08	13,796	0.47	179	0.37	4,264	0.33	23,821
Pennsylvania	589	2.71	118,882	0.94	1,899	1.03	33,953	0.60	17,879
Rhode Island	50	2.63	11,842	1.12	183	1.01	3,808	0.81	20,809
South Carolina	40	0.86	9,906	0.32	129	0.26	3,960	0.28	30,698
South Dakota	14	1.45	1,774	0.31	40	0.44	469	0.18	11,725
Tennessee	90	1.09	23,034	0.34	316	0.32	7,343	0.26	23,237
Texas	382	1.28	104,569	0.46	1,235	0.36	32,935	0.36	26,668
Utah	44	1.44	9,326	0.51	173	0.56	2,737	0.36	15,821
Vermont	9	0.97	1,157	0.29	19	0.25	228	0.14	12,000
Virginia	164	1.68	40,402	0.60	602	0.59	15,965	0.53	26,520
Washington	146	1.58	31,204	0.58	445	0.51	8,482	0.36	19,061

[Continued]

★ 371 ★

Offices and Clinics of Podiatrists by State: 1992

[Continued]

Area	Establishments		Revenues		Employment		Payroll		
	Number	% of HS[1] in area	Total ($000)	% of HS[1] in area	Number	% of HS[1] in area	Total ($000)	% of HS[1] in area	Payroll per employee
West Virginia	26	0.97	5,602	0.31	75	0.26	1,103	0.16	14,707
Wisconsin	119	1.65	27,720	0.59	430	0.51	9,869	0.42	22,951
Wyoming	5	0.70	1,035	0.32	16	0.28	142	0.10	8,875

Source: U.S. Department of Commerce. Bureau of the Census. *1992 Economic Census Report Series,* CD-ROM 1i, Washington, DC, October 1996. *Notes:* - means no data reported. 1. HS stands for total health service establishments, revenues, employment, or payroll.

★ 372 ★

Establishment Data

Offices of Dentists by Major Metro Areas: 1992

Area	Establishments		Revenues		Employment		Payroll		
	Number	% of HS[1] in area	Total ($000)	% of HS[1] in area	Number	% of HS[1] in area	Total ($000)	% of HS[1] in area	Payroll per employee
United States	108,200	24.50	35,171,784	11.76	549,357	12.34	12,900,793	9.99	23,483
Atlanta, GA MSA	1,333	21.88	492,116	10.21	7,080	11.83	192,223	9.52	27,150
Boston – Worcester – Lawrence, MA – NH – ME – CT CMSA	2,707	27.71	-	-	-	-	-	-	-
Chicago – Gary – Kenosha, IL – IN – WI CMSA	3,998	27.46	-	-	-	-	-	-	-
Cincinnati – Hamilton, OH – KY – IN CMSA	741	23.63	-	-	-	-	-	-	-
Cleveland – Akron, OH CMSA	1,421	26.46	-	-	-	-	-	-	-
Dallas – Fort Worth, TX CMSA	1,787	21.48	607,704	9.31	8,571	9.96	218,443	8.24	25,486
Denver – Boulder – Greeley, CO CMSA	1,206	27.58	-	-	-	-	-	-	-
Detroit – Ann Arbor – Flint, MI CMSA	2,555	27.12	-	-	-	-	-	-	-
Houston – Galveston – Brazoria, TX CMSA	1,469	20.80	-	-	-	-	-	-	-
Indianapolis, IN MSA	655	25.77	-	-	-	-	-	-	-
Kansas City, MO – KS MSA	765	26.80	-	-	-	-	-	-	-
Los Angeles – Riverside – Orange County, CA CMSA	6,599	21.58	2,407,029	10.25	33,734	12.15	851,053	9.31	25,228
Miami – Fort Lauderdale, FL CMSA	1,532	16.76	-	-	-	-	-	-	-
Milwaukee – Racine, WI CMSA	832	27.46	-	-	-	-	-	-	-
Minneapolis – St. Paul, MN – WI MSA	1,193	32.04	-	-	-	-	-	-	-
New York – Northern New Jersey – Long Island, NY – NJ – CT- CMSA	10,468	25.78	3,541,941	13.56	46,503	13.94	1,169,101	10.70	25,140
Orlando, FL MSA	502	19.82	187,799	9.87	2,742	10.87	73,596	8.99	26,840
Philadelphia – Wilmington – Atlantic City, PA – NJ – DE – MD CMSA	2,555	22.03	-	-	-	-	-	-	-
Phoenix – Mesa, AZ MSA	976	20.30	334,378	10.63	4,943	12.83	131,548	9.58	26,613
Pittsburgh, PA MSA	1,258	26.41	-	-	-	-	-	-	-
Portland – Salem, OR – WA CMSA	1,012	28.55	-	-	-	-	-	-	-
Sacramento – Yolo, CA CMSA	829	28.68	320,682	16.63	4,453	17.86	113,760	13.78	25,547
St. Louis, MO – IL MSA	1,100	24.72	-	-	-	-	-	-	-
San Diego, CA MSA	1,191	24.16	447,750	13.71	6,273	15.06	161,961	12.03	25,819
San Francisco – Oakland – San Jose, CA CMSA	3,952	28.14	1,521,383	16.88	21,607	19.02	552,167	14.62	25,555
Seattle – Tacoma – Bremerton, WA CMSA	1,791	29.56	738,394	20.74	10,916	20.14	290,747	18.71	26,635

[Continued]

★ 372 ★

Offices of Dentists by Major Metro Areas: 1992
[Continued]

Area	Establishments		Revenues		Employment		Payroll		
	Number	% of HS[1] in area	Total ($000)	% of HS[1] in area	Number	% of HS[1] in area	Total ($000)	% of HS[1] in area	Payroll per employee
Tampa – St. Petersburg – Clearwater, FL MSA	801	16.22	309,140	7.09	4,597	7.51	126,159	7.31	27,444
Washington – Baltimore, DC – MD – VA – WV CMSA	3,173	24.53	-	-	-	-	-	-	-
West Palm Beach – Boca Raton, FL MSA	510	18.97	186,464	9.43	2,523	10.27	69,657	8.26	27,609

Source: U.S. Department of Commerce. Bureau of the Census. *1992 Economic Census Report Series,* CD-ROM 1i, Washington, DC, October 1996. *Notes:* - means no data reported. 1. HS stands for total health service establishments, revenues, employment, or payroll.

★ 373 ★

Establishment Data

Offices of Dentists by State: 1992

Area	Establishments		Revenues		Employment		Payroll		
	Number	% of HS[1] in area	Total ($000)	% of HS[1] in area	Number	% of HS[1] in area	Total ($000)	% of HS[1] in area	Payroll per employee
United States	108,200	24.50	35,171,784	11.76	549,357	12.34	12,900,793	9.99	23,483
Alabama	1,325	24.01	421,914	8.57	6,804	8.80	150,960	7.15	22,187
Alaska	258	30.07	-	-	-	-	-	-	-
Arizona	1,506	21.19	499,480	10.93	7,498	12.76	186,542	9.56	24,879
Arkansas	817	22.92	225,146	9.24	3,761	8.81	76,239	7.16	20,271
California	14,702	23.92	5,439,637	12.65	76,927	14.35	1,935,492	11.22	25,160
Colorado	1,903	27.14	-	-	-	-	-	-	-
Connecticut	1,735	26.30	666,282	13.57	9,360	12.95	258,816	11.03	27,651
Delaware	215	17.93	102,416	12.97	1,566	13.48	48,229	13.26	30,798
District of Columbia	345	25.02	-	-	-	-	-	-	-
Florida	5,340	18.04	1,882,193	8.08	28,460	9.03	731,633	7.60	25,707
Georgia	2,335	21.06	825,745	9.57	12,479	10.31	318,073	8.67	25,489
Hawaii	626	28.13	210,269	16.04	3,130	20.01	82,661	14.02	26,409
Idaho	454	26.18	-	-	-	-	-	-	-
Illinois	5,130	27.43	1,501,011	12.13	24,817	13.23	571,474	10.21	23,028
Indiana	2,167	24.89	635,763	10.44	10,961	10.27	226,103	8.23	20,628
Iowa	1,146	27.39	319,586	13.66	5,744	12.77	116,871	10.51	20,347
Kansas	997	25.78	304,697	10.00	5,107	9.55	112,230	8.48	21,976
Kentucky	1,458	26.45	338,834	8.23	6,160	9.19	113,284	6.37	18,390
Louisiana	1,541	22.59	402,853	7.29	7,011	8.12	135,330	6.22	19,303
Maine	457	21.17	-	-	-	-	-	-	-
Maryland	2,184	23.88	708,316	12.55	11,250	14.08	272,093	10.90	24,186
Massachusetts	2,930	27.64	988,899	12.97	15,621	12.28	365,093	10.30	23,372
Michigan	4,318	27.45	1,460,758	16.78	25,573	18.15	606,808	14.74	23,728
Minnesota	1,998	33.82	-	-	-	-	-	-	-
Mississippi	778	25.21	196,695	9.44	3,204	8.70	64,942	7.39	20,269
Missouri	2,045	24.28	-	-	-	-	-	-	-

[Continued]

★ 373 ★

Offices of Dentists by State: 1992
[Continued]

Area	Establishments		Revenues		Employment		Payroll		
	Number	% of HS[1] in area	Total ($000)	% of HS[1] in area	Number	% of HS[1] in area	Total ($000)	% of HS[1] in area	Payroll per employee
Montana	395	26.51	-	-	-	-	-	-	-
Nebraska	745	31.61	-	-	-	-	-	-	-
Nevada	477	20.56	-	-	-	-	-	-	-
New Hampshire	514	27.97	167,595	14.11	2,667	13.89	61,188	11.28	22,943
New Jersey	4,023	24.38	1,411,079	13.56	20,194	15.82	518,516	11.73	25,677
New Mexico	528	22.01	158,720	10.74	2,793	11.81	57,607	9.31	20,625
New York	8,522	26.30	2,748,875	13.83	38,073	13.68	866,335	10.51	22,755
North Carolina	2,150	24.23	747,172	11.22	11,840	11.04	296,557	9.94	25,047
North Dakota	248	32.00	-	-	-	-	-	-	-
Ohio	4,489	24.18	1,333,612	11.45	23,609	11.83	524,618	9.42	22,221
Oklahoma	1,220	22.87	335,728	10.25	5,593	9.47	115,715	8.19	20,689
Oregon	1,548	27.44	507,029	17.14	8,195	17.02	186,253	14.36	22,728
Pennsylvania	5,295	24.36	1,565,659	12.39	25,673	13.92	543,054	9.59	21,153
Rhode Island	403	21.23	-	-	-	-	-	-	-
South Carolina	1,150	24.76	-	-	-	-	-	-	-
South Dakota	257	26.55	78,580	13.94	1,317	14.46	25,697	9.86	19,512
Tennessee	1,984	24.12	572,138	8.48	9,013	8.99	189,445	6.60	21,019
Texas	6,201	20.71	1,903,991	8.31	28,443	8.21	671,847	7.29	23,621
Utah	969	31.73	256,246	13.88	4,628	14.97	83,804	11.10	18,108
Vermont	244	26.24	-	-	-	-	-	-	-
Virginia	2,517	25.81	810,173	12.13	12,845	12.57	324,823	10.73	25,288
Washington	2,636	28.58	1,070,379	19.82	16,162	18.47	413,599	17.36	25,591
West Virginia	561	20.84	-	-	-	-	-	-	-
Wisconsin	2,212	30.64	692,908	14.63	12,809	15.07	283,129	12.08	22,104
Wyoming	202	28.33	52,712	16.25	941	16.72	18,054	13.34	19,186

Source: U.S. Department of Commerce. Bureau of the Census. *1992 Economic Census Report Series,* CD-ROM 1i, Washington, DC, October 1996. *Notes:* - means no data reported. 1. HS stands for total health service establishments, revenues, employment, or payroll.

★ 374 ★

Establishment Data

Offices of Doctors of Medicine by Major Metro Areas: 1992

Area	Establishments		Revenues		Employment		Payroll		
	Number	% of HS[1] in area	Total ($000)	% of HS[1] in area	Number	% of HS[1] in area	Total ($000)	% of HS[1] in area	Payroll per employee
United States	192,965	43.69	128,838,689	43.08	1,231,342	27.65	63,659,757	49.31	51,699
Albany – Schenectady – Troy, NY MSA	615	46.98	388,007	48.04	3,942	29.85	187,900	51.71	47,666
Albuquerque, NM MSA	394	36.93	-	-	-	-	-	-	-
Allentown – Bethlehem – Easton, PA MSA	549	44.35	372,136	54.10	3,492	37.35	192,928	63.08	55,249
Anchorage, AK MSA	205	42.18	-	-	-	-	-	-	-
Appleton – Oshkosh – Neenah, WI MSA	180	34.55	199,389	55.12	2,301	40.14	108,178	59.61	47,013
Atlanta, GA MSA	2,704	44.38	2,270,566	47.12	18,853	31.50	1,103,857	54.69	58,551

[Continued]

★ 374 ★

Offices of Doctors of Medicine by Major Metro Areas: 1992
[Continued]

Area	Establishments		Revenues		Employment		Payroll		
	Number	% of HS[1] in area	Total ($000)	% of HS[1] in area	Number	% of HS[1] in area	Total ($000)	% of HS[1] in area	Payroll per employee
Augusta – Aiken, GA – SC MSA	354	49.79	244,325	38.00	2,273	24.56	138,419	49.13	60,897
Austin – San Marcos, TX MSA	629	40.04	460,149	38.45	4,473	24.08	216,354	44.57	48,369
Bakersfield, CA MSA	347	45.72	238,493	43.73	2,305	28.23	100,452	45.84	43,580
Baton Rouge, LA MSA	372	42.03	341,093	45.98	2,908	26.36	155,544	51.29	53,488
Beaumont – Port Arthur, TX MSA	373	51.59	218,775	38.01	2,128	20.82	109,208	45.34	51,320
Birmingham, AL MSA	651	47.28	695,059	45.99	6,345	31.42	377,197	58.81	59,448
Boise City, ID MSA	254	42.40	-	-	-	-	-	-	-
Boston – Worcester – Lawrence, MA – NH – ME – CT CMSA	4,094	41.91	2,784,234	39.38	27,980	24.30	1,409,556	43.30	50,377
Buffalo – Niagara Falls, NY MSA	989	49.62	546,957	49.42	6,343	29.29	258,637	51.80	40,775
Canton – Massillon, OH MSA	270	38.96	191,931	46.50	1,981	27.78	112,979	53.58	57,031
Charleston – North Charleston, SC MSA	393	48.16	272,328	46.00	2,963	32.52	124,172	53.11	41,908
Charlotte – Gastonia – Rock Hill, NC – SC MSA	625	38.99	625,786	44.76	5,923	29.10	363,116	55.21	61,306
Chattanooga, TN – GA MSA	350	45.99	282,750	39.41	2,610	26.17	155,064	50.74	59,411
Chicago – Gary – Kenosha, IL – IN – WI CMSA	6,742	46.31	-	-	-	-	-	-	-
Cincinnati – Hamilton, OH – KY – IN CMSA	1,446	46.11	-	-	-	-	-	-	-
Cleveland – Akron, OH CMSA	2,364	44.02	1,616,403	49.68	13,936	27.16	853,035	55.51	61,211
Colorado Springs, CO MSA	318	35.81	192,272	43.29	1,947	29.47	105,648	52.47	54,262
Columbia, SC MSA	342	45.91	268,301	55.56	2,583	36.01	154,955	64.53	59,990
Columbus, OH MSA	969	39.86	718,316	40.82	6,821	24.23	400,562	49.34	58,725
Corpus Christi, TX MSA	392	52.20	245,385	42.48	2,104	24.88	111,518	49.39	53,003
Dallas – Fort Worth, TX CMSA	3,738	44.93	2,434,142	37.31	20,033	23.27	1,211,432	45.72	60,472
Davenport – Moline – Rock Island, IA – IL MSA	249	36.73	154,796	42.85	1,706	28.44	81,885	51.80	47,998
Dayton – Springfield, OH MSA	662	40.17	568,630	49.68	5,539	31.25	332,046	58.90	59,947
Daytona Beach, FL MSA	309	41.76	-	-	-	-	-	-	-
Denver – Boulder – Greeley, CO CMSA	1,665	38.08							
Des Moines, IA MSA	275	37.26	280,138	55.08	2,296	32.26	164,540	62.02	71,664
Detroit – Ann Arbor – Flint, MI CMSA	3,545	37.63	-	-	-	-	-	-	-
El Paso, TX MSA	409	51.38	248,198	31.95	2,322	21.67	117,276	40.16	50,506
Eugene – Springfield, OR MSA	233	39.90	175,735	52.33	2,235	41.31	90,979	58.48	40,706
Fort Myers – Cape Coral, FL MSA	322	45.10	292,280	43.96	2,434	29.58	178,641	57.69	73,394
Fort Pierce – Port St. Lucie, FL MSA	242	46.63	155,041	34.56	1,361	22.03	82,745	44.34	60,797
Fort Wayne, IN MSA	275	39.23	275,849	49.85	2,934	31.10	140,859	55.03	48,009
Fresno, CA MSA	690	46.59	388,294	44.71	3,916	31.81	179,417	48.36	45,816
Grand Rapids – Muskegon – Holland, MI MSA	496	32.52	406,959	45.32	4,504	31.38	236,956	54.76	52,610
Greensboro – Winston-Salem – High Point, NC MSA	649	43.01	518,813	43.71	5,399	31.59	273,903	51.90	50,732
Greenville – Spartanburg – Anderson, SC MSA	547	46.51	410,145	52.59	4,323	36.05	229,882	60.99	53,176
Harrisburg – Lebanon – Carlisle, PA MSA	341	34.55	281,171	43.09	2,853	29.96	157,891	51.16	55,342
Hartford, CT MSA	1,002	44.16	-	-	-	-	-	-	-
Honolulu, HI MSA	789	46.91	409,510	39.47	3,886	32.28	197,171	41.31	50,739
Houston – Galveston – Brazoria, TX CMSA	3,520	49.84	-	-	-	-	-	-	-
Huntsville, AL MSA	247	46.34	-	-	-	-	-	-	-
Indianapolis, IN MSA	1,095	43.08	862,791	43.04	8,042	25.00	476,714	50.65	59,278
Jackson, MS MSA	306	48.04	251,424	49.62	2,108	29.23	117,771	56.27	55,869
Jacksonville, FL MSA	869	49.01	645,638	49.38	5,248	30.66	292,817	52.63	55,796
Johnson City – Kingsport – Bristol, TN – VA MSA	322	46.67	261,983	42.88	2,862	29.06	147,165	54.07	51,420

[Continued]

★ 374 ★

Offices of Doctors of Medicine by Major Metro Areas: 1992
[Continued]

Area	Establishments		Revenues		Employment		Payroll		
	Number	% of HS[1] in area	Total ($000)	% of HS[1] in area	Number	% of HS[1] in area	Total ($000)	% of HS[1] in area	Payroll per employee
Kalamazoo – Battle Creek, MI MSA	321	43.50	-	-	-	-	-	-	-
Kansas City, MO – KS MSA	1,047	36.67	889,971	40.72	8,986	26.60	496,042	50.09	55,202
Knoxville, TN MSA	560	46.82	461,251	56.81	4,376	41.04	259,761	66.47	59,360
Lafayette, LA MSA	299	46.87	189,383	42.12	1,762	24.99	94,915	51.70	53,868
Lakeland – Winter Haven, FL MSA	204	41.89	213,202	53.07	2,364	37.20	96,041	57.33	40,626
Lancaster, PA MSA	205	33.94	190,559	50.10	2,135	33.74	112,733	58.99	52,802
Lansing – East Lansing, MI MSA	207	28.32	145,638	36.38	1,450	23.04	80,932	42.53	55,815
Las Vegas, NV – AZ MSA	727	46.72	599,660	35.51	4,542	24.62	305,258	44.81	67,208
Lexington, KY MSA	371	45.75	303,962	51.31	3,174	35.14	170,615	61.87	53,754
Little Rock – North Little Rock, AR MSA	520	50.00	411,991	52.98	3,884	34.72	231,482	62.98	59,599
Los Angeles – Riverside – Orange County, CA CMSA	14,921	48.78	9,444,325	40.21	77,229	27.81	4,028,171	44.06	52,159
Louisville, KY – IN MSA	852	49.53	670,283	39.93	6,541	25.32	341,998	47.91	52,285
Macon, GA MSA	274	50.37	-	-	-	-	-	-	-
Madison, WI MSA	137	26.45	307,075	59.31	2,816	39.12	141,698	60.45	50,319
Melbourne – Titusville – Palm Bay, FL MSA	368	45.26	299,175	55.12	2,707	37.24	155,281	62.01	57,363
Memphis, TN – AR – MS MSA	790	47.97	639,288	51.47	6,047	37.02	333,360	62.01	55,128
Miami – Fort Lauderdale, FL CMSA	4,492	49.14	2,710,742	39.62	24,437	28.11	1,344,732	47.93	55,029
Milwaukee – Racine, WI CMSA	1,282	42.31	1,011,576	49.52	10,509	30.77	581,070	55.91	55,293
Minneapolis – St. Paul, MN – WI MSA	1,002	26.91	1,373,381	47.39	13,847	27.74	810,244	54.01	58,514
Mobile, AL MSA	273	42.52	255,471	45.52	2,531	26.48	147,694	56.24	58,354
Modesto, CA MSA	272	40.30	197,105	32.65	1,836	22.90	93,603	37.80	50,982
Montgomery, AL MSA	261	53.16	-	-	-	-	-	-	-
Nashville, TN MSA	882	45.39	671,566	36.23	5,735	22.66	347,397	44.75	60,575
New Orleans, LA MSA	1,231	50.78	942,375	43.07	8,908	30.08	411,982	48.99	46,249
New York – Northern New Jersey – Long Island, NY – NJ – CT- CMSA	19,764	48.68	-	-	-	-	-	-	-
Norfolk – Virginia Beach – Newport News, VA – NC MSA	1,109	49.16	738,374	54.44	7,861	35.92	396,724	61.32	50,467
Oklahoma City, OK MSA	850	43.15	572,381	44.07	5,263	26.88	292,745	52.22	55,623
Omaha, NE – IA MSA	444	44.00	375,700	45.80	3,602	28.96	203,772	54.55	56,572
Orlando, FL MSA	1,150	45.40	806,956	42.43	7,607	30.16	421,880	51.55	55,459
Pensacola, FL MSA	249	47.25	-	-	-	-	-	-	-
Peoria – Pekin, IL MSA	211	41.54	-	-	-	-	-	-	-
Philadelphia – Wilmington – Atlantic City, PA – NJ – DE – MD CMSA	4,977	42.92	3,268,012	44.73	31,358	31.41	1,656,863	50.89	52,837
Phoenix – Mesa, AZ MSA	2,120	44.08	1,353,256	43.03	11,717	30.41	692,595	50.42	59,110
Pittsburgh, PA MSA	2,087	43.81	1,458,934	53.68	13,486	35.36	804,285	64.36	59,639
Portland, ME MSA	195	36.04	160,315	41.83	1,429	24.29	89,999	50.21	62,980
Portland – Salem, OR – WA CMSA	1,329	37.49	-	-	-	-	-	-	-
Providence – Fall River – Warwick, RI – MA MSA	981	47.30	517,894	43.91	5,452	27.48	249,720	47.16	45,803
Raleigh – Durham – Chapel Hill, NC MSA	525	36.51	425,601	35.04	4,270	24.82	231,990	45.93	54,330
Reno, NV MSA	293	43.93	228,172	43.77	1,710	28.72	118,139	54.21	69,087
Richmond – Petersburg, VA MSA	761	47.59	578,311	36.95	5,935	26.71	323,775	48.95	54,553
Rochester, NY MSA	702	45.85	-	-	-	-	-	-	-
Rockford, IL MSA	170	35.64	-	-	-	-	-	-	-
Sacramento – Yolo, CA CMSA	1,065	36.84	-	-	-	-	-	-	-
Saginaw – Bay City – Midland, MI MSA	283	41.50	189,125	49.44	1,926	29.99	109,075	55.19	56,633
St. Louis, MO – IL MSA	1,880	42.26	1,216,048	42.51	11,618	26.64	645,194	51.93	55,534
Salinas, CA MSA	263	43.26	-	-	-	-	-	-	-
Salt Lake City – Ogden, UT MSA	854	41.48	-	-	-	-	-	-	-
San Antonio, TX MSA	1,325	50.50	739,612	41.06	6,812	23.69	349,114	46.78	51,250
San Diego, CA MSA	2,110	42.81	1,244,091	38.11	10,892	26.15	553,915	41.15	50,855

[Continued]

★ 374 ★

Offices of Doctors of Medicine by Major Metro Areas: 1992
[Continued]

Area	Establishments		Revenues		Employment		Payroll		
	Number	% of HS[1] in area	Total ($000)	% of HS[1] in area	Number	% of HS[1] in area	Total ($000)	% of HS[1] in area	Payroll per employee
San Francisco – Oakland – San Jose, CA CMSA	5,609	39.94	-	-	-	-	-	-	-
Santa Barbara – Santa Maria – Lompoc, CA MSA	344	41.15	-	-	-	-	-	-	-
Sarasota – Bradenton, FL MSA	563	45.88	377,919	38.50	3,515	24.34	191,622	47.02	54,516
Scranton – Wilkes-Barre – Hazleton, PA MSA	491	42.92	280,061	44.36	2,862	26.95	132,933	50.74	46,448
Seattle – Tacoma – Bremerton, WA CMSA	2,232	36.84	1,440,429	40.47	15,486	28.57	709,835	45.69	45,837
Shreveport – Bossier City, LA MSA	312	48.60	240,248	42.03	2,224	26.16	121,062	52.26	54,434
Spokane, WA MSA	279	37.96	268,342	52.58	2,605	33.23	141,128	60.38	54,176
Springfield, MO MSA	140	30.43	-	-	-	-	-	-	-
Springfield, MA MSA	358	39.56	248,376	37.17	2,501	20.70	130,548	40.68	52,198
Stockton – Lodi, CA MSA	377	45.15	-	-	-	-	-	-	-
Syracuse, NY MSA	548	50.18	382,043	55.35	3,451	35.22	193,929	61.61	56,195
Tallahassee, FL MSA	187	47.10	-	-	-	-	-	-	-
Tampa – St. Petersburg – Clearwater, FL MSA	2,373	48.06	1,556,532	35.71	13,264	21.68	726,510	42.10	54,773
Toledo, OH MSA	495	43.96	375,722	48.25	3,881	30.90	215,150	54.22	55,437
Tucson, AZ MSA	510	40.44	408,709	41.38	3,783	27.78	195,982	48.72	51,806
Tulsa, OK MSA	474	34.65	405,199	42.65	3,639	25.49	215,831	50.74	59,311
Washington – Baltimore, DC – MD – VA – WV CMSA	6,569	50.78	-	-	-	-	-	-	-
West Palm Beach – Boca Raton, FL MSA	1,234	45.91	807,570	40.86	6,539	26.61	415,421	49.28	63,530
Wichita, KS MSA	285	37.25	402,944	41.62	3,878	28.67	210,504	50.69	54,282
Youngstown – Warren, OH MSA	496	41.23	319,186	45.93	3,046	24.78	165,942	51.71	54,479

Source: U.S. Department of Commerce. Bureau of the Census. *1992 Economic Census Report Series,* CD-ROM 1i, Washington, DC, October 1996. *Notes:* - means no data reported. 1. HS stands for total health service establishments, revenues, employment, or payroll.

★ 375 ★

Establishment Data

Offices of Doctors of Medicine by State: 1992

Area	Establishments		Revenues		Employment		Payroll		
	Number	% of HS[1] in area	Total ($000)	% of HS[1] in area	Number	% of HS[1] in area	Total ($000)	% of HS[1] in area	Payroll per employee
United States	192,965	43.69	128,838,689	43.08	1,231,342	27.65	63,659,757	49.31	51,699
Alabama	2,554	46.28	2,126,195	43.17	20,857	26.97	1,117,431	52.95	53,576
Alaska	343	39.98	246,773	45.55	2,281	40.34	117,488	54.10	51,507
Arizona	3,048	42.88	1,970,662	43.14	17,751	30.22	983,969	50.44	55,432
Arkansas	1,618	45.40	1,070,213	43.92	11,559	27.08	566,225	53.20	48,986
California	27,645	44.98	16,441,864	38.24	144,290	26.92	7,107,711	41.22	49,260
Colorado	2,623	37.41	1,716,611	45.94	16,728	30.26	874,907	53.30	52,302
Connecticut	2,996	45.42	2,196,334	44.74	19,320	26.73	1,147,701	48.92	59,405
Delaware	572	47.71	365,843	46.32	3,302	28.42	182,434	50.17	55,250
District of Columbia	763	55.33	432,805	54.22	3,606	37.17	201,847	58.20	55,975
Florida	14,075	47.55	9,420,257	40.42	84,478	26.80	4,640,600	48.18	54,933

[Continued]

★ 375 ★

Offices of Doctors of Medicine by State: 1992
[Continued]

Area	Establishments		Revenues		Employment		Payroll		
	Number	% of HS[1] in area	Total ($000)	% of HS[1] in area	Number	% of HS[1] in area	Total ($000)	% of HS[1] in area	Payroll per employee
Georgia	5,099	45.98	3,930,297	45.57	35,033	28.95	1,975,810	53.84	56,399
Hawaii	1,019	45.80	539,094	41.12	5,434	34.74	252,714	42.87	46,506
Idaho	716	41.29	424,741	43.04	4,834	28.57	216,532	52.08	44,794
Illinois	8,235	44.03	5,927,252	47.91	54,643	29.12	3,084,310	55.13	56,445
Indiana	3,656	42.00	2,720,346	44.67	28,082	26.32	1,403,224	51.11	49,969
Iowa	1,285	30.71	1,106,531	47.31	12,121	26.95	604,214	54.33	49,849
Kansas	1,314	33.98	1,172,314	38.46	13,628	25.50	606,023	45.82	44,469
Kentucky	2,526	45.83	1,823,070	44.26	18,844	28.10	931,576	52.39	49,436
Louisiana	3,213	47.10	2,308,539	41.77	21,828	25.29	1,037,704	47.68	47,540
Maine	902	41.78	485,378	41.23	4,919	22.36	244,322	45.85	49,669
Maryland	4,652	50.87	2,832,632	50.20	27,152	33.99	1,349,122	54.06	49,688
Massachusetts	4,434	41.82	3,018,954	39.59	30,453	23.93	1,525,380	43.04	50,090
Michigan	5,798	36.86	3,619,096	41.57	38,414	27.26	1,981,402	48.14	51,580
Minnesota	1,434	24.27	1,896,402	46.19	20,783	27.42	1,100,605	52.84	52,957
Mississippi	1,419	45.98	934,900	44.87	9,742	26.45	442,938	50.37	45,467
Missouri	3,140	37.27	2,205,251	40.13	21,615	22.80	1,186,561	48.54	54,895
Montana	588	39.46	328,527	50.43	3,595	33.32	144,145	55.53	40,096
Nebraska	863	36.61	719,883	46.29	7,639	28.32	386,611	53.96	50,610
Nevada	1,052	45.34	841,579	37.40	6,394	25.32	427,293	46.64	66,827
New Hampshire	724	39.39	424,199	35.72	4,847	25.24	218,248	40.22	45,027
New Jersey	7,600	46.06	4,813,553	46.27	40,663	31.87	2,289,016	51.80	56,292
New Mexico	1,003	41.81	-	-	-	-	-	-	-
New York	16,048	49.53	9,611,405	48.36	82,163	29.53	4,143,310	50.25	50,428
North Carolina	3,723	41.95	2,918,542	43.84	30,544	28.47	1,549,016	51.93	50,714
North Dakota	238	30.71	415,021	66.11	5,031	55.04	225,584	74.26	44,839
Ohio	7,810	42.07	5,433,429	46.67	53,317	26.71	2,975,290	53.40	55,804
Oklahoma	2,003	37.54	1,305,771	39.87	12,936	21.90	655,929	46.42	50,706
Oregon	2,202	39.04	1,408,725	47.61	15,625	32.46	679,028	52.35	43,458
Pennsylvania	9,211	42.37	5,992,889	47.44	59,016	32.01	3,151,170	55.65	53,395
Rhode Island	877	46.21	445,344	42.01	4,682	25.77	210,382	44.99	44,934
South Carolina	2,154	46.37	1,433,616	45.76	15,422	30.82	764,833	54.84	49,594
South Dakota	335	34.61	293,017	51.97	3,047	33.46	155,717	59.75	51,105
Tennessee	3,747	45.55	2,793,826	41.40	27,128	27.05	1,461,149	50.89	53,861
Texas	14,026	46.84	8,773,546	38.28	78,430	22.65	4,175,694	45.29	53,241
Utah	1,232	40.34	663,827	35.95	7,263	23.50	345,423	45.76	47,559
Vermont	386	41.51	183,410	45.24	2,025	26.84	76,100	46.14	37,580
Virginia	4,649	47.67	3,087,077	46.21	32,953	32.25	1,671,374	55.21	50,720
Washington	3,360	36.43	2,274,703	42.12	25,631	29.30	1,129,676	47.42	44,075
West Virginia	1,308	48.59	808,496	45.21	8,060	27.91	368,392	52.32	45,706
Wisconsin	2,458	34.05	2,297,426	48.50	25,970	30.56	1,259,130	53.73	48,484
Wyoming	289	40.53	-	-	-	-	-	-	-

Source: U.S. Department of Commerce. Bureau of the Census. *1992 Economic Census Report Series*, CD-ROM 1i, Washington, DC, October 1996. *Notes:* - means no data reported. 1. HS stands for total health service establishments, revenues, employment, or payroll.

★ 376 ★

Establishment Data

Offices of Osteopathic Physicians by Major Metro Areas: 1992

Area	Establishments		Revenues		Employment		Payroll		
	Number	% of HS[1] in area	Total ($000)	% of HS[1] in area	Number	% of HS[1] in area	Total ($000)	% of HS[1] in area	Payroll per employee
United States	8,391	1.90	3,493,717	1.17	44,883	1.01	1,583,840	1.23	35,288
Atlanta, GA MSA	78	1.28	27,772	0.58	364	0.61	12,450	0.62	34,203
Boston – Worcester – Lawrence, MA – NH – ME – CT CMSA	35	0.36	11,030	0.16	149	0.13	4,633	0.14	31,094
Chicago – Gary – Kenosha, IL – IN – WI CMSA	140	0.96	56,114	0.58	690	0.51	27,134	0.62	39,325
Cincinnati – Hamilton, OH – KY – IN CMSA	31	0.99	-	-	-	-	-	-	-
Cleveland – Akron, OH CMSA	180	3.35	73,517	2.26	883	1.72	37,134	2.42	42,054
Dallas – Fort Worth, TX CMSA	373	4.48	-	-	-	-	-	-	-
Denver – Boulder – Greeley, CO CMSA	101	2.31	-	-	-	-	-	-	-
Detroit – Ann Arbor – Flint, MI CMSA	712	7.56	405,930	7.45	5,259	6.26	214,953	8.43	40,873
Houston – Galveston – Brazoria, TX CMSA	62	0.88	-	-	-	-	-	-	-
Indianapolis, IN MSA	31	1.22	-	-	-	-	-	-	-
Kansas City, MO – KS MSA	102	3.57	44,268	2.03	634	1.88	21,912	2.21	34,562
Los Angeles – Riverside – Orange County, CA CMSA	166	0.54	-	-	-	-	-	-	-
Miami – Fort Lauderdale, FL CMSA	194	2.12	86,069	1.26	975	1.12	37,931	1.35	38,904
Milwaukee – Racine, WI CMSA	59	1.95	23,346	1.14	334	0.98	11,344	1.09	33,964
Minneapolis – St. Paul, MN – WI MSA	6	0.16	-	-	-	-	-	-	-
New York – Northern New Jersey – Long Island, NY – NJ – CT – CMSA	289	0.71	124,710	0.48	1,410	0.42	51,664	0.47	36,641
Orlando, FL MSA	68	2.68	30,206	1.59	343	1.36	14,533	1.78	42,370
Philadelphia – Wilmington – Atlantic City, PA – NJ – DE – MD CMSA	819	7.06	-	-	-	-	-	-	-
Phoenix – Mesa, AZ MSA	217	4.51	-	-	-	-	-	-	-
Pittsburgh, PA MSA	53	1.11	-	-	-	-	-	-	-
Portland – Salem, OR – WA CMSA	73	2.06	23,487	1.18	326	1.05	8,858	1.00	27,172
Sacramento – Yolo, CA CMSA	12	0.42	5,084	0.26	60	0.24	1,497	0.18	24,950
St. Louis, MO – IL MSA	98	2.20	43,908	1.53	553	1.27	21,563	1.74	38,993
San Diego, CA MSA	36	0.73	16,497	0.51	230	0.55	9,971	0.74	43,352
San Francisco – Oakland – San Jose, CA CMSA	44	0.31	-	-	-	-	-	-	-
Seattle – Tacoma – Bremerton, WA CMSA	91	1.50	-	-	-	-	-	-	-
Tampa – St. Petersburg – Clearwater, FL MSA	214	4.33	88,364	2.03	1,002	1.64	41,152	2.38	41,070
Washington – Baltimore, DC – MD – VA – WV CMSA	26	0.20	9,494	0.12	101	0.09	3,807	0.11	37,693
West Palm Beach – Boca Raton, FL MSA	78	2.90	-	-	-	-	-	-	-

Source: U.S. Department of Commerce. Bureau of the Census. *1992 Economic Census Report Series,* CD-ROM 1i, Washington, DC, October 1996. *Notes:* - means no data reported. 1. HS stands for total health service establishments, revenues, employment, or payroll.

★ 377 ★

Establishment Data

Offices of Osteopathic Physicians by State: 1992

Area	Establishments		Revenues		Employment		Payroll		
	Number	% of HS[1] in area	Total ($000)	% of HS[1] in area	Number	% of HS[1] in area	Total ($000)	% of HS[1] in area	Payroll per employee
United States	8,391	1.90	3,493,717	1.17	44,883	1.01	1,583,840	1.23	35,288
Alabama	31	0.56	-	-	-	-	-	-	-
Alaska	11	1.28	5,757	1.06	31	0.55	1,959	0.90	63,194
Arizona	311	4.38	139,657	3.06	1,593	2.71	65,312	3.35	40,999
Arkansas	25	0.70	-	-	-	-	-	-	-
California	304	0.49	119,368	0.28	1,294	0.24	51,390	0.30	39,714
Colorado	200	2.85	66,918	1.79	953	1.72	28,119	1.71	29,506
Connecticut	13	0.20	-	-	-	-	-	-	-
Delaware	47	3.92	-	-	-	-	-	-	-
District of Columbia	1	0.07	-	-	-	-	-	-	-
Florida	737	2.49	315,100	1.35	3,712	1.18	143,409	1.49	38,634
Georgia	124	1.12	42,184	0.49	549	0.45	18,258	0.50	33,257
Hawaii	10	0.45	-	-	-	-	-	-	-
Idaho	10	0.58	-	-	-	-	-	-	-
Illinois	164	0.88	56,223	0.45	715	0.38	25,711	0.46	35,959
Indiana	135	1.55	52,427	0.86	753	0.71	23,625	0.86	31,375
Iowa	180	4.30	72,013	3.08	968	2.15	31,859	2.86	32,912
Kansas	86	2.22	36,598	1.20	595	1.11	17,055	1.29	28,664
Kentucky	37	0.67	-	-	-	-	-	-	-
Louisiana	6	0.09	1,804	0.03	17	0.02	390	0.02	22,941
Maine	118	5.47	-	-	-	-	-	-	-
Maryland	16	0.17	4,765	0.08	56	0.07	1,147	0.05	20,482
Massachusetts	40	0.38	10,746	0.14	149	0.12	4,069	0.11	27,309
Michigan	1,158	7.36	565,600	6.50	7,573	5.37	287,732	6.99	37,994
Minnesota	16	0.27	-	-	-	-	-	-	-
Mississippi	20	0.65	8,865	0.43	154	0.42	3,634	0.41	23,597
Missouri	425	5.05	153,822	2.80	2,077	2.19	68,624	2.81	33,040
Montana	12	0.81	3,003	0.46	54	0.50	1,005	0.39	18,611
Nebraska	2	0.08	-	-	-	-	-	-	-
Nevada	39	1.68	-	-	-	-	-	-	-
New Hampshire	9	0.49	2,867	0.24	34	0.18	1,340	0.25	39,412
New Jersey	391	2.37	204,967	1.97	2,546	2.00	101,548	2.30	39,885
New Mexico	57	2.38	18,596	1.26	277	1.17	7,202	1.16	26,000
New York	196	0.60	73,847	0.37	903	0.32	29,308	0.36	32,456
North Carolina	16	0.18	-	-	-	-	-	-	-
North Dakota	2	0.26	-	-	-	-	-	-	-
Ohio	790	4.26	364,229	3.13	4,885	2.45	186,091	3.34	38,094
Oklahoma	311	5.83	120,520	3.68	1,469	2.49	46,125	3.26	31,399
Oregon	104	1.84	-	-	-	-	-	-	-
Pennsylvania	1,039	4.78	439,324	3.48	5,753	3.12	197,606	3.49	34,348
Rhode Island	54	2.85	-	-	-	-	-	-	-
South Carolina	21	0.45	6,489	0.21	70	0.14	2,221	0.16	31,729
South Dakota	9	0.93	3,914	0.69	92	1.01	1,244	0.48	13,522
Tennessee	49	0.60	22,004	0.33	279	0.28	8,710	0.30	31,219
Texas	682	2.28	277,375	1.21	3,248	0.94	110,596	1.20	34,050

[Continued]

★ 377 ★

Offices of Osteopathic Physicians by State: 1992
[Continued]

Area	Establishments		Revenues		Employment		Payroll		
	Number	% of HS[1] in area	Total ($000)	% of HS[1] in area	Number	% of HS[1] in area	Total ($000)	% of HS[1] in area	Payroll per employee
Utah	9	0.29	-	-	-	-	-	-	-
Vermont	6	0.65	1,074	0.26	19	0.25	412	0.25	21,684
Virginia	38	0.39	-	-	-	-	-	-	-
Washington	144	1.56	45,243	0.84	640	0.73	16,374	0.69	25,584
West Virginia	85	3.16	35,230	1.97	488	1.69	10,974	1.56	22,488
Wisconsin	91	1.26	34,962	0.74	530	0.62	16,449	0.70	31,036
Wyoming	10	1.40	2,617	0.81	41	0.73	1,212	0.90	29,561

Source: U.S. Department of Commerce. Bureau of the Census. *1992 Economic Census Report Series,* CD-ROM 1i, Washington, DC, October 1996. *Notes:* - means no data reported. 1. HS stands for total health service establishments, revenues, employment, or payroll.

★ 378 ★

Establishment Data

Osteopathic Clinics by Major Metro Areas: 1992

Area	Establishments		Revenues		Employment		Payroll		
	Number	% of HS[1] in area	Total ($000)	% of HS[1] in area	Number	% of HS[1] in area	Total ($000)	% of HS[1] in area	Payroll per employee
United States	317	0.07	144,427	0.05	2,146	0.05	66,441	0.05	30,960
Atlanta, GA MSA	0	0.00	0	0.00	0	0.00	0	0.00	0
Boston – Worcester – Lawrence, MA – NH – ME – CT CMSA	0	0.00	0	0.00	0	0.00	0	0.00	0
Chicago – Gary – Kenosha, IL – IN – WI CMSA	7	0.05	-	-	-	-	-	-	-
Cincinnati – Hamilton, OH – KY – IN CMSA	0	0.00	0	0.00	0	0.00	0	0.00	0
Cleveland – Akron, OH CMSA	5	0.09	942	0.03	18	0.04	575	0.04	31,944
Dallas – Fort Worth, TX CMSA	7	0.08	-	-	-	-	-	-	-
Denver – Boulder – Greeley, CO CMSA	5	0.11	-	-	-	-	-	-	-
Detroit – Ann Arbor – Flint, MI CMSA	24	0.25	21,046	0.39	295	0.35	10,738	0.42	36,400
Houston – Galveston – Brazoria, TX CMSA	7	0.10	-	-	-	-	-	-	-
Indianapolis, IN MSA	1	0.04	-	-	-	-	-	-	-
Kansas City, MO – KS MSA	7	0.25	2,121	0.10	27	0.08	1,273	0.13	47,148
Los Angeles – Riverside – Orange County, CA CMSA	9	0.03	-	-	-	-	-	-	-
Miami – Fort Lauderdale, FL CMSA	13	0.14	3,817	0.06	45	0.05	1,508	0.05	33,511
Milwaukee – Racine, WI CMSA	2	0.07	-	-	-	-	-	-	-
Minneapolis – St. Paul, MN – WI MSA	0	0.00	0	0.00	0	0.00	0	0.00	0
New York – Northern New Jersey – Long Island, NY – NJ – CT- CMSA	6	0.01	3,267	0.01	47	0.01	1,346	0.01	28,638
Orlando, FL MSA	3	0.12	2,983	0.16	40	0.16	985	0.12	24,625
Philadelphia – Wilmington – Atlantic City, PA – NJ – DE – MD CMSA	14	0.12	8,113	0.11	103	0.10	4,220	0.13	40,971
Phoenix – Mesa, AZ MSA	3	0.06	-	-	-	-	-	-	-

[Continued]

★ 378 ★

Osteopathic Clinics by Major Metro Areas: 1992

[Continued]

Area	Establishments		Revenues		Employment		Payroll		
	Number	% of HS[1] in area	Total ($000)	% of HS[1] in area	Number	% of HS[1] in area	Total ($000)	% of HS[1] in area	Payroll per employee
Pittsburgh, PA MSA	2	0.04	-	-	-	-	-	-	-
Portland – Salem, OR – WA CMSA	3	0.08	1,116	0.06	11	0.04	536	0.06	48,727
Sacramento – Yolo, CA CMSA	0	0.00	0	0.00	0	0.00	0	0.00	0
St. Louis, MO – IL MSA	6	0.13	1,391	0.05	23	0.05	651	0.05	28,304
San Diego, CA MSA	0	0.00	0	0.00	0	0.00	0	0.00	0
San Francisco – Oakland – San Jose, CA CMSA	5	0.04	-	-	-	-	-	-	-
Seattle – Tacoma – Bremerton, WA CMSA	4	0.07	-	-	-	-	-	-	-
Tampa – St. Petersburg – Clearwater, FL MSA	5	0.10	1,452	0.03	30	0.05	541	0.03	18,033
Washington – Baltimore, DC – MD – VA – WV CMSA	2	0.02	-	-	-	-	-	-	-
West Palm Beach – Boca Raton, FL MSA	1	0.04	-	-	-	-	-	-	-

Source: U.S. Department of Commerce. Bureau of the Census. *1992 Economic Census Report Series,* CD-ROM 1i, Washington, DC, October 1996. *Notes:* - means no data reported. 1. HS stands for total health service establishments, revenues, employment, or payroll.

★ 379 ★

Establishment Data

Osteopathic Clinics by State: 1992

Area	Establishments		Revenues		Employment		Payroll		
	Number	% of HS[1] in area	Total ($000)	% of HS[1] in area	Number	% of HS[1] in area	Total ($000)	% of HS[1] in area	Payroll per employee
United States	317	0.07	144,427	0.05	2,146	0.05	66,441	0.05	30,960
Alabama	1	0.02	-	-	-	-	-	-	-
Alaska	0	0.00	0	0.00	0	0.00	0	0.00	0
Arizona	6	0.08	1,725	0.04	25	0.04	901	0.05	36,040
Arkansas	1	0.03	-	-	-	-	-	-	-
California	18	0.03	9,423	0.02	129	0.02	3,778	0.02	29,287
Colorado	7	0.10	1,288	0.03	29	0.05	434	0.03	14,966
Connecticut	1	0.02	-	-	-	-	-	-	-
Delaware	3	0.25	-	-	-	-	-	-	-
District of Columbia	1	0.07	-	-	-	-	-	-	-
Florida	25	0.08	10,422	0.04	140	0.04	4,235	0.04	30,250
Georgia	0	0.00	0	0.00	0	0.00	0	0.00	0
Hawaii	1	0.04	-	-	-	-	-	-	-
Idaho	3	0.17	-	-	-	-	-	-	-
Illinois	9	0.05	6,558	0.05	63	0.03	3,718	0.07	59,016
Indiana	7	0.08	2,167	0.04	43	0.04	990	0.04	23,023
Iowa	13	0.31	5,472	0.23	69	0.15	2,428	0.22	35,188
Kansas	11	0.28	3,230	0.11	50	0.09	1,499	0.11	29,980
Kentucky	1	0.02	-	-	-	-	-	-	-

[Continued]

★ 379 ★

Osteopathic Clinics by State: 1992
[Continued]

Area	Establishments		Revenues		Employment		Payroll		
	Number	% of HS[1] in area	Total ($000)	% of HS[1] in area	Number	% of HS[1] in area	Total ($000)	% of HS[1] in area	Payroll per employee
Louisiana	0	0.00	0	0.00	0	0.00	0	0.00	0
Maine	2	0.09	-	-	-	-	-	-	-
Maryland	0	0.00	0	0.00	0	0.00	0	0.00	0
Massachusetts	0	0.00	0	0.00	0	0.00	0	0.00	0
Michigan	43	0.27	27,739	0.32	431	0.31	13,598	0.33	31,550
Minnesota	0	0.00	0	0.00	0	0.00	0	0.00	0
Mississippi	0	0.00	0	0.00	0	0.00	0	0.00	0
Missouri	21	0.25	6,490	0.12	113	0.12	3,097	0.13	27,407
Montana	0	0.00	0	0.00	0	0.00	0	0.00	0
Nebraska	0	0.00	0	0.00	0	0.00	0	0.00	0
Nevada	2	0.09	-	-	-	-	-	-	-
New Hampshire	0	0.00	0	0.00	0	0.00	0	0.00	0
New Jersey	8	0.05	8,232	0.08	107	0.08	4,611	0.10	43,093
New Mexico	0	0.00	0	0.00	0	0.00	0	0.00	0
New York	5	0.02	1,108	0.01	9	0.00	253	0.00	28,111
North Carolina	3	0.03	-	-	-	-	-	-	-
North Dakota	0	0.00	0	0.00	0	0.00	0	0.00	0
Ohio	31	0.17	21,774	0.19	288	0.14	10,400	0.19	36,111
Oklahoma	17	0.32	6,740	0.21	114	0.19	3,163	0.22	27,746
Oregon	8	0.14	-	-	-	-	-	-	-
Pennsylvania	23	0.11	8,002	0.06	129	0.07	3,182	0.06	24,667
Rhode Island	1	0.05	-	-	-	-	-	-	-
South Carolina	0	0.00	0	0.00	0	0.00	0	0.00	0
South Dakota	0	0.00	0	0.00	0	0.00	0	0.00	0
Tennessee	3	0.04	584	0.01	17	0.02	252	0.01	14,824
Texas	25	0.08	9,305	0.04	139	0.04	3,264	0.04	23,482
Utah	1	0.03	-	-	-	-	-	-	-
Vermont	0	0.00	0	0.00	0	0.00	0	0.00	0
Virginia	1	0.01	-	-	-	-	-	-	-
Washington	5	0.05	1,079	0.02	15	0.02	232	0.01	15,467
West Virginia	5	0.19	2,436	0.14	54	0.19	984	0.14	18,222
Wisconsin	5	0.07	1,094	0.02	25	0.03	734	0.03	29,360
Wyoming	0	0.00	0	0.00	0	0.00	0	0.00	0

Source: U.S. Department of Commerce. Bureau of the Census. *1992 Economic Census Report Series,* CD-ROM 1i, Washington, DC, October 1996.
Notes: - means no data reported. 1. HS stands for total health service establishments, revenues, employment, or payroll.

★ 380 ★

Establishment Data

Other Health Services by Major Metro Areas, Non-Taxed Establishments: 1992

Area	Establish-ments	Revenues in $1,000	Employ-ment	Payroll in $1,000	Payroll per employee
United States	8,707	12,836,201	342,635	6,411,250	18,712
Albany – Schenectady – Troy, NY MSA	35	-	-	-	-
Albuquerque, NM MSA	16	23,335	755	11,243	14,891
Allentown – Bethlehem – Easton, PA MSA	30	-	-	-	-
Atlanta, GA MSA	40	78,638	1,361	35,870	26,356
Austin – San Marcos, TX MSA	20	22,018	1,501	10,366	6,906
Baton Rouge, LA MSA	8	-	-	-	-
Birmingham, AL MSA	16	37,407	598	14,461	24,182
Boston – Worcester – Lawrence, MA – NH – ME – CT CMSA	285	617,458	14,263	304,045	21,317
Buffalo – Niagara Falls, NY MSA	38	-	-	-	-
Charlotte – Gastonia – Rock Hill, NC – SC MSA	22	-	-	-	-
Chicago – Gary – Kenosha, IL – IN – WI CMSA	233	-	-	-	-
Cincinnati – Hamilton, OH – KY – IN CMSA	76	-	-	-	-
Cleveland – Akron, OH CMSA	94	162,195	3,100	72,108	23,261
Columbus, OH MSA	55	54,893	1,459	25,179	17,258
Dallas – Fort Worth, TX CMSA	60	181,972	5,530	84,605	15,299
Dayton – Springfield, OH MSA	27	-	-	-	-
Denver – Boulder – Greeley, CO CMSA	115	119,421	3,077	55,491	18,034
Des Moines, IA MSA	15	-	-	-	-
Detroit – Ann Arbor – Flint, MI CMSA	183	-	-	-	-
Fresno, CA MSA	17	18,265	369	8,005	21,694
Grand Rapids – Muskegon – Holland, MI MSA	33	59,412	1,501	34,264	22,827
Greensboro – Winston-Salem – High Point, NC MSA	16	-	-	-	-
Greenville – Spartanburg – Anderson, SC MSA	17	23,437	526	10,174	19,342
Harrisburg – Lebanon – Carlisle, PA MSA	31	29,322	630	12,692	20,146
Hartford, CT MSA	50	96,663	2,699	55,760	20,660
Honolulu, HI MSA	26	-	-	-	-
Houston – Galveston – Brazoria, TX CMSA	68	-	-	-	-
Indianapolis, IN MSA	65	82,027	1,850	37,594	20,321
Jacksonville, FL MSA	38	54,475	1,503	28,609	19,035
Kalamazoo – Battle Creek, MI MSA	22	29,230	659	14,395	21,844
Kansas City, MO – KS MSA	46	78,233	1,843	38,446	20,861
Knoxville, TN MSA	22	42,451	723	17,514	24,224
Lansing – East Lansing, MI MSA	14	-	-	-	-

[Continued]

★ 380 ★

Other Health Services by Major Metro Areas, Non-Taxed Establishments: 1992

[Continued]

Area	Establish- ments	Revenues in $1,000	Employ- ment	Payroll in $1,000	Payroll per employee
Lexington, KY MSA	39	33,938	746	13,674	18,330
Little Rock – North Little Rock, AR MSA	14	25,611	585	11,176	19,104
Los Angeles – Riverside – Orange County, CA CMSA	251	-	-	-	-
Louisville, KY – IN MSA	39	76,572	1,820	36,502	20,056
Madison, WI MSA	13	-	-	-	-
Memphis, TN – AR – MS MSA	38	91,021	2,041	44,436	21,772
Miami – Fort Lauderdale, FL CMSA	71	170,653	2,760	59,878	21,695
Milwaukee – Racine, WI CMSA	63	-	-	-	-
Minneapolis – St. Paul, MN – WI MSA	82	190,890	4,082	78,847	19,316
Nashville, TN MSA	33	49,732	1,089	21,165	19,435
New Orleans, LA MSA	19	-	-	-	-
New York – Northern New Jersey – Long Island, NY – NJ – CT- CMSA	670	-	-	-	-
Norfolk – Virginia Beach – Newport News, VA – NC MSA	14	-	-	-	-
Oklahoma City, OK MSA	46	48,435	1,033	21,130	20,455
Omaha, NE – IA MSA	17	-	-	-	-
Orlando, FL MSA	46	71,833	1,633	30,835	18,882
Philadelphia – Wilmington – Atlantic City, PA – NJ – DE – MD CMSA	209	439,844	9,855	208,491	21,156
Phoenix – Mesa, AZ MSA	81	88,269	1,985	44,875	22,607
Pittsburgh, PA MSA	91	174,727	3,760	78,873	20,977
Portland – Salem, OR – WA CMSA	44	-	-	-	-
Providence – Fall River – Warwick, RI – MA MSA	58	121,556	3,022	64,960	21,496
Raleigh – Durham – Chapel Hill, NC MSA	29	44,110	1,165	20,926	17,962
Richmond – Petersburg, VA MSA	27	37,403	1,027	17,533	17,072
Rochester, NY MSA	33	102,822	2,632	52,037	19,771
Sacramento – Yolo, CA CMSA	30	-	-	-	-
St. Louis, MO – IL MSA	85	139,378	3,311	63,649	19,223
Salt Lake City – Ogden, UT MSA	9	-	-	-	-
San Antonio, TX MSA	31	35,707	1,441	16,368	11,359
San Diego, CA MSA	68	100,507	2,176	41,929	19,269
San Francisco – Oakland – San Jose, CA CMSA	194	-	-	-	-
Santa Barbara – Santa Maria – Lompoc, CA MSA	15	-	-	-	-
Scranton – Wilkes-Barre – Hazleton, PA MSA	53	62,062	1,668	33,667	20,184
Seattle – Tacoma – Bremerton, WA CMSA	117	-	-	-	-
Springfield, MA MSA	37	44,882	1,460	25,551	17,501

[Continued]

★ 380 ★

Other Health Services by Major Metro Areas, Non-Taxed Establishments: 1992

[Continued]

Area	Establish-ments	Revenues in $1,000	Employ-ment	Payroll in $1,000	Payroll per employee
Syracuse, NY MSA	19	-	-	-	-
Tampa–St. Petersburg–Clearwater, FL MSA	62	101,465	2,227	47,938	21,526
Toledo, OH MSA	24	-	-	-	-
Tucson, AZ MSA	47	45,810	982	18,263	18,598
Tulsa, OK MSA	20	22,238	580	10,237	17,650
Washington–Baltimore, DC–MD–VA–WV CMSA	155	-	-	-	-
West Palm Beach–Boca Raton, FL MSA	26	35,628	914	17,355	18,988
Wichita, KS MSA	21	-	-	-	-
Youngstown–Warren, OH MSA	31	-	-	-	-

Source: U.S. Department of Commerce. Bureau of the Census. *1992 Economic Census Report Series,* CD-ROM 1i, Washington, DC, October 1996. *Notes:* - means no data reported. 1. HS stands for total health service establishments, revenues, employment, or payroll.

★ 381 ★

Establishment Data

Other Health Services by State, Non-Taxed Establishments: 1992

Area	Establish-ments	Revenues in $1,000	Employ-ment	Payroll in $1,000	Payroll per employee
United States	8,707	12,836,201	342,635	6,411,250	18,712
Alabama	122	151,071	4,284	75,896	17,716
Alaska	29	31,456	653	15,812	24,214
Arizona	155	150,243	3,267	69,042	21,133
Arkansas	91	79,926	2,436	36,362	14,927
California	656	953,978	18,896	437,681	23,163
Colorado	197	150,060	4,160	71,221	17,120
Connecticut	165	257,174	7,118	142,991	20,089
Delaware	22	55,178	1,436	27,665	19,265
District of Columbia	38	90,029	1,647	38,294	23,251
Florida	462	692,340	15,008	301,428	20,084
Georgia	125	173,342	3,550	75,977	21,402
Hawaii	41	39,946	910	21,388	23,503
Idaho	16	12,203	301	5,293	17,585
Illinois	386	470,416	12,572	234,629	18,663
Indiana	295	263,170	6,460	129,964	20,118
Iowa	151	103,607	3,064	52,018	16,977
Kansas	82	77,837	1,881	38,737	20,594
Kentucky	280	209,711	5,236	100,010	19,100

[Continued]

★ 381 ★

Other Health Services by State, Non-Taxed Establishments: 1992

[Continued]

Area	Establish-ments	Revenues in $1,000	Employ-ment	Payroll in $1,000	Payroll per employee
Louisiana	51	52,456	933	18,419	19,742
Maine	94	79,250	2,421	43,391	17,923
Maryland	101	119,093	2,422	54,880	22,659
Massachusetts	315	658,707	15,678	331,756	21,161
Michigan	334	529,022	11,483	251,467	21,899
Minnesota	188	253,045	5,937	112,637	18,972
Mississippi	65	100,534	2,087	44,741	21,438
Missouri	147	226,088	5,633	104,828	18,610
Montana	88	46,366	2,682	25,701	9,583
Nebraska	40	38,576	784	17,500	22,321
Nevada	21	27,420	466	9,064	19,451
New Hampshire	110	117,406	3,272	59,057	18,049
New Jersey	227	403,735	10,537	203,769	19,338
New Mexico	76	56,725	2,045	27,931	13,658
New York	645	2,439,727	71,721	1,426,664	19,892
North Carolina	147	219,441	5,978	110,239	18,441
North Dakota	12	9,757	191	3,020	15,812
Ohio	467	505,360	12,497	239,795	19,188
Oklahoma	100	90,771	2,063	39,398	19,097
Oregon	82	94,562	2,519	42,030	16,685
Pennsylvania	560	765,864	18,870	372,530	19,742
Rhode Island	54	-	-	-	-
South Carolina	49	57,060	1,328	26,314	19,815
South Dakota	42	31,389	1,077	13,403	12,445
Tennessee	230	289,928	6,453	135,720	21,032
Texas	422	631,492	32,543	308,717	9,486
Utah	15	20,968	584	10,905	18,673
Vermont	76	80,822	2,595	45,501	17,534
Virginia	109	122,422	3,107	58,188	18,728
Washington	205	360,589	9,578	182,910	19,097
West Virginia	83	116,743	2,981	51,230	17,186
Wisconsin	205	201,337	6,178	97,579	15,795
Wyoming	34	-	-	-	-

Source: U.S. Department of Commerce. Bureau of the Census. *1992 Economic Census Report Series,* CD-ROM 1i, Washington, DC, October 1996. *Notes:* - means no data reported. 1. HS stands for total health service establishments, revenues, employment, or payroll.

★ 382 ★

Establishment Data

Physical Fitness Facilities by Major Metro Areas: 1992

	Establish ments	Revenues ($ 000)	Employ- ment	Payroll ($ 000)	Payroll per employee
United States	9,216	3,823,566	129,925	1,043,229	8,029
Albany – Schenectady – Troy, NY MSA	29	10,445	359	3,367	9,379
Albuquerque, NM MSA	21	5,984	290	1,481	5,107
Allentown – Bethlehem – Easton, PA MSA	19	8,367	373	2,527	6,775
Anchorage, AK MSA	11	8,700	388	1,933	4,982
Appleton – Oshkosh – Neenah, WI MSA	14	2,141	143	552	3,860
Atlanta, GA MSA	129	62,081	2,185	17,518	8,017
Augusta – Aiken, GA – SC MSA	13	4,714	201	1,393	6,930
Austin – San Marcos, TX MSA	29	18,707	546	6,078	11,132
Bakersfield, CA MSA	12	3,936	138	966	7,000
Baton Rouge, LA MSA	22	7,743	341	2,502	7,337
Beaumont – Port Arthur, TX MSA	11	2,242	84	325	3,869
Birmingham, AL MSA	32	8,583	356	2,568	7,213
Boise City, ID MSA	16	6,625	201	1,543	7,677
Boston – Worcester – Lawrence, MA – NH – ME – CT CMSA	284	119,372	4,102	33,908	8,266
Buffalo – Niagara Falls, NY MSA	32	13,011	493	3,649	7,402
Canton – Massillon, OH MSA	12	4,718	145	1,285	8,862
Charleston – North Charleston, SC MSA	17	11,017	305	2,784	9,128
Charlotte – Gastonia – Rock Hill, NC – SC MSA	37	10,555	416	2,577	6,195
Chattanooga, TN – GA MSA	13	2,053	74	590	7,973
Chicago – Gary – Kenosha, IL – IN – WI CMSA	262	179,309	5,289	48,259	9,124
Cincinnati – Hamilton, OH – KY – IN CMSA	58	-	-	-	-
Cleveland – Akron, OH CMSA	83	35,208	1,366	7,921	5,799
Colorado Springs, CO MSA	17	9,314	343	2,345	6,837
Columbia, SC MSA	13	3,988	226	1,237	5,473
Columbus, OH MSA	45	21,187	833	5,280	6,339
Corpus Christi, TX MSA	9	942	43	211	4,907
Dallas – Fort Worth, TX CMSA	144	85,772	2,491	20,999	8,430
Davenport – Moline – Rock Island, IA – IL MSA	14	2,419	151	786	5,205
Dayton – Springfield, OH MSA	38	12,459	413	3,107	7,523
Daytona Beach, FL MSA	17	2,848	102	1,101	10,794
Denver – Boulder – Greeley, CO CMSA	119	73,023	3,049	19,414	6,367
Des Moines, IA MSA	9	5,443	221	2,687	12,158
Detroit – Ann Arbor – Flint, MI CMSA	160	71,095	1,607	14,611	9,092
El Paso, TX MSA	11	1,852	98	557	5,684
Eugene – Springfield, OR MSA	15	7,088	304	2,468	8,118
Fort Myers – Cape Coral, FL MSA	13	2,613	153	1,093	7,144
Fort Pierce – Port St. Lucie, FL MSA	8	2,154	55	444	8,073
Fort Wayne, IN MSA	17	2,904	121	965	7,975

[Continued]

★ 382 ★

Physical Fitness Facilities by Major Metro Areas: 1992

[Continued]

	Establish ments	Revenues ($ 000)	Employ- ment	Payroll ($ 000)	Payroll per employee
Fresno, CA MSA	24	9,789	312	2,422	7,763
Grand Rapids – Muskegon – Holland, MI MSA	41	15,352	650	4,419	6,798
Greensboro – Winston-Salem – High Point, NC MSA	39	8,270	435	2,475	5,690
Greenville – Spartanburg – Anderson, SC MSA	31	8,624	336	3,310	9,851
Harrisburg – Lebanon – Carlisle, PA MSA	31	6,761	367	2,105	5,736
Hartford, CT MSA	50	-	-	-	-
Honolulu, HI MSA	23	13,059	278	3,577	12,867
Houston – Galveston – Brazoria, TX CMSA	134	92,875	2,244	20,822	9,279
Huntsville, AL MSA	14	1,921	128	835	6,523
Indianapolis, IN MSA	61	23,457	912	6,631	7,271
Jackson, MS MSA	8	3,394	90	817	9,078
Jacksonville, FL MSA	36	13,016	553	4,420	7,993
Johnson City – Kingsport – Bristol, TN – VA MSA	12	2,520	163	949	5,822
Kalamazoo – Battle Creek, MI MSA	26	5,016	328	1,320	4,024
Kansas City, MO – KS MSA	54	24,679	946	6,737	7,122
Knoxville, TN MSA	22	8,620	340	2,270	6,676
Lafayette, LA MSA	8	6,633	204	1,929	9,456
Lakeland – Winter Haven, FL MSA	9	728	18	142	7,889
Lancaster, PA MSA	12	2,415	101	650	6,436
Lansing – East Lansing, MI MSA	11	8,174	234	2,091	8,936
Las Vegas, NV – AZ MSA	41	22,804	449	6,157	13,713
Lexington, KY MSA	19	5,688	319	1,307	4,097
Little Rock – North Little Rock, AR MSA	23	7,966	428	2,406	5,621
Los Angeles – Riverside – Orange County, CA CMSA	502	421,736	10,586	97,760	9,235
Louisville, KY – IN MSA	37	6,900	452	2,522	5,580
Macon, GA MSA	6	1,874	63	489	7,762
Madison, WI MSA	18	8,909	423	2,779	6,570
Melbourne – Titusville – Palm Bay, FL MSA	22	6,029	194	1,629	8,397
Memphis, TN – AR – MS MSA	29	8,993	301	2,590	8,605
Miami – Fort Lauderdale, FL CMSA	144	69,373	1,617	17,017	10,524
Milwaukee – Racine, WI CMSA	45	27,135	920	6,903	7,503
Minneapolis – St. Paul, MN – WI MSA	86	58,737	2,105	19,562	9,293
Mobile, AL MSA	14	2,468	115	829	7,209
Modesto, CA MSA	16	4,379	165	1,215	7,364
Montgomery, AL MSA	7	1,352	75	358	4,773
Nashville, TN MSA	43	19,019	551	5,582	10,131

[Continued]

★ 382 ★

Physical Fitness Facilities by Major Metro Areas: 1992
[Continued]

	Establish ments	Revenues ($ 000)	Employ- ment	Payroll ($ 000)	Payroll per employee
New Orleans, LA MSA	40	13,337	545	4,641	8,516
New York – Northern New Jersey – Long Island, NY – NJ – CT- CMSA	844	-	-	-	-
Norfolk – Virginia Beach – Newport News, VA – NC MSA	47	29,470	1,065	6,819	6,403
Oklahoma City, OK MSA	51	15,040	864	5,489	6,353
Omaha, NE – IA MSA	25	8,953	392	2,377	6,064
Orlando, FL MSA	61	21,559	494	3,997	8,091
Pensacola, FL MSA	17	3,313	181	1,208	6,674
Peoria – Pekin, IL MSA	14	8,118	268	2,558	9,545
Philadelphia – Wilmington – Atlantic City, PA – NJ – DE – MD CMSA	240	103,859	3,055	28,772	9,418
Phoenix – Mesa, AZ MSA	88	39,385	1,158	10,613	9,165
Pittsburgh, PA MSA	66	25,516	799	5,886	7,367
Portland, ME MSA	13	4,726	106	1,138	10,736
Portland – Salem, OR – WA CMSA	78	-	-	-	-
Providence – Fall River – Warwick, RI – MA MSA	48	13,378	476	3,602	7,567
Raleigh – Durham – Chapel Hill, NC MSA	38	17,440	642	4,434	6,907
Reno, NV MSA	19	8,432	380	3,107	8,176
Richmond – Petersburg, VA MSA	27	11,454	615	3,294	5,356
Rochester, NY MSA	48	15,732	661	4,424	6,693
Rockford, IL MSA	13	2,805	123	628	5,106
Sacramento – Yolo, CA CMSA	80	39,245	1,223	10,858	8,878
Saginaw – Bay City – Midland, MI MSA	9	984	20	199	9,950
St. Louis, MO – IL MSA	97	32,032	1,280	8,639	6,749
Salinas, CA MSA	12	3,610	123	879	7,146
Salt Lake City – Ogden, UT MSA	40	17,623	696	4,889	7,024
San Antonio, TX MSA	44	21,241	720	5,741	7,974
San Diego, CA MSA	110	78,050	2,179	22,921	10,519
San Francisco – Oakland – San Jose, CA CMSA	337	198,078	6,940	61,718	8,893
Santa Barbara – Santa Maria – Lompoc, CA MSA	18	9,529	392	2,743	6,997
Sarasota – Bradenton, FL MSA	15	6,736	320	2,883	9,009
Scranton – Wilkes-Barre – Hazleton, PA MSA	20	4,168	147	1,161	7,898
Seattle – Tacoma – Bremerton, WA CMSA	164	105,027	3,133	29,123	9,296
Shreveport – Bossier City, LA MSA	15	2,825	116	1,002	8,638
Spokane, WA MSA	16	4,961	199	1,214	6,101
Springfield, MO MSA	11	4,092	231	1,433	6,203
Springfield, MA MSA	26	5,853	277	1,919	6,928
Stockton – Lodi, CA MSA	17	6,961	293	1,976	6,744
Syracuse, NY MSA	23	9,481	253	2,323	9,182

[Continued]

★ 382 ★

Physical Fitness Facilities by Major Metro Areas: 1992
[Continued]

	Establish ments	Revenues ($ 000)	Employ- ment	Payroll ($ 000)	Payroll per employee
Tallahassee, FL MSA	9	3,771	201	1,241	6,174
Tampa–St. Petersburg–Clearwater, FL MSA	73	31,768	688	5,776	8,395
Toledo, OH MSA	23	8,225	271	1,887	6,963
Tucson, AZ MSA	21	13,494	727	4,382	6,028
Tulsa, OK MSA	25	9,753	315	2,547	8,086
Washington–Baltimore, DC–MD–VA–WV CMSA	302	-	-	-	-
West Palm Beach–Boca Raton, FL MSA	35	37,627	644	5,698	8,848
Wichita, KS MSA	11	2,172	146	764	5,233
Youngstown–Warren, OH MSA	21	3,716	134	799	5,963

Source: U.S. Department of Commerce. Bureau of the Census. *1992 Economic Census Report Series,* CD-ROM 1i, Washington, DC, October 1996. *Note:* - means no data reported.

★ 383 ★

Establishment Data

Physical Fitness Facilities by State: 1992

	Establish ments	Revenues ($ 000)	Employ- ment	Payroll ($ 000)	Payroll per employee
United States	9,216	3,823,566	129,925	1,043,229	8,029
Alabama	126	22,650	1,102	7,520	6,824
Alaska	25	12,887	546	3,279	6,005
Arizona	130	57,257	2,114	16,273	7,698
Arkansas	75	12,757	686	3,568	5,201
California	1,218	799,672	23,431	209,947	8,960
Colorado	188	99,374	4,305	28,823	6,695
Connecticut	174	65,919	2,251	22,434	9,966
Delaware	26	9,154	265	2,539	9,581
District of Columbia	24	13,327	257	3,544	13,790
Florida	525	213,388	5,837	50,032	8,572
Georgia	226	82,177	3,099	23,242	7,500
Hawaii	37	18,257	456	5,225	11,458
Idaho	49	14,094	643	3,857	5,998
Illinois	378	197,841	6,384	53,458	8,374
Indiana	185	44,121	1,980	13,062	6,597
Iowa	74	16,089	860	6,310	7,337
Kansas	83	20,910	1,105	6,293	5,695
Kentucky	115	19,313	1,103	5,614	5,090
Louisiana	130	37,306	1,556	12,044	7,740
Maine	60	10,197	362	2,606	7,199

[Continued]

★ 383 ★

Physical Fitness Facilities by State: 1992
[Continued]

	Establish ments	Revenues ($ 000)	Employ- ment	Payroll ($ 000)	Payroll per employee
Maryland	199	81,142	2,809	22,012	7,836
Massachusetts	309	123,653	4,202	35,100	8,353
Michigan	307	107,027	3,173	24,641	7,766
Minnesota	136	66,383	2,570	21,941	8,537
Mississippi	46	9,266	299	2,266	7,579
Missouri	178	47,709	2,082	13,148	6,315
Montana	48	9,812	581	2,936	5,053
Nebraska	49	14,716	701	4,119	5,876
Nevada	64	31,315	837	9,311	11,124
New Hampshire	51	12,012	731	3,860	5,280
New Jersey	361	145,022	4,709	41,255	8,761
New Mexico	59	13,198	528	3,190	6,042
New York	663	347,856	9,878	93,231	9,438
North Carolina	214	52,136	2,356	14,165	6,012
North Dakota	26	2,842	241	799	3,315
Ohio	362	114,976	4,384	28,210	6,435
Oklahoma	106	27,688	1,372	8,982	6,547
Oregon	123	51,090	1,745	15,680	8,986
Pennsylvania	402	138,425	4,831	38,606	7,991
Rhode Island	45	12,790	477	3,764	7,891
South Carolina	97	32,159	1,142	9,997	8,754
South Dakota	19	2,612	210	913	4,348
Tennessee	158	44,610	1,595	13,069	8,194
Texas	529	246,948	7,457	62,697	8,408
Utah	63	26,269	1,080	7,347	6,803
Vermont	35	9,151	481	3,224	6,703
Virginia	235	97,829	4,064	26,818	6,599
Washington	250	127,667	4,269	35,915	8,413
West Virginia	48	6,640	301	1,876	6,233
Wisconsin	161	49,674	2,197	13,340	6,072
Wyoming	25	4,259	281	1,147	4,082

Source: U.S. Department of Commerce. Bureau of the Census. *1992 Economic Census Report Series,* CD-ROM 1i, Washington, DC, October 1996. *Note:* - means no data reported.

★ 384 ★

Establishment Data

Psychiatric Hospitals by Major Metro Areas: 1992

Area	Establishments		Revenues		Employment		Payroll		
	Number	% of HS[1] in area	Total ($000)	% of HS[1] in area	Number	% of HS[1] in area	Total ($000)	% of HS[1] in area	Payroll per employee
United States	492	0.11	4,396,163	1.47	69,669	1.56	1,609,727	1.25	23,105
Atlanta, GA MSA	7	0.11	102,307	2.12	1,453	2.43	30,484	1.51	20,980
Boston – Worcester – Lawrence, MA – NH – ME – CT CMSA	12	0.12	124,691	1.76	2,168	1.88	54,436	1.67	25,109
Chicago – Gary – Kenosha, IL – IN – WI CMSA	14	0.10	191,466	1.97	2,814	2.06	73,721	1.68	26,198
Cincinnati – Hamilton, OH – KY – IN CMSA	0	0.00	0	0.00	0	0.00	0	0.00	0
Cleveland – Akron, OH CMSA	2	0.04	-	-	-	-	-	-	-
Dallas – Fort Worth, TX CMSA	25	0.30	160,631	2.46	3,033	3.52	64,816	2.45	21,370
Denver – Boulder – Greeley, CO CMSA	5	0.11	-	-	-	-	-	-	-
Detroit – Ann Arbor – Flint, MI CMSA	5	0.05	-	-	-	-	-	-	-
Houston – Galveston – Brazoria, TX CMSA	18	0.25	180,270	3.07	2,298	3.08	52,933	2.26	23,034
Indianapolis, IN MSA	6	0.24	47,493	2.37	693	2.15	15,598	1.66	22,508
Kansas City, MO – KS MSA	7	0.25	55,026	2.52	861	2.55	19,320	1.95	22,439
Los Angeles – Riverside – Orange County, CA CMSA	38	0.12	314,935	1.34	4,595	1.65	117,703	1.29	25,615
Miami – Fort Lauderdale, FL CMSA	11	0.12	94,840	1.39	1,573	1.81	35,069	1.25	22,294
Milwaukee – Racine, WI CMSA	3	0.10	-	-	-	-	-	-	-
Minneapolis – St. Paul, MN – WI MSA	1	0.03	-	-	-	-	-	-	-
New York – Northern New Jersey – Long Island, NY – NJ – CT- CMSA	10	0.02	217,821	0.83	3,449	1.03	98,542	0.90	28,571
Orlando, FL MSA	4	0.16	30,655	1.61	441	1.75	10,011	1.22	22,701
Philadelphia – Wilmington – Atlantic City, PA – NJ – DE – MD CMSA	9	0.08	-	-	-	-	-	-	-
Phoenix – Mesa, AZ MSA	5	0.10	-	-	-	-	-	-	-
Pittsburgh, PA MSA	2	0.04	-	-	-	-	-	-	-
Portland – Salem, OR – WA CMSA	4	0.11	-	-	-	-	-	-	-
Sacramento – Yolo, CA CMSA	4	0.14	-	-	-	-	-	-	-
St. Louis, MO – IL MSA	1	0.02	-	-	-	-	-	-	-
San Diego, CA MSA	6	0.12	-	-	-	-	-	-	-
San Francisco – Oakland – San Jose, CA CMSA	13	0.09	81,617	0.91	1,353	1.19	33,706	0.89	24,912
Seattle – Tacoma – Bremerton, WA CMSA	1	0.02	-	-	-	-	-	-	-
Tampa – St. Petersburg – Clearwater, FL MSA	9	0.18	91,668	2.10	1,371	2.24	32,684	1.89	23,840
Washington – Baltimore, DC – MD – VA – WV CMSA	7	0.05	-	-	-	-	-	-	-
West Palm Beach – Boca Raton, FL MSA	5	0.19	-	-	-	-	-	-	-

Source: U.S. Department of Commerce. Bureau of the Census. *1992 Economic Census Report Series,* CD-ROM 1i, Washington, DC, October 1996. *Notes:* - means no data reported. 1. HS stands for total health service establishments, revenues, employment, or payroll.

★ 385 ★
Establishment Data

Psychiatric Hospitals by Major Metro Areas, Non-Taxed Establishments: 1992

Area	Establish-ments	Revenues in $1,000	Employ-ment	Payroll in $1,000	Payroll per employee
United States	427	10,932,256	247,738	7,296,493	29,452
Albany – Schenectady – Troy, NY MSA	1	-	-	-	-
Atlanta, GA MSA	6	-	-	-	-
Boston – Worcester – Lawrence, MA – NH – ME – CT CMSA	15	492,401	9,768	312,517	31,994
Buffalo – Niagara Falls, NY MSA	3	-	-	-	-
Chicago – Gary – Kenosha, IL – IN – WI CMSA	8	-	-	-	-
Cincinnati – Hamilton, OH – KY – IN CMSA	4	48,377	1,039	36,339	34,975
Cleveland – Akron, OH CMSA	5	-	-	-	-
Columbus, OH MSA	2	-	-	-	-
Dallas – Fort Worth, TX CMSA	2	-	-	-	-
Denver – Boulder – Greeley, CO CMSA	3	-	-	-	-
Detroit – Ann Arbor – Flint, MI CMSA	13	-	-	-	-
Hartford, CT MSA	7	-	-	-	-
Houston – Galveston – Brazoria, TX CMSA	1	-	-	-	-
Indianapolis, IN MSA	3	-	-	-	-
Kansas City, MO – KS MSA	4	-	-	-	-
Los Angeles – Riverside – Orange County, CA CMSA	9	-	-	-	-
Miami – Fort Lauderdale, FL CMSA	1	-	-	-	-
Milwaukee – Racine, WI CMSA	5	-	-	-	-
Minneapolis – St. Paul, MN – WI MSA	2	-	-	-	-
New York – Northern New Jersey – Long Island, NY – NJ – CT- CMSA	44	1,715,523	36,883	1,246,341	33,792
Philadelphia – Wilmington – Atlantic City, PA – NJ – DE – MD CMSA	14	-	-	-	-
Phoenix – Mesa, AZ MSA	5	-	-	-	-
Pittsburgh, PA MSA	7	-	-	-	-
Portland – Salem, OR – WA CMSA	2	-	-	-	-
Providence – Fall River – Warwick, RI – MA MSA	5	87,705	1,806	51,263	28,385
Sacramento – Yolo, CA CMSA	1	-	-	-	-
St. Louis, MO – IL MSA	4	85,000	1,996	47,289	23,692
San Diego, CA MSA	4	-	-	-	-
San Francisco – Oakland – San Jose, CA CMSA	2	-	-	-	-
Seattle – Tacoma – Bremerton, WA CMSA	3	-	-	-	-
Tampa – St. Petersburg – Clearwater, FL MSA	2	-	-	-	-

[Continued]

★ 385 ★

Psychiatric Hospitals by Major Metro Areas, Non-Taxed Establishments: 1992

[Continued]

Area	Establish-ments	Revenues in $1,000	Employ-ment	Payroll in $1,000	Payroll per employee
Washington – Baltimore, DC – MD – VA – WV CMSA	10	417,657	8,220	247,496	30,109

Source: U.S. Department of Commerce. Bureau of the Census. *1992 Economic Census Report Series,* CD-ROM 1i, Washington, DC, October 1996. *Notes:* - means no data reported. 1. HS stands for total health service establishments, revenues, employment, or payroll.

★ 386 ★

Establishment Data

Psychiatric Hospitals by State: 1992

Area	Establishments		Revenues		Employment		Payroll		
	Number	% of HS[1] in area	Total ($000)	% of HS[1] in area	Number	% of HS[1] in area	Total ($000)	% of HS[1] in area	Payroll per employee
United States	492	0.11	4,396,163	1.47	69,669	1.56	1,609,727	1.25	23,105
Alabama	5	0.09	48,509	0.98	626	0.81	15,198	0.72	24,278
Alaska	2	0.23	-	-	-	-	-	-	-
Arizona	12	0.17	-	-	-	-	-	-	-
Arkansas	7	0.20	50,262	2.06	761	1.78	17,724	1.67	23,290
California	68	0.11	519,437	1.21	7,932	1.48	197,008	1.14	24,837
Colorado	7	0.10	57,505	1.54	803	1.45	18,528	1.13	23,073
Connecticut	2	0.03	-	-	-	-	-	-	-
Delaware	2	0.17	-	-	-	-	-	-	-
District of Columbia	1	0.07	-	-	-	-	-	-	-
Florida	47	0.16	372,066	1.60	5,778	1.83	131,425	1.36	22,746
Georgia	16	0.14	191,366	2.22	2,536	2.10	55,584	1.51	21,918
Hawaii	1	0.04	-	-	-	-	-	-	-
Idaho	6	0.35	-	-	-	-	-	-	-
Illinois	14	0.07	193,915	1.57	2,850	1.52	73,768	1.32	25,884
Indiana	17	0.20	153,981	2.53	1,998	1.87	45,625	1.66	22,835
Iowa	0	0.00	0	0.00	0	0.00	0	0.00	0
Kansas	7	0.18	-	-	-	-	-	-	-
Kentucky	7	0.13	-	-	-	-	-	-	-
Louisiana	26	0.38	167,996	3.04	3,106	3.60	55,875	2.57	17,989
Maine	1	0.05	-	-	-	-	-	-	-
Maryland	5	0.05	-	-	-	-	-	-	-
Massachusetts	9	0.08	82,885	1.09	1,444	1.13	39,831	1.12	27,584
Michigan	7	0.04	49,969	0.57	869	0.62	17,270	0.42	19,873
Minnesota	1	0.02	-	-	-	-	-	-	-
Mississippi	6	0.19	-	-	-	-	-	-	-
Missouri	9	0.11	65,166	1.19	1,202	1.27	25,421	1.04	21,149
Montana	3	0.20	-	-	-	-	-	-	-

[Continued]

★ 386 ★

Psychiatric Hospitals by State: 1992
[Continued]

Area	Establishments		Revenues		Employment		Payroll		
	Number	% of HS[1] in area	Total ($000)	% of HS[1] in area	Number	% of HS[1] in area	Total ($000)	% of HS[1] in area	Payroll per employee
Nebraska	2	0.08	-	-	-	-	-	-	-
Nevada	4	0.17	-	-	-	-	-	-	-
New Hampshire	4	0.22	48,500	4.08	845	4.40	19,501	3.59	23,078
New Jersey	2	0.01	-	-	-	-	-	-	-
New Mexico	8	0.33	70,074	4.74	1,055	4.46	22,031	3.56	20,882
New York	12	0.04	-	-	-	-	-	-	-
North Carolina	12	0.14	-	-	-	-	-	-	-
North Dakota	0	0.00	0	0.00	0	0.00	0	0.00	0
Ohio	8	0.04	51,460	0.44	902	0.45	19,671	0.35	21,808
Oklahoma	10	0.19	-	-	-	-	-	-	-
Oregon	4	0.07	-	-	-	-	-	-	-
Pennsylvania	11	0.05	-	-	-	-	-	-	-
Rhode Island	0	0.00	0	0.00	0	0.00	0	0.00	0
South Carolina	6	0.13	-	-	-	-	-	-	-
South Dakota	1	0.10	-	-	-	-	-	-	-
Tennessee	10	0.12	-	-	-	-	-	-	-
Texas	78	0.26	595,839	2.60	9,469	2.73	207,929	2.26	21,959
Utah	6	0.20	42,435	2.30	721	2.33	16,405	2.17	22,753
Vermont	0	0.00	0	0.00	0	0.00	0	0.00	0
Virginia	14	0.14	154,562	2.31	2,691	2.63	52,750	1.74	19,602
Washington	2	0.02	-	-	-	-	-	-	-
West Virginia	2	0.07	-	-	-	-	-	-	-
Wisconsin	6	0.08	-	-	-	-	-	-	-
Wyoming	2	0.28	-	-	-	-	-	-	-

Source: U.S. Department of Commerce. Bureau of the Census. *1992 Economic Census Report Series*, CD-ROM 1i, Washington, DC, October 1996. *Notes:* - means no data reported. 1. HS stands for total health service establishments, revenues, employment, or payroll.

★ 387 ★

Establishment Data

Psychiatric Hospitals by State, Non-Taxed Establishments: 1992

Area	Establish-ments	Revenues in $1,000	Employ-ment	Payroll in $1,000	Payroll per employee
United States	427	10,932,256	247,738	7,296,493	29,452
Alabama	5	151,379	3,934	102,433	26,038
Alaska	1	-	-	-	-
Arizona	6	-	-	-	-
Arkansas	2	-	-	-	-
California	19	615,132	12,559	422,725	33,659

[Continued]

★ 387 ★

Psychiatric Hospitals by State, Non-Taxed Establishments: 1992
[Continued]

Area	Establish-ments	Revenues in $1,000	Employ-ment	Payroll in $1,000	Payroll per employee
Colorado	6	136,615	3,185	95,261	29,909
Connecticut	19	325,085	5,545	204,901	36,952
Delaware	1	-	-	-	-
District of Columbia	1	-	-	-	-
Florida	16	286,940	7,666	197,048	25,704
Georgia	17	388,126	9,843	239,407	24,323
Hawaii	2	-	-	-	-
Idaho	2	-	-	-	-
Illinois	14	364,382	9,357	274,817	29,370
Indiana	17	245,440	6,310	183,919	29,147
Iowa	6	-	-	-	-
Kansas	7	146,987	3,711	100,002	26,947
Kentucky	6	92,248	2,301	48,266	20,976
Louisiana	8	111,986	2,854	64,359	22,550
Maine	3	-	-	-	-
Maryland	9	239,701	5,423	147,460	27,192
Massachusetts	20	579,527	11,415	368,606	32,291
Michigan	20	546,323	9,909	347,721	35,091
Minnesota	7	196,637	4,024	142,598	35,437
Mississippi	2	-	-	-	-
Missouri	11	201,534	6,138	119,517	19,472
Montana	2	-	-	-	-
Nebraska	5	-	-	-	-
Nevada	1	-	-	-	-
New Hampshire	1	-	-	-	-
New Jersey	14	522,997	11,705	368,481	31,481
New Mexico	3	-	-	-	-
New York	34	1,574,063	34,831	1,169,167	33,567
North Carolina	8	301,584	6,789	189,881	27,969
North Dakota	1	-	-	-	-
Ohio	21	390,655	8,713	298,280	34,234
Oklahoma	7	101,377	2,391	62,644	26,200
Oregon	3	-	-	-	-
Pennsylvania	29	936,739	17,754	576,886	32,493
Rhode Island	3	-	-	-	-
South Carolina	4	91,069	2,110	50,925	24,135
South Dakota	0	0	0	0	0
Tennessee	9	120,690	3,605	84,047	23,314
Texas	19	421,873	14,269	291,931	20,459
Utah	2	-	-	-	-
Vermont	2	-	-	-	-
Virginia	10	195,443	5,674	131,775	23,224
Washington	5	-	-	-	-
West Virginia	3	-	-	-	-

[Continued]

★ 387 ★

Psychiatric Hospitals by State, Non-Taxed Establishments: 1992

[Continued]

Area	Establish-ments	Revenues in $1,000	Employ-ment	Payroll in $1,000	Payroll per employee
Wisconsin	12	292,229	6,228	163,712	26,286
Wyoming	2	-	-	-	-

Source: U.S. Department of Commerce. Bureau of the Census. *1992 Economic Census Report Series*, CD-ROM 1i, Washington, DC, October 1996. *Notes:* - means no data reported. 1. HS stands for total health service establishments, revenues, employment, or payroll.

★ 388 ★

Establishment Data

Psychiatric Hospitals, Government by Major Metro Areas, Non-Taxed Establishments: 1992

Area	Establish-ments	Revenues in $1,000	Employ-ment	Payroll in $1,000	Payroll per employee
United States	282	9,109,683	210,779	6,341,826	30,088
Albany – Schenectady – Troy, NY MSA	1	-	-	-	-
Atlanta, GA MSA	2	-	-	-	-
Boston – Worcester – Lawrence, MA – NH – ME – CT CMSA	11	-	-	-	-
Buffalo – Niagara Falls, NY MSA	3	-	-	-	-
Chicago – Gary – Kenosha, IL – IN – WI CMSA	6	-	-	-	-
Cincinnati – Hamilton, OH – KY – IN CMSA	2	-	-	-	-
Cleveland – Akron, OH CMSA	4	-	-	-	-
Columbus, OH MSA	1	-	-	-	-
Dallas – Fort Worth, TX CMSA	1	-	-	-	-
Denver – Boulder – Greeley, CO CMSA	1	-	-	-	-
Detroit – Ann Arbor – Flint, MI CMSA	7	-	-	-	-
Hartford, CT MSA	4	-	-	-	-
Houston – Galveston – Brazoria, TX CMSA	1	-	-	-	-
Indianapolis, IN MSA	2	-	-	-	-
Kansas City, MO – KS MSA	2	-	-	-	-
Los Angeles – Riverside – Orange County, CA CMSA	4	-	-	-	-
Miami – Fort Lauderdale, FL CMSA	1	-	-	-	-
Milwaukee – Racine, WI CMSA	1	-	-	-	-
Minneapolis – St. Paul, MN – WI MSA	1	-	-	-	-
New York – Northern New Jersey – Long Island, NY – NJ – CT- CMSA	31	-	-	-	-

[Continued]

★ 388 ★

Psychiatric Hospitals, Government by Major Metro Areas, Non-Taxed Establishments: 1992
[Continued]

Area	Establish-ments	Revenues in $1,000	Employ-ment	Payroll in $1,000	Payroll per employee
Philadelphia – Wilmington – Atlantic City, PA – NJ – DE – MD CMSA	7	-	-	-	-
Phoenix – Mesa, AZ MSA	1	-	-	-	-
Pittsburgh, PA MSA	4	173,530	3,424	108,622	31,724
Portland – Salem, OR – WA CMSA	2	-	-	-	-
Providence – Fall River – Warwick, RI – MA MSA	2	-	-	-	-
Sacramento – Yolo, CA CMSA	0	0	0	0	0
St. Louis, MO – IL MSA	3	-	-	-	-
San Diego, CA MSA	2	-	-	-	-
San Francisco – Oakland – San Jose, CA CMSA	1	-	-	-	-
Seattle – Tacoma – Bremerton, WA CMSA	1	-	-	-	-
Tampa – St. Petersburg – Clearwater, FL MSA	1	-	-	-	-
Washington – Baltimore, DC – MD – VA – WV CMSA	6	-	-	-	-

Source: U.S. Department of Commerce. Bureau of the Census. *1992 Economic Census Report Series,* CD-ROM 1i, Washington, DC, October 1996. *Notes:* - means no data reported. 1. HS stands for total health service establishments, revenues, employment, or payroll.

★ 389 ★

Establishment Data

Psychiatric Hospitals, Government by State, Non-Taxed Establishments: 1992

Area	Establish-ments	Revenues in $1,000	Employ-ment	Payroll in $1,000	Payroll per employee
United States	282	9,109,683	210,779	6,341,826	30,088
Alabama	5	151,379	3,934	102,433	26,038
Alaska	1	-	-	-	-
Arizona	1	-	-	-	-
Arkansas	1	-	-	-	-
California	8	502,446	10,443	365,069	34,958
Colorado	4	-	-	-	-
Connecticut	10	241,326	3,905	159,166	40,760
Delaware	1	-	-	-	-
District of Columbia	1	-	-	-	-
Florida	6	227,879	6,159	164,858	26,767
Georgia	9	322,369	8,341	207,983	24,935
Hawaii	2	-	-	-	-

[Continued]

★ 389 ★

Psychiatric Hospitals, Government by State, Non-Taxed Establishments: 1992

[Continued]

Area	Establish-ments	Revenues in $1,000	Employ-ment	Payroll in $1,000	Payroll per employee
Idaho	2	-	-	-	-
Illinois	13	-	-	-	-
Indiana	8	179,679	4,717	149,072	31,603
Iowa	6	-	-	-	-
Kansas	3	-	-	-	-
Kentucky	3	61,397	1,579	34,786	22,030
Louisiana	6	-	-	-	-
Maine	2	-	-	-	-
Maryland	6	-	-	-	-
Massachusetts	14	-	-	-	-
Michigan	12	395,231	7,075	279,605	39,520
Minnesota	6	-	-	-	-
Mississippi	2	-	-	-	-
Missouri	8	-	-	-	-
Montana	1	-	-	-	-
Nebraska	3	-	-	-	-
Nevada	1	-	-	-	-
New Hampshire	1	-	-	-	-
New Jersey	10	459,809	10,255	330,518	32,230
New Mexico	3	-	-	-	-
New York	30	1,411,844	31,957	1,078,340	33,743
North Carolina	6	-	-	-	-
North Dakota	1	-	-	-	-
Ohio	16	325,168	7,182	263,448	36,682
Oklahoma	5	-	-	-	-
Oregon	3	-	-	-	-
Pennsylvania	16	609,804	12,187	408,171	33,492
Rhode Island	1	-	-	-	-
South Carolina	3	-	-	-	-
South Dakota	0	0	0	0	0
Tennessee	6	-	-	-	-
Texas	13	376,525	12,909	269,373	20,867
Utah	1	-	-	-	-
Vermont	1	-	-	-	-
Virginia	8	-	-	-	-
Washington	2	-	-	-	-
West Virginia	2	-	-	-	-
Wisconsin	7	257,085	5,460	146,128	26,763
Wyoming	2	-	-	-	-

Source: U.S. Department of Commerce. Bureau of the Census. *1992 Economic Census Report Series*, CD-ROM 1i, Washington, DC, October 1996. *Notes:* - means no data reported. 1. HS stands for total health service establishments, revenues, employment, or payroll.

★ 390 ★

Establishment Data

Psychiatric Hospitals, Nongovernment by Major Metro Areas, Non-Taxed Establishments: 1992

Area	Establish-ments	Revenues in $1,000	Employ-ment	Payroll in $1,000	Payroll per employee
United States	145	1,822,573	36,959	954,667	25,830
Albany – Schenectady – Troy, NY MSA	0	0	0	0	0
Atlanta, GA MSA	4	45,229	996	21,479	21,565
Boston – Worcester – Lawrence, MA – NH – ME – CT CMSA	4	-	-	-	-
Buffalo – Niagara Falls, NY MSA	0	0	0	0	0
Chicago – Gary – Kenosha, IL – IN – WI CMSA	2	-	-	-	-
Cincinnati – Hamilton, OH – KY – IN CMSA	2	-	-	-	-
Cleveland – Akron, OH CMSA	1	-	-	-	-
Columbus, OH MSA	1	-	-	-	-
Dallas – Fort Worth, TX CMSA	1	-	-	-	-
Denver – Boulder – Greeley, CO CMSA	2	-	-	-	-
Detroit – Ann Arbor – Flint, MI CMSA	6	-	-	-	-
Hartford, CT MSA	3	-	-	-	-
Houston – Galveston – Brazoria, TX CMSA	0	0	0	0	0
Indianapolis, IN MSA	1	-	-	-	-
Kansas City, MO – KS MSA	2	-	-	-	-
Los Angeles – Riverside – Orange County, CA CMSA	5	-	-	-	-
Miami – Fort Lauderdale, FL CMSA	0	0	0	0	0
Milwaukee – Racine, WI CMSA	4	-	-	-	-
Minneapolis – St. Paul, MN – WI MSA	1	-	-	-	-
New York – Northern New Jersey – Long Island, NY – NJ – CT- CMSA	13	-	-	-	-
Philadelphia – Wilmington – Atlantic City, PA – NJ – DE – MD CMSA	7	124,149	2,271	66,365	29,223
Phoenix – Mesa, AZ MSA	4	-	-	-	-
Pittsburgh, PA MSA	3	-	-	-	-
Portland – Salem, OR – WA CMSA	0	0	0	0	0
Providence – Fall River – Warwick, RI – MA MSA	3	-	-	-	-
Sacramento – Yolo, CA CMSA	1	-	-	-	-
St. Louis, MO – IL MSA	1	-	-	-	-
San Diego, CA MSA	2	-	-	-	-
San Francisco – Oakland – San Jose, CA CMSA	1	-	-	-	-
Seattle – Tacoma – Bremerton, WA CMSA	2	-	-	-	-
Tampa – St. Petersburg – Clearwater, FL MSA	1	-	-	-	-

[Continued]

★ 390 ★

Psychiatric Hospitals, Nongovernment by Major Metro Areas, Non-Taxed Establishments: 1992

[Continued]

Area	Establish-ments	Revenues in $1,000	Employ-ment	Payroll in $1,000	Payroll per employee
Washington – Baltimore, DC – MD – VA – WV CMSA	4	-	-	-	-

Source: U.S. Department of Commerce. Bureau of the Census. *1992 Economic Census Report Series,* CD-ROM 1i, Washington, DC, October 1996. *Notes:* - means no data reported. 1. HS stands for total health service establishments, revenues, employment, or payroll.

★ 391 ★

Establishment Data

Psychiatric Hospitals, Nongovernment by State, Non-Taxed Establishments: 1992

Area	Establish-ments	Revenues in $1,000	Employ-ment	Payroll in $1,000	Payroll per employee
United States	145	1,822,573	36,959	954,667	25,830
Alabama	0	0	0	0	0
Alaska	0	0	0	0	0
Arizona	5	-	-	-	-
Arkansas	1	-	-	-	-
California	11	112,686	2,116	57,656	27,248
Colorado	2	-	-	-	-
Connecticut	9	83,759	1,640	45,735	27,887
Delaware	0	0	0	0	0
District of Columbia	0	0	0	0	0
Florida	10	59,061	1,507	32,190	21,360
Georgia	8	65,757	1,502	31,424	20,921
Hawaii	0	0	0	0	0
Idaho	0	0	0	0	0
Illinois	1	-	-	-	-
Indiana	9	65,761	1,593	34,847	21,875
Iowa	0	0	0	0	0
Kansas	4	-	-	-	-
Kentucky	3	30,851	722	13,480	18,670
Louisiana	2	-	-	-	-
Maine	1	-	-	-	-
Maryland	3	-	-	-	-
Massachusetts	6	-	-	-	-
Michigan	8	151,092	2,834	68,116	24,035
Minnesota	1	-	-	-	-
Mississippi	0	0	0	0	0
Missouri	3	-	-	-	-

[Continued]

★ 391 ★

Psychiatric Hospitals, Nongovernment by State, Non-Taxed Establishments: 1992
[Continued]

Area	Establish-ments	Revenues in $1,000	Employ-ment	Payroll in $1,000	Payroll per employee
Montana	1	-	-	-	-
Nebraska	2	-	-	-	-
Nevada	0	0	0	0	0
New Hampshire	0	0	0	0	0
New Jersey	4	63,188	1,450	37,963	26,181
New Mexico	0	0	0	0	0
New York	4	162,219	2,874	90,827	31,603
North Carolina	2	-	-	-	-
North Dakota	0	0	0	0	0
Ohio	5	65,487	1,531	34,832	22,751
Oklahoma	2	-	-	-	-
Oregon	0	0	0	0	0
Pennsylvania	13	326,935	5,567	168,715	30,306
Rhode Island	2	-	-	-	-
South Carolina	1	-	-	-	-
South Dakota	0	0	0	0	0
Tennessee	3	-	-	-	-
Texas	6	45,348	1,360	22,558	16,587
Utah	1	-	-	-	-
Vermont	1	-	-	-	-
Virginia	2	-	-	-	-
Washington	3	-	-	-	-
West Virginia	1	-	-	-	-
Wisconsin	5	35,144	768	17,584	22,896
Wyoming	0	0	0	0	0

Source: U.S. Department of Commerce. Bureau of the Census. *1992 Economic Census Report Series*, CD-ROM 1i, Washington, DC, October 1996. *Notes:* - means no data reported. 1. HS stands for total health service establishments, revenues, employment, or payroll.

★ 392 ★

Establishment Data

Skilled Nursing Care Facilities by Major Metro Areas: 1992

Area	Establishments		Revenues		Employment		Payroll		
	Number	% of HS[1] in area	Total ($000)	% of HS[1] in area	Number	% of HS[1] in area	Total ($000)	% of HS[1] in area	Payroll per employee
United States	10,242	2.32	28,797,807	9.63	937,907	21.06	13,520,962	10.47	14,416
Albany – Schenectady – Troy, NY MSA	14	1.07	72,563	8.98	2,242	16.98	37,000	10.18	16,503
Albuquerque, NM MSA	14	1.31	50,325	6.03	1,694	13.39	20,819	5.52	12,290
Allentown – Bethlehem – Easton, PA MSA	18	1.45	67,847	9.86	1,819	19.45	29,204	9.55	16,055
Anchorage, AK MSA	0	0.00	0	0.00	0	0.00	0	0.00	0
Appleton – Oshkosh – Neenah, WI MSA	13	2.50	-	-	-	-	-	-	-

[Continued]

Skilled Nursing Care Facilities by Major Metro Areas: 1992

[Continued]

Area	Establishments		Revenues		Employment		Payroll		
	Number	% of HS[1] in area	Total ($000)	% of HS[1] in area	Number	% of HS[1] in area	Total ($000)	% of HS[1] in area	Payroll per employee
Atlanta, GA MSA	99	1.62	264,075	5.48	9,343	15.61	124,277	6.16	13,302
Augusta – Aiken, GA – SC MSA	21	2.95	43,543	6.77	1,585	17.13	20,433	7.25	12,891
Austin – San Marcos, TX MSA	41	2.61	82,620	6.90	3,204	17.25	37,973	7.82	11,852
Bakersfield, CA MSA	15	1.98	-	-	-	-	-	-	-
Baton Rouge, LA MSA	19	2.15	51,758	6.98	2,147	19.47	21,988	7.25	10,241
Beaumont – Port Arthur, TX MSA	19	2.63	32,761	5.69	1,342	13.13	14,483	6.01	10,792
Birmingham, AL MSA	33	2.40	-	-	-	-	-	-	-
Boise City, ID MSA	13	2.17	38,310	10.16	1,375	23.54	16,117	9.49	11,721
Boston – Worcester – Lawrence, MA – NH – ME – CT CMSA	313	3.20	1,209,070	17.10	33,261	28.89	633,876	19.47	19,058
Buffalo – Niagara Falls, NY MSA	28	1.40	-	-	-	-	-	-	-
Canton – Massillon, OH MSA	25	3.61	59,650	14.45	1,969	27.61	26,034	12.35	13,222
Charleston – North Charleston, SC MSA	14	1.72	-	-	-	-	-	-	-
Charlotte – Gastonia – Rock Hill, NC – SC MSA	42	2.62	126,552	9.05	4,342	21.33	60,730	9.23	13,987
Chattanooga, TN – GA MSA	12	1.58	-	-	-	-	-	-	-
Chicago – Gary – Kenosha, IL – IN – WI CMSA	237	1.63	-	-	-	-	-	-	-
Cincinnati – Hamilton, OH – KY – IN CMSA	114	3.64	282,122	13.91	9,247	26.58	137,693	13.55	14,891
Cleveland – Akron, OH CMSA	127	2.36	470,262	14.45	15,107	29.44	218,469	14.22	14,461
Colorado Springs, CO MSA	9	1.01	28,007	6.31	873	13.21	11,719	5.82	13,424
Columbia, SC MSA	12	1.61	-	-	-	-	-	-	-
Columbus, OH MSA	55	2.26	218,465	12.41	6,918	24.58	98,829	12.17	14,286
Corpus Christi, TX MSA	17	2.26	-	-	-	-	-	-	-
Dallas – Fort Worth, TX CMSA	181	2.18	397,365	6.09	14,139	16.42	181,377	6.85	12,828
Davenport – Moline – Rock Island, IA – IL MSA	9	1.33	23,900	6.62	938	15.64	10,376	6.56	11,062
Dayton – Springfield, OH MSA	45	2.73	128,629	11.24	4,025	22.71	54,083	9.59	13,437
Daytona Beach, FL MSA	26	3.51	-	-	-	-	-	-	-
Denver – Boulder – Greeley, CO CMSA	68	1.56	-	-	-	-	-	-	-
Des Moines, IA MSA	10	1.36	21,141	4.16	811	11.40	10,485	3.95	12,928
Detroit – Ann Arbor – Flint, MI CMSA	154	1.63	-	-	-	-	-	-	-
El Paso, TX MSA	9	1.13	-	-	-	-	-	-	-
Eugene – Springfield, OR MSA	12	2.05	25,886	7.71	876	16.19	12,772	8.21	14,580
Fort Myers – Cape Coral, FL MSA	10	1.40	-	-	-	-	-	-	-
Fort Pierce – Port St. Lucie, FL MSA	9	1.73	-	-	-	-	-	-	-
Fort Wayne, IN MSA	34	4.85	54,652	9.88	1,919	20.34	23,425	9.15	12,207
Fresno, CA MSA	35	2.36	-	-	-	-	-	-	-
Grand Rapids – Muskegon – Holland, MI MSA	27	1.77	58,781	6.55	2,215	15.43	27,480	6.35	12,406
Greensboro – Winston-Salem – High Point, NC MSA	38	2.52	106,667	8.99	3,841	22.47	53,938	10.22	14,043
Greenville – Spartanburg – Anderson, SC MSA	36	3.06	-	-	-	-	-	-	-
Harrisburg – Lebanon – Carlisle, PA MSA	13	1.32	56,388	8.64	1,671	17.55	27,760	9.00	16,613
Hartford, CT MSA	78	3.44	374,313	21.27	10,009	36.65	199,048	23.43	19,887
Honolulu, HI MSA	9	0.54	-	-	-	-	-	-	-
Houston – Galveston – Brazoria, TX CMSA	98	1.39	223,932	3.81	8,240	11.03	97,364	4.15	11,816
Huntsville, AL MSA	8	1.50	-	-	-	-	-	-	-
Indianapolis, IN MSA	108	4.25	302,304	15.08	9,704	30.17	136,675	14.52	14,084
Jackson, MS MSA	16	2.51	-	-	-	-	-	-	-
Jacksonville, FL MSA	31	1.75	108,638	8.31	3,148	18.39	45,157	8.12	14,345

[Continued]

★ 392 ★

Skilled Nursing Care Facilities by Major Metro Areas: 1992
[Continued]

Area	Establishments		Revenues		Employment		Payroll		
	Number	% of HS[1] in area	Total ($000)	% of HS[1] in area	Number	% of HS[1] in area	Total ($000)	% of HS[1] in area	Payroll per employee
Johnson City – Kingsport – Bristol, TN – VA MSA	12	1.74	34,969	5.72	1,267	12.87	14,469	5.32	11,420
Kalamazoo – Battle Creek, MI MSA	16	2.17	-	-	-	-	-	-	-
Kansas City, MO – KS MSA	106	3.71	197,637	9.04	7,848	23.24	91,354	9.23	11,640
Knoxville, TN MSA	19	1.59	-	-	-	-	-	-	-
Lafayette, LA MSA	17	2.66	36,202	8.05	1,588	22.52	16,126	8.78	10,155
Lakeland – Winter Haven, FL MSA	16	3.29	-	-	-	-	-	-	-
Lancaster, PA MSA	14	2.32	44,426	11.68	1,375	21.73	20,314	10.63	14,774
Lansing – East Lansing, MI MSA	7	0.96	14,614	3.65	560	8.90	6,742	3.54	12,039
Las Vegas, NV – AZ MSA	18	1.16	60,677	3.59	1,705	9.24	30,216	4.44	17,722
Lexington, KY MSA	17	2.10	-	-	-	-	-	-	-
Little Rock – North Little Rock, AR MSA	34	3.27	68,445	8.80	2,813	25.14	32,196	8.76	11,445
Los Angeles – Riverside – Orange County, CA CMSA	557	1.82	1,534,186	6.53	44,440	16.00	686,340	7.51	15,444
Louisville, KY – IN MSA	41	2.38	128,664	7.66	4,581	17.73	56,998	7.98	12,442
Macon, GA MSA	18	3.31	33,620	5.95	1,457	19.32	14,999	6.62	10,294
Madison, WI MSA	15	2.90	38,025	7.34	1,402	19.47	19,030	8.12	13,573
Melbourne – Titusville – Palm Bay, FL MSA	14	1.72	44,256	8.15	1,307	17.98	19,169	7.66	14,666
Memphis, TN – AR – MS MSA	22	1.34	59,670	4.80	2,189	13.40	26,714	4.97	12,204
Miami – Fort Lauderdale, FL CMSA	129	1.41	342,491	5.01	8,956	10.30	144,815	5.16	16,170
Milwaukee – Racine, WI CMSA	51	1.68	-	-	-	-	-	-	-
Minneapolis – St. Paul, MN – WI MSA	108	2.90	389,502	13.44	13,195	26.43	205,052	13.67	15,540
Mobile, AL MSA	19	2.96	48,287	8.60	1,813	18.97	22,269	8.48	12,283
Modesto, CA MSA	21	3.11	-	-	-	-	-	-	-
Montgomery, AL MSA	12	2.44	-	-	-	-	-	-	-
Nashville, TN MSA	29	1.49	79,280	4.28	2,515	9.94	35,189	4.53	13,992
New Orleans, LA MSA	31	1.28	90,249	4.12	3,175	10.72	36,052	4.29	11,355
New York – Northern New Jersey – Long Island, NY – NJ – CT- CMSA	457	1.13	2,868,210	10.98	62,457	18.72	1,366,156	12.51	21,874
Norfolk – Virginia Beach – Newport News, VA – NC MSA	20	0.89	55,921	4.12	1,993	9.11	25,635	3.96	12,863
Oklahoma City, OK MSA	37	1.88	68,710	5.29	3,010	15.37	30,092	5.37	9,997
Omaha, NE – IA MSA	23	2.28	49,742	6.06	1,835	14.75	25,122	6.73	13,690
Orlando, FL MSA	33	1.30	110,073	5.79	3,028	12.00	47,268	5.78	15,610
Pensacola, FL MSA	10	1.90	-	-	-	-	-	-	-
Peoria – Pekin, IL MSA	13	2.56	36,430	10.05	1,207	20.64	15,092	8.02	12,504
Philadelphia – Wilmington – Atlantic City, PA – NJ – DE – MD CMSA	153	1.32	-	-	-	-	-	-	-
Phoenix – Mesa, AZ MSA	52	1.08	189,904	6.04	5,769	14.97	86,155	6.27	14,934
Pittsburgh, PA MSA	78	1.64	198,893	7.32	5,942	15.58	84,302	6.75	14,187
Portland, ME MSA	5	0.92	10,597	2.77	327	5.56	5,631	3.14	17,220
Portland – Salem, OR – WA CMSA	79	2.23	-	-	-	-	-	-	-
Providence – Fall River – Warwick, RI – MA MSA	74	3.57	238,738	20.24	7,360	37.10	123,667	23.36	16,803
Raleigh – Durham – Chapel Hill, NC MSA	30	2.09	85,992	7.08	3,006	17.47	46,486	9.20	15,464
Reno, NV MSA	8	1.20	38,290	7.35	875	14.70	15,492	7.11	17,705
Richmond – Petersburg, VA MSA	19	1.19	60,765	3.88	2,193	9.87	29,128	4.40	13,282
Rochester, NY MSA	28	1.83	97,486	11.78	3,050	21.88	45,076	12.86	14,779
Rockford, IL MSA	10	2.10	32,196	8.89	1,207	22.22	14,343	8.72	11,883
Sacramento – Yolo, CA CMSA	54	1.87	128,610	6.67	4,252	17.06	64,330	7.79	15,129
Saginaw – Bay City – Midland, MI MSA	10	1.47	27,824	7.27	1,110	17.28	13,886	7.03	12,510
St. Louis, MO – IL MSA	128	2.88	322,508	11.27	11,525	26.43	146,496	11.79	12,711
Salinas, CA MSA	10	1.64	-	-	-	-	-	-	-
Salt Lake City – Ogden, UT MSA	32	1.55	88,877	6.44	3,147	14.25	41,069	7.15	13,050

[Continued]

413

★ 392 ★

Skilled Nursing Care Facilities by Major Metro Areas: 1992

[Continued]

Area	Establishments		Revenues		Employment		Payroll		
	Number	% of HS[1] in area	Total ($000)	% of HS[1] in area	Number	% of HS[1] in area	Total ($000)	% of HS[1] in area	Payroll per employee
San Antonio, TX MSA	46	1.75	109,295	6.07	3,956	13.76	46,300	6.20	11,704
San Diego, CA MSA	72	1.46	212,228	6.50	6,643	15.95	99,800	7.41	15,023
San Francisco – Oakland – San Jose, CA CMSA	251	1.79	641,686	7.12	18,769	16.52	323,229	8.56	17,221
Santa Barbara – Santa Maria – Lompoc, CA MSA	7	0.84	-	-	-	-	-	-	-
Sarasota – Bradenton, FL MSA	29	2.36	-	-	-	-	-	-	-
Scranton – Wilkes-Barre – Hazleton, PA MSA	29	2.53	85,700	13.58	2,593	24.41	36,742	14.02	14,170
Seattle – Tacoma – Bremerton, WA CMSA	120	1.98	-	-	-	-	-	-	-
Shreveport – Bossier City, LA MSA	24	3.74	56,056	9.81	2,170	25.53	22,436	9.69	10,339
Spokane, WA MSA	18	2.45	50,937	9.98	1,690	21.56	23,227	9.94	13,744
Springfield, MO MSA	24	5.22	34,698	9.02	1,540	22.42	15,987	8.07	10,381
Springfield, MA MSA	41	4.53	159,406	23.85	4,838	40.05	83,604	26.05	17,281
Stockton – Lodi, CA MSA	28	3.35	-	-	-	-	-	-	-
Syracuse, NY MSA	12	1.10	-	-	-	-	-	-	-
Tallahassee, FL MSA	7	1.76	18,903	5.47	560	11.88	8,699	5.71	15,534
Tampa – St. Petersburg – Clearwater, FL MSA	115	2.33	387,036	8.88	11,147	18.22	168,138	9.74	15,084
Toledo, OH MSA	27	2.40	85,557	10.99	2,667	21.24	36,746	9.26	13,778
Tucson, AZ MSA	15	1.19	-	-	-	-	-	-	-
Tulsa, OK MSA	25	1.83	-	-	-	-	-	-	-
Washington – Baltimore, DC – MD – VA – WV CMSA	151	1.17	-	-	-	-	-	-	-
West Palm Beach – Boca Raton, FL MSA	41	1.53	135,294	6.84	3,340	13.59	58,450	6.93	17,500
Wichita, KS MSA	18	2.35	33,022	3.41	1,383	10.23	16,192	3.90	11,708
Youngstown – Warren, OH MSA	44	3.66	130,549	18.79	4,551	37.03	61,450	19.15	13,503

Source: U.S. Department of Commerce. Bureau of the Census. *1992 Economic Census Report Series,* CD-ROM 1i, Washington, DC, October 1996. *Notes:* - means no data reported. 1. HS stands for total health service establishments, revenues, employment, or payroll.

★ 393 ★

Establishment Data

Skilled Nursing Care Facilities by Major Metro Areas, Non-Taxed Establishments: 1992

Area	Establish-ments	Revenues in $1,000	Employ-ment	Payroll in $1,000	Payroll per employee
United States	2,723	11,683,096	367,161	5,821,838	15,856
Albany – Schenectady – Troy, NY MSA	17	94,112	3,038	48,712	16,034
Atlanta, GA MSA	10	36,699	1,277	18,883	14,787
Boston – Worcester – Lawrence, MA – NH – ME – CT CMSA	65	-	-	-	-
Buffalo – Niagara Falls, NY MSA	23	121,689	4,153	63,893	15,385
Chicago – Gary – Kenosha, IL – IN – WI CMSA	70	300,530	8,882	142,940	16,093
Cincinnati – Hamilton, OH – KY – IN CMSA	33	-	-	-	-

[Continued]

★ 393 ★

Skilled Nursing Care Facilities by Major Metro Areas, Non-Taxed Establishments: 1992

[Continued]

Area	Establish- ments	Revenues in $1,000	Employ- ment	Payroll in $1,000	Payroll per employee
Cleveland – Akron, OH CMSA	24	138,402	4,625	74,164	16,035
Columbus, OH MSA	19	82,734	2,650	38,933	14,692
Dallas – Fort Worth, TX CMSA	16	-	-	-	-
Denver – Boulder – Greeley, CO CMSA	13	-	-	-	-
Detroit – Ann Arbor – Flint, MI CMSA	50	226,374	7,094	105,952	14,935
Hartford, CT MSA	16	-	-	-	-
Houston – Galveston – Brazoria, TX CMSA	3	15,917	385	7,107	18,460
Indianapolis, IN MSA	11	52,079	1,572	26,066	16,581
Kansas City, MO – KS MSA	14	60,813	2,274	32,403	14,249
Los Angeles – Riverside – Orange County, CA CMSA	56	-	-	-	-
Miami – Fort Lauderdale, FL CMSA	12	111,580	2,600	47,686	18,341
Milwaukee – Racine, WI CMSA	34	-	-	-	-
Minneapolis – St. Paul, MN – WI MSA	65	338,580	11,690	172,949	14,795
New York – Northern New Jersey – Long Island, NY – NJ – CT- CMSA	202	2,118,874	45,032	1,107,119	24,585
Philadelphia – Wilmington – Atlantic City, PA – NJ – DE – MD CMSA	98	606,631	16,386	278,120	16,973
Phoenix – Mesa, AZ MSA	29	124,836	3,447	51,928	15,065
Pittsburgh, PA MSA	33	183,243	5,148	74,606	14,492
Portland – Salem, OR – WA CMSA	16	-	-	-	-
Providence – Fall River – Warwick, RI – MA MSA	24	98,732	3,125	55,358	17,715
Sacramento – Yolo, CA CMSA	16	-	-	-	-
St. Louis, MO – IL MSA	28	105,550	3,360	46,335	13,790
San Diego, CA MSA	11	-	-	-	-
San Francisco – Oakland – San Jose, CA CMSA	33	-	-	-	-
Seattle – Tacoma – Bremerton, WA CMSA	26	136,269	4,229	73,207	17,311
Tampa – St. Petersburg – Clearwater, FL MSA	18	74,804	2,142	31,235	14,582
Washington – Baltimore, DC – MD – VA – WV CMSA	51	-	-	-	-

Source: U.S. Department of Commerce. Bureau of the Census. *1992 Economic Census Report Series*, CD-ROM 1i, Washington, DC, October 1996. *Notes:* - means no data reported. 1. HS stands for total health service establishments, revenues, employment, or payroll.

★ 394 ★

Establishment Data

Skilled Nursing Care Facilities by State: 1992

Area	Establishments		Revenues		Employment		Payroll		
	Number	% of HS[1] in area	Total ($000)	% of HS[1] in area	Number	% of HS[1] in area	Total ($000)	% of HS[1] in area	Payroll per employee
United States	10,242	2.32	28,797,807	9.63	937,907	21.06	13,520,962	10.47	14,416
Alabama	187	3.39	474,408	9.63	18,483	23.90	225,772	10.70	12,215
Alaska	0	0.00	0	0.00	0	0.00	0	0.00	0
Arizona	87	1.22	304,722	6.67	9,235	15.72	136,534	7.00	14,784
Arkansas	176	4.94	318,950	13.09	14,058	32.93	149,071	14.01	10,604
California	1,136	1.85	3,018,953	7.02	90,955	16.97	1,420,680	8.24	15,620
Colorado	130	1.85	383,621	10.27	11,742	21.24	167,185	10.19	14,238
Connecticut	191	2.90	957,378	19.50	24,806	34.32	508,731	21.68	20,508
Delaware	26	2.17	84,093	10.65	3,030	26.08	39,152	10.77	12,921
District of Columbia	6	0.44	47,391	5.94	817	8.42	17,510	5.05	21,432
Florida	554	1.87	1,723,918	7.40	49,363	15.66	737,844	7.66	14,947
Georgia	296	2.67	649,798	7.53	26,198	21.65	305,447	8.32	11,659
Hawaii	10	0.45	56,653	4.32	1,063	6.80	25,878	4.39	24,344
Idaho	42	2.42	96,979	9.83	3,732	22.05	45,431	10.93	12,173
Illinois	410	2.19	1,298,126	10.49	41,446	22.09	551,829	9.86	13,314
Indiana	391	4.49	946,839	15.55	31,542	29.56	422,999	15.41	13,411
Iowa	135	3.23	206,161	8.82	9,275	20.62	103,426	9.30	11,151
Kansas	169	4.37	256,699	8.42	11,142	20.84	130,044	9.83	11,672
Kentucky	135	2.45	319,563	7.76	12,050	17.97	145,438	8.18	12,070
Louisiana	201	2.95	460,535	8.33	18,269	21.16	189,472	8.71	10,371
Maine	53	2.45	114,779	9.75	4,145	18.84	58,409	10.96	14,091
Maryland	136	1.49	536,185	9.50	15,825	19.81	255,722	10.25	16,159
Massachusetts	389	3.67	1,521,089	19.95	41,973	32.99	801,285	22.61	19,090
Michigan	293	1.86	776,024	8.91	28,867	20.48	376,841	9.16	13,054
Minnesota	197	3.33	591,538	14.41	21,331	28.14	314,375	15.09	14,738
Mississippi	126	4.08	247,936	11.90	10,010	27.18	118,500	13.48	11,838
Missouri	387	4.59	688,754	12.53	28,686	30.26	316,862	12.96	11,046
Montana	39	2.62	83,317	12.79	3,050	28.27	38,098	14.68	12,491
Nebraska	77	3.27	151,339	9.73	5,970	22.13	78,735	10.99	13,188
Nevada	32	1.38	111,678	4.96	3,110	12.31	52,799	5.76	16,977
New Hampshire	23	1.25	88,771	7.47	2,357	12.27	41,338	7.62	17,538
New Jersey	225	1.36	1,090,471	10.48	26,493	20.76	500,636	11.33	18,897
New Mexico	36	1.50	90,253	6.11	3,335	14.10	39,157	6.33	11,741
New York	326	1.01	2,144,190	10.79	48,914	17.58	1,004,669	12.19	20,539
North Carolina	284	3.20	735,695	11.05	27,657	25.78	373,855	12.53	13,518
North Dakota	9	1.16	-	-	-	-	-	-	-
Ohio	617	3.32	1,774,992	15.24	59,954	30.03	821,808	14.75	13,707
Oklahoma	168	3.15	220,769	6.74	10,161	17.20	101,369	7.17	9,976
Oregon	118	2.09	246,448	8.33	8,539	17.74	118,142	9.11	13,836
Pennsylvania	380	1.75	1,243,818	9.85	35,786	19.41	548,299	9.68	15,322
Rhode Island	72	3.79	223,466	21.08	6,912	38.05	111,829	23.91	16,179
South Carolina	140	3.01	320,384	10.23	12,609	25.20	150,555	10.80	11,940
South Dakota	35	3.62	51,630	9.16	2,299	25.25	26,346	10.11	11,460
Tennessee	163	1.98	426,188	6.31	14,658	14.61	176,727	6.16	12,057
Texas	901	3.01	1,645,949	7.18	65,468	18.90	752,874	8.17	11,500

[Continued]

★ 394 ★

Skilled Nursing Care Facilities by State: 1992

[Continued]

Area	Establishments		Revenues		Employment		Payroll		
	Number	% of HS[1] in area	Total ($000)	% of HS[1] in area	Number	% of HS[1] in area	Total ($000)	% of HS[1] in area	Payroll per employee
Utah	53	1.74	122,761	6.65	4,654	15.06	55,543	7.36	11,934
Vermont	24	2.58	70,235	17.33	2,433	32.24	34,339	20.82	14,114
Virginia	129	1.32	367,375	5.50	12,821	12.55	169,627	5.60	13,230
Washington	239	2.59	685,252	12.69	23,187	26.50	354,670	14.89	15,296
West Virginia	55	2.04	128,536	7.19	4,821	16.70	55,948	7.95	11,605
Wisconsin	218	3.02	637,876	13.47	22,518	26.50	322,177	13.75	14,308
Wyoming	16	2.24	-	-	-	-	-	-	-

Source: U.S. Department of Commerce. Bureau of the Census. *1992 Economic Census Report Series,* CD-ROM 1i, Washington, DC, October 1996. *Notes:* - means no data reported. 1. HS stands for total health service establishments, revenues, employment, or payroll.

★ 395 ★

Establishment Data

Skilled Nursing Care Facilities by State, Non-Taxed Establishments: 1992

Area	Establish-ments	Revenues in $1,000	Employ-ment	Payroll in $1,000	Payroll per employee
United States	2,723	11,683,096	367,161	5,821,838	15,856
Alabama	16	43,038	1,994	20,750	10,406
Alaska	7	38,818	835	18,254	21,861
Arizona	37	146,720	4,306	64,417	14,960
Arkansas	18	27,263	1,116	12,291	11,013
California	137	485,380	13,452	231,493	17,209
Colorado	30	92,009	3,326	44,185	13,285
Connecticut	45	323,736	8,132	174,885	21,506
Delaware	8	36,468	1,173	17,417	14,848
District of Columbia	4	30,174	661	16,559	25,051
Florida	102	527,859	14,379	213,159	14,824
Georgia	35	104,530	4,012	50,106	12,489
Hawaii	5	27,823	665	14,029	21,096
Idaho	8	21,970	890	10,208	11,470
Illinois	154	517,908	17,870	250,698	14,029
Indiana	47	155,932	5,128	74,674	14,562
Iowa	67	-	-	-	-
Kansas	60	130,448	5,456	65,604	12,024
Kentucky	45	150,361	5,638	73,436	13,025
Louisiana	22	-	-	-	-
Maine	10	37,010	1,231	18,345	14,903
Maryland	48	295,455	8,480	143,635	16,938
Massachusetts	84	452,431	12,714	246,589	19,395

[Continued]

★ 395 ★

Skilled Nursing Care Facilities by State, Non-Taxed Establishments: 1992
[Continued]

Area	Establish-ments	Revenues in $1,000	Employ-ment	Payroll in $1,000	Payroll per employee
Michigan	104	420,082	13,869	195,416	14,090
Minnesota	171	637,327	24,531	334,672	13,643
Mississippi	11	24,466	1,029	12,371	12,022
Missouri	67	206,424	8,022	101,182	12,613
Montana	17	32,980	1,402	18,076	12,893
Nebraska	48	114,308	5,044	62,597	12,410
Nevada	0	0	0	0	0
New Hampshire	4	-	-	-	-
New Jersey	81	427,466	11,316	218,668	19,324
New Mexico	17	45,093	1,745	23,038	13,202
New York	227	2,257,139	52,919	1,171,999	22,147
North Carolina	40	151,676	5,803	75,721	13,049
North Dakota	61	147,291	6,729	82,367	12,241
Ohio	130	558,365	18,545	272,390	14,688
Oklahoma	13	-	-	-	-
Oregon	28	90,997	3,452	47,659	13,806
Pennsylvania	289	1,257,828	37,431	571,366	15,265
Rhode Island	21	81,061	2,595	45,069	17,368
South Carolina	14	37,095	1,308	19,260	14,725
South Dakota	45	86,357	4,326	47,754	11,039
Tennessee	27	98,543	3,684	43,983	11,939
Texas	79	246,350	8,564	117,459	13,715
Utah	7	24,601	889	12,653	14,233
Vermont	6	12,477	467	6,950	14,882
Virginia	26	110,081	3,632	51,843	14,274
Washington	52	217,696	7,254	115,804	15,964
West Virginia	12	39,822	1,525	20,772	13,621
Wisconsin	132	455,323	18,685	259,400	13,883
Wyoming	5	-	-	-	-

Source: U.S. Department of Commerce. Bureau of the Census. *1992 Economic Census Report Series,* CD-ROM 1i, Washington, DC, October 1996. *Notes:* - means no data reported. 1. HS stands for total health service establishments, revenues, employment, or payroll.

★ 396 ★
Establishment Data

Specialty Hospitals by Major Metro Areas: 1992

Area	Establishments		Revenues		Employment		Payroll		
	Number	% of HS[1] in area	Total ($000)	% of HS[1] in area	Number	% of HS[1] in area	Total ($000)	% of HS[1] in area	Payroll per employee
United States	699	0.16	6,920,685	2.31	105,009	2.36	2,543,515	1.97	24,222
Albany – Schenectady – Troy, NY MSA	3	0.23	54,368	6.73	944	7.15	25,843	7.11	27,376
Albuquerque, NM MSA	5	0.47	-	-	-	-	-	-	-
Allentown – Bethlehem – Easton, PA MSA	0	0.00	0	0.00	0	0.00	0	0.00	0
Anchorage, AK MSA	2	0.41	-	-	-	-	-	-	-
Appleton – Oshkosh – Neenah, WI MSA	0	0.00	0	0.00	0	0.00	0	0.00	0
Atlanta, GA MSA	10	0.16	130,313	2.70	1,806	3.02	40,033	1.98	22,167
Augusta – Aiken, GA – SC MSA	3	0.42	-	-	-	-	-	-	-
Austin – San Marcos, TX MSA	12	0.76	-	-	-	-	-	-	-
Bakersfield, CA MSA	2	0.26	-	-	-	-	-	-	-
Baton Rouge, LA MSA	4	0.45	-	-	-	-	-	-	-
Beaumont – Port Arthur, TX MSA	2	0.28	-	-	-	-	-	-	-
Birmingham, AL MSA	4	0.29	35,764	2.37	521	2.58	13,788	2.15	26,464
Boise City, ID MSA	3	0.50	-	-	-	-	-	-	-
Boston – Worcester – Lawrence, MA – NH – ME – CT CMSA	21	0.21	309,796	4.38	5,543	4.81	153,883	4.73	27,762
Buffalo – Niagara Falls, NY MSA	1	0.05	-	-	-	-	-	-	-
Canton – Massillon, OH MSA	0	0.00	0	0.00	0	0.00	0	0.00	0
Charleston – North Charleston, SC MSA	3	0.37	-	-	-	-	-	-	-
Charlotte – Gastonia – Rock Hill, NC – SC MSA	3	0.19	-	-	-	-	-	-	-
Chattanooga, TN – GA MSA	4	0.53	32,012	4.46	521	5.22	12,111	3.96	23,246
Chicago – Gary – Kenosha, IL – IN – WI CMSA	18	0.12	287,850	2.96	3,862	2.83	108,218	2.46	28,021
Cincinnati – Hamilton, OH – KY – IN CMSA	2	0.06	-	-	-	-	-	-	-
Cleveland – Akron, OH CMSA	3	0.06	-	-	-	-	-	-	-
Colorado Springs, CO MSA	3	0.34	-	-	-	-	-	-	-
Columbia, SC MSA	2	0.27	-	-	-	-	-	-	-
Columbus, OH MSA	0	0.00	0	0.00	0	0.00	0	0.00	0
Corpus Christi, TX MSA	4	0.53	-	-	-	-	-	-	-
Dallas – Fort Worth, TX CMSA	38	0.46	-	-	-	-	-	-	-
Davenport – Moline – Rock Island, IA – IL MSA	0	0.00	0	0.00	0	0.00	0	0.00	0
Dayton – Springfield, OH MSA	2	0.12	-	-	-	-	-	-	-
Daytona Beach, FL MSA	1	0.14	-	-	-	-	-	-	-
Denver – Boulder – Greeley, CO CMSA	7	0.16	-	-	-	-	-	-	-
Des Moines, IA MSA	0	0.00	0	0.00	0	0.00	0	0.00	0
Detroit – Ann Arbor – Flint, MI CMSA	7	0.07	53,879	0.99	1,031	1.23	21,438	0.84	20,793
El Paso, TX MSA	2	0.25	-	-	-	-	-	-	-
Eugene – Springfield, OR MSA	0	0.00	0	0.00	0	0.00	0	0.00	0
Fort Myers – Cape Coral, FL MSA	2	0.28	-	-	-	-	-	-	-
Fort Pierce – Port St. Lucie, FL MSA	2	0.39	-	-	-	-	-	-	-
Fort Wayne, IN MSA	1	0.14	-	-	-	-	-	-	-
Fresno, CA MSA	3	0.20	-	-	-	-	-	-	-
Grand Rapids – Muskegon – Holland, MI MSA	1	0.07	-	-	-	-	-	-	-
Greensboro – Winston-Salem – High Point, NC MSA	2	0.13	-	-	-	-	-	-	-
Greenville – Spartanburg – Anderson, SC MSA	1	0.09	-	-	-	-	-	-	-
Harrisburg – Lebanon – Carlisle, PA MSA	1	0.10	-	-	-	-	-	-	-
Hartford, CT MSA	1	0.04	-	-	-	-	-	-	-
Honolulu, HI MSA	1	0.06	-	-	-	-	-	-	-

[Continued]

★ 396 ★

Specialty Hospitals by Major Metro Areas: 1992
[Continued]

Area	Establishments		Revenues		Employment		Payroll		
	Number	% of HS[1] in area	Total ($000)	% of HS[1] in area	Number	% of HS[1] in area	Total ($000)	% of HS[1] in area	Payroll per employee
Houston – Galveston – Brazoria, TX CMSA	26	0.37	294,022	5.01	3,857	5.16	95,463	4.07	24,751
Huntsville, AL MSA	2	0.38	-	-	-	-	-	-	-
Indianapolis, IN MSA	7	0.28	-	-	-	-	-	-	-
Jackson, MS MSA	3	0.47	-	-	-	-	-	-	-
Jacksonville, FL MSA	4	0.23	-	-	-	-	-	-	-
Johnson City – Kingsport – Bristol, TN – VA MSA	3	0.43	-	-	-	-	-	-	-
Kalamazoo – Battle Creek, MI MSA	0	0.00	0	0.00	0	0.00	0	0.00	0
Kansas City, MO – KS MSA	11	0.39	-	-	-	-	-	-	-
Knoxville, TN MSA	1	0.08	-	-	-	-	-	-	-
Lafayette, LA MSA	2	0.31	-	-	-	-	-	-	-
Lakeland – Winter Haven, FL MSA	1	0.21	-	-	-	-	-	-	-
Lancaster, PA MSA	0	0.00	0	0.00	0	0.00	0	0.00	0
Lansing – East Lansing, MI MSA	1	0.14	-	-	-	-	-	-	-
Las Vegas, NV – AZ MSA	4	0.26	50,003	2.96	577	3.13	12,348	1.81	21,400
Lexington, KY MSA	1	0.12	-	-	-	-	-	-	-
Little Rock – North Little Rock, AR MSA	5	0.48	-	-	-	-	-	-	-
Los Angeles – Riverside – Orange County, CA CMSA	41	0.13	-	-	-	-	-	-	-
Louisville, KY – IN MSA	3	0.17	38,448	2.29	633	2.45	12,653	1.77	19,989
Macon, GA MSA	3	0.55	40,133	7.11	514	6.81	11,541	5.10	22,453
Madison, WI MSA	1	0.19	-	-	-	-	-	-	-
Melbourne – Titusville – Palm Bay, FL MSA	2	0.25	-	-	-	-	-	-	-
Memphis, TN – AR – MS MSA	3	0.18	-	-	-	-	-	-	-
Miami – Fort Lauderdale, FL CMSA	15	0.16	167,924	2.45	2,626	3.02	63,132	2.25	24,041
Milwaukee – Racine, WI CMSA	4	0.13	-	-	-	-	-	-	-
Minneapolis – St. Paul, MN – WI MSA	1	0.03	-	-	-	-	-	-	-
Mobile, AL MSA	1	0.16	-	-	-	-	-	-	-
Modesto, CA MSA	1	0.15	-	-	-	-	-	-	-
Montgomery, AL MSA	1	0.20	-	-	-	-	-	-	-
Nashville, TN MSA	7	0.36	-	-	-	-	-	-	-
New Orleans, LA MSA	14	0.58	99,432	4.54	1,813	6.12	34,333	4.08	18,937
New York – Northern New Jersey – Long Island, NY – NJ – CT- CMSA	15	0.04	297,205	1.14	4,367	1.31	122,165	1.12	27,975
Norfolk – Virginia Beach – Newport News, VA – NC MSA	7	0.31	65,949	4.86	1,441	6.58	25,987	4.02	18,034
Oklahoma City, OK MSA	4	0.20	-	-	-	-	-	-	-
Omaha, NE – IA MSA	1	0.10	-	-	-	-	-	-	-
Orlando, FL MSA	4	0.16	30,655	1.61	441	1.75	10,011	1.22	22,701
Pensacola, FL MSA	2	0.38	-	-	-	-	-	-	-
Peoria – Pekin, IL MSA	0	0.00	0	0.00	0	0.00	0	0.00	0
Philadelphia – Wilmington – Atlantic City, PA – NJ – DE – MD CMSA	15	0.13	-	-	-	-	-	-	-
Phoenix – Mesa, AZ MSA	7	0.15	-	-	-	-	-	-	-
Pittsburgh, PA MSA	3	0.06	-	-	-	-	-	-	-
Portland, ME MSA	2	0.37	-	-	-	-	-	-	-
Portland – Salem, OR – WA CMSA	4	0.11	-	-	-	-	-	-	-
Providence – Fall River – Warwick, RI – MA MSA	0	0.00	0	0.00	0	0.00	0	0.00	0
Raleigh – Durham – Chapel Hill, NC MSA	3	0.21	-	-	-	-	-	-	-
Reno, NV MSA	2	0.30	-	-	-	-	-	-	-
Richmond – Petersburg, VA MSA	5	0.31	60,553	3.87	884	3.98	18,839	2.85	21,311
Rochester, NY MSA	0	0.00	0	0.00	0	0.00	0	0.00	0

[Continued]

★ 396 ★

Specialty Hospitals by Major Metro Areas: 1992
[Continued]

Area	Establishments		Revenues		Employment		Payroll		
	Number	% of HS[1] in area	Total ($000)	% of HS[1] in area	Number	% of HS[1] in area	Total ($000)	% of HS[1] in area	Payroll per employee
Rockford, IL MSA	1	0.21	-	-	-	-	-	-	-
Sacramento – Yolo, CA CMSA	5	0.17	33,155	1.72	468	1.88	12,325	1.49	26,335
Saginaw – Bay City – Midland, MI MSA	0	0.00	0	0.00	0	0.00	0	0.00	0
St. Louis, MO – IL MSA	3	0.07	-	-	-	-	-	-	-
Salinas, CA MSA	0	0.00	0	0.00	0	0.00	0	0.00	0
Salt Lake City – Ogden, UT MSA	7	0.34	-	-	-	-	-	-	-
San Antonio, TX MSA	11	0.42	98,930	5.49	1,530	5.32	34,468	4.62	22,528
San Diego, CA MSA	8	0.16	81,589	2.50	1,288	3.09	33,435	2.48	25,959
San Francisco – Oakland – San Jose, CA CMSA	18	0.13	-	-	-	-	-	-	-
Santa Barbara – Santa Maria – Lompoc, CA MSA	1	0.12	-	-	-	-	-	-	-
Sarasota – Bradenton, FL MSA	4	0.33	-	-	-	-	-	-	-
Scranton – Wilkes-Barre – Hazleton, PA MSA	1	0.09	-	-	-	-	-	-	-
Seattle – Tacoma – Bremerton, WA CMSA	3	0.05	-	-	-	-	-	-	-
Shreveport – Bossier City, LA MSA	4	0.62	45,604	7.98	415	4.88	11,626	5.02	28,014
Spokane, WA MSA	1	0.14	-	-	-	-	-	-	-
Springfield, MO MSA	1	0.22	-	-	-	-	-	-	-
Springfield, MA MSA	2	0.22	-	-	-	-	-	-	-
Stockton – Lodi, CA MSA	0	0.00	0	0.00	0	0.00	0	0.00	0
Syracuse, NY MSA	1	0.09	-	-	-	-	-	-	-
Tallahassee, FL MSA	1	0.25	-	-	-	-	-	-	-
Tampa – St. Petersburg – Clearwater, FL MSA	12	0.24	165,184	3.79	2,315	3.78	57,803	3.35	24,969
Toledo, OH MSA	1	0.09	-	-	-	-	-	-	-
Tucson, AZ MSA	7	0.56	-	-	-	-	-	-	-
Tulsa, OK MSA	4	0.29	-	-	-	-	-	-	-
Washington – Baltimore, DC – MD – VA – WV CMSA	12	0.09	-	-	-	-	-	-	-
West Palm Beach – Boca Raton, FL MSA	6	0.22	60,972	3.08	820	3.34	19,950	2.37	24,329
Wichita, KS MSA	4	0.52	-	-	-	-	-	-	-
Youngstown – Warren, OH MSA	1	0.08	-	-	-	-	-	-	-

Source: U.S. Department of Commerce. Bureau of the Census. *1992 Economic Census Report Series*, CD-ROM 1i, Washington, DC, October 1996. *Notes:* - means no data reported. 1. HS stands for total health service establishments, revenues, employment, or payroll.

★ 397 ★

Establishment Data

Specialty Hospitals by Major Metro Areas, Non-Taxed Establishments: 1992

Area	Establish- ments	Revenues in $1,000	Employ- ment	Payroll in $1,000	Payroll per employee
United States	797	25,344,022	478,431	14,065,221	29,399
Albany – Schenectady – Troy, NY MSA	2	-	-	-	-
Albuquerque, NM MSA	6	-	-	-	-
Allentown – Bethlehem – Easton, PA MSA	2	-	-	-	-
Atlanta, GA MSA	12	576,791	8,899	239,767	26,943

[Continued]

★ 397 ★

Specialty Hospitals by Major Metro Areas, Non-Taxed Establishments: 1992
[Continued]

Area	Establish- ments	Revenues in $1,000	Employ- ment	Payroll in $1,000	Payroll per employee
Austin – San Marcos, TX MSA	1	-	-	-	-
Baton Rouge, LA MSA	3	99,886	1,592	43,751	27,482
Birmingham, AL MSA	2	-	-	-	-
Boston – Worcester – Lawrence, MA – NH – ME – CT CMSA	36	1,525,283	26,051	825,819	31,700
Buffalo – Niagara Falls, NY MSA	5	-	-	-	-
Charlotte – Gastonia – Rock Hill, NC – SC MSA	4	117,327	2,114	70,613	33,403
Chicago – Gary – Kenosha, IL – IN – WI CMSA	17	-	-	-	-
Cincinnati – Hamilton, OH – KY – IN CMSA	8	-	-	-	-
Cleveland – Akron, OH CMSA	10	-	-	-	-
Columbus, OH MSA	6	-	-	-	-
Dallas – Fort Worth, TX CMSA	7	-	-	-	-
Dayton – Springfield, OH MSA	4	123,634	2,391	63,218	26,440
Denver – Boulder – Greeley, CO CMSA	10	-	-	-	-
Des Moines, IA MSA	1	-	-	-	-
Detroit – Ann Arbor – Flint, MI CMSA	18	-	-	-	-
Fresno, CA MSA	1	-	-	-	-
Grand Rapids – Muskegon – Holland, MI MSA	3	70,688	1,645	38,768	23,567
Greensboro – Winston-Salem – High Point, NC MSA	6	54,860	1,291	33,972	26,314
Greenville – Spartanburg – Anderson, SC MSA	4	-	-	-	-
Harrisburg – Lebanon – Carlisle, PA MSA	3	-	-	-	-
Hartford, CT MSA	10	-	-	-	-
Honolulu, HI MSA	5	-	-	-	-
Houston – Galveston – Brazoria, TX CMSA	6	-	-	-	-
Indianapolis, IN MSA	6	94,853	2,005	61,151	30,499
Jacksonville, FL MSA	2	-	-	-	-
Kalamazoo – Battle Creek, MI MSA	5	146,572	2,857	104,555	36,596
Kansas City, MO – KS MSA	6	171,319	3,997	100,845	25,230
Knoxville, TN MSA	3	-	-	-	-
Lansing – East Lansing, MI MSA	0	0	0	0	0
Lexington, KY MSA	3	-	-	-	-
Little Rock – North Little Rock, AR MSA	3	-	-	-	-
Los Angeles – Riverside – Orange County, CA CMSA	21	-	-	-	-
Louisville, KY – IN MSA	3	64,034	1,418	31,542	22,244
Madison, WI MSA	2	-	-	-	-

[Continued]

★ 397 ★

Specialty Hospitals by Major Metro Areas, Non-Taxed Establishments: 1992

[Continued]

Area	Establish- ments	Revenues in $1,000	Employ- ment	Payroll in $1,000	Payroll per employee
Memphis, TN – AR – MS MSA	3	-	-	-	-
Miami – Fort Lauderdale, FL CMSA	4	223,475	3,312	96,649	29,181
Milwaukee – Racine, WI CMSA	11	-	-	-	-
Minneapolis – St. Paul, MN – WI MSA	8	-	-	-	-
Nashville, TN MSA	2	-	-	-	-
New Orleans, LA MSA	4	132,234	2,197	53,604	24,399
New York – Northern New Jersey – Long Island, NY – NJ – CT- CMSA	72	-	-	-	-
Norfolk – Virginia Beach – Newport News, VA – NC MSA	3	-	-	-	-
Oklahoma City, OK MSA	5	66,161	1,445	37,798	26,158
Omaha, NE – IA MSA	4	105,838	1,789	51,449	28,759
Orlando, FL MSA	4	-	-	-	-
Philadelphia – Wilmington – Atlantic City, PA – NJ – DE – MD CMSA	32	-	-	-	-
Phoenix – Mesa, AZ MSA	6	-	-	-	-
Pittsburgh, PA MSA	14	-	-	-	-
Portland – Salem, OR – WA CMSA	4	-	-	-	-
Providence – Fall River – Warwick, RI – MA MSA	7	-	-	-	-
Raleigh – Durham – Chapel Hill, NC MSA	4	71,472	1,598	43,298	27,095
Richmond – Petersburg, VA MSA	5	-	-	-	-
Rochester, NY MSA	3	141,184	3,244	97,314	29,998
Sacramento – Yolo, CA CMSA	1	-	-	-	-
St. Louis, MO – IL MSA	11	-	-	-	-
Salt Lake City – Ogden, UT MSA	4	-	-	-	-
San Antonio, TX MSA	7	156,209	3,373	81,827	24,259
San Diego, CA MSA	7	197,961	3,718	95,411	25,662
San Francisco – Oakland – San Jose, CA CMSA	10	614,612	10,233	364,450	35,615
Santa Barbara – Santa Maria – Lompoc, CA MSA	1	-	-	-	-
Scranton – Wilkes-Barre – Hazleton, PA MSA	6	70,728	1,525	34,555	22,659
Seattle – Tacoma – Bremerton, WA CMSA	7	356,588	4,618	153,121	33,157
Springfield, MA MSA	5	108,635	2,111	66,886	31,685
Syracuse, NY MSA	1	-	-	-	-
Tampa – St. Petersburg – Clearwater, FL MSA	5	211,070	3,211	84,580	26,341
Toledo, OH MSA	1	-	-	-	-
Tucson, AZ MSA	3	-	-	-	-
Tulsa, OK MSA	3	-	-	-	-
Washington – Baltimore, DC – MD – VA – WV CMSA	24	1,161,180	19,461	592,030	30,421

[Continued]

★ 397 ★

Specialty Hospitals by Major Metro Areas, Non-Taxed Establishments: 1992

[Continued]

Area	Establish-ments	Revenues in $1,000	Employ-ment	Payroll in $1,000	Payroll per employee
West Palm Beach – Boca Raton, FL MSA	2	-	-	-	-
Wichita, KS MSA	1	-	-	-	-
Youngstown – Warren, OH MSA	2	-	-	-	-

Source: U.S. Department of Commerce. Bureau of the Census. *1992 Economic Census Report Series,* CD-ROM 1i, Washington, DC, October 1996. *Notes:* - means no data reported. 1. HS stands for total health service establishments, revenues, employment, or payroll.

★ 398 ★

Establishment Data

Specialty Hospitals by State: 1992

Area	Establishments		Revenues		Employment		Payroll		
	Number	% of HS[1] in area	Total ($000)	% of HS[1] in area	Number	% of HS[1] in area	Total ($000)	% of HS[1] in area	Payroll per employee
United States	699	0.16	6,920,685	2.31	105,009	2.36	2,543,515	1.97	24,222
Alabama	11	0.20	120,478	2.45	1,389	1.80	37,125	1.76	26,728
Alaska	2	0.23	-	-	-	-	-	-	-
Arizona	16	0.23	145,929	3.19	2,111	3.59	55,806	2.86	26,436
Arkansas	11	0.31	108,717	4.46	1,570	3.68	38,183	3.59	24,320
California	85	0.14	715,132	1.66	10,640	1.99	271,738	1.58	25,539
Colorado	10	0.14	-	-	-	-	-	-	-
Connecticut	3	0.05	-	-	-	-	-	-	-
Delaware	3	0.25	23,651	2.99	396	3.41	9,317	2.56	23,528
District of Columbia	1	0.07	-	-	-	-	-	-	-
Florida	65	0.22	671,519	2.88	9,474	3.01	227,611	2.36	24,025
Georgia	22	0.20	240,442	2.79	3,204	2.65	72,226	1.97	22,542
Hawaii	1	0.04	-	-	-	-	-	-	-
Idaho	7	0.40	-	-	-	-	-	-	-
Illinois	18	0.10	290,299	2.35	3,898	2.08	108,265	1.94	27,774
Indiana	21	0.24	193,529	3.18	2,527	2.37	58,052	2.11	22,973
Iowa	0	0.00	0	0.00	0	0.00	0	0.00	0
Kansas	12	0.31	-	-	-	-	-	-	-
Kentucky	9	0.16	83,171	2.02	1,279	1.91	28,772	1.62	22,496
Louisiana	32	0.47	268,043	4.85	4,325	5.01	89,293	4.10	20,646
Maine	2	0.09	-	-	-	-	-	-	-
Maryland	10	0.11	-	-	-	-	-	-	-
Massachusetts	17	0.16	-	-	-	-	-	-	-
Michigan	10	0.06	79,682	0.92	1,428	1.01	30,033	0.73	21,032
Minnesota	1	0.02	-	-	-	-	-	-	-
Mississippi	7	0.23	65,645	3.15	970	2.63	21,657	2.46	22,327
Missouri	13	0.15	96,433	1.75	1,563	1.65	37,700	1.54	24,120
Montana	3	0.20	-	-	-	-	-	-	-

[Continued]

★ 398 ★

Specialty Hospitals by State: 1992

[Continued]

Area	Establishments		Revenues		Employment		Payroll		
	Number	% of HS[1] in area	Total ($000)	% of HS[1] in area	Number	% of HS[1] in area	Total ($000)	% of HS[1] in area	Payroll per employee
Nebraska	2	0.08	-	-	-	-	-	-	-
Nevada	6	0.26	-	-	-	-	-	-	-
New Hampshire	10	0.54	-	-	-	-	-	-	-
New Jersey	5	0.03	113,124	1.09	1,582	1.24	35,195	0.80	22,247
New Mexico	11	0.46	-	-	-	-	-	-	-
New York	16	0.05	284,316	1.43	4,758	1.71	133,098	1.61	27,974
North Carolina	15	0.17	170,997	2.57	2,425	2.26	58,181	1.95	23,992
North Dakota	0	0.00	0	0.00	0	0.00	0	0.00	0
Ohio	10	0.05	-	-	-	-	-	-	-
Oklahoma	13	0.24	109,704	3.35	1,737	2.94	38,808	2.75	22,342
Oregon	4	0.07	-	-	-	-	-	-	-
Pennsylvania	24	0.11	-	-	-	-	-	-	-
Rhode Island	0	0.00	0	0.00	0	0.00	0	0.00	0
South Carolina	9	0.19	68,542	2.19	949	1.90	24,953	1.79	26,294
South Dakota	2	0.21	-	-	-	-	-	-	-
Tennessee	16	0.19	170,453	2.53	2,742	2.73	62,060	2.16	22,633
Texas	114	0.38	1,091,524	4.76	16,117	4.65	382,517	4.15	23,734
Utah	9	0.29	66,568	3.60	1,066	3.45	24,045	3.19	22,556
Vermont	0	0.00	0	0.00	0	0.00	0	0.00	0
Virginia	21	0.22	186,980	2.80	3,353	3.28	67,599	2.23	20,161
Washington	4	0.04	22,626	0.42	428	0.49	9,363	0.39	21,876
West Virginia	7	0.26	70,401	3.94	1,075	3.72	24,101	3.42	22,420
Wisconsin	7	0.10	-	-	-	-	-	-	-
Wyoming	2	0.28	-	-	-	-	-	-	-

Source: U.S. Department of Commerce. Bureau of the Census. *1992 Economic Census Report Series,* CD-ROM 1i, Washington, DC, October 1996. *Notes:* - means no data reported. 1. HS stands for total health service establishments, revenues, employment, or payroll.

★ 399 ★

Establishment Data

Specialty Hospitals by State, Non-Taxed Establishments: 1992

Area	Establish- ments	Revenues in $1,000	Employ- ment	Payroll in $1,000	Payroll per employee
United States	797	25,344,022	478,431	14,065,221	29,399
Alabama	9	297,941	6,426	167,177	26,016
Alaska	1	-	-	-	-
Arizona	9	161,314	2,715	70,561	25,989
Arkansas	5	170,471	3,556	80,395	22,608
California	46	2,060,987	33,557	1,174,870	35,011

[Continued]

★ 399 ★

Specialty Hospitals by State, Non-Taxed Establishments: 1992
[Continued]

Area	Establish-ments	Revenues in $1,000	Employ-ment	Payroll in $1,000	Payroll per employee
Colorado	14	432,764	7,843	233,593	29,784
Connecticut	24	468,742	8,007	293,020	36,595
Delaware	2	-	-	-	-
District of Columbia	5	517,864	8,533	259,335	30,392
Florida	30	813,001	15,410	409,001	26,541
Georgia	25	902,240	17,581	447,097	25,431
Hawaii	8	209,220	3,806	105,680	27,767
Idaho	5	46,557	1,237	29,998	24,251
Illinois	24	762,641	15,872	468,440	29,514
Indiana	21	294,549	7,218	208,114	28,833
Iowa	8	171,504	4,300	137,469	31,970
Kansas	11	222,931	6,085	156,223	25,673
Kentucky	10	143,425	3,491	75,576	21,649
Louisiana	15	328,221	6,247	159,890	25,595
Maine	5	85,593	2,052	61,391	29,918
Maryland	20	663,398	11,505	349,666	30,393
Massachusetts	46	1,662,719	28,802	909,897	31,591
Michigan	30	969,497	16,339	523,493	32,039
Minnesota	16	506,623	9,538	307,167	32,205
Mississippi	3	104,275	3,570	63,912	17,903
Missouri	22	638,053	13,283	305,566	23,004
Montana	2	-	-	-	-
Nebraska	10	183,939	4,103	103,646	25,261
Nevada	1	-	-	-	-
New Hampshire	3	-	-	-	-
New Jersey	29	894,728	18,089	561,571	31,045
New Mexico	9	137,382	3,596	81,031	22,534
New York	53	2,971,465	54,843	1,862,801	33,966
North Carolina	23	447,652	9,610	267,169	27,801
North Dakota	4	42,232	1,210	30,276	25,021
Ohio	37	1,164,189	21,629	644,825	29,813
Oklahoma	13	158,960	3,676	91,553	24,906
Oregon	8	89,013	1,979	70,398	35,573
Pennsylvania	60	2,214,881	36,569	1,107,505	30,285
Rhode Island	5	186,050	3,516	99,450	28,285
South Carolina	10	120,369	2,865	66,876	23,342
South Dakota	1	-	-	-	-
Tennessee	14	408,960	8,150	199,710	24,504
Texas	37	1,785,463	32,606	864,433	26,511
Utah	6	-	-	-	-
Vermont	2	-	-	-	-
Virginia	19	433,780	11,581	256,211	22,123
Washington	11	408,643	5,754	185,969	32,320
West Virginia	4	76,095	1,866	41,818	22,411

[Continued]

★ 399 ★

Specialty Hospitals by State, Non-Taxed Establishments: 1992

[Continued]

Area	Establish-ments	Revenues in $1,000	Employ-ment	Payroll in $1,000	Payroll per employee
Wisconsin	20	496,038	10,137	252,742	24,933
Wyoming	2	-	-	-	-

Source: U.S. Department of Commerce. Bureau of the Census. *1992 Economic Census Report Series,* CD-ROM 1i, Washington, DC, October 1996. *Notes:* - means no data reported. 1. HS stands for total health service establishments, revenues, employment, or payroll.

★ 400 ★

Establishment Data

Specialty Hospitals, Except Psychiatric by Major Metro Areas: 1992

Area	Establishments		Revenues		Employment		Payroll		
	Number	% of HS[1] in area	Total ($000)	% of HS[1] in area	Number	% of HS[1] in area	Total ($000)	% of HS[1] in area	Payroll per employee
United States	207	0.05	2,524,522	0.84	35,340	0.79	933,788	0.72	26,423
Atlanta, GA MSA	3	0.05	28,006	0.58	353	0.59	9,549	0.47	27,051
Boston – Worcester – Lawrence, MA – NH – ME – CT CMSA	9	0.09	185,105	2.62	3,375	2.93	99,447	3.05	29,466
Chicago – Gary – Kenosha, IL – IN – WI CMSA	4	0.03	96,384	0.99	1,048	0.77	34,497	0.78	32,917
Cincinnati – Hamilton, OH – KY – IN CMSA	2	0.06	-	-	-	-	-	-	-
Cleveland – Akron, OH CMSA	1	0.02	-	-	-	-	-	-	-
Dallas – Fort Worth, TX CMSA	13	0.16	-	-	-	-	-	-	-
Denver – Boulder – Greeley, CO CMSA	2	0.05	-	-	-	-	-	-	-
Detroit – Ann Arbor – Flint, MI CMSA	2	0.02	-	-	-	-	-	-	-
Houston – Galveston – Brazoria, TX CMSA	8	0.11	113,752	1.94	1,559	2.09	42,530	1.81	27,280
Indianapolis, IN MSA	1	0.04	-	-	-	-	-	-	-
Kansas City, MO – KS MSA	4	0.14	-	-	-	-	-	-	-
Los Angeles – Riverside – Orange County, CA CMSA	3	0.01	-	-	-	-	-	-	-
Miami – Fort Lauderdale, FL CMSA	4	0.04	73,084	1.07	1,053	1.21	28,063	1.00	26,651
Milwaukee – Racine, WI CMSA	1	0.03	-	-	-	-	-	-	-
Minneapolis – St. Paul, MN – WI MSA	0	0.00	0	0.00	0	0.00	0	0.00	0
New York – Northern New Jersey – Long Island, NY – NJ – CT- CMSA	5	0.01	79,384	0.30	918	0.28	23,623	0.22	25,733
Orlando, FL MSA	0	0.00	0	0.00	0	0.00	0	0.00	0
Philadelphia – Wilmington – Atlantic City, PA – NJ – DE – MD CMSA	6	0.05	-	-	-	-	-	-	-
Phoenix – Mesa, AZ MSA	2	0.04	-	-	-	-	-	-	-
Pittsburgh, PA MSA	1	0.02	-	-	-	-	-	-	-
Portland – Salem, OR – WA CMSA	0	0.00	0	0.00	0	0.00	0	0.00	0
Sacramento – Yolo, CA CMSA	1	0.03	-	-	-	-	-	-	-
St. Louis, MO – IL MSA	2	0.04	-	-	-	-	-	-	-
San Diego, CA MSA	2	0.04	-	-	-	-	-	-	-
San Francisco – Oakland – San Jose, CA CMSA	5	0.04	-	-	-	-	-	-	-
Seattle – Tacoma – Bremerton, WA CMSA	2	0.03	-	-	-	-	-	-	-

[Continued]

★ 400 ★

Specialty Hospitals, Except Psychiatric by Major Metro Areas: 1992

[Continued]

Area	Establishments		Revenues		Employment		Payroll		
	Number	% of HS[1] in area	Total ($000)	% of HS[1] in area	Number	% of HS[1] in area	Total ($000)	% of HS[1] in area	Payroll per employee
Tampa – St. Petersburg – Clearwater, FL MSA	3	0.06	73,516	1.69	944	1.54	25,119	1.46	26,609
Washington – Baltimore, DC – MD – VA – WV CMSA	5	0.04	-	-	-	-	-	-	-
West Palm Beach – Boca Raton, FL MSA	1	0.04	-	-	-	-	-	-	-

Source: U.S. Department of Commerce. Bureau of the Census. *1992 Economic Census Report Series,* CD-ROM 1i, Washington, DC, October 1996. *Notes:* - means no data reported. 1. HS stands for total health service establishments, revenues, employment, or payroll.

★ 401 ★

Establishment Data

Specialty Hospitals, Except Psychiatric by Major Metro Areas, Non-Taxed Establishments: 1992

Area	Establish- ments	Revenues in $1,000	Employ- ment	Payroll in $1,000	Payroll per employee
United States	370	14,411,766	230,693	6,768,728	29,341
Albany – Schenectady – Troy, NY MSA	1	-	-	-	-
Atlanta, GA MSA	6	-	-	-	-
Boston – Worcester – Lawrence, MA – NH – ME – CT CMSA	21	1,032,882	16,283	513,302	31,524
Buffalo – Niagara Falls, NY MSA	2	-	-	-	-
Chicago – Gary – Kenosha, IL – IN – WI CMSA	9	-	-	-	-
Cincinnati – Hamilton, OH – KY – IN CMSA	4	-	-	-	-
Cleveland – Akron, OH CMSA	5	167,491	2,564	76,173	29,709
Columbus, OH MSA	4	-	-	-	-
Dallas – Fort Worth, TX CMSA	5	-	-	-	-
Denver – Boulder – Greeley, CO CMSA	7	-	-	-	-
Detroit – Ann Arbor – Flint, MI CMSA	5	-	-	-	-
Hartford, CT MSA	3	-	-	-	-
Houston – Galveston – Brazoria, TX CMSA	5	-	-	-	-
Indianapolis, IN MSA	3	-	-	-	-
Kansas City, MO – KS MSA	2	-	-	-	-
Los Angeles – Riverside – Orange County, CA CMSA	12	-	-	-	-
Miami – Fort Lauderdale, FL CMSA	3	-	-	-	-
Milwaukee – Racine, WI CMSA	6	-	-	-	-
Minneapolis – St. Paul, MN – WI MSA	6	205,442	3,006	94,055	31,289
New York – Northern New Jersey – Long Island, NY – NJ – CT- CMSA	28	-	-	-	-

[Continued]

★ 401 ★

Specialty Hospitals, Except Psychiatric by Major Metro Areas, Non-Taxed Establishments: 1992

[Continued]

Area	Establish-ments	Revenues in $1,000	Employ-ment	Payroll in $1,000	Payroll per employee
Philadelphia – Wilmington – Atlantic City, PA – NJ – DE – MD CMSA	18	-	-	-	-
Phoenix – Mesa, AZ MSA	1	-	-	-	-
Pittsburgh, PA MSA	7	389,220	5,747	171,184	29,787
Portland – Salem, OR – WA CMSA	2	-	-	-	-
Providence – Fall River – Warwick, RI – MA MSA	2	-	-	-	-
Sacramento – Yolo, CA CMSA	0	0	0	0	0
St. Louis, MO – IL MSA	7	-	-	-	-
San Diego, CA MSA	3	-	-	-	-
San Francisco – Oakland – San Jose, CA CMSA	8	-	-	-	-
Seattle – Tacoma – Bremerton, WA CMSA	4	-	-	-	-
Tampa – St. Petersburg – Clearwater, FL MSA	3	-	-	-	-
Washington – Baltimore, DC – MD – VA – WV CMSA	14	743,523	11,241	344,534	30,650

Source: U.S. Department of Commerce. Bureau of the Census. *1992 Economic Census Report Series*, CD-ROM 1i, Washington, DC, October 1996. Notes: - means no data reported. 1. HS stands for total health service establishments, revenues, employment, or payroll.

★ 402 ★

Establishment Data

Specialty Hospitals, Except Psychiatric by State: 1992

Area	Establishments		Revenues		Employment		Payroll		
	Number	% of HS[1] in area	Total ($000)	% of HS[1] in area	Number	% of HS[1] in area	Total ($000)	% of HS[1] in area	Payroll per employee
United States	207	0.05	2,524,522	0.84	35,340	0.79	933,788	0.72	26,423
Alabama	6	0.11	71,969	1.46	763	0.99	21,927	1.04	28,738
Alaska	0	0.00	0	0.00	0	0.00	0	0.00	0
Arizona	4	0.06	-	-	-	-	-	-	-
Arkansas	4	0.11	58,455	2.40	809	1.90	20,459	1.92	25,289
California	17	0.03	195,695	0.46	2,708	0.51	74,730	0.43	27,596
Colorado	3	0.04	-	-	-	-	-	-	-
Connecticut	1	0.02	-	-	-	-	-	-	-
Delaware	1	0.08	-	-	-	-	-	-	-
District of Columbia	0	0.00	0	0.00	0	0.00	0	0.00	0
Florida	18	0.06	299,453	1.28	3,696	1.17	96,186	1.00	26,024
Georgia	6	0.05	49,076	0.57	668	0.55	16,642	0.45	24,913
Hawaii	0	0.00	0	0.00	0	0.00	0	0.00	0

[Continued]

★ 402 ★

Specialty Hospitals, Except Psychiatric by State: 1992
[Continued]

Area	Establishments		Revenues		Employment		Payroll		
	Number	% of HS[1] in area	Total ($000)	% of HS[1] in area	Number	% of HS[1] in area	Total ($000)	% of HS[1] in area	Payroll per employee
Idaho	1	0.06	-	-	-	-	-	-	-
Illinois	4	0.02	96,384	0.78	1,048	0.56	34,497	0.62	32,917
Indiana	4	0.05	39,548	0.65	529	0.50	12,427	0.45	23,491
Iowa	0	0.00	0	0.00	0	0.00	0	0.00	0
Kansas	5	0.13	63,376	2.08	720	1.35	23,536	1.78	32,689
Kentucky	2	0.04	-	-	-	-	-	-	-
Louisiana	6	0.09	100,047	1.81	1,219	1.41	33,418	1.54	27,414
Maine	1	0.05	-	-	-	-	-	-	-
Maryland	5	0.05	-	-	-	-	-	-	-
Massachusetts	8	0.08	-	-	-	-	-	-	-
Michigan	3	0.02	29,713	0.34	559	0.40	12,763	0.31	22,832
Minnesota	0	0.00	0	0.00	0	0.00	0	0.00	0
Mississippi	1	0.03	-	-	-	-	-	-	-
Missouri	4	0.05	31,267	0.57	361	0.38	12,279	0.50	34,014
Montana	0	0.00	0	0.00	0	0.00	0	0.00	0
Nebraska	0	0.00	0	0.00	0	0.00	0	0.00	0
Nevada	2	0.09	-	-	-	-	-	-	-
New Hampshire	6	0.33	-	-	-	-	-	-	-
New Jersey	3	0.02	-	-	-	-	-	-	-
New Mexico	3	0.13	-	-	-	-	-	-	-
New York	4	0.01	-	-	-	-	-	-	-
North Carolina	3	0.03	-	-	-	-	-	-	-
North Dakota	0	0.00	0	0.00	0	0.00	0	0.00	0
Ohio	2	0.01	-	-	-	-	-	-	-
Oklahoma	3	0.06	-	-	-	-	-	-	-
Oregon	0	0.00	0	0.00	0	0.00	0	0.00	0
Pennsylvania	13	0.06	-	-	-	-	-	-	-
Rhode Island	0	0.00	0	0.00	0	0.00	0	0.00	0
South Carolina	3	0.06	-	-	-	-	-	-	-
South Dakota	1	0.10	-	-	-	-	-	-	-
Tennessee	6	0.07	-	-	-	-	-	-	-
Texas	36	0.12	495,685	2.16	6,648	1.92	174,588	1.89	26,262
Utah	3	0.10	24,133	1.31	345	1.12	7,640	1.01	22,145
Vermont	0	0.00	0	0.00	0	0.00	0	0.00	0
Virginia	7	0.07	32,418	0.49	662	0.65	14,849	0.49	22,431
Washington	2	0.02	-	-	-	-	-	-	-
West Virginia	5	0.19	-	-	-	-	-	-	-
Wisconsin	1	0.01	-	-	-	-	-	-	-
Wyoming	0	0.00	0	0.00	0	0.00	0	0.00	0

Source: U.S. Department of Commerce. Bureau of the Census. *1992 Economic Census Report Series,* CD-ROM 1i, Washington, DC, October 1996. *Notes:* - means no data reported. 1. HS stands for total health service establishments, revenues, employment, or payroll.

★ 403 ★

Establishment Data

Specialty Hospitals, Except Psychiatric by State, Non-Taxed Establishments: 1992

Area	Establish-ments	Revenues in $1,000	Employ-ment	Payroll in $1,000	Payroll per employee
United States	370	14,411,766	230,693	6,768,728	29,341
Alabama	4	146,562	2,492	64,744	25,981
Alaska	0	0	0	0	0
Arizona	3	-	-	-	-
Arkansas	3	-	-	-	-
California	27	1,445,855	20,998	752,145	35,820
Colorado	8	296,149	4,658	138,332	29,698
Connecticut	5	143,657	2,462	88,119	35,792
Delaware	1	-	-	-	-
District of Columbia	4	-	-	-	-
Florida	14	526,061	7,744	211,953	27,370
Georgia	8	514,114	7,738	207,690	26,840
Hawaii	6	-	-	-	-
Idaho	3	-	-	-	-
Illinois	10	398,259	6,515	193,623	29,720
Indiana	4	49,109	908	24,195	26,646
Iowa	2	-	-	-	-
Kansas	4	75,944	2,374	56,221	23,682
Kentucky	4	51,177	1,190	27,310	22,950
Louisiana	7	216,235	3,393	95,531	28,155
Maine	2	-	-	-	-
Maryland	11	423,697	6,082	202,206	33,247
Massachusetts	26	1,083,192	17,387	541,291	31,132
Michigan	10	423,174	6,430	175,772	27,336
Minnesota	9	309,986	5,514	164,569	29,846
Mississippi	1	-	-	-	-
Missouri	11	436,519	7,145	186,049	26,039
Montana	0	0	0	0	0
Nebraska	5	-	-	-	-
Nevada	0	0	0	0	0
New Hampshire	2	-	-	-	-
New Jersey	15	371,731	6,384	193,090	30,246
New Mexico	6	-	-	-	-
New York	19	1,397,402	20,012	693,634	34,661
North Carolina	15	146,068	2,821	77,288	27,397
North Dakota	3	-	-	-	-
Ohio	16	773,534	12,916	346,545	26,831
Oklahoma	6	57,583	1,285	28,909	22,497
Oregon	5	-	-	-	-
Pennsylvania	31	1,278,142	18,815	530,619	28,202
Rhode Island	2	-	-	-	-
South Carolina	6	29,300	755	15,951	21,127
South Dakota	1	-	-	-	-
Tennessee	5	288,270	4,545	115,663	25,448

[Continued]

★ 403 ★

Specialty Hospitals, Except Psychiatric by State, Non-Taxed Establishments: 1992

[Continued]

Area	Establish-ments	Revenues in $1,000	Employ-ment	Payroll in $1,000	Payroll per employee
Texas	18	1,363,590	18,337	572,502	31,221
Utah	4	-	-	-	-
Vermont	0	0	0	0	0
Virginia	9	238,337	5,907	124,436	21,066
Washington	6	-	-	-	-
West Virginia	1	-	-	-	-
Wisconsin	8	203,809	3,909	89,030	22,776
Wyoming	0	0	0	0	0

Source: U.S. Department of Commerce. Bureau of the Census. *1992 Economic Census Report Series,* CD-ROM 1i, Washington, DC, October 1996. *Notes:* - means no data reported. 1. HS stands for total health service establishments, revenues, employment, or payroll.

★ 404 ★

Establishment Data

Specialty Hospitals, Except Psychiatric; Government by Major Metro Areas, Non-Taxed Establishments: 1992

Area	Establish-ments	Revenues in $1,000	Employ-ment	Payroll in $1,000	Payroll per employee
United States	92	3,051,876	59,006	1,721,840	29,181
Albany – Schenectady – Troy, NY MSA	0	0	0	0	0
Atlanta, GA MSA	0	0	0	0	0
Boston – Worcester – Lawrence, MA – NH – ME – CT CMSA	8	-	-	-	-
Buffalo – Niagara Falls, NY MSA	1	-	-	-	-
Chicago – Gary – Kenosha, IL – IN – WI CMSA	0	0	0	0	0
Cincinnati – Hamilton, OH – KY – IN CMSA	0	0	0	0	0
Cleveland – Akron, OH CMSA	1	-	-	-	-
Columbus, OH MSA	1	-	-	-	-
Dallas – Fort Worth, TX CMSA	0	0	0	0	0
Denver – Boulder – Greeley, CO CMSA	0	0	0	0	0
Detroit – Ann Arbor – Flint, MI CMSA	0	0	0	0	0
Hartford, CT MSA	1	-	-	-	-
Houston – Galveston – Brazoria, TX CMSA	1	-	-	-	-
Indianapolis, IN MSA	0	0	0	0	0
Kansas City, MO – KS MSA	0	0	0	0	0

[Continued]

★ 404 ★

Specialty Hospitals, Except Psychiatric; Government by Major Metro Areas, Non-Taxed Establishments: 1992
[Continued]

Area	Establish- ments	Revenues in $1,000	Employ- ment	Payroll in $1,000	Payroll per employee
Los Angeles – Riverside – Orange County, CA CMSA	1	-	-	-	-
Miami – Fort Lauderdale, FL CMSA	0	0	0	0	0
Milwaukee – Racine, WI CMSA	0	0	0	0	0
Minneapolis – St. Paul, MN – WI MSA	0	0	0	0	0
New York – Northern New Jersey – Long Island, NY – NJ – CT- CMSA	7	-	-	-	-
Philadelphia – Wilmington – Atlantic City, PA – NJ – DE – MD CMSA	1	-	-	-	-
Phoenix – Mesa, AZ MSA	0	0	0	0	0
Pittsburgh, PA MSA	0	0	0	0	0
Portland – Salem, OR – WA CMSA	0	0	0	0	0
Providence – Fall River – Warwick, RI – MA MSA	1	-	-	-	-
Sacramento – Yolo, CA CMSA	0	0	0	0	0
St. Louis, MO – IL MSA	0	0	0	0	0
San Diego, CA MSA	0	0	0	0	0
San Francisco – Oakland – San Jose, CA CMSA	3	-	-	-	-
Seattle – Tacoma – Bremerton, WA CMSA	1	-	-	-	-
Tampa – St. Petersburg – Clearwater, FL MSA	0	0	0	0	0
Washington – Baltimore, DC – MD – VA – WV CMSA	3	-	-	-	-

Source: U.S. Department of Commerce. Bureau of the Census. *1992 Economic Census Report Series,* CD-ROM 1i, Washington, DC, October 1996. *Notes:* - means no data reported. 1. HS stands for total health service establishments, revenues, employment, or payroll.

★ 405 ★
Establishment Data

Specialty Hospitals, Except Psychiatric; Government by State, Non-Taxed Establishments: 1992

Area	Establish- ments	Revenues in $1,000	Employ- ment	Payroll in $1,000	Payroll per employee
United States	92	3,051,876	59,006	1,721,840	29,181
Alabama	0	0	0	0	0
Alaska	0	0	0	0	0
Arizona	1	-	-	-	-
Arkansas	0	0	0	0	0
California	5	379,126	7,135	273,279	38,301

[Continued]

★ 405 ★

Specialty Hospitals, Except Psychiatric; Government by State, Non-Taxed Establishments: 1992

[Continued]

Area	Establish-ments	Revenues in $1,000	Employ-ment	Payroll in $1,000	Payroll per employee
Colorado	0	0	0	0	0
Connecticut	2	-	-	-	-
Delaware	0	0	0	0	0
District of Columbia	0	0	0	0	0
Florida	2	-	-	-	-
Georgia	1	-	-	-	-
Hawaii	3	-	-	-	-
Idaho	1	-	-	-	-
Illinois	1	-	-	-	-
Indiana	1	-	-	-	-
Iowa	2	-	-	-	-
Kansas	3	-	-	-	-
Kentucky	0	0	0	0	0
Louisiana	3	58,831	972	30,419	31,295
Maine	1	-	-	-	-
Maryland	4	-	-	-	-
Massachusetts	11	153,973	3,732	95,123	25,488
Michigan	1	-	-	-	-
Minnesota	3	104,544	2,508	70,514	28,116
Mississippi	0	0	0	0	0
Missouri	1	-	-	-	-
Montana	0	0	0	0	0
Nebraska	1	-	-	-	-
Nevada	0	0	0	0	0
New Hampshire	0	0	0	0	0
New Jersey	3	92,551	1,949	55,476	28,464
New Mexico	5	65,857	1,807	33,919	18,771
New York	7	422,819	8,045	233,097	28,974
North Carolina	6	53,774	1,109	29,567	26,661
North Dakota	1	-	-	-	-
Ohio	4	112,410	1,737	39,957	23,003
Oklahoma	3	-	-	-	-
Oregon	1	-	-	-	-
Pennsylvania	2	-	-	-	-
Rhode Island	1	-	-	-	-
South Carolina	1	-	-	-	-
South Dakota	0	0	0	0	0
Tennessee	1	-	-	-	-
Texas	3	-	-	-	-
Utah	0	0	0	0	0
Vermont	0	0	0	0	0
Virginia	4	117,826	3,871	73,967	19,108
Washington	2	-	-	-	-
West Virginia	0	0	0	0	0

[Continued]

★ 405 ★

Specialty Hospitals, Except Psychiatric; Government by State, Non-Taxed Establishments: 1992
[Continued]

Area	Establish-ments	Revenues in $1,000	Employ-ment	Payroll in $1,000	Payroll per employee
Wisconsin	1	-	-	-	-
Wyoming	0	0	0	0	0

Source: U.S. Department of Commerce. Bureau of the Census. *1992 Economic Census Report Series,* CD-ROM 1i, Washington, DC, October 1996. *Notes:* - means no data reported. 1. HS stands for total health service establishments, revenues, employment, or payroll.

★ 406 ★

Establishment Data

Specialty Hospitals, Except Psychiatric; Nongovernment by Major Metro Areas, Non-Taxed Establishments: 1992

Area	Establish-ments	Revenues in $1,000	Employ-ment	Payroll in $1,000	Payroll per employee
United States	278	11,359,890	171,687	5,046,888	29,396
Albany – Schenectady – Troy, NY MSA	1	-	-	-	-
Atlanta, GA MSA	6	-	-	-	-
Boston – Worcester – Lawrence, MA – NH – ME – CT CMSA	13	-	-	-	-
Buffalo – Niagara Falls, NY MSA	1	-	-	-	-
Chicago – Gary – Kenosha, IL – IN – WI CMSA	9	-	-	-	-
Cincinnati – Hamilton, OH – KY – IN CMSA	4	-	-	-	-
Cleveland – Akron, OH CMSA	4	-	-	-	-
Columbus, OH MSA	3	-	-	-	-
Dallas – Fort Worth, TX CMSA	5	-	-	-	-
Denver – Boulder – Greeley, CO CMSA	7	-	-	-	-
Detroit – Ann Arbor – Flint, MI CMSA	5	-	-	-	-
Hartford, CT MSA	2	-	-	-	-
Houston – Galveston – Brazoria, TX CMSA	4	-	-	-	-
Indianapolis, IN MSA	3	-	-	-	-
Kansas City, MO – KS MSA	2	-	-	-	-
Los Angeles – Riverside – Orange County, CA CMSA	11	-	-	-	-
Miami – Fort Lauderdale, FL CMSA	3	-	-	-	-
Milwaukee – Racine, WI CMSA	6	-	-	-	-
Minneapolis – St. Paul, MN – WI MSA	6	205,442	3,006	94,055	31,289
New York – Northern New Jersey – Long Island, NY – NJ – CT- CMSA	21	-	-	-	-

[Continued]

★ 406 ★

Specialty Hospitals, Except Psychiatric; Nongovernment by Major Metro Areas, Non-Taxed Establishments: 1992

[Continued]

Area	Establish-ments	Revenues in $1,000	Employ-ment	Payroll in $1,000	Payroll per employee
Philadelphia – Wilmington – Atlantic City, PA – NJ – DE – MD CMSA	17	-	-	-	-
Phoenix – Mesa, AZ MSA	1	-	-	-	-
Pittsburgh, PA MSA	7	389,220	5,747	171,184	29,787
Portland – Salem, OR – WA CMSA	2	-	-	-	-
Providence – Fall River – Warwick, RI – MA MSA	1	-	-	-	-
Sacramento – Yolo, CA CMSA	0	0	0	0	0
St. Louis, MO – IL MSA	7	-	-	-	-
San Diego, CA MSA	3	-	-	-	-
San Francisco – Oakland – San Jose, CA CMSA	5	-	-	-	-
Seattle – Tacoma – Bremerton, WA CMSA	3	-	-	-	-
Tampa – St. Petersburg – Clearwater, FL MSA	3	-	-	-	-
Washington – Baltimore, DC – MD – VA – WV CMSA	11	-	-	-	-

Source: U.S. Department of Commerce. Bureau of the Census. *1992 Economic Census Report Series,* CD-ROM 1i, Washington, DC, October 1996. *Notes:* - means no data reported. 1. HS stands for total health service establishments, revenues, employment, or payroll.

★ 407 ★

Establishment Data

Specialty Hospitals, Except Psychiatric; Nongovernment by State, Non-Taxed Establishments: 1992

Area	Establish-ments	Revenues in $1,000	Employ-ment	Payroll in $1,000	Payroll per employee
United States	278	11,359,890	171,687	5,046,888	29,396
Alabama	4	146,562	2,492	64,744	25,981
Alaska	0	0	0	0	0
Arizona	2	-	-	-	-
Arkansas	3	-	-	-	-
California	22	1,066,729	13,863	478,866	34,543
Colorado	8	296,149	4,658	138,332	29,698
Connecticut	3	-	-	-	-
Delaware	1	-	-	-	-
District of Columbia	4	-	-	-	-
Florida	12	-	-	-	-
Georgia	7	-	-	-	-
Hawaii	3	-	-	-	-

[Continued]

★ 407 ★

Specialty Hospitals, Except Psychiatric; Nongovernment by State, Non-Taxed Establishments: 1992

[Continued]

Area	Establish- ments	Revenues in $1,000	Employ- ment	Payroll in $1,000	Payroll per employee
Idaho	2	-	-	-	-
Illinois	9	-	-	-	-
Indiana	3	-	-	-	-
Iowa	0	0	0	0	0
Kansas	1	-	-	-	-
Kentucky	4	51,177	1,190	27,310	22,950
Louisiana	4	157,404	2,421	65,112	26,895
Maine	1	-	-	-	-
Maryland	7	-	-	-	-
Massachusetts	15	929,219	13,655	446,168	32,674
Michigan	9	-	-	-	-
Minnesota	6	205,442	3,006	94,055	31,289
Mississippi	1	-	-	-	-
Missouri	10	-	-	-	-
Montana	0	0	0	0	0
Nebraska	4	92,506	1,708	44,552	26,084
Nevada	0	0	0	0	0
New Hampshire	2	-	-	-	-
New Jersey	12	279,180	4,435	137,614	31,029
New Mexico	1	-	-	-	-
New York	12	974,583	11,967	460,537	38,484
North Carolina	9	92,294	1,712	47,721	27,874
North Dakota	2	-	-	-	-
Ohio	12	661,124	11,179	306,588	27,425
Oklahoma	3	-	-	-	-
Oregon	4	-	-	-	-
Pennsylvania	29	-	-	-	-
Rhode Island	1	-	-	-	-
South Carolina	5	-	-	-	-
South Dakota	1	-	-	-	-
Tennessee	4	-	-	-	-
Texas	15	-	-	-	-
Utah	4	-	-	-	-
Vermont	0	0	0	0	0
Virginia	5	120,511	2,036	50,469	24,788
Washington	4	-	-	-	-
West Virginia	1	-	-	-	-
Wisconsin	7	-	-	-	-
Wyoming	0	0	0	0	0

Source: U.S. Department of Commerce. Bureau of the Census. *1992 Economic Census Report Series,* CD-ROM 1i, Washington, DC, October 1996. *Notes:* - means no data reported. 1. HS stands for total health service establishments, revenues, employment, or payroll.

Establishments: Ratios

★ 408 ★

Clinics of Doctors of Medicine and Dentists, Ratios, Non-Taxed Establishments, by State: 1992

Area	Sales per establish- ment	Sales per employee	Payroll per employee	Employees per establish- ment	% change in sales 1987 to 1992	% change in payroll 1987 to 1992
United States	5,033,886	105,363	33,569	48	121.10	157.30
Alabama	3,085,200	80,005	32,343	39	134.40	106.10
Alaska	1,137,909	46,705	24,011	24	34.40	42.50
Arizona	2,587,073	89,942	25,749	29	219.20	105.40
Arkansas	644,143	51,239	22,129	13	100.00	99.70
California	10,406,537	237,660	31,181	44	86.60	107.20
Colorado	5,531,508	129,500	26,656	43	-	-
Connecticut	4,603,824	102,508	31,860	45	32.30	49.30
Delaware	680,250	46,119	27,661	15	-	-
District of Columbia	12,812,167	146,518	59,517	87	-	-
Florida	2,257,263	77,093	32,209	29	155.10	217.70
Georgia	2,582,630	73,289	24,186	35	272.70	218.00
Hawaii	-	-	-	-	-	-
Idaho	646,158	45,303	22,358	14	90.80	176.20
Illinois	4,041,932	106,113	32,041	38	73.80	85.50
Indiana	2,009,386	94,464	29,101	21	56.80	20.80
Iowa	2,012,947	60,708	19,763	33	179.60	119.40
Kansas	2,298,700	78,187	21,677	29	142.60	107.90
Kentucky	1,300,763	66,082	23,210	20	130.20	114.10
Louisiana	1,365,412	60,764	24,236	22	150.20	199.20
Maine	771,244	47,766	24,914	16	237.90	221.00
Maryland	7,417,308	101,500	33,995	73	135.10	186.30
Massachusetts	8,818,525	89,347	43,571	99	85.20	175.10
Michigan	4,951,065	98,789	34,559	50	65.90	86.50
Minnesota	14,924,526	73,703	40,623	202	-	-
Mississippi	972,600	53,967	21,676	18	214.80	157.30
Missouri	3,083,882	85,850	34,528	36	140.10	103.50
Montana	474,385	30,530	14,059	16	26.60	9.40
Nebraska	1,951,889	55,946	32,642	35	124.80	298.50
Nevada	-	-	-	-	-	-
New Hampshire	-	-	-	-	-	-
New Jersey	2,671,286	81,798	28,462	33	70.50	70.70
New Mexico	736,870	40,257	18,222	18	190.50	221.80
New York	5,170,765	78,510	34,488	66	170.20	218.70
North Carolina	3,021,038	112,523	19,786	27	232.30	79.30
North Dakota	560,556	55,440	29,571	10	-	-
Ohio	4,351,420	114,131	25,246	38	124.40	123.50
Oklahoma	2,108,765	51,656	26,928	41	77.90	80.00
Oregon	-	-	-	-	-	-

[Continued]

★ 408 ★

Clinics of Doctors of Medicine and Dentists, Ratios, Non-Taxed Establishments, by State: 1992

[Continued]

Area	Sales per establish-ment	Sales per employee	Payroll per employee	Employees per establish-ment	% change in sales 1987 to 1992	% change in payroll 1987 to 1992
Pennsylvania	2,361,422	85,863	40,175	28	233.40	343.10
Rhode Island	-	-	-	-	-	-
South Carolina	970,881	52,145	24,574	19	175.50	153.90
South Dakota	740,000	39,917	23,266	19	47.80	66.70
Tennessee	687,226	50,724	27,748	14	-15.80	-3.20
Texas	1,688,248	61,921	19,888	27	65.40	92.90
Utah	419,750	60,687	21,566	7	-6.30	-12.40
Vermont	1,988,367	97,310	34,625	20	86.60	73.70
Virginia	4,188,092	101,562	29,569	41	86.00	110.50
Washington	8,304,162	88,270	34,134	94	232.50	178.30
West Virginia	1,056,808	52,705	23,455	20	61.90	31.00
Wisconsin	7,515,565	100,082	39,551	75	-	-
Wyoming	-	-	-	-	-	-

Source: U.S. Department of Commerce. Bureau of the Census. *1992 Economic Census Report Series,* CD-ROM 1i, Washington, DC, October 1996. *Note:* - means no data reported.

★ 409 ★

Establishments: Ratios

Commercial Economic, Sociological, and Educational Research Establishments, Ratios by State: 1992

Area	Sales per establish-ment	Sales per employee	Payroll per employee	Employees per establish-ment	% change in sales 1987 to 1992	% change in payroll 1987 to 1992
United States	1,188,445	60,939	22,225	20	34.10	41.80
Alabama	478,148	43,763	17,478	11	25.70	14.00
Alaska	440,867	75,148	29,432	6	96.50	113.00
Arizona	1,084,857	43,372	17,218	25	124.20	107.10
Arkansas	367,000	22,442	7,194	16	103.30	54.90
California	946,623	68,084	24,101	14	25.50	35.00
Colorado	842,210	58,019	20,654	15	39.60	23.50
Connecticut	1,746,871	141,121	41,747	12	88.00	64.90
Delaware	-	-	-	-	-	-
District of Columbia	1,444,083	94,293	38,875	15	55.40	49.80
Florida	1,056,677	59,701	18,095	18	28.10	48.90
Georgia	830,731	43,396	14,155	19	59.60	59.20
Hawaii	-	-	-	-	-	-
Idaho	-	-	-	-	-	-
Illinois	1,564,522	63,947	25,376	24	68.50	94.80

[Continued]

★ 409 ★

Commercial Economic, Sociological, and Educational Research Establishments, Ratios by State: 1992
[Continued]

Area	Sales per establish-ment	Sales per employee	Payroll per employee	Employees per establish-ment	% change in sales 1987 to 1992	% change in payroll 1987 to 1992
Indiana	1,243,649	52,277	21,605	24	45.50	47.70
Iowa	1,283,289	41,858	17,245	31	-46.40	-19.50
Kansas	593,955	14,773	6,648	40	174.90	191.40
Kentucky	902,000	41,797	16,773	22	78.10	130.10
Louisiana	247,407	19,086	7,563	13	-63.50	-45.80
Maine	235,150	38,549	12,902	6	-11.90	-15.90
Maryland	2,337,396	67,915	23,704	34	28.90	50.60
Massachusetts	2,013,463	80,996	31,532	25	118.40	128.40
Michigan	1,505,186	35,867	13,568	42	82.70	110.50
Minnesota	860,630	52,483	19,059	16	68.80	56.10
Mississippi	409,091	42,453	23,406	10	3.50	52.90
Missouri	646,262	38,887	14,241	17	7.10	18.30
Montana	-	-	-	-	-	-
Nebraska	-	-	-	-	-	-
Nevada	-	-	-	-	-	-
New Hampshire	361,286	69,606	24,872	5	44.80	64.00
New Jersey	2,067,690	96,238	29,234	21	92.00	53.60
New Mexico	313,652	24,790	9,529	13	19.30	-5.90
New York	1,392,317	82,333	29,628	17	13.10	21.90
North Carolina	758,724	55,516	18,101	14	141.20	139.70
North Dakota	-	-	-	-	-	-
Ohio	1,418,274	53,693	18,886	26	73.30	63.20
Oklahoma	383,548	25,848	9,209	15	-66.80	-68.10
Oregon	457,963	34,491	13,372	13	86.00	71.20
Pennsylvania	1,375,589	50,144	22,577	27	-11.40	9.90
Rhode Island	-	-	-	-	-	-
South Carolina	291,607	33,463	11,934	9	-11.30	-8.30
South Dakota	-	-	-	-	-	-
Tennessee	-	-	-	-	-	-
Texas	845,638	51,966	20,492	16	4.50	13.90
Utah	380,536	11,494	6,073	33	129.40	135.90
Vermont	413,300	52,987	25,795	8	402.20	488.30
Virginia	1,008,669	50,595	19,550	20	64.10	58.90
Washington	496,651	47,780	17,750	10	11.60	24.70
West Virginia	599,818	25,087	9,236	24	297.00	450.80
Wisconsin	487,866	24,819	10,305	20	120.00	153.10
Wyoming	156,500	96,308	38,923	2	-	-

Source: U.S. Department of Commerce. Bureau of the Census. *1992 Economic Census Report Series,* CD-ROM 1i, Washington, DC, October 1996. *Note:* - means no data reported.

★ 410 ★

Establishments: Ratios

Commercial Economic, Sociological, and Educational Research Establishments, Ratios, Non-Taxed, by State: 1992

Area	Sales per establish-ment	Sales per employee	Payroll per employee	Employees per establish-ment	% change in sales 1987 to 1992	% change in payroll 1987 to 1992
United States	657,414	74,782	28,488	9	112.60	90.70
Alabama	62,750	62,750	17,250	1	-	-
Alaska	-	-	-	-	-	-
Arizona	228,900	67,324	19,500	3	-	-
Arkansas	-	-	-	-	-	-
California	-	-	-	-	-	-
Colorado	-	-	-	-	-	-
Connecticut	360,333	52,732	17,683	7	-	-
Delaware	0	0	0	0	0.00	0.00
District of Columbia	1,016,154	128,669	38,250	8	-	-
Florida	-	-	-	-	-	-
Georgia	373,667	70,063	24,125	5	-	-
Hawaii	-	-	-	-	-	-
Idaho	-	-	-	-	-	-
Illinois	1,672,786	49,722	21,048	34	94.80	81.30
Indiana	-	-	-	-	-	-
Iowa	290,400	58,080	14,480	5	-	-
Kansas	-	-	-	-	-	-
Kentucky	-	-	-	-	-	-
Louisiana	89,000	33,375	15,500	3	-	-
Maine	-	-	-	-	-	-
Maryland	-	-	-	-	-	-
Massachusetts	-	-	-	-	-	-
Michigan	-	-	-	-	-	-
Minnesota	-	-	-	-	-	-
Mississippi	-	-	-	-	-	-
Missouri	279,250	22,796	13,071	12	-	-
Montana	438,571	53,860	21,860	8	406.60	311.20
Nebraska	-	-	-	-	-	-
Nevada	-	-	-	-	-	-
New Hampshire	-	-	-	-	-	-
New Jersey	357,636	60,523	22,585	6	-	-
New Mexico	-	-	-	-	-	-
New York	-	-	-	-	-	-
North Carolina	208,222	50,649	17,568	4	-	-
North Dakota	-	-	-	-	-	-
Ohio	217,182	50,830	21,298	4	-	-
Oklahoma	-	-	-	-	-	-
Oregon	1,080,077	88,867	36,557	12	-	-
Pennsylvania	-	-	-	-	-	-
Rhode Island	-	-	-	-	-	-
South Carolina	-	-	-	-	-	-
South Dakota	-	-	-	-	-	-

[Continued]

★ 410 ★

Commercial Economic, Sociological, and Educational Research Establishments, Ratios, Non-Taxed, by State: 1992

[Continued]

Area	Sales per establish-ment	Sales per employee	Payroll per employee	Employees per establish-ment	% change in sales 1987 to 1992	% change in payroll 1987 to 1992
Tennessee	-	-	-	-	-	-
Texas	-	-	-	-	-	-
Utah	231,000	72,947	29,053	3	-	-
Vermont	-	-	-	-	-	-
Virginia	-	-	-	-	-	-
Washington	-	-	-	-	-	-
West Virginia	-	-	-	-	-	-
Wisconsin	-	-	-	-	-	-
Wyoming	-	-	-	-	-	-

Source: U.S. Department of Commerce. Bureau of the Census. *1992 Economic Census Report Series,* CD-ROM 1i, Washington, DC, October 1996. *Note:* - means no data reported.

★ 411 ★

Establishments: Ratios

Commercial Physical and Biological Research Establishments, Ratios by State: 1992

Area	Sales per establish-ment	Sales per employee	Payroll per employee	Employees per establish-ment	% change in sales 1987 to 1992	% change in payroll 1987 to 1992
United States	3,081,114	106,083	44,904	29	63.50	65.50
Alabama	2,530,214	88,282	41,874	29	31.10	59.40
Alaska	569,250	84,333	34,556	7	368.20	428.10
Arizona	2,392,481	191,104	41,366	13	231.80	108.00
Arkansas	514,077	37,335	24,911	14	152.50	182.90
California	2,854,248	111,035	50,461	26	60.00	73.90
Colorado	1,832,376	95,496	48,114	19	59.10	71.60
Connecticut	1,885,948	130,375	50,184	14	28.40	14.40
Delaware	-	-	-	-	-	-
District of Columbia	-	-	-	-	-	-
Florida	1,112,813	65,045	31,744	17	108.70	146.40
Georgia	787,837	90,620	39,190	9	81.60	87.70
Hawaii	-	-	-	-	-	-
Idaho	-	-	-	-	-	-
Illinois	2,464,432	94,827	44,114	26	201.30	240.60
Indiana	943,371	63,741	25,195	15	98.30	93.20
Iowa	408,923	73,833	24,611	6	23.10	-1.30
Kansas	922,154	67,538	31,699	14	25.40	179.60
Kentucky	565,391	68,442	31,095	8	581.20	816.00

[Continued]

★ 411 ★

Commercial Physical and Biological Research Establishments, Ratios by State: 1992
[Continued]

Area	Sales per establishment	Sales per employee	Payroll per employee	Employees per establishment	% change in sales 1987 to 1992	% change in payroll 1987 to 1992
Louisiana	416,538	83,953	36,597	5	-35.60	-39.50
Maine	343,692	56,557	19,861	6	-7.30	-2.20
Maryland	3,632,319	94,978	39,786	38	79.80	75.90
Massachusetts	3,045,681	126,698	50,899	24	75.10	61.30
Michigan	3,040,053	105,403	41,951	29	121.50	125.00
Minnesota	815,878	101,813	40,757	8	80.90	41.70
Mississippi	479,714	84,655	34,479	6	668.40	469.90
Missouri	1,634,881	138,438	46,510	12	220.40	142.00
Montana	-	-	-	-	-	-
Nebraska	-	-	-	-	-	-
Nevada	12,753,920	102,425	41,985	125	-	-
New Hampshire	783,821	109,735	51,065	7	82.80	115.90
New Jersey	4,966,429	129,442	59,807	38	86.00	111.40
New Mexico	1,983,741	68,568	37,347	29	32.60	57.20
New York	3,525,648	118,246	46,720	30	23.20	15.10
North Carolina	1,410,137	94,009	37,960	15	185.50	166.50
North Dakota	-	-	-	-	-	-
Ohio	4,448,220	100,199	41,029	44	45.40	33.80
Oklahoma	219,947	54,273	21,078	4	70.00	55.90
Oregon	544,305	80,285	35,940	7	119.00	90.90
Pennsylvania	5,080,696	118,656	48,036	43	20.70	19.50
Rhode Island	891,333	76,839	44,851	12	-	-
South Carolina	266,278	106,511	40,644	3	46.40	80.20
South Dakota	-	-	-	-	-	-
Tennessee	-	-	-	-	-	-
Texas	2,280,611	92,274	43,573	25	137.70	110.80
Utah	1,075,525	72,548	33,943	15	29.70	57.90
Vermont	495,778	114,410	42,231	4	481.70	339.20
Virginia	2,311,723	96,484	41,592	24	23.00	23.30
Washington	6,578,247	112,088	41,932	59	89.40	66.50
West Virginia	806,077	105,848	34,354	8	-	-
Wisconsin	2,415,333	105,014	37,117	23	21.60	-0.30
Wyoming	126,600	158,250	51,500	1	-	-

Source: U.S. Department of Commerce. Bureau of the Census. *1992 Economic Census Report Series,* CD-ROM 1i, Washington, DC, October 1996. *Note:* - means no data reported.

.

★412★

Establishments: Ratios

Commercial Physical and Biological Research Establishments Ratios, Non-Taxed Establishments, by State: 1992

Area	Sales per establish- ment	Sales per employee	Payroll per employee	Employees per establish- ment	% change in sales 1987 to 1992	% change in payroll 1987 to 1992
United States	14,472,308	103,777	43,607	139	30.30	30.00
Alabama	-	-	-	-	-	-
Alaska	0	0	0	0	0.00	0.00
Arizona	-	-	-	-	-	-
Arkansas	0	0	0	0	0.00	0.00
California	6,034,855	94,027	45,627	64	-	-
Colorado	-	-	-	-	-	-
Connecticut	-	-	-	-	-	-
Delaware	0	0	0	0	-	-
District of Columbia	2,538,857	103,930	39,135	24	-	-
Florida	1,795,429	80,051	43,739	22	46.70	103.90
Georgia	-	-	-	-	-	-
Hawaii	-	-	-	-	-	-
Idaho	-	-	-	-	-	-
Illinois	74,448,778	78,376	37,743	950	47.50	42.70
Indiana	-	-	-	-	-	-
Iowa	-	-	-	-	-	-
Kansas	-	-	-	-	-	-
Kentucky	-	-	-	-	-	-
Louisiana	-	-	-	-	-	-
Maine	0	0	0	0	-	-
Maryland	23,631,160	126,614	46,670	187	-	-
Massachusetts	36,336,250	100,689	50,354	361	-5.20	26.20
Michigan	-	-	-	-	-	-
Minnesota	317,500	84,667	35,067	4	-	-
Mississippi	2,484,250	52,856	28,027	47	-	-
Missouri	-	-	-	-	-	-
Montana	0	0	0	0	0.00	0.00
Nebraska	-	-	-	-	-	-
Nevada	0	0	0	0	-	-
New Hampshire	-	-	-	-	-	-
New Jersey	-	-	-	-	-	-
New Mexico	2,973,000	47,644	37,003	62	23.00	48.10
New York	11,877,179	81,791	45,260	145	11.80	14.70
North Carolina	-	-	-	-	-	-
North Dakota	0	0	0	0	-	-
Ohio	-	-	-	-	-	-
Oklahoma	-	-	-	-	-	-
Oregon	-	-	-	-	-	-
Pennsylvania	2,801,115	93,132	32,350	30	107.50	122.60
Rhode Island	485,500	55,486	26,143	9	-	-
South Carolina	-	-	-	-	-	-
South Dakota	0	0	0	0	0.00	0.00

[Continued]

★ 412 ★

Commercial Physical and Biological Research Establishments Ratios, Non-Taxed Establishments, by State: 1992

[Continued]

Area	Sales per establish-ment	Sales per employee	Payroll per employee	Employees per establish-ment	% change in sales 1987 to 1992	% change in payroll 1987 to 1992
Tennessee	-	-	-	-	-	-
Texas	-	-	-	-	-	-
Utah	973,750	41,882	19,731	23	-	-
Vermont	0	0	0	0	0.00	0.00
Virginia	34,444,125	114,957	51,912	300	83.40	87.50
Washington	1,872,857	87,400	31,547	21	66.20	60.90
West Virginia	-	-	-	-	-	-
Wisconsin	-	-	-	-	-	-
Wyoming	-	-	-	-	-	-

Source: U.S. Department of Commerce. Bureau of the Census. *1992 Economic Census Report Series,* CD-ROM 1i, Washington, DC, October 1996. *Note:* - means no data reported.

★ 413 ★

Establishments: Ratios

Dental Laboratories, Ratios by State: 1992

Area	Sales per establish-ment	Sales per employee	Payroll per employee	Employees per establish-ment	% change in sales 1987 to 1992	% change in payroll 1987 to 1992
United States	258,863	49,825	21,079	5	22.10	20.60
Alabama	251,183	45,868	20,084	5	24.30	22.30
Alaska	287,917	56,639	23,131	5	-	-
Arizona	220,513	52,337	21,593	4	36.80	30.90
Arkansas	319,372	49,938	18,800	6	44.60	22.40
California	247,017	57,276	20,850	4	25.20	17.20
Colorado	210,734	48,762	20,574	4	35.40	36.70
Connecticut	313,092	59,344	25,763	5	3.60	2.10
Delaware	452,636	38,898	20,789	12	-	-
District of Columbia	147,000	70,304	28,870	2	19.40	21.60
Florida	202,593	46,052	19,786	4	33.00	30.10
Georgia	309,634	46,908	21,652	7	20.10	23.30
Hawaii	276,947	53,694	23,628	5	29.40	42.10
Idaho	203,255	61,237	21,083	3	67.70	46.80
Illinois	271,601	49,029	22,939	6	5.80	21.30
Indiana	295,753	41,400	18,528	7	12.20	10.50
Iowa	276,732	42,528	19,690	7	23.50	20.10
Kansas	610,946	50,686	21,376	12	51.30	37.90
Kentucky	195,792	51,630	20,781	4	36.00	27.20
Louisiana	219,907	44,084	17,984	5	15.10	1.30

[Continued]

★ 413 ★

Dental Laboratories, Ratios by State: 1992

[Continued]

Area	Sales per establish-ment	Sales per employee	Payroll per employee	Employees per establish-ment	% change in sales 1987 to 1992	% change in payroll 1987 to 1992
Maine	287,647	40,413	18,711	7	-1.40	19.50
Maryland	253,708	43,769	21,261	6	-2.20	1.20
Massachusetts	244,345	50,432	22,212	5	4.00	2.50
Michigan	276,401	49,800	22,015	6	23.60	25.10
Minnesota	393,622	47,363	22,668	8	31.60	28.10
Mississippi	206,961	44,536	17,460	5	35.60	27.80
Missouri	295,342	44,545	20,680	7	29.30	29.80
Montana	144,867	73,661	23,034	2	75.10	75.10
Nebraska	278,500	43,135	19,340	6	27.00	23.40
Nevada	194,136	58,109	22,306	3	19.30	2.70
New Hampshire	261,242	51,623	20,880	5	9.80	7.80
New Jersey	301,252	59,826	26,986	5	16.30	25.90
New Mexico	187,500	52,273	17,206	4	31.80	6.10
New York	334,615	53,562	22,635	6	7.70	5.70
North Carolina	190,906	44,896	20,032	4	36.90	51.80
North Dakota	469,833	40,561	22,353	12	17.60	15.20
Ohio	234,098	41,562	18,668	6	13.50	20.90
Oklahoma	208,746	47,810	19,100	4	23.30	14.50
Oregon	228,443	55,521	21,199	4	27.70	25.40
Pennsylvania	262,539	45,504	19,631	6	15.20	17.00
Rhode Island	245,194	63,342	30,217	4	42.60	47.60
South Carolina	195,324	45,177	20,333	4	24.90	27.80
South Dakota	196,440	45,055	13,826	4	59.90	39.30
Tennessee	240,735	52,187	19,975	5	33.00	20.80
Texas	229,130	48,876	19,693	5	32.70	25.70
Utah	261,627	48,256	16,791	5	92.60	68.40
Vermont	169,200	49,765	18,569	3	44.20	35.30
Virginia	213,728	46,657	21,599	5	12.10	16.50
Washington	227,102	55,884	21,493	4	42.60	31.60
West Virginia	327,037	47,219	21,610	7	28.10	41.70
Wisconsin	351,217	43,006	21,159	8	10.90	14.90
Wyoming	91,143	42,533	11,300	2	40.20	3.40

Source: U.S. Department of Commerce. Bureau of the Census. *1992 Economic Census Report Series,* CD-ROM 1i, Washington, DC, October 1996. *Note:* - means no data reported.

★ 414 ★

Establishments: Ratios

General Medical and Surgical Hospitals, Ratios by State: 1992

Area	Sales per establish- ment	Sales per employee	Payroll per employee	Employees per establish- ment	% change in sales 1987 to 1992	% change in payroll 1987 to 1992
United States	34,321,435	74,773	24,797	459	-	-
Alabama	31,291,677	72,554	21,476	431	-	-
Alaska	-	-	-	-	-	-
Arizona	39,755,000	69,930	21,963	569	-	-
Arkansas	21,394,769	68,573	19,633	312	-	-
California	33,987,719	78,210	29,338	435	-	-
Colorado	-	-	-	-	-	-
Connecticut	0	0	0	0	-	-
Delaware	0	0	0	0	-	-
District of Columbia	0	0	0	0	-	-
Florida	43,409,884	76,415	24,765	568	-	-
Georgia	30,769,861	78,807	22,300	390	-	-
Hawaii	-	-	-	-	-	-
Idaho	-	-	-	-	-	-
Illinois	47,578,400	65,916	26,310	722	-	-
Indiana	33,800,400	61,522	20,947	549	-	-
Iowa	-	-	-	-	-	-
Kansas	-	-	-	-	-	-
Kentucky	31,771,217	68,485	23,262	464	-	-
Louisiana	23,520,300	74,449	24,456	316	-	-
Maine	0	0	0	0	-	-
Maryland	-	-	-	-	-	-
Massachusetts	-	-	-	-	-	-
Michigan	0	0	0	0	-	-
Minnesota	0	0	0	0	-	-
Mississippi	15,611,643	59,586	19,923	262	-	-
Missouri	33,962,364	67,131	21,882	506	-	-
Montana	-	-	-	-	-	-
Nebraska	-	-	-	-	-	-
Nevada	-	-	-	-	-	-
New Hampshire	-	-	-	-	-	-
New Jersey	0	0	0	0	-	-
New Mexico	-	-	-	-	-	-
New York	47,331,077	67,423	32,692	702	-	-
North Carolina	29,480,417	69,434	21,954	425	-	-
North Dakota	-	-	-	-	-	-
Ohio	-	-	-	-	-	-
Oklahoma	28,456,364	66,685	21,323	427	-	-
Oregon	-	-	-	-	-	-
Pennsylvania	-	-	-	-	-	-
Rhode Island	0	0	0	0	-	-
South Carolina	37,497,417	71,130	21,394	527	-	-
South Dakota	0	0	0	0	-	-
Tennessee	20,958,271	69,643	22,534	301	-	-
Texas	35,181,382	80,293	24,628	438	-	-

[Continued]

★ 414 ★

General Medical and Surgical Hospitals, Ratios by State: 1992
[Continued]

Area	Sales per establish-ment	Sales per employee	Payroll per employee	Employees per establish-ment	% change in sales 1987 to 1992	% change in payroll 1987 to 1992
Utah	31,927,500	66,395	20,022	481	-	-
Vermont	0	0	0	0	-	-
Virginia	63,116,385	79,863	23,350	790	-	-
Washington	22,549,200	73,355	24,849	307	-	-
West Virginia	18,003,100	64,993	21,462	277	-	-
Wisconsin	-	-	-	-	-	-
Wyoming	-	-	-	-	-	-

Source: U.S. Department of Commerce. Bureau of the Census. *1992 Economic Census Report Series,* CD-ROM 1i, Washington, DC, October 1996. *Note:* - means no data reported.

★ 415 ★
Establishments: Ratios

General Medical and Surgical Hospitals, Ratios, Non-Taxed, by State: 1992

Area	Sales per establish-ment	Sales per employee	Payroll per employee	Employees per establish-ment	% change in sales 1987 to 1992	% change in payroll 1987 to 1992
United States	51,705,531	62,230	27,431	831	-	-
Alabama	41,867,831	61,430	24,688	682	-	-
Alaska	-	-	-	-	-	-
Arizona	51,332,015	67,744	27,461	758	-	-
Arkansas	28,007,877	54,718	22,637	512	-	-
California	77,719,632	76,589	32,250	1,015	-	-
Colorado	44,099,411	63,962	27,149	689	-	-
Connecticut	97,092,615	65,010	32,142	1,494	-	-
Delaware	-	-	-	-	-	-
District of Columbia	182,203,750	73,267	34,044	2,487	-	-
Florida	78,559,353	68,109	28,664	1,153	-	-
Georgia	45,897,291	59,852	25,385	767	-	-
Hawaii	54,336,579	65,858	31,786	825	-	-
Idaho	17,528,103	57,726	23,068	304	-	-
Illinois	64,324,659	60,471	26,142	1,064	-	-
Indiana	51,153,371	58,675	24,343	872	-	-
Iowa	23,140,358	48,577	21,074	476	-	-
Kansas	16,115,761	49,278	22,630	327	-	-
Kentucky	37,538,640	55,585	23,051	675	-	-
Louisiana	41,652,333	57,963	25,078	719	-	-
Maine	30,164,125	53,539	25,283	563	-	-
Maryland	87,314,830	59,006	27,016	1,480	-	-

[Continued]

★ 415 ★

General Medical and Surgical Hospitals, Ratios, Non-Taxed, by State: 1992
[Continued]

Area	Sales per establish- ment	Sales per employee	Payroll per employee	Employees per establish- ment	% change in sales 1987 to 1992	% change in payroll 1987 to 1992
Massachusetts	81,891,358	62,105	28,301	1,319	-	-
Michigan	58,073,419	60,837	27,118	955	-	-
Minnesota	27,751,007	54,141	25,120	513	-	-
Mississippi	23,821,372	54,103	22,575	440	-	-
Missouri	47,359,612	56,170	24,431	843	-	-
Montana	-	-	-	-	-	-
Nebraska	16,786,165	52,047	23,322	323	-	-
Nevada	-	-	-	-	-	-
New Hampshire	-	-	-	-	-	-
New Jersey	87,474,812	64,727	30,138	1,351	-	-
New Mexico	26,310,881	57,929	26,205	454	-	-
New York	97,751,619	63,614	32,470	1,537	-	-
North Carolina	51,907,661	60,555	26,373	857	-	-
North Dakota	15,401,000	49,438	22,071	312	-	-
Ohio	65,745,886	60,199	25,767	1,092	-	-
Oklahoma	23,455,115	52,993	22,798	443	-	-
Oregon	43,380,467	62,643	27,495	693	-	-
Pennsylvania	67,620,769	61,006	27,081	1,108	-	-
Rhode Island	66,982,688	55,930	29,471	1,198	-	-
South Carolina	51,530,226	64,927	26,352	794	-	-
South Dakota	-	-	-	-	-	-
Tennessee	53,455,887	61,403	25,212	871	-	-
Texas	41,404,987	65,321	27,416	634	-	-
Utah	-	-	-	-	-	-
Vermont	-	-	-	-	-	-
Virginia	60,138,517	61,202	26,315	983	-	-
Washington	46,967,909	65,354	29,247	719	-	-
West Virginia	37,580,784	59,128	24,926	636	-	-
Wisconsin	36,509,403	55,553	23,085	657	-	-
Wyoming	-	-	-	-	-	-

Source: U.S. Department of Commerce. Bureau of the Census. *1992 Economic Census Report Series,* CD-ROM 1i, Washington, DC, October 1996. *Note:* - means no data reported.

★416★
Establishments: Ratios

General Medical Clinics, Ratios by State: 1992

Area	Sales per establish-ment	Sales per employee	Payroll per employee	Employees per establish-ment	% change in sales 1987 to 1992	% change in payroll 1987 to 1992
United States	2,658,450	100,448	40,466	26	89.30	87.30
Alabama	1,193,070	59,135	16,919	20	48.20	16.60
Alaska	1,845,667	96,296	27,617	19	110.70	69.00
Arizona	3,798,049	115,024	40,962	33	56.00	44.00
Arkansas	2,483,065	88,406	34,292	28	39.30	47.30
California	6,510,821	107,207	46,545	61	96.30	99.40
Colorado	1,430,173	88,647	31,959	16	40.40	13.30
Connecticut	1,587,023	79,536	31,308	20	58.20	57.90
Delaware	2,415,533	81,606	32,189	30	10.70	58.80
District of Columbia	686,300	149,196	71,304	5	14.60	8.40
Florida	2,283,075	100,141	32,092	23	122.90	122.50
Georgia	1,441,330	72,540	25,483	20	256.50	283.30
Hawaii	1,746,447	121,425	88,139	14	104.50	134.60
Idaho	896,000	68,484	18,611	13	67.20	61.30
Illinois	1,718,466	83,130	30,109	21	52.60	42.60
Indiana	1,241,261	95,232	40,622	13	151.30	132.60
Iowa	983,328	80,995	37,743	12	277.90	336.30
Kansas	1,432,265	79,897	30,476	18	180.00	182.70
Kentucky	1,130,949	81,831	39,028	14	69.80	78.10
Louisiana	1,288,375	90,731	33,334	14	87.40	109.50
Maine	709,917	74,728	38,281	10	71.20	73.00
Maryland	2,052,046	76,579	32,698	27	185.40	170.60
Massachusetts	943,022	104,522	45,313	9	18.10	8.80
Michigan	2,047,635	125,515	31,644	16	57.60	17.30
Minnesota	1,476,522	66,263	32,887	22	32.70	37.80
Mississippi	861,795	93,621	32,240	9	-21.30	-44.50
Missouri	2,553,971	115,901	35,988	22	208.20	243.80
Montana	758,000	75,117	21,090	10	133.10	83.00
Nebraska	1,327,565	71,009	30,686	19	83.10	47.50
Nevada	2,404,386	96,880	33,923	25	134.10	121.00
New Hampshire	2,360,833	126,927	91,715	19	-	-
New Jersey	2,255,034	105,887	43,584	21	255.00	279.60
New Mexico	-	-	-	-	-	-
New York	1,593,455	90,938	39,864	18	65.50	89.20
North Carolina	2,447,039	123,009	37,945	20	187.00	114.30
North Dakota	1,407,400	101,986	20,072	14	77.80	-25.20
Ohio	1,393,124	87,663	37,405	16	43.80	39.40
Oklahoma	1,230,286	66,173	34,056	19	73.30	85.40
Oregon	1,362,820	74,894	31,486	18	121.10	117.90
Pennsylvania	1,404,088	104,063	43,717	13	11.70	0.40
Rhode Island	1,087,917	62,167	23,771	18	100.50	85.70
South Carolina	886,615	79,162	33,834	11	54.70	79.40
South Dakota	867,214	89,272	24,081	10	-	-
Tennessee	1,441,710	86,558	30,536	17	132.80	65.20
Texas	2,097,191	123,131	45,973	17	75.50	63.90

[Continued]

★ 416 ★

General Medical Clinics, Ratios by State: 1992
[Continued]

Area	Sales per establish-ment	Sales per employee	Payroll per employee	Employees per establish-ment	% change in sales 1987 to 1992	% change in payroll 1987 to 1992
Utah	5,281,724	80,616	23,921	66	122.30	155.60
Vermont	592,429	60,985	40,176	10	141.80	153.00
Virginia	1,599,560	71,923	22,755	22	186.80	130.80
Washington	1,355,115	131,589	42,009	10	43.80	52.50
West Virginia	1,253,438	54,945	22,752	23	28.50	97.70
Wisconsin	1,343,784	83,512	47,338	16	54.50	95.20
Wyoming	-	-	-	-	-	-

Source: U.S. Department of Commerce. Bureau of the Census. *1992 Economic Census Report Series,* CD-ROM 1i, Washington, DC, October 1996. *Note:* - means no data reported.

★ 417 ★

Establishments: Ratios

Health Services Establishments, Ratios by State: 1992

Area	Sales per establish-ment	Sales per employee	Payroll per employee	Employees per establish-ment	% change in sales 1987 to 1992	% change in payroll 1987 to 1992
United States	677,073	67,168	28,993	10	64.10	63.80
Alabama	892,387	63,683	27,286	14	71.30	70.40
Alaska	631,478	95,827	38,406	7	46.80	43.90
Arizona	642,693	77,772	33,211	8	77.70	78.60
Arkansas	683,645	57,081	24,932	12	60.80	61.30
California	699,482	80,220	32,176	9	53.50	49.00
Colorado	532,887	67,599	29,694	8	53.70	60.40
Connecticut	744,315	67,919	32,456	11	74.10	80.80
Delaware	658,687	67,984	31,304	10	58.80	62.20
District of Columbia	578,893	82,290	35,749	7	41.40	42.40
Florida	787,358	73,951	30,564	11	80.70	78.50
Georgia	777,831	71,281	30,330	11	81.30	81.10
Hawaii	589,160	83,800	37,688	7	76.50	89.00
Idaho	569,074	58,313	24,571	10	71.70	72.90
Illinois	661,529	65,946	29,821	10	70.20	69.30
Indiana	699,589	57,082	25,735	12	66.90	69.90
Iowa	558,968	52,001	24,728	11	49.20	55.70
Kansas	788,274	57,027	24,745	14	69.40	67.80
Kentucky	747,286	61,429	26,520	12	68.60	75.40
Louisiana	810,155	64,028	25,211	13	64.20	60.90
Maine	545,324	53,521	24,223	10	76.20	79.40
Maryland	616,997	70,639	31,244	9	66.10	64.70
Massachusetts	719,316	59,937	27,856	12	62.90	68.70

[Continued]

★ 417 ★

Health Services Establishments, Ratios by State: 1992

[Continued]

Area	Sales per establish-ment	Sales per employee	Payroll per employee	Employees per establish-ment	% change in sales 1987 to 1992	% change in payroll 1987 to 1992
Michigan	553,510	61,783	29,204	9	40.00	43.70
Minnesota	694,879	54,161	27,478	13	43.90	51.90
Mississippi	675,179	56,570	23,875	12	68.20	67.50
Missouri	652,295	57,972	25,787	11	59.20	56.40
Montana	437,217	60,381	24,060	7	54.20	54.00
Nebraska	659,812	57,657	26,563	11	58.00	62.20
Nevada	969,901	89,095	36,272	11	89.60	95.50
New Hampshire	646,186	61,846	28,255	10	57.10	71.40
New Jersey	630,461	81,529	34,628	8	78.40	75.50
New Mexico	616,119	62,511	26,173	10	52.30	58.40
New York	613,339	71,417	29,628	9	61.00	60.60
North Carolina	750,123	62,044	27,804	12	85.90	79.70
North Dakota	810,023	68,684	33,236	12	38.50	47.40
Ohio	627,191	58,319	27,909	11	59.00	57.60
Oklahoma	613,955	55,451	23,919	11	59.80	57.40
Oregon	524,551	61,466	26,945	9	53.30	51.80
Pennsylvania	581,089	68,511	30,707	8	57.90	57.90
Rhode Island	558,548	58,361	25,745	10	56.00	62.00
South Carolina	674,498	62,607	27,869	11	76.50	83.80
South Dakota	582,442	61,916	28,622	9	56.10	61.80
Tennessee	820,467	67,288	28,623	12	77.70	74.20
Texas	765,334	66,177	26,622	12	69.80	68.90
Utah	604,676	59,740	24,418	10	83.10	79.90
Vermont	435,891	53,721	21,857	8	63.60	59.90
Virginia	684,965	65,379	29,626	10	66.50	72.30
Washington	585,543	61,735	27,231	9	63.40	70.00
West Virginia	664,235	61,924	24,383	11	64.80	58.90
Wisconsin	656,214	55,750	27,580	12	46.50	45.70
Wyoming	454,892	57,629	24,041	8	49.50	49.40

Source: U.S. Department of Commerce. Bureau of the Census. *1992 Economic Census Report Series,* CD-ROM 1i, Washington, DC, October 1996. *Note:* - means no data reported.

★ 418 ★

Establishments: Ratios

Home Health Care Services Establishments, Ratios by State: 1992

Area	Sales per establish- ment	Sales per employee	Payroll per employee	Employees per establish- ment	% change in sales 1987 to 1992	% change in payroll 1987 to 1992
United States	1,294,449	30,460	14,195	42	244.40	207.50
Alabama	1,272,873	28,101	13,692	45	351.20	335.70
Alaska	-	-	-	-	-	-
Arizona	1,247,147	41,804	16,504	30	332.40	204.90
Arkansas	965,958	34,550	12,377	28	366.20	291.40
California	1,354,398	44,770	18,266	30	202.20	142.40
Colorado	826,339	28,612	12,793	29	201.40	168.30
Connecticut	1,533,000	27,922	14,428	55	226.70	231.40
Delaware	703,143	20,900	11,361	34	97.20	64.80
District of Columbia	-	-	-	-	-	-
Florida	1,339,286	36,985	15,748	36	301.30	249.70
Georgia	1,269,521	46,520	20,050	27	388.70	407.70
Hawaii	-	-	-	-	-	-
Idaho	607,700	20,123	11,572	30	358.00	498.10
Illinois	1,736,308	34,612	15,041	50	399.40	290.40
Indiana	1,143,447	26,418	13,295	43	394.60	394.50
Iowa	639,379	22,877	10,505	28	345.80	255.30
Kansas	1,028,598	34,427	13,677	30	650.70	413.10
Kentucky	1,433,059	31,338	14,044	46	270.20	232.30
Louisiana	979,928	38,843	18,688	25	460.40	499.80
Maine	976,341	28,471	11,674	34	749.50	463.90
Maryland	1,460,031	50,959	20,230	29	327.30	252.40
Massachusetts	1,690,607	27,669	12,804	61	160.10	134.50
Michigan	844,315	25,477	13,279	33	161.30	138.90
Minnesota	1,313,111	22,561	12,221	58	328.80	281.10
Mississippi	1,181,065	37,807	17,510	31	765.90	749.40
Missouri	1,102,776	29,771	12,373	37	223.40	150.70
Montana	497,667	38,119	16,149	13	289.00	373.20
Nebraska	1,373,857	29,627	11,803	46	351.60	381.30
Nevada	1,571,886	43,092	18,856	36	525.60	385.50
New Hampshire	595,917	29,030	14,318	21	289.10	241.30
New Jersey	1,455,250	39,005	17,645	37	83.30	94.70
New Mexico	645,696	21,776	10,269	30	328.70	250.90
New York	2,315,517	23,543	13,666	98	175.80	164.40
North Carolina	1,039,439	27,333	14,147	38	382.80	448.80
North Dakota	574,133	21,056	10,423	27	155.10	136.20
Ohio	1,036,677	26,706	12,258	39	238.90	225.90
Oklahoma	1,227,565	42,398	17,707	29	457.50	333.10
Oregon	616,178	26,228	12,790	23	251.70	220.80
Pennsylvania	1,059,582	28,454	12,907	37	158.60	124.10
Rhode Island	796,280	23,614	11,203	34	121.30	119.50
South Carolina	835,319	28,667	14,018	29	-	-
South Dakota	218,286	7,242	3,853	30	77.10	89.50
Tennessee	1,535,597	47,369	19,962	32	349.10	288.40
Texas	1,324,390	21,215	10,040	62	253.90	194.70

[Continued]

★ 418 ★

Home Health Care Services Establishments, Ratios by State: 1992
[Continued]

Area	Sales per establish-ment	Sales per employee	Payroll per employee	Employees per establish-ment	% change in sales 1987 to 1992	% change in payroll 1987 to 1992
Utah	1,113,186	27,557	13,040	40	777.00	788.60
Vermont	520,182	21,271	12,394	24	-	-
Virginia	950,670	23,071	11,615	41	180.60	160.30
Washington	1,223,267	29,548	13,407	41	177.90	161.70
West Virginia	831,417	28,164	12,241	30	242.80	237.10
Wisconsin	1,034,524	20,869	12,077	50	108.00	116.10
Wyoming	276,824	16,512	8,986	17	208.40	303.90

Source: U.S. Department of Commerce. Bureau of the Census. *1992 Economic Census Report Series,* CD-ROM 1i, Washington, DC, October 1996. *Note:* - means no data reported.

★ 419 ★

Establishments: Ratios

Home Health Care Services Establishments, Ratios, Non-Taxed, by State: 1992

Area	Sales per establish-ment	Sales per employee	Payroll per employee	Employees per establish-ment	% change in sales 1987 to 1992	% change in payroll 1987 to 1992
United States	2,579,640	29,541	16,733	87	171.70	160.70
Alabama	1,742,091	28,903	16,073	60	131.60	162.50
Alaska	-	-	-	-	-	-
Arizona	2,476,667	31,251	16,865	79	-	-
Arkansas	1,325,500	22,215	10,971	60	594.60	513.00
California	2,718,953	41,931	24,182	65	164.70	206.00
Colorado	1,253,951	28,658	15,203	44	290.20	224.90
Connecticut	2,523,875	33,291	18,984	76	103.90	91.50
Delaware	2,690,667	30,460	18,150	88	161.00	163.30
District of Columbia	-	-	-	-	-	-
Florida	3,075,400	50,260	20,748	61	271.40	208.80
Georgia	1,594,291	48,472	23,004	33	155.60	171.70
Hawaii	1,136,600	30,719	20,978	37	437.10	501.20
Idaho	-	-	-	-	-	-
Illinois	1,665,200	30,825	17,165	54	214.10	189.80
Indiana	1,516,104	29,874	17,477	51	187.00	174.80
Iowa	896,295	28,230	14,807	32	317.40	229.00
Kansas	1,006,091	33,587	16,865	30	171.20	154.10
Kentucky	1,339,333	43,453	19,950	31	240.70	204.10
Louisiana	908,000	47,169	23,558	19	10.00	5.50
Maine	1,230,947	29,756	17,495	41	115.10	121.80
Maryland	1,650,538	37,743	22,344	44	180.00	225.40

[Continued]

★ 419 ★

Home Health Care Services Establishments, Ratios, Non-Taxed, by State: 1992
[Continued]

Area	Sales per establish-ment	Sales per employee	Payroll per employee	Employees per establish-ment	% change in sales 1987 to 1992	% change in payroll 1987 to 1992
Massachusetts	2,847,701	36,561	19,580	78	200.90	185.40
Michigan	2,224,258	40,552	20,190	55	254.70	215.20
Minnesota	2,039,129	28,864	16,463	71	-	-
Mississippi	3,677,417	38,880	21,933	95	75.10	102.00
Missouri	1,640,184	30,197	16,444	54	55.90	58.10
Montana	1,948,250	8,932	6,319	218	204.10	241.20
Nebraska	-	-	-	-	-	-
Nevada	-	-	-	-	-	-
New Hampshire	938,674	23,210	14,025	40	184.70	166.20
New Jersey	3,693,763	33,487	18,157	110	202.10	191.60
New Mexico	1,045,864	18,160	11,232	58	285.00	252.20
New York	8,942,889	29,370	18,953	304	155.80	146.90
North Carolina	2,277,393	31,420	16,691	72	468.50	469.60
North Dakota	-	-	-	-	-	-
Ohio	1,726,452	33,408	17,133	52	159.50	134.90
Oklahoma	-	-	-	-	-	-
Oregon	3,254,933	39,122	15,486	83	-	-
Pennsylvania	1,773,715	35,100	18,350	51	109.80	101.60
Rhode Island	3,079,650	41,035	22,544	75	199.40	171.80
South Carolina	1,821,444	39,406	20,822	46	71.90	75.90
South Dakota	-	-	-	-	-	-
Tennessee	2,007,718	39,209	18,617	51	284.80	273.50
Texas	2,175,326	10,721	6,433	203	167.60	144.80
Utah	-	-	-	-	-	-
Vermont	-	-	-	-	-	-
Virginia	1,891,968	32,085	17,006	59	234.10	198.90
Washington	2,232,804	25,138	15,086	89	207.70	202.00
West Virginia	1,683,625	34,894	15,842	48	397.50	338.20
Wisconsin	1,517,554	22,358	12,837	68	-	-
Wyoming	-	-	-	-	-	-

Source: U.S. Department of Commerce. Bureau of the Census. *1992 Economic Census Report Series,* CD-ROM 1i, Washington, DC, October 1996. *Note:* - means no data reported.

★ 420 ★

Establishments: Ratios

Hospitals, Ratios by State: 1992

Area	Sales per establish-ment	Sales per employee	Payroll per employee	Employees per establish-ment	% change in sales 1987 to 1992	% change in payroll 1987 to 1992
United States	22,154,651	72,598	24,656	305	57.60	60.40
Alabama	25,964,762	73,888	21,970	351	92.70	88.20
Alaska	-	-	-	-	-	-
Arizona	19,332,042	69,675	23,381	277	141.30	112.50
Arkansas	16,118,708	68,761	20,941	234	103.30	105.30
California	23,063,980	76,265	28,666	302	32.60	45.40
Colorado	17,229,769	78,592	26,232	219	-19.00	-13.50
Connecticut	-	-	-	-	-	-
Delaware	7,883,667	59,725	23,528	132	-	-
District of Columbia	-	-	-	-	-	-
Florida	29,971,613	75,588	24,654	397	69.00	74.90
Georgia	23,244,086	78,109	22,345	298	77.50	67.60
Hawaii	-	-	-	-	-	-
Idaho	15,037,700	64,072	21,086	235	125.90	89.50
Illinois	27,360,107	68,917	26,823	397	114.00	122.40
Indiana	13,943,500	68,739	21,918	203	124.90	132.00
Iowa	-	-	-	-	-	-
Kansas	27,871,412	72,984	24,711	382	95.40	67.10
Kentucky	25,434,656	68,115	23,180	373	41.40	52.20
Louisiana	16,789,653	71,268	23,485	236	50.40	58.10
Maine	-	-	-	-	-	-
Maryland	12,447,750	54,180	22,632	230	4.60	13.10
Massachusetts	14,336,263	55,409	28,750	259	29.60	45.40
Michigan	7,968,200	55,800	21,032	143	46.80	27.40
Minnesota	-	-	-	-	-	-
Mississippi	13,533,714	61,278	20,426	221	103.40	101.00
Missouri	19,584,125	65,940	22,373	297	78.90	64.30
Montana	4,943,000	61,788	24,991	80	57.90	62.70
Nebraska	-	-	-	-	-	-
Nevada	46,970,167	94,650	28,055	496	54.60	70.30
New Hampshire	14,222,333	56,196	22,089	253	36.20	60.80
New Jersey	22,624,800	71,507	22,247	316	7.90	-5.80
New Mexico	19,724,750	60,879	22,536	324	29.90	48.90
New York	31,021,379	64,795	31,075	479	29.10	38.20
North Carolina	19,435,630	69,782	22,611	279	67.50	59.30
North Dakota	-	-	-	-	-	-
Ohio	11,207,308	55,167	21,368	203	201.50	186.60
Oklahoma	17,613,500	65,732	21,598	268	70.70	63.10
Oregon	13,067,636	61,905	22,227	211	48.80	20.80
Pennsylvania	12,776,480	62,300	24,741	205	44.70	60.90
Rhode Island	0	0	0	0	0.00	0.00
South Carolina	24,691,000	71,273	22,033	346	92.60	85.90
South Dakota	-	-	-	-	-	-
Tennessee	18,382,031	68,450	22,550	269	49.90	55.00
Texas	22,864,278	77,400	24,422	295	71.00	73.00

[Continued]

★ 420 ★

Hospitals, Ratios by State: 1992
[Continued]

Area	Sales per establish- ment	Sales per employee	Payroll per employee	Employees per establish- ment	% change in sales 1987 to 1992	% change in payroll 1987 to 1992
Utah	18,940,471	65,538	20,572	289	191.20	142.30
Vermont	0	0	0	0	0.00	0.00
Virginia	29,632,147	73,934	22,565	401	44.70	50.00
Washington	15,041,333	68,892	24,202	218	11.40	-0.20
West Virginia	14,731,294	65,132	21,730	226	86.00	72.60
Wisconsin	7,131,500	55,337	18,260	129	117.00	55.60
Wyoming	-	-	-	-	-	-

Source: U.S. Department of Commerce. Bureau of the Census. *1992 Economic Census Report Series,* CD-ROM 1i, Washington, DC, October 1996. *Note:* - means no data reported.

★ 421 ★

Establishments: Ratios

Hospitals, Ratios, Non-Taxed Establishments, by State: 1992

Area	Sales per establish- ment	Sales per employee	Payroll per employee	Employees per establish- ment	% change in sales 1987 to 1992	% change in payroll 1987 to 1992
United States	48,930,424	61,261	27,638	799	62.60	53.30
Alabama	41,063,041	59,987	24,815	685	75.40	63.50
Alaska	22,950,115	78,102	35,908	294	56.00	46.00
Arizona	47,375,776	67,322	27,386	704	55.80	51.00
Arkansas	28,398,026	54,128	22,635	525	65.30	58.70
California	73,981,074	75,309	32,483	982	57.60	44.60
Colorado	41,977,253	62,778	27,504	669	72.70	57.80
Connecticut	67,545,302	64,228	32,680	1,052	65.30	56.30
Delaware	67,646,462	62,307	29,048	1,086	96.10	71.30
District of Columbia	159,077,000	70,471	33,232	2,257	55.60	50.40
Florida	69,424,562	66,763	28,478	1,040	75.30	65.60
Georgia	44,284,184	58,547	25,392	756	71.40	55.10
Hawaii	45,985,741	63,731	31,001	722	67.30	75.20
Idaho	16,594,386	55,826	23,180	297	80.00	66.40
Illinois	60,913,520	59,628	26,370	1,022	50.10	41.40
Indiana	45,462,336	57,485	24,642	791	63.80	53.60
Iowa	23,036,397	47,983	21,819	480	54.00	49.30
Kansas	16,430,641	47,737	23,001	344	52.80	43.40
Kentucky	35,122,375	54,763	22,971	641	78.50	62.60
Louisiana	39,050,895	57,525	25,119	679	64.90	58.00
Maine	28,714,622	52,552	25,669	546	59.10	56.60
Maryland	72,480,603	58,834	27,448	1,232	65.40	54.70
Massachusetts	66,967,362	61,287	28,916	1,093	53.90	43.50

[Continued]

★ 421 ★

Hospitals, Ratios, Non-Taxed Establishments, by State: 1992
[Continued]

Area	Sales per establish-ment	Sales per employee	Payroll per employee	Employees per establish-ment	% change in sales 1987 to 1992	% change in payroll 1987 to 1992
Michigan	54,376,263	60,706	27,547	896	49.40	40.70
Minnesota	28,128,157	54,028	25,902	521	50.00	45.30
Mississippi	24,159,629	52,126	22,204	463	65.90	49.00
Missouri	44,685,053	55,284	24,276	808	55.00	50.40
Montana	13,853,115	54,554	23,745	254	52.60	52.80
Nebraska	16,945,347	51,162	23,560	331	64.30	62.40
Nevada	36,665,000	74,712	29,301	491	86.80	56.40
New Hampshire	37,248,310	60,867	26,576	612	73.60	59.50
New Jersey	74,843,723	62,941	30,244	1,189	81.30	73.80
New Mexico	24,361,549	54,801	25,623	445	64.40	63.00
New York	90,312,660	62,410	32,661	1,447	61.80	58.70
North Carolina	46,831,306	59,397	26,492	788	92.40	81.40
North Dakota	15,055,071	48,428	22,276	311	48.30	50.80
Ohio	60,231,065	59,606	26,144	1,010	50.60	37.20
Oklahoma	22,296,730	52,325	22,942	426	43.70	37.90
Oregon	39,585,897	61,840	27,862	640	59.40	60.30
Pennsylvania	61,245,803	60,951	27,484	1,005	57.50	51.80
Rhode Island	59,893,952	55,462	29,287	1,080	44.00	44.90
South Carolina	46,045,042	63,667	26,186	723	91.50	68.70
South Dakota	13,304,397	48,635	22,050	274	62.50	50.60
Tennessee	50,398,027	60,415	25,150	834	70.80	59.00
Texas	42,133,374	63,822	27,287	660	77.80	62.20
Utah	33,458,564	57,761	24,818	579	51.50	50.20
Vermont	30,315,333	55,784	25,843	543	65.00	57.80
Virginia	53,575,074	58,425	25,825	917	72.90	61.30
Washington	45,986,055	65,778	29,477	699	84.20	78.00
West Virginia	36,231,182	58,129	24,789	623	58.70	38.80
Wisconsin	34,937,926	54,846	23,282	637	62.40	48.10
Wyoming	12,060,207	48,799	23,178	247	35.70	28.10

Source: U.S. Department of Commerce. Bureau of the Census. *1992 Economic Census Report Series,* CD-ROM 1i, Washington, DC, October 1996. *Note:* - means no data reported.

★ 422 ★

Establishments: Ratios

Intermediate Care Facilities, Ratios by State: 1992

Area	Sales per establish-ment	Sales per employee	Payroll per employee	Employees per establish-ment	% change in sales 1987 to 1992	% change in payroll 1987 to 1992
United States	1,246,546	25,543	12,189	49	92.10	91.70
Alabama	1,106,364	25,041	10,019	44	26.50	6.80
Alaska	0	0	0	0	0.00	0.00
Arizona	936,900	44,403	16,370	21	53.50	11.50
Arkansas	1,492,500	21,497	10,566	69	20.60	29.90
California	675,068	26,512	13,904	25	45.00	62.50
Colorado	531,963	25,740	12,446	21	29.20	28.80
Connecticut	1,995,974	41,672	19,502	48	53.00	37.70
Delaware	-	-	-	-	-	-
District of Columbia	-	-	-	-	-	-
Florida	1,658,012	31,117	13,882	53	112.80	112.80
Georgia	1,042,958	26,404	12,455	40	40.80	30.70
Hawaii	3,467,857	38,654	17,524	90	-	-
Idaho	-	-	-	-	-	-
Illinois	1,504,252	27,802	11,063	54	183.00	147.10
Indiana	1,290,870	27,550	12,419	47	128.20	130.00
Iowa	1,173,825	20,413	10,713	58	85.90	101.10
Kansas	1,104,857	20,162	10,564	55	76.10	83.50
Kentucky	1,978,203	25,739	11,941	77	83.40	96.40
Louisiana	1,773,861	24,964	10,183	71	91.80	69.40
Maine	2,068,271	26,482	14,065	78	255.00	237.40
Maryland	1,471,818	27,487	13,704	54	39.80	30.80
Massachusetts	1,438,679	29,438	16,861	49	72.50	81.60
Michigan	819,628	23,590	12,534	35	60.70	65.10
Minnesota	441,919	20,679	11,656	21	39.50	47.40
Mississippi	2,677,000	25,770	10,416	104	160.70	114.80
Missouri	764,736	20,456	9,294	37	73.20	63.80
Montana	-	-	-	-	-	-
Nebraska	-	-	-	-	-	-
Nevada	760,143	25,705	11,019	30	-	-
New Hampshire	-	-	-	-	-	-
New Jersey	1,599,000	35,732	16,673	45	-4.70	-6.00
New Mexico	2,145,333	28,352	12,969	76	88.60	91.90
New York	1,570,759	30,695	14,823	51	28.90	47.30
North Carolina	883,639	24,786	12,109	36	126.90	122.10
North Dakota	-	-	-	-	-	-
Ohio	1,390,192	26,808	13,123	52	43.20	39.60
Oklahoma	1,175,282	20,574	9,778	57	112.80	124.90
Oregon	1,378,060	22,407	13,236	62	101.50	151.60
Pennsylvania	1,212,526	31,716	14,907	38	84.00	99.30
Rhode Island	-	-	-	-	-	-
South Carolina	865,444	29,729	12,901	29	0.50	-12.90
South Dakota	-	-	-	-	-	-
Tennessee	2,071,165	24,852	10,627	83	237.90	246.30
Texas	969,312	23,851	10,923	41	55.50	52.80

[Continued]

★ 422 ★

Intermediate Care Facilities, Ratios by State: 1992
[Continued]

Area	Sales per establish-ment	Sales per employee	Payroll per employee	Employees per establish-ment	% change in sales 1987 to 1992	% change in payroll 1987 to 1992
Utah	-	-	-	-	-	-
Vermont	1,068,923	22,818	11,833	47	63.00	53.60
Virginia	2,497,676	26,725	13,650	93	163.50	212.90
Washington	1,259,905	29,075	14,496	43	28.30	23.20
West Virginia	1,533,261	26,824	11,612	57	521.20	477.30
Wisconsin	668,907	26,836	14,772	25	44.50	45.00
Wyoming	-	-	-	-	-	-

Source: U.S. Department of Commerce. Bureau of the Census. *1992 Economic Census Report Series,* CD-ROM 1i, Washington, DC, October 1996. *Note:* - means no data reported.

★ 423 ★

Establishments: Ratios

Kidney Dialysis Centers, Ratios by State: 1992

Area	Sales per establish-ment	Sales per employee	Payroll per employee	Employees per establish-ment	% change in sales 1987 to 1992	% change in payroll 1987 to 1992
United States	1,841,164	97,205	26,332	19	149.80	129.40
Alabama	1,949,188	104,479	22,002	19	254.40	166.50
Alaska	0	0	0	0	0.00	0.00
Arizona	1,322,842	79,790	21,143	17	155.10	184.40
Arkansas	814,176	87,601	24,753	9	151.50	264.50
California	1,794,528	91,474	28,537	20	91.80	83.50
Colorado	1,909,167	83,309	33,364	23	128.90	133.90
Connecticut	2,595,600	100,605	32,357	26	-	-
Delaware	-	-	-	-	-	-
District of Columbia	2,096,091	92,972	26,581	23	-	-
Florida	1,330,496	89,106	23,014	15	143.50	120.70
Georgia	1,378,450	101,731	22,185	14	92.60	58.20
Hawaii	0	0	0	0	0.00	0.00
Idaho	0	0	0	0	0.00	0.00
Illinois	1,656,921	80,618	25,119	21	80.20	131.10
Indiana	2,537,231	151,303	26,670	17	-	-
Iowa	-	-	-	-	-	-
Kansas	2,309,429	95,657	24,225	24	191.90	98.80
Kentucky	1,757,273	93,835	21,549	19	-	-
Louisiana	1,382,643	100,687	24,049	14	124.60	79.30
Maine	2,962,000	113,923	23,577	26	-	-
Maryland	1,659,182	91,714	26,236	18	212.20	180.10
Massachusetts	-	-	-	-	-	-

[Continued]

★ 423 ★

Kidney Dialysis Centers, Ratios by State: 1992

[Continued]

Area	Sales per establish-ment	Sales per employee	Payroll per employee	Employees per establish-ment	% change in sales 1987 to 1992	% change in payroll 1987 to 1992
Michigan	2,563,143	98,854	24,873	26	-	-
Minnesota	-	-	-	-	-	-
Mississippi	1,207,692	81,771	25,292	15	249.20	218.00
Missouri	1,543,563	107,847	27,166	14	185.90	191.90
Montana	0	0	0	0	0.00	0.00
Nebraska	0	0	0	0	0.00	0.00
Nevada	-	-	-	-	-	-
New Hampshire	-	-	-	-	-	-
New Jersey	-	-	-	-	-	-
New Mexico	1,412,222	101,680	29,008	14	86.00	142.10
New York	3,141,290	87,967	30,890	36	154.30	124.90
North Carolina	2,003,234	110,119	24,710	18	236.80	164.30
North Dakota	0	0	0	0	0.00	0.00
Ohio	2,280,200	109,275	26,326	21	309.20	238.70
Oklahoma	967,429	114,780	29,746	8	216.40	142.70
Oregon	1,878,833	109,447	29,922	17	-	-
Pennsylvania	2,007,935	88,923	25,266	23	101.90	87.50
Rhode Island	-	-	-	-	-	-
South Carolina	1,459,655	87,459	22,184	17	92.30	88.10
South Dakota	0	0	0	0	0.00	0.00
Tennessee	3,911,000	91,038	27,443	43	779.20	815.10
Texas	2,241,936	121,264	28,159	18	251.90	192.80
Utah	-	-	-	-	-	-
Vermont	0	0	0	0	0.00	0.00
Virginia	1,342,182	98,921	24,739	14	128.80	98.50
Washington	-	-	-	-	-	-
West Virginia	-	-	-	-	-	-
Wisconsin	2,058,800	110,688	32,075	19	-	-
Wyoming	-	-	-	-	-	-

Source: U.S. Department of Commerce. Bureau of the Census. *1992 Economic Census Report Series,* CD-ROM 1i, Washington, DC, October 1996. *Note:* - means no data reported.

★ 424 ★

Establishments: Ratios

Medical Equipment Rental and Leasing Establishments, Ratios by State: 1992

Area	Sales per establish-ment	Sales per employee	Payroll per employee	Employees per establish-ment	% change in sales 1987 to 1992	% change in payroll 1987 to 1992
United States	949,281	100,117	24,684	9	107.40	119.90
Alabama	452,452	77,492	16,102	6	46.90	45.60
Alaska	-	-	-	-	-	-
Arizona	922,041	106,306	27,812	9	149.50	131.40
Arkansas	512,803	94,014	19,858	5	128.90	115.10
California	1,382,595	118,041	28,033	12	114.90	111.20
Colorado	1,224,250	98,645	23,771	12	294.40	311.30
Connecticut	1,231,813	96,377	24,244	13	546.70	570.00
Delaware	937,000	137,122	24,902	7	-	-
District of Columbia	0	0	0	0	-	-
Florida	583,612	96,223	23,524	6	148.30	122.80
Georgia	669,415	87,517	23,765	8	93.50	96.90
Hawaii	1,857,333	132,667	24,738	14	160.90	225.20
Idaho	432,500	86,500	23,250	5	-	-
Illinois	1,161,624	117,194	27,634	10	-6.90	10.20
Indiana	1,524,424	102,561	20,893	15	129.90	86.20
Iowa	673,952	107,627	21,783	6	59.50	26.90
Kansas	1,034,032	101,120	20,319	10	105.50	93.70
Kentucky	531,440	81,279	20,286	7	258.90	246.80
Louisiana	615,154	86,221	18,941	7	97.80	73.90
Maine	685,900	83,646	24,067	8	81.80	125.80
Maryland	1,506,956	114,356	30,047	13	139.10	244.80
Massachusetts	1,297,349	152,203	27,291	9	214.00	125.70
Michigan	1,006,612	100,273	26,596	10	120.50	108.00
Minnesota	1,449,606	99,041	21,781	15	66.00	75.10
Mississippi	492,643	89,571	18,208	6	116.40	128.30
Missouri	1,097,235	94,446	22,191	12	124.00	101.30
Montana	336,882	64,348	18,697	5	88.60	104.40
Nebraska	716,552	88,803	20,444	8	157.60	111.30
Nevada	869,480	109,231	24,980	8	239.50	258.90
New Hampshire	630,368	114,067	25,448	6	185.30	81.20
New Jersey	2,665,934	113,064	36,812	24	155.10	333.50
New Mexico	624,609	117,754	20,721	5	41.30	39.90
New York	940,292	93,854	27,434	10	99.10	153.10
North Carolina	806,125	96,542	24,099	8	189.30	189.60
North Dakota	817,444	74,313	17,465	11	178.70	285.10
Ohio	1,131,018	94,811	22,768	12	153.30	138.10
Oklahoma	547,250	85,843	17,977	6	60.80	66.50
Oregon	904,923	92,630	21,043	10	269.30	245.30
Pennsylvania	1,105,739	86,688	23,731	13	112.60	120.20
Rhode Island	-	-	-	-	-	-
South Carolina	668,387	92,089	21,924	7	127.10	188.80
South Dakota	-	-	-	-	-	-

[Continued]

★ 424 ★

Medical Equipment Rental and Leasing Establishments, Ratios by State: 1992

[Continued]

Area	Sales per establish- ment	Sales per employee	Payroll per employee	Employees per establish- ment	% change in sales 1987 to 1992	% change in payroll 1987 to 1992
Tennessee	656,559	89,651	22,228	7	125.10	97.90
Texas	752,853	88,773	22,053	8	13.90	38.60
Utah	1,053,714	142,761	21,948	7	543.10	551.70
Vermont	514,800	73,543	18,571	7	-18.40	-4.10
Virginia	628,872	77,705	21,421	8	179.80	231.00
Washington	1,295,686	90,698	21,810	14	200.30	204.90
West Virginia	954,889	114,282	22,181	8	72.80	84.50
Wisconsin	835,360	123,574	22,417	7	193.00	141.00
Wyoming	398,105	75,640	17,420	5	290.70	213.30

Source: U.S. Department of Commerce. Bureau of the Census. *1992 Economic Census Report Series,* CD-ROM 1i, Washington, DC, October 1996. *Note:* - means no data reported.

★ 425 ★

Establishments: Ratios

Medical Laboratories, Ratios by State: 1992

Area	Sales per establish- ment	Sales per employee	Payroll per employee	Employees per establish- ment	% change in sales 1987 to 1992	% change in payroll 1987 to 1992
United States	1,483,440	90,165	28,682	16	126.70	111.30
Alabama	1,456,302	80,443	25,808	18	95.40	97.80
Alaska	736,133	107,204	35,825	7	177.70	211.40
Arizona	1,237,591	100,623	34,331	12	90.10	115.20
Arkansas	1,002,318	87,504	26,935	11	145.40	116.00
California	1,596,122	99,652	31,833	16	124.40	97.30
Colorado	1,078,480	84,688	26,808	13	154.60	133.10
Connecticut	1,208,477	87,344	30,641	14	131.90	186.90
Delaware	873,828	85,323	28,049	10	-	-
District of Columbia	1,032,000	177,375	84,313	6	169.10	328.90
Florida	1,000,233	89,720	24,219	11	146.30	123.70
Georgia	1,430,500	99,802	30,250	14	111.20	99.40
Hawaii	2,096,030	86,246	29,918	24	113.10	100.50
Idaho	915,560	86,701	24,470	11	49.90	33.10
Illinois	1,215,039	86,470	26,697	14	97.70	73.30
Indiana	1,392,744	86,232	32,179	16	110.50	118.80
Iowa	1,228,980	78,822	27,427	16	57.90	35.10
Kansas	3,230,321	105,974	30,449	30	142.30	186.00
Kentucky	1,630,128	86,915	25,303	19	186.70	154.00
Louisiana	1,138,610	80,109	24,577	14	129.40	108.10

[Continued]

★ 425 ★

Medical Laboratories, Ratios by State: 1992
[Continued]

Area	Sales per establish-ment	Sales per employee	Payroll per employee	Employees per establish-ment	% change in sales 1987 to 1992	% change in payroll 1987 to 1992
Maine	1,424,750	108,111	23,485	13	232.60	126.20
Maryland	1,587,439	74,932	27,467	21	129.40	128.50
Massachusetts	1,998,369	97,407	32,011	21	93.80	93.70
Michigan	1,879,964	75,800	25,965	25	90.90	97.90
Minnesota	1,572,115	104,579	32,683	15	98.80	107.80
Mississippi	1,184,036	73,501	21,015	16	113.40	77.80
Missouri	1,264,080	109,192	33,093	12	53.00	20.50
Montana	589,286	84,760	30,856	7	52.50	80.30
Nebraska	1,372,111	73,506	30,526	19	72.70	69.40
Nevada	2,382,420	100,950	30,437	24	278.90	200.00
New Hampshire	951,974	64,681	23,228	15	155.10	149.10
New Jersey	2,571,931	115,841	34,949	22	207.20	168.90
New Mexico	1,208,032	85,696	24,286	14	99.10	78.40
New York	1,431,118	89,706	29,502	16	105.40	131.00
North Carolina	3,866,485	91,530	21,957	42	324.20	253.40
North Dakota	1,384,813	130,335	42,294	11	144.90	106.10
Ohio	1,388,540	73,439	23,158	19	164.80	131.90
Oklahoma	1,110,258	81,587	33,406	14	172.10	147.40
Oregon	1,215,914	68,974	30,614	18	71.70	65.30
Pennsylvania	1,312,331	89,257	25,616	15	96.70	68.10
Rhode Island	669,141	70,517	29,879	9	122.20	124.20
South Carolina	1,101,400	89,951	25,731	12	-	-
South Dakota	3,317,000	114,379	59,204	29	111.60	112.80
Tennessee	2,357,154	92,914	31,208	25	153.70	98.10
Texas	1,237,830	91,452	28,253	14	106.80	98.30
Utah	1,787,295	72,816	25,145	25	106.10	98.60
Vermont	546,875	71,721	19,918	8	58.50	6.40
Virginia	1,550,699	72,734	26,233	21	105.00	105.00
Washington	1,407,105	81,609	29,440	17	94.20	96.90
West Virginia	1,043,327	111,423	24,225	9	223.40	103.00
Wisconsin	1,735,238	69,509	25,763	25	210.50	209.20
Wyoming	429,800	93,435	21,022	5	108.90	50.90

Source: U.S. Department of Commerce. Bureau of the Census. *1992 Economic Census Report Series,* CD-ROM 1i, Washington, DC, October 1996. *Note:* - means no data reported.

★ 426 ★

Establishments: Ratios

Nursing and Personal Care Facilities Establishments, Ratios, Non-Taxed, by State: 1992

Area	Sales per establish-ment	Sales per employee	Payroll per employee	Employees per establish-ment	% change in sales 1987 to 1992	% change in payroll 1987 to 1992
United States	2,568,859	30,570	15,246	84	85.60	78.00
Alabama	1,626,333	20,484	9,902	79	74.70	79.90
Alaska	2,856,200	43,232	21,031	66	85.20	74.30
Arizona	2,334,671	33,462	15,049	70	72.50	67.40
Arkansas	1,036,844	26,271	11,082	39	165.00	103.00
California	2,327,352	34,656	16,620	67	43.40	33.30
Colorado	2,773,268	28,519	13,589	97	-	-
Connecticut	4,259,446	39,634	21,312	107	140.00	135.80
Delaware	3,312,875	30,710	14,969	108	97.20	76.40
District of Columbia	3,305,733	42,309	21,654	78	-	-
Florida	4,155,870	35,907	14,979	116	94.10	92.70
Georgia	2,249,929	26,745	13,046	84	94.30	79.60
Hawaii	-	-	-	-	-	-
Idaho	1,418,292	26,224	12,700	54	130.10	109.00
Illinois	2,319,399	29,084	13,908	80	88.60	80.20
Indiana	2,137,237	27,885	13,585	77	129.30	124.20
Iowa	1,904,016	21,491	11,516	89	83.10	87.10
Kansas	1,689,347	23,579	11,851	72	78.50	72.80
Kentucky	2,663,708	26,230	12,951	102	71.20	78.70
Louisiana	1,176,805	24,074	10,604	49	133.90	118.70
Maine	1,601,722	27,293	14,628	59	78.80	75.70
Maryland	2,900,000	34,106	16,183	85	104.50	99.30
Massachusetts	3,043,006	34,984	19,003	87	103.70	98.40
Michigan	1,672,113	29,475	14,012	57	127.00	101.00
Minnesota	2,256,128	25,278	13,389	89	76.80	64.80
Mississippi	2,103,063	26,812	13,967	78	150.30	145.40
Missouri	2,456,017	25,044	12,202	98	54.10	40.20
Montana	1,299,000	22,674	12,384	57	83.40	77.80
Nebraska	2,130,284	22,764	12,618	94	30.90	30.50
Nevada	-	-	-	-	-	-
New Hampshire	-	-	-	-	-	-
New Jersey	3,746,333	37,547	19,099	100	81.50	87.10
New Mexico	2,707,462	26,776	13,702	101	88.60	89.70
New York	4,072,362	39,994	20,802	102	76.60	70.80
North Carolina	2,116,287	25,855	13,067	82	87.90	90.40
North Dakota	1,676,566	21,492	11,769	78	81.50	76.00
Ohio	2,182,193	28,736	14,446	76	70.80	70.60
Oklahoma	1,469,000	23,841	11,933	62	32.50	39.20
Oregon	2,486,080	27,135	14,135	92	81.30	79.90
Pennsylvania	2,907,320	32,290	14,851	90	106.80	92.00
Rhode Island	1,647,431	32,364	16,427	51	-	-
South Carolina	1,071,758	29,454	14,415	36	131.20	124.20
South Dakota	1,705,712	19,834	10,907	86	62.40	62.40

[Continued]

★ 426 ★

Nursing and Personal Care Facilities Establishments, Ratios, Non-Taxed, by State: 1992

[Continued]

Area	Sales per establish-ment	Sales per employee	Payroll per employee	Employees per establish-ment	% change in sales 1987 to 1992	% change in payroll 1987 to 1992
Tennessee	2,278,328	26,264	11,569	87	81.60	63.20
Texas	1,892,478	27,890	13,225	68	57.70	40.40
Utah	2,234,267	22,737	11,537	98	209.30	196.60
Vermont	1,258,625	26,638	14,817	47	84.60	94.70
Virginia	3,192,452	29,058	14,117	110	147.70	136.90
Washington	3,662,619	30,139	15,986	122	88.90	85.40
West Virginia	2,525,500	25,026	12,477	101	98.70	110.80
Wisconsin	2,657,737	24,689	13,887	108	46.50	53.60
Wyoming	2,405,500	20,257	11,743	119	96.20	89.90

Source: U.S. Department of Commerce. Bureau of the Census. *1992 Economic Census Report Series,* CD-ROM 1i, Washington, DC, October 1996. *Note:* - means no data reported.

★ 427 ★

Establishments: Ratios

Offices and Clinics of Chiropractors, Ratios by State: 1992

Area	Sales per establish-ment	Sales per employee	Payroll per employee	Employees per establish-ment	% change in sales 1987 to 1992	% change in payroll 1987 to 1992
United States	216,543	69,844	19,499	3	80.70	83.60
Alabama	180,833	59,366	16,581	3	74.90	95.40
Alaska	308,465	96,480	29,599	3	22.40	31.80
Arizona	198,021	69,982	20,468	3	62.60	64.80
Arkansas	166,097	61,412	16,922	3	60.70	63.10
California	222,766	77,130	19,374	3	54.50	40.90
Colorado	170,879	65,826	17,988	3	30.70	26.30
Connecticut	293,876	84,486	22,790	3	-	-
Delaware	273,320	66,663	30,024	4	68.30	120.40
District of Columbia	316,077	82,180	22,000	4	-	-
Florida	240,524	70,104	23,270	3	93.70	116.40
Georgia	202,738	66,016	19,282	3	67.00	93.90
Hawaii	326,286	95,167	31,613	3	121.70	128.50
Idaho	167,687	68,926	12,957	2	45.60	32.90
Illinois	202,772	62,826	18,353	3	77.50	80.60
Indiana	225,140	69,030	20,293	3	89.50	109.60
Iowa	152,897	50,401	12,769	3	64.00	75.10
Kansas	183,776	59,348	18,348	3	64.20	86.20
Kentucky	190,019	59,784	17,899	3	132.00	163.90
Louisiana	206,007	62,707	17,772	3	3.70	8.30

[Continued]

★ 427 ★

Offices and Clinics of Chiropractors, Ratios by State: 1992
[Continued]

Area	Sales per establish-ment	Sales per employee	Payroll per employee	Employees per establish-ment	% change in sales 1987 to 1992	% change in payroll 1987 to 1992
Maine	212,532	62,568	17,720	3	67.70	57.40
Maryland	330,303	72,460	23,341	5	226.30	204.10
Massachusetts	284,991	82,513	24,607	3	127.00	146.40
Michigan	165,984	60,534	16,710	3	39.20	37.00
Minnesota	195,381	60,343	17,742	3	60.40	71.00
Mississippi	169,938	54,246	14,590	3	52.80	66.60
Missouri	149,386	57,933	15,361	3	46.10	52.80
Montana	139,402	62,731	11,604	2	58.00	18.90
Nebraska	184,503	64,815	17,246	3	88.10	95.50
Nevada	287,090	91,472	28,361	3	96.80	85.10
New Hampshire	200,815	67,564	18,181	3	79.40	73.50
New Jersey	262,418	83,006	22,259	3	141.40	140.30
New Mexico	185,395	62,474	15,734	3	58.40	64.90
New York	223,060	75,820	17,322	3	113.40	102.70
North Carolina	225,777	71,564	22,435	3	74.00	77.60
North Dakota	166,578	65,183	18,100	3	68.30	83.30
Ohio	273,225	68,720	21,792	4	95.50	102.00
Oklahoma	210,304	74,253	20,027	3	58.70	70.30
Oregon	140,713	60,833	15,249	2	-10.10	-19.30
Pennsylvania	223,703	68,263	18,171	3	134.90	156.30
Rhode Island	227,430	81,668	24,191	3	148.40	171.80
South Carolina	188,981	71,091	20,542	3	141.50	162.30
South Dakota	177,178	65,131	12,975	3	120.40	120.30
Tennessee	208,183	69,590	18,502	3	97.80	98.00
Texas	232,411	65,954	19,364	4	131.40	143.80
Utah	181,137	55,207	12,896	3	65.30	78.60
Vermont	162,554	61,075	11,821	3	100.50	77.20
Virginia	240,518	72,115	23,242	3	141.50	155.50
Washington	183,056	70,792	16,607	3	51.10	39.70
West Virginia	232,781	62,352	18,852	4	84.20	104.50
Wisconsin	214,678	62,205	20,405	3	110.30	115.40
Wyoming	169,902	67,631	14,951	3	49.30	31.50

Source: U.S. Department of Commerce. Bureau of the Census. *1992 Economic Census Report Series,* CD-ROM 1i, Washington, DC, October 1996. *Note:* - means no data reported.

★ 428 ★

Establishments: Ratios

Offices and Clinics of Optometrists, Ratios by State: 1992

Area	Sales per establish-ment	Sales per employee	Payroll per employee	Employees per establish-ment	% change in sales 1987 to 1992	% change in payroll 1987 to 1992
United States	288,271	72,009	18,966	4	43.20	45.60
Alabama	286,498	72,898	18,497	4	66.40	53.20
Alaska	388,909	96,678	28,107	4	39.50	43.90
Arizona	260,132	73,162	18,440	4	38.30	32.70
Arkansas	280,554	61,869	16,299	5	54.20	64.20
California	316,674	79,695	19,115	4	41.60	42.20
Colorado	284,961	64,581	19,736	4	58.10	78.50
Connecticut	324,386	81,544	20,237	4	37.80	35.60
Delaware	321,825	63,414	20,443	5	56.20	113.50
District of Columbia	384,000	82,286	24,759	5	-	-
Florida	259,110	75,189	23,814	3	52.80	69.40
Georgia	274,383	69,528	21,718	4	48.70	50.70
Hawaii	279,263	83,779	19,824	3	87.50	97.90
Idaho	261,777	68,927	13,902	4	52.00	54.50
Illinois	306,209	67,275	18,857	5	32.60	15.70
Indiana	287,384	69,157	18,696	4	38.40	56.20
Iowa	292,719	65,752	17,998	4	36.60	53.70
Kansas	317,291	71,053	17,923	4	48.70	55.40
Kentucky	292,944	71,576	18,300	4	75.90	91.40
Louisiana	246,903	65,132	18,129	4	41.60	71.50
Maine	287,374	78,900	17,536	4	45.30	58.70
Maryland	332,357	65,966	20,689	5	37.70	29.10
Massachusetts	264,273	73,741	20,452	4	26.90	36.30
Michigan	335,802	74,013	21,735	5	26.00	25.90
Minnesota	255,125	66,813	17,399	4	43.50	37.50
Mississippi	254,426	69,092	16,070	4	71.80	93.50
Missouri	293,983	66,784	18,966	4	36.70	47.10
Montana	237,233	67,875	16,194	3	37.00	31.00
Nebraska	320,041	64,114	18,555	5	56.80	60.70
Nevada	335,673	73,408	22,193	5	77.70	78.90
New Hampshire	271,257	73,798	17,772	4	41.40	39.50
New Jersey	269,047	76,751	18,576	4	41.60	49.90
New Mexico	289,337	71,645	15,769	4	49.60	41.30
New York	286,903	76,695	19,801	4	37.30	30.90
North Carolina	294,279	72,407	21,043	4	78.20	118.70
North Dakota	338,047	64,970	18,550	5	39.40	57.50
Ohio	261,493	66,386	17,754	4	24.70	20.60
Oklahoma	240,719	70,265	16,475	3	51.90	43.50
Oregon	232,455	67,458	14,673	3	3.80	1.60
Pennsylvania	283,344	69,931	17,711	4	49.00	55.80
Rhode Island	293,097	74,046	16,274	4	47.80	48.40
South Carolina	293,399	71,720	20,847	4	-	-
South Dakota	239,563	67,246	17,053	4	26.90	38.10
Tennessee	278,566	73,530	16,600	4	68.60	88.30
Texas	299,358	73,569	19,280	4	47.20	47.90

[Continued]

★ 428 ★

Offices and Clinics of Optometrists, Ratios by State: 1992

[Continued]

Area	Sales per establish-ment	Sales per employee	Payroll per employee	Employees per establish-ment	% change in sales 1987 to 1992	% change in payroll 1987 to 1992
Utah	270,914	64,352	16,956	4	92.70	116.00
Vermont	235,360	86,529	14,647	3	49.10	53.80
Virginia	265,493	67,299	19,058	4	46.90	41.40
Washington	279,760	70,508	16,497	4	42.60	47.80
West Virginia	285,987	74,584	14,883	4	34.30	22.80
Wisconsin	272,138	61,479	16,273	4	25.20	14.30
Wyoming	291,000	71,104	17,371	4	23.60	20.00

Source: U.S. Department of Commerce. Bureau of the Census. *1992 Economic Census Report Series,* CD-ROM 1i, Washington, DC, October 1996. Note: - means no data reported.

★ 429 ★

Establishments: Ratios

Offices and Clinics of Podiatrists, Ratios by State: 1992

Area	Sales per establish-ment	Sales per employee	Payroll per employee	Employees per establish-ment	% change in sales 1987 to 1992	% change in payroll 1987 to 1992
United States	241,580	72,650	23,618	3	50.30	54.40
Alabama	324,694	69,476	29,480	5	31.40	23.40
Alaska	444,400	105,810	13,190	4	44.30	22.00
Arizona	231,091	69,213	26,069	3	34.20	63.70
Arkansas	250,850	70,662	26,310	4	4.40	42.10
California	233,981	81,652	24,485	3	19.50	20.00
Colorado	215,682	64,339	21,542	3	46.00	49.40
Connecticut	321,250	87,041	31,383	4	88.40	105.50
Delaware	272,040	73,924	32,598	4	32.20	29.00
District of Columbia	255,656	73,703	26,712	3	27.00	31.50
Florida	260,936	70,686	25,167	4	75.00	77.60
Georgia	342,446	83,072	32,408	4	103.70	125.10
Hawaii	241,938	90,023	22,558	3	181.90	139.50
Idaho	310,765	67,731	21,218	5	96.00	128.60
Illinois	252,375	77,186	26,190	3	65.80	76.30
Indiana	251,759	66,022	26,139	4	91.70	151.30
Iowa	199,973	55,548	18,689	4	56.60	64.10
Kansas	220,127	61,770	21,031	4	39.80	29.40
Kentucky	223,891	62,418	17,842	4	53.60	36.20
Louisiana	289,083	78,841	23,188	4	44.30	14.40
Maine	179,556	68,766	17,894	3	52.70	65.20
Maryland	267,199	72,281	28,873	4	43.30	29.70
Massachusetts	208,490	73,007	21,242	3	57.70	78.20

[Continued]

★ 429 ★

Offices and Clinics of Podiatrists, Ratios by State: 1992

[Continued]

Area	Sales per establish-ment	Sales per employee	Payroll per employee	Employees per establish-ment	% change in sales 1987 to 1992	% change in payroll 1987 to 1992
Michigan	282,178	67,185	27,446	4	33.00	38.80
Minnesota	207,333	66,170	23,064	3	20.60	30.40
Mississippi	211,167	55,897	13,103	4	45.60	91.20
Missouri	249,612	69,297	24,756	4	46.70	61.10
Montana	215,063	90,553	20,211	2	59.40	35.90
Nebraska	206,471	63,818	24,345	3	-	-
Nevada	285,536	90,852	27,136	3	136.30	126.10
New Hampshire	215,833	75,072	26,913	3	94.60	180.90
New Jersey	231,457	80,003	20,066	3	70.60	54.60
New Mexico	248,939	56,655	17,579	4	41.10	16.20
New York	222,875	77,371	19,495	3	42.40	38.60
North Carolina	250,229	66,348	23,616	4	97.20	109.40
North Dakota	197,429	53,154	16,308	4	101.50	196.50
Ohio	223,886	65,222	22,746	3	53.30	62.90
Oklahoma	285,577	71,053	24,431	4	38.30	40.80
Oregon	226,164	77,073	23,821	3	32.20	53.20
Pennsylvania	201,837	62,602	17,879	3	55.20	68.60
Rhode Island	236,840	64,710	20,809	4	28.50	22.20
South Carolina	247,650	76,791	30,698	3	-	-
South Dakota	126,714	44,350	11,725	3	25.70	43.90
Tennessee	255,933	72,892	23,237	4	70.60	79.30
Texas	273,741	84,671	26,668	3	70.90	75.40
Utah	211,955	53,908	15,821	4	47.70	39.20
Vermont	128,556	60,895	12,000	2	33.40	15.70
Virginia	246,354	67,113	26,520	4	51.00	60.10
Washington	213,726	70,121	19,061	3	38.40	36.80
West Virginia	215,462	74,693	14,707	3	58.50	36.70
Wisconsin	232,941	64,465	22,951	4	36.60	33.10
Wyoming	207,000	64,688	8,875	3	11.30	-29.70

Source: U.S. Department of Commerce. Bureau of the Census. *1992 Economic Census Report Series,* CD-ROM 1i, Washington, DC, October 1996. *Note:* - means no data reported.

★ 430 ★

Establishments: Ratios

Offices of Doctors of Medicine, Ratios by State: 1992

Area	Sales per establish-ment	Sales per employee	Payroll per employee	Employees per establish-ment	% change in sales 1987 to 1992	% change in payroll 1987 to 1992
United States	667,679	104,633	51,699	6	53.70	54.70
Alabama	832,496	101,942	53,576	8	55.50	58.00
Alaska	719,455	108,186	51,507	7	32.60	37.20
Arizona	646,543	111,017	55,432	6	67.50	76.90
Arkansas	661,442	92,587	48,986	7	47.90	51.20
California	594,750	113,950	49,260	5	37.60	29.80
Colorado	654,446	102,619	52,302	6	57.70	68.40
Connecticut	733,089	113,682	59,405	6	70.70	80.50
Delaware	639,586	110,794	55,250	6	68.20	63.80
District of Columbia	567,241	120,024	55,975	5	33.60	31.80
Florida	669,290	111,511	54,933	6	68.80	65.80
Georgia	770,798	112,188	56,399	7	72.80	77.60
Hawaii	529,042	99,208	46,506	5	51.30	64.60
Idaho	593,214	87,865	44,794	7	56.60	66.20
Illinois	719,763	108,472	56,445	7	62.00	64.10
Indiana	744,077	96,872	49,969	8	58.30	59.60
Iowa	861,114	91,290	49,849	9	44.80	53.80
Kansas	892,172	86,022	44,469	10	50.20	53.50
Kentucky	721,722	96,745	49,436	7	65.30	71.30
Louisiana	718,500	105,760	47,540	7	52.00	45.60
Maine	538,113	98,674	49,669	5	61.50	73.70
Maryland	608,906	104,325	49,688	6	53.60	51.30
Massachusetts	680,865	99,135	50,090	7	60.50	65.10
Michigan	624,197	94,213	51,580	7	34.20	40.50
Minnesota	1,322,456	91,248	52,957	14	41.60	53.90
Mississippi	658,844	95,966	45,467	7	54.00	55.70
Missouri	702,309	102,024	54,895	7	47.00	47.60
Montana	558,719	91,384	40,096	6	48.30	50.80
Nebraska	834,163	94,238	50,610	9	47.20	54.70
Nevada	799,980	131,620	66,827	6	85.70	90.40
New Hampshire	585,910	87,518	45,027	7	-	-
New Jersey	633,362	118,377	56,292	5	70.30	66.90
New Mexico	-	-	-	-	-	-
New York	598,916	116,980	50,428	5	60.00	57.40
North Carolina	783,922	95,552	50,714	8	61.10	58.70
North Dakota	1,743,786	82,493	44,839	21	32.80	50.10
Ohio	695,702	101,908	55,804	7	46.10	48.40
Oklahoma	651,908	100,941	50,706	6	42.60	39.50
Oregon	639,748	90,158	43,458	7	59.80	60.00
Pennsylvania	650,623	101,547	53,395	6	49.30	52.80
Rhode Island	507,804	95,118	44,934	5	48.30	59.40
South Carolina	665,560	92,959	49,594	7	65.90	80.10
South Dakota	874,678	96,166	51,105	9	-	-
Tennessee	745,617	102,987	53,861	7	63.90	66.10
Texas	625,520	111,865	53,241	6	55.30	56.90

[Continued]

★ 430 ★

Offices of Doctors of Medicine, Ratios by State: 1992

[Continued]

Area	Sales per establish-ment	Sales per employee	Payroll per employee	Employees per establish-ment	% change in sales 1987 to 1992	% change in payroll 1987 to 1992
Utah	538,821	91,398	47,559	6	48.20	54.60
Vermont	475,155	90,573	37,580	5	59.70	61.10
Virginia	664,030	93,681	50,720	7	62.90	69.60
Washington	676,995	88,748	44,075	8	59.80	68.50
West Virginia	618,116	100,310	45,706	6	44.90	43.80
Wisconsin	934,673	88,465	48,484	11	33.30	32.50
Wyoming	-	-	-	-	-	-

Source: U.S. Department of Commerce. Bureau of the Census. *1992 Economic Census Report Series,* CD-ROM 1i, Washington, DC, October 1996. *Note:* - means no data reported.

★ 431 ★

Establishments: Ratios

Other Health Services Establishments, Ratios, Non-Taxed, by State: 1992

Area	Sales per establish-ment	Sales per employee	Payroll per employee	Employees per establish-ment	% change in sales 1987 to 1992	% change in payroll 1987 to 1992
United States	1,474,239	37,463	18,712	39	114.50	110.60
Alabama	1,238,287	35,264	17,716	35	71.60	93.10
Alaska	1,084,690	48,172	24,214	23	124.40	109.40
Arizona	969,310	45,988	21,133	21	164.70	133.90
Arkansas	878,308	32,810	14,927	27	200.30	180.70
California	1,454,235	50,486	23,163	29	120.80	125.80
Colorado	761,726	36,072	17,120	21	71.20	68.80
Connecticut	1,558,630	36,130	20,089	43	77.80	72.40
Delaware	2,508,091	38,425	19,265	65	-	-
District of Columbia	2,369,184	54,662	23,251	43	144.50	135.20
Florida	1,498,571	46,131	20,084	32	155.50	126.80
Georgia	1,386,736	48,829	21,402	28	147.20	159.50
Hawaii	974,293	43,897	23,503	22	137.90	201.80
Idaho	762,688	40,542	17,585	19	90.00	118.20
Illinois	1,218,694	37,418	18,663	33	109.70	90.30
Indiana	892,102	40,738	20,118	22	95.70	83.60
Iowa	686,139	33,814	16,977	20	115.70	100.90
Kansas	949,232	41,381	20,594	23	95.20	128.00
Kentucky	748,968	40,052	19,100	19	128.90	132.20
Louisiana	1,028,549	56,223	19,742	18	123.00	90.60
Maine	843,085	32,734	17,923	26	83.00	79.50
Maryland	1,179,139	49,171	22,659	24	103.40	87.70

[Continued]

★ 431 ★

Other Health Services Establishments, Ratios, Non-Taxed, by State: 1992

[Continued]

Area	Sales per establish-ment	Sales per employee	Payroll per employee	Employees per establish-ment	% change in sales 1987 to 1992	% change in payroll 1987 to 1992
Massachusetts	2,091,133	42,015	21,161	50	130.20	116.20
Michigan	1,583,898	46,070	21,899	34	122.70	142.50
Minnesota	1,345,984	42,622	18,972	32	-	-
Mississippi	1,546,677	48,172	21,438	32	92.20	80.20
Missouri	1,538,014	40,136	18,610	38	143.60	127.10
Montana	526,886	17,288	9,583	30	110.50	155.70
Nebraska	964,400	49,204	22,321	20	214.00	185.30
Nevada	1,305,714	58,841	19,451	22	266.40	239.70
New Hampshire	1,067,327	35,882	18,049	30	104.30	91.40
New Jersey	1,778,568	38,316	19,338	46	103.70	100.20
New Mexico	746,382	27,738	13,658	27	139.20	127.80
New York	3,782,522	34,017	19,892	111	110.00	114.90
North Carolina	1,492,796	36,708	18,441	41	268.90	273.90
North Dakota	813,083	51,084	15,812	16	-	-
Ohio	1,082,141	40,439	19,188	27	95.20	92.10
Oklahoma	907,710	44,000	19,097	21	169.40	127.50
Oregon	1,153,195	37,539	16,685	31	-	-
Pennsylvania	1,367,614	40,586	19,742	34	71.20	75.90
Rhode Island	-	-	-	-	-	-
South Carolina	1,164,490	42,967	19,815	27	102.20	102.30
South Dakota	747,357	29,145	12,445	26	143.40	138.40
Tennessee	1,260,557	44,929	21,032	28	101.70	104.60
Texas	1,496,427	19,405	9,486	77	165.90	141.40
Utah	1,397,867	35,904	18,673	39	112.10	61.90
Vermont	1,063,447	31,145	17,534	34	106.50	107.10
Virginia	1,123,138	39,402	18,728	29	106.30	170.10
Washington	1,758,971	37,648	19,097	47	95.90	83.80
West Virginia	1,406,542	39,162	17,186	36	224.60	162.30
Wisconsin	982,132	32,589	15,795	30	-	-
Wyoming	-	-	-	-	-	-

Source: U.S. Department of Commerce. Bureau of the Census. *1992 Economic Census Report Series,* CD-ROM 1i, Washington, DC, October 1996. *Note:* - means no data reported.

★ 432 ★

Establishments: Ratios

Physical Fitness Facilities, Ratios by State: 1992

Area	Sales per establish- ment	Sales per employee	Payroll per employee	Employees per establish- ment	% change in sales 1987 to 1992	% change in payroll 1987 to 1992
United States	414,883	29,429	8,029	14	48.70	40.10
Alabama	179,762	20,554	6,824	9	35.90	32.20
Alaska	515,480	23,603	6,005	22	25.70	28.50
Arizona	440,438	27,085	7,698	16	88.80	94.50
Arkansas	170,093	18,596	5,201	9	89.20	95.00
California	656,545	34,129	8,960	19	100.80	74.60
Colorado	528,585	23,083	6,695	23	90.30	83.30
Connecticut	378,845	29,284	9,966	13	36.00	82.40
Delaware	352,077	34,543	9,581	10	-	-
District of Columbia	555,292	51,856	13,790	11	-	-
Florida	406,453	36,558	8,572	11	43.60	13.70
Georgia	363,615	26,517	7,500	14	58.70	50.10
Hawaii	493,432	40,037	11,458	12	115.20	143.40
Idaho	287,633	21,919	5,998	13	90.90	78.60
Illinois	523,389	30,990	8,374	17	51.90	77.00
Indiana	238,492	22,283	6,597	11	47.00	33.80
Iowa	217,419	18,708	7,337	12	30.00	80.20
Kansas	251,928	18,923	5,695	13	24.30	22.70
Kentucky	167,939	17,510	5,090	10	31.70	16.70
Louisiana	286,969	23,976	7,740	12	14.30	26.20
Maine	169,950	28,169	7,199	6	43.80	8.40
Maryland	407,749	28,886	7,836	14	10.50	31.80
Massachusetts	400,172	29,427	8,353	14	51.10	43.00
Michigan	348,622	33,731	7,766	10	18.70	-8.50
Minnesota	488,110	25,830	8,537	19	6.30	29.40
Mississippi	201,435	30,990	7,579	7	76.30	72.10
Missouri	268,028	22,915	6,315	12	-1.40	-7.20
Montana	204,417	16,888	5,053	12	69.30	86.80
Nebraska	300,327	20,993	5,876	14	43.90	20.20
Nevada	489,297	37,413	11,124	13	172.10	138.70
New Hampshire	235,529	16,432	5,280	14	-2.10	0.70
New Jersey	401,723	30,797	8,761	13	39.70	43.70
New Mexico	223,695	24,996	6,042	9	21.40	-12.10
New York	524,670	35,215	9,438	15	43.40	37.10
North Carolina	243,626	22,129	6,012	11	35.70	15.30
North Dakota	109,308	11,793	3,315	9	-37.10	-30.00
Ohio	317,613	26,226	6,435	12	8.50	-1.90
Oklahoma	261,208	20,181	6,547	13	71.40	83.70
Oregon	415,366	29,278	8,986	14	135.70	131.50
Pennsylvania	344,341	28,653	7,991	12	33.10	28.80
Rhode Island	284,222	26,813	7,891	11	4.10	24.70
South Carolina	331,536	28,160	8,754	12	89.00	70.50
South Dakota	137,474	12,438	4,348	11	-32.60	-35.10
Tennessee	282,342	27,969	8,194	10	60.90	41.80
Texas	466,820	33,116	8,408	14	22.70	0.40

[Continued]

★ 432 ★

Physical Fitness Facilities, Ratios by State: 1992
[Continued]

Area	Sales per establish-ment	Sales per employee	Payroll per employee	Employees per establish-ment	% change in sales 1987 to 1992	% change in payroll 1987 to 1992
Utah	416,968	24,323	6,803	17	78.20	75.70
Vermont	261,457	19,025	6,703	14	27.80	40.70
Virginia	416,294	24,072	6,599	17	42.90	47.90
Washington	510,668	29,906	8,413	17	64.90	36.90
West Virginia	138,333	22,060	6,233	6	-6.90	-14.60
Wisconsin	308,534	22,610	6,072	14	22.90	28.60
Wyoming	170,360	15,157	4,082	11	38.60	28.70

Source: U.S. Department of Commerce. Bureau of the Census. *1992 Economic Census Report Series,* CD-ROM 1i, Washington, DC, October 1996. *Note:* - means no data reported.

★ 433 ★

Establishments: Ratios

Selected Health Services Establishments, Ratios, Non-Taxed, by State: 1992

Area	Sales per establish-ment	Sales per employee	Payroll per employee	Employees per establish-ment	% change in sales 1987 to 1992	% change in payroll 1987 to 1992
United States	13,716,706	58,299	26,147	235	69.10	58.90
Alabama	13,440,643	58,071	24,215	231	77.70	66.60
Alaska	8,438,506	71,558	33,232	118	56.40	46.40
Arizona	11,394,713	64,169	26,069	178	61.80	55.00
Arkansas	10,021,945	51,878	21,766	193	69.30	62.20
California	20,625,519	79,821	31,464	258	61.80	47.90
Colorado	10,990,387	61,790	26,042	178	73.80	59.90
Connecticut	14,558,238	59,922	30,386	243	68.30	61.00
Delaware	18,005,618	57,128	26,831	315	98.70	74.90
District of Columbia	34,937,989	71,889	33,498	486	62.40	59.40
Florida	14,681,915	62,774	26,765	234	83.30	73.10
Georgia	18,863,681	57,262	24,797	329	74.60	58.10
Hawaii	13,778,048	61,769	29,953	223	66.30	77.90
Idaho	7,657,010	52,758	22,143	145	82.00	70.40
Illinois	14,790,713	56,107	24,835	264	53.50	45.00
Indiana	10,864,512	54,647	23,560	199	68.30	57.80
Iowa	7,215,129	42,301	19,581	171	59.20	55.00
Kansas	7,320,035	44,331	21,298	165	56.80	47.90
Kentucky	7,941,605	51,298	21,808	155	81.10	67.10
Louisiana	15,090,648	55,062	23,987	274	67.30	60.10
Maine	6,365,479	48,298	23,910	132	63.10	60.70
Maryland	17,218,877	57,523	26,386	299	71.20	60.90

[Continued]

★ 433 ★

Selected Health Services Establishments, Ratios, Non-Taxed, by State: 1992

[Continued]

Area	Sales per establish-ment	Sales per employee	Payroll per employee	Employees per establish-ment	% change in sales 1987 to 1992	% change in payroll 1987 to 1992
Massachusetts	15,686,227	59,482	28,443	264	61.10	55.60
Michigan	12,989,732	58,740	26,407	221	55.20	47.50
Minnesota	9,189,398	50,438	25,117	182	62.20	61.70
Mississippi	11,306,879	51,342	21,952	220	69.00	52.10
Missouri	15,861,271	52,577	23,185	302	57.90	52.30
Montana	4,859,285	46,543	20,761	104	55.70	57.40
Nebraska	8,530,615	46,869	22,007	182	63.60	62.40
Nevada	16,296,745	73,073	28,640	223	89.20	58.80
New Hampshire	8,310,886	60,550	24,540	137	108.60	75.40
New Jersey	20,654,347	59,825	28,806	345	81.90	75.30
New Mexico	7,052,533	49,789	23,422	142	69.40	68.30
New York	17,945,433	56,704	29,745	316	68.30	65.70
North Carolina	15,739,842	56,992	25,129	276	97.60	84.80
North Dakota	5,817,420	40,287	19,061	144	53.60	55.80
Ohio	12,875,045	56,647	24,595	227	54.80	41.50
Oklahoma	10,614,535	50,862	22,405	209	45.90	40.00
Oregon	12,563,364	59,095	26,089	213	67.40	64.20
Pennsylvania	12,818,756	56,669	25,692	226	63.20	58.00
Rhode Island	9,160,365	52,481	27,261	175	50.10	52.30
South Carolina	15,464,573	61,652	25,543	251	93.20	71.10
South Dakota	5,535,723	41,472	19,231	133	64.10	53.80
Tennessee	13,799,683	57,542	24,158	240	71.70	60.60
Texas	14,716,978	56,973	24,479	258	79.50	64.30
Utah	14,725,161	55,186	23,863	267	53.40	51.90
Vermont	4,840,243	50,719	23,812	95	71.30	65.70
Virginia	17,649,929	57,018	24,905	310	78.60	67.90
Washington	13,376,539	62,975	28,037	212	98.00	87.20
West Virginia	9,385,421	54,609	23,466	172	63.70	43.20
Wisconsin	10,414,755	51,207	22,230	203	75.10	63.10
Wyoming	5,051,947	44,635	21,604	113	34.00	29.10

Source: U.S. Department of Commerce. Bureau of the Census. *1992 Economic Census Report Series*, CD-ROM 1i, Washington, DC, October 1996. *Note:* - means no data reported.

★ 434 ★

Establishments: Ratios

Skilled Nursing Care Facilities, Ratios by State: 1992

Area	Sales per establish-ment	Sales per employee	Payroll per employee	Employees per establish-ment	% change in sales 1987 to 1992	% change in payroll 1987 to 1992
United States	2,811,737	30,704	14,416	92	70.00	69.10
Alabama	2,536,941	25,667	12,215	99	90.90	94.30
Alaska	0	0	0	0	0.00	0.00
Arizona	3,502,552	32,996	14,784	106	125.20	96.40
Arkansas	1,812,216	22,688	10,604	80	77.00	83.10
California	2,657,529	33,192	15,620	80	75.70	68.70
Colorado	2,950,931	32,671	14,238	90	76.10	68.30
Connecticut	5,012,450	38,595	20,508	130	68.90	71.80
Delaware	3,234,346	27,753	12,921	117	92.30	106.90
District of Columbia	7,898,500	58,006	21,432	136	47.20	41.40
Florida	3,111,765	34,923	14,947	89	107.60	102.40
Georgia	2,195,264	24,803	11,659	89	75.80	69.30
Hawaii	5,665,300	53,295	24,344	106	111.50	91.10
Idaho	2,309,024	25,986	12,173	89	112.40	94.00
Illinois	3,166,161	31,321	13,314	101	67.50	60.50
Indiana	2,421,583	30,018	13,411	81	57.50	63.50
Iowa	1,527,119	22,228	11,151	69	6.40	16.60
Kansas	1,518,929	23,039	11,672	66	52.70	64.20
Kentucky	2,367,133	26,520	12,070	89	62.10	72.40
Louisiana	2,291,219	25,209	10,371	91	130.60	113.00
Maine	2,165,642	27,691	14,091	78	11.80	11.10
Maryland	3,942,537	33,882	16,159	116	51.90	63.40
Massachusetts	3,910,254	36,240	19,090	108	70.50	82.20
Michigan	2,648,546	26,883	13,054	99	47.90	46.70
Minnesota	3,002,731	27,731	14,738	108	39.10	38.60
Mississippi	1,967,746	24,769	11,838	79	88.20	98.60
Missouri	1,779,726	24,010	11,046	74	52.30	55.50
Montana	2,136,333	27,317	12,491	78	80.40	80.70
Nebraska	1,965,442	25,350	13,188	78	61.40	73.80
Nevada	3,489,938	35,909	16,977	97	-	-
New Hampshire	3,859,609	37,663	17,538	102	43.40	44.30
New Jersey	4,846,538	41,161	18,897	118	87.00	82.00
New Mexico	2,507,028	27,062	11,741	93	126.50	127.20
New York	6,577,270	43,836	20,539	150	50.80	43.60
North Carolina	2,590,475	26,601	13,518	97	118.70	132.70
North Dakota	-	-	-	-	-	-
Ohio	2,876,810	29,606	13,707	97	87.90	81.10
Oklahoma	1,314,101	21,727	9,976	60	32.20	39.40
Oregon	2,088,542	28,861	13,836	72	50.00	44.60
Pennsylvania	3,273,205	34,757	15,322	94	53.10	55.30
Rhode Island	3,103,694	32,330	16,179	96	57.30	59.90
South Carolina	2,288,457	25,409	11,940	90	-	-
South Dakota	1,475,143	22,458	11,460	66	33.70	38.40
Tennessee	2,614,650	29,075	12,057	90	66.10	51.50
Texas	1,826,802	25,141	11,500	73	88.00	90.40

[Continued]

★ 434 ★

Skilled Nursing Care Facilities, Ratios by State: 1992

[Continued]

Area	Sales per establish-ment	Sales per employee	Payroll per employee	Employees per establish-ment	% change in sales 1987 to 1992	% change in payroll 1987 to 1992
Utah	2,316,245	26,378	11,934	88	104.50	105.40
Vermont	2,926,458	28,868	14,114	101	95.60	62.10
Virginia	2,847,868	28,654	13,230	99	40.20	49.40
Washington	2,867,163	29,553	15,296	97	85.00	93.60
West Virginia	2,337,018	26,662	11,605	88	41.50	34.30
Wisconsin	2,926,037	28,327	14,308	103	46.70	50.80
Wyoming	-	-	-	-	-	-

Source: U.S. Department of Commerce. Bureau of the Census. *1992 Economic Census Report Series,* CD-ROM 1i, Washington, DC, October 1996. *Note:* - means no data reported.

★ 435 ★

Establishments: Ratios

Specialty Hospitals, Ratios by State: 1992

Area	Sales per establish-ment	Sales per employee	Payroll per employee	Employees per establish-ment	% change in sales 1987 to 1992	% change in payroll 1987 to 1992
United States	9,900,837	65,906	24,222	150	-	-
Alabama	10,952,545	86,737	26,728	126	-	-
Alaska	-	-	-	-	-	-
Arizona	9,120,563	69,128	26,436	132	-	-
Arkansas	9,883,364	69,246	24,320	143	-	-
California	8,413,318	67,212	25,539	125	-	-
Colorado	-	-	-	-	-	-
Connecticut	-	-	-	-	-	-
Delaware	7,883,667	59,725	23,528	132	-	-
District of Columbia	-	-	-	-	-	-
Florida	10,331,062	70,880	24,025	146	-	-
Georgia	10,929,182	75,044	22,542	146	-	-
Hawaii	-	-	-	-	-	-
Idaho	-	-	-	-	-	-
Illinois	16,127,722	74,474	27,774	217	-	-
Indiana	9,215,667	76,584	22,973	120	-	-
Iowa	0	0	0	0	-	-
Kansas	-	-	-	-	-	-
Kentucky	9,241,222	65,028	22,496	142	-	-
Louisiana	8,376,344	61,975	20,646	135	-	-
Maine	-	-	-	-	-	-
Maryland	-	-	-	-	-	-
Massachusetts	-	-	-	-	-	-

[Continued]

★ 435 ★

Specialty Hospitals, Ratios by State: 1992

[Continued]

Area	Sales per establish-ment	Sales per employee	Payroll per employee	Employees per establish-ment	% change in sales 1987 to 1992	% change in payroll 1987 to 1992
Michigan	7,968,200	55,800	21,032	143	-	-
Minnesota	-	-	-	-	-	-
Mississippi	9,377,857	67,675	22,327	139	-	-
Missouri	7,417,923	61,697	24,120	120	-	-
Montana	-	-	-	-	-	-
Nebraska	-	-	-	-	-	-
Nevada	-	-	-	-	-	-
New Hampshire	-	-	-	-	-	-
New Jersey	22,624,800	71,507	22,247	316	-	-
New Mexico	-	-	-	-	-	-
New York	17,769,750	59,755	27,974	297	-	-
North Carolina	11,399,800	70,514	23,992	162	-	-
North Dakota	0	0	0	0	-	-
Ohio	-	-	-	-	-	-
Oklahoma	8,438,769	63,157	22,342	134	-	-
Oregon	-	-	-	-	-	-
Pennsylvania	-	-	-	-	-	-
Rhode Island	0	0	0	0	-	-
South Carolina	7,615,778	72,226	26,294	105	-	-
South Dakota	-	-	-	-	-	-
Tennessee	10,653,313	62,164	22,633	171	-	-
Texas	9,574,772	67,725	23,734	141	-	-
Utah	7,396,444	62,447	22,556	118	-	-
Vermont	0	0	0	0	-	-
Virginia	8,903,810	55,765	20,161	160	-	-
Washington	5,656,500	52,864	21,876	107	-	-
West Virginia	10,057,286	65,489	22,420	154	-	-
Wisconsin	-	-	-	-	-	-
Wyoming	-	-	-	-	-	-

Source: U.S. Department of Commerce. Bureau of the Census. *1992 Economic Census Report Series,* CD-ROM 1i, Washington, DC, October 1996. *Note:* - means no data reported.

★ 436 ★

Establishments: Ratios

Specialty Hospitals, Ratios, Non-Taxed Establishments, by State: 1992

Area	Sales per establish-ment	Sales per employee	Payroll per employee	Employees per establish-ment	% change in sales 1987 to 1992	% change in payroll 1987 to 1992
United States	31,799,275	52,973	29,399	600	-	-
Alabama	33,104,556	46,365	26,016	714	-	-
Alaska	-	-	-	-	-	-
Arizona	17,923,778	59,416	25,989	302	-	-
Arkansas	34,094,200	47,939	22,608	711	-	-
California	44,804,065	61,417	35,011	730	-	-
Colorado	30,911,714	55,178	29,784	560	-	-
Connecticut	19,530,917	58,542	36,595	334	-	-
Delaware	-	-	-	-	-	-
District of Columbia	103,572,800	60,690	30,392	1,707	-	-
Florida	27,100,033	52,758	26,541	514	-	-
Georgia	36,089,600	51,319	25,431	703	-	-
Hawaii	26,152,500	54,971	27,767	476	-	-
Idaho	9,311,400	37,637	24,251	247	-	-
Illinois	31,776,708	48,049	29,514	661	-	-
Indiana	14,026,143	40,808	28,833	344	-	-
Iowa	21,438,000	39,885	31,970	538	-	-
Kansas	20,266,455	36,636	25,673	553	-	-
Kentucky	14,342,500	41,084	21,649	349	-	-
Louisiana	21,881,400	52,541	25,595	416	-	-
Maine	17,118,600	41,712	29,918	410	-	-
Maryland	33,169,900	57,662	30,393	575	-	-
Massachusetts	36,146,065	57,729	31,591	626	-	-
Michigan	32,316,567	59,336	32,039	545	-	-
Minnesota	31,663,938	53,116	32,205	596	-	-
Mississippi	34,758,333	29,209	17,903	1,190	-	-
Missouri	29,002,409	48,035	23,004	604	-	-
Montana	-	-	-	-	-	-
Nebraska	18,393,900	44,830	25,261	410	-	-
Nevada	-	-	-	-	-	-
New Hampshire	-	-	-	-	-	-
New Jersey	30,852,690	49,463	31,045	624	-	-
New Mexico	15,264,667	38,204	22,534	400	-	-
New York	56,065,377	54,181	33,966	1,035	-	-
North Carolina	19,463,130	46,582	27,801	418	-	-
North Dakota	10,558,000	34,902	25,021	303	-	-
Ohio	31,464,568	53,825	29,813	585	-	-
Oklahoma	12,227,692	43,243	24,906	283	-	-
Oregon	11,126,625	44,979	35,573	247	-	-
Pennsylvania	36,914,683	60,567	30,285	609	-	-
Rhode Island	37,210,000	52,915	28,285	703	-	-
South Carolina	12,036,900	42,014	23,342	287	-	-
South Dakota	-	-	-	-	-	-
Tennessee	29,211,429	50,179	24,504	582	-	-
Texas	48,255,757	54,759	26,511	881	-	-

[Continued]

★ 436 ★

Specialty Hospitals, Ratios, Non-Taxed Establishments, by State: 1992

[Continued]

Area	Sales per establish- ment	Sales per employee	Payroll per employee	Employees per establish- ment	% change in sales 1987 to 1992	% change in payroll 1987 to 1992
Utah	-	-	-	-	-	-
Vermont	-	-	-	-	-	-
Virginia	22,830,526	37,456	22,123	610	-	-
Washington	37,149,364	71,019	32,320	523	-	-
West Virginia	19,023,750	40,780	22,411	467	-	-
Wisconsin	24,801,900	48,933	24,933	507	-	-
Wyoming	-	-	-	-	-	-

Source: U.S. Department of Commerce. Bureau of the Census. *1992 Economic Census Report Series,* CD-ROM 1i, Washington, DC, October 1996. *Note:* - means no data reported.

Health Maintenance Organizations

★ 437 ★

Financial Profile of Leading HMOs: 1995

HMO	Members (millions)	Cash and investments (millions)	Cash per share	Stock price
Kaiser Permanente	6.6	$1,347	N.A.	N.A.
United HealthCare	3.2	2,600	$16.00	$45.75
U.S. Healthcare	1.9	1,164	7.00	42.50
Humana	1.8	887	5.50	22.00
FHP International	1.7	456	8.00	26.13
Health Systems	1.4	475	9.50	23.50
PacifiCare	1.4	711	25.00	67.00
HIP	1.2	334	N.A.	N.A.
Foundation Health	1.0	645	13.00	31.13
WellPoint	0.7	1,918	19.00	28.38

Source: "Money Machines: HMOs Pile Up Billions in Cash As Analysts Wonder What They Will Do With It." *Wall Street Journal,* 21 December 1994, p. A12. Primary source: Salomon Brothers Inc.; Sanford C. Bernstein & Co. *Note:* "N.A." represents "Not Applicable."

★ 438 ★

Health Maintenance Organizations

Leading HMOs: 1996

The table lists the leading HMOs according to their prevention score, which summarizes how well they meet national standards in five areas: immunization rates, prenatal care, mammography rates, pap test rates, and cholesterol testing rates.

HMO	Score
Fallon Community Health Plan (MA)	45
Harvard Community Health Plan (MA, NJ, RI)	43
Wellborn Health Plans (IN)	41
Columbia Medical Plan (MD)	40
Kaiser Foundation Health Plan of the Mid-Atlantic States (DC, MD, VA)	29
Group Health Cooperative of South Central Wisconsin	27
HMO Blue (MA)	27
Health Care Plan (NY)	25
Tufts Associated Health Plan (MA, ME, NH)	25
Finger Lakes Health Insurance (NY)	23
Matthew Thornton Health Plan (MA, ME, NH, VT)	23
Providence Health Plan of Oregon (OR, WA)	23
Rochester Area HMO (Preferred Care) (NY)	23
Pilgrim Health Care (MA, RI)	22
HealthPartners (MN)	21
Healthsource CMHC (MA)	21
Healthsource Maine	21
Group Health Cooperative of Eau Claire (WI)	19
Prudential HealthCare-Orlando (FL)	19
CIGNA HealthCare of Arizona-Phoenix	18
HMO Maine	18

Source: Rubin, Rita. "Rating the HMOs." *U.S. News & World Report,* 2 September 1996, p. 54.

Home Health Care

★ 439 ★

Home Health and Hospice Care Agencies, by Selected Characteristics: 1994

In percent, except total in thousands. Based on the 1994 National Home and Hospice Care Surveys. Home health care is provided to individuals and families in their place of residence. Hospice care is available in both the home and inpatient settings. Agencies which provide both types of care are classified according to how the majority of their patients are cared for. See source for details.

ITEM	AGENCIES			CURRENT PATIENTS[1]			DISCHARGES[2]		
	Total	Home health agency	Hospice	Total	Home health agency	Hospice	Total	Home health agency	Hospice
Total (1,000)	10.9	9.8	1.1	1,950.3	1,889.4	61.0	5,600.2	5,272.2	328.0
PERCENT DISTRIBUTION Ownership:									
Proprietary	40.2	43.8	7.3	29.7	30.3	11.0	26.9	28.0	10.2
Voluntary nonprofit	42.0	36.8	90.4	59.8	59.0	86.3	66.6	65.4	87.0
Government and other	17.8	19.5	2.3	10.5	10.7	2.7	6.4	6.7	2.8
Certification:									
Medicare	79.4	80.0	69.2	88.1	87.9	84.3	94.9	95.1	87.6
Medicaid	38.0	79.4	59.9	87.9	87.9	80.8	91.5	91.5	85.3
Region:									
Northeast	18.0	18.1	16.9	33.4	33.7	25.2	36.9	37.1	33.5
Midwest	26.8	26.8	27.0	19.5	19.4	23.4	20.4	20.2	22.4
South	41.1	41.7	35.9	34.0	34.0	34.2	26.8	26.7	29.8
West	14.0	13.3	20.3	13.1	12.9	17.2	15.9	16.0	14.3

Source: 1996 Statistical Abstract of the United States on CD-ROM [machine-readable datafiles]. CD-8A-97. Washington, DC: U.S. Department of Commerce, Economics and Statistics Administration, Bureau of the Census, Data User Services Division, January 1997. Primary source: U.S. National Center for Health Statistics, *Advance Data*, No. 274, April 24, 1996. *Notes:* 1. Patients on the rolls of the agency as of midnight the day prior to the survey. 2. Patients removed from the rolls of the agency during the 12 months prior to the day of the survey. A patient could be included more than once if the individual had more than one episode of care during the year.

★ 440 ★

Home Health Care

Services Provided Through Home Health Care, by Type: 1995

According to the source, the number of home health care agencies grew to more than 15,000 in 1995, up from fewer than 13,500 in 1994. The table shows each type of service and its percentage of all services provided.

Services	Percentage
Nursing care	96.0
Home health aides	87.9
Physical therapy	77.7
Speech therapy	68.8
Occupational therapy	66.7
Medical social service	65.8
IV and infusion therapy	63.4
Durable Medical Equipment	39.2
Pharmaceutical services	34.3
Nutritional guidance	31.1
Lab services	25.7
Vocational guidance	17.9
Respiratory therapy	16.7
Other services	12.7

Source: "Continuum of Care: Home Health's Growth Spurt." *Hospitals & Health Networks,* 20 June 1996, p. 18. Primary source: SMG Marketing Group, Chicago.

Hospices

★ 441 ★

National Hospice Usage

This table shows national usage of hospices by client age, gender, and race.

Characteristic	Percent
Age	
Under 45 years	8.5
45-54 years	6.4
55-64 years	12.3
65 years and over	71.5
65-69 years	10.8
70-74 years	18.2
75-79 years	12.9
80-84 years	15.0

[Continued]

★ 441 ★

National Hospice Usage
[Continued]

Characteristic	Percent
85 years and over	14.6
Gender	
Male	41.1
Female	58.9
Race	
White	84.5
Black	10.4
Hispanic	3.5
Asian	1.3
Native American	0.4

Source: "National Hospice Usage, by Client Age, Gender, and Race." *Caring Magazine* (November 1995), p. 14. Primary sources: NCHS Sample Survey, 1993; Race data: Catholic University of America, National Catholic School of Social Services, "Hospice Care for Substance Abusing AIDS Patients." Final report, January 1995.

Hospitals

★ 442 ★

Hospital Care Expenditures: 1991-1994

Data in the tables show expenditures for hospital care and the percent distribution by source of funds for the years shown. Data were compiled by the Health Care Financing Administration.

Service and year	Total in billions	Out-of-pocket payments	Private health insurance	Other private funds	Government		
					Total[1]	Medicaid	Medicare
Hospital care[2]							
1991	282.3	4.0	35.5	4.1	56.4	13.5	27.0
1992	305.3	3.5	34.7	3.9	57.9	14.2	28.4
1993	324.2	3.1	34.9	4.1	58.0	14.5	28.6
1994	338.5	2.9	34.2	4.0	59.0	14.6	30.0

Source: U.S. Department of Health and Human Services. Public Health Service. Centers for Disease Control and Prevention. National Center for Health Statistics. *Health, United States, 1995.* Hyattsville, MD: Public Health Service, 1996. p. 250. Primary source: Office of National Health Statistics, Office of the Actuary. National Health Expenditures, 1994. *Health Care Financing Review,* vol. 17, no. 3. *Notes:* These data include revisions in health expenditures and in population back to 1960 and differ from previous editions of *Health, United States.* 1. Includes other government expenditures for these health care services, for example, care funded by the Department of Veterans Affairs and State and locally financed subsidies to hospitals. 2. Includes expenditures for hospital-based nursing home care and home health agency care.

★ 443 ★

Hospitals

Hospital Days Covered by Insurers, by Procedure and Insurer: 1995

Carrier	Vaginal delivery	Caesarean section	Abdominal hysterectomy	Vaginal hysterectomy
Chartered Health	2	4	4	4
Cigna, Equitable	1	3	2	2
D.C. Medicaid	1	3	3	2
M.D. IPA	1	3	2	1
New York Life	2	4	3	3
Principle Healthcare HMO	1	3	3	2
Aetna	1	3	3	2
Blue Cross/Blue Shield, D.C.	1	2	2	1

Source: "How Hospital Stays Differ." *USA TODAY*, 5 September 1995, p. 12A.

★ 444 ★

Hospitals

Hospital Emergency Room Visits: 1994

An emergency room is a hospital facility staffed by physicians for the provision of providing outpatient services to patients whose conditions require immediate attention and is staffed 24 hours a day. Data are for non-Federal short stay, or general hospitals. Based on the annual National Hospital Ambulatory Care Surveys and subject to sampling error; see source for details.

CHARACTERISTIC	NUMBER OF VISITS (1,000)				VISITS PER 100 PERSONS			
	Total	Urgent[1]	Non-urgent	Injury-related	Total	Urgent[1]	Non-urgent	Injury-related
1992								
All visits[2]	93,402	44,091	49,311	39,640	36.0	17.0	19.0	15.6
Age:								
Under 15 years old	23,751	9,985	13,766	9,839	40.2	16.9	23.3	16.6
15 to 24 years old	15,411	6,532	8,879	7,632	42.7	18.1	24.5	21.1
25 to 44 years old	28,219	12,241	15,978	13,250	34.0	14.8	19.3	16.0
45 to 64 years old	13,011	6,949	6,062	5,105	25.8	13.8	12.0	10.1
65 to 74 years old	5,797	3,576	2,221	1,586	30.3	19.6	10.7	8.7
75 years old and over	7,214	4,808	2,406	2,229	56.5	37.6	18.8	17.5
Sex:								
Male	44,666	21,622	23,044	21,776	35.3	17.1	18.2	17.6
Female	48,736	22,469	26,267	17,863	36.6	16.9	19.7	13.7

[Continued]

★ 444 ★

Hospital Emergency Room Visits: 1994
[Continued]

CHARACTERISTIC	NUMBER OF VISITS (1,000)				VISITS PER 100 PERSONS			
	Total	Urgent[1]	Non-urgent	Injury-related	Total	Urgent[1]	Non-urgent	Injury-related
Race:								
White	72,337	34,839	37,498	31,857	33.7	16.2	17.5	14.9
Black	18,603	8,158	10,445	6,842	56.3	24.7	31.6	20.7

Source: 1996 Statistical Abstract of the United States on CD-ROM [machine-readable datafiles]. CD-8A-97. Washington, DC: U.S. Department of Commerce, Economics and Statistics Administration, Bureau of the Census, Data User Services Division, January 1997. Primary source: U.S. National Center for Health Statistics, Advance Data, No. 275, May 17, 1996. Notes: 1. Patient requires immediate attention. 2. Includes other races, not shown separately.

★ 445 ★

Hospitals

Hospital Outpatient Department Visits: 1994

An outpatient department is a hospital facility where nonurgent ambulatory care is provided under the supervision of a physician. Data exclude clinics where only ancillary services, such as radiology, are provided. Based on the annual National Hospital Ambulatory Care Surveys and subject to sampling error; see source for details.

CHARACTERISTIC	Number of visits (1,000)	Per-cent distri-bution	Visits per 100 per-sons
All visits	66,345	100.0	25.6
Age:			
Under 15 years old	13,516	20.4	22.9
15 to 24 years old	7,834	11.8	21.7
25 to 44 years old	19,815	29.9	23.9
45 to 64 years old	14,306	21.6	28.4
65 to 74 years old	5,955	9.0	32.6
75 years old and over	4,920	7.4	38.5
Sex:			
Male	25,746	38.8	20.4
Female	40,599	61.2	30.5
Race:			
White	49,701	74.9	23.2
Black	15,132	22.8	45.8
Asian/Pacific Islander	1,283	1.9	(NA)
American Indian/Eskimo/Aleut	228	0.3	(NA)
Visit status:			
Old patient	52,180	78.7	(X)
Old problem	42,258	63.7	(X)
New problem	9,922	15.0	(X)
New patient	14,165	21.4	(X)

[Continued]

★ 445 ★

Hospital Outpatient Department Visits: 1994

[Continued]

CHARACTERISTIC	Number of visits (1,000)	Per-cent distri-bution	Visits per 100 per-sons
Expected source of payment:[1]			
Medicaid	20,029	30.2	(X)
Private/commercial insurance	18,411	27.8	(X)
Medicare	11,867	17.9	(X)
Patient paid	7,323	11.0	(X)
HMO/other prepaid	7,680	11.6	(X)
Other government	2,342	3.5	(X)
No charge	923	1.4	(X)
Other and unknown	6,080	9.2	(X)
Disposition:[1]			
Return to clinic:			
By appointment	42,821	64.5	(X)
As needed	13,135	19.8	(X)
Refer to other clinic/physician	5,045	7.6	(X)
Return to referring physician	2,004	3.0	(X)
No followup	4,122	6.2	(X)
Telephone follow-up	2,044	3.1	(X)
Admit to hospital	938	1.4	(X)
Other	1,659	2.5	(X)

Source: 1996 Statistical Abstract of the United States on CD-ROM [machine-readable datafiles]. CD-8A-97. Washington, DC: U.S. Department of Commerce, Economics and Statistics Administration, Bureau of the Census, Data User Services Division, January 1997. Primary source: U.S. National Center for Health Statistics, Advance Data, No. 276, June 11, 1996. Notes: NA indicates "not available." X indicates "not applicable." 1. More than one source of payment or disposition may be reported.

★ 446 ★

Hospitals

Hospital Utilization and Expenditures

Item	Calendar year				1996	
	1992	1993	1994	1995	Q1	Q2
Utilization						
All Ages						
Admissions in Thousands	32,411	32,652	32,938	33,389	8,511	8,267
Admissions Per 1,000 population[1]	121	121	121	122	123	119
Inpatient Days in Thousands	206,440	202,078	196,117	190,377	48,051	45,532
Adult Length of Stay	6.4	6.2	6.0	5.7	5.6	5.5
65 Years of Age or Over						
Admissions in Thousands	11,860	12,209	12,456	12,820	3,324	3,204
Admissions Per 1,000 population	360	366	369	375	387	372

[Continued]

★ 446 ★

Hospital Utilization and Expenditures
[Continued]

Item	Calendar year				1996	
	1992	1993	1994	1995	Q1	Q2
Inpatient Days in Thousands	98,920	97,042	94,877	91,164	22,972	21,445
Adult Length of Stay	8.3	7.9	7.6	7.1	6.9	6.7
Under 65 Years of Age						
Admissions in Thousands	20,551	20,443	20,483	20,569	5,187	5,063
Admissions Per 1,000 population	88	87	86	85	86	84
Inpatient Days in Thousands	107,520	105,036	101,240	99,213	25,078	24,087
Adult Length of Stay	5.2	5.1	4.9	4.8	4.8	4.8
Surgical Operations in Thousands	22,463	22,710	23,286	23,739	5,948	6,087
Outpatient Visits in Thousands	366,243	390,188	417,684	452,558	116,335	119,874
Adjusted Patient Days in Thousands[2]	281,525	278,938	276,209	273,638	69,232	67,394
Beds in Thousands	908	902	891	874	862	859
Adult Occupancy Rate[3]	62.1	61.4	60.3	59.7	61.2	58.3
Total Hospital Revenues[4]	$275,430	$295,035	$309,354	$324,961	$84,280	$84,396
Total Patient Revenues	262,034	280,414	293,285	307,228	79,710	79,349
Inpatient Revenue	192,163	203,167	208,262	213,771	55,322	53,609
Outpatient Revenue	69,870	77,248	85,023	93,457	24,387	25,740
Total Expenses						
Total Hospital Expenses	$260,994	$278,880	$292,801	$308,411	$79,361	$79,958
Labor in Millions	140,112	149,733	156,826	163,842	41,873	41,935
Non-Labor in Millions	120,882	129,147	135,975	144,569	37,488	38,023
Inpatient Expense in Millions[5]	$191,385	$202,035	$207,897	$214,570	$55,081	$54,020
Amount per Patient Day	927	1,000	1,060	1,127	1,146	1,186
Amount per Admission	5,905	6,188	6,312	6,426	6,472	6,534
Outpatient Expense in Millions	$69,609	$76,845	$84,903	$93,841	$24,281	$25,937
Amount per Outpatient	190	197	203	207	209	216

Source: American Hospital Association; Trend Analysis Group: National Hospital Panel Survey Reports. Chicago. Monthly reports for January 1992 - June 1996. *Notes:* 1. Admissions per 1,000 population is calculated using population estimates prepared by the Social Security Administration. 2. Adjusted patient days is an aggregate figure reflecting the number of days of inpatient care, plus an estimate of the volume of outpatient services, expressed in units equivalent to an inpatient day in terms of level of effort. It is derived by multiplying the number of outpatient visits by the ratio of outpatient revenue per outpatient visit to inpatient revenue per inpatient day, and adding the product to the number of inpatient days. 3. The adult occupancy rate is calculated by the Office of National Health Statistics. The AHA does not publish this statistic. Adult occupancy rate is the ratio of average daily census to average number of beds maintained during the reporting period. 4. Total hospital revenue is the sum of total patient revenue and all other operating revenue. Total patient revenue is the sum of inpatient revenue and outpatient revenue. 5. Inpatient Expense and Outpatient Expense are calculated by the Office of National Health Statistics. These statistics are calculated by applying the ratio of inpatient or outpatient revenue to total patient revenue multiplied by total hospital expenses. The AHA does not publish these statistics. Q designates quarter of year. Quarterly data are not seasonally adjusted.

★ 447 ★
Hospitals

Hospital Utilization Rates: 1970 to 1993

Represents estimates of inpatients discharged from noninstitutional, short-stay hospitals, exclusive of Federal hospitals. Excludes newborn infants. Based on sample data collected from the National Hospital Discharge Survey, a sample survey of hospital records of patients discharged in year shown; subject to sampling variability.

SELECTED CHARACTERISTIC	Patients dis-charged (1,000)	PATIENTS DISCHARGED PER 1,000 PERSONS[1]			DAYS OF CARE PER 1,000 PERSONS[1]			AVERAGE STAY (days)		
		Total	Male	Female	Total	Male	Female	Total	Male	Female
1970	29,127	144	118	169	1,122	982	1,251	8.0	8.7	7.6
1980	37,832	168	139	194	1,217	1,068	1,356	7.3	7.7	7.0
1983	38,783	167	139	193	1,155	1,024	1,278	6.9	7.4	6.6
1984	37,162	159	132	184	1,044	924	1,155	6.6	7.0	6.3
1985	35,056	148	124	171	954	849	1,053	6.5	6.9	6.2
1986	34,256	143	121	164	913	817	1,003	6.4	6.8	6.1
1987	33,387	138	116	159	889	806	968	6.4	6.9	6.1
1988[2]	31,146	128	107	147	834	757	907	6.5	7.1	6.2
1989[2]	30,947	126	105	145	815	741	884	6.5	7.0	6.1
1990[2]	30,788	124	102	144	792	704	875	6.4	6.9	6.1
1991[2]	31,098	124	103	144	795	715	869	6.4	7.0	6.0
1992[2]	30,951	122	101	142	751	680	818	6.2	6.7	5.8
1993,[2] total	30,825	120	98	141	720	644	792	6.0	6.5	5.6
Age:										
Under 1 year old	710	181	206	156	1,155	1,265	1,041	6.4	6.1	6.7
1 to 4 years old	654	41	46	37	163	169	157	3.9	3.7	4.3
5 to 14 years old	777	21	22	20	108	110	105	5.1	5.1	5.2
15 to 24 years old	3,088	87	37	138	309	204	416	3.5	5.5	3.0
25 to 34 years old	4,655	113	53	171	446	313	575	4.0	5.9	3.4
35 to 44 years old	3,457	85	72	99	431	424	438	5.1	5.9	4.4
45 to 64 years old	6,283	127	132	123	785	831	742	6.2	6.3	6.1
65 to 74 years old	4,890	262	284	245	1,927	2,033	1,844	7.4	7.2	7.5
75 years old and over	6,310	446	476	430	3,665	3,764	3,609	8.2	7.9	8.4
Region:										
Northeast	6,965	136	119	152	952	876	1,023	7.0	7.4	6.7
Midwest	7,097	116	98	134	706	638	771	6.1	6.5	5.8
South	11,580	131	104	156	749	658	834	5.7	6.3	5.4
West	5,183	93	72	114	473	419	527	5.1	5.8	4.6

Source: 1996 Statistical Abstract of the United States on CD-ROM [machine-readable datafiles]. CD-8A-97. Washington, DC: U.S. Department of Commerce, Economics and Statistics Administration, Bureau of the Census, Data User Services Division, January 1997. Primary source: U.S. National Center for Health Statistics, *Vital and Health Statistics*, series 13; and unpublished data. *Notes:* 1. Based on Bureau of the Census estimated civilian population as of July 1. Estimates for 1980-90 do not reflect revisions based on the 1990 Census of Population. 2. Comparisons beginning 1988 with data for earlier years should be made with caution as estimates of change may reflect improvements in the design rather than true changes in hospital use.

★ 448 ★

Hospitals

Hospitals: Decline in Length of Stay, 1969 to 1993

This table shows the decline in the number of days spent in the hospital between 1969 and 1993.

Diagnosis/Procedure	Percent decline in hospital stay
Single-term newborn	43.6
Infectious mononucleosis	53.9
Delivery without complications	57.5
Acute myocardial infarction	61.4
Otosclerosis	63.6
Cataract	77.9
Detachment of retina	81.1

Source: "The Week in Medicine: Shorter Stays." *American Medical News,* 7 October 1996, p. 2. Primary source: HCIA, Inc.

★ 449 ★

Hospitals

Hospitals: Surgical and Nonsurgical Procedures for Discharges from Short-Stay Hospitals: Both Sexes

This table shows the number of all listed surgical and nonsurgical procedures for discharges from short-stay hospitals, both sexes, by age, and procedure category: United States, 1980, 1985, 1990, and 1991. Data are based on a sample of hospital records.

Age and procedure category	Procedures in thousands			
	1980	1985	1990[1,2]	1991[1,2]
Both sexes, all ages				
All procedures[3,4]	31,412	36,760	40,506	43,922
All surgical procedures[3]	24,494	24,799	23,051	23,403
All nonsurgical procedures[3,4]	6,918	11,961	17,455	20,519
Lens extraction	467	211	66	86
Bronchoscopy with or without biopsy	269	292	298	309
Removal of coronary artery obstruction	*6	82	285	331
Coronary artery bypass graft[5]	137	230	392	407
Cardiac catheterization	348	681	995	1,000
Insertion, replacement, removal, and revision of pacemaker leads or device	187	223	259	300
Endoscopy of small intestine with or without biopsy	282	537	785	804
Endoscopy of large intestine with or without biopsy	535	614	548	574
Cholecystectomy	458	475	522	571
Prostatectomy	335	367	364	363
Open reduction of fracture with internal fixation	301	393	391	418
Total and partial hip replacement	109	171	210	207

[Continued]

★ 449 ★

Hospitals: Surgical and Nonsurgical Procedures for Discharges from Short-Stay Hospitals: Both Sexes
[Continued]

Age and procedure category	Procedures in thousands			
	1980	1985	1990[1,2]	1991[1,2]
Total knee replacement[6]	127	160	129	160
Mastectomy	109	116	122	118
Miscellaneous diagnostic and therapeutic procedures[3,4]	3,930	8,819	11,890	14,785
Computerized axial tomography	306	1,378	1,506	1,459
Arteriography and angiocardiography using contrast material	569	1,117	1,735	1,718
Diagnostic ultrasound	318	1,234	1,608	1,592
Circulatory monitoring	76	635	724	703
Radioisotope scan	525	838	603	539
Respiratory therapy	*7	62	1,164	1,214
Other miscellaneous diagnostic and therapeutic procedures	2,128	3,556	4,549	7,560
Both sexes, 55-64 years				
All procedures[3,4]	4,022	5,036	5,059	5,339
All surgical procedures[3]	2,773	2,982	2,777	2,711
All nonsurgical procedures[3,4]	1,249	2,054	2,282	2,628
Lens extraction	83	32	*7	*9
Bronchoscopy with or without biopsy	65	68	59	60
Removal of coronary artery obstruction	*	27	87	97
Coronary artery bypass graft[5]	54	83	111	118
Cardiac catheterization	106	210	273	275
Insertion, replacement, removal, and revision of pacemaker leads or device	27	33	35	34
Endoscopy of small intestine with or without biopsy	55	90	118	117
Endoscopy of large intestine with or without biopsy	108	100	83	79
Cholecystectomy	86	88	85	97
Prostatectomy	71	72	69	61
Open reduction of fracture with internal fixation	29	45	40	40
Total and partial hip replacement	16	26	26	31
Total knee replacement[6]	19	22	24	29
Mastectomy	24	25	28	22
Miscellaneous diagnostic and therapeutic procedures[3,4]	739	1,561	1,850	2,183
Computerized axial tomography	52	215	179	184
Arteriography and angiocardiography using contrast material	165	322	449	443
Diagnostic ultrasound	55	175	203	198
Circulatory monitoring	12	106	101	109
Radioisotope scan	101	147	93	86
Respiratory therapy	*	*7	144	157
Other miscellaneous diagnostic and therapeutic procedures	353	588	681	1,007
Both sexes, 65-74 years				
All procedures[3,4]	3,916	5,788	6,777	7,421
All surgical procedures[3]	2,644	3,211	3,528	3,651
All nonsurgical procedures[3,4]	1,272	2,578	3,249	3,770
Lens extraction	153	61	21	27
Bronchoscopy with or without biopsy	74	83	79	84
Removal of coronary artery obstruction	*	20	89	98
Coronary artery bypass graft[5]	33	68	140	146

[Continued]

★ 449 ★

Hospitals: Surgical and Nonsurgical Procedures for Discharges from Short-Stay Hospitals: Both Sexes
[Continued]

Age and procedure category	Procedures in thousands			
	1980	1985	1990[1,2]	1991[1,2]
Cardiac catheterization	71	178	296	296
Insertion, replacement, removal, and revision of pacemaker leads or device	55	63	70	85
Endoscopy of small intestine with or without biopsy	49	114	170	186
Endoscopy of large intestine with or without biopsy	119	145	132	137
Cholecystectomy	83	83	81	107
Prostatectomy	139	150	159	158
Open reduction of fracture with internal fixation	33	44	50	50
Total and partial hip replacement	33	51	59	63
Total knee replacement[6]	16	31	62	72
Mastectomy	26	28	31	32
Miscellaneous diagnostic and therapeutic procedures[3,4]	724	1,950	2,627	3,129
Computerized axial tomography	58	300	309	285
Arteriography and angiocardiography using contrast material	140	320	514	506
Diagnostic ultrasound	55	235	319	314
Circulatory monitoring	18	175	180	166
Radioisotope scan	127	214	153	129
Respiratory therapy	*	15	248	250
Other miscellaneous diagnostic and therapeutic procedures	325	691	905	1,479
Both sexes, 75-84 years				
All procedures[3,4]	2,412	4,006	4,879	5,581
All surgical procedures[3]	1,610	2,129	2,324	2,525
All nonsurgical procedures[3,4]	802	1,877	2,555	3,055
Lens extraction	146	75	24	28
Bronchoscopy with or without biopsy	35	47	52	53
Removal of coronary artery obstruction	-	*	24	40
Coronary artery bypass graft[5]	*	21	61	58
Cardiac catheterization	11	47	118	135
Insertion, replacement, removal, and revision of pacemaker leads or device	64	75	87	110
Endoscopy of small intestine with or without biopsy	32	97	174	184
Endoscopy of large intestine with or without biopsy	76	123	139	152
Cholecystectomy	37	54	52	60
Prostatectomy	90	110	103	114
Open reduction of fracture with internal fixation	42	64	65	68
Total and partial hip replacement	34	52	74	63
Total knee replacement[6]	11	24	29	44
Mastectomy	16	16	18	22
Miscellaneous diagnostic and therapeutic procedures[3,4]	461	1,397	2,020	2,521
Computerized axial tomography	51	265	309	282
Arteriography and angiocardiography using contrast material	43	131	208	255
Diagnostic ultrasound	39	197	308	301
Circulatory monitoring	18	164	158	152
Radioisotope scan	97	158	120	100
Respiratory therapy	*	14	224	220

[Continued]

★ 449 ★

Hospitals: Surgical and Nonsurgical Procedures for Discharges from Short-Stay Hospitals: Both Sexes
[Continued]

Age and procedure category	Procedures in thousands			
	1980	1985	1990[1,2]	1991[1,2]
Other miscellaneous diagnostic and therapeutic procedures	212	468	692	1,211
Both sexes, 65 years and over				
All procedures[3,4]	6,969	11,027	13,308	15,073
All surgical procedures[3]	4,704	5,969	6,569	6,960
All nonsurgical procedures[3,4]	2,265	5,058	6,739	8,112
Lens extraction	335	157	51	68
Bronchoscopy with or without biopsy	115	141	144	152
Removal of coronary artery obstruction	*	23	115	143
Coronary artery bypass graft[5]	38	89	204	206
Cardiac catheterization	84	227	421	446
Insertion, replacement, removal, and revision of pacemaker leads or device	146	167	199	244
Endoscopy of small intestine with or without biopsy	89	241	414	446
Endoscopy of large intestine with or without biopsy	217	322	329	353
Cholecystectomy	129	150	146	185
Prostatectomy	251	284	284	295
Open reduction of fracture with internal fixation	109	150	163	170
Total and partial hip replacement	81	128	162	158
Total knee replacement[6]	28	58	95	121
Mastectomy	47	48	56	58
Miscellaneous diagnostic and therapeutic procedures[3,4]	1,289	3,801	5,371	6,715
Computerized axial tomography	120	650	745	702
Arteriography and angiocardiography using contrast material	187	463	742	791
Diagnostic ultrasound	103	506	734	739
Circulatory monitoring	41	403	409	390
Radioisotope scan	248	421	318	270
Respiratory therapy	*	33	565	588
Other miscellaneous diagnostic and therapeutic procedures	586	1,324	1,858	3,234
Both sexes, 75 years and over				
All procedures[3,4]	3,053	5,239	6,531	7,652
All surgical procedures[3]	2,060	2,759	3,041	3,310
All nonsurgical procedures[3,4]	993	2,480	3,490	4,342
Lens extraction	182	96	30	41
Bronchoscopy with or without biopsy	41	58	65	68
Removal of coronary artery obstruction	-	*	26	45
Coronary artery bypass graft[5]	*	21	64	60
Cardiac catheterization	13	50	125	150
Insertion, replacement, removal, and revision of pacemaker leads or device	90	104	129	160
Endoscopy of small intestine with or without biopsy	40	127	244	260
Endoscopy of large intestine with or without biopsy	98	176	198	216
Cholecystectomy	46	67	66	77
Prostatectomy	112	134	125	138
Open reduction of fracture with internal fixation	76	106	113	120
Total and partial hip replacement	48	77	103	95

[Continued]

★ 449 ★

Hospitals: Surgical and Nonsurgical Procedures for Discharges from Short-Stay Hospitals: Both Sexes
[Continued]

Age and procedure category	Procedures in thousands			
	1980	1985	1990[1,2]	1991[1,2]
Total knee replacement[6]	12	27	33	50
Mastectomy	21	20	25	26
Miscellaneous diagnostic and therapeutic procedures[3,4]	564	1,851	2,744	3,587
Computerized axial tomography	62	349	435	417
Arteriography and angiocardiography using contrast material	47	143	228	285
Diagnostic ultrasound	49	272	416	426
Circulatory monitoring	23	228	230	224
Radioisotope scan	121	207	166	142
Respiratory therapy	*	18	317	338
Other miscellaneous diagnostic and therapeutic procedures	261	633	952	1,755
Both sexes, 85 years and over				
All procedures[3,4]	641	1,233	1,652	2,071
All surgical procedures[3]	450	629	717	785
All nonsurgical procedures[3,4]	191	603	936	1,287
Lens extraction	36	21	*7	*12
Bronchoscopy with or without biopsy	*6	*10	13	15
Removal of coronary artery obstruction	-	-	*	*
Coronary artery bypass graft[5]	-	-	*	*
Cardiac catheterization	*	*	*7	14
Insertion, replacement, removal, and revision of pacemaker leads or device	26	29	42	50
Endoscopy of small intestine with or without biopsy	*8	30	70	76
Endoscopy of large intestine with or without biopsy	22	53	58	64
Cholecystectomy	*9	13	14	17
Prostatectomy	22	25	22	23
Open reduction of fracture with internal fixation	33	42	47	52
Total and partial hip replacement	15	25	29	32
Total knee replacement[6]	*	*	*	*5
Mastectomy	*	*	*6	*4
Miscellaneous diagnostic and therapeutic procedures[3,4]	104	454	724	1,065
Computerized axial tomography	11	84	126	135
Arteriography and angiocardiography using contrast material	*	*12	20	30
Diagnostic ultrasound	*10	74	108	125
Circulatory monitoring	*	64	71	71
Radioisotope scan	24	50	46	41

[Continued]

★ 449 ★

Hospitals: Surgical and Nonsurgical Procedures for Discharges from Short-Stay Hospitals: Both Sexes

[Continued]

Age and procedure category	Procedures in thousands			
	1980	1985	1990[1,2]	1991[1,2]
Respiratory therapy	*	*	92	119
Other miscellaneous diagnostic and therapeutic procedures	49	165	261	544

Source: Cohen, R.A., and J.F. Van Nostrand. *Trends in the Health of Older Americans: United States, 1994*. National Center for Health Statistics. Vital and Health Statistics 3(30). 1995. U.S. Department of Health and Human Services, Public Health Service, Centers for Disease Control and Prevention. Data are from the National Hospital Discharge Survey. *Notes:* 1. Comparisons of data for 1990 and 1991 with earlier years should be made with caution, as estimates of change may reflect improvements in the design rather than true changes in hospital use. 2. Beginning in 1989, the definitions of some surgical and diagnostic and other nonsurgical procedures were revised, thus causing a discontinuity in the trends for the totals and selected surgical procedures. 3. Includes procedures not listed on the table. 4. Inpatients discharged from short-stay hospitals had an estimated 20,519,000 nonsurgical procedures in 1991. In 1990, only 17,450,000 nonsurgical procedures were reported. The main reason for this increase was that 1991 was the first year in which all ICD-9-CM procedure codes were used in the National Hospital Discharge Survey. In previous years, selected codes were excluded, primarily codes for certain miscellaneous diagnostic and therapeutic procedures. 5. In 1991, there were 407,000 all-listed coronary artery bypass graft procedures performed on only 265,000 discharged patients. 6. For 1980 and 1985, this category is arthroplasty and replacement of knee. *Estimates based on fewer than 30 discharges are not shown; estimates based on 30-59 discharges are to be used with caution and are preceded by an asterisk. Discharges are from non-Federal hospitals. Discharges exclude newborn infants. Data do not reflect total use of surgical and diagnostic procedures because surgical and diagnostic procedures for outpatients are not included in the National Hospital Discharge Survey. In recent years, for example, lens extractions are frequently performed on outpatients. Surgical and nonsurgical procedure categories are based on the *International Classification of Diseases, 9th Revision, Clinical Modification* (ICD-9-CM).

★ 450 ★

Hospitals

Hospitals: Surgical and Nonsurgical Procedures for Discharges from Short-Stay Hospitals: Females

This table shows the number of all listed surgical and nonsurgical procedures for discharges from short-stay hospitals, females, by age, and procedure category: United States, 1980, 1985, 1990, and 1991. Data are based on a sample of hospital records.

Age and procedure category	Procedures in thousands			
	1980	1985	1990[1,2]	1991[1,2]
All ages				
All procedures[3,4]	19,521	22,066	24,590	26,658
All surgical procedures[3]	15,989	15,994	14,513	14,711
All nonsurgical procedures[3,4]	3,532	6,072	10,077	11,947
Lens extraction	274	132	39	57
Bronchoscopy with or without biopsy	102	111	123	123
Removal of coronary artery obstruction	*	24	85	107
Coronary artery bypass graft[5]	29	58	106	111
Cardiac catheterization	120	241	376	397
Insertion, replacement, removal, and revision of pacemaker leads or device	85	105	121	155
Endoscopy of small intestine with or without biopsy	164	287	428	413
Endoscopy of large intestine with or without biopsy	307	345	336	340
Cholecystectomy	336	327	375	404
Prostatectomy	...	...	...	...
Open reduction of fracture with internal fixation	149	215	214	225
Total and partial hip replacement	75	117	143	136
Total knee replacement[6]	56	75	83	100

[Continued]

★ 450 ★

Hospitals: Surgical and Nonsurgical Procedures for Discharges from Short-Stay Hospitals: Females
[Continued]

Age and procedure category	Procedures in thousands			
	1980	1985	1990[1,2]	1991[1,2]
Mastectomy	103	114	121	117
Miscellaneous diagnostic and therapeutic procedures[3,4]	2,036	4,540	6,048	7,804
Computerized axial tomography	154	707	770	757
Arteriography and angiocardiography using contrast material	215	425	685	729
Diagnostic ultrasound	204	756	941	940
Circulatory monitoring	37	303	380	364
Radioisotope scan	289	463	335	311
Respiratory therapy	*	27	578	618
Other miscellaneous diagnostic and therapeutic procedures	1,134	1,858	2,358	4,084
55-64 years				
All procedures[3,4]	2,021	2,425	2,389	2,523
All surgical procedures[3]	1,442	1,497	1,307	1,264
All nonsurgical procedures[3,4]	580	928	1,081	1,259
Lens extraction	44	17	*4	*5
Bronchoscopy with or without biopsy	27	29	25	21
Removal of coronary artery obstruction	-	*8	26	28
Coronary artery bypass graft[5]	*11	20	24	31
Cardiac catheterization	34	68	94	95
Insertion, replacement, removal, and revision of pacemaker leads or device	*10	11	12	15
Endoscopy of small intestine with or without biopsy	31	41	60	57
Endoscopy of large intestine with or without biopsy	57	54	46	46
Cholecystectomy	55	57	59	65
Prostatectomy	...	...	...	...
Open reduction of fracture with internal fixation	19	29	25	25
Total and partial hip replacement	*10	17	14	16
Total knee replacement[6]	*11	11	13	17
Mastectomy	23	25	28	21
Miscellaneous diagnostic and therapeutic procedures[3,4]	360	712	876	1,047
Computerized axial tomography	25	101	88	97
Arteriography and angiocardiography using contrast material	59	109	167	168
Diagnostic ultrasound	27	90	97	106
Circulatory monitoring	*5	44	52	51
Radioisotope scan	55	75	47	51
Respiratory therapy	*	*	73	70
Other miscellaneous diagnostic and therapeutic procedures	187	291	352	504
65-74 years				
All procedures[3,4]	1,899	2,883	3,282	3,633
All surgical procedures[3]	1,315	1,647	1,679	1,746
All nonsurgical procedures[3,4]	584	1,236	1,603	1,887
Lens extraction	91	36	12	17
Bronchoscopy with or without biopsy	25	30	30	36
Removal of coronary artery obstruction	*	*9	31	38
Coronary artery bypass graft[5]	*10	23	40	41
Cardiac catheterization	25	76	126	127

[Continued]

★ 450 ★

Hospitals: Surgical and Nonsurgical Procedures for Discharges from Short-Stay Hospitals: Females
[Continued]

Age and procedure category	Procedures in thousands			
	1980	1985	1990[1,2]	1991[1,2]
Insertion, replacement, removal, and revision of pacemaker leads or device	23	27	32	42
Endoscopy of small intestine with or without biopsy	27	56	96	88
Endoscopy of large intestine with or without biopsy	68	80	81	77
Cholecystectomy	52	49	48	66
Prostatectomy	...	...	...	...
Open reduction of fracture with internal fixation	22	32	35	33
Total and partial hip replacement	22	32	38	41
Total knee replacement[6]	12	20	40	47
Mastectomy	24	28	31	32
Miscellaneous diagnostic and therapeutic procedures[3,4]	370	983	1,319	1,595
Computerized axial tomography	30	156	165	140
Arteriography and angiocardiography using contrast material	57	140	222	232
Diagnostic ultrasound	29	121	167	159
Circulatory monitoring	*8	80	85	79
Radioisotope scan	73	116	85	79
Respiratory therapy	*	*7	124	126
Other miscellaneous diagnostic and therapeutic procedures	172	362	470	780
75-84 years				
All procedures[3,4]	1,294	2,185	2,646	3,084
All surgical procedures[3]	875	1,171	1,253	1,369
All nonsurgical procedures[3,4]	419	1,014	1,393	1,716
Lens extraction	93	54	16	22
Bronchoscopy with or without biopsy	14	18	24	22
Removal of coronary artery obstruction	-	*	10	19
Coronary artery bypass graft[5]	*	*8	25	21
Cardiac catheterization	*6	24	55	75
Insertion, replacement, removal, and revision of pacemaker leads or device	32	41	42	52
Endoscopy of small intestine with or without biopsy	22	61	102	100
Endoscopy of large intestine with or without biopsy	49	76	89	90
Cholecystectomy	24	31	27	38
Prostatectomy	...	...	...	...
Open reduction of fracture with internal fixation	32	48	53	53
Total and partial hip replacement	24	39	59	47
Total knee replacement[6]	*9	16	22	28
Mastectomy	16	16	18	22
Miscellaneous diagnostic and therapeutic procedures[3,4]	262	787	1,128	1,456
Computerized axial tomography	29	162	181	167
Arteriography and angiocardiography using contrast material	21	58	103	139
Diagnostic ultrasound	24	119	176	168
Circulatory monitoring	*9	82	86	82
Radioisotope scan	57	94	73	60
Respiratory therapy	*	*	117	121
Other miscellaneous diagnostic and therapeutic procedures	122	265	392	720

[Continued]

★ 450 ★

Hospitals: Surgical and Nonsurgical Procedures for Discharges from Short-Stay Hospitals: Females

[Continued]

Age and procedure category	Procedures in thousands			
	1980	1985	1990[1,2]	1991[1,2]
65 years and over				
All procedures[3,4]	3,587	5,833	6,982	8,078
All surgical procedures[3]	2,480	3,208	3,385	3,612
All nonsurgical procedures[3,4]	1,107	2,626	3,596	4,466
Lens extraction	211	104	33	48
Bronchoscopy with or without biopsy	42	52	63	64
Removal of coronary artery obstruction	*	*10	43	59
Coronary artery bypass graft[5]	12	31	67	63
Cardiac catheterization	32	101	185	211
Insertion, replacement, removal, and revision of pacemaker leads or device	70	86	99	128
Endoscopy of small intestine with or without biopsy	55	136	243	240
Endoscopy of large intestine with or without biopsy	131	190	211	212
Cholecystectomy	83	89	83	115
Prostatectomy	...	...	...	...
Open reduction of fracture with internal fixation	82	116	124	130
Total and partial hip replacement	58	92	118	113
Total knee replacement[6]	21	38	65	79
Mastectomy	45	48	55	58
Miscellaneous diagnostic and therapeutic procedures[3,4]	695	2,067	2,920	3,785
Computerized axial tomography	66	370	436	408
Arteriography and angiocardiography using contrast material	80	205	336	391
Diagnostic ultrasound	62	294	415	412
Circulatory monitoring	21	204	220	210
Radioisotope scan	143	244	189	167
Respiratory therapy	*	16	295	320
Other miscellaneous diagnostic and therapeutic procedures	322	733	1,029	1,877
75 years and over				
All procedures[3,4]	1,689	2,950	3,700	4,445
All surgical procedures[3]	1,165	1,561	1,706	1,866
All nonsurgical procedures[3,4]	523	1,389	1,993	2,579
Lens extraction	120	68	21	31
Bronchoscopy with or without biopsy	16	22	33	28
Removal of coronary artery obstruction	-	*	12	21
Coronary artery bypass graft[5]	*	*8	27	22
Cardiac catheterization	*7	26	59	84
Insertion, replacement, removal, and revision of pacemaker leads or device	47	59	67	85
Endoscopy of small intestine with or without biopsy	27	81	148	151
Endoscopy of large intestine with or without biopsy	63	110	130	135
Cholecystectomy	32	40	36	49
Prostatectomy	...	...	...	...
Open reduction of fracture with internal fixation	60	84	89	97
Total and partial hip replacement	36	60	80	72
Total knee replacement[6]	*9	19	24	33

[Continued]

★ 450 ★

Hospitals: Surgical and Nonsurgical Procedures for Discharges from Short-Stay Hospitals: Females
[Continued]

Age and procedure category	Procedures in thousands			
	1980	1985	1990[1,2]	1991[1,2]
Mastectomy	21	20	25	26
Miscellaneous diagnostic and therapeutic procedures[3,4]	326	1,084	1,601	2,190
Computerized axial tomography	36	215	270	268
Arteriography and angiocardiography using contrast material	23	66	114	159
Diagnostic ultrasound	32	173	248	254
Circulatory monitoring	13	124	135	131
Radioisotope scan	70	128	104	88
Respiratory therapy	*	*9	171	194
Other miscellaneous diagnostic and therapeutic procedures	151	371	559	1,096
85 years and over				
All procedures[3,4]	395	766	1,053	1,360
All surgical procedures[3]	291	390	453	497
All nonsurgical procedures[3,4]	104	376	600	863
Lens extraction	27	15	*5	*8
Bronchoscopy with or without biopsy	*	*	10	*7
Removal of coronary artery obstruction	-	-	*	*
Coronary artery bypass graft[5]	-	-	*	*
Cardiac catheterization	*	*	*	9
Insertion, replacement, removal, and revision of pacemaker leads or device	15	18	25	33
Endoscopy of small intestine with or without biopsy	*6	20	46	51
Endoscopy of large intestine with or without biopsy	14	35	42	45
Cholecystectomy	*7	*9	8	11
Prostatectomy	...	...	...	...
Open reduction of fracture with internal fixation	28	35	36	44
Total and partial hip replacement	12	21	21	25
Total knee replacement[6]	*	*	*	*
Mastectomy	*	*	*6	*4
Miscellaneous diagnostic and therapeutic procedures[3,4]	64	297	473	733
Computerized axial tomography	*7	52	89	100
Arteriography and angiocardiography using contrast material	*	*7	11	20
Diagnostic ultrasound	*8	53	72	86
Circulatory monitoring	*	42	49	49
Radioisotope scan	14	34	32	28

[Continued]

★ 450 ★

Hospitals: Surgical and Nonsurgical Procedures for Discharges from Short-Stay Hospitals: Females
[Continued]

Age and procedure category	Procedures in thousands			
	1980	1985	1990[1,2]	1991[1,2]
Respiratory therapy	*	*	54	73
Other miscellaneous diagnostic and therapeutic procedures	29	106	167	376

Source: Cohen, R.A., and J.F. Van Nostrand. *Trends in the Health of Older Americans: United States, 1994.* National Center for Health Statistics. Vital and Health Statistics 3(30). 1995. U.S. Department of Health and Human Services, Public Health Service, Centers for Disease Control and Prevention. Data are from the National Hospital Discharge Survey. *Notes:* ...means "not applicable." 1. Comparisons of data for 1990 and 1991 with earlier years should be made with caution, as estimates of change may reflect improvements in the design rather than true changes in hospital use. 2. Beginning in 1989, the definitions of some surgical and diagnostic and other nonsurgical procedures were revised, thus causing a discontinuity in the trends for the totals and selected surgical procedures. 3. Includes procedures not listed on the table. 4. Inpatients discharged from short-stay hospitals had an estimated 20,519,000 nonsurgical procedures in 1991. In 1990, only 17,450,000 nonsurgical procedures were reported. The main reason for this increase was that 1991 was the first year in which all ICD-9-CM procedure codes were used in the National Hospital Discharge Survey. In previous years, selected codes were excluded, primarily codes for certain miscellaneous diagnostic and therapeutic procedures. 5. In 1991, there were 407,000 all-listed coronary artery bypass graft procedures performed on only 265,000 discharged patients. 6. For 1980 and 1985, this category is arthroplasty and replacement of knee. *Estimates based on fewer than 30 discharges are not shown; estimates based on 30-59 discharges are to be used with caution and are preceded by an asterisk. Discharges are from non-Federal hospitals. Discharges exclude newborn infants. Data do not reflect total use of surgical and diagnostic procedures because surgical and diagnostic procedures for outpatients are not included in the National Hospital Discharge Survey. In recent years, for example, lens extractions are frequently performed on outpatients. Surgical and nonsurgical procedure categories are based on the *International Classification of Diseases, 9th Revision, Clinical Modification* (ICD-9-CM).

★ 451 ★
Hospitals

Hospitals: Surgical and Nonsurgical Procedures for Discharges from Short-Stay Hospitals: Males

This table shows the number of all listed surgical and nonsurgical procedures for discharges from short-stay hospitals, males, by age, and procedure category: United States, 1980, 1985, 1990, and 1991. Data are based on a sample of hospital records.

Age, and procedure category	Procedures in thousands			
	1980	1985	1990[1,2]	1991[1,2]
All ages				
All procedures[3,4]	11,891	14,694	15,916	17,264
All surgical procedures[3]	8,505	8,805	8,538	8,692
All nonsurgical procedures[3,4]	3,386	5,889	7,378	8,572
Lens extraction	194	79	26	30
Bronchoscopy with or without biopsy	167	181	175	186
Removal of coronary artery obstruction	*5	58	200	223
Coronary artery bypass graft[5]	108	172	286	296
Cardiac catheterization	228	439	620	603
Insertion, replacement, removal, and revision of pacemaker leads or device	102	118	138	145
Endoscopy of small intestine with or without biopsy	117	250	357	391
Endoscopy of large intestine with or without biopsy	228	269	212	234
Cholecystectomy	122	147	147	166
Prostatectomy	335	367	364	363
Open reduction of fracture with internal fixation	153	178	177	193
Total and partial hip replacement	34	54	66	71
Total knee replacement[6]	71	86	46	60

[Continued]

★ 451 ★

Hospitals: Surgical and Nonsurgical Procedures for Discharges from Short-Stay Hospitals: Males
[Continued]

Age, and procedure category	Procedures in thousands			
	1980	1985	1990[1,2]	1991[1,2]
Mastectomy	*6	*	*	*
Miscellaneous diagnostic and therapeutic procedures[3,4]	1,894	4,279	5,842	6,981
Computerized axial tomography	152	671	736	702
Arteriography and angiocardiography using contrast material	355	693	1,051	989
Diagnostic ultrasound	114	478	667	652
Circulatory monitoring	39	332	344	339
Radioisotope scan	236	375	268	228
Respiratory therapy	*	34	586	596
Other miscellaneous diagnostic and therapeutic procedures	994	1,697	2,191	3,476
55-64 years				
All procedures[3,4]	2,000	2,611	2,670	2,816
All surgical procedures[3]	1,331	1,485	1,469	1,446
All nonsurgical procedures[3,4]	669	1,126	1,201	1,370
Lens extraction	39	15	*	*
Bronchoscopy with or without biopsy	38	39	34	38
Removal of coronary artery obstruction	*	20	61	69
Coronary artery bypass graft[5]	43	63	88	87
Cardiac catheterization	72	142	179	180
Insertion, replacement, removal, and revision of pacemaker leads or device	17	22	23	19
Endoscopy of small intestine with or without biopsy	24	49	59	60
Endoscopy of large intestine with or without biopsy	51	46	37	32
Cholecystectomy	30	31	26	32
Prostatectomy	71	72	69	61
Open reduction of fracture with internal fixation	10	16	16	15
Total and partial hip replacement	*6	*9	12	15
Total knee replacement[6]	*8	*11	11	12
Mastectomy	*	*	*	*
Miscellaneous diagnostic and therapeutic procedures[3,4]	380	848	973	1,136
Computerized axial tomography	27	114	91	86
Arteriography and angiocardiography using contrast material	106	213	282	275
Diagnostic ultrasound	28	85	106	92
Circulatory monitoring	*7	61	48	58
Radioisotope scan	45	72	46	35
Respiratory therapy	*	*	71	87
Other miscellaneous diagnostic and therapeutic procedures	166	297	329	502
65-74 years				
All procedures[3,4]	2,017	2,906	3,495	3,787
All surgical procedures[3]	1,329	1,564	1,849	1,904
All nonsurgical procedures[3,4]	689	1,342	1,646	1,883
Lens extraction	62	25	9	*10
Bronchoscopy with or without biopsy	49	53	48	48
Removal of coronary artery obstruction	*	*11	58	60
Coronary artery bypass graft[5]	24	45	100	105
Cardiac catheterization	46	102	170	169

[Continued]

★ 451 ★

Hospitals: Surgical and Nonsurgical Procedures for Discharges from Short-Stay Hospitals: Males
[Continued]

Age, and procedure category	Procedures in thousands			
	1980	1985	1990[1,2]	1991[1,2]
Insertion, replacement, removal, and revision of pacemaker leads or device	32	37	38	43
Endoscopy of small intestine with or without biopsy	22	58	74	98
Endoscopy of large intestine with or without biopsy	51	66	51	60
Cholecystectomy	31	34	33	41
Prostatectomy	139	150	159	158
Open reduction of fracture with internal fixation	*11	12	15	17
Total and partial hip replacement	11	19	21	21
Total knee replacement[6]	*	*11	22	25
Mastectomy	*	*	*	*
Miscellaneous diagnostic and therapeutic procedures[3,4]	355	967	1,308	1,534
Computerized axial tomography	29	145	144	145
Arteriography and angiocardiography using contrast material	83	180	291	274
Diagnostic ultrasound	25	114	151	155
Circulatory monitoring	*10	95	94	87
Radioisotope scan	54	97	68	50
Respiratory therapy	*	*8	124	124
Other miscellaneous diagnostic and therapeutic procedures	153	329	435	699
75-84 years				
All procedures[3,4]	1,119	1,821	2,233	2,496
All surgical procedures[3]	735	958	1,071	1,156
All nonsurgical procedures[3,4]	383	863	1,162	1,340
Lens extraction	53	21	8	*6
Bronchoscopy with or without biopsy	21	30	29	31
Removal of coronary artery obstruction	-	*	14	21
Coronary artery bypass graft[5]	*	12	36	38
Cardiac catheterization	*6	23	63	60
Insertion, replacement, removal, and revision of pacemaker leads or device	32	34	44	58
Endoscopy of small intestine with or without biopsy	*10	36	72	84
Endoscopy of large intestine with or without biopsy	27	48	50	62
Cholecystectomy	13	23	24	22
Prostatectomy	90	110	103	114
Open reduction of fracture with internal fixation	*10	15	13	15
Total and partial hip replacement	*9	13	15	17
Total knee replacement[6]	*	*8	8	16
Mastectomy	*	*	*	*
Miscellaneous diagnostic and therapeutic procedures[3,4]	199	610	892	1,065
Computerized axial tomography	22	103	128	115
Arteriography and angiocardiography using contrast material	22	73	105	116
Diagnostic ultrasound	14	78	132	133
Circulatory monitoring	*9	82	72	70
Radioisotope scan	41	64	47	41
Respiratory therapy	*	*7	108	99
Other miscellaneous diagnostic and therapeutic procedures	90	204	299	491

[Continued]

★ 451 ★

Hospitals: Surgical and Nonsurgical Procedures for Discharges from Short-Stay Hospitals: Males
[Continued]

Age, and procedure category	Procedures in thousands			
	1980	1985	1990[1,2]	1991[1,2]
65 years and over				
All procedures[3,4]	3,382	5,194	6,326	6,994
All surgical procedures[3]	2,224	2,762	3,184	3,348
All nonsurgical procedures[3,4]	1,158	2,432	3,143	3,646
Lens extraction	124	53	18	20
Bronchoscopy with or without biopsy	73	89	80	88
Removal of coronary artery obstruction	*	13	72	84
Coronary artery bypass graft[5]	27	57	137	144
Cardiac catheterization	52	126	236	235
Insertion, replacement, removal, and revision of pacemaker leads or device	75	82	100	117
Endoscopy of small intestine with or without biopsy	35	104	171	207
Endoscopy of large intestine with or without biopsy	86	131	118	141
Cholecystectomy	45	61	63	70
Prostatectomy	251	284	284	295
Open reduction of fracture with internal fixation	27	34	39	40
Total and partial hip replacement	23	36	45	45
Total knee replacement[6]	*7	20	31	42
Mastectomy	*	*	*	*
Miscellaneous diagnostic and therapeutic procedures[3,4]	593	1,734	2,451	2,931
Computerized axial tomography	54	280	309	294
Arteriography and angiocardiography using contrast material	107	258	406	401
Diagnostic ultrasound	42	213	319	327
Circulatory monitoring	20	199	189	180
Radioisotope scan	105	177	129	104
Respiratory therapy	*	17	269	268
Other miscellaneous diagnostic and therapeutic procedures	264	591	829	1,358
75 years and over				
All procedures[3,4]	1,364	2,288	2,831	3,207
All surgical procedures[3]	894	1,198	1,335	1,444
All nonsurgical procedures[3,4]	469	1,091	1,497	1,763
Lens extraction	62	27	9	*10
Bronchoscopy with or without biopsy	25	36	32	40
Removal of coronary artery obstruction	-	*	15	24
Coronary artery bypass graft[5]	*	12	37	39
Cardiac catheterization	*6	24	66	66
Insertion, replacement, removal, and revision of pacemaker leads or device	43	45	62	74
Endoscopy of small intestine with or without biopsy	13	47	97	109
Endoscopy of large intestine with or without biopsy	35	66	67	81
Cholecystectomy	15	27	30	29
Prostatectomy	112	134	125	138
Open reduction of fracture with internal fixation	16	22	24	23
Total and partial hip replacement	*12	17	23	24
Total knee replacement[6]	*	*8	9	17

[Continued]

★ 451 ★

Hospitals: Surgical and Nonsurgical Procedures for Discharges from Short-Stay Hospitals: Males
[Continued]

Age, and procedure category	Procedures in thousands			
	1980	1985	1990[1,2]	1991[1,2]
Mastectomy	*	*	*	*
Miscellaneous diagnostic and therapeutic procedures[3,4]	239	767	1,143	1,397
Computerized axial tomography	26	135	165	149
Arteriography and angiocardiography using contrast material	24	78	115	127
Diagnostic ultrasound	16	99	168	172
Circulatory monitoring	*10	104	95	93
Radioisotope scan	51	80	61	54
Respiratory therapy	*	*10	146	144
Other miscellaneous diagnostic and therapeutic procedures	111	262	393	659
85 years and over				
All procedures[3,4]	246	467	599	711
All surgical procedures[3]	159	239	264	288
All nonsurgical procedures[3,4]	86	228	335	424
Lens extraction	*9	*7	*	*
Bronchoscopy with or without biopsy	*	*	*3	8
Removal of coronary artery obstruction	-	-	*	*
Coronary artery bypass graft[5]	-	-	*	*
Cardiac catheterization	*	*	*	*5
Insertion, replacement, removal, and revision of pacemaker leads or device	*11	11	18	17
Endoscopy of small intestine with or without biopsy	*	*10	25	25
Endoscopy of large intestine with or without biopsy	*8	18	17	19
Cholecystectomy	*	*	*6	*6
Prostatectomy	22	25	22	23
Open reduction of fracture with internal fixation	*6	*7	11	8
Total and partial hip replacement	*	*	*8	*7
Total knee replacement[6]	*	*	*	*
Mastectomy	-	-	*	*
Miscellaneous diagnostic and therapeutic procedures[3,4]	40	157	251	332
Computerized axial tomography	*	32	37	34
Arteriography and angiocardiography using contrast material	*	*	9	10
Diagnostic ultrasound	*	21	36	39
Circulatory monitoring	*	22	23	23
Radioisotope scan	*10	16	14	13

[Continued]

★ 451 ★

Hospitals: Surgical and Nonsurgical Procedures for Discharges from Short-Stay Hospitals: Males
[Continued]

Age, and procedure category	Procedures in thousands			
	1980	1985	1990[1,2]	1991[1,2]
Respiratory therapy	*	*	38	45
Other miscellaneous diagnostic and therapeutic procedures	20	58	94	168

Source: Cohen, R.A., and J.F. Van Nostrand. *Trends in the Health of Older Americans: United States, 1994.* National Center for Health Statistics. Vital and Health Statistics 3(30). 1995. U.S. Department of Health and Human Services, Public Health Service, Centers for Disease Control and Prevention. Data are from the National Hospital Discharge Survey. *Notes:* 1. Comparisons of data for 1990 and 1991 with earlier years should be made with caution, as estimates of change may reflect improvements in the design rather than true changes in hospital use. 2. Beginning in 1989, the definitions of some surgical and diagnostic and other nonsurgical procedures were revised, thus causing a discontinuity in the trends for the totals and selected surgical procedures. 3. Includes procedures not listed on the table. 4. Inpatients discharged from short-stay hospitals had an estimated 20,519,000 nonsurgical procedures in 1991. In 1990, only 17,450,000 nonsurgical procedures were reported. The main reason for this increase was that 1991 was the first year in which all ICD-9-CM procedure codes were used in the National Hospital Discharge Survey. In previous years, selected codes were excluded, primarily codes for certain miscellaneous diagnostic and therapeutic procedures. 5. In 1991, there were 407,000 all-listed coronary artery bypass graft procedures performed on only 265,000 discharged patients. 6. For 1980 and 1985, this category is arthroplasty and replacement of knee. *Estimates based on fewer than 30 discharges are not shown; estimates based on 30-59 discharges are to be used with caution and are preceded by an asterisk. Discharges are from non-Federal hospitals. Discharges exclude newborn infants. Data do not reflect total use of surgical and diagnostic procedures because surgical and diagnostic procedures for outpatients are not included in the National Hospital Discharge Survey. In recent years, for example, lens extractions are frequently performed on outpatients. Surgical and nonsurgical procedure categories are based on the *International Classification of Diseases, 9th Revision, Clinical Modification* (ICD-9-CM).

★ 452 ★
Hospitals

Hospitals: Surgical and Nonsurgical Procedures for Discharges from Short-Stay Hospitals: Rates for Both Sexes

This table shows the rate of all listed surgical and nonsurgical procedures for discharges from short-stay hospitals, both sexes, by age, and procedure category: United States, 1980, 1985, 1990, and 1991. Data are based on a sample of hospital records. Rates are per 100,000 population.

Sex, age, and procedure category	Rate per 100,000 population			
	1980	1985	1990[1,2]	1991[1,2]
Both Sexes, all Ages				
All procedures[3,4]	13,922.3	15,561.8	16,347.8	17,529.3
All surgical procedures[3]	10,856.1	10,498.3	9,303.0	9,340.1
All nonsurgical procedures[3,4]	3,066.1	5,063.5	7,044.7	8,189.2
Lens extraction	207.2	89.5	26.5	34.4
Bronchoscopy with or without biopsy	119.2	123.6	120.2	123.4
Removal of coronary artery obstruction	*2.6	34.7	115.2	131.9
Coronary artery bypass graft[5]	60.8	97.5	158.3	162.6
Cardiac catheterization	154.4	288.1	401.8	399.1
Insertion, replacement, removal, and revision of pacemaker leads or device	83.0	94.6	104.5	119.6
Endoscopy of small intestine with or without biopsy	124.8	227.4	316.7	320.9
Endoscopy of large intestine with or without biopsy	237.2	260.1	221.1	229.0
Cholecystectomy	203.0	201.0	210.7	227.8
Prostatectomy	148.5	155.3	146.8	145.1
Open reduction of fracture with internal fixation	133.6	166.4	157.8	166.7
Total and partial hip replacement	48.4	72.4	84.6	82.5
Total knee replacement[6]	56.4	67.9	52.1	64.0

[Continued]

★ 452 ★

Hospitals: Surgical and Nonsurgical Procedures for Discharges from Short-Stay Hospitals: Rates for Both Sexes

[Continued]

Sex, age, and procedure category	Rate per 100,000 population			
	1980	1985	1990[1,2]	1991[1,2]
Mastectomy	48.2	49.1	49.2	47.2
Miscellaneous diagnostic and therapeutic procedures[3,4]	1,741.8	3,733.4	4,798.6	5,900.5
Computerized axial tomography	135.6	583.2	607.7	582.4
Arteriography and angiocardiography using contrast material	252.3	472.9	700.3	685.8
Diagnostic ultrasound	141.2	522.3	649.2	635.2
Circulatory monitoring	33.7	268.8	292.3	280.5
Radioisotope scan	232.6	354.8	243.4	215.0
Respiratory therapy	*3.3	26.1	469.8	484.5
Other miscellaneous diagnostic and therapeutic procedures	943.2	1,505.3	1,835.9	3,017.1
Both sexes, 55-64 years				
All procedures[3,4]	18,487.6	22,754.5	23,987.7	25,419.2
All surgical procedures[3]	12,745.9	13,474.3	13,166.2	12,905.4
All nonsurgical procedures[3,4]	5,741.6	9,280.2	10,821.5	12,513.8
Lens extraction	381.8	143.8	*34.5	42.0
Bronchoscopy with or without biopsy	299.0	306.5	278.2	284.2
Removal of coronary artery obstruction	*	123.4	412.3	461.5
Coronary artery bypass graft[5]	247.7	373.8	528.1	562.6
Cardiac catheterization	487.0	950.4	1,294.7	1,309.6
Insertion, replacement, removal, and revision of pacemaker leads or device	124.2	148.9	167.3	162.0
Endoscopy of small intestine with or without biopsy	253.1	407.4	561.5	557.5
Endoscopy of large intestine with or without biopsy	497.5	452.9	392.7	373.9
Cholecystectomy	393.3	397.0	403.4	463.5
Prostatectomy	327.5	326.0	328.1	288.1
Open reduction of fracture with internal fixation	134.2	204.1	191.9	191.5
Total and partial hip replacement	72.1	116.0	122.6	147.7
Total knee replacement[6]	86.8	100.8	114.2	137.8
Mastectomy	111.4	114.2	134.0	102.9
Miscellaneous diagnostic and therapeutic procedures[3,4]	3,399.2	7,052.1	8,770.2	10,394.0
Computerized axial tomography	240.4	972.4	847.7	873.7
Arteriography and angiocardiography using contrast material	757.0	1,456.8	2,127.3	2,109.4
Diagnostic ultrasound	251.9	790.2	964.7	942.1
Circulatory monitoring	55.7	477.4	478.0	518.6
Radioisotope scan	462.1	663.9	441.8	410.2
Respiratory therapy	*	*33.3	681.3	747.4
Other miscellaneous diagnostic and therapeutic procedures	1,623.3	2,658.0	3,229.5	4,792.6
Both sexes, 65-74 years				
All procedures[3,4]	25,021.7	34,335.2	37,446.9	40,594.6
All surgical procedures[3]	16,891.6	19,045.7	19,494.6	19,970.5
All nonsurgical procedures[3,4]	8,130.1	15,289.4	17,952.3	20,624.2
Lens extraction	978.5	364.4	116.1	147.9
Bronchoscopy with or without biopsy	473.7	495.2	433.8	459.3
Removal of coronary artery obstruction	*	118.4	490.3	536.5
Coronary artery bypass graft[5]	213.3	402.8	773.3	798.7
Cardiac catheterization	454.3	1,055.1	1,637.0	1,620.5

[Continued]

★ 452 ★

Hospitals: Surgical and Nonsurgical Procedures for Discharges from Short-Stay Hospitals: Rates for Both Sexes
[Continued]

Sex, age, and procedure category	Rate per 100,000 population			
	1980	1985	1990[1,2]	1991[1,2]
Insertion, replacement, removal, and revision of pacemaker leads or device	351.8	375.8	384.9	464.1
Endoscopy of small intestine with or without biopsy	312.9	675.5	939.7	1,019.4
Endoscopy of large intestine with or without biopsy	758.8	863.0	728.7	747.0
Cholecystectomy	527.1	494.3	445.6	587.5
Prostatectomy	889.5	888.8	878.4	862.4
Open reduction of fracture with internal fixation	210.4	260.7	276.6	273.7
Total and partial hip replacement	211.0	304.5	326.5	342.7
Total knee replacement[6]	100.4	184.2	342.5	392.5
Mastectomy	165.9	167.8	170.5	176.4
Miscellaneous diagnostic and therapeutic procedures[3,4]	4,627.1	11,568.1	14,517.2	17,115.5
Computerized axial tomography	373.4	1,782.4	1,709.3	1,558.1
Arteriography and angiocardiography using contrast material	896.9	1,898.4	2,838.9	2,769.4
Diagnostic ultrasound	350.0	1,391.9	1,761.1	1,715.8
Circulatory monitoring	116.6	1,038.1	992.0	907.8
Radioisotope scan	808.7	1,269.1	844.5	704.6
Respiratory therapy	*	88.5	1,368.9	1,368.4
Other miscellaneous diagnostic and therapeutic procedures	2,073.8	4,099.7	5,002.5	8,091.5
Both sexes, 75-84 years				
All procedures[3,4]	30,984.9	45,057.3	48,419.5	54,107.4
All surgical procedures[3]	20,681.9	23,948.4	23,067.7	24,482.5
All nonsurgical procedures[3,4]	10,303.0	21,108.9	25,351.8	29,624.9
Lens extraction	1,875.2	838.1	233.8	275.7
Bronchoscopy with or without biopsy	446.2	534.2	519.9	515.1
Removal of coronary artery obstruction	-	*	239.5	385.5
Coronary artery bypass graft[5]	*	232.7	605.0	566.3
Cardiac catheterization	144.7	528.4	1,167.7	1,313.6
Insertion, replacement, removal, and revision of pacemaker leads or device	824.2	848.4	859.1	1,064.8
Endoscopy of small intestine with or without biopsy	410.0	1,093.2	1,726.2	1,782.6
Endoscopy of large intestine with or without biopsy	975.4	1,388.2	1,382.5	1,476.2
Cholecystectomy	478.9	603.9	513.2	585.6
Prostatectomy	1,155.1	1,235.0	1,021.4	1,109.9
Open reduction of fracture with internal fixation	545.0	714.7	649.6	661.9
Total and partial hip replacement	433.3	582.5	738.5	615.4
Total knee replacement[6]	145.2	270.5	291.0	428.2
Mastectomy	210.7	179.8	183.2	214.3
Miscellaneous diagnostic and therapeutic procedures[3,4]	5,918.9	15,712.0	20,045.5	24,446.6
Computerized axial tomography	650.4	2,984.0	3,067.8	2,738.3
Arteriography and angiocardiography using contrast material	553.8	1,470.9	2,066.8	2,471.8
Diagnostic ultrasound	498.1	2,220.8	3,056.5	2,917.2
Circulatory monitoring	225.2	1,844.7	1,571.9	1,475.7
Radioisotope scan	1,251.8	1,771.8	1,190.4	971.5
Respiratory therapy	*	152.0	2,227.7	2,129.5
Other miscellaneous diagnostic and therapeutic procedures	2,728.9	5,268.0	6,864.4	11,742.6

[Continued]

★ 452 ★

Hospitals: Surgical and Nonsurgical Procedures for Discharges from Short-Stay Hospitals: Rates for Both Sexes

[Continued]

Sex, age, and procedure category	Rate per 100,000 population			
	1980	1985	1990[1,2]	1991[1,2]
Both sexes, 65 years and over				
All procedures[3,4]	27,108.7	38,805.8	42,621.0	47,467.2
All surgical procedures[3]	18,297.1	21,007.1	21,038.3	21,919.9
All nonsurgical procedures[3,4]	8,811.6	17,798.7	21,582.7	25,547.3
Lens extraction	1,304.1	553.1	164.0	213.2
Bronchoscopy with or without biopsy	448.4	496.7	459.8	479.0
Removal of coronary artery obstruction	*	82.4	368.3	449.1
Coronary artery bypass graft[5]	149.6	311.6	653.5	650.2
Cardiac catheterization	326.5	799.8	1,348.6	1,404.8
Insertion, replacement, removal, and revision of pacemaker leads or device	566.1	589.0	636.4	769.8
Endoscopy of small intestine with or without biopsy	347.3	847.3	1,326.6	1,405.6
Endoscopy of large intestine with or without biopsy	842.6	1,130.8	1,055.1	1,111.1
Cholecystectomy	501.2	528.2	468.8	581.9
Prostatectomy	976.8	1,000.0	909.6	930.0
Open reduction of fracture with internal fixation	422.9	527.1	521.5	535.6
Total and partial hip replacement	316.2	450.8	519.7	497.8
Total knee replacement[6]	107.1	204.1	305.1	382.3
Mastectomy	182.3	168.6	178.1	184.0
Miscellaneous diagnostic and therapeutic procedures[3,4]	5,012.4	13,368.7	17,200.6	21,148.5
Computerized axial tomography	467.3	2,285.7	2,384.5	2,210.6
Arteriography and angiocardiography using contrast material	728.5	1,629.2	2,376.4	2,492.2
Diagnostic ultrasound	402.3	1,781.0	2,351.7	2,328.6
Circulatory monitoring	159.5	1,417.1	1,310.7	1,226.9
Radioisotope scan	964.8	1,482.0	1,019.8	851.8
Respiratory therapy	*	117.2	1,808.0	1,853.0
Other miscellaneous diagnostic and therapeutic procedures	2,279.6	4,659.4	5,949.4	10,185.6
Both sexes, 75 years and over				
All procedures[3,4]	30,356.6	45,327.0	49,754.6	56,791.1
All surgical procedures[3]	20,484.5	23,868.0	23,166.6	24,564.8
All nonsurgical procedures[3,4]	9,872.2	21,458.9	26,588.0	32,226.3
Lens extraction	1,810.8	827.8	230.1	301.9
Bronchoscopy with or without biopsy	409.0	498.8	495.5	505.7
Removal of coronary artery obstruction	-	*	200.0	330.5
Coronary artery bypass graft[5]	*	178.7	488.2	448.7
Cardiac catheterization	127.7	428.0	950.9	1,112.1
Insertion, replacement, removal, and revision of pacemaker leads or device	899.5	899.4	983.1	1,184.6
Endoscopy of small intestine with or without biopsy	400.7	1,097.6	1,860.1	1,929.6
Endoscopy of large intestine with or without biopsy	972.9	1,520.7	1,505.2	1,604.9
Cholecystectomy	460.9	577.4	500.8	574.2
Prostatectomy	1,112.7	1,161.9	952.7	1,021.8
Open reduction of fracture with internal fixation	753.6	915.1	859.0	890.8
Total and partial hip replacement	479.8	664.1	786.1	708.2
Total knee replacement[6]	117.4	233.1	253.5	368.4

[Continued]

★ 452 ★

Hospitals: Surgical and Nonsurgical Procedures for Discharges from Short-Stay Hospitals: Rates for Both Sexes

[Continued]

Sex, age, and procedure category	Rate per 100,000 population			
	1980	1985	1990[1,2]	1991[1,2]
Mastectomy	207.9	169.8	188.6	194.4
Miscellaneous diagnostic and therapeutic procedures[3,4]	5,612.0	15,990.9	20,900.3	26,619.9
Computerized axial tomography	613.6	3,018.8	3,315.5	3,095.8
Arteriography and angiocardiography using contrast material	466.4	1,237.1	1,738.8	2,116.1
Diagnostic ultrasound	483.7	2,347.8	3,165.9	3,159.9
Circulatory monitoring	226.3	1,969.1	1,750.2	1,659.8
Radioisotope scan	1,207.8	1,792.0	1,261.5	1,051.5
Respiratory therapy	*	158.9	2,413.4	2,510.4
Other miscellaneous diagnostic and therapeutic procedures	2,600.0	5,475.7	7,254.9	13,026.6
Both sexes, 85 years and over				
All procedures[3,4]	28,203.4	46,225.7	54,165.7	65,550.7
All surgical procedures[3]	19,807.8	23,600.2	23,493.5	24,833.2
All nonsurgical procedures[3,4]	8,395.6	22,625.5	30,672.2	40,717.6
Lens extraction	1,590.1	793.8	*217.6	387.3
Bronchoscopy with or without biopsy	*281.5	*381.9	414.7	475.0
Removal of coronary artery obstruction	-	-	*	151.0
Coronary artery bypass graft[5]	*	*	*	64.6
Cardiac catheterization	*	*	*234.9	454.3
Insertion, replacement, removal, and revision of pacemaker leads or device	1,157.6	1,068.3	1,393.1	1,575.6
Endoscopy of small intestine with or without biopsy	*368.8	1,112.1	2,302.2	2,409.5
Endoscopy of large intestine with or without biopsy	964.4	1,959.4	1,910.5	2,025.2
Cholecystectomy	*399.5	489.8	459.8	536.9
Prostatectomy	967.7	919.8	725.9	734.3
Open reduction of fracture with internal fixation	1,468.5	1,578.4	1,551.1	1,637.9
Total and partial hip replacement	639.1	936.1	943.4	1,011.1
Total knee replacement[6]	*	*	*	173.0
Mastectomy	*	*	*206.8	129.2
Miscellaneous diagnostic and therapeutic procedures[3,4]	4,560.3	16,914.2	23,733.0	33,713.5
Computerized axial tomography	487.4	3,133.9	4,133.8	4,262.8
Arteriography and angiocardiography using contrast material	*	*463.3	655.2	954.8
Diagnostic ultrasound	*434.1	2,768.2	3,527.4	3,951.7
Circulatory monitoring	*	2,381.2	2,339.2	2,260.6
Radioisotope scan	1,057.3	1,859.1	1,496.4	1,312.5

[Continued]

★ 452 ★

Hospitals: Surgical and Nonsurgical Procedures for Discharges from Short-Stay Hospitals: Rates for Both Sexes
[Continued]

Sex, age, and procedure category	Rate per 100,000 population			
	1980	1985	1990[1,2]	1991[1,2]
Respiratory therapy	*	*	3,027.2	3,753.8
Other miscellaneous diagnostic and therapeutic procedures	2,158.1	6,167.9	8,544.9	17,217.3

Source: Cohen, R.A., and J.F. Van Nostrand. *Trends in the Health of Older Americans: United States, 1994.* National Center for Health Statistics. Vital and Health Statistics 3(30). 1995. U.S. Department of Health and Human Services, Public Health Service, Centers for Disease Control and Prevention. Data are from the National Hospital Discharge Survey. *Notes:* 1. Comparisons of data for 1990 and 1991 with earlier years should be made with caution, as estimates of change may reflect improvements in the design rather than true changes in hospital use. 2. Beginning in 1989, the definitions of some surgical and diagnostic and other nonsurgical procedures were revised, thus causing a discontinuity in the trends for the totals and selected surgical procedures. 3. Includes procedures not listed on the table. 4. Inpatients discharged from short-stay hospitals had an estimated 20,519,000 nonsurgical procedures in 1991. In 1990, only 17,450,000 nonsurgical procedures were reported. The main reason for this increase was that 1991 was the first year in which all ICD-9-CM procedure codes were used in the National Hospital Discharge Survey. In previous years, selected codes were excluded, primarily codes for certain miscellaneous diagnostic and therapeutic procedures. 5. In 1991, there were 407,000 all-listed coronary artery bypass graft procedures performed on only 265,000 discharged patients. 6. For 1980 and 1985, this category is arthroplasty and replacement of knee. *Estimates based on fewer than 30 discharges are not shown; estimates based on 30-59 discharges are to be used with caution and are preceded by an asterisk. Discharges are from non-Federal hospitals. Discharges exclude newborn infants. Data do not reflect total use of surgical and diagnostic procedures because surgical and diagnostic procedures for outpatients are not included in the National Hospital Discharge Survey. In recent years, for example, lens extractions are frequently performed on outpatients. Surgical and nonsurgical procedure categories are based on the *International Classification of Diseases, 9th Revision, Clinical Modification* (ICD-9-CM).

★ 453 ★

Hospitals

Hospitals: Surgical and Nonsurgical Procedures for Discharges from Short-Stay Hospitals: Rates for Females

This table shows the rate of all listed surgical and nonsurgical procedures for discharges from short-stay hospitals, females, by age, and procedure category: United States, 1980, 1985, 1990, and 1991. Data are based on a sample of hospital records. Rates are per 100,000 population.

Age and procedure category	Rate per 100,000 population			
	1980	1985	1990[1,2]	1991[1,2]
All ages				
All procedures[3,4]	16,727.7	18,082.0	19,264.6	20,661.1
All surgical procedures[3]	13,701.4	13,106.5	11,370.1	11,401.4
All nonsurgical procedures[3,4]	3,026.3	4,975.5	7,894.6	9,259.7
Lens extraction	234.4	108.4	30.6	44.0
Bronchoscopy with or without biopsy	87.6	90.7	96.2	95.2
Removal of coronary artery obstruction	*	19.9	66.6	83.3
Coronary artery bypass graft[5]	25.1	47.4	83.0	86.4
Cardiac catheterization	102.9	197.8	294.4	307.9
Insertion, replacement, removal, and revision of pacemaker leads or device	72.7	86.3	94.8	119.9
Endoscopy of small intestine with or without biopsy	140.7	235.5	335.2	320.0
Endoscopy of large intestine with or without biopsy	263.0	282.7	263.3	263.4
Cholecystectomy	287.6	268.3	293.5	313.4
Prostatectomy	...	...	...	...
Open reduction of fracture with internal fixation	127.5	176.1	167.9	174.6
Total and partial hip replacement	64.4	96.3	112.3	105.0
Total knee replacement[6]	48.3	61.2	65.4	77.8
Mastectomy	88.2	93.7	94.7	90.9

[Continued]

★ 453 ★

Hospitals: Surgical and Nonsurgical Procedures for Discharges from Short-Stay Hospitals: Rates for Females
[Continued]

Age and procedure category	Rate per 100,000 population			
	1980	1985	1990[1,2]	1991[1,2]
Miscellaneous diagnostic and therapeutic procedures[3,4]	1,744.7	3,720.0	4,737.9	6,048.2
Computerized axial tomography	132.3	579.3	603.5	587.0
Arteriography and angiocardiography using contrast material	183.8	347.9	536.3	565.3
Diagnostic ultrasound	175.1	619.6	737.5	728.5
Circulatory monitoring	31.9	248.3	297.7	282.0
Radioisotope scan	247.6	379.8	262.4	241.0
Respiratory therapy	*	22.4	453.1	479.1
Other miscellaneous diagnostic and therapeutic procedures	971.4	1,522.8	1,847.4	3,166.6
55-64 years				
All procedures[3,4]	17,457.2	20,638.6	21,445.8	22,783.8
All surgical procedures[3]	12,450.5	12,742.1	11,737.3	11,416.1
All nonsurgical procedures[3,4]	5,006.7	7,896.5	9,708.5	11,367.7
Lens extraction	380.8	142.8	*34.8	*45.2
Bronchoscopy with or without biopsy	230.8	248.8	225.2	194.0
Removal of coronary artery obstruction	-	*65.1	231.2	253.9
Coronary artery bypass graft[5]	*93.7	170.5	211.2	279.1
Cardiac catheterization	289.6	578.4	841.2	857.0
Insertion, replacement, removal, and revision of pacemaker leads or device	*82.6	93.5	107.5	132.1
Endoscopy of small intestine with or without biopsy	268.0	352.3	535.6	511.6
Endoscopy of large intestine with or without biopsy	493.8	459.9	408.9	416.5
Cholecystectomy	478.8	485.3	532.6	587.3
Prostatectomy	...	...	...	...
Open reduction of fracture with internal fixation	162.5	249.1	222.3	223.6
Total and partial hip replacement	84.5	145.1	127.6	141.0
Total knee replacement[6]	*91.2	92.5	120.7	154.0
Mastectomy	199.6	213.0	248.3	191.3
Miscellaneous diagnostic and therapeutic procedures[3,4]	3,106.9	6,062.6	7,868.3	9,457.6
Computerized axial tomography	220.0	858.9	789.5	878.0
Arteriography and angiocardiography using contrast material	506.8	929.5	1,500.3	1,517.9
Diagnostic ultrasound	235.3	763.0	874.0	955.4
Circulatory monitoring	*42.1	378.4	470.6	460.8
Radioisotope scan	476.8	640.6	420.4	459.5
Respiratory therapy	*	*	656.1	632.2
Other miscellaneous diagnostic and therapeutic procedures	1,618.4	2,476.4	3,157.5	4,553.9
65-74 years				
All procedures[3,4]	21,422.6	30,283.3	32,285.9	35,421.9
All surgical procedures[3]	14,836.9	17,299.2	16,517.5	17,025.7
All nonsurgical procedures[3,4]	6,585.7	12,984.1	15,768.4	18,396.3
Lens extraction	1,031.9	378.3	119.3	163.8
Bronchoscopy with or without biopsy	286.8	319.8	296.7	348.4
Removal of coronary artery obstruction	*	*91.5	306.8	372.1
Coronary artery bypass graft[5]	*110.3	242.2	393.5	397.7
Cardiac catheterization	286.1	796.6	1,241.3	1,240.8

[Continued]

★ 453 ★

Hospitals: Surgical and Nonsurgical Procedures for Discharges from Short-Stay Hospitals: Rates for Females
[Continued]

Age and procedure category	Rate per 100,000 population			
	1980	1985	1990[1,2]	1991[1,2]
Insertion, replacement, removal, and revision of pacemaker leads or device	261.3	282.0	314.4	411.6
Endoscopy of small intestine with or without biopsy	307.6	587.5	943.6	861.8
Endoscopy of large intestine with or without biopsy	769.6	837.0	793.6	748.8
Cholecystectomy	583.3	517.2	467.7	648.0
Prostatectomy	...	...	...	...
Open reduction of fracture with internal fixation	247.5	337.5	345.4	321.3
Total and partial hip replacement	247.8	339.8	371.9	403.2
Total knee replacement[6]	133.7	206.8	395.2	454.6
Mastectomy	274.8	295.7	302.8	312.2
Miscellaneous diagnostic and therapeutic procedures[3,4]	4,169.3	10,325.7	12,978.9	15,548.6
Computerized axial tomography	334.9	1,635.6	1,627.6	1,367.6
Arteriography and angiocardiography using contrast material	644.6	1,469.3	2,188.0	2,263.2
Diagnostic ultrasound	332.3	1,271.6	1,646.7	1,546.2
Circulatory monitoring	*94.6	843.3	838.2	772.6
Radioisotope scan	818.7	1,223.6	835.3	768.4
Respiratory therapy	*	*76.0	1,219.5	1,224.9
Other miscellaneous diagnostic and therapeutic procedures	1,935.8	3,806.3	4,623.6	7,605.9
75-84 years				
All procedures[3,4]	26,416.0	39,022.3	41,995.6	47,997.8
All surgical procedures[3]	17,860.8	20,914.0	19,889.1	21,299.7
All nonsurgical procedures[3,4]	8,555.2	18,108.3	22,106.5	26,698.1
Lens extraction	1,900.4	959.6	254.7	349.3
Bronchoscopy with or without biopsy	277.6	316.8	373.4	336.6
Removal of coronary artery obstruction	-	*	165.9	291.0
Coronary artery bypass graft[5]	*	*149.5	403.7	321.3
Cardiac catheterization	*115.8	420.0	867.9	1,168.3
Insertion, replacement, removal, and revision of pacemaker leads or device	656.6	737.7	671.4	810.5
Endoscopy of small intestine with or without biopsy	441.6	1,087.7	1,617.5	1,557.3
Endoscopy of large intestine with or without biopsy	992.0	1,350.8	1,410.6	1,398.3
Cholecystectomy	498.7	554.8	436.3	590.4
Prostatectomy	...	...	...	...
Open reduction of fracture with internal fixation	662.4	862.9	838.1	828.2
Total and partial hip replacement	495.4	692.7	935.0	729.8
Total knee replacement[6]	*182.8	286.3	345.6	441.6
Mastectomy	331.4	283.7	291.4	338.0
Miscellaneous diagnostic and therapeutic procedures[3,4]	5,352.1	14,053.6	17,900.5	22,665.6
Computerized axial tomography	588.3	2,898.2	2,875.0	2,606.3
Arteriography and angiocardiography using contrast material	433.3	1,040.0	1,632.4	2,156.1
Diagnostic ultrasound	496.0	2,128.9	2,796.9	2,609.2
Circulatory monitoring	*178.3	1,465.9	1,364.6	1,278.0
Radioisotope scan	1,157.3	1,677.8	1,153.3	928.1
Respiratory therapy	*	*	1,854.3	1,883.5
Other miscellaneous diagnostic and therapeutic procedures	2,493.2	4,724.9	6,224.0	11,204.4

[Continued]

★ 453 ★

Hospitals: Surgical and Nonsurgical Procedures for Discharges from Short-Stay Hospitals: Rates for Females
[Continued]

Age and procedure category	Rate per 100,000 population			
	1980	1985	1990[1,2]	1991[1,2]
65 years and over				
All procedures[3,4]	23,380.3	34,265.8	37,400.4	42,599.9
All surgical procedures[3]	16,165.0	18,843.1	18,135.0	19,049.7
All nonsurgical procedures[3,4]	7,215.4	15,422.7	19,265.4	23,550.2
Lens extraction	1,376.7	612.3	179.1	251.4
Bronchoscopy with or without biopsy	272.5	306.5	338.8	336.9
Removal of coronary artery obstruction	*	*60.5	228.7	310.3
Coronary artery bypass graft[5]	76.3	184.4	357.3	329.8
Cardiac catheterization	208.4	594.9	991.1	1,114.2
Insertion, replacement, removal, and revision of pacemaker leads or device	457.2	503.4	530.4	672.4
Endoscopy of small intestine with or without biopsy	356.8	800.7	1,304.0	1,264.0
Endoscopy of large intestine with or without biopsy	853.4	1,115.4	1,130.9	1,118.6
Cholecystectomy	543.3	523.1	446.1	606.7
Prostatectomy	...	...	...	...
Open reduction of fracture with internal fixation	535.3	679.6	664.0	686.7
Total and partial hip replacement	380.2	540.9	630.4	595.9
Total knee replacement[6]	136.5	225.9	345.6	418.4
Mastectomy	293.9	279.9	296.9	304.9
Miscellaneous diagnostic and therapeutic procedures[3,4]	4,531.7	12,128.1	15,643.3	20,246.2
Computerized axial tomography	429.0	2,173.0	2,333.5	2,183.6
Arteriography and angiocardiography using contrast material	521.4	1,205.8	1,799.8	2,089.9
Diagnostic ultrasound	402.6	1,723.6	2,224.2	2,204.9
Circulatory monitoring	137.4	1,197.2	1,177.7	1,123.7
Radioisotope scan	931.9	1,433.7	1,014.0	892.7
Respiratory therapy	*	92.9	1,581.5	1,712.0
Other miscellaneous diagnostic and therapeutic procedures	2,100.8	4,306.3	5,512.6	9,896.6
75 years and over				
All procedures[3,4]	26,058.2	39,318.1	43,515.3	51,058.2
All surgical procedures[3]	17,981.5	20,801.7	20,068.9	21,434.8
All nonsurgical procedures[3,4]	8,076.7	18,516.3	23,446.4	29,623.4
Lens extraction	1,848.3	908.3	250.7	354.5
Bronchoscopy with or without biopsy	253.0	289.7	389.2	323.3
Removal of coronary artery obstruction	-	*	135.3	237.5
Coronary artery bypass graft[5]	*	*111.2	314.1	249.8
Cardiac catheterization	*102.1	339.6	691.9	965.1
Insertion, replacement, removal, and revision of pacemaker leads or device	725.2	783.5	788.8	979.8
Endoscopy of small intestine with or without biopsy	424.1	1,070.5	1,734.9	1,738.0
Endoscopy of large intestine with or without biopsy	968.1	1,467.7	1,534.1	1,554.4
Cholecystectomy	488.5	530.7	420.2	558.0
Prostatectomy	...	...	...	...
Open reduction of fracture with internal fixation	929.0	1,112.5	1,044.8	1,117.2
Total and partial hip replacement	561.4	795.9	939.5	823.0
Total knee replacement[6]	*140.4	250.0	286.4	375.8

[Continued]

★ 453 ★

Hospitals: Surgical and Nonsurgical Procedures for Discharges from Short-Stay Hospitals: Rates for Females
[Continued]

Age and procedure category	Rate per 100,000 population			
	1980	1985	1990[1,2]	1991[1,2]
Mastectomy	320.0	259.9	290.0	296.2
Miscellaneous diagnostic and therapeutic procedures[3,4]	5,027.4	14,409.2	18,828.8	25,958.9
Computerized axial tomography	557.8	2,853.1	3,177.5	3,175.8
Arteriography and angiocardiography using contrast material	352.9	872.3	1,335.6	1,879.2
Diagnostic ultrasound	498.7	2,295.6	2,914.7	3,006.1
Circulatory monitoring	196.0	1,645.2	1,583.6	1,550.7
Radioisotope scan	1,086.6	1,699.7	1,227.6	1,043.8
Respiratory therapy	*	*114.3	2,014.4	2,304.3
Other miscellaneous diagnostic and therapeutic procedures	2,326.3	4,940.7	6,575.4	12,595.8
85 years and over				
All procedures[3,4]	24,951.4	40,186.9	47,867.0	59,687.8
All surgical procedures[3]	18,354.9	20,472.1	20,584.0	21,815.7
All nonsurgical procedures[3,4]	6,596.5	19,714.8	27,283.0	37,872.1
Lens extraction	1,687.0	759.0	*239.4	*369.4
Bronchoscopy with or without biopsy	*	*	434.4	*285.8
Removal of coronary artery obstruction	-	-	*	*
Coronary artery bypass graft[5]	-	-	*	*
Cardiac catheterization	*	*	*	392.2
Insertion, replacement, removal, and revision of pacemaker leads or device	937.2	916.9	1,124.8	1,457.2
Endoscopy of small intestine with or without biopsy	*369.7	1,020.7	2,071.1	2,247.6
Endoscopy of large intestine with or without biopsy	894.3	1,807.8	1,887.8	1,994.6
Cholecystectomy	*457.0	*460.5	374.2	466.9
Prostatectomy	...	...	...	...
Open reduction of fracture with internal fixation	1,753.7	1,838.7	1,636.8	1,932.0
Total and partial hip replacement	765.5	1,099.0	952.6	1,085.5
Total knee replacement[6]	*	*	*	*
Mastectomy	*	*	*285.8	*178.5
Miscellaneous diagnostic and therapeutic procedures[3,4]	4,023.0	15,443.7	21,487.0	32,169.5
Computerized axial tomography	*463.3	2,722.0	4,043.8	4,405.5
Arteriography and angiocardiography using contrast material	*	*384.4	485.8	875.6
Diagnostic ultrasound	*507.0	2,780.5	3,252.0	3,769.0
Circulatory monitoring	*	2,166.8	2,210.9	2,136.0
Radioisotope scan	867.7	1,763.7	1,440.3	1,246.5

[Continued]

★ 453 ★

Hospitals: Surgical and Nonsurgical Procedures for Discharges from Short-Stay Hospitals: Rates for Females

[Continued]

Age and procedure category	Rate per 100,000 population			
	1980	1985	1990[1,2]	1991[1,2]
Respiratory therapy	*	*	2,472.7	3,217.7
Other miscellaneous diagnostic and therapeutic procedures	1,810.1	5,574.8	7,581.6	16,519.1

Source: Cohen, R.A., and J.F. Van Nostrand. *Trends in the Health of Older Americans: United States, 1994.* National Center for Health Statistics. Vital and Health Statistics 3(30). 1995. U.S. Department of Health and Human Services, Public Health Service, Centers for Disease Control and Prevention. Data are from the National Hospital Discharge Survey. *Notes:* 1. Comparisons of data for 1990 and 1991 with earlier years should be made with caution, as estimates of change may reflect improvements in the design rather than true changes in hospital use. 2. Beginning in 1989, the definitions of some surgical and diagnostic and other nonsurgical procedures were revised, thus causing a discontinuity in the trends for the totals and selected surgical procedures. 3. Includes procedures not listed on the table. 4. Inpatients discharged from short-stay hospitals had an estimated 20,519,000 nonsurgical procedures in 1991. In 1990, only 17,450,000 nonsurgical procedures were reported. The main reason for this increase was that 1991 was the first year in which all ICD-9-CM procedure codes were used in the National Hospital Discharge Survey. In previous years, selected codes were excluded, primarily codes for certain miscellaneous diagnostic and therapeutic procedures. 5. In 1991, there were 407,000 all-listed coronary artery bypass graft procedures performed on only 265,000 discharged patients. 6. For 1980 and 1985, this category is arthroplasty and replacement of knee. *Estimates based on fewer than 30 discharges are not shown; estimates based on 30-59 discharges are to be used with caution and are preceded by an asterisk. Discharges are from non-Federal hospitals. Discharges exclude newborn infants. Data do not reflect total use of surgical and diagnostic procedures because surgical and diagnostic procedures for outpatients are not included in the National Hospital Discharge Survey. In recent years, for example, lens extractions are frequently performed on outpatients. Surgical and nonsurgical procedure categories are based on the *International Classification of Diseases, 9th Revision, Clinical Modification* (ICD-9-CM).

★ 454 ★

Hospitals

Hospitals: Surgical and Nonsurgical Procedures for Discharges from Short-Stay Hospitals: Rates for Males

This table shows the rate of all listed surgical and nonsurgical procedures for discharges from short-stay hospitals, males, by age, and procedure category: United States, 1980, 1985, 1990, and 1991. Data are based on a sample of hospital records. Rates are per 100,000 population.

Age and procedure category	Rate per 100,000 population			
	1980	1985	1990[1,2]	1991[1,2]
All ages				
All procedures[3,4]	10,916.7	12,868.3	13,248.6	14,204.6
All surgical procedures[3]	7,807.8	7,710.8	7,106.8	7,151.9
All nonsurgical procedures[3,4]	3,108.8	5,157.4	6,141.8	7,052.7
Lens extraction	178.1	69.3	22.1	24.3
Bronchoscopy with or without biopsy	153.0	158.8	145.8	153.4
Removal of coronary artery obstruction	*4.6	50.4	166.8	183.5
Coronary artery bypass graft[5]	99.1	151.1	238.2	243.5
Cardiac catheterization	209.6	384.6	515.8	496.0
Insertion, replacement, removal, and revision of pacemaker leads or device	94.1	103.4	114.8	119.3
Endoscopy of small intestine with or without biopsy	107.7	218.7	297.2	321.9
Endoscopy of large intestine with or without biopsy	209.6	236.0	176.3	192.6
Cholecystectomy	112.4	129.1	122.7	136.9
Prostatectomy	307.5	321.2	302.8	299.1
Open reduction of fracture with internal fixation	140.2	156.1	147.0	158.4
Total and partial hip replacement	31.3	46.9	55.1	58.6
Total knee replacement[6]	65.1	75.1	37.9	49.4
Mastectomy	*5.4	*	*	0.9

[Continued]

★ 454 ★

Hospitals: Surgical and Nonsurgical Procedures for Discharges from Short-Stay Hospitals: Rates for Males
[Continued]

Age and procedure category	Rate per 100,000 population			
	1980	1985	1990[1,2]	1991[1,2]
Miscellaneous diagnostic and therapeutic procedures[3,4]	1,738.8	3,747.8	4,863.1	5,743.6
Computerized axial tomography	139.1	587.5	612.3	577.4
Arteriography and angiocardiography using contrast material	325.6	606.5	874.5	813.8
Diagnostic ultrasound	104.8	418.4	555.3	536.2
Circulatory monitoring	35.6	290.8	286.7	278.9
Radioisotope scan	216.5	328.1	223.1	187.5
Respiratory therapy	*	30.1	487.6	490.1
Other miscellaneous diagnostic and therapeutic procedures	913.0	1,486.5	1,823.7	2,858.4
55-64 years				
All procedures[3,4]	19,660.1	25,149.2	26,833.5	28,357.9
All surgical procedures[3]	13,082.1	14,303.0	14,765.9	14,566.2
All nonsurgical procedures[3,4]	6,578.0	10,846.2	12,067.5	13,791.8
Lens extraction	382.9	145.0	*	*
Bronchoscopy with or without biopsy	376.6	371.8	337.6	384.8
Removal of coronary artery obstruction	*	189.5	615.1	693.0
Coronary artery bypass graft[5]	422.9	603.8	882.9	878.6
Cardiac catheterization	711.7	1,371.5	1,802.5	1,814.3
Insertion, replacement, removal, and revision of pacemaker leads or device	171.6	211.7	234.3	195.3
Endoscopy of small intestine with or without biopsy	236.0	469.7	590.5	608.7
Endoscopy of large intestine with or without biopsy	501.8	444.9	374.5	326.4
Cholecystectomy	296.1	297.1	258.8	325.5
Prostatectomy	700.2	695.0	695.4	609.4
Open reduction of fracture with internal fixation	102.0	153.1	157.8	155.8
Total and partial hip replacement	*58.0	*82.9	116.9	155.2
Total knee replacement[6]	*81.8	*110.2	106.8	119.8
Mastectomy	*	*	*	*
Miscellaneous diagnostic and therapeutic procedures[3,4]	3,731.9	8,172.1	9,780.0	11,438.1
Computerized axial tomography	263.6	1,100.9	912.9	868.9
Arteriography and angiocardiography using contrast material	1,041.7	2,053.7	2,829.2	2,769.0
Diagnostic ultrasound	270.8	821.0	1,066.3	927.2
Circulatory monitoring	*71.1	589.5	486.2	583.1
Radioisotope scan	445.2	690.2	465.7	355.3
Respiratory therapy	*	*	709.6	875.8
Other miscellaneous diagnostic and therapeutic procedures	1,629.0	2,863.5	3,310.1	5,058.8
65-74 years				
All procedures[3,4]	29,721.6	39,591.3	44,060.7	47,208.7
All surgical procedures[3]	19,574.7	21,311.3	23,309.7	23,735.9
All nonsurgical procedures[3,4]	10,146.9	18,280.0	20,751.0	23,472.9
Lens extraction	908.8	346.3	111.9	127.5
Bronchoscopy with or without biopsy	717.9	722.7	609.6	601.0
Removal of coronary artery obstruction	*	*153.2	725.5	746.6
Coronary artery bypass graft[5]	347.8	611.2	1,260.1	1,311.3
Cardiac catheterization	673.8	1,390.5	2,144.1	2,106.0

[Continued]

★ 454 ★

Hospitals: Surgical and Nonsurgical Procedures for Discharges from Short-Stay Hospitals: Rates for Males

[Continued]

Age and procedure category	Rate per 100,000 population			
	1980	1985	1990[1,2]	1991[1,2]
Insertion, replacement, removal, and revision of pacemaker leads or device	469.9	497.6	475.3	531.3
Endoscopy of small intestine with or without biopsy	319.9	789.6	934.7	1,220.9
Endoscopy of large intestine with or without biopsy	744.7	896.7	645.5	744.8
Cholecystectomy	453.7	464.7	417.2	510.2
Prostatectomy	2,051.1	2,041.7	2,004.0	1,965.0
Open reduction of fracture with internal fixation	*161.8	161.0	188.4	212.8
Total and partial hip replacement	*163.0	258.7	268.3	265.4
Total knee replacement[6]	*	*154.9	275.0	313.2
Mastectomy	*	*	*	*
Miscellaneous diagnostic and therapeutic procedures[3,4]	5,225.0	13,179.8	16,488.5	19,119.0
Computerized axial tomography	423.6	1,972.9	1,814.0	1,801.6
Arteriography and angiocardiography using contrast material	1,226.3	2,454.9	3,673.1	3,416.6
Diagnostic ultrasound	373.1	1,547.9	1,907.7	1,932.8
Circulatory monitoring	*145.4	1,290.9	1,189.0	1,080.6
Radioisotope scan	795.6	1,328.2	856.3	623.0
Respiratory therapy	*	*104.7	1,560.4	1,551.9
Other miscellaneous diagnostic and therapeutic procedures	2,254.0	4,480.5	5,488.0	8,712.4
75-84 years				
All procedures[3,4]	38,731.1	55,319.7	59,142.5	64,205.5
All surgical procedures[3]	25,465.0	29,108.3	28,373.6	29,743.2
All nonsurgical procedures[3,4]	13,266.2	26,211.3	30,768.9	34,462.3
Lens extraction	1,832.5	631.4	199.0	154.2
Bronchoscopy with or without biopsy	732.0	903.8	764.5	810.1
Removal of coronary artery obstruction	-	*	362.2	541.7
Coronary artery bypass graft[5]	*	374.3	940.9	971.4
Cardiac catheterization	*193.6	712.8	1,668.0	1,553.9
Insertion, replacement, removal, and revision of pacemaker leads or device	1,108.3	1,036.7	1,172.3	1,485.0
Endoscopy of small intestine with or without biopsy	*356.3	1,102.7	1,907.8	2,155.0
Endoscopy of large intestine with or without biopsy	947.2	1,451.9	1,335.6	1,604.9
Cholecystectomy	445.3	687.4	641.4	577.8
Prostatectomy	3,113.3	3,335.1	2,726.3	2,944.4
Open reduction of fracture with internal fixation	*345.9	462.7	334.9	387.0
Total and partial hip replacement	*328.2	395.1	410.5	426.1
Total knee replacement[6]	*	*243.6	199.8	406.2
Mastectomy	*	*	*	*
Miscellaneous diagnostic and therapeutic procedures[3,4]	6,880.0	18,532.1	23,626.1	27,390.4
Computerized axial tomography	755.7	3,129.9	3,389.5	2,956.4
Arteriography and angiocardiography using contrast material	758.1	2,203.4	2,792.1	2,993.6
Diagnostic ultrasound	501.6	2,377.0	3,489.8	3,426.4
Circulatory monitoring	*304.7	2,488.8	1,918.1	1,802.6
Radioisotope scan	1,411.9	1,931.7	1,252.4	1,043.3
Respiratory therapy	*	*209.8	2,850.8	2,535.9
Other miscellaneous diagnostic and therapeutic procedures	3,128.5	6,191.5	7,933.4	12,632.1

[Continued]

★ 454 ★

Hospitals: Surgical and Nonsurgical Procedures for Discharges from Short-Stay Hospitals: Rates for Males
[Continued]

Age and procedure category	Rate per 100,000 population			
	1980	1985	1990[1,2]	1991[1,2]
65 years and over				
All procedures[3,4]	32,628.2	45,590.1	50,382.3	54,682.9
All surgical procedures[3]	21,453.6	24,240.8	25,354.5	26,175.0
All nonsurgical procedures[3,4]	11,174.6	21,349.3	25,027.8	28,507.9
Lens extraction	1,196.7	464.5	141.4	156.7
Bronchoscopy with or without biopsy	708.8	781.1	639.5	689.6
Removal of coronary artery obstruction	*	115.2	575.8	654.8
Coronary artery bypass graft[5]	257.9	501.9	1,093.7	1,125.0
Cardiac catheterization	501.3	1,106.4	1,880.1	1,835.5
Insertion, replacement, removal, and revision of pacemaker leads or device	727.2	717.1	793.9	914.2
Endoscopy of small intestine with or without biopsy	333.1	917.1	1,360.3	1,615.6
Endoscopy of large intestine with or without biopsy	826.5	1,153.8	942.5	1,099.9
Cholecystectomy	439.0	535.7	502.5	545.1
Prostatectomy	2,422.9	2,495.8	2,261.9	2,308.8
Open reduction of fracture with internal fixation	256.4	299.0	309.6	311.5
Total and partial hip replacement	221.4	316.1	355.1	352.3
Total knee replacement[6]	*63.4	171.6	244.8	328.7
Mastectomy	*	*	*	*
Miscellaneous diagnostic and therapeutic procedures[3,4]	5,724.1	15,224.4	19,515.8	22,913.4
Computerized axial tomography	524.1	2,454.4	2,460.4	2,296.7
Arteriography and angiocardiography using contrast material	1,035.0	2,262.4	3,233.8	3,132.6
Diagnostic ultrasound	401.8	1,866.9	2,541.1	2,558.4
Circulatory monitoring	192.3	1,746.1	1,508.5	1,403.6
Radioisotope scan	1,013.7	1,554.2	1,028.5	810.0
Respiratory therapy	*	153.5	2,144.8	2,098.2
Other miscellaneous diagnostic and therapeutic procedures	2,544.5	5,186.9	6,598.8	10,614.0
75 years and over				
All procedures[3,4]	38,143.5	56,451.0	61,225.9	67,255.8
All surgical procedures[3]	25,018.8	29,544.6	28,861.9	30,278.1
All nonsurgical procedures[3,4]	13,124.7	26,906.4	32,364.0	36,977.7
Lens extraction	1,742.9	678.4	192.1	205.8
Bronchoscopy with or without biopsy	691.6	886.8	690.9	838.6
Removal of coronary artery obstruction	-	*	319.1	500.2
Coronary artery bypass graft[5]	*	304.0	808.3	811.6
Cardiac catheterization	*173.9	592.0	1,427.3	1,380.4
Insertion, replacement, removal, and revision of pacemaker leads or device	1,215.3	1,114.5	1,340.5	1,558.3
Endoscopy of small intestine with or without biopsy	358.3	1,147.9	2,090.2	2,279.4
Endoscopy of large intestine with or without biopsy	981.6	1,619.2	1,452.0	1,697.2
Cholecystectomy	411.0	664.2	648.8	603.7
Prostatectomy	3,128.5	3,318.0	2,704.3	2,887.1
Open reduction of fracture with internal fixation	435.8	548.7	517.5	477.6
Total and partial hip replacement	332.1	420.1	503.9	498.6
Total knee replacement[6]	*	*201.8	193.0	354.9

[Continued]

★ 454 ★

Hospitals: Surgical and Nonsurgical Procedures for Discharges from Short-Stay Hospitals: Rates for Males

[Continued]

Age and procedure category	Rate per 100,000 population			
	1980	1985	1990[1,2]	1991[1,2]
Mastectomy	*	*	*	*
Miscellaneous diagnostic and therapeutic procedures[3,4]	6,671.1	18,926.2	24,708.7	29,296.3
Computerized axial tomography	714.7	3,326.1	3,569.0	3,129.6
Arteriography and angiocardiography using contrast material	672.1	1,914.0	2,480.2	2,654.8
Diagnostic ultrasound	456.4	2,444.6	3,627.8	3,610.7
Circulatory monitoring	*281.3	2,570.3	2,056.5	1,946.8
Radioisotope scan	1,427.5	1,963.3	1,323.9	1,124.5
Respiratory therapy	*	*241.8	3,147.2	3,017.0
Other miscellaneous diagnostic and therapeutic procedures	3,095.7	6,465.9	8,504.1	13,812.8
85 years and over				
All procedures[3,4]	35,678.7	61,343.2	70,486.2	80,717.2
All surgical procedures[3]	23,147.5	31,431.1	31,032.3	32,638.9
All nonsurgical procedures[3,4]	12,531.1	29,912.1	39,454.0	48,078.3
Lens extraction	*1367.5	*881.7	*	*
Bronchoscopy with or without biopsy	*	*	*363.7	964.5
Removal of coronary artery obstruction	---	---	*	*
Coronary artery bypass graft[5]	*	*	*	*
Cardiac catheterization	*	*	*	*614.9
Insertion, replacement, removal, and revision of pacemaker leads or device	*1664.3	1,450.9	2,088.4	1,881.9
Endoscopy of small intestine with or without biopsy	*	*1343.3	2,901.1	2,828.4
Endoscopy of large intestine with or without biopsy	*1125.5	2,342.7	1,969.3	2,104.5
Cholecystectomy	*	*	*681.7	*718.0
Prostatectomy	3,192.2	3,244.3	2,606.8	2,633.9
Open reduction of fracture with internal fixation	*812.9	*920.7	1,329.0	877.1
Total and partial hip replacement	*	*	*919.4	*818.5
Total knee replacement[6]	*	*	*	*
Mastectomy	---	---	*	*
Miscellaneous diagnostic and therapeutic procedures[3,4]	5,795.2	20,630.1	29,520.8	37,707.9
Computerized axial tomography	*	4,174.6	4,367.1	3,893.6
Arteriography and angiocardiography using contrast material	*	*	1,094.0	1,159.7
Diagnostic ultrasound	*	2,737.0	4,241.1	4,424.4
Circulatory monitoring	*	2,923.0	2,671.6	2,583.1
Radioisotope scan	*1,492.9	2,100.2	1,641.8	1,483.0

[Continued]

★ 454 ★

Hospitals: Surgical and Nonsurgical Procedures for Discharges from Short-Stay Hospitals: Rates for Males

[Continued]

Age and procedure category	Rate per 100,000 population			
	1980	1985	1990[1,2]	1991[1,2]
Respiratory therapy	*	*	4,464.2	5,140.5
Other miscellaneous diagnostic and therapeutic procedures	2,958.1	7,652.5	11,041.0	19,023.5

Source: Cohen, R.A., and J.F. Van Nostrand. Trends in the Health of Older Americans: United States, 1994. National Center for Health Statistics. Vital and Health Statistics 3(30). 1995. U.S. Department of Health and Human Services, Public Health Service, Centers for Disease Control and Prevention. Data are from the National Hospital Discharge Survey. Notes: 1. Comparisons of data for 1990 and 1991 with earlier years should be made with caution, as estimates of change may reflect improvements in the design rather than true changes in hospital use. 2. Beginning in 1989, the definitions of some surgical and diagnostic and other nonsurgical procedures were revised, thus causing a discontinuity in the trends for the totals and selected surgical procedures. 3. Includes procedures not listed on the table. 4. Inpatients discharged from short-stay hospitals had an estimated 20,519,000 nonsurgical procedures in 1991. In 1990, only 17,450,000 nonsurgical procedures were reported. The main reason for this increase was that 1991 was the first year in which all ICD-9-CM procedure codes were used in the National Hospital Discharge Survey. In previous years, selected codes were excluded, primarily codes for certain miscellaneous diagnostic and therapeutic procedures. 5. In 1991, there were 407,000 all-listed coronary artery bypass graft procedures performed on only 265,000 discharged patients. 6. For 1980 and 1985, this category is arthroplasty and replacement of knee. *Estimates based on fewer than 30 discharges are not shown; estimates based on 30-59 discharges are to be used with caution and are preceded by an asterisk. Discharges are from non-Federal hospitals. Discharges exclude newborn infants. Data do not reflect total use of surgical and diagnostic procedures because surgical and diagnostic procedures for outpatients are not included in the National Hospital Discharge Survey. In recent years, for example, lens extractions are frequently performed on outpatients. Surgical and nonsurgical procedure categories are based on the International Classification of Diseases, 9th Revision, Clinical Modification (ICD-9-CM).

★ 455 ★

Hospitals

Hospitals Use: Length of Stay Before Discharges from Short-Stay Hospitals: Both Sexes

This table shows the average length of stay before discharges from short-stay hospitals, both sexes, by age, and selected first-listed diagnosis: United States, 1970, 1980, 1985, 1990, and 1991. Data are based on a sample of hospital records.

Sex, age, and first-listed diagnosis	Average length of stay in days				
	1970	1980	1985	1990[1]	1991[1]
Both sexes, all ages					
All Conditions	7.8	7.3	6.5	6.4	6.4
Septicemia	---	14.3	11.9	13.3	11.6
Malignant neoplasms	13.9	11.9	8.9	9.4	9.2
Malignant neoplasms of colon and rectum	20.4	15.7	12.3	13.7	14.6
Malignant neoplasms of trachea, bronchus, and lung	14.2	12.8	9.2	8.5	8.6
Malignant neoplasms of the breast	13.2	10.9	7.2	4.6	4.4
Malignant neoplasms of the prostate	12.5	10.9	7.4	6.8	6.4
Diabetes mellitus	12.2	10.5	8.1	7.8	7.1
Volume depletion	---	8.9	6.2	6.5	7.5
Heart disease	12.3	9.5	7.3	6.9	6.8
Acute myocardial infarction	16.3	12.6	9.5	8.4	8.1
Coronary atherosclerosis	---	10.0	6.6	5.8	7.1
Other ischemic heart disease[2]	11.7	7.7	5.4	5.2	5.0
Cardiac dysrhythmias	7.6	7.6	6.2	5.8	5.3
Congestive heart failure	12.3	10.4	8.0	8.0	7.9
Cerebrovascular disease	14.2	12.7	10.5	9.5	9.3
Pneumonia	9.3	8.3	7.9	8.3	8.2
Cholelithiasis	11.2	9.3	7.5	5.8	5.0

[Continued]

★ 455 ★

Hospitals Use: Length of Stay Before Discharges from Short-Stay Hospitals:
Both Sexes
[Continued]

Sex, age, and first-listed diagnosis	Average length of stay in days				
	1970	1980	1985	1990[1]	1991[1]
Urinary tract infection, site unspecified	7.4	6.9	6.8	8.7	7.6
Hyperplasia of the prostate	12.1	8.9	6.4	4.9	5.3
Arthropathies and related disorders	10.8	9.4	7.7	7.8	7.4
Injury and poisoning	8.4	7.7	6.6	6.8	6.9
Fractures, all sites	11.6	10.8	8.7	8.3	8.4
Hip fracture	24.0	20.6	14.7	12.8	12.3
Both sexes, 55-64 years					
All Conditions	10.2	8.8	7.4	7.2	6.9
Septicemia	---	*	11.8	15.1	11.1
Malignant neoplasms	13.6	11.9	8.7	9.0	8.1
Malignant neoplasms of colon and rectum	19.5	15.7	10.6	12.9	9.9
Malignant neoplasms of trachea, bronchus, and lung	13.5	13.6	8.8	8.2	8.3
Malignant neoplasms of the breast	13.2	9.8	6.4	4.8	4.0
Malignant neoplasms of the prostate	11.0	10.4	7.1	7.6	5.6
Diabetes mellitus	11.8	10.2	8.7	9.0	8.0
Volume depletion	---	*	5.7	6.8	7.4
Heart disease	12.2	8.9	6.9	6.3	6.8
Acute myocardial infarction	16.8	12.0	9.6	7.9	7.5
Coronary atherosclerosis	---	8.5	5.5	5.3	10.0
Other ischemic heart disease[2]	10.8	7.6	5.1	5.0	4.5
Cardiac dysrhythmias	6.9	6.2	5.6	5.0	5.2
Congestive heart failure	12.2	10.5	7.5	7.0	7.4
Cerebrovascular disease	13.6	12.2	10.8	9.4	7.7
Pneumonia	11.0	9.7	9.1	8.6	8.1
Cholelithiasis	11.6	9.5	7.4	6.8	4.5
Urinary tract infection, site unspecified	*8.9	6.9	7.1	8.3	7.5
Hyperplasia of the prostate	11.1	7.5	5.8	4.4	6.0
Arthropathies and related disorders	11.6	11.0	8.4	8.1	7.5
Injury and poisoning	10.1	8.7	7.2	7.5	7.1
Fractures, all sites	12.2	11.2	8.1	7.8	8.4
Hip fracture	23.0	18.7	13.6	12.3	10.4
Both sexes, 65-74 years					
All Conditions	12.0	10.0	8.2	8.0	8.1
Septicemia	---	*16.4	17.9	15.9	11.4
Malignant neoplasms	15.3	12.2	9.2	9.4	9.9
Malignant neoplasms of colon and rectum	20.1	14.8	13.5	13.0	17.6
Malignant neoplasms of trachea, bronchus, and lung	14.1	12.2	8.7	9.2	9.1
Malignant neoplasms of the breast	14.0	13.0	8.7	4.5	4.0
Malignant neoplasms of the prostate	13.6	10.2	7.3	6.5	6.6
Diabetes mellitus	14.2	11.8	9.8	8.4	8.5
Volume depletion	---	9.7	7.2	7.1	6.8
Heart disease	12.9	10.3	7.5	7.0	6.9
Acute myocardial infarction	16.4	13.4	9.6	8.4	8.9
Coronary atherosclerosis	---	10.0	6.8	6.6	6.4
Other ischemic heart disease[2]	12.4	8.6	6.0	5.3	5.5

[Continued]

★ 455 ★

Hospitals Use: Length of Stay Before Discharges from Short-Stay Hospitals: Both Sexes

[Continued]

Sex, age, and first-listed diagnosis	Average length of stay in days				
	1970	1980	1985	1990[1]	1991[1]
Cardiac dysrhythmias	9.4	9.0	6.5	5.7	5.1
Congestive heart failure	12.7	10.1	8.1	8.4	7.5
Cerebrovascular disease	14.9	12.5	10.1	8.4	9.6
Pneumonia	12.1	10.0	9.6	9.5	8.6
Cholelithiasis	13.0	10.3	8.5	6.6	5.5
Urinary tract infection, site unspecified	11.3	8.5	8.2	8.0	8.2
Hyperplasia of the prostate	12.1	8.8	6.3	4.5	4.6
Arthropathies and related disorders	11.7	12.8	9.7	9.3	9.2
Injury and poisoning	13.0	11.5	8.7	8.7	8.9
Fractures, all sites	16.0	14.4	10.3	11.1	10.6
Hip fracture	21.1	19.0	14.2	15.5	12.6
Both sexes, 75-84 years					
All Conditions	13.2	11.2	9.1	9.1	9.0
Septicemia	---	13.6	12.0	12.1	12.8
Malignant neoplasms	15.1	14.1	10.0	10.4	10.3
Malignant neoplasms of colon and rectum	23.0	18.6	12.8	12.9	13.7
Malignant neoplasms of trachea, bronchus, and lung	14.9	14.2	10.8	9.5	10.4
Malignant neoplasms of the breast	16.5	12.1	8.5	5.8	5.2
Malignant neoplasms of the prostate	11.6	11.5	7.3	6.6	6.3
Diabetes mellitus	15.7	13.4	10.5	12.5	9.0
Volume depletion	---	9.8	7.8	8.1	10.6
Heart disease	13.3	10.4	8.1	8.0	7.3
Acute myocardial infarction	16.0	12.4	10.0	9.7	8.6
Coronary atherosclerosis	---	11.5	8.3	8.1	7.1
Other ischemic heart disease[2]	12.8	8.3	6.3	6.1	5.9
Cardiac dysrhythmias	9.8	8.6	6.8	6.6	5.7
Congestive heart failure	12.9	10.5	8.3	8.0	7.9
Cerebrovascular disease	15.2	12.9	10.6	10.4	10.0
Pneumonia	12.5	11.9	10.8	10.4	11.3
Cholelithiasis	13.8	12.4	9.8	8.5	7.4
Urinary tract infection, site unspecified	9.0	10.3	8.4	11.0	8.2
Hyperplasia of the prostate	13.8	10.8	6.9	6.0	4.9
Arthropathies and related disorders	13.4	13.5	11.9	10.4	9.7
Injury and poisoning	16.0	13.8	11.0	10.7	9.9
Fractures, all sites	19.7	16.7	13.3	11.0	11.2
Hip fracture	26.4	21.0	15.8	12.1	12.7
Both sexes, 65 years and over					
All Conditions	12.6	10.7	8.7	8.7	8.6
Septicemia	---	16.9	13.7	13.5	12.3
Malignant neoplasms	15.2	13.1	9.7	10.1	10.1
Malignant neoplasms of colon and rectum	20.8	16.7	13.1	14.2	16.1
Malignant neoplasms of trachea, bronchus, and lung	14.4	12.8	9.3	9.5	9.5
Malignant neoplasms of the breast	15.2	13.0	8.8	5.0	4.5
Malignant neoplasms of the prostate	13.0	11.0	7.5	6.7	6.5
Diabetes mellitus	14.7	12.8	10.1	9.7	8.9

[Continued]

★ 455 ★

Hospitals Use: Length of Stay Before Discharges from Short-Stay Hospitals: Both Sexes
[Continued]

Sex, age, and first-listed diagnosis	Average length of stay in days				
	1970	1980	1985	1990[1]	1991[1]
Volume depletion	---	10.2	7.7	8.5	9.8
Heart disease	13.1	10.5	7.9	7.6	7.2
Acute myocardial infarction	16.1	13.0	9.7	9.1	8.8
Coronary atherosclerosis	---	11.1	7.9	7.0	6.5
Other ischemic heart disease[2]	12.7	8.6	6.1	5.6	5.6
Cardiac dysrhythmias	9.9	8.8	6.8	6.5	5.6
Congestive heart failure	12.7	10.6	8.2	8.3	7.9
Cerebrovascular disease	14.7	12.9	10.4	9.5	9.7
Pneumonia	12.5	11.1	9.9	10.2	10.2
Cholelithiasis	13.7	11.4	9.5	7.7	6.4
Urinary tract infection, site unspecified	11.4	9.5	8.3	10.0	8.4
Hyperplasia of the prostate	12.8	9.8	6.7	5.2	4.8
Arthropathies and related disorders	12.6	12.8	10.5	9.8	9.4
Injury and poisoning	14.9	13.2	10.3	9.9	9.6
Fractures, all sites	18.5	16.2	12.4	11.1	11.3
Hip fracture	24.0	20.5	15.0	13.0	12.8
Both sexes, 75 years and over					
All Conditions	13.3	11.4	9.2	9.2	9.0
Septicemia	---	17.1	11.6	12.3	12.8
Malignant neoplasms	15.0	14.2	10.3	10.8	10.4
Malignant neoplasms of colon and rectum	21.7	18.4	12.8	15.0	14.5
Malignant neoplasms of trachea, bronchus, and lung	15.0	14.2	10.6	9.9	10.3
Malignant neoplasms of the breast	16.8	12.9	9.0	5.7	5.0
Malignant neoplasms of the prostate	12.4	11.8	7.6	6.8	6.3
Diabetes mellitus	15.4	14.0	10.6	11.6	9.4
Volume depletion	---	10.4	7.9	9.0	10.9
Heart disease	13.3	10.6	8.2	8.0	7.4
Acute myocardial infarction	15.7	12.5	9.9	9.7	8.8
Coronary atherosclerosis	---	11.9	9.0	7.9	6.8
Other ischemic heart disease[2]	13.0	8.6	6.2	5.9	5.8
Cardiac dysrhythmias	10.3	8.6	7.0	7.1	6.0
Congestive heart failure	12.7	10.9	8.3	8.2	8.0
Cerebrovascular disease	14.6	13.2	10.6	10.1	9.8
Pneumonia	12.9	11.9	10.1	14.5	11.0
Cholelithiasis	14.8	12.8	10.5	9.0	7.8
Urinary tract infection, site unspecified	11.5	10.1	8.3	10.7	8.4
Hyperplasia of the prostate	13.7	11.2	7.2	6.1	5.0
Arthropathies and related disorders	13.9	12.8	11.6	10.3	9.8
Injury and poisoning	16.5	14.3	11.3	10.7	10.1
Fractures, all sites	20.1	17.1	13.2	11.1	11.5
Hip fracture	25.0	21.0	15.3	12.3	12.8
Both sexes, 85 years and over					
All Conditions	13.8	12.0	9.6	9.6	9.2
Septicemia	---	*23.3	10.9	12.6	12.9
Malignant neoplasms	14.3	14.7	11.3	12.1	10.9

[Continued]

★ 455 ★

Hospitals Use: Length of Stay Before Discharges from Short-Stay Hospitals:
Both Sexes
[Continued]

Sex, age, and first-listed diagnosis	Average length of stay in days				
	1970	1980	1985	1990[1]	1991[1]
Malignant neoplasms of colon and rectum	*17.9	17.5	12.8	22.4	16.8
Malignant neoplasms of trachea, bronchus, and lung	*	*	*9.1	*12.6	*9.9
Malignant neoplasms of the breast	*	*16.0	*10.5	*5.3	*4.2
Malignant neoplasms of the prostate	*15.5	*13.2	*9.5	7.5	6.2
Diabetes mellitus	13.5	17.0	11.0	9.1	10.6
Volume depletion	---	11.1	8.0	10.1	11.4
Heart disease	13.4	11.3	8.4	8.1	7.7
Acute myocardial infarction	14.4	12.8	9.6	9.8	9.3
Coronary atherosclerosis	---	12.7	11.0	*6.2	*5.0
Other ischemic heart disease[2]	13.6	9.9	6.1	5.3	5.3
Cardiac dysrhythmias	*11.7	8.8	7.6	8.3	6.9
Congestive heart failure	12.4	11.5	8.2	8.6	8.2
Cerebrovascular disease	13.2	13.8	10.5	9.6	9.2
Pneumonia	13.7	11.8	9.1	10.9	10.5
Cholelithiasis	*18.8	14.4	13.4	10.3	9.2
Urinary tract infection, site unspecified	*	9.7	8.2	10.2	8.7
Hyperplasia of the prostate	13.7	*14.2	8.3	6.6	5.3
Arthropathies and related disorders	15.5	10.0	10.4	10.1	10.4
Injury and poisoning	17.7	15.2	11.9	10.7	10.4
Fractures, all sites	21.1	17.8	13.1	11.1	12.0
Hip fracture	22.7	21.0	14.5	12.7	13.0

Source: Cohen, R.A., and J.F. Van Nostrand. *Trends in the Health of Older Americans: United States, 1994.* National Center for Health Statistics. Vital and Health Statistics 3(30). 1995. U.S. Department of Health and Human Services, Public Health Service, Centers for Disease Control and Prevention. Data are from the National Hospital Discharge Survey. *Notes:* 1. Comparisons of data for 1990 and 1991 with data for earlier years should be made with caution, as estimates of change may reflect improvements in the design rather than true changes in hospital use. 2. For 1970 the classification "other ischemic heart disease" includes all diagnoses of ischemic heart disease. *Estimates based on fewer than 30 discharges are not shown; estimates based on 30-59 discharges are preceded by an asterisk. Data include races other than white and black. Discharges are from non-Federal hospitals. Discharges exclude newborn infants. Diagnostic grouping inclusions are based on the *International Classification of Diseases, 8th Revision, adapted for use in the United States* for 1970, and the *International Classification of Diseases, 9th Revision Clinical Modification* (ICD-9-CM) for 1980, 1985, 1990 and 1991.

★ 456 ★
Hospitals

Hospitals Use: Length of Stay Before Discharges from Short-Stay Hospitals: Females

This table shows the average length of stay before discharges from short-stay hospitals, females, by age, and selected first-listed diagnosis: United States, 1970, 1980, 1985, 1990, and 1991. Data are based on a sample of hospital records.

Age and first-listed diagnosis	Average length of stay in days				
	1970	1980	1985	1990[1]	1991[1]
All ages					
All Conditions	7.4	7.0	6.2	6.1	6.0
Septicemia	---	15.3	11.4	12.6	11.5
Malignant neoplasms	14.2	11.8	8.7	9.2	8.7
Malignant neoplasms of colon and rectum	22.3	16.5	12.4	14.4	12.4
Malignant neoplasms of trachea, bronchus, and lung	14.9	14.0	9.9	9.1	8.7
Malignant neoplasms of the breast	13.2	11.0	7.2	4.6	4.4
Malignant neoplasms of the prostate	...	...	...	...	...
Diabetes mellitus	12.2	10.7	8.2	8.1	7.3
Volume depletion	---	8.9	6.4	6.9	6.9
Heart disease	12.6	10.0	7.6	7.1	7.0
Acute myocardial infarction	17.4	13.1	10.3	8.4	9.1
Coronary atherosclerosis	---	10.8	7.9	6.2	6.5
Other ischemic heart disease[2]	12.2	8.0	5.6	5.3	5.1
Cardiac dysrhythmias	8.0	7.9	6.4	6.0	5.5
Congestive heart failure	12.6	10.6	8.2	8.4	8.4
Cerebrovascular disease	14.4	13.2	10.9	9.7	9.6
Pneumonia	9.6	8.4	8.1	8.4	8.5
Cholelithiasis	10.9	9.1	7.2	5.5	4.8
Urinary tract infection, site unspecified	7.0	6.6	6.4	9.2	7.2
Hyperplasia of the prostate	...	...	...	...	...
Arthropathies and related disorders	11.7	10.6	8.2	8.4	8.0
Injury and poisoning	9.5	8.7	7.3	7.6	7.6
Fractures, all sites	13.8	12.6	9.8	9.7	9.4
Hip fracture	23.9	20.8	14.1	13.3	12.8
55-64 years					
All Conditions	10.2	9.0	7.5	7.3	6.9
Septicemia	---	*	*10.5	15.5	11.1
Malignant neoplasms	14.2	12.0	8.4	8.8	7.9
Malignant neoplasms of colon and rectum	22.2	16.6	10.0	13.5	9.4
Malignant neoplasms of trachea, bronchus, and lung	13.6	14.8	8.7	9.0	7.9
Malignant neoplasms of the breast	13.2	9.9	6.4	4.9	4.0
Malignant neoplasms of the prostate	...	...	...	...	...
Diabetes mellitus	11.1	10.0	8.6	10.8	8.5
Volume depletion	---	*	5.8	6.2	6.2
Heart disease	12.1	9.0	6.9	6.5	6.6
Acute myocardial infarction	17.0	11.9	10.9	7.8	8.5
Coronary atherosclerosis	---	9.6	6.3	5.3	6.4
Other ischemic heart disease[2]	11.3	7.8	4.9	5.5	4.5
Cardiac dysrhythmias	7.0	6.8	6.1	5.2	6.1
Congestive heart failure	13.0	10.7	7.2	7.4	7.3
Cerebrovascular disease	14.3	13.9	11.7	10.0	8.0
Pneumonia	11.3	9.6	9.5	8.1	8.1

[Continued]

★ 456 ★

Hospitals Use: Length of Stay Before Discharges from Short-Stay Hospitals: Females
[Continued]

Age and first-listed diagnosis	Average length of stay in days				
	1970	1980	1985	1990[1]	1991[1]
Cholelithiasis	11.2	9.7	7.2	6.2	4.3
Urinary tract infection, site unspecified	*	7.0	*7.5	7.7	9.0
Hyperplasia of the prostate	...	...	...	...	...
Arthropathies and related disorders	12.3	11.7	8.1	8.5	7.9
Injury and poisoning	10.4	9.4	7.2	7.0	7.1
Fractures, all sites	12.9	11.8	7.6	8.0	8.1
Hip fracture	23.0	*19.5	*13.5	13.4	10.8
65-74 years					
All Conditions	12.3	10.2	8.3	8.1	8.2
Septicemia	---	*	15.9	14.4	11.0
Malignant neoplasms	16.9	12.5	9.4	9.0	8.8
Malignant neoplasms of colon and rectum	22.1	15.3	13.0	14.5	11.5
Malignant neoplasms of trachea, bronchus, and lung	*14.5	14.0	9.6	10.2	8.6
Malignant neoplasms of the breast	14.1	13.0	8.7	4.5	4.0
Malignant neoplasms of the prostate	...	...	...	...	...
Diabetes mellitus	15.2	11.8	9.7	8.0	7.9
Volume depletion	---	*10.4	6.8	7.2	6.9
Heart disease	13.3	10.6	7.6	7.0	7.0
Acute myocardial infarction	17.6	13.9	10.3	7.8	10.1
Coronary atherosclerosis	---	10.6	7.1	7.1	7.3
Other ischemic heart disease[2]	12.9	9.1	6.0	5.2	5.3
Cardiac dysrhythmias	10.3	9.6	6.3	5.8	5.5
Congestive heart failure	12.1	9.8	8.3	8.9	7.7
Cerebrovascular disease	14.5	13.0	10.3	8.5	10.6
Pneumonia	12.6	10.4	9.4	9.4	8.4
Cholelithiasis	12.8	10.5	8.1	6.4	5.0
Urinary tract infection, site unspecified	*11.1	8.0	6.7	8.4	7.1
Hyperplasia of the prostate	...	...	...	...	...
Arthropathies and related disorders	11.7	13.5	9.4	9.4	9.2
Injury and poisoning	13.9	12.2	9.1	9.3	9.3
Fractures, all sites	16.7	14.0	10.6	11.5	10.0
Hip fracture	21.3	19.4	13.9	16.7	12.1
75-84 years					
All Conditions	13.7	11.5	9.3	9.4	9.2
Septicemia	---	*15.8	11.5	11.5	13.1
Malignant neoplasms	16.7	14.3	10.4	11.7	11.1
Malignant neoplasms of colon and rectum	25.1	19.7	13.4	13.2	14.1
Malignant neoplasms of trachea, bronchus, and lung	*	12.0	14.4	9.4	12.5
Malignant neoplasms of the breast	16.5	12.1	8.5	5.8	5.2
Malignant neoplasms of the prostate	...	...	...	...	...
Diabetes mellitus	14.6	13.2	10.4	13.1	9.3
Volume depletion	---	9.2	7.7	7.8	8.3
Heart disease	13.8	10.9	8.3	7.8	7.1
Acute myocardial infarction	18.1	13.1	10.0	9.3	8.9
Coronary atherosclerosis	---	11.7	8.8	8.1	6.7

[Continued]

★ 456 ★

Hospitals Use: Length of Stay Before Discharges from Short-Stay Hospitals: Females
[Continued]

Age and first-listed diagnosis	Average length of stay in days				
	1970	1980	1985	1990[1]	1991[1]
Other ischemic heart disease[2]	13.0	8.0	6.3	5.9	5.4
Cardiac dysrhythmias	*10.2	8.8	7.2	6.7	5.5
Congestive heart failure	13.6	11.0	8.6	8.2	8.3
Cerebrovascular disease	15.4	13.6	11.0	10.6	9.6
Pneumonia	13.6	12.1	11.1	10.9	12.8
Cholelithiasis	13.7	12.2	9.0	8.8	6.7
Urinary tract infection, site unspecified	*9.2	11.2	8.5	12.3	8.5
Hyperplasia of the prostate	...	...	...	...	...
Arthropathies and related disorders	13.4	13.4	12.3	10.2	9.9
Injury and poisoning	16.5	14.1	10.9	10.6	10.1
Fractures, all sites	19.5	16.6	12.4	11.2	11.5
Hip fracture	26.2	21.0	14.3	12.5	13.1
65 years and over					
All Conditions	13.0	11.0	9.0	8.9	8.8
Septicemia	---	18.9	12.8	12.8	12.0
Malignant neoplasms	16.6	13.4	10.0	10.2	9.8
Malignant neoplasms of colon and rectum	22.5	17.7	13.1	14.9	13.0
Malignant neoplasms of trachea, bronchus, and lung	16.5	13.4	10.8	10.1	9.7
Malignant neoplasms of the breast	15.4	13.0	8.8	5.0	4.5
Malignant neoplasms of the prostate	...	...	...	...	...
Diabetes mellitus	15.0	12.8	10.1	9.6	8.6
Volume depletion	---	10.1	7.6	8.9	8.9
Heart disease	13.6	10.8	8.1	7.6	7.3
Acute myocardial infarction	17.8	13.6	10.1	8.9	9.6
Coronary atherosclerosis	---	11.4	8.8	7.4	6.9
Other ischemic heart disease[2]	13.1	8.8	6.1	5.5	5.3
Cardiac dysrhythmias	10.8	9.1	6.9	6.6	5.8
Congestive heart failure	12.9	10.8	8.4	8.6	8.1
Cerebrovascular disease	14.6	13.3	10.7	9.7	9.9
Pneumonia	13.4	11.2	9.9	10.4	10.7
Cholelithiasis	13.6	11.4	8.8	7.8	6.0
Urinary tract infection, site unspecified	12.4	9.8	8.1	10.8	8.1
Hyperplasia of the prostate	...	...	...	...	...
Arthropathies and related disorders	12.9	13.2	10.5	9.7	9.5
Injury and poisoning	15.8	13.7	10.6	10.2	10.0
Fractures, all sites	18.9	16.1	12.1	11.3	11.4
Hip fracture	24.3	20.6	14.2	13.3	13.1
75 years and over					
All Conditions	13.8	11.6	9.4	9.5	9.3
Septicemia	---	19.8	11.2	12.2	12.5
Malignant neoplasms	16.3	14.6	10.8	11.6	11.0
Malignant neoplasms of colon and rectum	23.1	20.0	13.1	15.1	14.1
Malignant neoplasms of trachea, bronchus, and lung	*	12.4	13.9	9.9	12.4
Malignant neoplasms of the breast	16.8	12.9	9.1	5.7	5.0
Malignant neoplasms of the prostate	...	...	...	...	...

[Continued]

★ 456 ★

Hospitals Use: Length of Stay Before Discharges from Short-Stay Hospitals: Females
[Continued]

Age and first-listed diagnosis	Average length of stay in days				
	1970	1980	1985	1990[1]	1991[1]
Diabetes mellitus	14.7	14.2	10.6	11.9	9.5
Volume depletion	---	10.0	7.9	9.5	9.7
Heart disease	13.8	11.0	8.4	8.0	7.4
Acute myocardial infarction	18.0	13.3	10.0	9.6	9.2
Coronary atherosclerosis	---	11.8	10.0	7.8	6.3
Other ischemic heart disease[2]	13.2	8.4	6.2	5.8	5.3
Cardiac dysrhythmias	11.3	8.7	7.3	7.0	6.0
Congestive heart failure	13.3	11.2	8.5	8.5	8.3
Cerebrovascular disease	14.7	13.5	10.9	10.2	9.5
Pneumonia	13.9	11.7	10.1	22.0	11.8
Cholelithiasis	14.9	12.8	9.6	9.4	7.3
Urinary tract infection, site unspecified	*13.7	10.7	8.6	11.6	8.4
Hyperplasia of the prostate	...	...	...	...	...
Arthropathies and related disorders	14.3	12.8	11.7	10.1	10.1
Injury and poisoning	17.2	14.5	11.3	10.6	10.4
Fractures, all sites	20.3	17.0	12.6	11.2	11.9
Hip fracture	25.3	20.9	14.3	12.5	13.3
85 years and over					
All Conditions	14.3	12.0	9.8	9.6	9.3
Septicemia	---	*	10.8	12.9	11.3
Malignant neoplasms	14.7	15.5	12.1	11.3	10.6
Malignant neoplasms of colon and rectum	*	*21.1	12.7	21.1	14.0
Malignant neoplasms of trachea, bronchus, and lung	*	*	*	*	*
Malignant neoplasms of the breast	*	*16.0	*11.0	*5.3	*4.2
Malignant neoplasms of the prostate	...	...	...	...	...
Diabetes mellitus	*14.8	18.5	*11.7	9.2	9.8
Volume depletion	---	10.9	8.0	11.3	11.5
Heart disease	13.7	11.1	8.8	8.2	7.9
Acute myocardial infarction	*17.5	14.0	10.2	10.3	9.9
Coronary atherosclerosis	---	12.1	12.5	*	*
Other ischemic heart disease[2]	13.6	9.7	5.9	5.7	5.0
Cardiac dysrhythmias	*	8.5	7.5	7.7	7.4
Congestive heart failure	*12.5	11.7	8.4	8.9	8.4
Cerebrovascular disease	12.8	13.4	10.8	9.5	9.4
Pneumonia	14.6	11.1	8.8	10.8	10.7
Cholelithiasis	*20.6	14.4	11.1	10.7	8.9
Urinary tract infection, site unspecified	*	9.8	8.9	10.7	8.2
Hyperplasia of the prostate	...	...	...	...	...
Arthropathies and related disorders	*17.8	10.2	*9.3	9.6	10.9
Injury and poisoning	18.8	15.3	12.0	10.6	10.8

[Continued]

★ 456 ★

Hospitals Use: Length of Stay Before Discharges from Short-Stay Hospitals: Females
[Continued]

Age and first-listed diagnosis	Average length of stay in days				
	1970	1980	1985	1990[1]	1991[1]
Fractures, all sites	21.8	17.7	12.9	11.1	12.4
Hip fracture	23.9	20.7	14.3	12.7	13.5

Source: Cohen, R.A., and J.F. Van Nostrand. *Trends in the Health of Older Americans: United States, 1994.* National Center for Health Statistics. Vital and Health Statistics 3(30). 1995. U.S. Department of Health and Human Services, Public Health Service, Centers for Disease Control and Prevention. Data are from the National Hospital Discharge Survey. *Notes:* 1. Comparisons of data for 1990 and 1991 with data for earlier years should be made with caution, as estimates of change may reflect improvements in the design rather than true changes in hospital use. 2. For 1970 the classification "other ischemic heart disease" includes all diagnoses of ischemic heart disease. *Estimates based on fewer than 30 discharges are not shown; estimates based on 30-59 discharges are preceded by an asterisk. Data include races other than white and black. Discharges are from non-Federal hospitals. Discharges exclude newborn infants. Diagnostic grouping inclusions are based on the *International Classification of Diseases, 8th Revision, adapted for use in the United States* for 1970, and the *International Classification of Diseases, 9th Revision Clinical Modification* (ICD-9-CM) for 1980, 1985, 1990 and 1991.

★ 457 ★

Hospitals

Hospitals Use: Length of Stay Before Discharges from Short-Stay Hospitals: Males

This table shows the average length of stay before discharges from short-stay hospitals, males, by age, and selected first-listed diagnosis: United States, 1970, 1980, 1985, 1990, and 1991. Data are based on a sample of hospital records.

Age and first-listed diagnosis	Average length of stay in days				
	1970	1980	1985	1990[1]	1991[1]
All ages					
All Conditions	8.4	7.7	6.9	6.9	7.0
Septicemia	---	13.1	12.6	14.0	11.7
Malignant neoplasms	13.5	12.0	9.1	9.5	9.7
Malignant neoplasms of colon and rectum	18.6	14.7	12.2	13.0	16.7
Malignant neoplasms of trachea, bronchus, and lung	14.0	12.3	8.8	8.0	8.5
Malignant neoplasms of the breast	*	*	*	*	*
Malignant neoplasms of the prostate	12.5	10.9	7.4	6.8	6.4
Diabetes mellitus	12.1	10.1	8.0	7.6	6.8
Volume depletion	---	9.0	5.9	6.1	8.5
Heart disease	12.0	9.1	7.0	6.7	6.7
Acute myocardial infarction	15.8	12.3	9.0	8.4	7.5
Coronary atherosclerosis	---	9.3	5.8	5.7	7.4
Other ischemic heart disease[2]	11.2	7.4	5.3	5.0	5.0
Cardiac dysrhythmias	7.1	7.3	5.9	5.5	5.0
Congestive heart failure	12.1	10.1	7.8	7.5	7.5
Cerebrovascular disease	14.0	12.1	10.0	9.2	9.1
Pneumonia	9.0	8.2	7.8	8.2	7.9
Cholelithiasis	11.9	9.9	8.3	6.6	5.3
Urinary tract infection, site unspecified	8.3	7.4	7.4	7.8	8.3
Hyperplasia of the prostate	12.1	8.9	6.4	4.9	5.3
Arthropathies and related disorders	9.3	7.5	7.0	7.0	6.6

[Continued]

★ 457 ★

Hospitals Use: Length of Stay Before Discharges from Short-Stay Hospitals: Males

[Continued]

Age and first-listed diagnosis	Average length of stay in days				
	1970	1980	1985	1990[1]	1991[1]
Injury and poisoning	7.5	6.9	6.1	6.1	6.3
Fractures, all sites	9.7	9.0	7.7	6.7	7.3
Hip fracture	24.4	20.1	16.6	11.7	10.9
55-64 years					
All Conditions	10.2	8.6	7.3	7.1	6.9
Septicemia	---	*	*13.0	14.6	11.0
Malignant neoplasms	13.0	11.9	9.0	9.3	8.3
Malignant neoplasms of colon and rectum	17.4	14.8	11.2	12.6	10.3
Malignant neoplasms of trachea, bronchus, and lung	13.5	12.9	8.8	7.7	8.5
Malignant neoplasms of the breast	*	*	*	*	*
Malignant neoplasms of the prostate	11.0	10.4	7.1	7.6	5.6
Diabetes mellitus	12.7	10.5	8.8	7.0	7.2
Volume depletion	---	*	*5.7	7.6	9.2
Heart disease	12.2	8.8	6.9	6.1	6.9
Acute myocardial infarction	16.8	12.0	9.2	7.9	7.1
Coronary atherosclerosis	---	8.0	5.2	5.3	11.1
Other ischemic heart disease[2]	10.5	7.4	5.2	4.8	4.5
Cardiac dysrhythmias	6.8	5.7	5.2	5.0	4.4
Congestive heart failure	11.7	10.3	7.7	6.8	7.4
Cerebrovascular disease	13.0	10.7	10.1	8.9	7.5
Pneumonia	10.6	9.9	8.7	8.9	8.0
Cholelithiasis	12.5	9.3	7.9	8.3	4.8
Urinary tract infection, site unspecified	*	*	*6.6	8.9	6.1
Hyperplasia of the prostate	11.1	7.5	5.8	4.4	6.0
Arthropathies and related disorders	10.6	9.6	8.9	7.5	6.9
Injury and poisoning	9.8	8.1	7.1	7.9	7.1
Fractures, all sites	11.2	10.0	8.9	7.4	8.9
Hip fracture	*	*	*	*11.5	*9.9
65-74 years					
All Conditions	11.7	9.7	8.1	7.8	7.9
Septicemia	---	*16.5	20.9	17.1	11.8
Malignant neoplasms	14.1	11.9	9.1	9.9	10.8
Malignant neoplasms of colon and rectum	18.2	14.2	14.0	11.4	22.2
Malignant neoplasms of trachea, bronchus, and lung	14.1	11.6	8.3	8.7	9.4
Malignant neoplasms of the breast	*	*	*	*	*
Malignant neoplasms of the prostate	13.6	10.2	7.3	6.5	6.6
Diabetes mellitus	12.3	11.7	9.9	9.1	9.8
Volume depletion	---	*8.7	7.7	7.0	6.6
Heart disease	12.5	9.9	7.4	7.0	6.7
Acute myocardial infarction	15.6	13.1	9.1	8.8	8.2
Coronary atherosclerosis	---	9.4	6.6	6.4	5.9
Other ischemic heart disease[2]	11.8	8.1	6.0	5.4	5.7
Cardiac dysrhythmias	8.5	8.5	6.6	5.6	4.7
Congestive heart failure	13.3	10.4	7.8	7.9	7.4
Cerebrovascular disease	15.2	12.0	9.8	8.3	8.6

[Continued]

★ 457 ★

Hospitals Use: Length of Stay Before Discharges from Short-Stay Hospitals:
Males
[Continued]

Age and first-listed diagnosis	Average length of stay in days				
	1970	1980	1985	1990[1]	1991[1]
Pneumonia	11.7	9.7	9.7	9.5	8.8
Cholelithiasis	13.5	10.1	9.2	6.9	6.2
Urinary tract infection, site unspecified	*11.5	9.3	9.9	7.2	9.7
Hyperplasia of the prostate	12.1	8.8	6.3	4.5	4.6
Arthropathies and related disorders	11.6	11.2	10.2	9.2	9.1
Injury and poisoning	11.6	10.6	8.2	7.9	8.4
Fractures, all sites	14.5	15.4	9.5	10.2	11.7
Hip fracture	*20.5	17.9	*15.2	11.8	13.5
75-84 years					
All Conditions	12.5	10.7	8.8	8.7	8.6
Septicemia	---	*11.0	12.7	12.9	12.2
Malignant neoplasms	13.6	13.8	9.7	9.3	9.5
Malignant neoplasms of colon and rectum	21.0	17.0	12.1	12.5	13.3
Malignant neoplasms of trachea, bronchus, and lung	13.5	15.0	9.6	9.6	9.4
Malignant neoplasms of the breast	*	*	*	*	*
Malignant neoplasms of the prostate	11.6	11.5	7.3	6.6	6.3
Diabetes mellitus	18.4	13.7	10.7	11.7	8.5
Volume depletion	---	*11.2	7.8	8.4	14.4
Heart disease	12.7	9.7	7.8	8.1	7.4
Acute myocardial infarction	14.1	11.4	10.0	10.1	8.3
Coronary atherosclerosis	---	11.2	7.8	8.1	7.4
Other ischemic heart disease[2]	12.5	8.5	6.3	6.5	6.7
Cardiac dysrhythmias	*9.3	8.3	6.2	6.5	6.1
Congestive heart failure	12.1	9.9	8.0	7.8	7.6
Cerebrovascular disease	14.8	11.9	10.1	10.0	10.7
Pneumonia	11.5	11.8	10.5	9.8	9.9
Cholelithiasis	14.0	12.8	10.8	8.0	8.6
Urinary tract infection, site unspecified	*8.9	8.9	8.3	8.1	7.7
Hyperplasia of the prostate	13.8	10.8	6.9	6.0	4.9
Arthropathies and related disorders	*13.4	13.7	10.8	10.8	9.4
Injury and poisoning	14.6	12.9	11.2	10.9	9.4
Fractures, all sites	20.4	17.3	16.6	10.0	9.9
Hip fracture	27.4	21.1	21.7	10.4	11.2
65 years and over					
All Conditions	12.1	10.3	8.4	8.3	8.3
Septicemia	---	14.5	15.2	14.5	12.7
Malignant neoplasms	13.9	12.7	9.4	9.9	10.4
Malignant neoplasms of colon and rectum	19.1	15.3	13.1	13.2	19.2
Malignant neoplasms of trachea, bronchus, and lung	13.9	12.6	8.7	9.1	9.3
Malignant neoplasms of the breast	*	*	*	*	*
Malignant neoplasms of the prostate	13.0	11.0	7.5	6.7	6.5
Diabetes mellitus	14.2	12.5	10.2	9.9	9.5
Volume depletion	---	10.4	7.8	7.7	11.4
Heart disease	12.6	10.0	7.6	7.5	7.1
Acute myocardial infarction	14.8	12.5	9.3	9.3	8.2

[Continued]

★ 457 ★

Hospitals Use: Length of Stay Before Discharges from Short-Stay Hospitals:
Males
[Continued]

Age and first-listed diagnosis	Average length of stay in days				
	1970	1980	1985	1990[1]	1991[1]
Coronary atherosclerosis	---	10.7	6.4	6.8	6.3
Other ischemic heart disease[2]	12.3	8.3	6.1	5.7	6.1
Cardiac dysrhythmias	8.7	8.5	6.6	6.4	5.4
Congestive heart failure	12.6	10.3	7.9	7.9	7.5
Cerebrovascular disease	14.9	12.3	9.9	9.2	9.5
Pneumonia	11.8	11.1	10.0	10.0	9.6
Cholelithiasis	14.0	11.2	10.6	7.6	7.2
Urinary tract infection, site unspecified	10.4	9.1	8.6	8.2	8.9
Hyperplasia of the prostate	12.8	9.8	6.7	5.2	4.8
Arthropathies and related disorders	11.8	12.0	10.6	9.8	9.2
Injury and poisoning	12.9	12.0	9.8	9.4	8.8
Fractures, all sites	17.2	16.7	13.4	10.4	10.7
Hip fracture	23.0	20.5	18.2	11.6	11.7
75 years and over					
All Conditions	12.6	11.1	8.8	8.8	8.7
Septicemia	---	*13.0	12.2	12.5	13.4
Malignant neoplasms	13.7	13.9	9.8	10.0	9.8
Malignant neoplasms of colon and rectum	20.2	16.3	12.3	15.0	15.2
Malignant neoplasms of trachea, bronchus, and lung	13.6	14.9	9.5	10.0	9.3
Malignant neoplasms of the breast	*	*	*	*	*
Malignant neoplasms of the prostate	12.4	11.8	7.6	6.8	6.3
Diabetes mellitus	17.0	13.6	10.5	11.0	9.2
Volume depletion	---	11.4	7.9	8.0	13.3
Heart disease	12.7	10.1	7.7	8.1	7.4
Acute myocardial infarction	13.7	11.4	9.7	9.9	8.3
Coronary atherosclerosis	---	11.9	7.6	8.0	7.2
Other ischemic heart disease[2]	12.8	8.7	6.3	6.0	6.5
Cardiac dysrhythmias	*8.9	8.5	6.5	7.2	6.1
Congestive heart failure	12.1	10.2	7.9	7.8	7.6
Cerebrovascular disease	14.6	12.6	10.0	9.9	10.2
Pneumonia	11.9	12.2	10.2	10.3	10.1
Cholelithiasis	14.6	13.0	12.1	8.3	8.8
Urinary tract infection, site unspecified	*9.6	9.1	7.8	8.6	8.5
Hyperplasia of the prostate	13.7	11.2	7.2	6.1	5.0
Arthropathies and related disorders	12.3	13.0	11.3	10.8	9.4
Injury and poisoning	14.5	13.5	11.3	10.9	9.3
Fractures, all sites	19.7	17.7	15.6	10.6	10.1
Hip fracture	24.0	21.7	19.2	11.5	11.1
85 years and over					
All Conditions	13.0	12.1	9.1	9.4	9.0
Septicemia	---	*	*11.0	11.8	16.0
Malignant neoplasms	13.9	14.0	10.3	13.4	11.1
Malignant neoplasms of colon and rectum	*	*14.3	*13.0	*25.0	*21.5
Malignant neoplasms of trachea, bronchus, and lung	*	*	*	*	*
Malignant neoplasms of the breast	*	*	*	*	*

[Continued]

★ 457 ★

Hospitals Use: Length of Stay Before Discharges from Short-Stay Hospitals:
Males
[Continued]

Age and first-listed diagnosis	Average length of stay in days				
	1970	1980	1985	1990[1]	1991[1]
Malignant neoplasms of the prostate	*15.5	*13.2	*9.5	7.5	6.2
Diabetes mellitus	*	*13.2	*	*	*
Volume depletion	---	*11.6	8.0	7.3	11.3
Heart disease	12.9	11.6	7.6	7.8	7.4
Acute myocardial infarction	*12.2	*11.5	8.5	8.9	8.3
Coronary atherosclerosis	---	14.0	*	*	*
Other ischemic heart disease[2]	13.6	*10.2	6.3	4.7	5.8
Cardiac dysrhythmia	*	*9.4	7.7	9.6	6.0
Congestive heart failure	*12.2	11.1	7.8	8.0	7.7
Cerebrovascular disease	13.9	14.5	9.9	9.6	8.8
Pneumonia	12.7	12.8	9.5	11.2	10.4
Cholelithiasis	*	*	*	*9.3	*10.0
Urinary tract infection, site unspecified	*	*9.4	*6.6	9.3	10.0
Hyperplasia of the prostate	13.7	*14.2	8.3	6.6	5.3
Arthropathies and related disorders	*	*	*	*	*
Injury and poisoning	14.1	14.6	11.4	10.9	9.0
Fractures, all sites	17.8	18.5	13.8	11.2	10.3
Hip fracture	*18.1	22.7	15.4	12.6	10.9

Source: Cohen, R.A., and J.F. Van Nostrand. *Trends in the Health of Older Americans: United States, 1994.* National Center for Health Statistics. Vital and Health Statistics 3(30). 1995. U.S. Department of Health and Human Services, Public Health Service, Centers for Disease Control and Prevention. Data are from the National Hospital Discharge Survey. *Notes:* 1. Comparisons of data for 1990 and 1991 with data for earlier years should be made with caution, as estimates of change may reflect improvements in the design rather than true changes in hospital use. 2. For 1970 the classification "other ischemic heart disease" includes all diagnoses of ischemic heart disease. *Estimates based on fewer than 30 discharges are not shown; estimates based on 30-59 discharges are preceded by an asterisk. Data include races other than white and black. Discharges are from non-Federal hospitals. Discharges exclude newborn infants. Diagnostic grouping inclusions are based on the *International Classification of Diseases, 8th Revision, adapted for use in the United States* for 1970, and the *International Classification of Diseases, 9th Revision Clinical Modification* (ICD-9-CM) for 1980, 1985, 1990 and 1991.

★ 458 ★
Hospitals

Hospitals Use: Number of Discharges from Short-Stay Hospitals: Both Sexes

This table shows the number of discharges from short-stay hospitals, both sexes, by selected first-listed diagnosis: United States, 1970, 1980, 1985, 1990, and 1991. Data are based on a sample of hospital records.

Sex, age, and first-listed diagnosis	Number of discharges in thousands				
	1970	1980	1985	1990[1]	1991[1]
Both sexes, all ages					
All conditions	29,127	37,832	35,056	30,788	31,098
Septicemia	---	59	149	216	240
Malignant neoplasms	1,142	1,873	1,911	1,571	1,594
Malignant neoplasms of colon and rectum	109	200	197	175	168
Malignant neoplasms of trachea, bronchus, and lung	122	277	315	231	236
Malignant neoplasms of the breast	128	213	208	164	158
Malignant neoplasms of the prostate	65	127	135	103	128
Diabetes mellitus	436	645	480	420	429

[Continued]

★ 458 ★

Hospitals Use: Number of Discharges from Short-Stay Hospitals: Both Sexes
[Continued]

Sex, age, and first-listed diagnosis	Number of discharges in thousands				
	1970	1980	1985	1990[1]	1991[1]
Volume depletion	---	100	239	319	329
Heart disease	1,869	3,201	3,584	3,556	3,704
Acute myocardial infarction	342	431	755	675	697
Coronary atherosclerosis	---	562	304	410	384
Other ischemic heart disease[2]	1,034	793	992	870	876
Cardiac dysrhythmias	112	389	511	483	536
Congestive heart failure	155	401	557	701	764
Cerebrovascular disease	519	796	916	812	835
Pneumonia	683	782	854	1,052	1,088
Cholelithiasis	396	458	474	506	552
Urinary tract infection, site unspecified	108	221	225	295	286
Hyperplasia of the prostate	214	276	246	259	229
Arthropathies and related disorders	365	543	465	479	526
Injury and poisoning	3,062	3,593	3,303	2,774	2,768
Fractures, all sites	1,077	1,163	1,129	1,017	1,034
Hip fracture	159	210	258	281	300
Both sexes, 55-64 years					
All conditions	3,274	4,685	4,312	3,412	3,378
Septicemia	---	*	17	18	26
Malignant neoplasms	278	453	434	345	311
Malignant neoplasms of colon and rectum	29	45	45	43	26
Malignant neoplasms of trachea, bronchus, and lung	42	86	92	72	68
Malignant neoplasms of the breast	32	57	47	33	31
Malignant neoplasms of the prostate	11	22	21	16	21
Diabetes mellitus	95	146	92	73	70
Volume depletion	---	*	23	31	26
Heart disease	414	705	761	691	696
Acute myocardial infarction	97	110	174	140	139
Coronary atherosclerosis	---	125	86	120	111
Other ischemic heart disease[2]	216	237	255	192	192
Cardiac dysrhythmias	26	76	87	87	86
Congestive heart failure	25	45	69	79	89
Cerebrovascular disease	84	126	142	111	103
Pneumonia	67	85	93	90	86
Cholelithiasis	71	89	82	78	95
Urinary tract infection, site unspecified	*9	21	18	21	23
Hyperplasia of the prostate	50	71	54	54	42
Arthropathies and related disorders	76	97	86	71	72
Injury and poisoning	280	301	317	251	250
Fractures, all sites	115	100	106	80	84
Hip fracture	14	14	19	16	20

[Continued]

★ 458 ★

Hospitals Use: Number of Discharges from Short-Stay Hospitals: Both Sexes
[Continued]

Sex, age, and first-listed diagnosis	Number of discharges in thousands				
	1970	1980	1985	1990[1]	1991[1]
Both sexes, 65-74 years					
All conditions	3,163	4,943	5,011	4,689	4,830
Septicemia	---	*11	31	49	56
Malignant neoplasms	298	523	566	436	486
Malignant neoplasms of colon and rectum	34	59	60	48	62
Malignant neoplasms of trachea, bronchus, and lung	39	98	114	77	83
Malignant neoplasms of the breast	23	50	49	40	41
Malignant neoplasms of the prostate	27	49	49	40	54
Diabetes mellitus	101	138	96	93	88
Volume depletion	---	18	38	47	52
Heart disease	491	854	983	1,000	1,063
Acute myocardial infarction	87	136	212	185	195
Coronary atherosclerosis	---	144	81	132	127
Other ischemic heart disease[2]	290	202	285	259	262
Cardiac dysrhythmias	24	106	134	124	159
Congestive heart failure	46	121	149	182	201
Cerebrovascular disease	161	240	279	222	231
Pneumonia	84	123	144	173	199
Cholelithiasis	65	81	80	79	99
Urinary tract infection, site unspecified	15	34	39	54	50
Hyperplasia of the prostate	84	114	99	113	97
Arthropathies and related disorders	76	93	102	137	155
Injury and poisoning	236	283	305	318	331
Fractures, all sites	117	124	121	120	116
Hip fracture	32	41	43	48	43
Both sexes, 75-84 years					
All conditions	2,099	3,611	3,969	3,949	4,136
Septicemia	---	14	38	54	68
Malignant neoplasms	179	319	338	300	315
Malignant neoplasms of colon and rectum	21	50	47	49	46
Malignant neoplasms of trachea, bronchus, and lung	16	39	49	36	35
Malignant neoplasms of the breast	16	29	24	24	27
Malignant neoplasms of the prostate	20	41	52	37	38
Diabetes mellitus	58	86	60	44	55
Volume depletion	---	25	60	67	80
Heart disease	402	694	804	865	912
Acute myocardial infarction	62	80	168	156	166
Coronary atherosclerosis	---	149	55	55	55
Other ischemic heart disease[2]	244	104	167	171	191
Cardiac dysrhythmias	15	85	137	133	149
Congestive heart failure	49	136	187	255	256
Cerebrovascular disease	154	234	294	258	274
Pneumonia	66	113	159	223	229

[Continued]

★ 458 ★

Hospitals Use: Number of Discharges from Short-Stay Hospitals: Both Sexes
[Continued]

Sex, age, and first-listed diagnosis	Number of discharges in thousands				
	1970	1980	1985	1990[1]	1991[1]
Cholelithiasis	31	43	60	48	53
Urinary tract infection, site unspecified	13	37	59	86	77
Hyperplasia of the prostate	48	63	66	69	69
Arthropathies and related disorders	43	71	66	83	91
Injury and poisoning	193	267	315	340	348
Fractures, all sites	121	152	180	195	197
Hip fracture	55	78	101	115	117
Both sexes, 65 years and over					
All conditions	5,897	9,864	10,508	10,333	10,806
Septicemia	---	33	91	144	159
Malignant neoplasms	520	921	991	812	883
Malignant neoplasms of colon and rectum	63	123	127	112	124
Malignant neoplasms of trachea, bronchus, and lung	57	142	169	119	125
Malignant neoplasms of the breast	43	86	81	72	73
Malignant neoplasms of the prostate	52	101	111	85	103
Diabetes mellitus	170	242	171	153	160
Volume depletion	---	65	143	171	189
Heart disease	1,021	1,808	2,111	2,200	2,361
Acute myocardial infarction	162	238	436	401	424
Coronary atherosclerosis	---	352	157	193	190
Other ischemic heart disease[2]	613	329	501	492	514
Cardiac dysrhythmias	45	225	324	308	361
Congestive heart failure	114	325	446	560	615
Cerebrovascular disease	372	585	686	610	640
Pneumonia	185	305	400	546	589
Cholelithiasis	105	138	157	145	168
Urinary tract infection, site unspecified	33	91	130	205	186
Hyperplasia of the prostate	145	188	179	195	180
Arthropathies and related disorders	131	181	183	237	261
Injury and poisoning	512	703	793	851	888
Fractures, all sites	294	375	419	448	452
Hip fracture	121	181	219	245	259
Both sexes, 75 years and over					
All conditions	2,734	4,921	5,497	5,644	5,976
Septicemia	---	22	61	95	104
Malignant neoplasms	222	398	425	377	397
Malignant neoplasms of colon and rectum	29	64	68	64	62
Malignant neoplasms of trachea, bronchus, and lung	18	44	56	42	42
Malignant neoplasms of the breast	19	36	31	33	32
Malignant neoplasms of the prostate	25	52	62	45	48
Diabetes mellitus	69	105	75	60	71
Volume depletion	---	48	105	124	137

[Continued]

★ 458 ★

Hospitals Use: Number of Discharges from Short-Stay Hospitals: Both Sexes
[Continued]

Sex, age, and first-listed diagnosis	Number of discharges in thousands				
	1970	1980	1985	1990[1]	1991[1]
Heart disease	530	954	1,128	1,199	1,298
Acute myocardial infarction	75	102	224	216	229
Coronary atherosclerosis	---	208	75	61	64
Other ischemic heart disease[2]	323	128	216	232	252
Cardiac dysrhythmias	21	119	190	184	202
Congestive heart failure	68	204	297	378	413
Cerebrovascular disease	211	344	407	388	409
Pneumonia	101	183	256	273	390
Cholelithiasis	40	57	76	66	69
Urinary tract infection, site unspecified	18	57	91	151	136
Hyperplasia of the prostate	61	74	80	82	83
Arthropathies and related disorders	55	88	81	100	107
Injury and poisoning	276	420	487	533	557
Fractures, all sites	177	251	298	328	336
Hip fracture	88	140	176	197	215
Both sexes, 85 years and over					
All conditions	635	1,310	1,528	1,694	1,840
Septicemia	---	*8	23	41	36
Malignant neoplasms	42	79	87	77	82
Malignant neoplasms of colon and rectum	*8	14	21	14	16
Malignant neoplasms of trachea, bronchus, and lung	*	*	*7	*6	*7
Malignant neoplasms of the breast	*	*7	*7	*9	*5
Malignant neoplasms of the prostate	*5	*11	*10	7	10
Diabetes mellitus	11	19	15	16	16
Volume depletion	---	23	44	57	57
Heart disease	128	260	324	335	386
Acute myocardial infarction	14	22	56	60	63
Coronary atherosclerosis	---	59	20	*6	*9
Other ischemic heart disease[2]	79	24	49	61	60
Cardiac dysrhythmias	*6	34	54	51	53
Congestive heart failure	19	68	109	123	157
Cerebrovascular disease	57	111	113	129	134
Pneumonia	35	70	98	150	161
Cholelithiasis	*8	13	16	18	16
Urinary tract infection, site unspecified	*	20	32	65	59
Hyperplasia of the prostate	12	*10	14	13	14
Arthropathies and related disorders	12	17	15	17	16
Injury and poisoning	83	153	172	193	209

[Continued]

★ 458 ★

Hospitals Use: Number of Discharges from Short-Stay Hospitals: Both Sexes
[Continued]

Sex, age, and first-listed diagnosis	Number of discharges in thousands				
	1970	1980	1985	1990[1]	1991[1]
Fractures, all sites	56	99	117	133	140
Hip fracture	33	62	76	82	98

Source: Cohen, R.A., and J.F. Van Nostrand. *Trends in the Health of Older Americans: United States, 1994.* National Center for Health Statistics. Vital and Health Statistics 3(30). 1995. U.S. Department of Health and Human Services, Public Health Service, Centers for Disease Control and Prevention. Data are from the National Hospital Discharge Survey. *Notes:* 1. Comparisons of data for 1990 and 1991 with data for earlier years should be made with caution, as estimates of change may reflect improvements in the design rather than true changes in hospital use. 2. For 1970 the classification "other ischemic heart disease" includes all diagnoses of ischemic heart disease. *Estimates based on fewer than 30 discharges are not shown; estimates based on 30-59 discharges are preceded by an asterisk. Data include races other than white and black. Discharges are from non-Federal hospitals. Discharges exclude newborn infants. Diagnostic grouping inclusions are based on the *International Classification of Diseases, 8th Revision, adapted for use in the United States* for 1970, and the *International Classification of Diseases, 9th Revision Clinical Modification* (ICD-9-CM) for 1980, 1985, 1990 and 1991.

★ 459 ★

Hospitals

Hospitals Use: Number of Discharges from Short-Stay Hospitals: Females

This table shows the number of discharges from short-stay hospitals, females, by selected first-listed diagnosis: United States, 1970, 1980, 1985, 1990, and 1991. Data are based on a sample of hospital records.

Age and first-listed diagnosis	Number of discharges in thousands				
	1970	1980	1985	1990[1]	1991[1]
All ages					
All conditions	17,696	22,686	20,896	18,508	18,620
Septicemia	---	32	85	116	137
Malignant neoplasms	617	994	1,019	841	812
Malignant neoplasms of colon and rectum	54	109	104	90	82
Malignant neoplasms of trachea, bronchus, and lung	27	84	110	90	89
Malignant neoplasms of the breast	126	212	207	163	156
Malignant neoplasms of the prostate	...	...	...	...	...
Diabetes mellitus	273	400	286	230	245
Volume depletion	---	65	147	192	208
Heart disease	854	1,513	1,674	1,643	1,727
Acute myocardial infarction	110	159	289	261	275
Coronary atherosclerosis	---	259	114	133	121
Other ischemic heart disease[2]	488	319	443	406	415
Cardiac dysrhythmias	59	204	267	239	287
Congestive heart failure	74	224	310	386	405
Cerebrovascular disease	279	425	500	452	466
Pneumonia	323	368	421	522	543
Cholelithiasis	298	342	334	374	393
Urinary tract infection, site unspecified	76	159	148	202	180
Hyperplasia of the prostate	...	...	...	...	...
Arthropathies and related disorders	226	328	276	283	298
Injury and poisoning	1,342	1,568	1,503	1,298	1,331
Fractures, all sites	512	580	579	551	553
Hip fracture	119	158	196	209	219

[Continued]

★ 459 ★

Hospitals Use: Number of Discharges from Short-Stay Hospitals: Females
[Continued]

Age and first-listed diagnosis	Number of discharges in thousands				
	1970	1980	1985	1990[1]	1991[1]
55-64 years					
All conditions	1,630	2,363	2,132	1,658	1,654
Septicemia	---	*	*8	11	16
Malignant neoplasms	145	247	226	180	150
Malignant neoplasms of colon and rectum	13	23	21	14	12
Malignant neoplasms of trachea, bronchus, and lung	10	30	39	31	25
Malignant neoplasms of the breast	32	56	47	33	30
Malignant neoplasms of the prostate	...	...	...	...	...
Diabetes mellitus	57	88	51	39	40
Volume depletion	---	*	12	18	15
Heart disease	154	264	281	260	251
Acute myocardial infarction	25	29	49	47	39
Coronary atherosclerosis	---	38	24	35	28
Other ischemic heart disease[2]	80	85	97	74	74
Cardiac dysrhythmias	13	34	37	33	39
Congestive heart failure	10	20	31	34	34
Cerebrovascular disease	39	59	62	51	46
Pneumonia	33	43	49	42	46
Cholelithiasis	49	58	56	55	63
Urinary tract infection, site unspecified	*	15	*10	10	11
Hyperplasia of the prostate	...	...	...	...	...
Arthropathies and related disorders	44	66	55	42	41
Injury and poisoning	140	146	160	118	123
Fractures, all sites	66	62	64	44	47
Hip fracture	11	*9	*13	7	11
65-74 years					
All conditions	1,651	2,585	2,623	2,421	2,478
Septicemia	---	*	19	21	28
Malignant neoplasms	131	240	281	214	225
Malignant neoplasms of colon and rectum	17	32	31	24	26
Malignant neoplasms of trachea, bronchus, and lung	*7	22	35	26	34
Malignant neoplasms of the breast	23	49	49	40	41
Malignant neoplasms of the prostate	...	...	...	...	...
Diabetes mellitus	69	94	64	59	60
Volume depletion	---	*10	21	29	34
Heart disease	243	418	470	453	496
Acute myocardial infarction	37	56	82	75	76
Coronary atherosclerosis	---	71	34	44	47
Other ischemic heart disease[2]	144	95	146	126	133
Cardiac dysrhythmias	12	51	72	57	81
Congestive heart failure	23	63	78	92	102
Cerebrovascular disease	79	120	143	114	115
Pneumonia	37	54	65	85	98

[Continued]

★ 459 ★

Hospitals Use: Number of Discharges from Short-Stay Hospitals: Females
[Continued]

Age and first-listed diagnosis	Number of discharges in thousands				
	1970	1980	1985	1990[1]	1991[1]
Cholelithiasis	46	54	49	49	60
Urinary tract infection, site unspecified	*8	20	21	37	28
Hyperplasia of the prostate	...	...	...	...	...
Arthropathies and related disorders	50	66	67	89	101
Injury and poisoning	145	172	188	179	186
Fractures, all sites	82	89	88	85	77
Hip fracture	25	29	33	36	29
75-84 years					
All conditions	1,191	2,140	2,312	2,289	2,387
Septicemia	---	*8	22	30	41
Malignant neoplasms	86	160	149	142	161
Malignant neoplasms of colon and rectum	10	29	24	29	25
Malignant neoplasms of trachea, bronchus, and lung	*	11	12	15	11
Malignant neoplasms of the breast	16	28	24	24	27
Malignant neoplasms of the prostate	...	...	...	...	...
Diabetes mellitus	41	59	40	27	35
Volume depletion	---	18	39	41	50
Heart disease	219	404	464	488	500
Acute myocardial infarction	29	46	92	73	86
Coronary atherosclerosis	---	89	30	25	25
Other ischemic heart disease[2]	139	53	102	107	113
Cardiac dysrhythmias	*8	48	79	76	88
Congestive heart failure	26	80	106	150	137
Cerebrovascular disease	92	137	176	154	166
Pneumonia	33	58	78	111	114
Cholelithiasis	21	28	36	28	33
Urinary tract infection, site unspecified	*6	23	37	61	48
Hyperplasia of the prostate	...	...	...	...	...
Arthropathies and related disorders	34	53	46	57	59
Injury and poisoning	139	197	223	244	242
Fractures, all sites	94	122	142	161	155
Hip fracture	43	62	80	95	91
65 years and over					
All conditions	3,230	5,596	5,975	5,861	6,098
Septicemia	---	18	56	80	93
Malignant neoplasms	239	440	478	401	428
Malignant neoplasms of colon and rectum	32	68	70	63	62
Malignant neoplasms of trachea, bronchus, and lung	11	35	48	44	48
Malignant neoplasms of the breast	42	85	80	72	73
Malignant neoplasms of the prostate	...	...	...	...	...
Diabetes mellitus	117	166	114	97	107
Volume depletion	---	43	94	109	124

[Continued]

Hospitals Use: Number of Discharges from Short-Stay Hospitals: Females
[Continued]

Age and first-listed diagnosis	Number of discharges in thousands				
	1970	1980	1985	1990[1]	1991[1]
Heart disease	541	995	1,158	1,164	1,254
Acute myocardial infarction	71	114	210	185	199
Coronary atherosclerosis	---	199	78	73	79
Other ischemic heart disease[2]	334	165	281	271	287
Cardiac dysrhythmias	25	124	186	167	205
Congestive heart failure	58	189	262	327	346
Cerebrovascular disease	208	331	396	362	377
Pneumonia	87	150	201	283	303
Cholelithiasis	73	93	97	90	105
Urinary tract infection, site unspecified	16	57	80	143	119
Hyperplasia of the prostate	...	...	...	...	...
Arthropathies and related disorders	92	133	125	158	173
Injury and poisoning	348	486	546	568	591
Fractures, all sites	221	295	328	350	346
Hip fracture	94	143	175	194	199
75 years and over					
All conditions	1,579	3,011	3,352	3,440	3,620
Septicemia	---	13	37	59	65
Malignant neoplasms	108	200	198	187	203
Malignant neoplasms of colon and rectum	15	36	40	39	36
Malignant neoplasms of trachea, bronchus, and lung	*	13	13	18	13
Malignant neoplasms of the breast	19	36	31	33	32
Malignant neoplasms of the prostate	...	...	...	...	...
Diabetes mellitus	48	72	49	39	47
Volume depletion	---	34	73	80	90
Heart disease	297	577	688	711	758
Acute myocardial infarction	34	58	127	110	123
Coronary atherosclerosis	---	128	44	29	31
Other ischemic heart disease[2]	190	70	135	145	154
Cardiac dysrhythmias	12	73	114	110	124
Congestive heart failure	35	126	184	235	245
Cerebrovascular disease	128	211	253	249	262
Pneumonia	50	96	136	98	206
Cholelithiasis	26	39	48	41	45
Urinary tract infection, site unspecified	*8	37	59	106	91
Hyperplasia of the prostate	...	...	...	...	...
Arthropathies and related disorders	42	67	58	68	71
Injury and poisoning	203	315	358	389	405
Fractures, all sites	139	206	240	265	269
Hip fracture	70	114	142	158	170
85 years and over					
All conditions	387	871	1,040	1,151	1,233

[Continued]

★ 459 ★

Hospitals Use: Number of Discharges from Short-Stay Hospitals: Females
[Continued]

Age and first-listed diagnosis	Number of discharges in thousands				
	1970	1980	1985	1990[1]	1991[1]
Septicemia	---	*	16	29	24
Malignant neoplasms	22	40	49	45	43
Malignant neoplasms of colon and rectum	*	*7	16	9	10
Malignant neoplasms of trachea, bronchus, and lung	*	*	*	*	*
Malignant neoplasms of the breast	*	*7	*6	*9	*5
Malignant neoplasms of the prostate	...	...	...	...	...
Diabetes mellitus	*7	13	*10	11	12
Volume depletion	---	16	33	40	41
Heart disease	78	172	223	223	258
Acute myocardial infarction	*6	12	36	37	37
Coronary atherosclerosis	---	39	15	*	*
Other ischemic heart disease[2]	51	17	33	38	41
Cardiac dysrhythmias	*	25	35	35	36
Congestive heart failure	*9	46	78	85	108
Cerebrovascular disease	36	74	77	95	96
Pneumonia	17	38	58	87	92
Cholelithiasis	*5	11	12	13	12
Urinary tract infection, site unspecified	*	13	22	45	43
Hyperplasia of the prostate	...	...	...	...	...
Arthropathies and related disorders	*9	13	*11	11	12
Injury and poisoning	64	118	136	145	163
Fractures, all sites	46	83	97	104	113
Hip fracture	26	52	62	63	79

Source: Cohen, R.A., and J.F. Van Nostrand. *Trends in the Health of Older Americans: United States, 1994.* National Center for Health Statistics. Vital and Health Statistics 3(30). 1995. U.S. Department of Health and Human Services, Public Health Service, Centers for Disease Control and Prevention. Data are from the National Hospital Discharge Survey. *Notes:* 1. Comparisons of data for 1990 and 1991 with data for earlier years should be made with caution, as estimates of change may reflect improvements in the design rather than true changes in hospital use. 2. For 1970 the classification "other ischemic heart disease" includes all diagnoses of ischemic heart disease. *Estimates based on fewer than 30 discharges are not shown; estimates based on 30-59 discharges are preceded by an asterisk. Data include races other than white and black. Discharges are from non-Federal hospitals. Discharges exclude newborn infants. Diagnostic grouping inclusions are based on the *International Classification of Diseases, 8th Revision, adapted for use in the United States* for 1970, and the *International Classification of Diseases, 9th Revision Clinical Modification* (ICD-9-CM) for 1980, 1985, 1990 and 1991.

★ 460 ★

Hospitals

Hospitals Use: Number of Discharges from Short-Stay Hospitals: Males

This table shows the number of discharges from short-stay hospitals, males, by selected first-listed diagnosis: United States, 1970, 1980, 1985, 1990, and 1991. Data are based on a sample of hospital records.

Age and first-listed diagnosis	Number of discharges in thousands				
	1970	1980	1985	1990[1]	1991[1]
All ages					
All conditions	11,431	15,145	14,160	12,280	12,478
Septicemia	---	28	64	99	103
Malignant neoplasms	525	878	892	730	781
Malignant neoplasms of colon and rectum	56	91	93	85	86

[Continued]

★ 460 ★

Hospitals Use: Number of Discharges from Short-Stay Hospitals: Males
[Continued]

Age and first-listed diagnosis	Number of discharges in thousands				
	1970	1980	1985	1990[1]	1991[1]
Malignant neoplasms of trachea, bronchus, and lung	95	193	206	141	147
Malignant neoplasms of the breast	*	*	*	*	*
Malignant neoplasms of the prostate	65	127	135	103	128
Diabetes mellitus	163	245	194	190	185
Volume depletion	---	35	93	127	121
Heart disease	1,015	1,688	1,910	1,913	1,977
Acute myocardial infarction	232	272	466	413	422
Coronary atherosclerosis	---	303	190	277	263
Other ischemic heart disease[2]	547	474	549	465	461
Cardiac dysrhythmias	54	185	244	244	249
Congestive heart failure	80	176	247	315	360
Cerebrovascular disease	241	371	416	359	370
Pneumonia	360	414	433	530	545
Cholelithiasis	98	115	140	132	159
Urinary tract infection, site unspecified	31	61	77	94	106
Hyperplasia of the prostate	214	276	246	259	229
Arthropathies and related disorders	139	215	188	197	228
Injury and poisoning	1,721	2,025	1,800	1,476	1,437
Fractures, all sites	565	582	550	466	481
Hip fracture	40	52	62	72	80
55-64 years					
All conditions	1,644	2,322	2,179	1,754	1,724
Septicemia	---	*	*9	7	10
Malignant neoplasms	134	206	208	166	161
Malignant neoplasms of colon and rectum	16	22	24	28	14
Malignant neoplasms of trachea, bronchus, and lung	33	56	53	41	43
Malignant neoplasms of the breast	*	*	*	*	*
Malignant neoplasms of the prostate	11	22	21	16	21
Diabetes mellitus	38	58	40	34	30
Volume depletion	---	*	*11	13	11
Heart disease	260	440	481	431	445
Acute myocardial infarction	72	80	125	92	100
Coronary atherosclerosis	---	88	62	85	84
Other ischemic heart disease[2]	136	152	158	117	118
Cardiac dysrhythmias	13	42	50	55	48
Congestive heart failure	15	25	38	46	56
Cerebrovascular disease	45	68	80	61	57
Pneumonia	34	42	44	48	40
Cholelithiasis	22	31	26	23	33
Urinary tract infection, site unspecified	*	*	*8	11	12
Hyperplasia of the prostate	50	71	54	54	42
Arthropathies and related disorders	31	31	31	29	31
Injury and poisoning	140	155	157	133	127
Fractures, all sites	49	38	42	35	37

[Continued]

★ 460 ★

Hospitals Use: Number of Discharges from Short-Stay Hospitals: Males
[Continued]

Age and first-listed diagnosis	Number of discharges in thousands				
	1970	1980	1985	1990[1]	1991[1]
Hip fracture	*	*	*	*10	*8
65-74 years					
All conditions	1,512	2,358	2,389	2,268	2,352
Septicemia	---	*6	12	27	27
Malignant neoplasms	167	283	285	222	261
Malignant neoplasms of colon and rectum	17	27	29	24	36
Malignant neoplasms of trachea, bronchus, and lung	32	76	79	50	49
Malignant neoplasms of the breast	*	*	*	*	*
Malignant neoplasms of the prostate	27	49	49	40	54
Diabetes mellitus	32	44	31	34	29
Volume depletion	---	*8	17	18	19
Heart disease	248	437	513	547	567
Acute myocardial infarction	50	80	129	110	118
Coronary atherosclerosis	---	74	48	87	80
Other ischemic heart disease[2]	145	106	140	133	129
Cardiac dysrhythmias	12	55	62	67	78
Congestive heart failure	23	58	72	90	99
Cerebrovascular disease	82	120	136	108	116
Pneumonia	47	69	79	88	101
Cholelithiasis	19	27	32	30	39
Urinary tract infection, site unspecified	*7	13	18	17	22
Hyperplasia of the prostate	84	114	99	113	97
Arthropathies and related disorders	26	27	35	48	53
Injury and poisoning	90	111	118	139	145
Fractures, all sites	35	35	33	36	39
Hip fracture	*8	13	*10	12	14
75-84 years					
All conditions	908	1,471	1,657	1,660	1,749
Septicemia	---	*6	17	24	27
Malignant neoplasms	94	159	189	158	155
Malignant neoplasms of colon and rectum	11	21	23	20	21
Malignant neoplasms of trachea, bronchus, and lung	13	28	36	22	24
Malignant neoplasms of the breast	*	*	*	*	*
Malignant neoplasms of the prostate	20	41	52	37	38
Diabetes mellitus	17	27	21	17	20
Volume depletion	---	*7	21	26	30
Heart disease	183	290	339	377	411
Acute myocardial infarction	33	34	77	83	80
Coronary atherosclerosis	---	59	25	29	29
Other ischemic heart disease[2]	105	50	64	65	79
Cardiac dysrhythmias	*7	37	57	58	61
Congestive heart failure	23	56	81	104	120

[Continued]

★ 460 ★

Hospitals Use: Number of Discharges from Short-Stay Hospitals: Males
[Continued]

Age and first-listed diagnosis	Number of discharges in thousands				
	1970	1980	1985	1990[1]	1991[1]
Cerebrovascular disease	62	96	118	104	108
Pneumonia	33	55	81	112	115
Cholelithiasis	10	16	24	20	20
Urinary tract infection, site unspecified	*7	14	22	25	29
Hyperplasia of the prostate	48	63	66	69	69
Arthropathies and related disorders	*9	18	20	26	32
Injury and poisoning	54	71	93	96	106
Fractures, all sites	27	29	38	35	41
Hip fracture	12	16	21	20	26
65 years and over					
All conditions	2,667	4,268	4,533	4,472	4,708
Septicemia	---	15	35	63	66
Malignant neoplasms	281	481	512	411	455
Malignant neoplasms of colon and rectum	31	55	57	49	62
Malignant neoplasms of trachea, bronchus, and lung	46	107	121	75	77
Malignant neoplasms of the breast	*	*	*	*	*
Malignant neoplasms of the prostate	52	101	111	85	103
Diabetes mellitus	54	77	57	56	52
Volume depletion	---	22	49	61	65
Heart disease	480	814	953	1,036	1,107
Acute myocardial infarction	91	124	226	216	225
Coronary atherosclerosis	---	153	79	120	112
Other ischemic heart disease[2]	278	164	220	221	227
Cardiac dysrhythmias	20	101	138	140	156
Congestive heart failure	55	136	184	233	268
Cerebrovascular disease	164	253	289	247	263
Pneumonia	97	156	199	264	286
Cholelithiasis	33	45	60	55	63
Urinary tract infection, site unspecified	17	34	50	62	67
Hyperplasia of the prostate	145	188	179	195	180
Arthropathies and related disorders	38	48	58	80	88
Injury and poisoning	163	217	247	283	297
Fractures, all sites	73	80	91	99	107
Hip fracture	26	39	45	51	59
75 years and over					
All conditions	1,155	1,910	2,144	2,203	2,356
Septicemia	---	*9	23	36	39
Malignant neoplasms	114	198	227	190	194
Malignant neoplasms of colon and rectum	14	28	28	25	27
Malignant neoplasms of trachea, bronchus, and lung	15	31	42	25	28
Malignant neoplasms of the breast	*	*	*	*	*
Malignant neoplasms of the prostate	25	52	62	45	48

[Continued]

★ 460 ★

Hospitals Use: Number of Discharges from Short-Stay Hospitals: Males
[Continued]

Age and first-listed diagnosis	Number of discharges in thousands				
	1970	1980	1985	1990[1]	1991[1]
Diabetes mellitus	21	33	26	21	24
Volume depletion	---	14	32	43	47
Heart disease	232	377	440	489	540
Acute myocardial infarction	41	44	97	106	106
Coronary atherosclerosis	---	80	31	32	32
Other ischemic heart disease[2]	133	58	80	88	98
Cardiac dysrhythmias	*9	46	76	74	78
Congestive heart failure	32	78	113	143	169
Cerebrovascular disease	83	133	154	139	147
Pneumonia	51	87	120	175	184
Cholelithiasis	14	17	28	25	24
Urinary tract infection, site unspecified	*9	21	32	45	45
Hyperplasia of the prostate	61	74	80	82	83
Arthropathies and related disorders	12	21	23	32	35
Injury and poisoning	73	106	129	144	152
Fractures, all sites	38	45	58	63	68
Hip fracture	18	26	34	39	45
85 years and over					
All conditions	247	439	488	543	607
Septicemia	---	*	*7	12	12
Malignant neoplasms	20	39	38	31	40
Malignant neoplasms of colon and rectum	*	*8	*5	*5	*6
Malignant neoplasms of trachea, bronchus, and lung	*	*	*	*	*
Malignant neoplasms of the breast	*	*	*	*	*
Malignant neoplasms of the prostate	*5	*11	*10	7	10
Diabetes mellitus	*	*5	*	*	*
Volume depletion	---	*7	11	17	16
Heart disease	49	87	101	112	128
Acute myocardial infarction	*8	*10	20	23	26
Coronary atherosclerosis	---	20	*	*	*
Other ischemic heart disease[2]	28	*7	16	23	19
Cardiac dysrhythmias	*	*9	19	16	17
Congestive heart failure	*9	22	32	38	49
Cerebrovascular disease	21	37	36	35	39
Pneumonia	18	31	40	64	69
Cholelithiasis	*	*	*	*6	*4
Urinary tract infection, site unspecified	*	*7	*10	20	17
Hyperplasia of the prostate	12	*10	14	13	14
Arthropathies and related disorders	*	*	*	*	*
Injury and poisoning	19	35	36	48	46

[Continued]

★ 460 ★

Hospitals Use: Number of Discharges from Short-Stay Hospitals: Males
[Continued]

Age and first-listed diagnosis	Number of discharges in thousands				
	1970	1980	1985	1990[1]	1991[1]
Fractures, all sites	11	16	20	28	27
Hip fracture	*7	10	14	19	19

Source: Cohen, R.A., and J.F. Van Nostrand. *Trends in the Health of Older Americans: United States, 1994.* National Center for Health Statistics. Vital and Health Statistics 3(30). 1995. U.S. Department of Health and Human Services, Public Health Service, Centers for Disease Control and Prevention. Data are from the National Hospital Discharge Survey. *Notes:* 1. Comparisons of data for 1990 and 1991 with data for earlier years should be made with caution, as estimates of change may reflect improvements in the design rather than true changes in hospital use. 2. For 1970 the classification "other ischemic heart disease" includes all diagnoses of ischemic heart disease. *Estimates based on fewer than 30 discharges are not shown; estimates based on 30-59 discharges are preceded by an asterisk. Data include races other than white and black. Discharges are from non-Federal hospitals. Discharges exclude newborn infants. Diagnostic grouping inclusions are based on the *International Classification of Diseases, 8th Revision, adapted for use in the United States* for 1970, and the *International Classification of Diseases, 9th Revision Clinical Modification* (ICD-9-CM) for 1980, 1985, 1990 and 1991.

★ 461 ★

Hospitals

Hospitals Use: Rate of Discharges from Short-Stay Hospitals: Both Sexes

This table shows the rate of discharges from short-stay hospitals, both sexes, by selected first-listed diagnosis: United States, 1970, 1980, 1985, 1990, and 1991. Data are based on a sample of hospital records.

Sex, age, and first-listed diagnosis	Discharges per 10,000 population				
	1970	1980	1985	1990[1]	1991[1]
Both sexes, all ages					
All conditions					
Septicemia	---	2.6	6.3	8.7	9.6
Malignant neoplasms	56.6	83.0	80.9	63.4	63.6
Malignant neoplasms of colon and rectum	5.4	8.9	8.3	7.1	6.7
Malignant neoplasms of trachea, bronchus, and lung	6.1	12.3	13.3	9.3	9.4
Malignant neoplasms of the breast	6.3	9.4	8.8	6.6	6.3
Malignant neoplasms of the prostate	3.2	5.6	5.7	4.2	5.1
Diabetes mellitus	21.6	28.6	20.3	17.0	17.1
Volume depletion	---	4.4	10.1	12.9	13.1
Heart disease	92.6	141.9	151.7	143.5	147.8
Acute myocardial infarction	16.9	19.1	31.9	27.2	27.8
Coronary atherosclerosis	---	24.9	12.9	16.5	15.3
Other ischemic heart disease[2]	51.2	35.1	42.0	35.1	35.0
Cardiac dysrhythmias	5.6	17.2	21.6	19.5	21.4
Congestive heart failure	7.7	17.8	23.6	28.3	30.5
Cerebrovascular disease	25.7	35.3	38.8	32.8	33.3
Pneumonia	33.8	34.7	36.2	42.4	43.4
Cholelithiasis	19.6	20.3	20.1	20.4	22.0
Urinary tract infection, site unspecified	5.3	9.8	9.5	11.9	11.4
Hyperplasia of the prostate	10.6	12.2	10.4	10.5	9.2
Arthropathies and related disorders	18.1	24.1	19.7	19.4	21.0
Injury and poisoning	151.7	159.2	139.8	111.9	110.5
Fractures, all sites	53.3	51.5	47.8	41.0	41.3
Hip fracture	7.9	9.3	10.9	11.3	12.0

[Continued]

★ 461 ★

Hospitals Use: Rate of Discharges from Short-Stay Hospitals: Both Sexes
[Continued]

Sex, age, and first-listed diagnosis	Discharges per 10,000 population				
	1970	1980	1985	1990[1]	1991[1]
Both sexes, 55-64 years					
All conditions					
Septicemia	---	*	7.8	8.5	12.3
Malignant neoplasms	149.0	208.0	196.0	163.7	148.0
Malignant neoplasms of colon and rectum	15.5	20.7	20.4	20.2	12.3
Malignant neoplasms of trachea, bronchus, and lung	22.7	39.7	41.7	34.2	32.5
Malignant neoplasms of the breast	17.2	26.1	21.3	15.8	14.6
Malignant neoplasms of the prostate	5.7	10.3	9.6	7.5	9.8
Diabetes mellitus	51.0	67.3	41.4	34.7	33.2
Volume depletion	---	*	10.3	14.5	12.2
Heart disease	221.6	324.0	344.0	327.5	331.5
Acute myocardial infarction	51.7	50.5	78.6	66.1	66.2
Coronary atherosclerosis	---	57.6	39.1	56.8	53.0
Other ischemic heart disease[2]	115.7	109.0	115.1	90.9	91.5
Cardiac dysrhythmias	13.8	35.0	39.4	41.5	41.1
Congestive heart failure	13.6	20.8	31.0	37.7	42.5
Cerebrovascular disease	45.2	58.1	64.1	52.7	49.0
Pneumonia	36.1	38.9	42.2	42.6	41.0
Cholelithiasis	38.0	40.7	37.2	37.1	45.3
Urinary tract infection, site unspecified	*10.0	9.8	8.0	10.0	11.0
Hyperplasia of the prostate	26.8	32.8	24.6	25.8	19.8
Arthropathies and related disorders	40.5	44.7	38.8	33.7	34.4
Injury and poisoning	149.9	138.3	143.1	118.8	119.0
Fractures, all sites	61.5	46.0	47.7	37.7	39.8
Hip fracture	7.7	6.5	8.4	7.7	9.3
Both sexes, 65-74 years					
All conditions					
Septicemia	---	*7.0	18.2	27.0	30.5
Malignant neoplasms	238.8	334.2	335.6	240.8	265.6
Malignant neoplasms of colon and rectum	27.0	38.0	35.3	26.4	33.7
Malignant neoplasms of trachea, bronchus, and lung	31.2	62.5	67.6	42.5	45.6
Malignant neoplasms of the breast	18.8	31.7	29.2	21.9	22.5
Malignant neoplasms of the prostate	21.3	31.6	28.9	22.0	29.7
Diabetes mellitus	81.1	87.9	56.8	51.4	48.3
Volume depletion	---	11.2	22.7	26.0	28.7
Heart disease	393.2	546.0	582.9	552.8	581.4
Acute myocardial infarction	69.7	87.1	125.5	102.3	106.5
Coronary atherosclerosis	---	92.2	48.3	72.8	69.4
Other ischemic heart disease[2]	232.0	128.9	169.2	143.2	143.3
Cardiac dysrhythmias	19.4	67.8	79.4	68.5	87.0
Congestive heart failure	36.8	77.3	88.6	100.6	110.2
Cerebrovascular disease	128.9	153.5	165.4	122.7	126.4
Pneumonia	67.1	78.3	85.3	95.8	108.9
Cholelithiasis	52.3	52.0	47.7	43.8	54.3
Urinary tract infection, site unspecified	12.2	21.5	23.1	29.9	27.3
Hyperplasia of the prostate	67.6	72.9	58.8	62.5	53.2

[Continued]

★ 461 ★

Hospitals Use: Rate of Discharges from Short-Stay Hospitals: Both Sexes
[Continued]

Sex, age, and first-listed diagnosis	Discharges per 10,000 population				
	1970	1980	1985	1990[1]	1991[1]
Arthropathies and related disorders	61.0	59.4	60.6	75.8	84.6
Injury and poisoning	188.6	180.7	181.1	175.7	180.8
Fractures, all sites	93.7	79.4	71.8	66.5	63.3
Hip fracture	26.0	26.5	25.7	26.5	23.8
Both sexes, 75-84 years					
All conditions					
Septicemia	---	18.5	42.8	53.4	65.6
Malignant neoplasms	290.1	410.0	380.5	297.5	305.6
Malignant neoplasms of colon and rectum	34.7	63.9	52.6	48.9	44.5
Malignant neoplasms of trachea, bronchus, and lung	25.8	49.5	54.6	36.1	33.9
Malignant neoplasms of the breast	25.8	36.8	27.5	23.5	26.5
Malignant neoplasms of the prostate	32.5	52.8	58.2	37.0	36.8
Diabetes mellitus	94.3	110.3	67.9	43.9	53.6
Volume depletion	---	31.8	67.7	66.2	77.4
Heart disease	650.3	891.5	903.9	858.3	883.8
Acute myocardial infarction	99.8	103.2	189.4	154.5	160.9
Coronary atherosclerosis	---	191.1	62.0	54.1	53.0
Other ischemic heart disease[2]	394.1	133.2	187.5	170.1	185.6
Cardiac dysrhythmias	24.4	109.1	153.8	132.1	144.6
Congestive heart failure	79.0	174.7	210.5	252.8	248.5
Cerebrovascular disease	248.6	300.0	330.9	256.5	266.1
Pneumonia	107.4	145.2	178.5	220.9	222.0
Cholelithiasis	50.8	55.7	68.0	47.2	51.6
Urinary tract infection, site unspecified	20.5	48.0	66.3	85.2	74.6
Hyperplasia of the prostate	77.8	81.4	74.4	68.4	66.4
Arthropathies and related disorders	69.0	91.2	74.1	82.8	87.9
Injury and poisoning	312.8	343.6	354.4	337.3	337.8
Fractures, all sites	195.6	194.6	203.0	193.9	190.6
Hip fracture	89.0	100.2	113.1	114.2	113.1
Both sexes, 65 years and over					
All conditions					
Septicemia	---	13.0	32.2	46.0	50.2
Malignant neoplasms	258.6	358.3	348.7	260.1	278.1
Malignant neoplasms of colon and rectum	31.2	48.0	44.7	35.7	39.0
Malignant neoplasms of trachea, bronchus, and lung	28.5	55.3	59.6	38.1	39.3
Malignant neoplasms of the breast	21.3	33.4	28.4	23.2	23.1
Malignant neoplasms of the prostate	25.8	39.4	38.9	27.1	32.4
Diabetes mellitus	84.7	94.2	60.1	49.1	50.3
Volume depletion	---	25.4	50.3	54.6	59.6
Heart disease	507.8	703.3	742.7	704.5	743.5
Acute myocardial infarction	80.7	92.7	153.3	128.5	133.5
Coronary atherosclerosis	---	137.0	55.1	61.7	60.0
Other ischemic heart disease[2]	304.7	128.1	176.3	157.4	161.7
Cardiac dysrhythmias	22.5	87.6	114.0	98.5	113.7
Congestive heart failure	56.5	126.4	157.0	179.3	193.6
Cerebrovascular disease	185.1	227.4	241.3	195.2	201.5

[Continued]

★ 461 ★

Hospitals Use: Rate of Discharges from Short-Stay Hospitals: Both Sexes
[Continued]

Sex, age, and first-listed diagnosis	Discharges per 10,000 population				
	1970	1980	1985	1990[1]	1991[1]
Pneumonia	91.9	118.7	140.8	175.0	185.5
Cholelithiasis	52.3	53.7	55.2	46.5	53.0
Urinary tract infection, site unspecified	16.4	35.4	45.7	65.8	58.7
Hyperplasia of the prostate	72.1	73.0	63.0	62.6	56.7
Arthropathies and related disorders	65.0	70.4	64.4	76.0	82.3
Injury and poisoning	254.4	273.5	278.9	272.5	279.5
Fractures, all sites	146.4	146.0	147.4	143.6	142.4
Hip fracture	59.9	70.6	77.2	78.5	81.4
Both sexes, 75 years and over					
All conditions					
Septicemia	---	22.3	52.5	72.2	77.0
Malignant neoplasms	291.2	395.9	367.6	286.8	294.9
Malignant neoplasms of colon and rectum	38.1	63.7	58.5	48.5	46.1
Malignant neoplasms of trachea, bronchus, and lung	24.0	44.0	48.1	32.1	30.8
Malignant neoplasms of the breast	25.5	35.9	27.3	24.9	24.0
Malignant neoplasms of the prostate	33.3	51.6	53.6	34.1	35.9
Diabetes mellitus	90.6	104.0	64.9	45.9	52.9
Volume depletion	---	47.5	90.5	94.1	101.5
Heart disease	695.7	948.3	975.8	913.8	963.3
Acute myocardial infarction	98.8	101.4	193.9	164.6	170.1
Coronary atherosclerosis	---	206.9	65.0	46.4	47.2
Other ischemic heart disease[2]	424.0	127.0	186.6	177.1	186.8
Cardiac dysrhythmias	27.7	118.4	164.7	139.9	150.0
Congestive heart failure	88.7	202.8	256.6	287.7	306.8
Cerebrovascular disease	277.4	342.5	352.0	295.3	303.4
Pneumonia	132.6	181.5	221.8	207.9	289.4
Cholelithiasis	52.3	56.2	66.1	50.2	51.3
Urinary tract infection, site unspecified	23.1	56.9	78.7	115.3	101.3
Hyperplasia of the prostate	79.6	73.2	69.1	62.7	61.4
Arthropathies and related disorders	71.7	87.6	70.0	76.3	79.2
Injury and poisoning	362.6	418.0	421.6	406.0	413.4
Fractures, all sites	233.0	249.5	257.7	249.9	249.7
Hip fracture	115.7	139.2	152.4	150.3	159.6
Both sexes, 85 years and over					
All conditions					
Septicemia	---	*35.3	84.9	134.4	114.4
Malignant neoplasms	296.1	347.8	324.9	251.7	259.8
Malignant neoplasms of colon and rectum	52.7	62.9	78.0	47.1	51.5
Malignant neoplasms of trachea, bronchus, and lung	*	*	*26.4	*18.9	*20.9
Malignant neoplasms of the breast	*	*32.8	*26.1	*29.8	*15.8
Malignant neoplasms of the prostate	*36.9	*47.7	*38.2	24.4	33.0
Diabetes mellitus	74.7	82.1	55.0	52.5	50.5
Volume depletion	---	101.4	166.3	186.2	180.2
Heart disease	892.4				
Acute myocardial infarction	94.7	94.9	208.8	198.0	200.1
Coronary atherosclerosis	---	260.8	75.2	*21.0	*28.1

[Continued]

★ 461 ★

Hospitals Use: Rate of Discharges from Short-Stay Hospitals: Both Sexes
[Continued]

Sex, age, and first-listed diagnosis	Discharges per 10,000 population				
	1970	1980	1985	1990[1]	1991[1]
Other ischemic heart disease[2]	553.4	105.8	183.7	200.1	190.4
Cardiac dysrhythmias	*41.9	150.3	200.8	165.7	167.6
Congestive heart failure	130.6	298.8	410.4	402.9	497.3
Cerebrovascular disease	401.9	488.0	422.4	423.3	425.2
Pneumonia	241.7	306.2	366.0	492.8	509.4
Cholelithiasis	*58.5	58.1	59.9	60.1	50.1
Urinary tract infection, site unspecified	*	87.6	120.0	214.5	188.2
Hyperplasia of the prostate	87.3	*44.9	51.4	44.0	45.1
Arthropathies and related disorders	83.5	75.1	56.0	54.9	50.7
Injury and poisoning	577.8	672.9	645.3	632.7	660.4
Fractures, all sites	394.6	437.5	439.9	435.0	442.7
Hip fracture	230.8	272.8	283.2	269.9	311.3

Source: Cohen, R.A., and J.F. Van Nostrand. *Trends in the Health of Older Americans: United States, 1994.* National Center for Health Statistics. Vital and Health Statistics 3(30). 1995. U.S. Department of Health and Human Services, Public Health Service, Centers for Disease Control and Prevention. Data are from the National Hospital Discharge Survey. *Notes:* 1. Comparisons of data for 1990 and 1991 with data for earlier years should be made with caution, as estimates of change may reflect improvements in the design rather than true changes in hospital use. 2. For 1970 the classification "other ischemic heart disease" includes all diagnoses of ischemic heart disease. *Estimates based on fewer than 30 discharges are not shown; estimates based on 30-59 discharges are preceded by an asterisk. Data include races other than white and black. Discharges are from non-Federal hospitals. Discharges exclude newborn infants. Diagnostic grouping inclusions are based on the *International Classification of Diseases, 8th Revision, adapted for use in the United States* for 1970, and the *International Classification of Diseases, 9th Revision Clinical Modification* (ICD-9-CM) for 1980, 1985, 1990 and 1991.

★ 462 ★

Hospitals

Hospitals Use: Rate of Discharges from Short-Stay Hospitals: Females

This table shows the rate of discharges from short-stay hospitals, females, by selected first-listed diagnosis: United States, 1970, 1980, 1985, 1990, and 1991. Data are based on a sample of hospital records.

Age and first-listed diagnosis	Discharges per 10,000 population				
	1970	1980	1985	1990[1]	1991[1]
All ages					
All conditions					
Septicemia	---	2.7	6.9	9.1	10.6
Malignant neoplasms	58.9	85.2	83.5	65.9	63.0
Malignant neoplasms of colon and rectum	5.1	9.3	8.5	7.1	6.4
Malignant neoplasms of trachea, bronchus, and lung	2.6	7.2	9.0	7.1	6.9
Malignant neoplasms of the breast	12.1	18.2	16.9	12.8	12.1
Malignant neoplasms of the prostate	...	...	...	...	...
Diabetes mellitus	26.0	34.3	23.4	18.0	19.0
Volume depletion	---	5.6	12.0	15.0	16.1
Heart disease	81.6	129.6	137.1	128.7	133.9
Acute myocardial infarction	10.5	13.6	23.7	20.5	21.3
Coronary atherosclerosis	---	22.2	9.3	10.4	9.3
Other ischemic heart disease[2]	46.6	27.3	36.3	31.8	32.1
Cardiac dysrhythmias	5.6	17.5	21.9	18.7	22.3
Congestive heart failure	7.1	19.2	25.4	30.2	31.4

[Continued]

★ 462 ★

Hospitals Use: Rate of Discharges from Short-Stay Hospitals: Females
[Continued]

Age and first-listed diagnosis	Discharges per 10,000 population				
	1970	1980	1985	1990[1]	1991[1]
Cerebrovascular disease	26.6	36.5	41.0	35.5	36.1
Pneumonia	30.9	31.5	34.5	40.9	42.1
Cholelithiasis	28.4	29.3	27.3	29.3	30.4
Urinary tract infection, site unspecified	7.3	13.7	12.1	15.8	14.0
Hyperplasia of the prostate	...	...	...	...	...
Arthropathies and related disorders	21.6	28.1	22.6	22.2	23.1
Injury and poisoning	128.2	134.4	123.2	101.7	103.2
Fractures, all sites	48.9	49.7	47.4	43.2	42.9
Hip fracture	11.4	13.6	16.1	16.4	17.0
55-64 years					
All conditions					
Septicemia	---	*	*7.2	10.1	14.7
Malignant neoplasms	146.8	213.0	192.4	161.2	135.8
Malignant neoplasms of colon and rectum	12.9	19.7	17.9	13.0	10.8
Malignant neoplasms of trachea, bronchus, and lung	9.7	25.9	33.0	28.2	22.5
Malignant neoplasms of the breast	32.2	48.7	40.1	29.4	27.3
Malignant neoplasms of the prostate	...	...	...	...	...
Diabetes mellitus	57.7	76.4	43.7	35.4	36.1
Volume depletion	---	*	10.2	16.1	13.5
Heart disease	155.9	228.4	239.0	233.0	226.7
Acute myocardial infarction	25.2	25.4	41.7	42.4	35.6
Coronary atherosclerosis	---	32.4	20.5	31.2	25.0
Other ischemic heart disease[2]	81.3	73.4	82.4	66.8	66.8
Cardiac dysrhythmias	12.7	29.6	31.4	29.4	35.0
Congestive heart failure	10.4	17.1	26.3	30.3	30.3
Cerebrovascular disease	39.8	50.7	52.9	45.4	41.3
Pneumonia	33.8	37.1	41.6	38.0	41.8
Cholelithiasis	50.1	49.8	48.0	49.7	56.5
Urinary tract infection, site unspecified	*	13.4	*8.1	9.3	9.8
Hyperplasia of the prostate	...	...	...	...	...
Arthropathies and related disorders	45.0	14.1	46.4	37.7	36.9
Injury and poisoning	142.2	126.1	136.3	105.8	111.1
Fractures, all sites	67.0	53.7	54.2	39.9	42.4
Hip fracture	11.2	*8.0	*11.0	6.0	10.1
65-74 years					
All conditions					
Septicemia	---	*	19.5	21.0	27.6
Malignant neoplasms	186.1	270.9	294.9	210.4	219.2
Malignant neoplasms of colon and rectum	23.8	36.6	32.2	23.7	25.4
Malignant neoplasms of trachea, bronchus, and lung	*10.2	24.9	36.3	26.0	33.6
Malignant neoplasms of the breast	32.5	55.8	51.5	38.9	39.8
Malignant neoplasms of the prostate	...	...	...	...	...
Diabetes mellitus	98.0	105.6	67.6	57.6	58.3
Volume depletion	---	*10.8	22.5	28.7	33.0
Heart disease	345.8	471.4	493.7	445.8	483.4
Acute myocardial infarction	52.0	63.6	86.5	73.7	74.5

[Continued]

★ 462 ★

Hospitals Use: Rate of Discharges from Short-Stay Hospitals: Females
[Continued]

Age and first-listed diagnosis	Discharges per 10,000 population				
	1970	1980	1985	1990[1]	1991[1]
Coronary atherosclerosis	---	79.8	35.3	43.6	46.2
Other ischemic heart disease[2]	205.4	107.7	153.0	123.7	129.3
Cardiac dysrhythmias	17.7	57.8	75.1	56.2	78.8
Congestive heart failure	32.3	70.9	81.8	90.6	99.4
Cerebrovascular disease	112.8	135.8	150.3	111.7	112.0
Pneumonia	52.8	60.4	68.1	83.7	95.2
Cholelithiasis	66.1	60.8	51.1	48.4	58.8
Urinary tract infection, site unspecified	*11.2	23.0	22.1	36.4	27.4
Hyperplasia of the prostate	...	...	...	...	...
Arthropathies and related disorders	71.0	74.4	70.3	87.7	98.9
Injury and poisoning	206.8	193.6	197.1	176.0	181.1
Fractures, all sites	116.9	100.8	92.6	83.4	75.1
Hip fracture	35.3	32.2	34.6	35.2	28.5
75-84 years					
All conditions					
Septicemia	---	*16.2	38.5	47.3	63.8
Malignant neoplasms	229.6	326.7	265.7	224.7	249.8
Malignant neoplasms of colon and rectum	28.0	59.6	43.0	46.7	39.5
Malignant neoplasms of trachea, bronchus, and lung	*	22.1	21.8	23.7	16.9
Malignant neoplasms of the breast	42.7	58.2	43.3	37.4	42.4
Malignant neoplasms of the prostate	...	...	...	...	...
Diabetes mellitus	110.3	120.1	70.7	43.5	54.8
Volume depletion	---	35.8	70.3	64.4	77.1
Heart disease	588.1	825.4	829.7	773.8	778.4
Acute myocardial infarction	77.1	94.8	163.5	115.3	133.3
Coronary atherosclerosis	---	182.7	52.9	40.4	39.4
Other ischemic heart disease[2]	371.9	108.8	182.9	169.3	175.8
Cardiac dysrhythmias	*22.3	98.8	141.6	119.8	137.1
Congestive heart failure	69.5	163.7	189.1	238.7	212.4
Cerebrovascular disease	246.8	280.2	314.6	244.6	259.0
Pneumonia	89.4	117.6	139.2	175.9	177.2
Cholelithiasis	57.2	56.9	65.0	44.4	51.2
Urinary tract infection, site unspecified	*14.9	48.0	66.6	96.5	75.4
Hyperplasia of the prostate	...	...	...	...	...
Arthropathies and related disorders	90.7	108.7	82.8	90.8	91.9
Injury and poisoning	373.1	401.8	397.5	387.4	377.3
Fractures, all sites	251.2	250.1	254.4	254.8	241.7
Hip fracture	116.4	126.5	143.0	150.5	141.7
65 years and over					
All conditions					
Septicemia	---	11.8	32.9	43.1	49.0
Malignant neoplasms	204.2	286.9	281.0	214.8	225.6
Malignant neoplasms of colon and rectum	27.1	44.6	41.3	33.7	32.5
Malignant neoplasms of trachea, bronchus, and lung	9.3	22.8	28.2	23.6	25.3
Malignant neoplasms of the breast	36.1	55.6	46.8	38.7	38.5
Malignant neoplasms of the prostate	...	...	...	...	...

[Continued]

★ 462 ★

Hospitals Use: Rate of Discharges from Short-Stay Hospitals: Females
[Continued]

Age and first-listed diagnosis	Discharges per 10,000 population				
	1970	1980	1985	1990[1]	1991[1]
Diabetes mellitus	99.7	107.9	66.7	52.2	56.6
Volume depletion	---	28.2	55.2	58.6	65.4
Heart disease	462.3	648.2	680.1	623.4	661.3
Acute myocardial infarction	60.8	74.5	123.2	99.0	105.0
Coronary atherosclerosis	---	129.7	45.8	39.2	41.5
Other ischemic heart disease[2]	285.7	107.7	165.1	144.9	151.2
Cardiac dysrhythmias	21.3	81.0	109.1	89.5	108.0
Congestive heart failure	49.7	123.1	153.7	175.2	182.7
Cerebrovascular disease	177.7	216.0	232.7	194.1	198.8
Pneumonia	74.7	97.5	118.0	151.5	159.9
Cholelithiasis	62.1	60.7	57.0	48.1	55.5
Urinary tract infection, site unspecified	13.8	37.1	47.2	76.6	62.9
Hyperplasia of the prostate	...	...	...	...	...
Arthropathies and related disorders	78.9	86.4	73.2	84.4	91.2
Injury and poisoning	297.9	317.0	320.8	304.3	311.6
Fractures, all sites	189.3	192.3	192.6	187.3	182.3
Hip fracture	80.7	93.0	102.7	103.9	105.2
75 years and over					
All conditions					
Septicemia	---	20.8	49.9	69.4	74.3
Malignant neoplasms	231.5	308.7	263.2	219.9	233.2
Malignant neoplasms of colon and rectum	32.1	55.4	52.8	45.6	40.9
Malignant neoplasms of trachea, bronchus, and lung	*	19.9	17.9	20.6	15.5
Malignant neoplasms of the breast	41.7	55.5	40.8	38.4	37.0
Malignant neoplasms of the prostate	...	...	...	...	...
Diabetes mellitus	102.3	111.1	65.6	45.7	54.5
Volume depletion	---	52.1	96.7	94.4	103.6
Heart disease	638.2	889.9	916.5	835.7	871.0
Acute myocardial infarction	74.0	89.5	169.8	129.2	141.0
Coronary atherosclerosis	---	198.1	59.1	33.8	36.1
Other ischemic heart disease[2]	406.8	107.8	180.4	170.4	176.9
Cardiac dysrhythmias	26.7	112.8	152.3	129.4	142.4
Congestive heart failure	75.9	194.5	244.9	276.3	280.9
Cerebrovascular disease	275.5	325.6	337.3	292.5	301.1
Pneumonia	107.9	148.2	181.2	114.8	236.1
Cholelithiasis	56.0	60.5	64.5	47.7	51.6
Urinary tract infection, site unspecified	17.8	56.4	79.1	124.7	104.7
Hyperplasia of the prostate	...	...	...	...	...
Arthropathies and related disorders	90.9	102.9	76.9	80.4	82.1
Injury and poisoning	435.4	485.8	477.6	457.7	465.4
Fractures, all sites	298.6	317.5	319.4	311.5	308.5
Hip fracture	149.3	176.2	189.2	186.0	195.6
85 years and over					
All conditions					
Septicemia	---	*	83.5	132.8	103.9
Malignant neoplasms	239.1	253.0	255.9	206.3	186.6

[Continued]

★ 462 ★

Hospitals Use: Rate of Discharges from Short-Stay Hospitals: Females
[Continued]

Age and first-listed diagnosis	Discharges per 10,000 population				
	1970	1980	1985	1990[1]	1991[1]
Malignant neoplasms of colon and rectum	*	*42.6	81.6	42.7	44.9
Malignant neoplasms of trachea, bronchus, and lung	*	*	*	*	*
Malignant neoplasms of the breast	*	*47.0	*33.5	*41.2	*21.8
Malignant neoplasms of the prostate	...	...	...	...	...
Diabetes mellitus	*70.2	83.4	50.5	52.2	53.9
Volume depletion	---	102.3	174.3	180.3	178.3
Heart disease	838.2				
Acute myocardial infarction	*61.7	72.8	188.3	169.0	162.5
Coronary atherosclerosis	---	245.5	77.3	*	*
Other ischemic heart disease[2]	546.1	104.8	173.0	173.4	180.1
Cardiac dysrhythmias	*	156.1	183.7	156.8	157.2
Congestive heart failure	*104.4	289.7	408.8	384.1	473.9
Cerebrovascular disease	390.1	466.1	403.8	429.8	419.8
Pneumonia	181.6	242.9	304.5	394.2	402.2
Cholelithiasis	*51.4	71.8	63.1	57.1	52.8
Urinary tract infection, site unspecified	*	82.4	115.8	205.3	187.2
Hyperplasia of the prostate	...	...	...	...	...
Arthropathies and related disorders	*91.8	84.9	*59.5	50.5	54.4
Injury and poisoning	684.1	745.5	712.9	658.7	714.0
Fractures, all sites	487.6	526.1	510.4	473.9	497.1
Hip fracture	280.7	330.0	325.1	287.7	347.7

Source: Cohen, R.A., and J.F. Van Nostrand. *Trends in the Health of Older Americans: United States, 1994*. National Center for Health Statistics. Vital and Health Statistics 3(30). 1995. U.S. Department of Health and Human Services, Public Health Service, Centers for Disease Control and Prevention. Data are from the National Hospital Discharge Survey. *Notes:* 1. Comparisons of data for 1990 and 1991 with data for earlier years should be made with caution, as estimates of change may reflect improvements in the design rather than true changes in hospital use. 2. For 1970 the classification "other ischemic heart disease" includes all diagnoses of ischemic heart disease. *Estimates based on fewer than 30 discharges are not shown; estimates based on 30-59 discharges are preceded by an asterisk. Data include races other than white and black. Discharges are from non-Federal hospitals. Discharges exclude newborn infants. Diagnostic grouping inclusions are based on the *International Classification of Diseases, 8th Revision, adapted for use in the United States* for 1970, and the *International Classification of Diseases, 9th Revision Clinical Modification* (ICD-9-CM) for 1980, 1985, 1990 and 1991.

★ 463 ★

Hospitals

Hospitals Use: Rate of Discharges from Short-Stay Hospitals: Males

This table shows the rate of discharges from short-stay hospitals, males, by selected first-listed diagnosis: United States, 1970, 1980, 1985, 1990, and 1991. Data are based on a sample of hospital records.

Age and first-listed diagnosis	Discharges per 10,000 population				
	1970	1980	1985	1990[1]	1991[1]
All ages					
All conditions					
Septicemia	---	2.5	5.6	8.3	8.5
Malignant neoplasms	54.0	80.6	78.1	60.8	64.3
Malignant neoplasms of colon and rectum	5.7	8.4	8.2	7.0	7.0
Malignant neoplasms of trachea, bronchus, and lung	9.8	17.7	18.0	11.8	12.1
Malignant neoplasms of the breast	*	*	*	*	*

[Continued]

★ 463 ★

Hospitals Use: Rate of Discharges from Short-Stay Hospitals: Males
[Continued]

Age and first-listed diagnosis	Discharges per 10,000 population				
	1970	1980	1985	1990[1]	1991[1]
Malignant neoplasms of the prostate	6.6	11.7	11.8	8.6	10.5
Diabetes mellitus	16.8	22.5	17.0	15.8	15.2
Volume depletion	---	3.2	8.1	10.6	10.0
Heart disease	104.3	155.0	167.3	159.3	162.6
Acute myocardial infarction	23.9	25.0	40.8	34.4	34.7
Coronary atherosclerosis	---	27.8	16.7	23.0	21.7
Other ischemic heart disease[2]	56.2	43.5	48.1	38.7	37.9
Cardiac dysrhythmias	5.5	17.0	21.4	20.3	20.5
Congestive heart failure	8.3	16.2	21.6	26.2	29.6
Cerebrovascular disease	24.7	34.0	36.4	29.9	30.4
Pneumonia	37.0	38.1	37.9	44.1	44.8
Cholelithiasis	10.1	10.6	12.3	11.0	13.1
Urinary tract infection, site unspecified	3.2	5.6	6.7	7.8	8.7
Hyperplasia of the prostate	22.0	25.3	21.5	21.6	18.9
Arthropathies and related disorders	14.3	19.8	16.5	16.4	18.7
Injury and poisoning	176.9	185.9	157.6	122.9	118.2
Fractures, all sites	58.1	53.5	48.2	38.8	39.6
Hip fracture	4.1	4.7	5.5	6.0	6.6
55-64 years					
All conditions					
Septicemia	---	*	*8.4	6.8	9.6
Malignant neoplasms	151.5	202.4	200.1	166.5	161.6
Malignant neoplasms of colon and rectum	18.4	21.7	23.2	28.2	13.8
Malignant neoplasms of trachea, bronchus, and lung	37.2	55.4	51.5	40.9	43.8
Malignant neoplasms of the breast	*	*	*	*	*
Malignant neoplasms of the prostate	12.0	22.0	20.5	16.0	20.7
Diabetes mellitus	43.5	56.9	38.8	34.0	30.0
Volume depletion	---	*	*10.4	12.7	10.7
Heart disease	294.8	432.8	462.9	433.4	448.4
Acute myocardial infarction	81.3	79.0	120.4	92.7	100.4
Coronary atherosclerosis	---	86.2	60.1	85.4	84.1
Other ischemic heart disease[2]	154.1	149.6	152.2	117.8	119.1
Cardiac dysrhythmias	14.9	41.1	48.4	55.0	47.9
Congestive heart failure	17.2	25.0	36.3	45.9	56.0
Cerebrovascular disease	51.3	66.6	76.8	60.9	57.7
Pneumonia	38.6	40.8	42.8	47.8	40.2
Cholelithiasis	24.5	30.3	25.0	23.1	32.8
Urinary tract infection, site unspecified	*	*	*7.8	10.6	12.3
Hyperplasia of the prostate	56.7	70.1	52.4	54.7	41.9
Arthropathies and related disorders	35.4	30.4	30.3	29.2	31.6
Injury and poisoning	158.4	152.1	150.8	133.3	127.9
Fractures, all sites	55.5	37.2	40.2	35.3	36.9
Hip fracture	*	*	*	*9.6	*8.4
65-74 years					
All conditions					
Septicemia	---	*9.4	16.7	34.7	34.0

[Continued]

★ 463 ★

Hospitals Use: Rate of Discharges from Short-Stay Hospitals: Males
[Continued]

Age and first-listed diagnosis	Discharges per 10,000 population				
	1970	1980	1985	1990[1]	1991[1]
Malignant neoplasms	306.6	416.7	388.4	279.6	325.1
Malignant neoplasms of colon and rectum	31.2	39.7	39.3	29.9	44.3
Malignant neoplasms of trachea, bronchus, and lung	58.3	111.7	108.1	63.5	60.9
Malignant neoplasms of the breast	*	*	*	*	*
Malignant neoplasms of the prostate	48.6	72.8	66.3	50.3	67.8
Diabetes mellitus	59.4	64.8	42.9	43.3	35.5
Volume depletion	---	*11.7	23.0	22.5	23.2
Heart disease	454.4	643.3	698.7	689.9	706.8
Acute myocardial infarction	92.4	117.8	176.2	138.9	147.5
Coronary atherosclerosis	---	108.4	65.2	110.2	99.2
Other ischemic heart disease[2]	266.1	156.5	190.2	168.2	161.1
Cardiac dysrhythmias	21.6	81.0	84.8	84.2	97.6
Congestive heart failure	42.7	85.7	97.5	113.4	124.0
Cerebrovascular disease	149.6	176.5	184.9	136.7	144.8
Pneumonia	85.6	101.7	107.7	111.3	126.5
Cholelithiasis	34.5	40.5	43.3	37.9	48.6
Urinary tract infection, site unspecified	*13.7	19.4	24.5	21.5	27.1
Hyperplasia of the prostate	154.6	168.0	135.1	142.6	121.2
Arthropathies and related disorders	48.1	39.7	48.1	60.6	66.2
Injury and poisoning	165.1	163.9	160.4	175.3	180.4
Fractures, all sites	63.9	51.5	44.8	44.9	48.2
Hip fracture	*14.0	19.0	*14.2	15.2	17.8
75-84 years					
All conditions					
Septicemia	---	*22.4	50.1	63.6	68.7
Malignant neoplasms	381.8	551.1	575.5	418.9	398.0
Malignant neoplasms of colon and rectum	45.0	71.3	69.0	52.7	52.8
Malignant neoplasms of trachea, bronchus, and lung	53.6	96.0	110.3	57.0	61.9
Malignant neoplasms of the breast	*	*	*	*	*
Malignant neoplasms of the prostate	81.8	142.3	157.1	98.7	97.6
Diabetes mellitus	70.0	93.9	63.1	44.7	51.8
Volume depletion	---	*25.0	63.4	69.3	77.9
Heart disease	744.6	*	*	999.4	*
Acute myocardial infarction	134.2	117.5	233.4	219.9	206.5
Coronary atherosclerosis	---	205.3	77.4	77.0	75.5
Other ischemic heart disease[2]	427.6	174.6	195.3	171.5	201.9
Cardiac dysrhythmias	*27.7	126.4	174.5	152.6	157.0
Congestive heart failure	93.5	193.5	246.8	276.5	308.0
Cerebrovascular disease	251.5	333.6	358.5	276.5	277.9
Pneumonia	134.7	191.9	245.2	296.0	296.1
Cholelithiasis	41.2	53.7	73.0	51.7	52.4
Urinary tract infection, site unspecified	*28.9	48.1	65.6	66.3	73.4
Hyperplasia of the prostate	195.9	219.5	200.9	182.5	176.2
Arthropathies and related disorders	*36.2	61.6	59.4	69.5	81.3
Injury and poisoning	221.2	244.8	281.3	253.7	272.5
Fractures, all sites	111.1	100.5	115.7	92.1	106.2

[Continued]

★ 463 ★

Hospitals Use: Rate of Discharges from Short-Stay Hospitals: Males
[Continued]

Age and first-listed diagnosis	Discharges per 10,000 population				
	1970	1980	1985	1990[1]	1991[1]
Hip fracture	47.6	55.6	62.4	53.4	65.9
65 years and over					
All conditions					
Septicemia	---	14.8	31.2	50.4	52.0
Malignant neoplasms	334.3	464.1	449.8	327.6	355.8
Malignant neoplasms of colon and rectum	36.9	53.1	49.9	38.7	48.6
Malignant neoplasms of trachea, bronchus, and lung	55.2	103.4	106.6	59.7	60.1
Malignant neoplasms of the breast	*	*	*	*	*
Malignant neoplasms of the prostate	61.7	97.8	97.1	67.4	80.3
Diabetes mellitus	63.9	73.8	50.3	44.4	40.9
Volume depletion	---	21.2	42.9	48.6	51.0
Heart disease	570.9	785.0	836.4	825.2	865.2
Acute myocardial infarction	108.4	119.6	198.3	172.3	175.8
Coronary atherosclerosis	---	147.9	69.0	95.3	87.3
Other ischemic heart disease[2]	331.0	158.4	193.0	176.0	177.4
Cardiac dysrhythmias	24.3	97.3	121.4	111.8	122.3
Congestive heart failure	65.9	131.2	161.8	185.3	209.8
Cerebrovascular disease	195.5	244.3	254.0	197.0	205.5
Pneumonia	115.8	150.1	175.0	209.9	223.5
Cholelithiasis	38.7	43.2	52.4	44.1	49.4
Urinary tract infection, site unspecified	19.9	32.8	43.5	49.7	52.5
Hyperplasia of the prostate	172.4	181.0	157.2	155.7	140.7
Arthropathies and related disorders	45.8	46.7	51.3	63.6	69.1
Injury and poisoning	194.0	209.2	216.4	225.2	231.9
Fractures, all sites	86.9	77.3	79.9	78.7	83.3
Hip fracture	31.0	37.3	39.1	40.8	46.1
75 years and over					
All conditions					
Septicemia	---	*25.1	57.4	77.3	82.1
Malignant neoplasms	385.4	553.9	560.9	409.8	407.4
Malignant neoplasms of colon and rectum	47.5	78.6	69.0	53.7	55.7
Malignant neoplasms of trachea, bronchus, and lung	49.4	87.7	103.9	53.3	58.9
Malignant neoplasms of the breast	*	*	*	*	*
Malignant neoplasms of the prostate	85.9	145.2	152.9	96.7	101.5
Diabetes mellitus	72.2	91.0	63.7	46.2	50.0
Volume depletion	---	39.3	79.0	93.6	97.7
Heart disease	786.6				
Acute myocardial infarction	138.0	122.9	238.5	229.7	223.3
Coronary atherosclerosis	---	222.8	76.0	69.6	67.4
Other ischemic heart disease[2]	451.1	161.8	198.2	189.5	204.7
Cardiac dysrhythmias	*29.3	128.4	187.5	159.2	163.9
Congestive heart failure	108.9	217.7	278.3	308.6	354.2
Cerebrovascular disease	280.5	373.0	379.3	300.4	307.7
Pneumonia	171.7	241.9	296.8	379.1	386.8
Cholelithiasis	46.4	48.5	69.0	54.7	50.7
Urinary tract infection, site unspecified	*31.5	58.0	77.8	97.9	95.1

[Continued]

★ 463 ★

Hospitals Use: Rate of Discharges from Short-Stay Hospitals: Males
[Continued]

Age and first-listed diagnosis	Discharges per 10,000 population				
	1970	1980	1985	1990[1]	1991[1]
Hyperplasia of the prostate	205.3	205.8	197.0	178.0	173.6
Arthropathies and related disorders	41.5	59.9	57.1	68.8	73.9
Injury and poisoning	247.5	295.1	317.9	310.9	318.5
Fractures, all sites	129.4	126.2	143.4	136.6	142.4
Hip fracture	62.6	72.1	84.1	84.7	93.9
85 years and over					
All conditions					
Septicemia	---	*	*88.6	138.5	141.6
Malignant neoplasms	403.3	565.7	497.7	369.1	449.2
Malignant neoplasms of colon and rectum	*	*109.5	*69.0	*58.4	*68.4
Malignant neoplasms of trachea, bronchus, and lung	*	*	*	*	*
Malignant neoplasms of the breast	*	*	*	*	*
Malignant neoplasms of the prostate	*106.3	*157.5	*134.6	87.5	118.4
Diabetes mellitus	*	*79.1	*	*	*
Volume depletion	---	*99.2	146.5	201.4	185.2
Heart disease	994.5				
Acute myocardial infarction	*157.0	*145.8	260.2	273.1	297.5
Coronary atherosclerosis	---	296.1	*	*	*
Other ischemic heart disease[2]	567.3	*108.4	210.5	269.2	217.0
Cardiac dysrhythmias	*	*136.9	243.5	188.8	194.4
Congestive heart failure	*185.6	319.6	414.5	451.4	557.9
Cerebrovascular disease	424.2	538.4	469.1	406.6	439.2
Pneumonia	354.7	451.5	520.1	748.4	786.7
Cholelithiasis	*	*	*	*67.9	*43.0
Urinary tract infection, site unspecified	*	*99.6	*130.4	238.4	190.9
Hyperplasia of the prostate	251.7	*148.0	180.2	158.0	161.8
Arthropathies and related disorders	*	*	*	*	*
Injury and poisoning	377.6	506.1	476.2	565.4	521.6
Fractures, all sites	219.6	233.9	263.3	334.4	302.0
Hip fracture	*136.8	141.3	178.2	223.5	217.2

Source: Cohen, R.A., and J.F. Van Nostrand. *Trends in the Health of Older Americans: United States, 1994.* National Center for Health Statistics. Vital and Health Statistics 3(30). 1995. U.S. Department of Health and Human Services, Public Health Service, Centers for Disease Control and Prevention. Data are from the National Hospital Discharge Survey. *Notes:* 1. Comparisons of data for 1990 and 1991 with data for earlier years should be made with caution, as estimates of change may reflect improvements in the design rather than true changes in hospital use. 2. For 1970 the classification "other ischemic heart disease" includes all diagnoses of ischemic heart disease. *Estimates based on fewer than 30 discharges are not shown; estimates based on 30-59 discharges are preceded by an asterisk. Data include races other than white and black. Discharges are from non-Federal hospitals. Discharges exclude newborn infants. Diagnostic grouping inclusions are based on the *International Classification of Diseases, 8th Revision, adapted for use in the United States* for 1970, and the *International Classification of Diseases, 9th Revision Clinical Modification* (ICD-9-CM) for 1980, 1985, 1990 and 1991.

★ 464 ★

Hospitals

Mark-Up by Hospitals on Orthopedic Items

According to the source, an analysis of hospital costs was conducted by Thomas M. Loeb, M.D., an alumnus of Duke University, when his patients complained about their hospital bills. Dr. Loeb analyzed bills related to common orthopedic procedures performed in both rural and urban hospitals in the Midwest, South, and Southeast. The largest markup Dr. Loeb cited was vitamin C caplets at 14,066% in one hospital.

Item	Hospital pays...	Hospital charges...
Knee splint	$20.00	$164
Skin staples	12.14	228.36
Knee prosthesis (total)	3050.00	8730.00
Hip prosthesis (total)	4570.00	7065.00
ACL graft knife	38.75	73.00
Ascorbic acid tablet	.06	8.50
Ethicon bone wax	2.20	214.20
Ace wrap	5.00	19.00
Toga space suit	50.00	600.00
Arthroscope shaver blade	30.00	98.00

Source: Stephenson, Michelle. "Hospital Cost Shifting: Surgeon Found Items Marked Up As Much As 14,000%." *Today's O.R. Nurse* (September/October 1995), p. 33.

★ 465 ★

Hospitals

Market Share of Catholic Hospitals, by State

This table shows Catholic hospital admissions by percentage in each state and the District of Columbia.

State	Percent of total admissions
Alabama	-10%
Alaska	25%+
Arizona	10-20%
Arkansas	20-25%
California	10-20%
Colorado	20-25%
Connecticut	20-25%
Delaware	10-20%
District of Columbia	10-20%
Florida	-10%
Georgia	-10%
Hawaii	-10%
Idaho	20-25%
Illinois	25%+

[Continued]

★ 465 ★

Market Share of Catholic Hospitals, by State
[Continued]

State	Percent of total admissions
Indiana	10-20%
Iowa	20-25%
Kansas	25%+
Kentucky	10-20%
Louisiana	10-20%
Maine	10-20%
Maryland	10-20%
Massachusetts	10-20%
Michigan	20-25%
Minnesota	20-25%
Mississippi	-10%
Missouri	25%+
Montana	25%+
Nebraska	10-20%
Nevada	10-20%
New Hampshire	20-25%
New Jersey	10-20%
New Mexico	10-20%
New York	10-20%
North Carolina	-10%
North Dakota	25%+
Ohio	10-20%
Oklahoma	20-25%
Oregon	25%+
Pennsylvania	10-20%
Rhode Island	-10%
South Carolina	-10%
South Dakota	25%+
Tennessee	-10%
Texas	10-20%
Utah	-10%
Vermont	-10%
Virginia	-10%
Washington	25%+
West Virginia	10-20%
Wisconsin	25%+
Wyoming	-10%

Source: Sexton, Kevin J. "The Ministry Change Imperative." *Health Progress* (March/April 1996), p. 21. Primary source: *Profile of Catholic Healthcare 1995,* Catholic Health Association, St. Louis.

★ 466 ★

Hospitals

Mental Health Hospital Beds

This table shows inpatient and residential treatment beds in mental health organizations and rate per 100,000 civilian population, according to type of organization. Data are for the United States for selected years, 1970-1992.

[Data are based on inventories of mental health organizations]

Organization	1970	1980	1984	1986	1988	1990	1992
Number							
All organizations	524,878	274,713	262,673	267,613	271,923	272,253	270,978
State and county mental hospitals	413,066	156,482	130,411	119,033	107,109	98,789	93,064
Private psychiatric hospitals	14,295	17,157	21,474	30,201	42,255	44,871	43,705
Non-Federal general hospital psychiatric services	22,394	29,384	46,045	45,808	48,421	53,479	52,059
Department of Veterans Affairs psychiatric services[1]	50,688	33,796	23,546	26,874	25,742	21,712	22,466
Federally funded community mental health centers	8,108	16,264	...	...	...	...	...
Residential treatment centers for emotionally disturbed children	15,129	20,197	16,745	24,547	25,173	29,756	30,059
All other[2]	1,198	1,433	24,452	21,150	23,223	23,646	29,625
Number per 100,000 civilian population							
All organizations	263.6	124.3	112.9	111.7	111.4	111.6	106.9
State and county mental hospitals	207.4	70.2	56.1	49.7	44.0	40.5	36.7
Private psychiatric hospitals	7.2	7.7	9.2	12.6	17.3	18.4	17.2
Non-Federal general hospital psychiatric services	11.2	13.7	19.8	19.1	19.8	21.9	20.5
Department of Veterans Affairs psychiatric services[1]	25.5	15.7	10.1	11.2	10.5	8.9	8.9
Federally funded community mental health centers	4.1	7.3	...	...	...	...	...
Residential treatment centers for emotionally disturbed children	7.6	9.1	7.2	10.3	10.3	12.2	11.9
All other[2]	0.6	0.6	10.5	8.8	9.5	9.7	11.7

Source: U.S. Department of Health and Human Services. Public Health Service. Centers for Disease Control and Prevention. National Center for Health Statistics. *Health, United States, 1995.* Hyattsville, MD: Public Health Service, 1996, p. 233. *Notes:* Changes in reporting procedures in 1970-80 and 1981-82 affect the comparability of data with those from previous years. 1. Includes Department of Veterans Affairs neuropsychiatric hospitals and general hospital psychiatric services. 2. Includes other multiservice mental health organizations with inpatient and residential treatment services that are not elsewhere classified. Beginning in 1983 a definitional change sharply increased the number of multiservice mental health organizations. See Appendix I.

★ 467 ★

Hospitals

Percent Change in Selected Community Hospital Statistics: 1992-96

Item	Calendar year				1996	
	1992	1993	1994	1995	Q1	Q2
Percent Change from the Same Period of Previous Year						
Utilization						
All Ages						
Admissions in Thousands	-0.8	0.7	0.9	1.4	-1.4	-0.2
Admissions Per 1,000 population	-1.8	-0.2	-0.1	0.4	-2.3	-1.1
Inpatient Days in Thousands	-2.4	-2.1	-2.9	-2.9	-4.6	-3.7
Adult Length of Stay	-1.6	-2.8	-3.8	-4.2	-3.2	-3.6
65 Years of Age or Over						
Admissions in Thousands	1.7	2.9	2.0	2.9	-1.6	0.5
Admissions Per 1,000 population	0.2	1.5	0.8	1.8	-2.7	-0.5
Inpatient Days in Thousands	-0.6	-1.9	-2.2	-3.9	-7.3	-6.0
Adult Length of Stay	-2.2	-4.7	-4.2	-6.6	-5.8	-6.5
Under 65 Years of Age						
Admissions in Thousands	-2.2	-0.5	0.2	0.4	-1.3	-0.6
Admissions Per 1,000 population	-3.1	-1.4	-0.7	-0.5	-2.2	-1.5
Inpatient Days in Thousands	-4.0	-2.3	-3.6	-2.0	-2.0	-1.6
Adult Length of Stay	-1.9	-1.8	-3.8	-2.4	-0.7	-1.0
Surgical Operations in Thousands	2.2	1.1	2.5	1.9	-1.3	2.1
Outpatient Visits in Thousands	6.4	6.5	7.0	8.3	4.7	5.4
Adjusted Patient Days in Thousands	-0.5	-0.9	-1.0	-0.9	-2.8	-1.1
Beds in Thousands	-0.5	-0.7	-1.2	-1.8	-2.1	-2.1
Adult Occupancy Rate[1]	-1.4	-0.7	-1.1	-0.7	-2.3	-1.0
Total Hospital Revenues	9.4	7.1	4.9	5.0	3.0	4.2
Total Patient Revenues	9.4	7.0	4.6	4.8	2.9	3.6
Inpatient Revenues	7.3	5.7	2.5	2.6	1.0	0.9
Outpatient Revenues	15.6	10.6	10.1	9.9	7.5	9.9
Operating Expenses						
Total in Millions	9.4	6.9	5.0	5.3	4.1	4.2
Labor in Millions	8.9	6.9	4.7	4.5	3.3	2.9
Non-Labor in Millions	10.0	6.8	5.3	6.3	4.9	5.7
Inpatient Expense in Millions	7.3	5.6	2.9	3.2	2.1	1.4
Amount per Patient Day	9.9	7.8	6.0	6.3	7.1	5.3
Amount per Admission	8.1	4.8	2.0	1.8	3.6	1.6

[Continued]

★ 467 ★

Percent Change in Selected Community Hospital Statistics: 1992-96

[Continued]

Item	Calendar year				1996	
	1992	1993	1994	1995	Q1	Q2
Outpatient Expense	15.6	10.4	10.5	10.5	8.8	10.5
Amount per Outpatient	8.6	3.6	3.2	2.0	3.9	4.8

Source: American Hospital Association; Trend Analysis Group: National Hospital Panel Survey Reports. Chicago. Monthly reports for January 1991 - June 1996. Q designates quarter of year. Quarterly data are not seasonally adjusted. *Note:* 1. Change in rate, rather than percent change.

★ 468 ★

Hospitals

Recommended Duration for Hospital Stay, by Illness or Procedure: 1995

Data refer to one set of guidelines set by insurers.

Condition	Hospital stay
Tonsillectomy	6-12 hours
Vaginal delivery	6-12 hours
Modified radical mastectomy	1 day
Gallbladder removal	1 day
Appendectomy	1 day
Removal of ruptured disc	1 day
Balloon angioplasty	1 day
Stroke	1 day
Cesarean delivery	2 days
Pneumonia	2 days
Hip replacement	4 days
Double bypass heart surgery	4 days
Heart attack	4 days

Source: "Shrinking Hospital Stays." *USA TODAY,* 5 September 1995, p. 12A. Primary source: Milliman & Robertson.

Insurance Carriers

★ 469 ★

Health Plan Coverage, by Region and Type of Plan: 1995

Region and Plan	Percentage
West	
HMO	40
PPO	25
POS	24
Indemnity	11
Midwest	
HMO	29
PPO	29
Indemnity	28
POS	14
South	
Indemnity	38
HMO	25
PPO	20
POS	17
Northeast	
HMO	31
Indemnity	31
POS	23
PPO	15

Source: "POS Takes A Big Slice of Every Pie." *Business & Health* (August 1996), p. 46. Primary source: KPMG Peat Marwick *Survey of Employer Sponsored Health Benefits,* 1995. *Notes:* HMO stands for Health Maintenance Organization. POS stands for Point of Service plan. PPO stands for Preferred Provider Organization.

★ 470 ★

Insurance Carriers

Leading Health Insurers, by Profit Growth: 1996

Company	% profit growth from '95
Foundation Health	200
Healthsouth	180
Tenet Healthcare	112
Oxford Health Plans	90
Living Centers	78

Source: "It's Red Ink for Health Care Investors." *Business & Health* (May 1997), p. 12. Primary source: *Fortune* magazine.

★ 471 ★

Insurance Carriers

Leading Health Insurers, by Revenues: 1996

Company	Revenues $ (in millions)
Columbia/HCA	$19,909
United Healthcare	10,074
Humana	6,788
Tenet Healthcare	5,559
Medpartners	4,813
Pacificare Health Systems	4,637
Allegiance	4,387
FHP International	4,179
Wellpoint Health Networks	4,170
Foundation Health	3,561

Source: "It's Red Ink for Health Care Investors." *Business & Health* (May 1997), p. 12. Primary source: *Fortune* magazine.

★ 472 ★

Insurance Carriers

Percentage of MSA Population Enrolled in HMOs: 1994 and 1995

Metropolitan statistical areas	1994 %	1995 %	Percentage change
Houston, TX	15	28	86.7
New York, NY	17	28	64.7
Boston, MA	36	55	52.8
Dallas, TX	18	27	50.0
Seattle, WA	24	34	41.7
Atlanta, GA	22	30	36.4
Washington, DC	36	44	22.2
Riverside, CA	37	45	21.6
Los Angeles, CA	38	42	10.5
Philadelphia, PA	40	43	7.5
San Diego, CA	41	44	7.3
Detroit, MI	24	25	4.2
San Francisco, CA	55	56	1.8
Minneapolis, MN	43	43	0
Chicago, IL	17	17	0

Source: "Managed Care: Where It's At." *Hospitals & Health Networks,* 20 January 1997, p. 19. Primary source: Medical Data International, 1996. *Note:* MSA represents "metropolitan statistical area."

Mergers and Acquisitions

★ 473 ★

Health Care Mergers and Acquisitions, by Sector, 1994-1995

Industry sector	Number of mergers and acquisitions		
	1995	1994	% change
Hospitals	144	100	44
Home health care	63	55	14
Long-term-care facilities	62	44	41
Laboratory and imaging/dialysis centers	52	49	6
Physician medical groups	103	65	58
Psychiatric hospitals	46	27	70
Rehabilitation	68	50	36
HMOs	32	42	-24

[Continued]

★ 473 ★

Health Care Mergers and Acquisitions, by Sector, 1994-1995
[Continued]

Industry sector	Number of mergers and acquisitions		
	1995	1994	% change
Other[1]	53	86	-38
Total	623	518	20

Source: "The Mad Pace of Health Care Mergers." *Business & Health* (April 1996), p. 17. Primary source: Levin Associates. Note: 1. Ambulance, outpatient surgery, institutional pharmacy.

★ 474 ★

Mergers and Acquisitions

Largest Medical Benefits Corporation Merger in the U.S.: 1996

The table profiles Aetna Life & Casualty Company and U.S. Healthcare Inc. According to the source, the combined entity, Aetna, Inc., will provide health care for 23 million people.

Profile	Aetna	U.S. Healthcare
1995 revenues	$13 billion	$3.6 billion
1995 net income	$474 million	$381 million
Employees	29,143	4,980
Managed-care enrollment	7.5 million	2.8 million
Number of physicians in network	200,000	54,000
Hospitals	2,200	441

Source: Smolowe, Jill. "A Healthy Merger?" *Time,* 15 April 1996, p. 77.

Nursing Homes

★ 475 ★

Number and Percent Distribution of Current Residents by Age, Sex, and Race, According to Selected Nursing Home Characteristics

Nursing home characteristic	All current residents Number	Percent distribution									
		Total	Age				Sex		Race		
			Under 65 yrs	65-74 yrs	75-84 yrs	85 yrs and over	Male	Female	White	Black and other	
										Total[2]	Black
All nursing homes	1,548,600	100.0	10.9	15.6	37.6	35.8	27.7	72.3	88.0	11.4	9.7
Ownership											
Proprietary	989,700	100.0	12.1	16.0	37.6	34.1	27.9	72.1	87.0	12.3	10.4
Voluntary nonprofit	420,800	100.0	6.2	13.7	38.0	42.1	24.5	75.5	90.3	9.3	8.0
Government and other	138,100	100.0	16.6	17.4	36.7	29.0	36.1	63.9	88.6	11.4	9.9
Certification											
Certified by Medicare and Medicaid	1,213,700	100.0	10.4	15.9	37.7	35.9	26.8	73.2	87.6	11.8	10.2
Certified by Medicare only	50,000	100.0	[1]	13.0[1]	37.8	44.3	26.7	73.3	96.1	[1]	[1]
Certified by Medicaid only	240,600	100.0	15.5	15.5	36.5	32.1	31.2	68.8	86.9	12.6	10.4
Not certified	44,300	100.0	8.8	11.4	39.9	39.9	33.3	66.7	93.5	5.9	4.2
Bed size											
Less than 50 beds	71,100	100.0	12.0	13.9	38.0	35.9	31.4	68.6	90.0	9.2	6.4
50-99 beds	378,300	100.0	11.0	13.7	36.5	38.5	28.5	71.5	90.5	9.3	7.6
100-199 beds	794,200	100.0	9.6	15.6	38.4	36.3	26.4	73.6	88.3	10.8	9.5
200 beds or more	305,000	100.0	13.1	18.2	37.1	31.3	28.5	71.5	83.8	15.9	13.7
Census Region											
Northeast	346,700	100.0	10.5	15.7	39.2	34.6	27.7	72.3	90.7	9.1	8.1
Midwest	494,900	100.0	10.0	15.2	36.3	38.2	27.1	72.9	93.0	6.9	6.3
South	495,000	100.0	11.2	16.0	38.7	34.0	27.3	72.7	82.4	16.4	15.5
West	212,000	100.0	12.8	15.2	35.8	35.9	30.0	70.0	85.0	14.1	7.6
Metropolitan statistical area (MSA)											
MSA	1,068,200	100.0	11.4	16.1	37.0	35.3	27.3	72.7	86.7	12.8	11.1
Not MSA	480,400	100.0	9.8	14.2	38.9	36.8	28.7	71.3	91.1	8.4	6.7

[Continued]

★ 475 ★

Number and Percent Distribution of Current Residents by Age, Sex, and Race, According to Selected Nursing Home Characteristics

[Continued]

Nursing home characteristic	All current residents Number	Percent distribution									
		Total	Age				Sex		Race		
			Under 65 yrs	65-74 yrs	75-84 yrs	85 yrs and over	Male	Fe-male	White	Black and other	
										Total[2]	Black
Affiliation[3]											
Chain	857,300	100.0	10.3	15.8	37.9	35.7	26.5	73.5	87.8	11.6	10.0
Independent	689,100	100.0	11.6	15.2	37.2	35.7	29.2	70.8	88.3	11.3	9.5

Source: Strahan, Genevieve. "An Overview of Nursing Homes and Their Current Residents: Data from the 1995 National Nursing Home Survey," Advance Data, Vital and Health Statistics, Centers for Disease Control and Prevention, National Center for Health Statistics, Number 280, January 23, 1997. *Notes:* Numbers may not add to totals because of rounding. - Quantity zero. 1. Figure does not meet standard of reliability or precision (sample size less than 30) and is therefore not reported. If shown with a number, it should not be assumed reliable because the sample size is between 30-59 or the sample size is greater than 60 but has a relative standard error over 30 percent. 2. Includes races other than white, black or unknown. 3. Excludes a small number of residents in nursing homes with unknown affiliation.

★ 476 ★

Nursing Homes

Number and Percent Distribution of Nursing Homes, and Number of Beds and Beds per Home, and of Current Residents and Occupancy Rate by Selected Facility Characteristics

Facility characteristic	Nursing homes		Beds		Current residents	
	Number	Percent distribution	Number	Beds per nursing home	Number	Occupancy rate[2]
All facilities	16,700	100.0	1,770,900	106.0	1,548,600	87.4
Ownership						
Proprietary	11,000	66.1	1,151,700	104.7	989,700	85.9
Voluntary nonprofit	4,300	25.7	468,100	108.9	420,800	89.9
Government and other	1,400	8.2	151,000	107.9	138,100	91.5
Certification						
Certified by Medicare and Medicaid	11,600	69.7	1,378,400	118.08	1,213,700	88.0
Certified by Medicare only	1,000[1]	6.1	59,600	59.6	50,000	83.9
Certified by Medicaid only	3,400	20.1	280,300	82.4	240,600	85.8
Not certified	700[1]	4.2	52,600	75.1	44,300	84.2
Bed size						
Less than 50 beds	2,800	16.8	87,300	31.2	71,100	81.4
50-99 beds	5,900	33.4	564,400	100.8	494,900	87.7
100-199 beds	6,700	40.1	902,500	134.7	794,200	88.0
200 beds or more	1,300	7.5	350,800	269.8	304,000	86.9

[Continued]

★ 476 ★

Number and Percent Distribution of Nursing Homes, and Number of Beds and Beds per Home, and of Current Residents and Occupancy Rate by Selected Facility Characteristics
[Continued]

Facility characteristic	Nursing homes		Beds		Current residents	
	Number	Percent distribution	Number	Beds per nursing home	Number	Occupancy rate[2]
Census region						
Northeast	2,900	17.1	378,800	130.6	346,700	91.5
Midwest	5,600	33.4	564,400	100.8	494,900	87.7
South	5,500	32.8	572,700	104.1	495,000	86.4
West	2,800	16.6	254,900	91.0	212,000	83.2
Metropolitan statistical area (MSA)						
MSA	10,300	61.5	1,217,500	118.2	1,068,200	87.7
Not MSA	6,400	38.5	553,400	86.5	480,400	86.8
Affiliation[3]						
Chain	9,100	54.3	978,000	107.5	857,300	87.7
Independent	7,600	45.5	788,200	90.7	689,100	87.4

Source: Strahan, Genevieve. "An Overview of Nursing Homes and Their Current Residents: Data from the 1995 National Nursing Home Survey," Advance Data, Vital and Health Statistics, Centers for Disease Control and Prevention, National Center for Health Statistics, Number 280, January 23, 1997. *Notes:* Figures may not add to totals because of rounding. 1. Figure should not be assumed reliable because the sample size is between 30-59 or the sample is greater than 60 but has a relative standard error over 30 percent. 2. Occupancy rate is calculated by dividing residents by available beds. 3. Excludes a small number of homes, beds, and residents with unknown affiliation.

★ 477 ★

Nursing Homes

Number and Percent of Facility Characteristics and Measures of Utilization for Nursing Homes by Survey Year: United States, 1973-74, 1977, 1985, and 1995

Admissions and admissions per 100 beds are for the calendar year prior to the survey year.

Survey year	Facility characteristic					Measures of utilization			
	Homes	Beds	Beds per nursing home	FTE[1,2]	FTE's per 100 beds[1,2]	Current residents	Admissions	Admissions per 100 beds	Occupancy rate[3]
1995	16,700	1,770,900	106.1	933,600	52.7	1,548,600	1,706,400	96.4	87.4
1985	19,100	1,624,200	85.0	793,600	48.9	1,491,400	1,299,200	80.5	91.8
1977	18,900	1,402,400	74.2	647,700	46.2	1,303,100	1,367,400	98.4	92.9
1973-74	15,700	1,177,300	75.0	485,400	41.2	1,075,800	1,110,800	95.3	91.4

Source: Strahan, Genevieve. "An Overview of Nursing Homes and Their Current Residents: Data from the 1995 National Nursing Home Survey", Advance Data, Vital and Health Statistics, Centers for Disease Control and Prevention, National Center for Health Statistics, Number 280, January 23, 1997. *Notes:* 1. FTE is full-time equivalent. 2. Includes only those providing direct patient care: administrative, medical, and therapeutic staff; registered nurses; licensed practical nurses; nurses' aides; and orderlies. 3. Occupancy rate is calculated by dividing current residents by beds.

★ 478 ★
Nursing Homes

Number and Percent of Facility Characteristics and Measures of Utilization for Nursing Homes by Survey Year: United States, 1973-74, 1977, 1985, and 1995

Admissions and admissions per 100 beds are for the calendar year prior to the survey year.

Survey year	Facility characteristic					Measures of utilization			
	Homes	Beds	Beds per nursing home	FTE[1,2]	FTE's per 100 beds[1,2]	Current residents	Admissions	Admissions per 100 beds	Occupancy rate[3]
1995	16,700	1,770,900	106.1	933,600	52.7	1,548,600	1,706,400	96.4	87.4
1985	19,100	1,624,200	85.0	793,600	48.9	1,491,400	1,299,200	80.5	91.8
1977	18,900	1,402,400	74.2	647,700	46.2	1,303,100	1,367,400	98.4	92.9
1973-74	15,700	1,177,300	75.0	485,400	41.2	1,075,800	1,110,800	95.3	91.4

Source: Strahan, Genevieve. "An Overview of Nursing Homes and Their Current Residents: Data from the 1995 National Nursing Home Survey," Advance Data, Vital and Health Statistics, Centers for Disease Control and Prevention, National Center for Health Statistics, Number 280, January 23, 1997. *Notes:* 1. FTE is full-time equivalent. 2. Includes only those providing direct patient care: administrative, medical, and therapeutic staff; registered nurses; licensed practical nurses; nurses' aides; and orderlies. 3. Occupancy rate is calculated by dividing current residents by beds.

★ 479 ★
Nursing Homes

Number and Rate per 100 Beds of Full-Time Equivalent Employees by Occupational Categories and Selected Nursing Home Characteristics: United States, 1995

Characteristic	Occupational category												
	All full-time equiv. empl.		Admin., medical, thera-peutic		Nursing								
					Total		Regis-tered nurse		Licens. practical nurse		Nurse's aide and orderly	
	No.	Rate per 100 beds	No.	Rate per 100 beds	No.	Rate per 100 beds	No.	Rate per 100 beds	No.	Rate per 100 beds	No.	Rate per 100 beds
Total	1,333,300	75.3	20,100	1.1	913,500	51.6	129,700	7.3	185,700	10.5	600,500	33.9
Ownership												
Proprietary	823,000	71.5	13,600	1.2	574,100	49.8	78,000	6.8	118,300	10.3	379,500	32.9
Voluntary nonprofit	383,100	81.8	4,900	1.0	254,300	54.3	38,300	9.0	15,900	10.5	56,300	37.3
Government and other	127,200	84.2	1,600	1.1	85,100	56.3	13,300	9.0	15,900	10.5	56,300	37.3
Certification												
Certified by Medicare and Medicaid	1,055,900	76.6	15,000	1.1	727,900	52.8	105,800	7.7	149,600	10.9	473,900	34.4
Medicare only	52,800	88.5	1,900	3.2	35,800	60.0	7,400	12.4	7,000	11.7	21,100	35.4
Medicaid only	191,600	68.4	2,800	1.0	127,500	45.5	13,600	4.8	24,300	8.7	90,400	32.3
Not certified	33,000	62.8	400	0.8	22,300	42.4	3,000	5.7	4,800	9.1	15,100	28.7
Bed size												
Less than 50 beds	73,000	83.7	4,700	5.4	49,600	56.8	10,700	12.3	11,100	12.8	29,000	33.3

[Continued]

★ 479 ★

Number and Rate per 100 Beds of Full-Time Equivalent Employees by Occupational Categories and Selected Nursing Home Characteristics: United States, 1995

[Continued]

Characteristic	All full-time equiv. empl.		Admin., medical, thera-peutic		Nursing									
					Total		Regis-tered nurse		Licens. practical nurse		Nurse's aide and orderly			
	No.	Rate per 100 beds	No.	Rate per 100 beds	No.	Rate per 100 beds	No.	Rate per 100 beds	No.	Rate per 100 beds	No.	Rate per 100 beds
50-99 beds	320,500	74.5	5,200	1.2	221,400	51.4	29,200	6.8	43,000	10.0	148,800	34.6
100-199 beds	674,500	74.7	8,400	0.9	468,500	51.9	63,700	7.1	96,500	10.7	310,100	34.4
200 beds or more	265,300	75.6	1,800	0.5	174,000	49.6	26,100	7.4	35,100	10.0	112,700	32.1
Census Region												
Northeast	310,400	81.9	4,200	1.1	214,500	56.6	38,000	10.0	39,300	10.4	136,600	36.0
Midwest	388,300	68.8	4,800	0.9	264,300	46.8	40,100	7.1	54,300	9.6	171,600	30.4
South	435,100	76.0	6,300	1.1	299,800	52.3	30,200	5.3	65,700	11.5	204,800	35.8
West	199,500	78.3	4,800	1.9	134,900	52.9	21,500	8.4	26,500	10.4	87,600	34.3

Source: Strahan, Genevieve. "An Overview of Nursing Homes and Their Current Residents: Data from the 1995 National Nursing Home Survey," Advance Data, Vital and Health Statistics, Centers for Disease Control and Prevention, National Center for Health Statistics, Number 280, January 23, 1997. *Note:* Figures may not add to totals because of rounding.

★ 480 ★

Nursing Homes

Number of Nursing Homes and Percent Change by Ownership and Affiliation: 1985 and 1995

Ownership and affiliation	1995	1985	Percent change
Ownership			
Proprietary	11,000	14,300	-23.1
Voluntary nonprofit	4,300	3,800	+13.2
Government and/or other	1,300	1,000	+30.0
Affiliation			
Chain	9,100	7,900	+15.2
Independent	7,600	11,100	-31.5

Source: Strahan, Genevieve. "An Overview of Nursing Homes and Their Current Residents: Data from the 1995 National Nursing Home Survey," Advance Data, Vital and Health Statistics, Centers for Disease Control and Prevention, National Center for Health Statistics, Number 280, January 23, 1997.

★ 481 ★

Nursing Homes

Nursing Home Expenditures: 1991-1994

Data in the table shows expenditures for nursing home care and the percent distribution by source of funds for the years shown. Data were compiled by the Health Care Financing Administration.

Year	Total in billions	Out-of-pocket payments	Private health insurance	Other private funds	Government Total[1]	Government Medicaid	Government Medicare
Nursing home care[2]							
1991	57.2	40.9	3.6	1.8	53.6	48.1	3.4
1992	62.3	39.0	3.4	1.9	55.7	48.5	5.1
1993	67.0	37.6	3.1	1.9	57.5	48.4	6.8
1994	72.3	37.2	3.0	1.9	57.9	47.4	8.2

Source: U.S. Department of Health and Human Services. Public Health Service. Centers for Disease Control and Prevention. National Center for Health Statistics. *Health, United States, 1995.* Hyattsville, MD: Public Health Service, 1996. p. 250. Primary source: Office of National Health Statistics, Office of the Actuary. National Health Expenditures, 1994. *Health Care Financing Review,* vol. 17, no. 3. *Notes:* These data include revisions in health expenditures and in population back to 1960 and differ from previous editions of *Health, United States.* 1. Includes other government expenditures for these health care services, for example, care funded by the Department of Veterans Affairs and State and locally financed subsidies to hospitals. 2. Includes expenditures for care in freestanding nursing homes. Expenditures for care in facility-based nursing homes are included with hospital care.

★ 482 ★

Nursing Homes

Nursing Homes: Bed and Resident Occupancy Rates, and Total Population 65 Years Old and Older: 1973-74, 1977, 1985, and 1995

[Bed rate is number of beds per nursing home; occupancy rate is number of residents per 1,000 persons 65 years old and older].

Survey year	Beds per 1,000 population 65 years and over	Residents 65 years and over per 1,000 population	Total U.S. resident population 65 years and over in thousands[1]
1995	52.6	41.3	33,648
1985	56.9	46.2	28,530
1977	59.7	47.1	23,494
1973-74	55.2	44.7	21,329

Source: Strahan, Genevieve. "An Overview of Nursing Homes and Their Current Residents: Data from the 1995 National Nursing Home Survey", Advance Data, Vital and Health Statistics, Centers for Disease Control and Prevention, National Center for Health Statistics, Number 280, January 23, 1997. *Notes:* 1. For 1995, U.S. Bureau of the Census: Population Projections of the United States, by age, sex, race and Hispanic origin, 1993-2020. *Current Population Reports,* Series P-25, No. 1111. Washington, U.S. Government Printing Office, 1996. For 1985, U.S. Bureau of the Census: Estimates of the population of the United States, by age, sex, and race, 1980 to 1985. *Current Population Reports.* Series P-25, No. 985. Washington, U.S. government Printing Office, 1986. For 1977 and 1973-74, U.S. Bureau of the Census: Estimates of the population of the United States, by age, sex, and race, 1970 to 1977. *Current Population Reports.* Series P-25. No. 721. Washington, U.S. Government Printing Office, 1978.

★ 483 ★
Nursing Homes

Nursing Homes Beds and Bed Rate by Regions and States

This table shows nursing homes with 3 or more beds, and bed rates, according to geographic division and state: United States, 1976, 1986, and 1991.

[Data are based on reporting by facilities]

Geographic division and State	Beds			Bed rate[1]		
	1976	1986	1991	1976	1986	1991
United States	1,298,968	1,504,683	1,559,394	685.3	542.1	494.5
New England	93,418	106,231	108,194	731.7	584.8	550.4
Maine	7,653	9,047	9,192	656.6	524.3	497.6
New Hampshire	6,110	6,901	7,493	761.6	550.5	545.7
Vermont	3,635	3,058	3,478	708.9	430.6	451.9
Massachusetts	46,436	50,675	50,133	732.4	580.2	540.3
Rhode Island	7,067	9,821	9,915	713.0	674.0	616.9
Connecticut	22,517	26,729	27,983	761.8	624.0	585.2
Middle Atlantic	178,323	211,274	220,241	527.4	447.7	423.9
New York	88,680	91,868	94,884	534.6	403.6	384.0
New Jersey	30,894	35,174	39,970	507.6	395.6	413.4
Pennsylvania	58,749	84,232	85,387	527.4	541.9	485.9
East North Central	288,352	324,442	331,278	806.5	654.6	602.1
Ohio	61,953	82,340	82,516	660.0	640.4	581.9
Indiana	36,029	47,081	55,701	752.3	721.3	759.1
Illinois	84,530	94,474	95,465	849.3	697.0	638.0
Michigan	56,858	50,552	48,886	824.5	511.3	446.7
Wisconsin	48,982	49,995	48,710	1,036.6	741.8	641.1
West North Central	163,231	182,256	187,639	803.2	663.5	610.4
Minnesota	41,313	43,574	42,001	932.9	685.0	600.3
Iowa	30,245	33,941	34,521	773.1	666.5	617.6
Missouri	32,677	48,262	51,652	605.0	665.3	619.7
North Dakota	6,015	5,904	6,056	845.9	625.2	519.3
South Dakota	8,154	7,800	8,448	909.5	643.1	626.6
Nebraska	22,484	17,288	17,846	1,097.6	634.4	599.3
Kansas	22,343	25,487	27,115	764.0	657.2	626.8
South Atlantic	140,161	187,935	210,534	531.3	428.4	393.0
Delaware	2,228	3,319	4,101	514.8	481.7	556.7
Maryland	18,804	24,330	27,163	695.0	573.6	567.6
District of Columbia	2,632	2,885	3,010	444.9	365.4	383.2
Virginia	23,251	24,440	26,324	680.3	463.1	426.0
West Virginia	5,152	7,753	9,792	298.0	334.1	376.9
North Carolina	19,891	26,159	28,259	541.5	432.2	387.3
South Carolina	8,224	13,471	13,122	501.8	496.0	410.3
Georgia	28,908	32,028	35,011	867.7	613.0	587.7
Florida	31,071	53,550	63,752	350.7	323.4	289.4
East South Central	65,037	86,124	93,932	562.1	517.2	490.5

[Continued]

★ 483 ★

Nursing Homes Beds and Bed Rate by Regions and States
[Continued]

Geographic division and State	Beds			Bed rate[1]		
	1976	1986	1991	1976	1986	1991
Kentucky	18,215	22,886	25,685	590.9	538.1	536.7
Tennessee	19,125	28,077	32,493	547.6	534.8	534.6
Alabama	19,188	12,685	21,323	646.1	505.3	426.6
Mississippi	8,509	13,476	14,431	420.1	471.0	439.1
West South Central	157,492	187,267	199,056	913.9	726.0	665.5
Arkansas	19,357	21,448	21,706	862.7	688.3	601.9
Louisiana	19,030	32,615	36,644	716.2	833.0	829.4
Oklahoma	25,890	29,570	32,421	874.2	731.5	691.8
Texas	93,215	103,634	108,285	994.8	704.0	629.6
Mountain	47,662	53,564	59,113	680.5	472.1	423.4
Montana	4,944	4,898	5,713	611.4	501.1	517.3
Idaho	4,567	4,694	4,887	640.8	463.1	408.3
Wyoming	1,721	2,165	2,243	584.4	517.4	485.6
Colorado	22,005	17,323	17,609	1,079.9	574.4	516.3
New Mexico	3,011	4,902	5,933	435.5	415.4	399.2
Arizona	5,884	11,240	13,265	406.2	374.7	329.3
Utah	4,233	5,655	6,292	574.7	482.2	434.0
Nevada	1,297	2,677	3,171	473.2	474.2	384.9
Pacific	165,292	165,590	149,407	668.8	441.6	361.1
Washington	28,436	27,986	26,506	807.3	454.3	457.8
Oregon	15,317	16,068	14,382	641.6	457.1	358.2
California	118,145	118,848	105,781	646.1	425.6	348.3
Alaska	770	1,082	780	1,285.5	950.0	591.8
Hawaii	2,624	1,606	1,958	571.6	197.6	184.2

Source: U.S. Department of Health and Human Services. Public Health Service. Centers for Disease Control and Prevention. National Center for Health Statistics. *Health, United States, 1995.* Hyattsville, MD: Public Health Service, 1996, p. 237. Primary source: Excludes hospital-based nursing homes. Data in this table are reported for nursing homes with three or more beds. Previous editions of *Health, United States* reported data for nursing homes with 25 beds or more. *Notes:* 1. Number of beds per 1,000 resident population 85 years of age and over.

★ 484 ★

Nursing Homes

Nursing Homes by Regions and States

This table shows nursing homes with 3 or more beds, according to geographic division and State: United States, 1976, 1986, and 1991.

[Data are based on reporting by facilities]

Geographic division and State	Nursing homes		
	1976	1986	1991
United States	16,091	16,388	14,744
New England	1,435	1,305	1,157
Maine	189	160	130
New Hampshire	99	92	79
Vermont	83	61	50
Massachusetts	694	641	554
Rhode Island	103	108	104
Connecticut	267	243	240
Middle Atlantic	1,607	1,643	1,497
New York	647	579	536
New Jersey	346	333	307
Pennsylvania	614	731	654
East North Central	3,184	3,254	3,029
Ohio	886	944	869
Indiana	466	454	528
Illinois	830	744	758
Michigan	543	690	469
Wisconsin	459	422	405
West North Central	2,185	2,139	2,108
Minnesota	456	400	399
Iowa	450	422	423
Missouri	439	575	525
North Dakota	80	67	70
South Dakota	133	115	122
Nebraska	264	209	209
Kansas	363	351	360
South Atlantic	1,749	2,150	1,883
Delaware	29	40	45
Maryland	183	207	212
District of Columbia	53	25	18
Virginia	244	235	217
West Virginia	102	95	107
North Carolina	414	357	283
South Carolina	108	182	132
Georgia	314	372	324
Florida	302	637	545
East South Central	867	970	890

[Continued]

★ 484 ★

Nursing Homes by Regions and States
[Continued]

Geographic division and State	Nursing homes		
	1976	1986	1991
Kentucky	258	331	271
Tennessee	267	279	275
Alabama	211	217	197
Mississippi	131	143	147
West South Central	1,758	1,889	1,935
Arkansas	212	231	221
Louisiana	203	276	298
Oklahoma	345	366	386
Texas	998	1,016	1,030
Mountain	630	642	611
Montana	89	63	70
Idaho	63	66	57
Wyoming	24	26	25
Colorado	225	197	176
New Mexico	46	63	62
Arizona	70	107	112
Utah	94	91	82
Nevada	19	29	27
Pacific	2,676	2,396	1,634
Washington	323	294	269
Oregon	233	199	183
California	2,031	1,831	1,133
Alaska	10	10	11
Hawaii	79	62	38

Source: U.S. Department of Health and Human Services. Public Health Service. Centers for Disease Control and Prevention. National Center for Health Statistics. *Health, United States, 1995.* Hyattsville, MD: Public Health Service, 1996, p. 237. Primary source: Excludes hospital-based nursing homes. Data in this table are reported for nursing homes with three or more beds. Previous editions of *Health, United States* reported data for nursing homes with 25 beds or more. *Notes:* 1. Number of beds per 1,000 resident population 85 years of age and over.

★ 485 ★
Nursing Homes

Nursing Homes: Full-Time Equivalent Employees Per 100 Beds, by Occupational Categories and Selected Facility Characteristics: 1995

	All full-time equiv. empl.		Admin., medical, thera-peutic		Occupational category							
					Nursing							
					Total		Regis-tered nurse		Licens. practical nurse		Nurse's aide and orderly	
	No.	Rate per 100 beds	No.	Rate per 100 beds	No.	Rate per 100 beds	No.	Rate per 100 beds	No.	Rate per 100 beds	No.	Rate per 100 beds
Total	1,333,300	75.3	20,100	1.1	913,500	51.6	129,700	7.3	185,700	10.5	600,500	33.9
Ownership												
Proprietary	823,000	71.5	13,600	1.2	574,100	49.8	78,000	6.8	118,300	10.3	379,500	32.9
Voluntary nonprofit	383,100	81.8	4,900	1.0	254,300	54.3	38,300	9.0	15,900	10.5	56,300	37.3
Government and other	127,200	84.2	1,600	1.1	85,100	56.3	13,300	9.0	15,900	10.5	56,300	37.3
Certification												
Certified by Medicare and Medicaid	1,055,900	76.6	15,000	1.1	727,900	52.8	105,800	7.7	149,600	10.9	473,900	34.4
Medicare only	52,800	88.5	1,900	3.2	35,800	60.0	7,400	12.4	7,000	11.7	21,100	35.4
Medicaid only	191,600	68.4	2,800	1.0	127,500	45.5	13,600	4.8	24,300	8.7	90,400	32.3
Not certified	33,000	62.8	400	0.8	22,300	42.4	3,000	5.7	4,800	9.1	15,100	28.7
Bed size												
Less than 50 beds	73,000	83.7	4,700	5.4	49,600	56.8	10,700	12.3	11,100	12.8	29,000	33.3
50-99 beds	320,500	74.5	5,200	1.2	221,400	51.4	29,200	6.8	43,000	10.0	148,800	34.6
100-199 beds	674,500	74.7	8,400	0.9	468,500	51.9	63,700	7.1	96,500	10.7	310,100	34.4
200 beds or more	265,300	75.6	1,800	0.5	174,000	49.6	26,100	7.4	35,100	10.0	112,700	32.1
Census Region												
Northeast	310,400	81.9	4,200	1.1	214,500	56.6	38,000	10.0	39,300	10.4	136,600	36.0
Midwest	388,300	68.8	4,800	0.9	264,300	46.8	40,100	7.1	54,300	9.6	171,600	30.4
South	435,100	76.0	6,300	1.1	299,800	52.3	30,200	5.3	65,700	11.5	204,800	35.8
West	199,500	78.3	4,800	1.9	134,900	52.9	21,500	8.4	26,500	10.4	87,600	34.3

Source: Strahan, Genevieve. "An Overview of Nursing Homes and Their Current Residents: Data from the 1995 National Nursing Home Survey", Advance Data, Vital and Health Statistics, Centers for Disease Control and Prevention, National Center for Health Statistics, Number 280, January 23, 1997. *Note:* Figures may not add to totals because of rounding.

★ 486 ★

Nursing Homes

Nursing Homes: Number and Percent, Beds and Bed Rates, Current Residents and Occupancy Rates, by Selected Facility Characteristics

[Bed rate is number of beds per nursing home]

Facility characteristic	Nursing homes		Beds		Current residents	
	Number	Percent distribution	Number	Beds per nursing home	Number	Occupancy rate[2]
All facilities	16,700	100.0	1,770,900	106.0	1,548,600	87.4
Ownership						
Proprietary	11,000	66.1	1,151,700	104.7	989,700	85.9
Voluntary nonprofit	4,300	25.7	468,100	108.9	420,800	89.9
Government and other	1,400	8.2	151,000	107.9	138,100	91.5
Certification						
Certified by Medicare and Medicaid	11,600	69.7	1,378,400	118.08	1,213,700	88.0
Certified by Medicare only	1,000[1]	6.1	59,600	59.6	50,000	83.9
Certified by Medicaid only	3,400	20.1	280,300	82.4	240,600	85.8
Not certified	700[1]	4.2	52,600	75.1	44,300	84.2
Bed size						
Less than 50 beds	2,800	16.8	87,300	31.2	71,100	81.4
50-99 beds	5,900	33.4	564,400	100.8	494,900	87.7
100-199 beds	6,700	40.1	902,500	134.7	794,200	88.0
200 beds or more	1,300	7.5	350,800	269.8	304,000	86.9
Census region						
Northeast	2,900	17.1	378,800	130.6	346,700	91.5
Midwest	5,600	33.4	564,400	100.8	494,900	87.7
South	5,500	32.8	572,700	104.1	495,000	86.4
West	2,800	16.6	254,900	91.0	212,000	83.2
Metropolitan statistical area (MSA)						
MSA	10,300	61.5	1,217,500	118.2	1,068,200	87.7
Not MSA	6,400	38.5	553,400	86.5	480,400	86.8
Affiliation[3]						
Chain	9,100	54.3	978,000	107.5	857,300	87.7
Independent	7,600	45.5	788,200	90.7	689,100	87.4

Source: Strahan, Genevieve. "An Overview of Nursing Homes and Their Current Residents: Data from the 1995 National Nursing Home Survey", Advance Data, Vital and Health Statistics, Centers for Disease Control and Prevention, National Center for Health Statistics, Number 280, January 23, 1997. *Notes:* Figures may not add to totals because of rounding. 1. Figure should not be assumed reliable because the sample size is between 30-59 or the sample is greater than 60 but has a relative standard error over 30 percent. 2. Occupancy rate is calculated by dividing residents by available beds. 3. Excludes a small number of homes, beds, and residents with unknown affiliation.

★ 487 ★

Nursing Homes

Nursing Homes: Number and Percent Change, by Ownership and Affiliation: 1985 and 1995

Ownership and affiliation	1995	1985	Percent change
Ownership			
Proprietary	11,000	14,300	-23.1
Voluntary nonprofit	4,300	3,800	+13.2
Government and/or other	1,300	1,000	+30.0
Affiliation			
Chain	9,100	7,900	+15.2
Independent	7,600	11,100	-31.5

Source: Strahan, Genevieve. "An Overview of Nursing Homes and Their Current Residents: Data from the 1995 National Nursing Home Survey", Advance Data, Vital and Health Statistics, Centers for Disease Control and Prevention, National Center for Health Statistics, Number 280, January 23, 1997.

★ 488 ★

Nursing Homes

Nursing Homes: Number and Percent of Current Residents, by Age, Sex, Race and Selected Facility Characteristics

Nursing home characteristic	All current residents Number	Percent distribution									
		Total	Age				Sex		Race		
			Under 65 yrs	65-74 yrs	75-84 yrs	85 yrs and over	Male	Female	White	Black and other Total[2]	Black
All nursing homes	1,548,600	100.0	10.9	15.6	37.6	35.8	27.7	72.3	88.0	11.4	9.7
Ownership											
Proprietary	989,700	100.0	12.1	16.0	37.6	34.1	27.9	72.1	87.0	12.3	10.4
Voluntary nonprofit	420,800	100.0	6.2	13.7	38.0	42.1	24.5	75.5	90.3	9.3	8.0
Government and other	138,100	100.0	16.6	17.4	36.7	29.0	36.1	63.9	88.6	11.4	9.9
Certification											
Certified by Medicare and Medicaid	1,213,700	100.0	10.4	15.9	37.7	35.9	26.8	73.2	87.6	11.8	10.2
Certified by Medicare only	50,000	100.0	[1]	13.0[1]	37.8	44.3	26.7	73.3	96.1	[1]	[1]
Certified by Medicaid only	240,600	100.0	15.5	15.5	36.5	32.1	31.2	68.8	86.9	12.6	10.4
Not certified	44,300	100.0	8.8	11.4	39.9	39.9	33.3	66.7	93.5	5.9	4.2
Bed size											
Less than 50 beds	71,100	100.0	12.0	13.9	38.0	35.9	31.4	68.6	90.0	9.2	6.4
50-99 beds	378,300	100.0	11.0	13.7	36.5	38.5	28.5	71.5	90.5	9.3	7.6

[Continued]

★ 488 ★

Nursing Homes: Number and Percent of Current Residents, by Age, Sex, Race and Selected Facility Characteristics
[Continued]

Nursing home characteristic	All current residents Number	Percent distribution									
		Total	Age				Sex		Race		
			Under 65 yrs	65-74 yrs	75-84 yrs	85 yrs and over	Male	Female	White	Black and other Total[2]	Black
100-199 beds	794,200	100.0	9.6	15.6	38.4	36.3	26.4	73.6	88.3	10.8	9.5
200 beds or more	305,000	100.0	13.1	18.2	37.1	31.3	28.5	71.5	83.8	15.9	13.7
Census Region											
Northeast	346,700	100.0	10.5	15.7	39.2	34.6	27.7	72.3	90.7	9.1	8.1
Midwest	494,900	100.0	10.0	15.2	36.3	38.2	27.1	72.9	93.0	6.9	6.3
South	495,000	100.0	11.2	16.0	38.7	34.0	27.3	72.7	82.4	16.4	15.5
West	212,000	100.0	12.8	15.2	35.8	35.9	30.0	70.0	85.0	14.1	7.6
Metropolitan statistical area (MSA)											
MSA	1,068,200	100.0	11.4	16.1	37.0	35.3	27.3	72.7	86.7	12.8	11.1
Not MSA	480,400	100.0	9.8	14.2	38.9	36.8	28.7	71.3	91.1	8.4	6.7
Affiliation[3]											
Chain	857,300	100.0	10.3	15.8	37.9	35.7	26.5	73.5	87.8	11.6	10.0
Independent	689,100	100.0	11.6	15.2	37.2	35.7	29.2	70.8	88.3	11.3	9.5

Source: Strahan, Genevieve. "An Overview of Nursing Homes and Their Current Residents: Data from the 1995 National Nursing Home Survey", Advance Data, Vital and Health Statistics, Centers for Disease Control and Prevention, National Center for Health Statistics, Number 280, January 23, 1997. *Notes:* Numbers may not add to totals because of rounding. - Quantity zero. 1. Figure does not meet standard of reliability or precision (sample size less than 30) and is therefore not reported. If shown with a number, it should not be assumed reliable because the sample size is between 30-59 or the sample size is greater than 60 but has a relative standard error over 30 percent. 2. Includes races other than white, black or unknown. 3. Excludes a small number of residents in nursing homes with unknown affiliation.

★ 489 ★

Nursing Homes

Nursing Homes: Number, by Ownership, Affiliation, and Certification Status: 1995

Ownership and affiliation	Total	Certification			Not certified
		Certified by Medicare and Medicaid	Certified by Medicare only	Certified by Medicaid only	
All facilities	16,700	11,600	1,000[1]	3,400	700[1]
Ownership					
Proprietary	11,000	7,100	[1]	2,200	300
Voluntary nonprofit	4,300	2,700	[1]	800[1]	300
Government and other	1,300	800	[1]	[1]	[1]

[Continued]

★ 489 ★

Nursing Homes: Number, by Ownership, Affiliation, and Certification Status: 1995
[Continued]

Ownership and affiliation	Total	Certification			Not certified
		Certified by Medicare and Medicaid	Certified by Medicare only	Certified by Medicaid only	
Affiliation					
Chain	9,100	7,100	600[1]	1,200	[1]
Independent	7,600	4,500	[1]	2,100	600[1]

Source: Strahan, Genevieve. "An Overview of Nursing Homes and Their Current Residents: Data from the 1995 National Nursing Home Survey", Advance Data, Vital and Health Statistics, Centers for Disease Control and Prevention, National Center for Health Statistics, Number 280, January 23, 1997. *Notes:* Numbers may not add to totals because of rounding. 1. Figure does not meet standard of reliability or precision (sample size less than 30) and is therefore not reported. If shown with a number, it should not be assumed reliable because the sample size is between 30-59 or the sample is greater than 60 but has a relative standard error over 30 percent.

★ 490 ★

Nursing Homes

Percent Change in Homes, Beds, and Residents Between Survey Years: United States, Selected Years 1973-95

Survey years	Homes	Beds	Residents
1985 and 1995	-12.6	+9.0	+3.8
1977 and 1985	+1.1	+15.8	+14.5
1973-74 and 1977	+20.4	+19.1	+21.1

Source: Strahan, Genevieve. "An Overview of Nursing Homes and Their Current Residents: Data from the 1995 National Nursing Home Survey," Advance Data, Vital and Health Statistics, Centers for Disease Control and Prevention, National Center for Health Statistics, Number 280, January 23, 1997.

Chapter 4
LIFESTYLES AND HEALTH

Diets

★ 491 ★

Low Fat-Airline Meals

Airline	Calories	Fats (grams)
Continental	529	3
Delta	517	13
United	460	4
Northwest	456	9
American	418	11
USAir	385	4

Source: Hobica, George. "Flying the Lowfat Skies: Special Order." *American Health* (November 1995), p. 96.

★ 492 ★
Diets

Per Capita Consumption of Major Food Commodities: 1970 to 1994

In pounds, retail weight except as indicated. Consumption represents the residual after exports, nonfood use and ending stocks are subtracted from the sum of beginning stocks, domestic production, and imports. Based on Bureau of the Census estimated population. Estimates reflect revisions based on the 1990 Census of Population.

COMMODITY	1970	1975	1980	1985	1990	1992	1993	1994
Red meat, total (boneless, trimmed weight) [1,2]	131.7	125.8	126.4	124.9	112.3	114.1	112.1	114.8
Beef	79.6	83.0	72.1	74.6	64.0	62.8	61.5	63.6
Veal	2.0	2.8	1.3	1.5	0.9	0.8	0.8	0.8
Lamb and mutton	2.1	1.3	1.0	1.1	1.0	1.0	1.0	0.9
Pork (excluding lard)	48.0	38.7	52.1	47.7	46.4	49.5	48.9	49.5
Fish and shellfish (edible weight) [3]	11.7	12.1	12.4	15.0	15.0	14.7	14.9	15.1
Fresh and frozen	6.9	7.5	7.8	9.7	9.6	9.8	10.1	10.3
Canned	4.4	4.2	4.3	5.0	5.1	4.6	4.5	4.5
Tuna	2.5	2.8	3.0	3.3	3.7	3.5	3.5	3.3
Cured	0.4	0.4	0.3	0.3	0.3	0.3	0.3	0.3
Poultry (boneless weight) [2,4]	33.8	32.9	40.8	45.5	56.3	60.9	62.6	63.7
Chicken	27.4	26.4	32.7	36.4	42.5	46.7	48.5	49.5
Turkey	6.4	6.5	8.1	9.1	13.8	14.2	14.1	14.2
Eggs (number)	308.9	276.0	271.1	254.7	234.3	235.0	235.5	237.6
Dairy products:								
Total (milk equivalent, milkfat basis) [5]	563.8	539.1	543.2	593.7	568.5	565.8	574.1	586.2
Fluid milk and cream [6]	275.1	261.4	245.6	241.0	233.4	230.9	226.8	225.7
Beverage milks	269.1	254.0	237.4	229.7	221.7	218.6	214.3	213.0
Plain whole milk	213.5	174.9	141.7	119.7	87.6	81.4	77.8	75.8
Plain lowfat milk	29.8	53.2	70.1	83.3	98.3	99.4	97.1	95.6
Plain skim milk	11.6	11.5	11.6	12.6	22.9	25.0	26.7	28.8
Flavored whole milk	5.6	6.3	4.7	3.7	2.8	2.7	2.7	2.7
Flavored lowfat and skim milks	3.0	3.3	5.3	6.0	6.6	6.9	6.9	7.1
Buttermilk	5.5	4.7	4.1	4.4	3.5	3.2	3.0	2.9
Yogurt (excl. frozen)	0.8	2.1	2.6	4.1	4.1	4.3	4.4	4.7
Cream [7]	3.8	3.3	3.4	4.4	4.6	4.8	4.9	4.9
Sour cream and dip	1.1	1.6	1.8	2.3	2.5	2.7	2.7	2.7
Condensed and evaporated milk:								
Whole milk	7.0	5.1	3.8	3.6	3.2	3.3	3.0	3.2
Skim milk	5.0	3.5	3.3	3.8	4.8	5.2	5.2	4.8
Cheese [8]	11.4	14.3	17.5	22.5	24.6	26.0	26.3	26.8
American	7.0	8.2	9.6	12.2	11.1	11.3	11.4	11.6
Cheddar	5.8	6.0	6.9	9.8	9.0	9.2	9.1	9.1
Italian	2.1	3.2	4.4	6.5	9.0	10.0	9.8	10.3
Mozzarella	1.2	2.1	3.0	4.6	6.9	7.7	7.6	7.9
Other [9]	2.3	2.9	3.4	3.9	4.5	4.7	5.0	5.0
Swiss	0.9	1.1	1.3	1.3	1.4	1.2	1.2	1.2
Cream and Neufchatel	0.6	0.7	1.0	1.2	1.7	2.0	2.1	2.2
Cottage cheese	5.2	4.6	4.5	4.1	3.4	3.1	2.9	2.8
Ice cream	17.8	18.6	17.5	18.1	15.8	16.3	16.1	16.1
Ice milk	7.7	7.6	7.1	6.9	7.7	7.1	6.9	7.6
Fats and oils:								
Total, fat content only [10]	52.6	52.6	57.2	64.3	62.2	65.7	68.4	66.9
Butter (product weight)	5.4	4.7	4.5	4.9	4.4	4.4	4.7	4.8
Margarine (product weight)	10.8	11.0	11.3	10.8	10.9	11.0	11.1	9.9

[Continued]

★ 492 ★

Per Capita Consumption of Major Food Commodities: 1970 to 1994
[Continued]

COMMODITY	1970	1975	1980	1985	1990	1992	1993	1994
Lard (direct use)	4.6	3.2	2.6	1.8	1.9	1.7	1.6	1.7
Edible tallow (direct use)	(NA)	(NA)	1.1	1.9	0.6	2.4	2.2	3.3
Shortening	17.3	17.0	18.2	22.9	22.2	22.4	25.1	24.1
Salad and cooking oils	15.4	17.9	21.2	23.5	24.2	25.6	25.1	24.3
Other edible fats and oils	2.3	2.0	1.5	1.6	1.2	1.4	1.7	1.6
Flour and cereal products	135.3	139.1	144.7	156.3	184.7	190.8	195.8	198.7
Wheat flour[11]	110.9	114.5	116.9	124.6	135.6	138.8	143.3	144.5
Rye flour	1.2	1.0	0.7	0.7	0.6	0.6	0.6	0.6
Rice, milled	6.7	7.6	9.4	9.0	16.3	17.5	17.6	19.0
Corn products	11.1	10.8	12.9	17.1	22.1	23.2	23.5	23.7
Oat products	4.7	4.4	3.9	4.0	8.7	9.0	9.2	9.2
Barley products	1.0	0.9	1.0	1.0	1.4	1.7	1.7	1.7
Caloric sweeteners, total[12]	122.3	118.0	123.0	128.8	137.0	141.2	144.4	147.6
Sugar, refined cane and beet	101.8	89.2	83.6	62.7	64.4	64.6	64.3	65.0
Corn sweeteners (dry weight)	19.1	27.4	38.2	64.8	71.2	75.3	78.7	81.3
Other:								
Cocoa beans	3.9	3.2	3.4	4.6	5.4	5.7	5.5	5.1
Coffee (green beans)	13.6	12.2	10.3	10.5	10.3	10.0	9.1	8.2
Peanuts (shelled)	5.5	6.0	4.8	6.3	6.0	6.2	6.0	5.8
Tree nuts (shelled)	1.7	1.9	1.8	2.5	2.4	2.2	2.2	2.3

Source: 1996 Statistical Abstract of the United States on CD-ROM [machine-readable datafiles]. CD-8A-97. Washington, DC: U.S. Department of Commerce, Economics and Statistics Administration, Bureau of the Census, Data User Services Division, January 1997. Primary source: U.S. Department of Agriculture, Economic Research Service, *Food Consumption, Prices, and Expenditures, 1996: Annual Data, 1970-1994.* Statistical Bulletin No. 928, April 1, 1996. *Notes:* NA Not available. 1. Excludes edible offals. 2. Excludes shipments to Puerto Rico and the other U.S. possessions. 3. Excludes consumption from recreational fishing, approximately 3 to 4 pounds per capita. 4. Includes backs, necks, skin, and giblets. 5. Includes other products, not shown separately. 6. Fluid milk figures are aggregates of commercial sales and milk produced and consumed on farms. 7. Heavy cream, light cream, and half and half. 8. Excludes cottage, pot, and baker's cheese. 9. Includes other cheeses not shown separately. 10. The fat content of butter and margarine is 80 percent of product weight. 11. White, whole wheat, semolina, and durum flour. 12. Dry weight. Includes edible syrups (maple, molasses, etc.) and honey not shown separately.

★ 493 ★

Diets

Per Capita Consumption of Selected Beverages, by Type: 1970 to 1994
[In gallons]

COMMODITY	1970	1975	1980	1985	1990	1991	1992	1993	1994
Nonalcoholic[1]	101.5	103.2	106.3	109.1	126.4	129.7	128.5	129.8	130.4
Milk (plain and flavored)	31.3	29.5	27.6	26.7	25.7	25.7	25.4	24.9	24.7
Whole	25.5	21.1	17.0	14.3	10.5	10.2	9.8	9.4	9.1
Lowfat	4.4	7.1	9.2	10.9	12.6	12.7	12.7	12.4	12.2
Skim	1.3	1.3	1.3	1.5	2.6	2.8	2.9	3.1	3.3
Tea	6.8	7.5	7.3	7.1	6.7	6.8	7.0	7.0	7.0
Coffee	33.4	31.4	26.7	27.4	26.9	26.8	25.9	23.5	21.1
Bottled water	(NA)	(NA)	2.4	4.5	8.0	8.0	8.2	9.4	10.5
Soft drinks	24.3	28.2	35.1	35.7	46.3	47.9	48.5	50.2	52.2
Diet	2.1	3.2	5.1	7.1	10.7	11.7	11.6	11.7	11.9
Regular	22.2	25.0	29.9	28.7	35.6	36.3	36.9	38.5	40.3

[Continued]

★ 493 ★

Per Capita Consumption of Selected Beverages, by Type: 1970 to 1994
[Continued]

COMMODITY	1970	1975	1980	1985	1990	1991	1992	1993	1994
Selected fruit juices	5.7	6.6	7.2	7.7	6.9	7.9	7.3	8.4	8.6
Fruit drinks, cocktails, and ades	(NA)	(NA)	(NA)	(NA)	5.8	6.4	6.0	6.0	5.7
Canned iced tea	(NA)	(NA)	(NA)	(NA)	0.1	0.2	0.2	0.4	0.6
Alcoholic (adult population)	35.7	39.7	42.8	40.7	40.0	37.8	37.3	36.7	36.4
Beer	30.6	33.9	36.6	34.6	34.9	33.2	32.6	32.3	32.0
Wine[2]	2.2	2.7	3.2	3.5	2.9	2.7	2.7	2.5	2.5
Distilled spirits	3.0	3.1	3.0	2.6	2.2	2.0	2.0	1.9	1.8

Source: 1996 Statistical Abstract of the United States on CD-ROM [machine-readable datafiles]. CD-8A-97. Washington, DC: U.S. Department of Commerce, Economics and Statistics Administration, Bureau of the Census, Data User Services Division, January 1997. Primary source: U.S. Dept. of Agriculture, Economic Research Service, *Food Consumption, Prices, and Expenditures 1996: Annual Data, 1970-1994.* Statistical Bulletin No. 928, April 1, 1996. *Notes:* NA Not available. 1. Excludes vegetable juices. 2. Beginning 1983, includes wine coolers.

★ 494 ★
Diets

Per Capita Utilization of Selected Commercially Produced Fresh Fruits and Vegetables: 1970 to 1994

In pounds, farm weight. Domestic food use of fresh fruits and vegetables reflects the fresh-market share of commodity production plus imports and minus exports. All data are on a calendar year basis except for citrus fruits, October or November; apples, August; grapes and pears, July.

COMMODITY	1970	1975	1980	1985	1990	1991	1992	1993	1994
Fresh fruits, total	101.2	101.8	104.8	110.6	116.5	113.2	123.6	124.9	126.7
Noncitrus	72.4	72.8	78.8	89.2	95.2	94.1	99.3	99.0	101.7
Bananas	17.4	17.6	20.8	23.5	24.4	25.1	27.3	26.8	28.1
Apples	17.0	19.5	19.2	17.3	19.6	18.2	19.2	19.2	19.5
Grapes	2.9	3.6	4.0	6.8	7.9	7.3	7.2	7.0	7.3
Nectarines and peaches	5.8	5.0	7.1	5.5	5.5	6.4	6.0	6.0	5.5
Pears	1.9	2.7	2.6	2.8	3.2	3.2	3.1	3.4	3.5
Strawberries	1.7	1.8	2.0	3.0	3.2	3.6	3.6	3.6	4.0
Pineapples	0.7	1.0	1.5	1.5	2.1	1.9	2.0	2.1	2.0
Plums and prunes	1.5	1.3	1.5	1.4	1.5	1.4	1.8	1.3	1.6
Selected melons	21.6	17.7	17.9	24.1	24.6	23.4	25.4	25.0	26.1
Watermelons	13.5	11.4	10.7	13.5	13.3	12.8	14.8	14.6	15.5
Cantaloupes	7.2	5.2	5.8	8.5	9.2	8.7	8.5	8.7	8.8
Honeydews	0.9	1.1	1.4	2.1	2.1	1.9	2.1	1.7	1.8
Other[1]	1.9	2.6	2.2	3.3	3.2	3.6	3.7	4.6	4.1
Citrus	28.9	29.0	26.1	21.5	21.4	19.1	24.4	26.0	24.9
Oranges	16.2	15.9	14.3	11.6	12.4	8.5	12.9	14.3	13.1
Grapefruit	8.2	8.4	7.3	5.5	4.4	5.9	5.9	6.2	6.1
Other[2]	4.5	4.7	4.5	4.4	4.6	4.7	5.6	5.6	5.7
Selected fresh vegetables	85.4	88.4	92.5	102.7	113.9	110.9	116.1	116.2	113.9
Asparagus	0.4	0.4	0.3	0.5	0.6	0.6	0.6	0.6	0.6
Broccoli	0.5	1.0	1.4	2.6	3.4	3.1	3.4	2.9	2.8
Cabbage	8.8	9.1	8.1	8.8	8.8	8.5	8.9	9.7	9.7

[Continued]

★ 494 ★

Per Capita Utilization of Selected Commercially Produced Fresh Fruits and Vegetables: 1970 to 1994
[Continued]

COMMODITY	1970	1975	1980	1985	1990	1991	1992	1993	1994
Carrots	6.0	6.4	6.2	6.5	8.3	7.7	8.3	8.2	7.9
Cauliflower	0.7	0.9	1.1	1.8	2.2	2.0	1.8	1.7	1.4
Celery	7.3	6.9	7.4	6.9	7.2	6.8	7.4	7.1	6.8
Corn	7.8	7.8	6.5	6.4	6.7	5.9	6.9	7.0	7.9
Cucumbers	2.8	2.8	3.9	4.4	4.7	4.6	5.0	5.3	5.3
Head lettuce	22.4	23.5	25.6	23.7	27.8	26.1	25.9	24.6	22.5
Onions	10.1	10.5	11.4	13.6	15.1	15.7	16.2	16.0	16.3
Snap beans	1.5	1.4	1.3	1.3	1.1	1.1	1.5	1.5	1.5
Bell peppers	2.2	2.5	2.9	3.8	4.5	5.1	5.7	6.2	6.6
Tomatoes	12.1	12.0	12.8	14.9	15.5	15.4	15.5	16.0	15.7
Other fresh vegetables[3]	2.8	3.2	3.6	7.5	8.0	8.3	9.0	9.4	8.9
Potatoes	121.7	121.9	114.7	122.4	127.7	130.4	132.4	137.1	141.0
Fresh	61.8	52.6	51.1	46.3	45.8	46.4	48.9	49.9	50.2
For freezing	28.5	37.1	35.4	45.4	50.2	51.3	51.0	54.5	57.8
For chips (shoestrings)	17.4	15.5	16.5	17.6	17.0	17.3	17.5	17.6	17.5
For dehydrating	12.0	14.7	9.8	11.2	12.8	13.7	13.2	13.4	13.8
For canning	2.0	2.0	1.9	1.9	1.9	1.7	1.8	1.7	1.7
Sweet potatoes[4]	5.4	5.4	4.4	5.4	4.6	4.0	4.3	3.9	4.7
Mushrooms, total	1.3	1.9	2.7	3.6	3.7	3.7	3.7	3.7	3.8
For fresh	0.3	0.7	1.2	1.8	2.0	1.9	2.0	2.0	2.0
For processing	1.0	1.2	1.5	1.8	1.7	1.8	1.7	1.7	1.8

Source: 1996 Statistical Abstract of the United States on CD-ROM [machine-readable datafiles]. CD-8A-97. Washington, DC: U.S. Department of Commerce, Economics and Statistics Administration, Bureau of the Census, Data User Services Division, January 1997. Primary source: U.S. Dept. of Agriculture, Economic Research Service, *Food Consumption, Prices, and Expenditures 1996: Annual Data, 1970-1994.* Statistical Bulletin No. 928, April 1, 1996. *Notes:* 1. Includes apricots, avocados, cherries, cranberries, kiwifruit, mangoes, and papayas. 2. Includes tangerines, tangelos, lemons, and limes. 3. Includes artichokes, Brussel sprouts, eggplant, escarole/endive, garlic, romaine and leaf lettuce (after 1984), radishes, and spinach. 4. Fresh and processed.

Fitness

★ 495 ★

Exercise Equipment Ownership and Use: 1995

Type	Percent	
	Have	Use
Exercise videos	33	21
Stationary bike	31	31
Free weights	29	39
Step machine	9	44
Treadmill	9	49
Home gym	8	45

[Continued]

★ 495 ★

Exercise Equipment Ownership and Use: 1995
[Continued]

Type	Percent	
	Have	Use
Cross-country ski machine	6	53
Rowing machine	6	20

Source: "Equipped for Fitness." *Workplace Vitality* (May 1995), p. 15. Primary source: U.S. News/CNN Poll; *U.S. News & World Report.*

★ 496 ★

Fitness

Most Popular Fitness Activities

This table shows Americans age 6 or older who participated in each activity at least once during the year, multiplied by their average number of days of participation. Data are for 1994.

[Total exercise person days per year]

Activity	Person days (millions)
Fitness walking	4,034
Free weights	2,779
Running/jogging	2,559
Stationary bikes	2,234
Fitness bicycling	1,483
Treadmills	1,418
Resistance machines	1,173
Fitness swimming	1,010
Stair-climbing machines	972
Low-impact aerobics	724

Source: Light, Larry. "Up Front: Walk, Don't Run." *Business Week,* 23 October 1995, p 6. Primary source: American Sports Data Inc.

★ 497 ★

Fitness

States With the Highest Percentages of Adults Who Do Not Exercise: 1996

Data refer to adults who report that they have had no leisure-time physical activity in the past month.

Area	Percentage
District of Columbia	49
Alabama	46
Kentucky	46
West Virginia	44
North Carolina	43

Source: "Washington Not Working Out." *USA TODAY,* 29 August 1996, p. 1D. Primary source: U.S. Centers for Disease Control and Prevention.

Obesity

★ 498 ★

Causes of Obesity

"British scientists have found the first direct evidence of two defective genes that can cause human obesity. The discoveries by Cambridge University researchers provide confirmation that losing weight isn't just a matter of willpower for some people, and is likely to set off a race for new drugs and other therapies."

Source: Wall Street Journal, 24 June 1997, p. 1.

★ 499 ★

Obesity

Overweight Adults, by City

A coalition of health and nutrition groups used numbers from the National Center for Health Statistics to come up with the percentages of people in 33 metropolitan areas considered to be obese.

City	Total %
New Orleans, LA	37.55
Norfolk, VA	33.94
San Antonio, TX	32.96
Kansas City, KS	31.66
Cleveland, OH	31.50
Detroit, MI	31.01
Columbus, OH	30.75
Cincinnati, OH	30.71
Pittsburgh, PA	29.99
Houston, TX	29.19
Philadelphia, PA	29.05
Milwaukee, WI	28.79
Buffalo, NY	28.43
Sacramento, CA	28.15
Dallas-Fort Worth, TX	27.46
Portland, OR	27.15
Chicago, IL	27.13
New York, NY	27.05
Miami, FL	26.95
Baltimore, MD	26.43
Boston, MA	26.17
Seattle, WA	25.87
Indianapolis, IN	25.77
Atlanta, GA	25.49
Los Angeles, CA	25.22
San Francisco, CA	25.16
Tampa, FL	24.91
St. Louis, MO	24.78
Phoenix, AZ	24.36
Washington, DC	23.84
San Diego, CA	22.91
Minneapolis, MN	22.63
Denver, CO	22.10

Source: "How Areas' Obese Weigh In." *USA TODAY,* 4 March 1997, p. 2D. Primary source: Centers for Disease Control and Prevention.

★ 500 ★

Obesity

Overweight Adults, by Selected Characteristics

This table shows overweight persons 20 years of age and over, according to sex, age, race, and Hispanic origin: United States, 1960-62, 1971-74, 1976-80, and 1988-91. Data are based on physical examinations of a sample of the civilian noninstitutionalized population.

Sex, age, race, and Hispanic origin[1]	1960-62	1971-74	1976-80[2]	1988-91
20-74 years, age adjusted				
Percent of population				
Both sexes	24.4	24.9	25.4	**33.0**
Male	22.9	23.6	24.0	**31.9**
Female[3]	25.6	25.9	26.5	**34.1**
White male	23.1	23.8	24.2	32.3
White female[3]	23.5	24.0	24.4	32.6
Black male	22.2	24.3	25.7	32.9
Black female[3]	41.7	42.9	44.3	49.6
White, non-Hispanic male	-	-	24.1	32.4
White, non-Hispanic female[3]	-	-	23.9	31.0
Black, non-Hispanic male	-	-	25.6	32.9
Black, non- Hispanic female[3]	-	-	44.1	49.8
Mexican- American male	-	-	31.0	39.9
Mexican- American female[3]	-	-	41.4	48.2
20-74 years, crude				
Both sexes	25.5	25.5	25.7	33.3
Male	23.4	24.0	24.2	31.9
Female[3]	27.4	27.0	27.1	34.6
White male	23.7	24.2	24.4	32.6
White female[3]	25.4	25.2	25.1	33.3
Black male	22.5	24.5	25.7	32.4
Black female[3]	43.0	43.2	43.7	48.6
White, non- Hispanic male	-	-	24.4	32.9
White, non- Hispanic female[3]	-	-	24.8	31.8
Black, non- Hispanic male	-	-	25.6	32.4
Black, non- Hispanic female[3]	-	-	43.4	49.0
Mexican- American male	-	-	29.5	35.4
Mexican- American female[3]	-	-	39.1	47.3
Male				
20-34 years	19.6	19.2	17.3	22.8
35-44 years	22.8	29.4	28.9	35.7
45-54 years	28.1	27.6	31.0	35.5
55-64 years	26.9	24.8	28.1	40.5
65-74 years	21.8	23.0	25.2	42.2
75 years and over	-	-	-	26.0
Female[3]				
20-34 years	13.2	14.8	16.8	24.5
35-44 years	24.1	27.3	27.0	35.1
45-54 years	30.7	32.3	32.5	39.8
55-64 years	43.2	38.5	37.0	48.7

[Continued]

★ 500 ★

Overweight Adults, by Selected Characteristics
[Continued]

Sex, age, race, and Hispanic origin[1]	1960-62	1971-74	1976-80[2]	1988-91
65-74 years	42.9	38.0	38.4	39.7
75 years and over	-	-	-	31.5

Source: U.S. Department of Health and Human Services. Public Health Service. Centers for Disease Control and Prevention. National Center for Health Statistics. Division of Health Examination Statistics. Hyattsville, MD: Public Health Service, 1995. Unpublished data. *Notes:* - Data not available. 1. The race groups, white and black, include persons of Hispanic and non-Hispanic origin. Conversely, persons of Hispanic origin may be of any race. 2. Data for Mexican Americans are for 1982-84. 3. Excludes pregnant women. Overweight is defined for men as body mass index greater than or equal to 27.8 kilograms/m. sq., and for women as body mass index greater than or equal to 27.3 kilograms/m. sq. These cut points were used because they represent the sex-specific 85th percentiles for persons 20-29 years of age in the 1976-80 National Health and Nutrition Examination Survey. Height was measured without shoes; 2 pounds are deducted from data for 1960-62 to allow for weight of clothing. Some data have been revised and differ from previous editions of Health, United States.

★ 501 ★
Obesity

Overweight Adults, by State

Men who have a body mass index of 27.8 or greater, and women who have a body mass index of 27.3 or greater, are considered overweight.

[In percentages]

State	Percent of overweight adults
Colorado	15-20
Hawaii	15-20
Washington	25.1-30
Oregon	25.1-30
Idaho	25.1-30
Nevada	25.1-30
Wyoming	25.1-30
North Dakota	25.1-30
South Dakota	25.1-30
Nebraska	25.1-30
Texas	25.1-30
Minnesota	25.1-30
Iowa	25.1-30
Montana	25.1-30
Arkansas	25.1-30
Louisiana	25.1-30
Indiana	25.1-30
Ohio	25.1-30
Kentucky	25.1-30
Tennessee	25.1-30
Maine	25.1-30
New York	25.1-30
Pennsylvania	25.1-30

[Continued]

★ 501 ★

Overweight Adults, by State
[Continued]

State	Percent of overweight adults
Virginia	25.1-30
North Carolina	25.1-30
South Carolina	25.1-30
Delaware	25.1-30
Maryland	25.1-30
District of Columbia	25.1-30
California	20.1-25
Montana	20.1-25
Utah	20.1-25
Arizona	20.1-25
New Mexico	20.1-25
Kansas	20.1-25
Oklahoma	20.1-25
Illinois	20.1-25
New Hampshire	20.1-25
Vermont	20.1-25
Massachusetts	20.1-25
Rhode Island	20.1-25
Connecticut	20.1-25
New Jersey	20.1-25
Georgia	20.1-25
Florida	20.1-25
Wisconsin	30.01
Michigan	30.01
West Virginia	30.01
Mississippi	30.01
Alabama	30.01

Source: "Notebook: The Fat of the Land." *Time,* 23 December 1996, p. 21. Primary source: Behavioral Risk Factor Surveillance System, 1994; American Cancer Society.

Safety

★ 502 ★

Seat Belt Wearing and Health Cost Relationships

Average costs to treat an injured motorist hospitalized after an accident for those wearing a seat belt versus not, by method of payment.

Program	Average cost of hospitalization	
	Belt worn	Not worn
Public (Medicaid, Medicare)	13,322	18,922
Private insurance/worker's comp.	8,581	14,058
Other (usually self payment)	8,180	10,534

Source: "Seat Belts Save Lives—and Money." *USA TODAY,* 25 March 1996, p. 1. Primary source: National Highway Traffic Safety Administration.

★ 503 ★
Safety

Use of Helmets When Riding a Bike

Based on estimates, there are 26 million young bicyclists. Of those, just over a quarter (26%) have helmets. But only 15% wear helmets most of the time.

Helmet is worn...	Percent of time helmet is worn while biking
Always or almost always	12.0
More than half of the time	3.0
Less than half of the time	7.0
Never or almost never	78.0

Source: "The Cutting Edge: Vital Statistics." *Washington Post,* 27 February 1996, p. 5. Primary source: Consumer Product Safety Commission.

Sex

★ 504 ★

Women Age 15-44 Who Had Premarital Voluntary First Sexual Intercourse and Used Contraceptive Methods, by Age: 1995

Age	Number in thousands	Used any method	Pill	Condom	Withdrawal	All other methods
All women[1]	53,588	59.0	19.5	29.2	6.8	3.5
Age at first intercourse						
Under 16 years	12,460	51.4	9.0	33.6	7.4	1.4
16 years	8,990	57.0	14.9	31.7	8.0	2.5
17 years	9,043	60.7	18.4	31.9	8.2	2.3
18 years	7,243	61.5	22.3	29.0	6.6	3.6
19 years	4,882	60.0	25.8	24.0	4.7	5.4
20 years and over	10,969	65.6	31.5	22.4	5.0	6.8

Source: Abma, J.C., A. Chandra, W.D. Mosher, L. Peterson, and L. Piccinino. *Fertility, Family Planning, and Women's Health: New Data from the 1995 National Survey of Family Growth.* National Center for Health Statistics. Vital Health Statistics 23(19), 1997. *Notes:* 1. Includes women of other race and origin groups not shown separately. Also, the total includes women who were never married.

★ 505 ★

Sex

Women Age 15-44 Who Had Premarital Voluntary First Sexual Intercourse and Used Contraceptive Methods, by Race/Ethnicity: 1995

Race and ethnicity	Number in thousands	Used any method	Pill	Condom	Withdrawal	All other methods
Hispanic	5,882	36.2	10.6	19.8	4.1	1.7
Non-Hispanic white	38,090	64.8	21.0	32.0	7.8	4.0
Non-Hispanic black	7,462	50.1	20.5	24.5	2.9	2.2

Source: Abma, J.C., A. Chandra, W.D. Mosher, L. Peterson, and L. Piccinino. *Fertility, Family Planning, and Women's Health: New Data from the 1995 National Survey of Family Growth.* National Center for Health Statistics. Vital Health Statistics 23(19), 1997. *Notes:* 1. Includes women of other race and origin groups not shown separately. Also, the total includes women who were never married.

★ 506 ★

Sex

Women Age 15-44 Who Had Premarital Voluntary First Sexual Intercourse and Used Contraceptive Methods, by Year of First Intercourse: 1995

Year of first intercourse	Number in thousands	Used any method	Pill	Condom	Withdrawal	All other methods
1990-95	9,140	75.9	15.5	54.3	4.4	1.6
1985-89	10,063	63.9	19.7	36.4	5.6	2.2
1980-84	10,514	59.4	21.9	25.1	8.0	4.4
Before 1980	23,871	50.2	19.9	18.3	7.6	4.4

Source: Abma, J.C., A. Chandra, W.D. Mosher, L. Peterson, and L. Piccinino. *Fertility, Family Planning, and Women's Health: New Data from the 1995 National Survey of Family Growth.* National Center for Health Statistics. Vital Health Statistics 23(19), 1997. *Notes:* 1. Includes women of other race and origin groups not shown separately. Also, the total includes women who were never married.

★ 507 ★

Sex

Women Age 15-44 Who Had Premarital Voluntary First Sexual Intercourse in 1990-1995 and Used Contraceptive Methods

Race and Ethnicity	Number in thousands	Used any method	Pill	Condom	Withdrawal	All other methods
All race and origin	9,140	75.9	15.5	54.3	4.4	1.6
Hispanic	1,333	53.1	10.3	38.4	3.8	0.5
Non-Hispanic white	6,002	82.7	17.6	60.2	3.4	1.5
Non-Hispanic black	1,331	72.2	15.2	50.5	4.3	2.2
Age at first intercourse						
Under 20 years[1]	7,134	76.9	11.3	60.4	4.4	0.9
Hispanic	930	52.8	5.4	42.3	5.2	...
Non-Hispanic white	4,774	83.0	11.8	67.1	3.4	0.7
Non-Hispanic black	1,193	72.1	14.5	51.2	3.9	2.5
20 years and over[1]	2,006	72.4	30.6	32.9	4.7	4.2
Hispanic	403	53.7	21.7	29.4	0.8	1.8
Non-Hispanic white	1,228	81.5	39.9	33.3	3.8	4.5
Non-Hispanic black	137	72.4	20.7	44.5	7.3	...

Source: Abma, J.C., A. Chandra, W.D. Mosher, L. Peterson, and L. Piccinino. *Fertility, Family Planning, and Women's Health: New Data from the 1995 National Survey of Family Growth.* National Center for Health Statistics. Vital Health Statistics 23(19), 1997. *Notes:* ... Category not applicable. 1. Includes women of other race and origin groups not shown separately. Also, the total includes women who were never married.

★ 508 ★

Sex

Women Age 15-44 Who Had Sexual Intercourse and Used Only Birth Control Pills for Contraception, by Age and Consistency of Use: 1995

Data refer to women who had intercourse and who used the pill in the three months preceding the interview.

Characteristic	Number in thousands	Percent distribution			
		Total	Never missed a pill	Missed one pill	Missed two or more pills
All women[1]	6,548	100.0	71.2	15.5	13.3
Age at interview					
15-19 years	462	100.0	69.8	13.3	16.9
15-17 years	131	100.0	58.4	13.6	28.0
18-19 years	331	100.0	74.3	13.2	12.5
20-24 years	1,774	100.0	67.2	19.3	13.5
25-29 years	1,713	100.0	68.9	16.1	15.0
30-44 years	2,599	100.0	75.7	12.8	11.5

Source: Abma, J.C., A. Chandra, W.D. Mosher, L. Peterson, and L. Piccinino. *Fertility, Family Planning, and Women's Health: New Data from the 1995 National Survey of Family Growth.* National Center for Health Statistics. Vital Health Statistics 23(19), 1997. *Note:* 1. Includes women of other race and origin groups not shown separately.

★ 509 ★

Sex

Women Age 15-44 Who Had Sexual Intercourse and Used Only Birth Control Pills for Contraception, by Educational Attainment and Consistency of Use: 1995

Data refer to women who had intercourse and who used the pill in the three months preceding the interview.

Characteristic	Number in thousands	Total	Never missed a pill	Missed one pill	Missed two or more pills
Education at interview[1]					
No high school diploma or GED[2]	343	100.0	83.0	6.7	10.2
High school diploma or GED	1,805	100.0	72.6	15.4	12.0
Some college, no bachelor's degree	1,624	100.0	71.9	13.6	14.5
Bachelor's degree or higher	1,685	100.0	70.6	16.2	13.2

Source: Abma, J.C., A. Chandra, W.D. Mosher, L. Peterson, and L. Piccinino. *Fertility, Family Planning, and Women's Health: New Data from the 1995 National Survey of Family Growth.* National Center for Health Statistics. Vital Health Statistics 23(19), 1997. *Notes:* 1. Limited to women 22-44 years of age at time of interview. 2. GED is general equivalency diploma.

★ 510 ★
Sex

Women Age 15-44 Who Had Sexual Intercourse and Used Only Birth Control Pills for Contraception, by Race/Ethnicity and Consistency of Use: 1995

Data refer to women who had intercourse and who used the pill in the three months preceding the interview.

Characteristic	Number in thousands	Total	Never missed a pill	Missed one pill	Missed two or more pills
Race and ethnicity					
Hispanic	538	100.0	70.6	7.4	22.0
Non-Hispanic white	5,256	100.0	71.5	17.0	11.5
Non-Hispanic black	585	100.0	70.1	11.4	18.6
Marital status					
Never married	2,288	100.0	70.4	16.4	13.2
Currently married	3,549	100.0	69.8	16.0	14.2
Formerly married	710	100.0	80.6	9.6	9.9
Poverty level income at interview[1]					
0-149 percent	793	100.0	76.3	11.2	12.5
150-299 percent	1,541	100.0	70.1	15.8	14.1

Source: Abma, J.C., A. Chandra, W.D. Mosher, L. Peterson, and L. Piccinino. *Fertility, Family Planning, and Women's Health: New Data from the 1995 National Survey of Family Growth.* National Center for Health Statistics. Vital Health Statistics 23(19), 1997. *Note:* 1. Limited to women 22-44 years of age at time of interview.

★ 511 ★
Sex

Women Age 15-44 Who Have Ever Had Sexual Intercourse (after Menarche), by Age and Marital Status: 1995

Age	All women		Never-married women	
	Number in thousands	Percent	Number in thousands	Percent
All women[1]	60,201	89.3	22,679	71.5
15 years	1,690	22.1	1,674	21.4
16 years	1,874	38.0	1,874	38.0
17 years	1,889	51.1	1,831	49.6
18 years	1,771	65.4	1,641	62.7
19 years	1,737	75.5	1,542	72.4
20-24 years	9,041	88.6	5,939	82.6

[Continued]

★ 511 ★

Women Age 15-44 Who Have Ever Had Sexual Intercourse (after Menarche), by Age and Marital Status: 1995

[Continued]

Age	All women		Never-married women	
	Number in thousands	Percent	Number in thousands	Percent
25-29 years	9,693	95.9	3,456	88.6
30-44 years	32,506	98.2	4,722	87.4

Source: Abma, J.C., A. Chandra, W.D. Mosher, L. Peterson, and L. Piccinino. *Fertility, Family Planning, and Women's Health: New Data from the 1995 National Survey of Family Growth.* National Center for Health Statistics. Vital Health Statistics 23(19), 1997. *Note:* 1. Includes women of other race and origin groups not shown separately.

★ 512 ★

Sex

Women Age 15-44 Who Have Ever Had Sexual Intercourse (after Menarche), by Age, Race, Ethnicity and Marital Status: 1995

Age, race and ethnicity	All women		Never-married women	
	Number in thousands	Percent	Number in thousands	Percent
15-19 years:				
Hispanic	1,150	55.0	1,078	52.0
Non-Hispanic white	5,962	49.5	5,693	47.1
Non-Hispanic black	1,392	59.5	1,351	58.3
15-17 years:				
Hispanic	688	50.0	673	48.8
Non-Hispanic white	3,534	34.9	3,485	33.9
Non-Hispanic black	853	48.2	853	48.2
18-19 years:				
Hispanic	462	62.5	405	57.2
Non-Hispanic white	2,428	70.7	2,208	67.8
Non-Hispanic black	538	77.4	498	75.5

Source: Abma, J.C., A. Chandra, W.D. Mosher, L. Peterson, and L. Piccinino. *Fertility, Family Planning, and Women's Health: New Data from the 1995 National Survey of Family Growth.* National Center for Health Statistics. Vital Health Statistics 23(19), 1997.

★ 513 ★

Sex

Women Age 15-44 Who Have Ever Had Voluntary Sexual Intercourse, by Age and Age of First Voluntary Partner: 1995

Age	Number in thousands	Total	Age of first voluntary partner in years					
			Under 16	16-17	18-19	20-22	23-24	25 and over
All women	53,416	100.0	5.8	23.4	26.3	22.3	8.4	13.9
Age at first intercourse								
Under 16 years	12,757	100.0	22.0	43.8	21.2	7.1	2.1	4.0
16 years	8,840	100.0	2.4	41.8	34.5	13.9	3.8	3.7
17 years	8,984	100.0	0.6	27.7	41.6	19.2	5.3	5.6
18 years	7,215	100.0	0.5	7.7	36.7	33.3	9.7	9.1
19 years	4,868	100.0	-	2.0	24.1	45.9	11.4	16.7
20-22 years	7,298	100.0	-	0.6	7.2	43.2	19.5	29.5
23-24 years	1,835	100.0	-	0.5	1.8	15.6	29.3	52.8
25 years and over	1,817	100.0	-	0.9	0.5	2.9	11.5	84.2

Source: Abma, J.C., A. Chandra, W.D. Mosher, L. Peterson, and L. Piccinino. *Fertility, Family Planning, and Women's Health: New Data from the 1995 National Survey of Family Growth.* National Center for Health Statistics. Vital Health Statistics 23(19), 1997. *Note:* - Quantity zero. Percents may not add to 100 due to rounding.

★ 514 ★

Sex

Women Age 15-44 Who Have Ever Had Voluntary Sexual Intercourse, by Selected Characteristics: 1995

Age, Race and Ethnicity	Number in thousands	Total	Age of first voluntary partner in years					
			Under 16	16-17	18-19	20-22	23-24	25 and over
Hispanic	5,887	100.0	4.7	17.9	21.1	25.8	10.3	20.3
Under 16 years	1,305	100.0	17.3	37.3	22.3	14.1	2.9	6.1
16-19 years	2,960	100.0	1.4	18.3	28.4	30.0	9.4	12.6
20 years and over	1,622	100.0	-	1.0	6.7	27.8	18.2	46.2
Non-Hispanic white	38,110	100.0	5.3	24.0	27.2	22.8	8.6	12.2
Under 16 years	8,411	100.0	21.2	45.9	20.8	6.6	2.0	3.5
16-19 years	22,166	100.0	1.1	23.5	37.1	24.7	6.9	6.7
20 years and over	7,534	100.0	-	0.7	5.4	35.3	20.7	38.1
Non-Hispanic black	7,462	100.0	9.7	27.5	28.9	18.2	5.4	10.3
Under 16 years	2,684	100.0	26.0	41.1	21.6	5.7	1.7	4.0
16-19 years	3,946	100.0	0.5	23.8	39.1	24.2	5.2	7.2
20 years and over	832	100.0	0.2	0.3	3.9	31.0	18.7	46.0

Source: Abma, J.C., A. Chandra, W.D. Mosher, L. Peterson, and L. Piccinino. *Fertility, Family Planning, and Women's Health: New Data from the 1995 National Survey of Family Growth.* National Center for Health Statistics. Vital Health Statistics 23(19), 1997. *Note:* - Quantity zero. Percents may not add to 100 due to rounding.

★515★

Sex

Women Age 18-44 Who Had Formal Instruction in Sex-Education Subjects Before Age 18, by Age: 1995

Data refer to women who had intercourse and who used the pill in the three months preceding the interview.

Characteristic	Number in thousands	Received any formal instruction	Type of formal instruction			
			Birth control methods	Sexually transmitted disease	Safe sex to prevent HIV[1]	How to say no to sex
All women	54,748	72.8	62.0	62.7	52.0	55.0
Age at interview						
18-19 years	3,508	95.9	86.9	93.2	91.3	89.9
20-24 years	9,041	89.2	80.9	82.1	64.1	80.1
25-29 years	9,692	80.4	71.7	71.1	27.0	62.0
30-34 years	11,065	73.0	62.3	60.8	11.6	49.3
35-39 years	11,211	65.0	53.7	55.5	...	41.5
40-44 years	10,230	51.4	36.2	37.0	...	35.2

Source: Abma, J.C., A. Chandra, W.D. Mosher, L. Peterson, and L. Piccinino. *Fertility, Family Planning, and Women's Health: New Data from the 1995 National Survey of Family Growth.* National Center for Health Statistics. Vital Health Statistics 23(19), 1997. *Notes:* ... Category not applicable. Percents do not add to 100 because respondents could report more than one type of formal instruction. 1. Limited to women 15-30 years of age at interview. HIV is human immunodeficiency virus.

★516★

Sex

Women Age 18-44 Who Had Formal Instruction in Sex-Education Subjects Before Age 18, by Mother's Education and Poverty Status: 1995

Characteristic	Number in thousands	Received any formal instruction	Type of formal instruction			
			Birth control methods	Sexually transmitted disease	Safe sex to prevent HIV[1]	How to say no to sex
Mother's education						
0-11 years	16,454	64.9	54.1	53.9	49.0	49.0
12 years	23,251	74.2	63.0	64.3	51.9	55.9
13-15 years	7,480	79.6	69.0	69.5	56.1	59.6
16 years or more	7,210	79.6	69.0	70.8	51.9	61.2
No mother-figure identified	353	74.2	67.0	65.1	61.7	60.1
Poverty level income at interview[2]						
0-149 percent	10,072	65.8	57.0	56.8	39.5	51.0
0-99 percent	5,992	64.2	55.7	54.7	38.2	50.6

[Continued]

★ 516 ★

Women Age 18-44 Who Had Formal Instruction in Sex-Education Subjects Before Age 18, by Mother's Education and Poverty Status: 1995
[Continued]

Characteristic	Number in thousands	Received any formal instruction	Type of formal instruction			
			Birth control methods	Sexually transmitted disease	Safe sex to prevent HIV[1]	How to say no to sex
150-299 percent	14,932	70.3	59.6	59.4	38.5	51.4
300 percent or higher	22,736	70.9	58.3	59.2	33.2	49.1

Source: Abma, J.C., A. Chandra, W.D. Mosher, L. Peterson, and L. Piccinino. *Fertility, Family Planning, and Women's Health: New Data from the 1995 National Survey of Family Growth.* National Center for Health Statistics. Vital Health Statistics 23(19), 1997. *Notes:* Percents do not add to 100 because respondents could report more than one type of formal instruction. 1. Limited to women 15-30 years of age at interview. HIV is human immunodeficiency virus. 2. Limited to women 22-44 years of age at time of interview.

★ 517 ★

Sex

Women Age 18-44 Who Had Formal Instruction in Sex-Education Subjects Before Age 18, by Race and Ethnicity: 1995

Characteristic	Number in thousands	Received any formal instruction	Type of formal instruction			
			Birth control methods	Sexually transmitted disease	Safe sex to prevent HIV[1]	How to say no to sex
Race and ethnicity						
Hispanic	6,015	64.8	56.8	55.4	50.2	49.3
Non-Hispanic white	38,987	74.0	62.2	63.6	50.9	55.0
Non-Hispanic black	7,357	76.1	67.1	67.8	59.9	62.5
Non-Hispanic other	2,390	63.1	55.7	51.0	47.4	46.5

Source: Abma, J.C., A. Chandra, W.D. Mosher, L. Peterson, and L. Piccinino. *Fertility, Family Planning, and Women's Health: New Data from the 1995 National Survey of Family Growth.* National Center for Health Statistics. Vital Health Statistics 23(19), 1997. *Notes:* Percents do not add to 100 because respondents could report more than one type of formal instruction. 1. Limited to women 15-30 years of age at interview. HIV is human immunodeficiency virus.

★518★

Sex

Women Age 18-44 Who Had Formal Instruction in Sex-Education Subjects Before Age 18, by Residence and Family Background: 1995

Characteristic	Number in thousands	Received any formal instruction	Type of formal instruction			
			Birth control methods	Sexually transmitted disease	Safe sex to prevent HIV[1]	How to say no to sex
Family background						
Both parents from birth[2]	34,610	71.7	60.0	61.2	51.1	53.7
Single parent from birth	1,760	70.5	61.0	60.2	55.7	57.6
Both parents, then one parent	6,979	74.6	65.3	64.6	53.5	57.5
Stepparent[3]	7,386	76.3	66.6	67.5	52.4	58.6
Other	4,013	73.9	65.1	64.9	52.4	54.2

Source: Abma, J.C., A. Chandra, W.D. Mosher, L. Peterson, and L. Piccinino. *Fertility, Family Planning, and Women's Health: New Data from the 1995 National Survey of Family Growth.* National Center for Health Statistics. Vital Health Statistics 23(19), 1997. *Notes:* Percents do not add to 100 because respondents could report more than one type of formal instruction. 1. Limited to women 15-30 years of age at interview. HIV is human immunodeficiency virus. 2. Includes women who lived with either both biological or both adoptive parents until they left home. 3. Parents separated or divorced, then custodial parent remarried.

Smoking and Tobacco

★519★

Comparison of Advertising to Brand Preference in Adolescents and Adults: 1993[1]

Category	Value
Advertising ($ mil.)	
Marlboro	75
Camel	43
Newport	35
Kool	21
Winston	17
Benson & Hedges	4
Salem	3
Adolescent Brand Preference (%)	
Marlboro	60.0
Camel	13.3
Newport	12.7
Kool	1.2
Winston	1.2
Salem	1.0

[Continued]

★519★

Comparison of Advertising to Brand Preference in Adolescents and Adults: 1993

[Continued]

Category	Value
Benson & Hedges	0.3
Adult Brand Preference[2](%)	
Marlboro	23.5
Winston	6.7
Newport	4.8
Camel	3.9
Salem	3.9
Kool	3.0
Benson & Hedges	2.5

Source: 1993 TAPS II, The Maxwell Consumer Report 1994, Ad $ Summary 1993. *Notes:* 1. Among name brands from 1993 TAPS II. 2. Over all marketshare used as an estimate.

★520★

Smoking and Tobacco

Current Smoking Status Among Adults

This table presents the percentage of adults 18 years and older who used cigars, pipes, chewing tobacco, snuff, or any form of tobacco, by Hispanic origin, race, and sex, National Health Interview Surveys, 1987, 1991 (combined)—United States.

Category	Non-Hispanic[1]					Hispanic[1]					Total[1]
	White	Black	Asian/ Pacific Islander	American Indian/ Alaska Native	All	Mexican American	Puerto Rican American	Cuban American	Other	All	
Cigar smoking											
Male	4.8	3.9	2.2	5.3	4.6	1.3	1.5	2.5	3.8	2.1	4.4
Female	0.1	0.1	0.1	0.2	0.1	0.1	.	.	0.2	0.1	0.1
Total	2.3	1.8	1.1	2.7	2.2	0.7	0.6	1.0	1.9	1.1	2.1
Pipe smoking											
Male	2.9	2.4	2.3	6.9	2.8	0.2	1.5	2.6	1.7	1.0	2.7
Female	0.1	.	.	.	0.0	.	.	.	.	.	0.0
Total	1.4	1.1	1.2	3.5	1.4	0.1	0.7	1.1	0.8	0.5	1.3
Cigar or pipe smoking											
Male	6.7	5.6	3.3	9.8	6.5	1.5	2.7	5.1	4.3	2.7	6.2
Female	0.1	0.1	0.1	0.2	0.1	0.1	.	.	0.2	0.1	0.1
Total	3.3	2.5	1.7	4.9	3.1	0.8	1.2	2.1	2.1	1.3	3.0
Any tobacco smoking											
Male	33.2	40.2	24.0	37.3	33.7	29.4	31.9	30.8	27.2	29.3	33.4
Female	26.3	26.5	7.8	35.6	25.9	14.8	23.1	16.9	16.9	16.8	25.2
Total	29.6	32.6	16.0	36.4	29.6	22.1	26.8	22.5	21.7	22.7	29.1

[Continued]

★ 520 ★

Current Smoking Status Among Adults

[Continued]

Category	Non-Hispanic[1]					Hispanic[1]					Total[1]
	White	Black	Asian/ Pacific Islander	American Indian/ Alaska Native	All	Mexican American	Puerto Rican American	Cuban American	Other	All	
Chewing tobacco use											
Male	4.1	2.7	0.4	5.3	3.8	0.8	0.3	.	1.1	0.7	3.5
Female	0.1	1.5	.	0.8	0.3	0.1	.	.	0.1	0.1	0.3
Total	2.0	2.0	0.2	3.1	2.0	0.4	0.1	.	0.5	0.4	1.8
Snuff use											
Male	3.8	0.9	0.9	3.2	3.4	1.0	0.6	0.3	1.6	1.0	3.2
Female	0.3	1.9	.	0.4	0.5	0.2	.	.	0.0	0.1	0.4
Total	1.9	1.4	0.5	1.8	1.8	0.6	0.3	0.1	0.8	0.5	1.7
Chewing tobacco or snuff use											
Male	6.8	3.1	1.2	7.8	6.2	1.5	0.6	0.3	2.3	1.5	5.9
Female	0.3	2.9	.	1.2	0.6	0.3	.	.	0.1	0.1	0.6
Total	3.4	3.0	0.6	4.5	3.3	0.9	0.3	0.1	1.1	0.8	3.1
Any tobacco use											
Male	38.0	42.4	25.6	43.9	38.2	30.7	32.8	31.2	28.4	30.4	37.6
Female	26.8	29.3	7.9	36.6	26.7	15.1	23.3	17.0	17.1	17.0	26.0
Total	32.2	35.2	16.8	40.2	32.2	22.9	27.4	22.7	22.4	23.4	31.5

Source: National Health Interview Surveys: 1987 and 1991 (combined). Obtained from the Centers for Disease Control and Prevention Tobacco Information & Prevention Sourcepage. See http://www.cdc.gov. *Notes:* Current use identified those persons who, for cigars, had smoked greater than or equal to 50 cigars and currently smoked cigars; for pipes, had smoked a pipe greater than or equal to 50 times and currently smoked a pipe; for cigars or pipes, were current users of cigars or pipes; for any tobacco smoking, were current users of cigarettes (i.e., had smoked greater than or equal to 100 cigarettes and currently smoked cigarettes), cigars, or pipes; for chewing tobacco, had used chewing tobacco greater than or equal to 20 times and currently used chewing tobacco; for snuff, had used snuff greater than or equal to 20 times and currently used snuff; for chewing tobacco or snuff, were current users of chewing tobacco or snuff; for any tobacco use, were current users of cigarettes, cigars, pipes, chewing tobacco, or snuff. 0.0 Indicates a value >0 and <0.05. A . indicates a value of zero. 1. Includes other, unknown, and multiple race and unknown Hispanic origin.

★ 521 ★

Smoking and Tobacco

Mothers Who Smoked During Pregnancy, by Race/ Ethnicity, Educational Attainment, and Age: 1993

Characteristic of mother	Percent[2]
Race of mother[1]	
All races	15.8
White	16.8
Black	12.7
American Indian or Alaskan Native	21.6
Asian or Pacific Islander[3]	4.3
Chinese	1.1

[Continued]

★ 521 ★

Mothers Who Smoked During Pregnancy, by Race/ Ethnicity, Educational Attainment, and Age: 1993

[Continued]

Characteristic of mother	Percent[2]
Japanese	6.7
Filipino	4.3
Hawaiian and part Hawaiian	17.2
Other Asian or Pacific Islander	3.2
Hispanic origin of mother[4]	
Hispanic origin	5.0
Mexican American	3.7
Puerto Rican	11.2
Cuban	5.0
Central and South American	2.3
Other and unknown Hispanic	9.3
White, non-Hispanic	18.6
Black, non-Hispanic	12.7
Education of mother[5]	
0-8 years	15.2
9-11 years	29.0
12 years	19.3
13-15 years	11.3
16 years or more	3.1
Age of mother[2]	
10-14 years	7.0
16-19 years	17.5
15-17 years	14.8
18-19 years	19.1
20-24 years	19.2
25-29 years	14.8
30-34 years	13.4
35-39 years	12.8
40-49 years	11.0

Source: U.S. Department of Health and Human Services. Public Health Service. Centers for Disease Control and Prevention. National Center for Health Statistics. *Health, United States, 1995.* Hyattsville, MD: Public Health Service, 1996, p. 89. Primary source: Centers for Disease Control and Prevention. National Center for Health Statistics. Data computed by the Division of Health and Utilization Analysis from data compiled by the Division of Vital Statistics. *Notes:* The race groups, white and black, include persons of Hispanic and non-Hispanic origin. Conversely, persons of Hispanic origin may be of any race. 1. Includes data for 47 states and DC in 1993. Excludes data for California, Indiana, New York, and South Dakota, which did not require the reporting of mother's tobacco use during pregnancy on the birth certificate. 2. Excludes live births for whom smoking status of mother is unknown. 3. Maternal tobacco use during pregnancy was not reported. 4. Includes data for 46 states and DC in 1993. Excludes data for California, Indiana, New York, and South Dakota, which did not require the reporting of mother's tobacco use during pregnancy on the birth certificate. 5. Includes data for 46 states and DC in 1993. Excludes data for California, Indiana, New York, and South Dakota, which did not require the reporting of mother's tobacco use during pregnancy on the birth certificate.

★ 522 ★

Smoking and Tobacco

Projected Smokers and Smoking-Related Deaths, by State: 1996

State	Projected smokers	Projected number of deaths
Alabama	260,639	83,404
Alaska	56,246	17,999
Arizona	307,864	98,516
Arkansas	155,690	49,821
California	1,446,550	462,896
Colorado	271,694	86,942
Connecticut	175,501	56,160
Delaware	51,806	16,578
District of Columbia	15,398	4,927
Florida	928,464	297,108
Georgia	409,726	131,112
Hawaii	64,574	20,664
Idaho	76,230	24,394
Illinois	813,670	260,374
Indiana	439,515	140,645
Iowa	167,507	53,602
Kansas	153,862	49,236
Kentucky	274,693	87,902
Louisiana	331,366	106,037
Maine	97,536	31,211
Maryland	267,876	85,720
Massachusetts	330,186	105,659
Michigan	721,572	230,903
Minnesota	303,153	97,009
Mississippi	152,610	48,835
Missouri	372,052	119,057
Montana	47,014	15,045
Nebraska	110,913	35,492
Nevada	98,770	31,606
New Hampshire	74,303	23,777
New Jersey	423,728	135,593
New Mexico	104,271	33,367
New York	1,179,584	377,467
North Carolina	517,786	165,692
North Dakota	38,350	12,272
Ohio	891,129	285,161
Oklahoma	199,490	63,837
Oregon	191,688	61,340
Pennsylvania	857,371	274,359
Rhode Island	73,446	23,503
South Carolina	208,142	66,606
South Dakota	45,705	14,626
Tennessee	329,147	105,327
Texas	1,158,389	370,685

[Continued]

★ 522 ★

Projected Smokers and Smoking-Related Deaths, by State: 1996

[Continued]

State	Projected smokers	Projected number of deaths
Utah	108,883	34,843
Vermont	38,613	12,356
Virginia	423,288	135,452
Washington	336,871	107,799
West Virginia	120,443	38,542
Wisconsin	365,907	117,090
Wyoming	31,669	10,134

Source: Levy, Doug. "The Toll Smoking Will Take on Today's Youth: 16.6M Will Get Hooked and 5M Will Die." *USA TODAY,* 8 November 1996, p. 6D. Primary source: U.S. Centers for Disease Control and Prevention.

★ 523 ★

Smoking and Tobacco

Smokeless Tobacco: Boys Using

This table shows past month smokeless tobacco use among boys, grades 9-12.

State	Prevalence (Percentage)
District of Columbia	2.7
Hawaii	8.9
Utah	11.9
New Jersey	13.3
Delaware	15.0
Illinois	16.2
Massachusetts	17.0
Georgia	17.6
Maine	18.8
Nevada	19.0
New York	19.4
New Hampshire	19.5
South Carolina	20.4
North Carolina	20.5
Wisconsin	21.0
Ohio	22.5
New Mexico	24.1
Mississippi	24.2
Louisiana	25.1
Oregon	25.5
Arkansas	26.2
Nebraska	26.5
Idaho	26.7

[Continued]

★ 523 ★

Smokeless Tobacco: Boys Using
[Continued]

State	Prevalence (Percentage)
Wyoming	32.6
Tennessee	33.8
Montana	36.5
South Dakota	37.9
Kentucky	39.0
West Virginia	40.3
Northeastern Region	15.5
Western Region	18.6
Southern Region	19.0
Midwestern Region	25.2
United States	20.4

Source: Youth Risk Behavior Survey (YRBS), 1993. Obtained from the Centers for Disease Control and Prevention Tobacco Information & Prevention Sourcepage. See http://www.cdc.gov. In 1993, past month cigarette smoking among youth was measured in 28 states and DC using the Youth Risk Behavior Surveillance System.

★ 524 ★

Smoking and Tobacco

Smokeless Tobacco: Men Using

This table shows current smokeless tobacco use among men aged 18 years and older.

State	Prevalence (Percentage)	Rank
Connecticut	0.1	1
New Jersey	0.4	2
Rhode Island	0.4	2
District of Columbia	0.5	4
Massachusetts	0.5	4
New York	1.0	6
Hawaii	1.2	7
Maryland	1.3	8
Delaware	1.5	9
California	1.6	10
Maine	1.7	11
New Hampshire	1.7	11
Illinois	2.1	13
Florida	2.3	14
Vermont	2.5	15
Nevada	2.6	16
Utah	2.6	16
Michigan	2.8	18

[Continued]

★ 524 ★

Smokeless Tobacco: Men Using
[Continued]

State	Prevalence (Percentage)	Rank
Ohio	3.6	19
Wisconsin	3.7	20
Washington	4.0	21
Minnesota	4.1	22
Arizona	4.3	23
Pennsylvania	4.4	24
South Carolina	4.4	24
Indiana	4.9	26
New Mexico	5.2	27
Colorado	5.3	28
Virginia	5.3	28
Nebraska	5.7	30
Oregon	5.7	30
Missouri	6.0	32
North Dakota	6.0	32
Iowa	6.1	34
Alaska	6.3	35
Texas	6.3	35
Kansas	6.5	37
Louisiana	6.7	38
Georgia	6.8	39
North Carolina	6.8	39
Idaho	7.7	41
Oklahoma	8.0	42
South Dakota	8.2	43
Kentucky	8.5	44
Alabama	9.0	45
Tennessee	9.0	45
Arkansas	11.1	47
Mississippi	11.1	47
Montana	11.9	49
Wyoming	13.5	50
West Virginia	15.6	51
United States	4.0	-

Source: Current Population Survey (CPS), 1992-1993. Obtained from the Centers for Disease Control and Prevention Tobacco Information & Prevention Sourcepage. See http://www.cdc.gov.

★ 525 ★

Smoking and Tobacco

Smokers by Characteristic

Current cigarette smoking by persons 18 years of age and over, according to sex, race, and age: United States, selected years 1965-93. Data are based on household interviews of a sample of the civilian noninstitutionalized population.

Sex, race, and age	1965	1974	1979	1983	1985	1987	1988	1990	1991	1992	1993
All persons											
18 years and over, age adjusted	42.3	37.2	33.5	32.2	30.0	28.7	27.9	25.4	25.4	26.4	25.0
18 years and over, crude	42.4	37.1	33.5	32.1	30.1	28.8	28.1	25.5	25.6	26.5	25.0
All males											
18 years and over, age adjusted	51.6	42.9	37.2	34.7	32.1	31.0	30.1	28.0	27.5	28.2	27.5
18 years and over, crude	51.9	43.1	37.5	35.1	32.6	31.2	30.8	28.4	28.1	28.6	27.7
18-24 years	54.1	42.1	35.0	32.9	28.0	28.2	25.5	26.6	23.5	28.0	28.8
25-34 years	60.7	50.5	43.9	38.8	38.2	34.8	36.2	31.6	32.8	32.8	30.2
35-44 years	58.2	51.0	41.8	41.0	37.6	36.6	36.5	34.5	33.1	32.9	32.0
45-64 years	51.9	42.6	39.3	35.9	33.4	33.5	31.3	29.3	29.3	28.6	29.2
65 years and over	28.5	24.8	20.9	22.0	19.6	17.2	18.0	14.6	15.1	16.1	13.5
White:											
18 years and over, age adjusted	50.8	41.7	36.5	34.1	31.3	30.4	29.5	27.6	27.0	28.0	27.0
18 years and over, crude	51.1	41.9	36.8	34.5	31.7	30.5	30.1	28.0	27.4	28.2	27.0
18-24 years	53.0	40.8	34.3	32.5	28.4	29.2	26.7	27.4	25.1	30.0	30.4
25-34 years	60.1	49.5	43.6	38.6	37.3	33.8	35.4	31.6	32.1	33.5	29.9
35-44 years	57.3	50.1	41.3	40.8	36.6	36.2	35.8	33.5	32.1	30.9	31.2
45-64 years	51.3	41.2	38.3	35.0	32.1	32.4	30.0	28.7	28.0	28.1	27.8
65 years and over	27.7	24.3	20.5	20.6	18.9	16.0	16.9	13.7	14.2	14.9	12.5
Black:											
18 years and over, age adjusted	59.2	54.0	44.1	41.3	39.9	39.0	36.5	32.2	34.7	32.0	33.2
18 years and over, crude	60.4	54.3	44.1	40.6	39.9	39.0	36.5	32.5	35.0	32.2	32.7
18-24 years	62.8	54.9	40.2	34.2	27.2	24.9	18.6	21.3	15.0	16.2	19.9
25-34 years	68.4	58.5	47.5	39.9	45.6	44.9	41.6	33.8	39.4	29.5	30.7
35-44 years	67.3	61.5	48.6	45.5	45.0	44.0	42.5	42.0	44.4	47.5	36.9
45-64 years	57.9	57.8	50.0	44.8	46.1	44.3	43.2	36.7	42.0	35.4	42.4
65 years and over	36.4	29.7	26.2	38.9	27.7	30.3	29.8	21.5	24.3	28.3	27.9

[Continued]

★ 525 ★

Smokers by Characteristic
[Continued]

Sex, race, and age	1965	1974	1979	1983	1985	1987	1988	1990	1991	1992	1993
All females											
18 years and over, age adjusted	34.0	32.5	30.3	29.9	28.2	26.7	26.0	23.1	23.6	24.8	22.7
18 years and over, crude	33.9	32.1	29.9	29.5	27.9	26.5	25.7	22.8	23.5	24.6	22.5
18-24 years	38.1	34.1	33.8	35.5	30.4	26.1	26.3	22.5	22.4	24.9	22.9
25-34 years	43.7	38.8	33.7	32.6	32.0	31.8	31.3	28.2	28.4	30.1	27.3
35-44 years	43.7	39.8	37.0	33.8	31.5	29.6	27.8	24.8	27.6	27.3	27.4
45-64 years	32.0	33.4	30.7	31.0	29.9	28.6	27.7	24.8	24.6	26.1	23.0
65 years and over	9.6	12.0	13.2	13.1	13.5	13.7	12.8	11.5	12.0	12.4	10.5
White:											
18 years and over, age adjusted	34.3	32.3	30.6	30.1	28.3	27.2	26.2	23.9	24.2	25.7	23.7
18 years and over, crude	34.0	31.7	30.1	29.4	27.7	26.7	25.7	23.4	23.7	25.1	23.1
18-24 years	38.4	34.0	34.5	36.5	31.8	27.8	27.5	25.4	25.1	28.5	26.8
25-34 years	43.4	38.6	34.1	32.2	32.0	31.9	31.0	28.5	28.4	31.5	28.4
35-44 years	43.9	39.3	37.2	34.8	31.0	29.2	28.3	25.0	27.0	27.6	27.3
45-64 years	32.7	33.0	30.6	30.6	29.7	29.0	27.7	25.4	25.3	25.8	23.4
65 years and over	9.8	12.3	13.8	13.2	13.3	13.9	12.6	11.5	12.1	12.6	10.5
Black:											
18 years and over, age adjusted	32.1	35.9	30.8	31.8	30.7	27.2	27.1	20.4	23.1	23.9	19.8
18 years and over, crude	33.7	36.4	31.1	32.2	31.0	28.0	27.8	21.2	24.4	24.2	20.8
18-24 years	37.1	35.6	31.8	32.0	23.7	20.4	21.8	10.0	11.8	10.3	8.2
25-34 years	47.8	42.2	35.2	38.0	36.2	35.8	37.2	29.1	32.4	26.9	24.7
35-44 years	42.8	46.4	37.7	32.7	40.2	35.3	27.6	25.5	35.3	32.4	31.5
45-64 years	25.7	38.9	34.2	36.3	33.4	28.4	29.5	22.6	23.4	30.9	21.3
65 years and over	7.1	8.9	8.5	13.1	14.5	11.7	14.8	11.1	9.6	11.1	10.2

Source: U.S. Department of Health and Human Services. Public Health Service. Centers for Disease Control and Prevention. National Center for Health Statistics. Division of Health Interview Statistics: Data from the National Health Interview Survey; data computed by the Division of Health and Utilization Analysis from data compiled by the Division of Health Interview Statistics. National Center for Health Statistics. *Health, United States, 1995.* Hyattsville, MD: Public Health Service, p 173. 1996. *Notes:* Estimates for 1992 and beyond are not strictly comparable with those for earlier years, and estimates for 1992 and 1993 are not strictly comparable with each other due to a change in the definition of current smoker in 1992 and the use of a split sample in 1992.

★ 526 ★

Smoking and Tobacco

Smokers: Current and Former

This table shows the percentage of adults[1] who were current, former, or never smokers,[2] overall and by sex, race, Hispanic origin, age, and education, National Health Interview Surveys, selected years—United States, 1980-1993.

Smoking Status	1980	1983	1985	1987	1988	1990	1991	1992	1993
Total population									
Current	33.2	32.1	30.1	28.8	28.1	25.5	25.7	26.5	25.0
Former	21.3	21.8	24.2	22.8	23.8	24.6	24.1	23.4	24.6
Never	45.5	46.1	45.8	48.4	48.1	49.9	50.2	50.1	50.5
Sex									
Male									
Current	37.6	35.1	32.6	31.2	30.8	28.4	28.1	28.6	27.7
Former	28.1	28.3	30.9	28.9	29.6	30.3	29.9	28.8	29.9
Never	34.4	36.6	36.5	39.9	39.6	41.3	42.1	42.6	42.4
Female									
Current	29.3	29.5	27.9	26.5	25.7	22.8	23.5	24.6	22.5
Former	15.1	15.9	18.1	17.4	18.6	19.5	19.0	18.5	19.7
Never	55.5	54.6	54.0	56.0	55.8	57.7	57.6	57.0	57.8
Race									
White									
Current	32.9	31.8	29.6	28.5	27.8	25.6	25.5	26.6	24.9
Former	22.2	22.8	25.5	24.2	25.3	25.9	25.7	24.9	26.2
Never	44.9	45.3	44.9	47.3	47.0	48.5	48.9	48.6	48.9
Black									
Current	36.9	35.9	34.9	32.9	31.7	26.2	29.1	27.8	26.1
Former	13.8	14.2	15.9	14.8	15.2	16.7	14.6	15.9	15.7
Never	49.4	49.9	49.2	52.3	53.1	57.1	56.2	56.3	58.2
Hispanic origin									
Hispanic									
Current	30.0	25.3	25.9	23.6	23.6	23.0	20.2	20.7	20.4
Former	15.1	15.7	17.2	16.1	19.2	17.0	16.9	16.4	16.2
Never	54.9	59.0	56.9	60.4	57.3	60.0	63.0	62.9	63.4
Non-Hispanic									
Current	33.4	32.6	30.3	29.2	28.4	25.7	26.1	27.0	25.4
Former	21.6	22.2	24.6	23.4	24.1	25.3	24.8	24.0	25.2
Never	45.0	45.3	45.1	47.5	47.4	49.0	49.0	49.1	49.4
Age (years)									
18-24									
Current	33.3	34.2	29.3	27.1	25.9	24.5	22.9	26.4	25.8
Former	10.5	9.3	10.1	8.0	9.3	9.5	7.7	6.1	7.2
Never	56.2	56.5	60.6	64.9	64.8	66.0	69.3	67.4	67.0
25-44									
Current	37.8	36.3	34.8	33.2	32.9	29.7	30.4	30.8	29.2
Former	19.8	19.0	21.4	19.6	19.2	20.0	19.4	18.1	18.6
Never	42.5	44.7	43.8	47.2	47.9	50.3	50.2	51.1	52.2
45-64									
Current	35.6	33.3	31.6	30.9	29.4	27.0	26.9	27.3	26.0
Former	26.6	28.8	31.2	29.9	32.9	32.9	32.9	32.7	33.9
Never	37.9	37.9	37.3	39.3	37.6	40.1	40.2	40.1	40.1

[Continued]

★ 526 ★

Smokers: Current and Former

[Continued]

Smoking Status	1980	1983	1985	1987	1988	1990	1991	1992	1993
> =65									
Current	17.2	16.7	16.0	15.2	14.9	12.8	13.3	14.0	11.8
Former	27.9	30.7	34.0	34.1	34.5	36.6	36.4	36.5	38.4
Never	54.9	52.6	50.0	50.7	50.6	50.6	50.3	49.5	49.8
Education (years)[3]									
<12									
Current	35.1	34.7	34.2	34.2	32.9	30.8	31.4	30.9	29.7
Former	21.7	23.2	26.3	24.8	25.8	26.3	25.3	27.0	27.1
Never	43.2	42.2	39.6	41.0	41.3	42.9	43.3	42.2	43.3
12									
Current	35.4	34.9	33.4	32.9	32.7	30.1	30.6	31.3	29.2
Former	22.8	23.7	25.1	24.7	25.0	26.2	26.1	25.1	26.8
Never	41.8	41.4	41.5	42.5	42.3	43.7	43.3	43.6	44.1
13-15									
Current	33.9	32.1	30.6	28.2	28.1	24.6	25.5	25.5	25.0
Former	24.9	25.1	27.5	26.1	27.2	27.5	28.1	27.7	28.2
Never	41.2	42.8	42.0	45.7	44.7	47.9	46.4	46.8	46.8
> =16									
Current	24.5	20.6	19.0	16.6	16.3	13.9	13.9	15.5	13.5
Former	27.6	26.5	30.3	27.2	28.2	28.7	27.6	25.2	26.9
Never	47.9	52.9	50.7	56.2	55.5	57.4	58.5	59.3	59.5

Source: National Health Interview Surveys: 1980, 1983, 1985, 1987, 1988, 1990, 1991, 1992, 1993. Obtained from the Centers for Disease Control and Prevention Tobacco Information & Prevention Sourcepage. See http://www.cdc.gov. For any year, 95% confidence intervals do not exceed 1.2% for the total population, 1.8% for men, 1.4% for women, 1.2% for whites, 3.9% for blacks, 4.7% for Hispanics, 1.2% for non-Hispanics, 2.4% for persons ages 18-24 years, 1.8% for persons ages 25-44 years, 1.8% for persons ages 45-64 years, 2.5% for persons ages 65 years, 2.1% for <12 years of education, 1.9% for 12 years of education, 3.2% for 13-15 years of education, and 2.9% for 16 years of education. *Notes:* NA=Data not available. 1. Persons > =18 years of age. 2. Current smokers reported smoking > =100 cigarettes and currently smoked. Former smokers reported smoking > =100 cigarettes and did not currently smoke. Never smokers reported that they had smoked <100 cigarettes. 3. Data on education are presented for persons > =25 years of age.

★ 527 ★

Smoking and Tobacco

Smokers: Current and Former: Young Adults

This table shows the percentage of young adults[1] who were current, former, or never smokers,[2] overall and by sex, race, Hispanic origin, age, and education, National Health Interview Surveys, selected years—United States, 1980-1993.

Smoking Status	1980	1983	1985	1987	1988	1990	1991	1992	1993
Total population									
Current	33.3	34.2	29.3	27.1	25.9	24.5	22.9	26.4	25.8
Former	10.5	9.3	10.1	8.0	9.3	9.5	7.7	6.1	7.2
Never	56.2	56.5	60.6	64.9	64.8	66.0	69.3	67.4	67.0
Sex									
Male									
Current	35.4	32.9	28.1	28.2	25.5	26.6	23.5	28.0	28.8

[Continued]

★ 527 ★

Smokers: Current and Former: Young Adults
[Continued]

Smoking Status	1980	1983	1985	1987	1988	1990	1991	1992	1993
Former	10.5	8.1	10.7	6.7	9.6	9.1	8.0	6.9	6.9
Never	54.1	59.0	61.3	65.2	64.9	64.4	68.4	65.1	64.3
Female									
Current	31.4	35.5	30.4	26.2	26.3	22.5	22.4	24.9	22.9
Former	10.4	10.4	9.6	9.2	9.0	9.9	7.5	5.4	7.4
Never	58.2	54.1	60.0	64.7	64.7	67.6	70.2	69.7	69.7
Race									
White									
Current	33.1	34.6	30.1	28.5	27.1	26.4	25.1	29.3	28.6
Former	11.3	9.9	10.9	8.8	10.6	10.6	8.4	6.6	8.2
Never	55.7	55.5	58.9	62.8	62.3	63.1	66.5	64.2	63.2
Black									
Current	35.6	33.0	25.3	22.4	20.3	15.2	13.3	13.0	13.7
Former	5.2	6.2	6.0	3.7	3.4	5.2	3.9	4.5	1.2
Never	59.3	60.8	68.7	73.8	76.3	79.6	82.8	82.5	85.1
Education[3]									
Sex									
Male									
Current	51.0	49.1	43.0	43.8	40.1	37.3	34.5	40.4	38.3
Former	10.5	10.3	11.6	7.4	11.4	10.2	11.0	8.6	8.3
Never	38.5	40.6	45.4	48.8	48.6	52.4	54.5	51.1	53.4
Female									
Current	40.3	45.5	43.6	37.6	37.0	33.4	30.6	34.8	33.3
Former	12.5	11.7	11.8	10.8	11.5	11.7	9.0	5.7	10.8
Never	47.2	42.8	44.6	51.6	51.4	54.9	60.5	59.6	55.9
> =13 years									
Sex									
Male									
Current	20.1	16.2	15.5	16.3	12.1	16.1	12.2	17.6	19.6
Former	14.7	7.1	10.9	8.4	9.8	10.3	9.2	6.6	8.0
Never	65.3	76.7	73.7	75.4	78.1	73.7	78.6	75.8	72.4
Female									
Current	20.0	22.9	17.2	15.1	16.2	13.8	14.6	18.4	16.0
Former	8.3	9.4	9.7	10.0	8.9	8.5	7.6	5.2	6.0
Never	71.8	67.7	73.2	74.9	74.9	77.8	77.8	76.4	78.0

Source: National Health Interview Surveys: 1980, 1983, 1985, 1987, 1988, 1990, 1991, 1992, 1993. Obtained from the Centers for Disease Control and Prevention Tobacco Information & Prevention Sourcepage. See http://www.cdc.gov. For any year, 95% confidence intervals do not exceed 1.2% for the total population, 1.8% for men, 1.4% for women, 1.2% for whites, 3.9% for blacks, 4.7% for Hispanics, 1.2% for non-Hispanics, 2.4% for persons ages 18-24 years, 1.8% for persons ages 25-44 years, 1.8% for persons ages 45-64 years, 2.5% for persons ages 65 years, 2.1% for <12 years of education, 1.9% for 12 years of education, 3.2% for 13-15 years of education, and 2.9% for 16 years of education. *Notes:* NA=Data not available. 1. Persons 18-24 years of age. 2. Current smokers reported smoking > =100 cigarettes and currently smoked. Former smokers reported smoking > =100 cigarettes and did not currently smoke. Never smokers reported that they had smoked <100 cigarettes. 3. Data on education are presented for persons > =25 years of age.

★ 528 ★

Smoking and Tobacco

Smokers: Percent Who Smoked in Last 30 Days

This table shows the percentage of people who smoked 1 or more cigarettes per day during the previous 30 days.

Year	Total	Sex		Race	
		Males	Females	Whites	Blacks
1976	28.8	28.0	28.8	28.8	26.8
1977	28.9	27.2	30.1	29.0	23.7
1978	27.5	25.9	28.3	27.8	22.2
1979	25.4	22.3	27.9	25.8	19.3
1980	21.4	18.5	23.5	21.8	15.7
1981	20.3	18.1	21.7	20.9	13.6
1982	21.0	18.2	23.2	22.4	12.4
1983	21.1	19.2	22.1	21.9	12.6
1984	18.7	16.0	20.5	20.1	9.0
1985	19.5	17.8	20.6	20.7	10.8
1986	18.7	16.9	19.8	20.4	7.8
1987	18.7	16.4	20.6	20.6	8.1
1988	18.1	17.4	18.1	20.5	6.7
1989	18.9	17.9	19.4	21.7	6.0
1990	19.1	18.7	19.3	21.8	5.4
1991	18.4	18.8	17.9	21.1	4.9
1992	17.2	17.2	16.7	19.9	3.7
1993	19.0	19.4	18.2	22.9	4.4
1994	19.4	20.4	18.1	23.0	5.4
1995	21.6	21.7	20.8	24.9	6.9
1996	22.2	22.2	21.8	26.1	7.0
Percentage point difference					
1976-1996	-6.6	-5.8	-7.0	-2.7	-19.8
1976-1984	-10.1	-12.0	-8.3	-8.7	-17.8
1984-1996	+3.5	+6.2	+1.3	+6.0	-2.0
Percentage change					
1976-1996	-22.9	-20.7	-24.3	-9.4	-73.9
1976-1984	-35.1	-42.9	-28.8	-30.2	-66.4
1984-1996	+18.7	+38.8	+6.3	+29.9	-22.2

Source: Smoking status of high school seniors—United States, Monitoring the Future Project, 1976-1996, University of Michigan. Obtained from the Centers for Disease Control and Prevention Tobacco Information & Prevention Sourcepage. See http://www.cdc.gov. *Notes:* NA=Data not available. 1. Persons >=18 years of age. 2. Current smokers reported smoking >=100 cigarettes and currently smoked. Former smokers reported smoking >=100 cigarettes and did not currently smoke. Never smokers reported that they had smoked <100 cigarettes. 3. Data on education are presented for persons >=25 years of age.

★ 529 ★
Smoking and Tobacco

Smokers: Percentage Distribution

This table shows the percentage distribution of adult[1] current cigarette smokers,[2] by number of cigarettes smoked per day, and percentage of adult current cigarette smokers who smoked > =25 cigarettes per day, by sex, race, Hispanic origin, age, and education, National Health Interview Surveys, selected years—United States, 1974-1993.

	1974	1978	1979	1980	1983	1985	1987	1988	1990	1991	1992	1993
Current smokers												
Number of cigarettes smoked per day												
<15	31.6	29.4	29.8	29.1	29.3	31.6	32.1	31.0	34.5	36.6	38.2	39.6
15-24	43.2	42.6	42.7	42.1	44.7	41.8	41.4	43.4	42.6	41.9	40.5	41.2
> =25	25.3	28.0	27.5	28.8	26.0	26.6	26.6	25.6	22.9	21.5	21.3	19.1
Mean	19.8	20.9	20.6	21.2	20.3	20.3	20.1	20.2	19.1	18.2	17.6	17.1
Percent smoking > =25 cigarettes per day												
Sex												
Male	31.1	34.5	32.4	33.7	32.3	32.4	32.8	30.5	28.5	26.4	27.0	24.2
Female	18.7	20.8	22.0	23.2	19.4	20.6	19.9	20.3	16.6	16.1	15.3	13.5
Race												
White	27.6	30.5	29.8	31.6	28.6	29.5	29.6	28.4	25.4	23.8	23.9	21.5
Black	8.7	9.7	10.5	9.4	9.2	9.3	8.2	9.0	6.0	8.6	5.4	6.0
Hispanic origin												
Hispanic	NA	16.3	12.0	13.4	9.2	15.8	12.0	9.7	6.8	5.3	7.3	4.9
Non-Hispanic	NA	28.7	28.4	29.6	26.8	27.2	27.5	26.6	24.1	22.5	22.1	20.0
Age (years)												
18-24	15.1	17.8	16.1	17.0	11.7	13.6	12.6	10.5	9.1	9.2	11.1	8.2
25-44	29.2	30.5	30.7	31.5	29.2	29.5	28.3	27.7	22.9	21.0	21.0	18.0
45-64	27.3	32.5	32.6	34.5	32.8	31.1	32.5	31.7	30.8	29.3	27.1	26.2
> =65	17.7	19.5	16.6	18.2	17.3	19.4	20.4	17.4	18.9	17.1	20.9	19.4
Education[3] (years)												
<12	25.8	28.5	27.9	29.4	29.1	29.0	28.8	29.1	24.5	27.4	26.1	22.7
12	27.8	30.7	30.7	31.6	29.1	29.0	29.8	28.1	25.7	22.9	23.4	21.4
13-15	32.5	33.1	33.1	32.7	30.3	29.3	28.1	27.9	25.5	20.0	21.5	19.4
> =16	27.3	30.9	30.8	33.3	28.4	28.7	26.9	25.0	22.6	20.1	16.6	17.2

Source: National Health Interview Surveys: 1980, 1983, 1985, 1987, 1988, 1990, 1991, 1992, 1993. Obtained from the Centers for Disease Control and Prevention Tobacco Information & Prevention Sourcepage. See http://www.cdc.gov. For any year, 95% confidence intervals do not exceed 1.2% for the total population, 1.8% for men, 1.4% for women, 1.2% for whites, 3.9% for blacks, 4.7% for Hispanics, 1.2% for non-Hispanics, 2.4% for persons ages 18-24 years, 1.8% for persons ages 25-44 years, 1.8% for persons ages 45-64 years, 2.5% for persons ages 65 years, 2.1% for <12 years of education, 1.9% for 12 years of education, 3.2% for 13-15 years of education, and 2.9% for 16 years of education. *Notes:* NA=Data not available. 1. Persons > =18 years of age. 2. Current smokers reported smoking > =100 cigarettes and currently smoked. 3. Data on education are presented for persons > =25 years of age.

★ 530 ★

Smoking and Tobacco

Smokers: Percentage Using Various Forms of Tobacco

This table shows the percentage of adults 18 years and older who used cigars, pipes, chewing tobacco, or snuff, by race, sex, and age, National Health Interview Surveys, 1970, 1987, and 1991—United States.

	White			Black			Total[1]		
	1970	1987	1991	1970	1987	1991	1970	1987	1991
Cigar smoking									
Male (age in years)									
18-24	7.4	1.8	1.0	3.2	0.4	.	6.8	1.6	0.8
25-34	17.3	5.3	2.4	11.8	2.4	2.2	16.7	4.9	2.3
35-44	19.5	7.5	4.9	16.5	5.5	3.0	19.0	7.1	4.6
45-64	18.8	7.4	5.2	22.0	4.2	6.9	19.0	7.0	5.5
>=65	16.7	4.2	2.7	23.8	10.7	6.6	17.2	4.8	3.0
Total	16.5	5.6	3.6	15.2	4.0	3.6	16.3	5.3	3.5
Female (age in years)									
18-24	0.2	0.0	.	0.1	0.1	.	0.2	0.0	.
25-34	0.2	0.1	0.1	0.6	.	0.2	0.2	0.1	0.1
35-44	0.3	0.0	0.1	0.1	.	.	0.3	0.0	0.1
45-64	0.2	0.1	0.1	.	0.2	0.1	0.2	0.1	0.1
>=65	0.1	0.0	.	1.0	0.2	.	0.2	0.1	0.0
Total	0.2	0.1	0.1	0.3	0.1	0.1	0.2	0.1	0.1
Pipe smoking									
Male (age in years)									
18-24	8.7	0.7	0.3	4.3	0.3	.	8.1	0.8	0.2
25-34	14.6	1.8	0.8	9.5	2.3	0.6	13.9	2.0	0.8
35-44	14.0	4.1	2.7	10.2	4.0	2.3	13.5	4.0	2.7
45-64	14.4	5.2	3.0	14.3	4.4	1.8	14.3	5.1	3.0
>=65	14.8	4.4	3.2	17.0	7.9	2.4	14.9	4.7	3.1
Total	13.5	3.4	2.1	10.8	3.4	1.4	13.1	3.4	2.0
Female (age in years)									
18-24	0.1	.	0.1	.	.	.	0.1	.	0.0
25-34	0.0	0.2	0.0	0.2	.	.	0.0	0.1	0.0
35-44	0.2	0.1	0.1	0.2	.	.	0.2	0.1	0.0
45-64	0.1	0.0	0.0	0.6	.	.	0.1	0.0	0.0
>=65	0.1	.	0.0	2.6	.	.	0.3	.	0.0
Total	0.1	0.1	0.0	0.5	.	.	0.1	0.1	0.0
Cigar or pipe smoking									
Male (age in years)									
18-24	13.8	2.2	1.2	6.4	0.7	.	12.9	2.1	1.0
25-34	25.9	6.4	3.1	17.6	4.4	2.6	24.9	6.1	3.0
35-44	27.1	10.0	6.5	22.3	7.9	5.2	26.4	9.5	6.4
45-64	26.8	10.8	7.3	29.5	7.5	8.4	26.9	10.3	7.5
>=65	25.7	7.4	5.3	33.3	15.2	8.5	26.1	8.1	5.5
Total	24.4	7.8	5.0	21.3	6.3	4.7	24.0	7.5	5.0
Female (age in years)									
18-24	0.4	0.0	0.1	0.1	0.1	.	0.3	0.0	0.0
25-34	0.2	0.3	0.1	0.6	.	0.2	0.2	0.2	0.1
35-44	0.4	0.1	0.1	0.2	.	.	0.4	0.1	0.1

[Continued]

★ 530 ★

Smokers: Percentage Using Various Forms of Tobacco
[Continued]

	White			Black			Total[1]		
	1970	1987	1991	1970	1987	1991	1970	1987	1991
45-64	0.2	0.1	0.1	0.6	0.2	0.1	0.3	0.1	0.1
> =65	0.2	0.0	0.1	2.9	0.2	.	0.4	0.1	0.1
Total	0.3	0.1	0.1	0.7	0.1	0.1	0.3	0.1	0.1
Chewing tobacco use									
Male (age in years)									
18-24	1.8	6.5	5.0	1.3	1.0	.	1.8	5.5	4.1
25-34	2.2	3.7	3.6	1.7	0.8	0.4	2.2	3.3	3.1
35-44	2.8	3.3	2.7	7.7	1.6	1.8	3.3	3.1	2.5
45-64	4.0	3.5	2.4	7.1	8.0	3.4	4.2	3.9	2.4
> =65	8.9	5.2	3.8	16.1	7.3	4.5	9.4	5.4	3.9
Total	3.8	4.2	3.3	5.9	3.4	1.8	3.9	4.1	3.1
Female (age in years)									
18-24	0.1	0.1	.	1.5	0.1	.	0.3	0.1	0.1
25-34	0.2	0.0	.	1.0	0.6	0.2	0.3	0.1	0.0
35-44	0.2	0.1	0.1	2.8	1.6	0.6	0.5	0.3	0.1
45-64	0.3	0.0	0.2	3.5	1.9	1.7	0.6	0.2	0.4
> =65	0.3	0.2	0.3	8.9	6.2	4.4	1.0	0.7	0.6
Total	0.2	0.1	0.1	3.1	1.7	1.2	0.5	0.3	0.3
Snuff use									
Male (age in years)									
18-24	0.7	7.3	7.5	0.7	0.7	.	0.7	6.4	6.2
25-34	0.5	4.1	5.5	.	0.1	0.5	0.5	3.6	4.8
35-44	0.7	2.7	3.3	1.1	0.7	0.4	0.8	2.5	2.9
45-64	1.8	1.6	1.6	2.0	2.0	0.5	1.8	1.6	1.4
> =65	3.4	2.1	2.1	11.4	3.5	1.8	4.0	2.2	2.2
Total	1.4	3.3	3.7	2.2	1.1	0.5	1.5	3.1	3.3
Female (age in years)									
18-24	0.1	0.3	0.2	0.6	0.2	.	0.2	0.3	0.2
25-34	0.2	0.1	0.0	1.2	0.4	0.0	0.3	0.1	0.1
35-44	0.3	0.1	0.1	2.7	0.9	0.2	0.6	0.2	0.1
45-64	1.2	0.2	0.1	7.9	2.6	2.2	1.8	0.4	0.3
> =65	3.1	0.8	0.8	15.8	9.6	6.9	4.0	1.5	1.3
Total	1.0	0.3	0.2	5.0	2.2	1.5	1.4	0.5	0.4
Chewing tobacco or									
snuff use									
Male (age in years)									
18-24	2.2	10.4	10.1	1.5	1.0	.	2.2	8.9	8.4
25-34	2.7	6.9	7.9	1.7	0.8	0.7	2.5	6.0	6.9
35-44	3.5	5.1	5.4	7.7	2.3	2.1	3.9	4.8	4.9
45-64	5.6	4.7	3.8	8.8	8.4	3.8	5.8	5.0	3.7
> =65	11.8	6.6	5.5	24.5	9.5	6.0	12.7	6.9	5.6
Total	5.0	6.4	6.2	7.4	3.8	2.2	5.2	6.1	5.6
Female (age in years)									
18-24	0.2	0.4	0.2	2.0	0.3	.	0.4	0.3	0.2

[Continued]

★ 530 ★

Smokers: Percentage Using Various Forms of Tobacco
[Continued]

	White			Black			Total[1]		
	1970	1987	1991	1970	1987	1991	1970	1987	1991
25-34	0.3	0.1	0.0	1.9	0.7	0.2	0.5	0.2	0.1
35-44	0.5	0.1	0.1	4.6	1.8	0.8	1.0	0.3	0.2
45-64	1.4	0.2	0.3	10.9	3.8	3.5	2.3	0.6	0.6
> =65	3.3	0.9	1.0	23.2	13.4	9.9	4.8	1.9	1.7
Total	1.2	0.3	0.3	7.5	3.2	2.4	1.8	0.6	0.6

Source: National Health Interview Surveys: 1970, 1987, and 1991. Surveillance for Selected Tobacco-Use Behaviors—United States, 1900-1994. Obtained from the Centers for Disease Control and Prevention Tobacco Information & Prevention Sourcepage. See http://www.cdc.gov. *Notes:* For 1970, current use identified those persons who, for cigars, had smoked greater than or equal to 50 cigars and currently smoked cigars; for pipes, had smoked greater than or equal to 3 packages of pipe tobacco and currently smoked a pipe; for cigars or pipes, were current users of cigars or pipes; for chewing tobacco, currently used chewing tobacco; for snuff, currently used snuff; for chewing tobacco or snuff, were current users of chewing tobacco or snuff. For 1987 and 1991, current use identified those persons who, for cigars, had smoked greater than or equal to 50 cigars and currently smoked cigars; for pipes, had smoked a pipe greater than or equal to 50 times and currently smoked a pipe; for cigars or pipes, were current users of cigars or pipes; for chewing tobacco, had used chewing tobacco greater than or equal to 20 times and currently used chewing tobacco; for snuff, had used snuff greater than or equal to 20 times and currently used snuff; for chewing tobacco or snuff, were current users of chewing tobacco or snuff. 0.0 indicates a value >zero and <0.05. A . indicates a value of zero. 1. Includes other, unknown, and multiple race.

★ 531 ★

Smoking and Tobacco

Smokers: Prevalence of Cessation

This table shows the percentage of adult[1] ever smokers who are former smokers[2] (prevalence of cessation), overall and by sex, race, Hispanic origin, age, and education, National Health Interview Surveys, selected years—United States, 1980-1993.

	1980	1983	1985	1987	1988	1990	1991	1992	1993
Total	39.0	40.4	44.5	44.3	45.8	49.1	48.5	46.9	49.6
Sex									
Male	42.8	44.6	48.7	48.0	49.0	51.6	51.6	50.1	51.9
Female	34.0	35.1	39.4	39.6	42.0	46.0	44.7	43.0	46.7
Race									
White	40.4	41.8	46.2	45.8	47.6	50.4	50.2	48.3	51.2
Black	27.2	28.3	31.3	31.0	32.4	38.9	33.4	36.4	37.6
Hispanic origin									
Hispanic	33.5	38.4	40.0	40.5	44.9	42.5	45.6	44.2	44.3
Non-Hispanic	39.3	40.5	44.8	44.5	45.9	49.5	48.7	47.1	49.9
Age (years)									
18-24	23.9	21.3	25.7	22.8	26.5	28.0	25.2	18.8	21.7
25-44	34.3	34.4	38.1	37.2	36.8	40.3	38.9	37.1	39.0
45-64	42.8	46.3	49.7	49.2	52.8	55.0	55.1	54.5	56.6
> =65	61.8	64.8	68.1	69.2	69.8	74.1	73.3	72.4	76.6
Education[3] (years)									
<12	38.2	40.1	43.5	42.1	44.0	46.1	44.6	46.6	47.7
12	39.2	40.4	42.9	42.9	43.3	46.5	46.0	44.5	47.9

[Continued]

★ 531 ★

Smokers: Prevalence of Cessation
[Continued]

	1980	1983	1985	1987	1988	1990	1991	1992	1993
13-15	42.4	43.9	47.4	48.1	49.2	52.8	52.3	52.1	53.0
> =16	52.9	56.2	61.5	62.1	63.4	67.3	66.5	61.8	66.6

Source: National Health Interview Surveys: 1980, 1983, 1985, 1987, 1988, 1990, 1991, 1992, 1993. Obtained from the Centers for Disease Control and Prevention Tobacco Information & Prevention Sourcepage. See http://www.cdc.gov. For any year, 95% confidence intervals do not exceed 1.2% for the total population, 1.8% for men, 1.4% for women, 1.2% for whites, 3.9% for blacks, 4.7% for Hispanics, 1.2% for non-Hispanics, 2.4% for persons ages 18-24 years, 1.8% for persons ages 25-44 years, 1.8% for persons ages 45-64 years, 2.5% for persons ages 365 years, 2.1% for <12 years of education, 1.9% for 12 years of education, 3.2% for 13-15 years of education, and 2.9% for 316 years of education. *Notes:* NA=Data not available. 1. Persons > =18 years of age. 2. Current smokers reported smoking > =100 cigarettes and currently smoked. Former smokers reported smoking > =100 cigarettes and did not currently smoke. Ever smokers include both current and former smokers. 3. Data on education are presented for persons > =25 years of age.

★ 532 ★

Smoking and Tobacco

Smoking: Cigarette Consumption Data

This table shows total and per capita manufactured cigarette consumption[1] and percentage change in per capita consumption—United States Department of Agriculture, 1900-1995.

Year	Total (Billion)	Per Capita[2] (>18 yrs)	% change in per capita consumption from previous year
1900	2.5	54	-
1901	2.5	53	-1.9
1902	2.8	60	+13.2
1903	3.1	64	+6.7
1904	3.3	66	+3.1
1905	3.6	70	+6.1
1906	4.5	86	+22.9
1907	5.3	99	+15.1
1908	5.7	105	+6.1
1909	7.0	125	+19.0
1910	8.6	151	+20.8
1911	10.1	173	+14.6
1912	13.2	223	+28.9
1913	15.8	260	+16.6
1914	16.5	267	+2.7
1915	17.9	285	+6.7
1916	25.2	395	+38.6
1917	35.7	551	+39.5
1918	45.6	697	+26.5
1919	48.0	727	+4.3
1920	44.6	665	-8.5
1921	50.7	742	+11.6

[Continued]

★ 532 ★

Smoking: Cigarette Consumption Data

[Continued]

Year	Total (Billion)	Per Capita[2] (>18 yrs)	% change in per capita consumption from previous year
1922	53.4	770	+3.8
1923	64.4	911	+18.3
1924	71.0	982	+7.8
1925	79.8	1,085	+10.5
1926	89.1	1,191	+9.8
1927	97.5	1,279	+7.4
1928	106.0	1,366	+6.8
1929	118.6	1,504	+10.1
1930	119.3	1,485	-1.3
1931	114.0	1,399	-5.8
1932	102.8	1,245	-11.0
1933	111.6	1,334	+7.1
1934	125.7	1,483	+11.2
1935	134.4	1,564	+5.5
1936	152.7	1,754	+12.1
1937	162.8	1,847	+5.3
1938	163.4	1,830	-0.9
1939	172.1	1,900	+3.8
1940	181.9	1,976	+4.0
1941	208.9	2,236	+13.2
1942	245.0	2,585	+15.6
1943	284.3	2,956	+14.4
1944	296.3	3,039	+2.8
1945	340.6	3,449	+13.5
1946	344.3	3,446	-0.1
1947	345.4	3,416	-0.9
1948	358.9	3,505	+2.6
1949	360.9	3,480	-0.7
1950	369.8	3,552	+2.1
1951	397.1	3,744	+5.4
1952	416.0	3,886	+3.8
1953	408.2	3,778	-2.8
1954	387.0	3,546	-6.1
1955	396.4	3,597	+1.4
1956	406.5	3,650	+1.5
1957	422.5	3,755	+2.9
1958	448.9	3,953	+5.3
1959	467.5	4,073	+3.0
1960	484.4	4,171	+2.4
1961	502.5	4,266	+2.3
1962	508.4	4,266	0.0
1963	523.9	4,345	+1.9
1964	511.3	4,194	-3.5

[Continued]

★ 532 ★

Smoking: Cigarette Consumption Data
[Continued]

Year	Total (Billion)	Per Capita[2] (>18 yrs)	% change in per capita consumption from previous year
1965	528.8	4,258	+1.5
1966	541.3	4,287	+0.7
1967	549.3	4,280	-0.2
1968	545.6	4,186	-2.2
1969	528.9	3,993	-4.6
1970	536.5	3,985	-0.2
1971	555.1	4,037	+1.3
1972	566.8	4,043	+0.1
1973	589.7	4,148	+2.6
1974	599.0	4,141	-0.2
1975	607.2	4,122	-0.5
1976	613.5	4,091	-0.8
1977	617.0	4,043	-1.2
1978	616.0	3,970	-1.8
1979	621.5	3,861	-2.7
1980	631.5	3,849	-0.3
1981	640.0	3,836	-0.3
1982	634.0	3,739	-2.5
1983	600.0	3,488	-6.7
1984	600.4	3,446	-1.2
1985	594.0	3,370	-2.2
1986	583.8	3,274	-2.8
1987	575.0	3,197	-2.4
1988	562.5	3,096	-3.3
1989	540.0	2,926	-5.5
1990	525.0	2,826	-3.4
1991	510.0	2,720	-3.8
1992	500.0	2,641	-2.9
1993	485.0	2,538	-3.9
1994	485.0	2,522	-0.6
1995[3]	487.0	2,515	-0.3

Source: Tobacco Situation and Outlook Report. U.S.D.A., April 1996 and September 1987. Miller, R. *U.S. cigarette consumption, 1900 to date.* In: Harr W, ed. Tobacco yearbook, 1981, page 53. *Notes:* 1. Includes overseas forces: "Total" consumption, 1917-1919 and 1940 to date, "Per Capita" consumption, 1930 to date. 2. 18 years and older. 3. Estimated.

★ 533 ★

Smoking and Tobacco

Smoking: Heart Attack Risks

This table shows smokers' vs. nonsmokers' risk of heart attack at a given age. The risk for nonsmokers is 1.

Age range	Risk (Nonsmoker = 1)
30-39	6.3
40-49	4.7
50-59	3.1
60-69	2.5
70-79	1.9

Source: "Heart Attacks and Cigarettes," *American Health* (November 1995), p. 11.

★ 534 ★

Smoking and Tobacco

Smoking: Prevalence Among U.S. Adults

This table shows the percentage of smoking prevalence among U.S. adults, 18 years of age and older, 1955-1994[1] In 1994, 48 million adults 18 years of age and older (25.3 million men, 22.7 million women) were current smokers in the United States. Smoking among adults decreased dramatically from 42% in 1965 to 26% in 1994. During this period, smoking among the adult male population declined from 52% to 28%; adult female smoking declined from 34% to 23%.

Year	Overall Population	Males	Females	Whites	Blacks
1955	--	56.9	28.4	--	--
1965	42.4	51.9	33.9	42.1	45.8
1966	42.6	52.5	33.9	42.4	45.9
1970	37.4	44.1	31.5	37.0	41.4
1974	37.1	43.1	32.1	36.4	44.0
1978	34.1	38.1	30.7	33.9	37.7
1979	33.5	37.5	29.9	33.3	36.9
1980	33.2	37.6	29.3	32.9	36.9
1983	32.1	35.1	29.5	31.8	35.9
1985	30.1	32.6	27.9	29.6	34.9
1987	28.8	31.2	26.5	28.5	32.9
1988	28.1	30.8	25.7	27.8	31.7
1990	25.5	28.4	22.8	25.6	26.2
1991	25.7	28.1	23.5	25.5	29.1
1992[1]	26.5	28.6	24.6	26.6	27.8

[Continued]

★ 534 ★

Smoking: Prevalence Among U.S. Adults
[Continued]

Year	Overall Population	Males	Females	Whites	Blacks
1993	25.0	27.7	22.5	24.9	26.1
1994	25.5	28.2	23.1	26.3	27.2

Source: Office on Smoking and Health, National Center for Chronic Disease Prevention and Health Promotion, Centers for Disease Control and Prevention, July 1996. The following references are cited: (1) Data compiled by the Centers for Disease Control and Prevention, Office on Smoking and Health, from the Current Population Survey, 1955, and the National Health Interview Surveys, 1965-1994. (2) Centers for Disease Control and Prevention. Cigarette smoking among adults-United States, 1994. Morbidity and Mortality Weekly Report 1996; 45 (27): 588-590. *Note:* 1. Estimates since 1992 incorporate people who smoke some days only.

★ 535 ★

Smoking and Tobacco

Smoking Status, by Number, 1965-1994

Table shows the number (in millions) of adults 18 years and older who were current, former, or never smokers, overall and by sex, race, Hispanic origin, age, and education, National Health Interview Surveys, selected years—United States, 1965-1994.

	1965	1970	1974	1979	1983	1988	1992	1993	1994
Smoking status									
Total population									
Current	50.1	48.1	48.9	51.1	53.5	49.4	48.4	46.4	48.0
Former	16.0	23.8	25.8	32.5	36.2	41.8	42.8	45.6	46.0
Never	52.0	56.8	57.3	68.9	76.8	84.5	91.6	93.7	93.9
Sex									
Male									
Current	28.9	26.4	25.8	26.9	27.6	25.6	25.0	24.5	25.3
Former	11.0	15.8	16.6	20.4	22.2	24.6	25.1	26.5	26.3
Never	15.8	17.8	17.5	24.5	28.8	33.0	37.1	37.5	38.0
Female									
Current	21.1	21.6	23.1	24.1	25.9	23.7	23.5	21.9	22.7
Former	5.0	8.0	9.1	12.1	14.0	17.1	17.7	19.2	19.6
Never	36.2	39.0	39.8	44.4	48.0	51.5	54.5	56.2	55.9
Race									
White									
Current	44.6	42.6	42.7	44.6	46.2	41.9	41.3	39.1	40.6
Former	15.0	22.3	24.1	29.9	33.1	38.1	38.6	41.0	41.6
Never	46.4	50.1	50.5	59.5	65.8	70.8	75.4	76.7	76.2
Black									
Current	5.0	5.1	5.8	5.8	6.4	6.1	5.7	5.5	5.8
Former	0.9	1.3	1.4	2.2	2.5	2.9	3.3	3.3	3.1
Never	5.0	5.9	6.0	7.8	8.9	10.3	11.6	12.2	12.5
Hispanic origin									
Hispanic									
Current	NA	NA	NA	2.7	2.6	2.8	2.8	2.9	3.1
Former	NA	NA	NA	1.6	1.6	2.3	2.2	2.3	2.6

[Continued]

★ 535 ★

Smoking Status, by Number, 1965-1994

[Continued]

	1965	1970	1974	1979	1983	1988	1992	1993	1994
Never	NA	NA	NA	4.9	6.0	6.8	8.5	9.0	10.3
Non-Hispanic									
Current	NA	NA	NA	48.1	50.6	46.4	45.5	43.3	44.7
Former	NA	NA	NA	30.8	34.5	39.4	40.4	43.0	43.2
Never	NA	NA	NA	63.6	70.4	77.4	82.7	84.4	83.2
Age (years)									
18-24									
Current	8.0	8.3	8.8	9.6	9.8	6.6	6.4	6.2	6.9
Former	1.2	2.0	2.2	2.9	2.6	2.4	1.5	1.7	1.8
Never	8.4	11.6	12.3	15.3	16.1	16.5	16.3	16.0	16.3
25-44									
Current	23.1	20.8	21.5	22.7	24.7	25.3	24.8	23.7	24.7
Former	6.1	8.8	8.9	11.4	12.9	14.7	14.6	15.1	14.9
Never	15.9	17.1	17.9	24.2	30.4	36.7	41.2	42.3	42.6
45-64									
Current	15.9	15.9	15.2	15.0	14.7	13.3	13.1	12.9	12.7
Former	6.1	8.9	10.0	11.7	12.7	14.9	15.6	16.9	17.0
Never	16.1	16.3	15.1	16.4	16.7	17.0	19.2	19.9	20.2
> =65									
Current	3.1	3.0	3.5	3.8	4.3	4.2	4.2	3.7	3.7
Former	2.6	4.0	4.7	6.4	7.9	9.8	11.1	11.9	12.3
Never	11.6	11.8	12.0	13.1	13.6	14.3	15.0	15.5	14.8
Education[1] (years)									
<12									
Current	NA	17.8	16.4	14.0	13.2	11.1	10.0	9.2	9.9
Former	NA	8.8	8.6	9.0	8.9	8.7	8.7	8.3	8.1
Never	NA	20.8	18.3	16.8	16.1	14.0	13.7	13.3	13.0
12									
Current	NA	13.7	14.3	16.0	17.8	18.5	18.4	17.6	17.5
Former	NA	6.9	7.7	10.3	12.0	14.2	14.8	16.2	15.4
Never	NA	14.3	14.9	19.0	21.1	24.0	25.6	26.7	25.7
13-15									
Current	NA	4.4	5.1	6.4	7.2	7.9	8.0	8.4	8.8
Former	NA	2.5	3.3	4.5	5.6	7.6	8.6	9.5	9.6
Never	NA	4.4	5.1	7.3	9.6	12.6	14.6	15.7	15.8
> =16									
Current	NA	3.4	4.0	4.7	5.3	5.1	5.6	4.9	4.6
Former	NA	3.3	3.9	5.5	6.8	8.8	9.0	9.8	10.6
Never	NA	5.1	6.0	9.6	13.6	17.3	21.2	21.7	22.6

Source: National Health Interview Surveys: 1965, 1970, 1974, 1979, 1983, 1988, 1992, 1993, 1994. Updated table, Surveillance for Selected Tobacco-Use Behaviors—United States, 1900-1994. Obtained from the Centers for Disease Control and Prevention Tobacco Information & Prevention Sourcepage. See http://www.cdc.gov. *Notes:* Current smokers reported smoking 100 or more cigarettes and currently smoked. Former smokers reported smoking 100 or more cigarettes and did not currently smoke. Newer smokers reported that they had smoked fewer than 100 cigarettes. 1. Data on education are presented for persons greater than or equal to 25 years of age.

★ 536 ★

Smoking and Tobacco

Smoking: Teen Smoking Trends

This table shows increase in smoking prevalence among teens between 1991 and 1994.

Grade	Percent who smoked in last 30 days		
	1991	1994	Percent increase 1991-1994
8th Grade	14.3	18.6	30.0
10th Grade	20.8	25.4	22.0
12th Grade	28.3	31.2	10.0

Source: Monitoring the Future Project, University of Michigan Survey Research Center, 1995. Primary source: *CQ Researcher,* 1 December 1995, p. 1072.

★ 537 ★

Smoking and Tobacco

States With the Highest Adult Smoking Rates: 1995

State	Rate
Kentucky	27.8
Indiana	27.2
Tennessee	26.5
Nevada	26.3
North Carolina	25.8

Source: Levy, Doug. "The Toll Smoking Will Take on Today's Youth: 16.6M Will Get Hooked and 5M Will Die." *USA TODAY,* 8 November 1996, p. 6D. Primary source: U.S. Centers for Disease Control and Prevention.

★ 538 ★

Smoking and Tobacco

States With the Lowest Adult Smoking Rates: 1995

State	Rate
Utah	13.2
California	15.5
Hawaii	17.8
New Jersey	19.2
Idaho	19.8

Source: Levy, Doug. "The Toll Smoking Will Take on Today's Youth: 16.6M Will Get Hooked and 5M Will Die." *USA TODAY,* 8 November 1996, p. 6D. Primary source: U.S. Centers for Disease Control and Prevention.

Substance Abuse

★ 539 ★

Alcohol and Breast Cancer

According to the source, women under the age of 45 who consume 14 or more drinks a week may double their chance of developing breast cancer... researchers think alcohol may raise the level of estrogen in blood, a hormone linked to the cancer.

Source: Cronin, Brian. "Health Report: The Bad News." *Time,* 28 April 1997, p. 26. Primary source: *Epidemiology;* Society of Behavioral Medicine meeting; Centers for Disease Control and Prevention.

★ 540 ★

Substance Abuse

Alcohol Use, by Full-Time Workers Age 18-49, by Industry Category: 1985-1993

Numbers appearing in parentheses in the table represent *Standard Industrial Classification* codes.

[In percentages]

Industry category	Heavy alcohol use					
	1985	1988	1990	1991	1992	1993
Total	9.7	7.0	7.5	7.4	6.8	7.4
Agriculture, forestry & fisheries (010-031)	11.0	[1]	[1]	8.1	6.5	9.9
Mining (040-050)	[1]	[1]	19.9	12.8	11.3	22.8
Construction (060)	18.4	20.7	21.5	15.2	11.8	13.6
Manufacturing, nondurable goods (100-222)	11.4	8.8	6.9	6.2	8.5	6.4
Manufacturing, durable goods (230-392)	N/A	4.5	5.9	7.7	9.4	6.1
Transportation, communication & other utilities (400-472)	17.4	3.8	11.7	7.9	6.4	8.2
Wholesale trade, durable goods (500-532)	11.2	[1]	[1]	8.0	[1]	10.2
Wholesale trade, nondurable goods (540-571)	N/A	[1]	[1]	10.5	11.1	13.8
Retail trade (580-691)	5.2	7.6	7.3	8.7	8.1	10.1
Finance, insurance & real estate (700-712)	4.0	9.3	5.0	5.6	3.1	4.9
Business & repair services (721-760)	12.9	5.7	5.0	7.8	8.9	12.4
Personal services (761-791)	[1]	[1]	5.5	6.8	7.3	3.8
Entertainment & recreation (800-802)	[1]	[1]	[1]	8.7	4.4	7.1
Professional & related services (812-892)	3.9	3.0	4.7	4.1	2.9	2.8
Public administration (900-932)	10.7	5.2	5.9	7.0	4.6	9.0

Source: U.S. Department of Health and Human Services. Public Health Service. Substance Abuse and Mental Health Services Administration. Office of Applied Studies. *Drug Use Among U.S. Workers: Prevalence and Trends by Occupation and Industry Categories.* Rockville, Maryland: SAMHSA, May 1996, DHHS pub. no. (SMA) 96-3089, p. 12. *Notes:* Numbers in parentheses refer to Standard Industrial Classifications. N/A indicates "not available." 1. Low precision; no estimate reported.

★ 541 ★

Substance Abuse

Drug/Alcohol Use and Rock Concerts

Data were collected from first-aid stations at the concerts.

Concert	Drug use %	Alcohol use %
Grateful Dead	55	86
Rolling Stones	28	7
Pink Floyd	17	7

Source: Montague, Jim. "Currents: Drinking, Drugs and Rock 'n' Roll." *Hospitals & Health Networks,* 5 September 1996, p. 22. Primary source: *Annals of Emergency Medicine,* 1996.

★ 542 ★

Substance Abuse

Drug Use, (Current) by Full-Time Workers Age 18-49, by Industry Category: 1985-1993

Numbers appearing in parentheses in the table represent *Standard Industrial Classification* codes.

[In percentages]

Industry category	Current illicit drug use					
	1985	1988	1990	1991	1992	1993
Total	16.7	9.9	8.2	7.5	7.0	7.3
Agriculture, forestry & fisheries (010-031)	9.0	8.9	14.5	6.3	4.7	7.8
Mining (040-050)	1	1	1	1	1	1
Construction (060)	23.1	18.5	16.9	12.7	12.2	11.6
Manufacturing, nondurable goods (100-222)	17.4	9.0	8.8	6.0	6.0	8.7
Manufacturing, durable goods (230-392)	N/A	8.3	5.2	7.1	6.3	6.7
Transportation, communication & other utilities (400-472)	18.7	7.8	8.7	4.3	7.3	5.4
Wholesale trade, durable goods (500-532)	15.0	1	1	10.3	6.1	1
Wholesale trade, nondurable goods (540-571)	N/A	1	1	7.3	10.4	3.7
Retail trade (580-691)	19.2	10.6	11.7	11.4	9.5	11.7
Finance, insurance & real estate (700-712)	12.3	6.6	7.1	6.9	4.0	5.3
Business & repair services (721-760)	11.5	16.1	9.7	11.1	10.5	11.7
Personal services (761-791)	1	1	6.0	10.2	7.9	12.4
Entertainment & recreation (800-802)	1	1	1	18.3	9.7	1
Professional & related services (812-892)	12.8	8.6	5.3	4.4	4.7	3.6
Public administration (900-932)	1	7.3	4.6	5.3	3.1	2.1

Source: U.S. Department of Health and Human Services. Public Health Service. Substance Abuse and Mental Health Services Administration. Office of Applied Studies. *Drug Use Among U.S. Workers: Prevalence and Trends by Occupation and Industry Categories.* Rockville, Maryland: SAMHSA, May 1996, DHHS pub. no. (SMA) 96-3089, p. 12. *Notes:* N/A indicates "not available." 1. Low precision; no estimate reported.

★ 543 ★

Substance Abuse

Drug Use During Pregnancy, by Race/Ethnicity: 1992

Data are the latest available and are based on a national sample of 2,613 women who delivered babies in 52 urban and rural hospitals during 1992.

Drug use	Percentage
Blacks	
Illicit drug, any	11.3
Marijuana	4.6
Cocaine	4.5
Alcohol	15.8
Cigarettes	19.8

[Continued]

★ 543 ★

Drug Use During Pregnancy, by Race/Ethnicity: 1992

[Continued]

Drug use	Percentage
Whites	
Illicit drug, any	4.4
Marijuana	3.0
Cocaine	0.4
Alcohol	22.7
Cigarettes	24.4
Hispanics	
Illicit drug, any	4.5
Marijuana	1.5
Cocaine	0.7
Alcohol	8.7
Cigarettes	5.8

Source: Mathias, Robert. "NIDA Survey Provides First National Data on Drug Use During Pregnancy." *NIDA Notes* (January/February 1995), p. 6.

★ 544 ★

Substance Abuse

Drug Use in Adults Age 26 and Older, 1976-1994: Lifetime

Drug (Unweighted N)	1976 (1,708)	1979 (3,015)	1982 (2,760)	1985 (3,979)	1988 (4,214)	1990 (5,030)	1991 (16,652)	1992 (13,857)	1993 (13,980)	1994 (2,351)
Any illicit drug use[1]	--	23.2	24.8	31.7	33.7	35.3	36.0	36.0	37.3	38.0
Marijuana/hashish	12.9	19.8	23.1	26.6	30.7	31.8	32.7	33.0	34.3	35.0
Cocaine	1.6	4.4	8.6	9.2	9.9	10.9	11.6	11.4	12.5	10.9
Inhalants	1.9	4.0	--	5.3	3.9	3.8	4.2	3.7	4.3	4.4
Hallucinogens	1.6	4.5	6.5	6.0	6.6	7.4	7.8	7.7	8.8	8.0
Heroin	0.5	1.0	1.1	1.1	1.1	0.9	1.5	0.9	1.3	1.3
Nonmedical use of any psychotherapeutic[2,3]	--	9.3	8.8	14.4	11.3	11.5	12.2	11.7	11.3	10.2
Stimulants	5.6	5.9	6.2	7.9	6.6	6.9	7.1	6.7	6.5	6.0
Sedatives	2.4	3.6	4.8	5.6	3.3	3.7	4.5	3.8	3.8	3.9
Tranquilizers	2.7	3.2	3.6	7.8	4.5	4.2	5.7	5.3	4.9	4.3
Analgesics	--	2.8	3.2	5.9	4.5	5.1	5.5	5.1	5.5	4.7

[Continued]

★ 544 ★

Drug Use in Adults Age 26 and Older, 1976-1994: Lifetime
[Continued]

Drug (Unweighted N)	1976 (1,708)	1979 (3,015)	1982 (2,760)	1985 (3,979)	1988 (4,214)	1990 (5,030)	1991 (16,652)	1992 (13,857)	1993 (13,980)	1994 (2,351)
Alcohol[3]	74.7	91.5	88.0	89.2	88.6	86.8	88.6	88.1	88.7	91.0
Cigarettes[4]	64.5	83.2	78.8	80.6	79.6	78.0	77.6	76.3	76.9	76.8

Source: U.S. Department of Health and Human Services. Public Health Service. Substance Abuse and Mental Health Services Administration. Office of Applied Studies. *National Household Survey on Drug Abuse: Main Findings 1994.* Primary source: Office of Applied Studies, SAMHSA, National Household Survey on Drug Abuse, 1976-1994-A. *Notes:*—Estimate not available. 1. Use of marijuana or hashish, cocaine (including crack), inhalants, hallucinogens (including PCP), heroin, or nonmedical use of psychotherapeutics at least once. 2. Nonmedical use of any prescription-type stimulant, sedative, tranquilizer or analgesic; does not include over-the-counter drugs. 3. Estimates before 1979 for alcohol and 1982 for psychotherapeutics may not be comparable to those for later years because of a change in methodology. 4. For 1979, includes only people who ever smoked at least five packs.

★ 545 ★

Substance Abuse

Drug Use in Middle Adults, 1993 and 1994: Lifetime

Trends in percentage of middle adults age 26-34 and older adults age 35 and older reporting drug use in their lifetime: 1993 and 1994.

Drug (Unweighted N)	26-34 Years		35+ Years		Total 26+ Years	
	1993 (8,342)	1994 (1,347)	1993 (5,638)	1994 (1,004)	1993 (13,980)	1994 (2,351)
Any illicit drug use[1]	61.1	58.9	29.9	31.8	37.3	38.0
Marijuana/hashish	59.2	56.9	26.6	28.4	34.3	35.0
Cocaine	25.6	22.9	8.5	7.3	12.5	10.9
Inhalants	9.4	9.5	2.8	2.9	4.3	4.4
Hallucinogens	15.9	14.2	6.6	6.2	8.8	8.0
Heroin	1.6	1.0[3]	1.2	1.4	1.3	1.3
Nonmedical use of any psychotherapeutic[2]	17.2	15.2	9.4	8.7	11.3	10.2
Stimulants	10.5	8.8	5.3	5.1	6.5	6.0
Sedatives	4.8	4.3	3.6	3.7	3.8	3.9
Tranquilizers	7.1	6.4	4.2	3.7	4.9	4.3
Analgesics	9.0	7.9	4.4	3.7	5.5	4.7
Alcohol	92.4	92.2	87.6	90.6	88.7	91.0
Cigarettes	74.0	72.0	77.9	78.3	76.9	76.8

Source: U.S. Department of Health and Human Services. Public Health Service. Substance Abuse and Mental Health Services Administration. Office of Applied Studies. *National Household Survey on Drug Abuse: Main Findings 1994.* Primary source: Office of Applied Studies, SAMHSA, National Household Survey on Drug Abuse, 1993 and 1994-A. *Notes:* 1. Use of marijuana or hashish, cocaine (including crack), inhalants, hallucinogens (including PCP), heroin, or nonmedical use of psychotherapeutics at least once. 2. Nonmedical use of any prescription-type stimulant, sedative, tranquilizer or analgesic; does not include over-the-counter drugs. 3. Difference between 1993 and 1994 statistically significant at the .05 level.

★ 546 ★

Substance Abuse

Drug Use in Young Adults Age 18-25, 1976-1994: Lifetime

Trends in percentage of young adults 18-25 reporting drug use in their lifetime: 1976-1994.

Drug (Unweighted N)	1976 (882)	1979 (2,044)	1982 (1,283)	1985 (1,812)	1988 (1,505)	1990 (2,052)	1991 (7,937)	1992 (7,721)	1993 (5,531)	1994 (902)
Any illicit drug use[1]	--	69.8	64.5	63.7	58.9	55.8	54.7	51.7	50.9	47.0
Marijuana/hashish	52.9	68.1	63.3	59.4	56.4	52.2	50.5	48.1	47.4	43.4
Cocaine	13.4	27.3	27.6	24.4	19.7	19.4	17.9	15.8	12.5	9.6
Inhalants	9.0	16.3	--	13.0	12.5	10.4	10.9	9.8	9.9	8.3
Hallucinogens	17.3	24.9	20.5	11.6	13.8	12.0	13.1	13.4	12.5	11.7
Heroin	3.9	3.4	1.2	1.3	0.3	0.6	0.8	1.3	0.7	0.2[5]
Nonmedical use of any psychotherapeutic[2,3]	--	29.4	27.6	26.6	17.6	15.6	17.9	15.4	14.2	11.9
Stimulants	16.6	18.0	17.3	17.5	11.3	9.0	9.4	6.8	6.4	5.3
Sedatives	11.9	16.9	17.9	11.8	5.5	4.0	4.3	3.2	2.7	1.9
Tranquilizers	9.1	15.7	14.5	12.6	7.8	5.9	7.4	6.8	5.4	4.5
Analgesics	--	11.6	11.9	11.5	9.4	8.1	10.2	8.7	8.7	7.1
Alcohol[3]	83.6	95.1	94.4	92.0	90.3	88.2	90.2	86.3	87.1	86.8
Cigarettes[4]	70.1	82.9	76.5	75.2	74.9	70.5	71.2	68.7	66.7	68.6

Source: U.S. Department of Health and Human Services. Public Health Service. Substance Abuse and Mental Health Services Administration. Office of Applied Studies. *National Household Survey on Drug Abuse: Main Findings 1994.* Primary source: Office of Applied Studies, SAMHSA, National Household Survey on Drug Abuse, 1976-1994-A. *Notes:*—Estimate not available. 1. Use of marijuana or hashish, cocaine (including crack), inhalants, hallucinogens (including PCP), heroin, or nonmedical use of psychotherapeutics at least once. 2. Nonmedical use of any prescription-type stimulant, sedative, tranquilizer or analgesic; does not include over-the-counter drugs. 3. Estimates before 1979 for alcohol and 1982 for psychotherapeutics may not be comparable to those for later years because of a change in methodology. 4. For 1979, includes only people who ever smoked at least five packs. 5. Difference between 1993 and 1994 statistically significant at the .05 level.

★ 547 ★

Substance Abuse

Drug Use in Youths, Age 12-17, 1976-1994: Lifetime

Trends in percentage of youth age 12-17 reporting drug use in their lifetime: 1976-1994.

Drug (Unweighted N)	1976 (986)	1979 (2,165)	1982 (1,581)	1985 (2,230)	1988 (3,095)	1990 (2,177)	1991 (8,005)	1992 (7,254)	1993 (6,978)	1994 (1,119)
Any illicit drug use[1]	--	34.4	28.0	29.7	24.7	22.7	20.1	16.5	17.9	22.2[5]
Marijuana/hashish	22.4	30.8	27.1	23.2	17.4	14.8	13.0	10.6	11.7	16.0[6]
Cocaine	3.4	5.6	6.5	4.8	3.4	2.6	2.4	1.7	1.1	1.3
Inhalants	8.1	9.9	--	9.6	8.8	7.8	7.0	5.7	5.9	6.2
Hallucinogens	5.1	7.2	5.0	3.2	3.5	3.3	3.3	2.6	2.9	4.0
Heroin	0.5	0.5	0.4	0.4	0.6	0.7	0.3	0.2	0.3	0.4
Nonmedical use of any psychotherapeutic[2,3]	--	7.3	10.3	12.1	7.7	10.2	7.5	5.5	5.9	6.5
Stimulants	4.4	3.5	6.7	5.5	4.2	4.5	3.0	2.1	2.1	2.6

[Continued]

★ 547 ★

Drug Use in Youths, Age 12-17, 1976-1994: Lifetime
[Continued]

Drug (Unweighted N)	1976 (986)	1979 (2,165)	1982 (1,581)	1985 (2,230)	1988 (3,095)	1990 (2,177)	1991 (8,005)	1992 (7,254)	1993 (6,978)	1994 (1,119)
Sedatives	2.8	3.2	5.8	4.1	2.3	3.3	2.4	1.5	1.4	3.2+
Tranquilizers	3.3	4.1	4.7	4.9	2.0	2.7	2.1	1.6	1.2	2.0
Analgesics	--	3.2	4.2	6.0	4.1	6.5	4.4	3.9	3.7	4.7
Alcohol[3]	53.6	69.9	64.8	55.4	50.2	48.2	46.4	39.3	41.3	41.5
Cigarettes[4]	45.5	54.0	49.4	45.3	42.3	40.2	37.9	33.7	34.5	33.5

Source: U.S. Department of Health and Human Services. Public Health Service. Substance Abuse and Mental Health Services Administration. Office of Applied Studies. *National Household Survey on Drug Abuse: Main Findings 1994.* Primary source: Office of Applied Studies, SAMHSA, National Household Survey on Drug Abuse, 1976-1994-A. *Notes:*—Estimate not available. 1. Use of marijuana or hashish, cocaine (including crack), inhalants, hallucinogens (including PCP), heroin, or nonmedical use of psychotherapeutics at least once. 2. Nonmedical use of any prescription-type stimulant, sedative, tranquilizer or analgesic; does not include over-the-counter drugs. 3. Estimates before 1979 for alcohol and 1982 for psychotherapeutics may not be comparable to those for later years because of a change in methodology. 4. For 1979, includes only people who ever smoked at least five packs. 5. Difference between 1993 and 1994 statistically significant at the .05 level. 6. Difference between 1993 and 1994 statistically significant at the .01 level.

★ 548 ★

Substance Abuse

Drug Use of Adults Age 26 and Older, 1976-1994: Past Month

Trends in percentage of adults age 26 and older reporting drug use in the past month: 1976-1994.

Drug (Unweighted N)	1976 (1,708)	1979 (3,015)	1982 (2,760)	1985 (3,979)	1988 (4,214)	1990 (5,030)	1991 (16,652)	1992 (13,857)	1993 (13,980)	1994 (2,351)
Any illicit drug use[1]	--	6.6	7.8	8.0	4.9	4.6	4.6	4.1	4.1	4.0
Marijuana/hashish	3.5	6.1	6.7	6.0	3.9	3.6	3.3	3.2	3.0	3.0
Cocaine	*	0.9	1.2	1.9	0.9	0.6	0.8	0.5	0.5	0.6
Inhalants	*	0.7	--	0.5	0.2	0.3	0.3	0.2	0.2	0.5
Hallucinogens	*	0.1	0.1	*	*	0.1	0.1	*	*	*
Heroin	*	*	0.1	*	*	*	*	*	*	0.1
Nonmedical use of any psychotherapeutic[2,3]	--	1.1	1.5	2.5	1.2	1.0	1.4	1.1	1.0	0.6
Stimulants	*	0.5	0.6	0.7	0.5	0.3	0.2	0.2	0.2	0.1[5]
Sedatives	0.5	0.4	0.4	0.6	0.3	0.1	0.3	0.3	0.2	*
Tranquilizers	*	0.3	0.4	1.0	0.6	0.2	0.5	0.4	0.2	0.1
Analgesics	--	0.1	0.4	0.9	0.4	0.6	0.5	0.7	0.5	0.4
Alcohol[3]	56.0	61.5	56.7	59.8	54.8	52.3	52.5	50.1	52.1	55.6
Cigarettes[4]	38.4	37.2	36.1	32.7	29.8	27.7	28.2	27.4	25.3	24.7

Source: U.S. Department of Health and Human Services. Public Health Service. Substance Abuse and Mental Health Services Administration. Office of Applied Studies. *National Household Survey on Drug Abuse: Main Findings 1994.* Primary source: Office of Applied Studies, SAMHSA, National Household Survey on Drug Abuse, 1976-1994-A. *Notes:*—Estimate not available. * Low precision; no estimate reported. 1. Use of marijuana or hashish, cocaine (including crack), inhalants, hallucinogens (including PCP), heroin, or nonmedical use of psychotherapeutics at least once. 2. Nonmedical use of any prescription-type stimulant, sedative, tranquilizer or analgesic; does not include over-the-counter drugs. 3. Estimates before 1979 for alcohol and 1982 for psychotherapeutics may not be comparable to those for later years because of a change in methodology. 4. For 1979, includes only people who ever smoked at least five packs. 5. Difference between 1993 and 1994 statistically significant at the .05 level.

★ 549 ★

Substance Abuse

Drug Use of Adults Age 26 and Older, 1976-1994: Past Year

Trends in percentage of adults age 26 and older reporting drug use in the past year: 1976-1994.

Drug (Unweighted N)	1976 (1,708)	1979 (3,015)	1982 (2,760)	1985 (3,979)	1988 (4,214)	1990 (5,030)	1991 (16,652)	1992 (13,857)	1993 (13,980)	1994 (2,351)
Any illicit drug use[1]	--	10.3	12.1	12.7	10.2	10.0	9.4	8.3	8.9	9.1
Marijuana/hashish	5.4	9.2	10.8	9.3	6.9	7.3	6.6	6.0	6.3	6.1
Cocaine	0.6	2.0	3.8	4.0	2.7	2.4	2.3	1.9	1.9	1.5
Inhalants	*	1.3	--	0.8	0.4	0.5	0.5	0.4	0.3	0.6
Hallucinogens	*	0.6	0.8	0.9	0.6	0.4	0.5	0.4	0.4	0.6
Heroin	*	0.1	0.1	*	0.2	0.1	0.2	0.1	0.1	0.1
Nonmedical use of any psychotherapeutic[2,3]	--	2.5	3.4	6.0	4.7	3.4	3.6	3.1	3.2	2.6
Stimulants	0.8	1.4	1.8	2.6	1.7	1.0	0.9	0.7	0.8	0.4[5]
Sedatives	0.6	0.8	1.5	2.0	1.2	0.8	0.9	0.7	0.7	0.6
Tranquilizers	1.2	0.9	1.2	2.8	1.8	1.0	1.5	1.3	1.2	1.0
Analgesics	--	0.6	1.1	2.8	2.1	1.9	1.9	1.9	1.9	1.2
Alcohol[3]	64.2	72.7	68.1	73.1	68.6	66.6	68.9	66.6	68.4	68.7
Cigarettes[4]	--	43.0	39.8	35.7	33.6	31.9	32.0	31.2	29.2	27.8

Source: U.S. Department of Health and Human Services. Public Health Service. Substance Abuse and Mental Health Services Administration. Office of Applied Studies. *National Household Survey on Drug Abuse: Main Findings 1994.* Primary source: Office of Applied Studies, SAMHSA, National Household Survey on Drug Abuse, 1976-1994-A. *Notes:*—Estimate not available. * Low precision; no estimate reported. 1. Use of marijuana or hashish, cocaine (including crack), inhalants, hallucinogens (including PCP), heroin, or nonmedical use of psychotherapeutics at least once. 2. Nonmedical use of any prescription-type stimulant, sedative, tranquilizer or analgesic; does not include over-the-counter drugs. 3. Estimates before 1979 for alcohol and 1982 for psychotherapeutics may not be comparable to those for later years because of a change in methodology. 4. For 1979, includes only people who ever smoked at least five packs. 5. Difference between 1993 and 1994 statistically significant at the .05 level.

★ 550 ★

Substance Abuse

Drug Use of Middle Adults, 1993-1994: Past Year

Trends in percentage of middle adults age 26-34 and older adults age 35 and older reporting drug use in the past year: 1993 and 1994.

Drug (Unweighted N)	Age Group (Years)/Survey Year					
	26-34 Years		35+ Years		Total 26+ Years	
	1993 (8,342)	1994 (1,347)	1993 (5,638)	1994 (1,004)	1993 (13,980)	1994 (2,351)
Any illicit drug use[1]	17.4	17.7	6.3	6.5	8.9	9.1
Marijuana/hashish	13.8	14.3	4.0	3.6	6.3	6.1
Cocaine	4.4	4.1	1.1	0.8	1.9	1.5
Inhalants	0.7	1.1	0.2	0.5	0.3	0.6
Hallucinogens	1.2	1.3	0.1	0.4	0.4	0.6
Heroin	0.1	0.1	0.1	0.2	0.1	0.1

[Continued]

★ 550 ★

Drug Use of Middle Adults, 1993-1994: Past Year
[Continued]

Drug (Unweighted N)	Age Group (Years)/Survey Year					
	26-34 Years		35+ Years		Total 26+ Years	
	1993 (8,342)	1994 (1,347)	1993 (5,638)	1994 (1,004)	1993 (13,980)	1994 (2,351)
Nonmedical use of any psychotherapeutic[2]	5.7	4.1	2.5	2.1	3.2	2.6
Stimulants	1.7	1.4	0.5	0.1[3]	0.8	0.4[3]
Sedatives	1.0	0.8	0.6	0.5	0.7	0.6
Tranquilizers	1.9	1.4	1.0	0.9	1.2	1.0
Analgesics	3.7	2.7	1.3	0.8	1.9	1.2
Alcohol	81.0	80.5	64.6	65.2	68.4	68.7
Cigarettes	35.1	32.7	27.4	26.3	29.2	27.8

Source: U.S. Department of Health and Human Services. Public Health Service. Substance Abuse and Mental Health Services Administration. Office of Applied Studies. *National Household Survey on Drug Abuse: Main Findings 1994.* Primary source: Office of Applied Studies, SAMHSA, National Household Survey on Drug Abuse, 1993 and 1994-A. *Notes:* 1. Use of marijuana or hashish, cocaine (including crack), inhalants, hallucinogens (including PCP), heroin, or nonmedical use of psychotherapeutics at least once. 2. Nonmedical use of any prescription-type stimulant, sedative, tranquilizer or analgesic; does not include over-the-counter drugs. 3. Difference between 1993 and 1994 statistically significant at the .05 level.

★ 551 ★

Substance Abuse

Drug Use of Middle Adults, 1993 and 1994: Past Month

Trends in percentage of middle adults age 26-34 and older adults age 35 and older reporting drug use in the past month: 1993 and 1994.

Drug (Unweighted N)	Age Group (Years)/Survey Year					
	26-34 Years		35+ Years		Total 26+ Years	
	1993 (8,342)	1994 (1,347)	1993 (5,638)	1994 (1,004)	1993 (13,980)	1994 (2,351)
Any illicit drug use[1]	8.5	7.8	2.8	2.9	4.1	4.0
Marijuana/hashish	6.7	6.3	1.9	2.0	3.0	3.0
Cocaine	1.0	1.5	0.4	0.3	0.5	0.6
Inhalants	0.4	0.7	0.1	0.4	0.2	0.5
Hallucinogens	0.1	*	*	*	*	*
Heroin	*	0.1	*	0.1	*	0.1
Nonmedical use of any psychotherapeutic[2]	1.9	1.3[3]	0.7	0.4	1.0	0.6
Stimulants	0.5	0.3	0.2	*	0.2	0.1[3]
Sedatives	0.3	0.1	0.1	*	0.2	*
Tranquilizers	0.5	0.4	0.1	*	0.2	0.1
Analgesics	1.0	0.4[3]	0.4	0.4	0.5	0.4

[Continued]

★ 551 ★

Drug Use of Middle Adults, 1993 and 1994: Past Month
[Continued]

Drug (Unweighted N)	Age Group (Years)/Survey Year					
	26-34 Years		35+ Years		Total 26+ Years	
	1993 (8,342)	1994 (1,347)	1993 (5,638)	1994 (1,004)	1993 (13,980)	1994 (2,351)
Alcohol	62.8	64.3	48.8	53.1	52.1	55.6
cigarettes	30.1	28.5	23.8	23.5	25.3	24.7

Source: U.S. Department of Health and Human Services. Public Health Service. Substance Abuse and Mental Health Services Administration. Office of Applied Studies. *National Household Survey on Drug Abuse: Main Findings 1994.* Primary source: Office of Applied Studies, SAMHSA, National Household Survey on Drug Abuse, 1993-1994-A. *Notes:* * Low precision; no estimate reported. 1. Use of marijuana or hashish, cocaine (including crack), inhalants, hallucinogens (including PCP), heroin, or nonmedical use of psychotherapeutics at least once. 2. Nonmedical use of any prescription-type stimulant, sedative, tranquilizer or analgesic; does not include over-the-counter drugs. 3. Difference between 1993 and 1994 statistically significant at the .05 level.

★ 552 ★

Substance Abuse

Drug Use of Young Adults Age 18-25, 1976-1994: Past Month

Trends in percentage of young adults age 18-25 reporting drug use in the past month: 1976-1994.

Drug (Unweighted N)	1976 (882)	1979 (2,044)	1982 (1,283)	1985 (1,812)	1988 (1,505)	1990 (2,052)	1991 (7,937)	1992 (7,721)	1993 (5,531)	1994 (902)
Any illicit drug use[1]	--	37.4	30.8	25.1	17.8	14.9	15.4	13.0	13.5	13.2
Marijuana/hashish	25.0	35.3	27.8	21.9	15.5	12.7	13.0	11.0	11.1	12.2
Cocaine	2.0	9.2	6.5	7.5	4.5	2.2	2.0	1.8	1.5	1.0
Inhalants	0.5	2.3	--	0.8	1.7	1.2	1.5	0.8	1.1	0.9
Hallucinogens	1.1	4.4	1.7	1.8	1.9	0.8	1.2	1.3	1.3	1.5
Heroin	*	0.4	0.1	0.3	*	0.1	0.1	0.2	0.1	0.1
Nonmedical use of any psychotherapeutic[2,3]	--	6.2	7.7	6.3	3.8	2.6	2.7	2.3	2.9	1.4[5]
Stimulants	4.7	3.5	5.0	3.8	2.4	1.2	0.8	0.7	0.9	0.3[5]
Sedatives	2.3	2.8	2.5	1.6	0.9	0.7	0.7	0.6	0.6	0.3
Tranquilizers	2.6	2.2	1.8	1.6	1.0	0.5	0.6	0.6	0.6	0.4
Analgesics	--	0.9	1.1	2.0	1.5	1.2	1.4	1.2	1.4	0.7
Alcohol[3]	69.0	75.7	67.2	70.7	65.3	63.3	63.6	59.2	59.3	63.8
Cigarettes[4]	49.4	42.6	40.2	36.6	35.2	31.5	32.2	31.9	29.0	26.5

Source: U.S. Department of Health and Human Services. Public Health Service. Substance Abuse and Mental Health Services Administration. Office of Applied Studies. *National Household Survey on Drug Abuse: Main Findings 1994.* Primary source: Office of Applied Studies, SAMHSA, National Household Survey on Drug Abuse, 1976-1994-A. *Notes:*—Estimate not available. * Low precision; no estimate reported. 1. Use of marijuana or hashish, cocaine (including crack), inhalants, hallucinogens (including PCP), heroin, or nonmedical use of psychotherapeutics at least once. 2. Nonmedical use of any prescription-type stimulant, sedative, tranquilizer or analgesic; does not include over-the-counter drugs. 3. Estimates before 1979 for alcohol and 1982 for psychotherapeutics may not be comparable to those for later years because of a change in methodology. 4. For 1979, includes only people who ever smoked at least five packs. 5. Difference between 1993 and 1994 statistically significant at the .05 level.

★ 553 ★
Substance Abuse

Drug Use of Young Adults Age 18-25, 1976-1994: Past Year

Trends in percentage of young adults age 18-25 reporting drug use in the past year: 1976-1994.

Drug (Unweighted N)	1976 (882)	1979 (2,044)	1982 (1,283)	1985 (1,812)	1988 (1,505)	1990 (2,052)	1991 (7,937)	1992 (7,721)	1993 (5,531)	1994 (902)
Any illicit drug use[1]	--	49.7	43.4	41.0	32.0	28.7	29.1	26.4	26.6	27.1
Marijuana/hashish	35.0	46.9	40.1	36.3	27.9	24.6	24.5	22.7	22.9	23.4
Cocaine	7.0	19.5	18.2	15.6	12.1	7.5	7.7	6.3	5.0	4.3
Inhalants	1.4	4.7	--	2.1	4.1	3.0	3.5	2.3	2.8	3.3
Hallucinogens	6.0	9.9	6.6	4.0	5.6	3.9	4.7	4.8	4.9	4.5
Heroin	0.6	0.8	0.4	0.6	0.3	0.5	0.3	0.5	0.3	0.1
Nonmedical use of any psychotherapeutic[2,3]	--	16.3	16.7	15.2	11.3	7.0	8.6	7.7	7.2	7.3
Stimulants	8.8	10.0	10.9	9.8	6.4	3.4	3.3	2.3	3.0	2.0
Sedatives	5.7	7.3	8.8	5.1	3.3	2.0	1.9	1.7	1.1	1.2
Tranquilizers	6.2	7.3	6.0	6.4	4.6	2.4	2.6	3.0	2.0	2.7
Analgesics	--	5.1	5.1	6.8	5.5	4.1	5.3	4.8	4.1	4.7
Alcohol[3]	77.9	86.9	82.9	86.4	81.7	80.2	82.8	77.7	79.0	80.8
Cigarettes[4]	--	56.3	48.1	43.9	44.7	39.7	41.2	41.1	38.3	36.0

Source: U.S. Department of Health and Human Services. Public Health Service. Substance Abuse and Mental Health Services Administration. Office of Applied Studies. *National Household Survey on Drug Abuse: Main Findings 1994.* Primary source: Office of Applied Studies, SAMHSA, National Household Survey on Drug Abuse, 1976-1994-A. *Notes:*—Estimate not available. 1. Use of marijuana or hashish, cocaine (including crack), inhalants, hallucinogens (including PCP), heroin, or nonmedical use of psychotherapeutics at least once. 2. Nonmedical use of any prescription-type stimulant, sedative, tranquilizer or analgesic; does not include over-the-counter drugs. 3. Estimates before 1979 for alcohol and 1982 for psychotherapeutics may not be comparable to those for later years because of a change in methodology. 4. For 1979, includes only people who ever smoked at least five packs.

★ 554 ★
Substance Abuse

Drug Use of Youth Age 12-17, 1976-1994: Past Month

Trends in percentage of youth age 12-17 reporting drug use in the past month: 1976-1994.

Drug (Unweighted N)	1976 (986)	1979 (2,165)	1982 (1,581)	1985 (2,230)	1988 (3,095)	1990 (2,177)	1991 (8,005)	1992 (7,254)	1993 (6,978)	1994 (1,119)
Any illicit drug use[1]	--	18.5	13.2	14.9	9.2	8.1	6.8	6.1	6.6	9.5[5]
Marijuana/hashish	12.3	16.8	11.9	11.9	6.4	5.2	4.3	4.0	4.9	7.3[5]
Cocaine	1.0	1.4	1.8	1.4	1.1	0.6	0.4	0.3	0.4	0.4
Inhalants	0.9	3.9	--	3.7	2.0	2.2	1.8	1.6	1.4	2.0
Hallucinogens	0.9	2.2	1.4	1.2	0.8	0.9	0.8	0.6	0.5	1.2
Heroin	*	0.2	0.1	0.1	*	*	0.1	0.1	*	*
Nonmedical use of any psychotherapeutic[2,3]	--	2.4	4.1	3.0	2.4	2.7	1.9	1.2	1.2	1.5
Stimulants	1.2	1.1	2.7	1.6	1.2	1.0	0.5	0.2	0.5	0.4
Sedatives	*	1.2	1.5	1.0	0.6	0.9	0.5	0.4	0.2	0.3

[Continued]

★ 554 ★

Drug Use of Youth Age 12-17, 1976-1994: Past Month
[Continued]

Drug (Unweighted N)	1976 (986)	1979 (2,165)	1982 (1,581)	1985 (2,230)	1988 (3,095)	1990 (2,177)	1991 (8,005)	1992 (7,254)	1993 (6,978)	1994 (1,119)
Tranquilizers	1.1	0.6	0.9	0.6	0.2	0.5	0.4	0.2	0.2	0.2
Analgesics	--	0.6	0.9	1.7	0.9	1.4	1.1	0.8	0.7	1.3
Alcohol[3]	32.4	37.3	26.3	31.0	25.2	24.5	20.3	15.7	18.0	16.3
Cigarettes[4]	23.4	12.0	15.0	15.3	11.8	11.6	10.8	9.6	9.6	9.8

Source: U.S. Department of Health and Human Services. Public Health Service. Substance Abuse and Mental Health Services Administration. Office of Applied Studies. *National Household Survey on Drug Abuse: Main Findings 1994.* Primary source: Office of Applied Studies, SAMHSA, National Household Survey on Drug Abuse, 1976-1994-A. *Notes:*—Estimate not available. * Low precision; no estimate reported. 1. Use of marijuana or hashish, cocaine (including crack), inhalants, hallucinogens (including PCP), heroin, or nonmedical use of psychotherapeutics at least once. 2. Nonmedical use of any prescription-type stimulant, sedative, tranquilizer or analgesic; does not include over-the-counter drugs. 3. Estimates before 1979 for alcohol and 1982 for psychotherapeutics may not be comparable to those for later years because of a change in methodology. 4. For 1979, includes only people who ever smoked at least five packs. 5. Difference between 1993 and 1994 statistically significant at the .05 level.

★ 555 ★

Substance Abuse

Drug Use of Youth Age 12-17, 1976-1994: Past Year

Trends in percentage of youth age 12-17 reporting drug use in the past year: 1976-1994.

Drug (Unweighted N)	1976 (986)	1979 (2,165)	1982 (1,581)	1985 (2,230)	1988 (3,095)	1990 (2,177)	1991 (8,005)	1992 (7,254)	1993 (6,978)	1994 (1,119)
Any illicit drug use[1]	--	27.3	22.2	23.3	16.8	15.9	14.8	11.7	13.6	17.6[5]
Marijuana/hashish	18.4	24.8	20.7	19.4	12.6	11.3	10.1	8.1	10.1	13.6[5]
Cocaine	2.3	4.2	4.2	3.9	2.9	2.2	1.5	1.1	0.8	1.1
Inhalants	2.9	6.1	--	5.3	3.9	4.0	4.0	3.4	3.6	3.5
Hallucinogens	2.8	4.8	3.5	2.6	2.8	2.4	2.1	1.9	2.1	3.2
Heroin	*	0.3	0.3	0.3	0.4	0.6	0.2	0.1	0.1	0.4
Nonmedical use of any psychotherapeutic[2,3]	--	5.7	8.3	8.2	5.4	7.0	5.4	3.6	3.5	4.5
Stimulants	2.2	2.9	5.6	4.1	2.8	3.0	1.9	1.3	1.6	1.3
Sedatives	1.2	2.2	4.0	2.8	1.7	2.2	1.3	1.0	0.8	2.1
Tranquilizers	1.8	2.7	3.4	3.4	1.5	1.2	1.3	1.0	0.7	1.1
Analgesics	--	2.2	3.8	4.0	3.0	4.8	3.3	2.4	2.2	3.2
Alcohol[3]	49.3	54.8	45.2	51.6	44.6	41.0	40.3	32.6	35.2	35.5
Cigarettes[4]	--	26.8	26.0	25.5	22.8	22.2	20.1	18.2	19.1	20.9

Source: U.S. Department of Health and Human Services. Public Health Service. Substance Abuse and Mental Health Services Administration. Office of Applied Studies. *National Household Survey on Drug Abuse: Main Findings 1994.* Primary source: Office of Applied Studies, SAMHSA, National Household Survey on Drug Abuse, 1976-1994-A. *Notes:*—Estimate not available. * Low precision; no estimate reported. 1. Use of marijuana or hashish, cocaine (including crack), inhalants, hallucinogens (including PCP), heroin, or nonmedical use of psychotherapeutics at least once. 2. Nonmedical use of any prescription-type stimulant, sedative, tranquilizer or analgesic; does not include over-the-counter drugs. 3. Estimates before 1979 for alcohol and 1982 for psychotherapeutics may not be comparable to those for later years because of a change in methodology. 4. For 1979, includes only people who ever smoked at least five packs. 5. Difference between 1993 and 1994 statistically significant at the .05 level.

★ 556 ★

Substance Abuse

Drug Use, (Past) by Full-Time Workers Age 18-49, by Industry Category: 1985-1993

Numbers appearing in parentheses in the table represent *Standard Industrial Classification* codes.

[In percentages]

Industry category	Past year illicit drug use					
	1985	1988	1990	1991	1992	1993
Total	26.3	19.5	18.5	15.3	14.3	15.3
Agriculture, forestry & fisheries (010-031)	15.9	1	1	19.1	10.1	1
Mining (040-050)	1	1	1	1	1	1
Construction (060)	34.7	33.7	31.9	20.5	19.6	21.8
Manufacturing, nondurable goods (100-222)	26.2	20.0	21.3	16.2	13.8	13.8
Manufacturing, durable goods (230-392)	N/A	17.9	16.7	17.2	14.0	12.8
Transportation, communication & other utilities (400-472)	27.0	15.9	16.4	13.1	19.9	15.0
Wholesale trade, durable goods (500-532)	27.2	1	1	16.4	14.7	18.1
Wholesale trade, nondurable goods (540-571)	N/A	1	1	13.5	18.1	13.1
Retail trade (580-691)	29.0	23.2	25.1	19.6	19.1	20.6
Finance, insurance & real estate (700-712)	26.2	13.3	17.5	17.0	11.8	14.9
Business & repair services (721-760)	23.0	23.4	17.1	20.4	18.2	21.0
Personal services (761-791)	1	1	1	18.0	20.8	19.2
Entertainment & recreation (800-802)	1	1	1	1	16.4	1
Professional & related services (812-892)	21.0	16.8	12.4	9.7	10.4	11.0
Public administration (900-932)	1	12.5	12.8	9.3	7.9	8.3

Source: U.S. Department of Health and Human Services. Public Health Service. Substance Abuse and Mental Health Services Administration. Office of Applied Studies. *Drug Use Among U.S. Workers: Prevalence and Trends by Occupation and Industry Categories.* Rockville, Maryland: SAMHSA, May 1996, DHHS pub. no. (SMA) 96-3089, p. 12. *Notes:* Numbers in parentheses refer to Standard Industrial Classifications. N/A indicates "not available." 1. Low precision; no estimate reported.

★ 557 ★

Substance Abuse

High School Students' Use of Substances

This table shows the percentages of high school students using substances as recorded in a report issued by the National Parents' Resource Institute for Drug Education (PRIDE).

Substance	% of high schoolers using substances	
	1991	1995
Beer	56.2	57.4
Liquor	48.7	51.5
Cigarettes	35.2	44.4
Marijuana	16.9	28.2
Uppers	7.6	9.3
Hallucinogens	4.9	7.7

[Continued]

★ 557 ★

High School Students' Use of Substances
[Continued]

Substance	% of high schoolers using substances	
	1991	1995
Inhalants	5.0	7.5
Downers	4.6	5.5
Cocaine	3.4	4.5

Source: "Teenagers and the 'Madness' of Drugs." *U.S. News & World Report,* 13 November 1995, p. 25. Primary source: National Parents' Resource Institute for Drug Education.

★ 558 ★

Substance Abuse

Occupations With the Highest Rates of Current Illicit Drug Use by Full-Time Workers Age 18-49: 1991-1993

Numbers appearing in parentheses in the table represent *Standard Industrial Classification* codes.

[In percentages]

Occupation category	Percentage reporting drug use
Other construction (563-566,573,588-599)	17.3
Construction supervisors (553-558)	17.2
Food preparation (436-444)	16.3
Waiters and waitresses (435)	15.4
Helpers and laborers (864-873)	13.1
Writers, designers, artists, and athletes (183,185-188,193-194,199)	13.1
Janitors (453)	13.0
Purchasing agents and buyers (028-033)	12.9
Auto mechanics (505)	12.8
Construction laborers (865,869)	12.8
Other laborers (889)	12.8

Source: U.S. Department of Health and Human Services. Public Health Service. Substance Abuse and Mental Health Services Administration. Office of Applied Studies. *Drug Use Among U.S. Workers: Prevalence and Trends by Occupation and Industry Categories.* Rockville, Maryland: SAMHSA, May 1996, DHHS pub. no. (SMA) 96-3089, p. 17.

★ 559 ★

Substance Abuse

Occupations With the Highest Rates of Heavy Alcohol Use by Full-Time Workers Age 18-49: 1991-1993

Numbers in parentheses in the table represent *Standard Industrial Classification* codes.

[In percentages]

Occupation category	Percentage
Other construction (563-566,573,588-599)	20.6
Construction laborers (865,869)	19.9
Helpers and laborers (864-873)	19.5
Auto mechanics (505)	16.3
Food preparation (436-444)	16.3
Truck drivers, light (805-806)	15.1
Vehicle and mobile equipment mechanics and repairers (505-519)	14.9
Painters, plasterers, and plumbers (579-587)	14.8
Carpenters (567-569)	13.8
Material moving operators (844-859)	13.8

Source: U.S. Department of Health and Human Services. Public Health Service. Substance Abuse and Mental Health Services Administration. Office of Applied Studies. *Drug Use Among U.S. Workers: Prevalence and Trends by Occupation and Industry Categories.* Rockville, Maryland: SAMHSA, May 1996, DHHS pub. no. (SMA) 96-3089, p. 19.

★ 560 ★

Substance Abuse

Occupations With the Lowest Rates of Current Illicit Drug Use by Full-Time Workers Age 18-49: 1991-1993

Numbers in parentheses in the table represent *Standard Industrial Classification* codes.

[In percentages]

Occupation category	Percentage
Police and detectives (418-424)	1.0
Administrative support (389)	2.2
Teachers (113-159)	2.3
Child care workers (406,468)	2.6
Dental and health aides (445-446)	2.8
Data clerks (384-386)	3.2
Records processing clerks (326-336)	3.5
Computer programmers and operators (229,308-309)	3.6

[Continued]

★ 560 ★

Occupations With the Lowest Rates of Current Illicit Drug Use by Full-Time Workers Age 18-49: 1991-1993

[Continued]

Occupation category	Percentage
Engineers (044-059)	3.9
Therapists (098-106)	4.0

Source: U.S. Department of Health and Human Services. Public Health Service. Substance Abuse and Mental Health Services Administration. Office of Applied Studies. *Drug Use Among U.S. Workers: Prevalence and Trends by Occupation and Industry Categories.* Rockville, Maryland: SAMHSA, May 1996, DHHS pub. no. (SMA) 96-3089, p. 17.

★ 561 ★

Substance Abuse

Occupations With the Lowest Rates of Heavy Alcohol Use by Full-Time Workers Age 18-49: 1991-1993

Numbers appearing in parentheses in the table represent *Standard Industrial Classification* codes.

[In percentages]

Occupation category	Percentage
Data clerks (384-386)	0.8
Personnel and training specialists (008,027)	1.1
Secretaries and typists (313-315)	1.4
Bank tellers (383)	1.5
Bookkeepers (337)	1.7
Clinical laboratory and technologists (203,208)	2.2
Teachers (113-159)	2.2
Dental and health aides (445-446)	2.3
Computer scientists and analysts (064-065)	2.4
Child care workers (406,408)	2.6

Source: U.S. Department of Health and Human Services. Public Health Service. Substance Abuse and Mental Health Services Administration. Office of Applied Studies. *Drug Use Among U.S. Workers: Prevalence and Trends by Occupation and Industry Categories.* Rockville, Maryland: SAMHSA, May 1996, DHHS pub. no. (SMA) 96-3089, p. 19.

★ 562 ★

Substance Abuse

Problems Affecting Teenagers: 1996

Data refer to the percentage of all survey respondents who were asked what issues trouble most teens.

Problem	Percentage
Drugs	31
Social pressures	14
Crime	14
Sexual issues	7

Source: Graff, James L. "High Times At New Trier High." *Time,* 9 December 1996, p. 33. Primary source: CASA survey of Teens and Adults.

★ 563 ★

Substance Abuse

Substance Use and Binge Drinking by High School Seniors and Eighth-Graders, by Sex and Race: 1995

Data on substance use pertain to use within the past month. Data on binge drinking pertain to drinking within the past two weeks.

Substance, sex, race, and grade in school	1995
Cigarettes	
All seniors	33.5
Male	34.5
Female	32.0
White	37.3
Black	15.0
All eighth-graders	19.1
Male	18.8
Female	19.0
White	21.7
Black	8.2
Marijuana	
All seniors	21.2
Male	24.6
Female	17.2
White	21.5
Black	17.8

[Continued]

★ 563 ★

Substance Use and Binge Drinking by High School Seniors and Eighth-Graders, by Sex and Race: 1995

[Continued]

Substance, sex, race, and grade in school	1995
All eighth-graders	9.1
Male	9.8
Female	8.2
White	9.0
Black	7.0
Cocaine	
All seniors	1.8
Male	2.2
Female	1.3
White	1.7
Black	0.4
All eighth-graders	1.2
Male	1.1
Female	1.2
White	1.0
Black	0.4
Inhalants	
All seniors	3.2
Male	3.9
Female	2.5
White	3.7
Black	1.1
All eighth-graders	6.1
Male	5.6
Female	6.6
White	7.0
Black	2.3
Alcohol[1]	
All seniors	51.3
Male	55.7
Female	47.0
White	54.8
Black	37.4

[Continued]

★ 563 ★

Substance Use and Binge Drinking by High School Seniors and Eighth-Graders, by Sex and Race: 1995

[Continued]

Substance, sex, race, and grade in school	1995
All eighth-graders	24.6
Male	25.0
Female	24.0
White	25.4
Black	17.3
Binge drinking[2]	
All seniors	29.8
Male	36.9
Female	23.0
White	32.9
Black	15.5
All eighth-graders	14.5
Male	15.1
Female	13.9
White	14.5
Black	10.0

Source: U.S. Department of Health and Human Services. Public Health Service. Centers for Disease Control and Prevention. National Center for Health Statistics. *Health, United States, 1995.* Hyattsville, MD: Public Health Service, 1996, p. 177. Primary source: National Institute on Drug Abuse. Monitoring the Future study. Annual surveys. *Notes:* Monitoring the Future Study excludes high school dropouts (about 15 percent of the age group during the 1980's) and absentees (about 16-19 percent of high school students). High school dropouts and absentees have higher drug usage than those included in the survey. Estimates of the use of substances from the National Household Survey on Drug Abuse and the Monitoring the Future Study differ because of different methodologies, sampling frames, and tabulation categories. Data for 1994 are based on 1994-A estimates. 1. In 1993 the alcohol question was changed to indicate that a "drink" meant "more than a few sips." 1993 data based on a half sample 2. Five or more drinks in a row at least once in the prior 2-week period.

★ 564 ★

Substance Abuse

Substance Use in the Past Month by Women Age 15-44, by Pregnancy and Parental Status: 1994

Sex/Parental status	Cigarettes	Moderate to heavy alcohol	Illicit drugs
No children and not pregnant	29.2	16.3	8.3
Pregnant	21.2	4.4	1.8
Have children under 18 years of age and not pregnant	31.6	9.7	6.7

Source: U.S. Department of Health and Human Services. Public Health Service. Centers for Disease Control and Prevention. National Center for Health Statistics. *Health, United States, 1995.* Hyattsville, MD: Public Health Service, 1996, p. 69. Primary source: Centers for Disease Control and Prevention, National Center for Health Statistics, National Home and Hospice Care Survey.

★ 565 ★

Substance Abuse

Substances Most Frequently Consumed

Data refer to people who report having used the substance within the last month.

Drug	Number of users
Heroin	200,000
Amphetamines	800,000
Cocaine/Crack	1,500,000
Marijuana	10,000,000
Alcohol	11,000,000[2]
Nicotine	61,000,000
Caffeine	130,000,000[1]

Source: Nash, J. Madeleine. "Addicted." *Time,* 5 May 1997, p. 72. Primary source: SAMHSA; National Coffee Association. *Notes:* 1. Coffee drinkers. 2. Number of abusers.

★ 566 ★

Substance Abuse

Users of Illicit Drugs, Alcohol and Tobacco, 1994: Lifetime

Percentage and estimated number of users (in thousands) of illicit drugs, alcohol and tobacco in the U.S. civilian, noninstitutionalized population age 12 and older in their lifetime, the past year and the past month: 1994.

| Drug | Time Period | | | | | |
| | Lifetime | | Past year | | Past month | |
	Percent	Number of users (in 1000s)	Percent	Number of users (in 1000s)	Percent	Number of users (in 1000s)
Any illicit drug user[1]	37.6	78,660	12.4	25,922	5.8	12,216
Marijuana/hashish	34.1	71,454	9.2	19,212	4.7	9,764
Cocaine	9.7	20,314	1.9	3,889	0.6	1,265
Crack	1.8	3,768	0.4	778	0.2	331
Inhalants	5.1	10,734	1.3	2,652	0.7	1,503
Hallucinogens	8.1	16,964	1.4	2,876	0.3	686
PCP	4.3	9,023	0.2	478	0.1	201
Heroin	1.1	2,215	0.2	349	0.1	191
Nonmedical use of any psychotherapeutic[2]	10.1	21,047	3.4	7,170	0.8	1,609
Stimulants	5.5	11,583	0.7	1,428	0.1	276
Sedatives	3.5	7,412	0.8	1,722	0.1	217
Tranquilizers	4.1	8,617	1.2	2,590	0.2	332
Analgesics	5.0	10,475	1.9	3,940	0.6	1,183
Alcohol	85.3	178,551	66.9	140,093	52.6	110,249
Cigarettes	71.2	149,161	28.1	58,931	23.4	48,939
Smokeless tobacco	15.0	31,510	4.7	9,755	3.0	6,351

Source: U.S. Department of Health and Human Services. Public Health Service. Substance Abuse and Mental Health Services Administration. Office of Applied Studies. *National Household Survey on Drug Abuse: Main Findings 1994.* Primary source: Office of Applied Studies, SAMHSA, National Household Survey on Drug Abuse, 1994-A. *Notes:* 1. Use of marijuana or hashish, cocaine (including crack), inhalants, hallucinogens (including PCP), heroin, or nonmedical use of psychotherapeutics at least once. 2. Nonmedical use of any prescription-type stimulant, sedative, tranquilizer or analgesic; does not include over-the-counter drugs.

Chapter 5
HEALTH IN THE WORKPLACE

Occupational Health and Safety: Disabilities

★ 567 ★

Carpal Tunnel Syndrome

"In 1993, 41,019 private industry workers missed days on the job because of CTS, up from 33,042 the previous year, according to the Bureau of Labor Statistics. Industries requiring long hours of repetitive motion work, such as dressmaking, meat packing, and telecommunications, see the most serious CTS problems."

Source: Zack Figura, Susannah. "Carpal Tunnel Syndrome: The Facts Behind the Hype." *Managing Office Technology* (March 1997), p. 28.

★ 568 ★

Occupational Health and Safety: Disabilities

Repetitive Strain Injuries

"The U.S. Department of Labor estimates that about half the nation's workforce will suffer some sort of cumulative trauma disorder by 2000. In 1993, the last year for which information is available, the Labor Department reported 302,400 cases of RSI injuries. That's up from 23,000 in 1981."

Source: Garner, Rochelle. "Painful Lessons." *Computerworld,* 20 January 1997, p. 87.

Occupational Health and Safety: Lost Work Time

★ 569 ★

Lost Work Time of Older and Younger Workers

"Workers age 55 and over are one-third less likely to be injured on the job seriously enough to lose time from work, according to the Bureau of Labor Statistics. However, when older workers are injured seriously, their recuperation time is usually double that of younger workers."

Source: "Here's One to Think About." *Risk Management* (July 1996), p. 9. Primary source: *Wall Street Journal,* 7 May 1996.

★ 570 ★

Occupational Health and Safety: Lost Work Time

Reasons for Lost Work Time, by Disability: 1995

Data refer to workers age 15 and older.

Type of disability	Percentage
Orthopedic	17
Cardiovascular	16
Sensory	12
Internal	10
Blood/skin	8
Respiratory	4
Neurological	4
Behavioral	2
Cancer	1

Source: Neuborne, Ellen. "Work Rules Stir Debate on Mental Health." *USA TODAY,* 21 May 1997, p. 4B.

Occupational Illnesses & Injuries

★ 571 ★

Blood Exposure Risks in the Health Care Field: 1995

According to the source, over one-third of infection control practitioners estimated that 50% or less of exposures to blood are actually reported at their facilities.

Percentage of blood exposures reported	Percentage of health care workers reporting
0-20	7
21-40	8
41-60	29
61-80	18
81-100	37

Source: "AJNNewsline: Many Aren't Reporting Exposures to Blood." *American Journal of Nursing* (May 1995), p. 72. Primary source: 3M Health Care.

★ 572 ★

Occupational Illnesses & Injuries

Cardiovascular Risks Among U.S. Employees: 1995

Table presents factors believed to adversely affect the cardiovascular health of employees.

Risk among employees	Percentage
Report high stress levels	21-35
High blood pressure	22-38
Overweight by 20% or more	26-40
Smoke cigarettes	18-45
High or borderline-high cholesterol	45-60
Exercise fewer than 3x per week	65-72
Drink alcoholic beverages	47-80

Source: "Snapshots of the Workplace Health Industry: Risk Takers." *Workplace Vitality* (July/ August 1996), p. 15. Primary source: Based on a survey of more than 75,000 employees in more than 100 workplaces.

★ 573 ★

Occupational Illnesses & Injuries

Dog Bites Sustained by Letter Carriers: 1995

Table presents the top danger zones for mail carriers. According to the source, of the estimated 4.7 million people bitten by dogs in 1995, children were usually the victims.

City	Number of letter carriers bitten
Houston, TX	117
Santa Ana, CA	101
San Jose, CA	75
Chicago, IL	75
San Antonio, TX	72

Source: "Notebook: Mail Handlers." *Time,* 24 June 1996, p. 20. Primary source: U.S. Postal Service; Humane Society of the U.S.

Chapter 6
HEALTH EXPENDITURES AND FUNDING

The U.S. health care establishment is said to be consuming an ever growing percentage of the Gross Domestic Product. In this chapter, tables present data on both the big picture and costs at the level of detail. Some financial information is also presented in Chapter 7 - Health Care Programs, so that all information on such topics as Medicaid and Medicare could be kept together. Topics covered in this chapter include costs, expenditures, prices, and trends in the movement of prices and costs. For international comparisons, please see Chapter 11.

Costs

★ 574 ★

Birth Defect Costs: Correctable Conditions

Correctable conditions	Cost per case	Total cost (millions)
Diaphragmatic hernia	250,000	364
Urinary tract obstruction	84,000	343
Colorectal/anal atresia[1]	123,000	219
Tracheo-esophageal fistula[2]	145,000	165
Omphalocele[3]	176,000	132

Source: "News & Trends: Addressing the High Cost of Birth Defects." *Business & Health* (November 1995), p. 16. Primary source: *Economic Costs of Congenital Abnormalities,* California Birth Defects Monitoring Program, 1995. *Notes:* 1. Absence of an anal opening. 2. Abnormal passage connecting the trachea to the esophagus. 3. Protrusion of the intestines or organs through the abdominal wall at the navel.

★ 575 ★
Costs

Birth Defect Costs: Disabling Conditions

Disabling conditions	Cost per case	Total cost (millions)
Cerebral palsy	503,000	2,425
Down's syndrome	451,000	1,848
Cleft lip/palate	101,000	697
Transposition of the great vessels[1]	267,000	515
Spina bifida	294,000	489

Source: "News & Trends: Addressing the High Cost of Birth Defects." *Business & Health* (November 1995), p. 16. Primary source: *Economic Costs of Congenital Abnormalities,* California Birth Defects Monitoring Program, 1995. *Note:* 1. Reversal of the aorta and pulmonary artery.

★ 576 ★
Costs

Cancer: Average Hospital Inpatient Costs by Month Prior to Death

Time in hospital	Average cost ($) when patient comes from --		
	Hospice	Home care	Other
Last month prior to death	765	5,747	6,423
Second month prior to death	602	2,535	4,661

Source: Amado, Anthony J., Virginia Grow, and James Nofziger. "An Evaluation of Hospice Care with Terminally Ill Cancer Patients." *Caring Magazine* (November 1995), p. 30.

★ 577 ★
Costs

Cancer: Average Total Cost for Last Month of Life

Type of care	Average Cost ($)
Hospice	5,058
Homecare	7,710
Other	8,839

Source: Amado, Anthony J., Virginia Grow, and James Nofziger. "An Evaluation of Hospice Care with Terminally Ill Cancer Patients." *Caring Magazine* (November 1995), p. 30.

★ 578 ★

Costs

Cost of Rehabilitation

Average costs of rehabilitation associated with selected medical cases.

Medical problem	Average cost ($) of rehabilitation per case
Spinal cord injury	46,409
Traumatic brain injury	36,161
Stroke	24,672
Lower extremity amputation	22,005
Cardiac	16,411
Joint replacement	15,104

Source: "Cost of Rehabilitation." *USA TODAY,* 18 September 1995, p. 1. Primary source: Medical Rehabilitation Education Foundation.

★ 579 ★

Costs

Direct Costs for TB in 1991

This table shows calculated direct costs for the treatment of tuberculosis, a resurgent disease.

	Costs ($ million)
Total	703.1
Contact investigations	3.4
Surveillance and outbreak investigations	3.6
Preventive therapy	17.9
Screening	72.1
Inpatient care	423.8
Outpatient care	182.3

Source: Research Activities, AHCPR, Rockville, MD (November/December 1995), p. 15.

★ 580 ★

Costs

Health Care as Leading Employment Benefit Cost

[In dollars per employee per year]

Benefits	$ per employee per year
Health care	3,500
Profit sharing	2,900
Retiree health care	2,800
Pension	2,700
Flexible benefits	2,400
ESOP	1,400
Salary reduction	1,200
Long-term disability insurance	330
Life insurance	250

Source: "Trends: Health Benefits Most Costly." *Corporate Cashflow* (January 1996), p. 12.

★ 581 ★

Costs

Health Insurance Costs per Enrollee, 1994-1995

Insurance plan	Cost ($) per enrollee	
	1994	1995
Indemnity	3,497	3,583
Preferred Provider Organization	3,100	3,083
Point of Service	3,051	3,194
Health Maintenance Organization	3,326	2,947

Source: "The Week in Medicine: Incredible Shrinking Indemnity Coverage." *American Medical News,* 23-30 September 1996, p. 2. Primary source: Johnson and Higgins, July 1996.

★ 582 ★

Costs

Monthly Costs for Treating Gastrointestinal Disorders, 1996, by Treatment: Antacids

Antacid	Cost per month ($)
Maalox ES	18
Mylanta DS	22
Riopan Plus	56
Tums	27

Source: "Direct Costs for GI Disorder Treatment Regimens." *Business & Health* (August 1996), p. 63. Primary source: *1996 Red Book* and *Physician's Desk Reference,* Medical Economics and Lewin Group, Fairfax, Virginia.

★ 583 ★

Costs

Monthly Costs for Treating Gastrointestinal Disorders, 1996, by Treatment: Prescription Drugs

Drug	Cost per month ($)
Omprazole	91
Lansoprazole	96
Tagamet HB 100 mg	51
Cimetidine 400 mg	43
Zantac 75	44
Ranitidine 150 mg	78
Pepcid AC	34
Famotidine 20 mg	76
Nizatidine 150 mg	86

Source: "Direct Costs for GI Disorder Treatment Regimens." *Business & Health* (August 1996), p. 63. Primary source: *1996 Red Book* and *Physician's Desk Reference,* Medical Economics and Lewin Group, Fairfax, Virginia.

★ 584 ★

Costs

Selected National Economic Indicators: 1992-1996

Item	Calendar year				1996	
	1992	1993	1994	1995	Q1	Q2
Gross Domestic Product						
Billions of Dollars	6,244	6,553	6,936	7,254	7,427	7,545
Billions of 1992 Chain Weighted Dollars	6,244	6,386	6,609	6,743	6,814	6,893
Implicit Price Deflator	100.0	102.6	104.9	107.6	109.0	109.5
Personal Income						
Personal Income in Billions	5,264	5,480	5,753	6,115	6,309	6,412
Disposable Income in Billions	4,614	4,790	5,022	5,321	5,484	5,542
Prices[1]						
Consumer Price Index, All	140.3	144.5	148.2	152.4	155.0	156.5
All Items Less Medical	137.5	141.2	144.7	148.6	151.0	152.5
Energy	103.0	104.2	104.6	105.2	105.3	112.0
Food and Beverages	138.7	141.6	144.9	148.9	151.6	152.8
Medical Care	190.1	201.4	211.0	220.5	226.0	227.4
Producer Price Index,[2] Finished Goods						
Consumer Goods	121.7	123.0	123.3	125.6	127.4	129.3
Energy	77.8	78.0	77.0	78.1	78.8	84.2
Food	123.3	125.6	126.8	129.0	131.1	132.1
Annual Percent Change or change from same period a year ago						
Gross Domestic Product						
Billions of Dollars	5.5	4.9	5.8	4.6	3.9	4.7
Billions of 1992 Chain Weighted Values	2.7	2.3	3.5	2.0	1.7	2.7
Implicit Price Deflator	2.7	2.6	2.3	2.5	2.1	2.0
Personal Income						
Personal Income in Billions	6.0	4.1	5.0	6.3	5.1	5.6
Disposable Income in Billions	6.2	3.8	4.8	6.0	4.8	5.1
Prices[1]						
Consumer Price Index, All	3.0	3.0	2.6	2.8	2.7	2.8
All Items Less Medical	2.7	2.7	2.5	2.7	2.7	2.8
Energy	0.5	1.1	0.5	0.6	1.6	5.2
Food and Beverages	1.4	2.1	2.3	2.8	2.5	2.8
Medical Care	7.4	6.0	4.8	4.5	3.8	3.7
Producer Price Index[2] Finished Goods						
Consumer Goods	1.0	1.1	0.2	1.9	2.3	2.9

[Continued]

★ 584 ★

Selected National Economic Indicators: 1992-1996
[Continued]

Item	Calendar year				1996	
	1992	1993	1994	1995	Q1	Q2
Energy	-0.4	0.3	-1.2	1.4	2.8	5.2
Food	-0.7	1.9	0.9	1.8	2.2	3.2

Source: U.S. Department of Commerce. Bureau of Economic Analysis: Survey of Current Business. Washington, DC: U.S. Government Printing Office. Monthly reports for January 1992-March 1996. *Notes:* 1. Base Period = 1982-84, unless noted. 2. Formerly called the "Wholesale Price Index." Q designates quarter of year. Unlike tables 1-5 quarterly data on GDP, personal income, and disposable personal income, are seasonally adjusted at annual rates.

Expenditures

★ 585 ★

Health Care Spending

Table shows where the nation's health care dollar came from and how it was spent.

Source	Percent of total
Where it came from	
Private health insurance	31
Medicare	19
Out-of-pocket payments	19
Medicaid	14
Other government programs	13
Other private	4
Where it went	
Hospital care	36
Other personal health care	25
Physician services	20
Other spending	11
Nursing home care	8

Source: "Health Care Finance. The Nation's Health Dollar: Calendar Year 1995." *Missouri Medicine,* vol. 94, no. 5 (May 1997), p. 223. Primary source: Health Care Financing Administration, Office of the Actuary: Data from the Office of National Health Statistics. *Notes:* 'Other private' includes industrial inplant health services, non-patient revenues, and privately financed construction. 'Other personal health care' includes dental services, other professional services, home health care, drugs and other non-durable medical products, vision products and other durable medical products, and other miscellaneous health care services. 'Other spending' covers program administration and the net cost of private health insurance, government public health, and research and construction.

★ 586 ★

Expenditures

Cancer: Research Funding

Table shows expenditures on research by type of cancer.

Cancer site	1995 Spending estimated (in mil.)	1996 Spending (in mil.)
Breast	$308.7	$336.7
Colorectal	96.5	99.3
Lung	13.9	116.9
Prostate	64.3	70.9

Source: Cancer Research Funding, Cancer Facts, U.S. Department of Health and Human Services, Public Health Service, National Institutes of Health, National Cancer Institute, September 1996.

★ 587 ★

Expenditures

Examples of Insurance Payment Final Use

Table shows examples of how monthly insurance payments are allocated to actual medical care and administrative costs/profits.

Organization	Medical care[1] (%)	Administration and profit (%)	Total monthly payment ($)
Blue Cross type old fee-for service programs (not-for-profit)	96.0	4.0	200
Kaiser Permanente (not-for-profit HMO)	94.0	6.0	145
Harvard Pilgrim (not-for-profit HMO)	89.0	11.0	150
HealthNet (for-profit HMO)	80.0	20.0	115

Source: Church, George J. "Backlash Against HMOs." *Time,* 14 April 1997, p. 32. Primary source: Company reports.

★ 588 ★

Expenditures

Expenditures for Health Care Plans by Employers and Employees, 1992

This table presents data on expenditures for health care in private industry and state and local governments, 1992, by industry, region, and establishment employment size; total and the share by employers and employees.

	Expenditures in billions of dollars				
	Total expenditure	Employer expenditure	Percent of total	Employee expenditure	Percent of total
Civilian workers[1]	$258.5	$221.4	86%	$37.2	14%
State and local government	54.8	46.6	85	8.3	15
Private industry	203.7	174.8	86	28.9	14
Goods-producing industries[2]	74.0	65.6	89	8.4	11
Construction	8.1	7.2	89	.9	11
Manufacturing	63.4	56.3	89	7.1	11
Service-producing industries	129.7	109.2	84	20.5	16
Transportation and utilities	22.4	20.9	93	1.5	7
Wholesale trade	17.1	14.6	86	2.4	14
Retail trade	20.2	15.6	77	4.6	23
Finance, insurance, and real estate	19.1	15.5	81	3.6	19
Services	50.9	42.5	84	8.4	17
Establishments employing:					
Fewer than 100 workers	92.2	78.1	85	14.2	15
100 workers or more	166.3	143.3	86	23.0	14
100-499 workers	53.5	45.0	84	8.5	16
500 workers or more	112.8	98.4	87	14.4	13
Region[3]:					
Northeast	67.0	59.3	89	7.7	12
South	72.5	58.7	81	13.8	19
Midwest	63.6	55.7	88	7.9	12
West	55.4	47.6	86	7.7	14

Source: U.S. Department of Labor. Press Release. December 20, 1993. The data presented are from a special survey of expenditures on health care plans conducted by the U.S. Department of Labor's Bureau of Labor Statistics for the Department of Health and Human Services' Health Care Financing Administration. Expenditures included employer and employee costs for health care plans, typically insurance premiums. *Notes:* Components may not sum to totals because of rounding. 1. Excludes agriculture, private households, and the federal government. 2. Includes mining in addition to industries shown. Mining is not shown separately because the standard errors on expenditure estimates are greater than 50 percent of those estimates. 3. The regional coverage is as follows: Northeast—Connecticut, Maine, Massachusetts, New Hampshire, New Jersey, New York, Pennsylvania, Rhode Island, and Vermont; South—Alabama, Arkansas, Delaware, District of Columbia, Florida, Georgia, Kentucky, Louisiana, Maryland, Mississippi, North Carolina, Oklahoma, South Carolina, Tennessee, Texas, Virginia, and West Virginia; Midwest—Illinois, Indiana, Iowa, Kansas, Michigan, Minnesota, Missouri, Nebraska, North Dakota, Ohio, South Dakota, and Wisconsin; and West—Alaska, Arizona, California, Colorado, Hawaii, Idaho, Montana, Nevada, New Mexico, Oregon, Utah, Washington, and Wyoming.

★ 589 ★

Expenditures

Expenditures on Hospital Care: 1980-1993

This table shows hospital care expenditures by geographic division and State and average annual percent change for the United States for selected years 1980-1993.

[Data are compiled by the Health Care Financing Administration]

Geographic division and State[1]	Amount in millions						Average annual percent change	
	1980	1985	1990	1991	1992	1993	1980-90	1990-93
United States[2]	$101,510	$166,545	$245,239	$279,820	$303,461	$323,919	9.6	8.4
New England	6,467	10,332	15,540	16,773	17,855	19,056	9.2	7.0
Maine	460	735	1,119	1,207	1,280	1,376	9.3	7.1
New Hampshire	313	590	1,056	1,102	1,233	1,388	12.9	9.5
Vermont	174	290	447	494	532	562	9.9	7.9
Massachusetts	3,646	5,628	8,159	8,826	9,380	10,034	8.4	7.1
Rhode Island	481	760	1,095	1,177	1,237	1,314	8.6	6.3
Connecticut	1,396	2,328	3,664	3,967	4,193	4,380	10.1	6.1
Middle Atlantic	18,361	29,462	45,472	49,673	53,779	57,854	9.5	8.4
New York	9,582	14,585	22,739	24,784	26,387	28,001	9.0	7.2
New Jersey	2,763	4,751	7,857	8,586	9,406	10,312	11.0	9.5
Pennsylvania	6,017	10,126	14,876	16,303	17,987	19,540	9.5	9.5
East North Central	19,590	30,093	42,984	47,026	50,835	54,172	8.2	8.0
Ohio	4,808	8,026	11,416	12,359	13,394	14,305	9.0	7.8
Indiana	2,125	3,399	5,288	5,918	6,473	6,998	9.5	9.8
Illinois	6,217	8,998	12,400	13,560	14,744	15,621	7.1	8.0
Michigan	4,482	6,882	9,500	10,309	11,008	11,711	7.8	7.2
Wisconsin	1,959	2,788	4,377	4,880	5,216	5,537	8.4	8.2
West North Central	7,810	12,261	18,012	19,664	21,116	22,252	8.7	7.3
Minnesota	1,740	2,716	4,094	4,473	4,674	4,796	8.9	5.4
Iowa	1,179	1,733	2,634	2,856	2,996	3,111	8.4	5.7
Missouri	2,532	4,172	5,986	6,527	7,077	7,652	9.0	8.5
North Dakota	313	524	717	786	853	903	8.6	8.0
South Dakota	275	450	694	786	863	920	9.7	9.9
Nebraska	681	1,060	1,587	1,749	1,881	2,003	8.8	8.1
Kansas	1,090	1,607	2,300	2,487	2,771	2,868	7.8	7.6
South Atlantic	15,588	26,925	44,077	48,917	52,971	56,711	11.0	8.8
Delaware	259	434	709	777	854	937	10.6	9.7
Maryland	2,034	2,980	4,655	5,097	5,516	5,926	8.6	8.4
District of Columbia	913	1,469	2,133	2,291	2,437	2,612	8.9	7.0
Virginia	2,077	3,530	5,661	6,240	6,618	7,031	10.5	7.5
West Virginia	831	1,219	1,763	1,977	2,190	2,346	7.8	10.0
North Carolina	1,963	3,250	5,901	6,658	7,311	7,801	11.6	9.8
South Carolina	978	1,753	3,108	3,588	3,962	4,221	12.3	10.7
Georgia	2,148	3,885	6,685	7,398	8,092	8,704	12.0	9.2
Florida	4,385	8,404	13,462	14,890	15,992	17,131	11.9	8.4

[Continued]

★ 589 ★

Expenditures on Hospital Care: 1980-1993
[Continued]

Geographic division and State[1]	Amount in millions						Average annual percent change	
	1980	1985	1990	1991	1992	1993	1980-90	1990-93
East South Central	5,713	9,673	15,149	16,955	18,715	19,921	10.2	9.6
Kentucky	1,230	2,157	3,437	3,900	4,268	4,515	10.8	9.5
Tennessee	2,027	3,483	5,511	6,146	6,671	7,208	10.5	9.4
Alabama	1,590	2,606	4,015	4,511	5,028	5,301	9.7	9.7
Mississippi	867	1,427	2,187	2,398	2,658	2,897	9.7	9.8
West South Central	9,210	16,230	25,344	28,335	31,236	33,601	10.7	9.9
Arkansas	746	1,313	2,109	2,336	2,546	2,723	11.0	8.9
Louisiana	1,744	3,155	4,627	5,164	5,575	5,956	10.2	8.8
Oklahoma	1,177	1,896	2,674	2,938	3,182	3,329	8.6	7.6
Texas	5,543	9,866	15,935	17,897	19,932	21,592	11.1	10.7
Mountain	4,255	7,652	11,748	13,092	14,223	15,095	10.7	8.7
Montana	264	438	679	764	841	894	9.9	9.6
Idaho	243	419	665	752	844	900	10.6	10.6
Wyoming	146	248	353	381	396	417	9.2	5.7
Colorado	1,218	2,087	3,101	3,480	3,776	3,932	9.8	8.2
New Mexico	451	873	1,364	1,538	1,703	1,848	11.7	10.7
Arizona	1,093	2,103	3,218	3,532	3,765	3,999	11.4	7.5
Utah	453	816	1,325	1,483	1,631	1,743	11.3	9.6
Nevada	387	667	1,043	1,162	1,267	1,362	10.4	9.3
Pacific	14,515	23,918	35,912	39,384	42,731	45,259	9.5	8.0
Washington	1,396	2,516	3,961	4,546	5,090	5,305	11.0	10.2
Oregon	928	1,486	2,297	2,403	2,714	2,966	9.5	8.9
California	11,632	18,883	27,949	30,554	32,880	34,827	9.2	7.6
Alaska	199	385	557	631	690	701	10.8	8.0
Hawaii	360	648	1,148	1,250	1,358	1,460	12.3	8.3

Source: U.S. Department of Health and Human Services. Public Health Service. Centers for Disease Control and Prevention. National Center for Health Statistics. *Health, United States, 1995.* Hyattsville, MD: Public Health Service, 1996, p. 268. *Notes:* Figures may not add up to totals due to rounding. 1. States where services were provided. 2. These estimates differ from National Health Expenditures estimates presented elsewhere in *Health, United States.*

★ 590 ★

Expenditures

Expenditures on Physician Services: 1980-1993

This table shows expenditures on physician services by geographic division and State and average annual percent change for the United States for selected years 1980-1993.

[Data are compiled by the Health Care Financing Administration]

Geographic division and State[1]	Amount in millions						Average annual percent change	
	1980	1985	1990	1991	1992	1993	1980-90	1990-93
United States[2]	$45,245	$83,636	$140,499	$150,318	$161,783	$171,226	12.0	6.8
New England	2,072	4,010	7,656	8,088	8,678	9,250	14.0	6.5
Maine	142	275	480	520	570	601	13.0	7.8
New Hampshire	130	281	491	583	719	780	14.2	16.7
Vermont	68	131	221	229	248	265	12.5	6.2
Massachusetts	978	1,890	3,766	3,892	4,130	4,442	14.4	5.7
Rhode Island	166	304	514	527	543	575	12.0	3.8
Connecticut	589	1,127	2,185	2,336	2,468	2,587	14.0	5.8
Middle Atlantic	6,636	12,255	20,470	22,035	24,044	25,238	11.9	7.2
New York	3,332	5,822	9,697	10,238	11,287	12,003	11.3	7.4
New Jersey	1,353	2,533	4,519	4,771	5,526	5,776	12.8	8.5
Pennsylvania	1,950	3,901	6,254	7,026	7,230	7,460	12.4	6.1
East North Central	8,078	13,646	21,823	23,280	24,837	26,275	10.4	6.4
Ohio	2,130	3,692	6,048	6,486	6,786	7,118	11.0	5.6
Indiana	891	1,607	2,680	2,821	3,061	3,263	11.6	6.8
Illinois	2,118	3,672	5,864	6,191	6,707	6,970	10.7	5.9
Michigan	2,002	3,080	4,668	5,017	5,224	5,562	8.8	6.0
Wisconsin	938	1,595	2,564	2,765	3,059	3,362	10.6	9.5
West North Central	3,286	5,739	9,125	9,594	10,395	10,987	10.8	6.4
Minnesota	944	1,765	2,957	3,202	3,322	3,617	12.1	6.9
Iowa	488	769	1,142	1,178	1,294	1,376	8.9	6.4
Missouri	877	1,537	2,485	2,581	2,879	2,958	11.0	6.0
North Dakota	139	288	368	371	433	445	10.2	6.5
South Dakota	102	173	274	280	319	342	10.4	7.7
Nebraska	276	433	688	700	785	825	9.6	6.2
Kansas	461	774	1,211	1,280	1,362	1,425	10.1	5.6
South Atlantic	7,141	14,169	25,449	26,853	28,585	30,041	13.6	5.7
Delaware	120	214	377	405	439	466	12.1	7.3
Maryland	835	1,702	2,968	3,249	3,498	3,704	13.5	7.7
District of Columbia	237	362	657	662	651	672	10.7	0.8
Virginia	886	1,772	3,172	3,462	3,565	3,769	13.6	5.9
West Virginia	330	642	856	882	973	988	10.0	4.9
North Carolina	866	1,543	3,005	3,213	3,458	3,717	13.2	7.3
South Carolina	399	734	1,325	1,423	1,552	1,685	12.8	8.3
Georgia	987	1,930	3,645	3,957	4,321	4,543	14.0	7.6
Florida	2,482	5,272	9,444	9,600	10,131	10,498	14.3	3.6

[Continued]

★ 590 ★

Expenditures on Physician Services: 1980-1993
[Continued]

Geographic division and State[1]	Amount in millions						Average annual percent change	
	1980	1985	1990	1991	1992	1993	1980-90	1990-93
East South Central	2,361	4,188	7,379	8,051	8,418	8,913	12.1	6.5
Kentucky	562	955	1,639	1,762	1,950	2,038	11.3	7.5
Tennessee	841	1,499	2,569	2,822	2,988	3,137	11.8	6.9
Alabama	632	1,167	2,247	2,477	2,466	2,631	13.5	5.4
Mississippi	327	568	925	990	1,015	1,107	11.0	6.2
West South Central	4,649	8,666	13,566	14,280	15,334	15,947	11.3	5.5
Arkansas	374	680	1,134	1,228	1,217	1,244	11.7	3.1
Louisiana	743	1,424	2,129	2,282	2,450	2,537	11.1	6.0
Oklahoma	536	972	1,382	1,432	1,558	1,640	9.9	5.9
Texas	2,996	5,590	8,920	9,340	10,108	10,526	11.5	5.7
Mountain	2,211	4,336	7,347	7,731	8,357	8,897	12.8	6.6
Montana	138	205	311	325	350	392	8.5	8.0
Idaho	140	235	374	410	453	485	10.3	9.1
Wyoming	64	118	146	142	152	160	8.6	3.1
Colorado	600	1,230	1,891	2,032	2,242	2,452	12.2	9.0
New Mexico	182	368	574	590	665	716	12.2	7.6
Arizona	635	1,287	2,500	2,559	2,676	2,799	14.7	3.8
Utah	244	472	739	794	832	864	11.7	5.3
Nevada	207	421	812	879	988	1,029	14.6	8.2
Pacific	8,811	16,627	27,682	30,406	33,132	35,677	12.1	8.8
Washington	909	1,667	2,834	3,155	3,413	3,720	12.0	9.5
Oregon	596	990	1,597	1,626	1,798	1,904	10.4	6.0
California	6,959	13,311	22,365	24,654	26,903	28,981	12.4	9.0
Alaska	97	214	258	265	276	301	10.3	5.3
Hawaii	249	444	629	706	742	771	9.7	7.0

Source: U.S. Department of Health and Human Services. Public Health Service. Centers for Disease Control and Prevention. National Center for Health Statistics. *Health, United States, 1995.* Hyattsville, MD: Public Health Service, 1996, p. 269. *Notes:* Figures may not add up to totals due to rounding. 1. States where services were provided. 2. These estimates differ from National Health Expenditures estimates presented elsewhere in *Health, United States.* See Appendix I.

★ 591 ★

Expenditures

Health Care Expenditures, by Type: 1993

Type	Percentage
Cardiovascular diseases	14
Injury and long-term effects	12
Cancer	9
Kidney/urinary/diabetes	9
Pregnancy and childbirth	7
Respiratory diseases	7

[Continued]

★ 591 ★

Health Care Expenditures, by Type: 1993
[Continued]

Type	Percentage
Digestive diseases	6
Musculoskeletal diseases	5
Circulatory disorders	3.5
Mental health	3.5
Wellcare	3
Congenital abnormalities	1
Medical errors	1
Miscellaneous	19

Source: "WV List: Who Ordered the Medical Errors?" *Workplace Vitality* (July/August 1996), p. 14. Primary source: The National Medical Expenditure Survey, conducted by the National Center for Health Statistics, U.S. Department of Health and Human Services.

★ 592 ★

Expenditures

Health Care Payments, by Type: 1993

Data are the latest figures available.

Health care bills	Percentage
Private health insurance	34
Consumer out of pocket	18
Medicare	17
Medicaid	13
Other government programs	13
Other private sources	5

Source: "How Health Care Bills Are Paid." *USA TODAY,* 13-15 January 1995, p. 1A. Primary source: Health Care Financing Administration.

★ 593 ★

Expenditures

Health-Care Spending Per Capita, by Segment: 1993

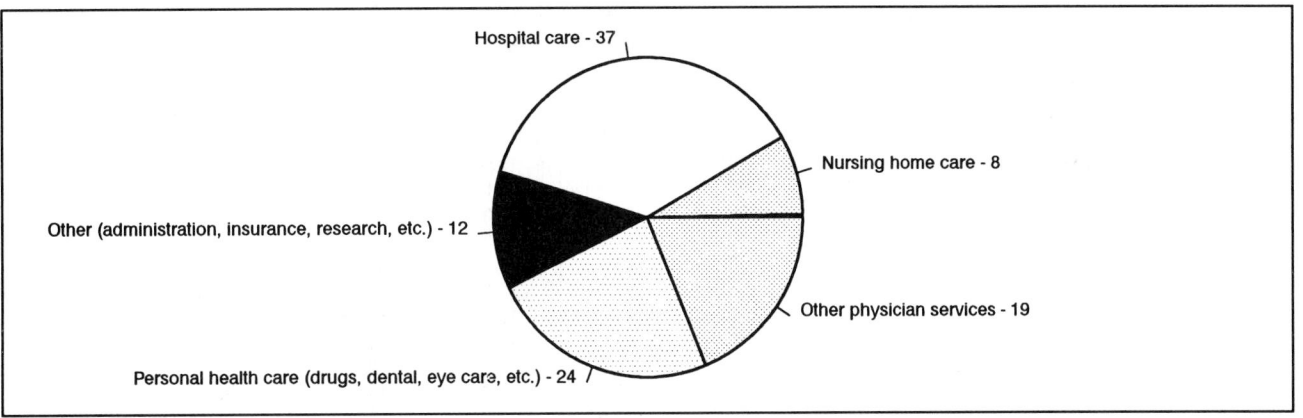

Hospital care - 37

Nursing home care - 8

Other (administration, insurance, research, etc.) - 12

Other physician services - 19

Personal health care (drugs, dental, eye care, etc.) - 24

According to the source, the average American spent $3,299 on health care in 1993.

Segment	Percentage
Hospital care	37
Personal health care (drugs, dental, eye care, etc.)	24
Other physician services	19
Other (administration, insurance, research, etc.)	12
Nursing home care	8

Source: "Paying for Health Care." *USA TODAY,* 12 January 1995, p. 1A. Primary source: Health Care Financing Administration.

★ 594 ★

Expenditures

Health Care: Total Expenditures, 1960-1991

This table shows gross domestic product, national health expenditures, and Federal, State, and local government expenditures: United States, selected years 1960-91.

Year	Gross domestic product in billions	National health expenditure			Federal government expenditure			State and local government expenditures		
		Amount in billions	Percent of gross domestic product	Amount per capita	Total in billions	Health in billions	Health as a percent of total	Total in billions	Health in billions	Health as a percent of total
1960	$513.4	$27.1	5.3	$143	$93.4	$2.9	3.1	$48.3	$3.7	7.8
1965	702.7	41.6	5.9	204	124.6	4.8	3.9	72.3	5.5	7.6
1966	769.8	45.9	6.0	222	144.9	7.5	5.2	81.1	6.1	7.5
1967	814.3	51.7	6.3	248	165.2	12.2	7.4	90.9	6.9	7.6
1968	889.3	58.5	6.6	278	181.5	14.1	7.8	102.6	7.7	7.5
1969	959.5	65.7	6.9	309	191.0	16.1	8.4	113.3	8.5	7.5
1970	1,010.7	74.4	7.4	346	208.5	17.7	8.5	127.2	9.9	7.8
1971	1,097.2	82.3	7.5	379	224.3	20.4	9.1	142.8	10.8	7.6
1972	1,207.0	92.3	7.6	421	249.3	22.9	9.2	156.3	12.2	7.8
1973	1,349.6	102.5	7.6	464	270.3	25.2	9.3	171.9	14.1	8.2

[Continued]

★ 594 ★

Health Care: Total Expenditures, 1960-1991
[Continued]

Year	Gross domestic product in billions	National health expenditure			Federal government expenditure			State and local government expenditures		
		Amount in billions	Percent of gross domestic product	Amount per capita	Total in billions	Health in billions	Health as a percent of total	Total in billions	Health in billions	Health as a percent of total
1974	1,458.6	116.1	8.0	521	305.6	30.5	10.0	193.5	16.1	8.3
1975	1,585.9	132.9	8.4	592	364.2	36.4	10.0	221.0	18.7	8.5
1976	1,768.4	152.2	8.6	672	392.7	42.9	10.9	239.3	19.5	8.1
1977	1,974.1	172.0	8.7	753	426.4	47.6	11.2	256.3	22.5	8.8
1978	2,232.7	193.7	8.7	840	469.3	54.3	11.6	278.2	25.5	9.1
1979	2,488.6	217.2	8.7	933	520.3	61.4	11.8	305.4	28.9	9.5
1980	2,708.0	250.1	9.2	1,064	613.1	72.0	11.7	336.6	33.2	9.9
1981	3,030.6	290.2	9.6	1,222	697.8	84.0	12.0	362.3	37.8	10.4
1982	3,149.6	326.1	10.4	1,359	770.9	93.3	12.1	382.1	41.5	10.9
1983	3,405.0	358.6	10.5	1,480	840.0	103.2	12.3	403.2	44.4	11.0
1984	3,777.2	389.6	10.3	1,592	892.7	112.6	12.6	434.1	47.0	10.8
1985	4,038.7	422.6	10.5	1,711	969.9	123.5	12.7	472.6	51.2	10.8
1986	4,268.6	454.9	10.7	1,824	1,028.2	132.5	12.9	517.0	57.2	11.1
1987	4,539.9	494.2	10.9	1,962	1,065.6	143.6	13.5	554.2	64.4	11.6
1988	4,900.4	546.1	11.1	2,146	1,109.0	156.6	14.1	593.0	70.5	11.9
1989	5,250.8	604.3	11.5	2,352	1,181.6	175.0	14.8	636.7	78.3	12.3
1990	5,522.2	675.0	12.2	2,601	1,273.6	194.5	15.3	699.2	90.5	12.9
1991	5,677.5	751.8	13.2	2,868	1,332.7	222.9	16.7	760.7	107.1	14.1

Source: Cohen, R.A., and J.F. Van Nostrand. *Trends in the Health of Older Americans: United States, 1994.* National Center for Health Statistics. Vital and Health Statistics 3(30). 1995. U.S. Department of Health and Human Services, Public Health Service, Centers for Disease Control and Prevention. Primary source: National Center for Health Statistics: *Health, United States, 1992.* Data are from the Office of National Health Statistics, Office of the Actuary: National Health Expenditures, 1991. *Health Care Financing Review.* Vol. 14, Number 2. HCFA Pub. No. 03335. Health Care Financing Administration. Washington: DC: U.S. Government Printing Office, 1992.

★ 595 ★

Expenditures

Health Services and Supplies – Per Capita Consumer Expenditures, by Object: 1980 to 1994

In dollars, except percent. Based on Social Security Administration estimates of total U.S. population as of July 1, including Armed Forces and Federal employees abroad and civilian population of outlying areas. Excludes research and construction.

OBJECT OF EXPENDITURE	1980	1985	1988	1989	1990	1991	1992	1993	1994
Total, national	1,002	1,668	2,118	2,336	2,593	2,807	3,040	3,222	3,398
Annual percent change[1]	13.9	9.3	10.6	10.3	11.0	8.3	8.3	6.0	5.5
Hospital care	437	682	832	902	988	1,076	1,151	1,210	1,251
Physician services	192	339	467	511	564	605	659	676	700
Dental services	57	88	108	115	122	127	140	146	156
Other professional services	27	67	105	116	134	146	159	173	183
Home health care	10	23	33	40	51	61	74	86	97
Drugs and other medical nondurables	92	150	193	209	231	250	269	281	290
Vision products and other medical durables	16	27	35	37	40	43	45	47	49
Nursing home care	75	124	156	175	196	218	235	250	267
Other health services	17	25	34	37	43	52	59	67	81
Net cost of insurance and administration	50	96	93	123	149	148	161	190	217
Government public health activities	29	47	61	70	76	82	88	96	107

[Continued]

★ 595 ★

Health Services and Supplies – Per Capita Consumer Expenditures, by Object: 1980 to 1994

[Continued]

OBJECT OF EXPENDITURE	1980	1985	1988	1989	1990	1991	1992	1993	1994
Total, private consumer[2]	553	943	1,197	1,324	1,467	1,551	1,663	1,739	1,805
Hospital care	178	274	337	370	402	425	439	459	464
Physician services	135	234	318	346	380	408	450	457	464
Dental services	54	85	105	112	118	123	134	139	149
Other professional services	19	50	79	86	98	105	114	122	128
Home health care	4	8	16	19	23	26	30	32	35
Drugs and other medical nondurables	85	138	175	188	206	221	238	246	254
Vision products and other medical durables	14	21	27	28	30	30	31	31	32
Nursing home care	32	58	75	80	93	97	100	102	107
Net cost of insurance	33	75	66	94	118	117	128	150	172

Source: 1996 Statistical Abstract of the United States on CD-ROM [machine-readable datafiles]. CD-8A-97. Washington, DC: U.S. Department of Commerce, Economics and Statistics Administration, Bureau of the Census, Data User Services Division, January 1997. Primary source: U.S. Health Care Financing Administration, *Health Care Financing Review,* spring 1996. *Notes:* 1. Change from immediate prior year. 2. Represents out-of-pocket payments and private health insurance.

★ 596 ★

Expenditures

HMO Revenue Allocations: 1994-1995

[In percentages]

HMO	Administrative costs and profit	Providing care
U.S. Healthcare	27.1	72.9
Wellpoint Health Networks	27.1	72.9
Health Systems International	22.1	77.9
United Healthcare	21.9	78.1
Foundation Health	21.5	78.5
Humana[1]	19.4	80.6
FHP International	17.3	82.7
Pacificare Health Systems	16.5	83.5

Source: Freudenheim, Milt. "A Bitter Pill for the HMOs." *New York Times,* 28 April 1995, p. C1. Primary source: Sherlock Company; Industry reports. *Notes:* 1. First quarter 1995 figures. Other figures are for the fourth quarter of 1994.

★ 597 ★

Expenditures

National Health Care Expenditures

Includes Puerto Rico and outlying areas.

YEAR	Total[1]			Health services and supplies						
					Private			Public		
				Total[3] (bil. dol.)	Out-of-pocket payments		Insur-ance premi-ums (bil. dol.)	Total (bil. dol.)	Medical payments	
	Total (bil. dol.)	Per capita (dol.)	Per-cent of GDP[2]		Total (bil. dol.)	Percent of total private			Medi-care (bil. dol.)	Public assist-ance (bil. dol.)
1960	26.9	141	5.1	19.5	13.1	67.2	5.9	5.7	(X)	0.5
1965	41.1	202	5.7	29.4	18.5	62.9	10.0	8.3	(X)	1.7
1970	73.2	341	7.1	43.0	24.9	57.9	16.3	24.9	7.7	6.3
1971	81.0	373	7.2	46.9	26.4	56.3	18.6	28.1	8.5	7.7
1972	90.9	415	7.4	52.5	29.0	55.2	21.3	31.8	9.4	8.9
1973	100.8	456	7.3	58.2	32.0	55.0	23.9	35.9	10.8	10.2
1974	114.3	513	7.6	64.3	34.8	54.1	26.8	42.7	13.5	11.9
1975	130.7	582	8.0	72.3	38.1	52.7	31.3	50.1	16.4	14.5
1976	149.9	662	8.2	83.8	41.9	50.0	37.9	56.7	19.8	16.4
1977	170.4	746	8.4	96.6	46.4	48.0	45.9	64.5	23.0	18.8
1978	190.6	827	8.3	107.4	49.7	46.3	52.5	73.3	26.8	20.9
1979	215.2	924	8.4	121.2	54.3	44.8	60.9	83.7	31.0	24.0
1980	247.2	1,052	8.9	138.0	60.3	43.7	69.7	97.6	37.5	28.0
1981	286.9	1,208	9.2	160.3	68.5	42.7	82.1	113.4	44.9	32.6
1982	322.9	1,346	10.0	181.8	75.5	41.5	95.3	126.4	52.5	34.6
1983	355.2	1,467	10.1	200.3	82.3	41.1	106.1	138.9	59.8	38.0
1984	389.7	1,594	10.0	222.4	90.8	40.8	118.8	150.9	66.5	41.1
1985	428.2	1,735	10.2	247.4	100.6	40.7	132.3	164.4	72.2	44.4
1986	460.9	1,849	10.4	264.4	108.0	40.8	140.1	179.7	76.9	49.0
1987	500.1	1,987	10.7	285.7	116.0	40.6	152.1	196.1	82.6	54.0
1988	559.6	2,201	11.1	324.5	129.2	39.8	175.1	213.9	90.4	58.9
1989	622.0	2,422	11.4	360.8	136.2	37.7	203.8	239.0	102.5	66.4
1990	697.5	2,688	12.1	402.9	148.4	36.8	232.4	270.0	112.1	80.4
1991	761.3	2,902	12.9	430.9	155.1	36.0	251.9	305.5	123.0	99.2
1992	833.6	3,144	13.3	465.9	164.4	35.3	276.6	340.1	138.7	112.4
1993	892.3	3,331	13.6	493.1	169.4	34.4	296.5	370.0	151.7	124.4
1994	949.4	3,510	13.7	517.1	174.9	33.8	313.3	402.2	169.2	134.8

Source: 1996 Statistical Abstract of the United States on CD-ROM [machine-readable datafiles]. CD-8A-97. Washington, DC: U.S. Department of Commerce, Economics and Statistics Administration, Bureau of the Census, Data User Services Division, January 1997. Primary source: U. S. Health Care Financing Administration, *Health Care Financing Review,* spring 1996. *Notes:* X indicates not applicable. 1. Includes medical research and medical facilities construction. 2. GDP=Gross domestic product 3. Includes other sources of funds not shown separately.

★ 598 ★

Expenditures

National Health Care Expenditures, 1995, by Type of Expenditure

This table shows expenditures by source of funds and type of expenditure for calendar year 1995.

[Amount in billions of dollars]

Year and Type of Expenditure	Total	All Private Funds	Total	Private Consumer Out of Pocket	Private Consumer Private Insurance	Private Consumer Other	Government Total	Government Federal	Government State and Local
1995									
National Health Expenditures	988.5	532.1	493.2	182.6	310.6	38.9	456.4	328.4	128.0
Health Services and Supplies	957.8	521.2	493.2	182.6	310.6	28.0	436.7	314.4	122.2
Personal Health Care	878.8	486.7	459.3	182.6	276.8	27.3	392.1	303.6	88.5
Hospital Care	350.1	135.8	124.5	11.4	113.1	11.3	214.3	175.3	39.0
Physician Services	201.6	137.6	133.9	36.9	97.0	3.7	64.0	50.9	13.1
Dental Services	45.8	44.0	43.8	21.8	22.0	0.2	1.8	1.0	0.8
Other Professional Services	52.6	39.9	36.0	20.2	15.8	3.9	12.7	9.6	3.1
Home Health Care	28.6	12.8	9.3	6.0	3.3	3.4	15.8	13.8	2.0
Drugs and Other Medical Nondurables	83.4	72.0	72.0	49.8	22.1	--	11.4	5.9	5.6
Vision Products and Other Medical Durables	13.8	8.7	8.7	7.8	0.9	--	5.1	5.0	0.1
Nursing Home Care	77.9	32.6	31.1	28.6	2.5	1.5	45.3	29.3	16.0
Other Personal Health Care	25.0	3.3	--	--	--	3.3	21.7	12.8	8.9
Program Administration and net									
Cost of Private Health Insurance	47.7	34.5	33.9	--	33.9	0.6	13.2	7.1	6.1
Government Public Health Activities	31.4	--	--	--	--	--	31.4	3.8	27.6
Research and Construction	30.7	10.9	--	--	--	10.9	19.7	14.0	5.7
Research	16.6	1.4	--	--	--	1.4	15.2	12.9	2.3
Construction	14.0	9.6	--	--	--	9.6	4.5	1.1	3.4

Source: Health Care Financing Administration, Office of the Actuary. *Notes:* Office of National Health Statistics Research and development expenditures of drug companies and other manufacturers and providers of medical equipment and supplies are excluded from research expenditures, but are included in the expenditure class in which the product falls. Numbers may not add to totals because of rounding.

★ 599 ★

Expenditures

National Health Care Expenditures, by Object

In billions of dollars. Includes Puerto Rico and outlying areas.

Object of Expenditure	1980	1985	1989	1990	1991	1992	1993	1994
Total	247.2	428.2	622.0	697.5	761.3	833.6	892.3	949.4
Spent by –								
Consumers	130.0	232.8	339.9	380.8	406.9	441.0	465.8	488.1
Government	104.8	174.3	252.2	284.3	320.3	356.5	387.2	420.8
Other[1]	12.5	21.1	29.9	32.3	34.0	36.0	39.2	40.4

[Continued]

★ 599 ★

National Health Care Expenditures, by Object

[Continued]

Object of Expenditure	1980	1985	1989	1990	1991	1992	1993	1994
Spent for –								
Health services and supplies	235.6	411.8	599.8	672.9	736.3	806.0	863.1	919.2
Personal health care expenses	217.0	376.4	550.1	614.7	676.2	739.8	786.5	831.7
Hospital care	102.7	168.3	231.6	256.4	282.3	305.3	324.2	338.5
Physician services	45.2	83.6	131.3	146.3	158.6	174.7	181.1	189.4
Dental services	13.3	21.7	29.5	31.6	33.3	37.0	39.2	42.2
Other professional services[2]	6.4	16.6	29.8	34.7	38.3	42.1	46.3	49.6
Home health care	2.4	5.6	10.2	13.1	16.1	19.6	23.0	26.2
Drugs/other medical nondurables	21.6	37.1	53.7	59.9	65.6	71.3	75.2	78.6
Vision products/other med. durables[3]	3.8	6.7	9.6	10.5	11.2	11.9	12.6	13.1
Nursing home care	17.6	30.7	44.9	50.9	57.2	62.3	67.0	72.3
Other health services	4.0	6.1	9.5	11.2	13.6	15.6	17.8	21.8
Net cost of insurance and admin.[4]	11.8	23.8	31.6	38.6	38.7	42.8	51.0	58.7
Government public health activities	6.7	11.6	18.1	19.6	21.4	23.4	25.7	28.8
Medical research	5.5	7.8	11.3	12.2	12.9	14.2	14.5	15.9
Medical facilities construction	6.2	8.5	11.0	12.3	12.0	13.4	14.7	14.3

Source: 1996 Statistical Abstract of the United States on CD-ROM [machine-readable datafiles]. CD-8A-97. Washington, DC: U.S. Department of Commerce, Economics and Statistics Administration, Bureau of the Census, Data User Services Division, January 1997. Primary source: U.S. Health Care Financing Administration, *Health Care Financing Review,* spring 1996. *Notes:* 1. Includes nonpatient revenues, privately funded construction, and industrial inplant. 2. Includes services of registered and practical nurses in private duty, podiatrists, optometrists, physical therapists, clinical psychologists, chiropractors, naturopaths, and Christian Science practitioners. 3. Includes expenditures for eyeglasses, hearing aids, orthopedic appliances, artificial limbs, crutches, wheelchairs, etc. 4. Includes administrative expenses of federally financed health programs.

★ 600 ★

Expenditures

National Health Care Expenditures, by Source of Funds

This table shows aggregate and per capita amounts, percent distribution, and average annual percent growth, by source of funds for selected years, 1960 to 1995.

Item	1960	1970	1980	1985	1990	1991	1992	1993	1994	1995
Amount in Billions										
National Health Expenditures	$26.9	$73.2	$247.2	$428.2	$697.5	$761.7	$834.2	$892.1	$937.1	$988.5
Private	20.2	45.5	142.5	253.9	413.1	441.4	478.8	505.5	517.2	532.1
Public	6.6	27.7	104.8	174.3	284.3	320.3	355.4	386.5	419.9	456.4
Federal	2.9	17.8	72.0	123.3	195.8	224.4	253.9	277.6	301.9	328.4
State and Local	3.7	9.9	32.8	51.0	88.5	95.9	101.6	108.9	118.0	128.0
Number in Millions										
U.S. Population[1]	190.1	214.8	235.1	247.1	260.0	262.6	265.2	267.9	270.4	273.0
Amount in Billions										
Gross Domestic Product	$527	$1,036	$2,784	$4,181	$5,744	$5,917	$6,244	$6,553	$6,936	$7,254
Per Capita Amount										
National Health Expenditures	$141	$341	$1,052	$1,733	$2,683	$2,901	$3,145	$3,330	$3,465	$3,621
Private	106	212	606	1,027	1,589	1,681	1,805	1,887	1,913	1,949

[Continued]

★ 600 ★

National Health Care Expenditures, by Source of Funds

[Continued]

Item	1960	1970	1980	1985	1990	1991	1992	1993	1994	1995
Public	35	129	446	705	1,094	1,220	1,340	1,443	1,553	1,672
Federal	15	83	306	499	753	855	957	1,036	1,116	1,203
State and Local	20	46	140	206	341	365	383	407	436	469
Percent Distribution										
National Health Expenditures	100.0	100.0	100.0	100.0	100.0	100.0	100.0	100.0	100.0	100.0
Private	75.2	62.2	57.6	59.3	59.2	58.0	57.4	56.7	55.2	53.8
Public	24.8	37.8	42.4	40.7	40.8	42.0	42.6	43.3	44.8	46.2
Federal	10.9	24.3	29.1	28.8	28.1	29.5	30.4	31.1	32.2	33.2
State and Local	13.9	13.5	13.3	11.9	12.7	12.6	12.2	12.2	12.6	12.9
Percent of Gross Domestic Product										
National Health Expenditures	5.1	7.1	8.9	10.2	12.1	12.9	13.4	13.6	13.5	13.6
Average Annual Percent Growth From Previous Year Shown										
National Health Expenditures	--	10.6	12.9	11.6	10.2	9.2	9.5	6.9	5.1	5.5
Private	--	8.5	12.1	12.3	10.2	6.8	8.5	5.6	2.3	2.9
Public	--	15.3	14.2	10.7	10.3	12.7	11.0	8.7	8.6	8.7
Federal	--	19.8	15.0	11.4	9.7	14.6	13.1	9.4	8.7	8.8
State and Local	--	10.2	12.7	9.2	11.6	8.3	6.0	7.2	8.4	8.4
U.S. Population	--	1.2	0.9	1.0	1.0	1.0	1.0	1.0	1.0	0.9
Gross Domestic Product	--	7.0	10.4	8.5	6.6	3.0	5.5	4.9	5.8	4.6

Source: Health Care Financing Administration, Office of the Actuary. Primary source: Office of National Health Statistics. *Notes:* 1. July 1 Social Security area population estimates for each year, 1960-95. Numbers and percents may not add to totals because of rounding.

★ 601 ★

Expenditures

National Health Care Expenditures, by Type

This table shows national health expenditures aggregate amounts and average annual percent change, by type of expenditure for selected years, 1960-1995.

Type of Expenditure	1960	1970	1980	1985	1990	1991	1992	1993	1994	1995
Amount in Billions										
National Health Expenditures	$26.9	$73.2	$247.2	$428.2	$697.5	$761.7	$834.2	$892.1	$937.1	$988.5
Health Services and Supplies	25.2	67.9	235.6	411.8	672.9	736.8	806.7	863.1	906.7	957.8
Personal Health Care	23.6	63.8	217.0	376.4	614.7	676.6	740.5	786.9	827.9	878.8
Hospital Care	9.3	28.0	102.7	168.3	256.4	282.3	305.4	323.3	335.0	350.1
Physician Services	5.3	13.6	45.2	83.6	146.3	159.2	175.7	182.7	190.6	201.6
Dental Services	2.0	4.7	13.3	21.7	31.6	33.3	37.0	39.2	42.1	45.8
Other Professional Services	0.6	1.4	6.4	16.6	34.7	38.3	42.1	46.3	49.1	52.6
Home Health Care	0.1	0.2	2.4	5.6	13.1	16.1	19.6	23.0	26.3	28.6
Drugs and Other Medical Nondurables	4.2	8.8	21.6	37.1	59.9	65.6	71.2	75.0	77.7	83.4
Vision Products and Other Medical Durables	0.6	1.6	3.8	6.7	10.5	11.2	11.9	12.5	12.9	13.8
Nursing Home Care	0.8	4.2	17.6	30.7	50.9	57.2	62.3	67.0	72.4	77.9
Other Personal Health Care	0.7	1.3	4.0	6.1	11.2	13.6	15.4	17.9	21.7	25.0
Program Administration and net Cost of Private Health Insurance	1.2	2.7	11.8	23.8	38.6	38.8	42.7	50.9	50.6	47.7

[Continued]

★ 601 ★

National Health Care Expenditures, by Type

[Continued]

Type of Expenditure	1960	1970	1980	1985	1990	1991	1992	1993	1994	1995
Government Public Health Activities	0.4	1.3	6.7	11.6	19.6	21.4	23.4	25.3	28.2	31.4
Research and Construction	1.7	5.3	11.6	16.4	24.5	24.9	27.5	29.0	30.4	30.7
Research[1]	0.7	2.0	5.5	7.8	12.2	12.9	14.2	14.5	15.8	16.6
Construction	1.0	3.4	6.2	8.5	12.3	12.0	13.4	14.5	14.6	14.0
Average Annual Percent Change From Previous Year Shown										
National Health Expenditures	--	10.6	12.9	11.6	10.2	9.2	9.5	6.9	5.1	5.5
Health Services and Supplies	--	10.4	13.2	11.8	10.3	9.5	9.5	7.0	5.1	5.6
Personal Health Care	--	10.5	13.0	11.6	10.3	10.1	9.5	6.3	5.2	6.1
Hospital Care	--	11.7	13.9	10.4	8.8	10.1	8.2	5.9	3.6	4.5
Physician Services	--	9.9	12.8	13.1	11.8	8.8	10.4	4.0	4.4	5.8
Dental Services	--	9.1	11.1	10.2	7.8	5.6	11.0	6.0	7.3	8.9
Other Professional Services	--	8.8	16.3	21.2	15.8	10.4	10.0	10.0	6.1	7.0
Home Health Care	--	14.5	26.9	18.9	18.4	22.4	22.3	17.1	14.4	8.6
Drugs and Other Medical Nondurables	--	7.6	9.4	11.4	10.1	9.4	8.6	5.4	3.6	7.3
Vision Products and Other Medical Durables	--	9.6	8.8	12.4	9.2	7.0	6.3	5.1	2.8	7.2
Nursing Home Care	--	17.4	15.4	11.7	10.7	12.2	9.0	7.6	8.1	7.5
Other Personal Health Care	--	6.5	12.0	8.8	12.9	20.7	13.3	16.4	21.6	14.9
Program Administration and net Cost of Private Health Insurance	--	8.9	15.8	15.0	10.2	0.4	10.2	19.1	-0.5	-5.8
Government Public Health Activities	--	13.9	17.5	11.5	11.0	9.2	9.3	7.9	11.6	11.3
Research and Construction	--	12.2	8.1	7.1	8.4	1.7	10.5	5.3	4.9	0.8
Research[1]	--	10.9	10.8	7.5	9.3	5.8	9.8	2.2	9.3	5.0
Construction	--	12.9	6.2	6.7	7.6	-2.4	11.2	8.7	0.5	-3.8

Source: Health Care Financing Administration, Office of the Actuary: Office of National Health Statistics. *Notes:* 1. Research and development expenditures of drug companies and other manufacturers and providers of medical equipment and supplies are excluded from research expenditures, but are included in the expenditure class in to which the product falls. Numbers may not add to totals because of rounding.

★ 602 ★

Expenditures

National Health Care Expenditures: Percent

Type of expenditure	1960	1965	1970	1975	1980	1985	1987	1988	1989	1990	1991
Amount in billions											
Total expenditures	$27.1	$41.6	$74.4	$132.9	$250.1	$422.6	$494.2	$546.1	$604.3	$675.0	$751.8
Percent distribution											
All expenditures	100.0	100.0	100.0	100.0	100.0	100.0	100.0	100.0	100.0	100.0	100.0
Health services and supplies	93.7	91.7	92.8	93.8	95.5	96.4	96.5	96.4	96.6	96.6	96.9
Personal health care	88.1	85.6	87.3	87.7	87.7	87.5	88.9	88.4	87.9	87.6	87.8
Hospital care	34.2	33.7	37.6	39.4	40.9	39.8	39.3	38.8	38.5	38.2	38.4
Physician services	19.5	19.7	18.3	17.5	16.7	17.5	18.8	19.3	19.2	19.1	18.9
Dentist services	7.2	6.7	6.3	6.2	5.7	5.5	5.5	5.4	5.2	5.0	4.9
Nursing home care	3.6	4.1	6.5	7.5	8.0	8.1	8.0	7.8	7.9	7.9	8.0
Other professional services	2.2	2.1	2.0	2.6	3.5	3.9	4.3	4.4	4.5	4.5	4.8
Home health care	0.1	0.1	0.2	0.3	0.5	0.9	0.8	0.8	0.9	1.1	1.3
Drugs and other medical nondurables	15.7	14.2	11.8	9.8	8.6	8.6	8.7	8.5	8.4	8.2	8.1
Vision products and other medical durables	3.0	3.0	2.7	2.3	1.8	1.7	1.8	1.9	1.7	1.7	1.6
Other personal health care	2.6	2.0	1.8	2.0	1.8	1.5	1.6	1.6	1.6	1.7	1.9

[Continued]

★ 602 ★

National Health Care Expenditures: Percent

[Continued]

Type of expenditure	1960	1965	1970	1975	1980	1985	1987	1988	1989	1990	1991
Program administration and net cost of health insurance	4.3	4.6	3.7	3.8	4.9	6.0	4.7	4.9	5.6	5.8	5.8
Government public health activities	1.4	1.5	1.9	2.3	2.9	2.9	3.0	3.0	3.1	3.3	3.3
Research and construction	6.3	8.3	7.2	6.2	4.5	3.6	3.5	3.6	3.4	3.4	3.1
Noncommercial research	2.6	3.7	2.6	2.5	2.2	1.8	1.8	1.9	1.8	1.8	1.7
Construction	3.7	4.6	4.5	3.7	2.3	1.8	1.7	1.7	1.6	1.6	1.4

Source: Cohen, R.A., and J.F. Van Nostrand. *Trends in the Health of Older Americans: United States, 1994.* National Center for Health Statistics. Vital and Health Statistics 3(30). 1995. U.S. Department of Health and Human Services, Public Health Service, Centers for Disease Control and Prevention. Primary source: National Center for Health Statistics: *Health, United States, 1992.* Data are from the Office of National Health Statistics, Office of the Actuary: National Health Expenditures, 1991. Health Care Financing Review. Vol. 14, Number 2. HCFA Pub. No. 03335. Health Care Financing Administration. Washington, DC: U.S. Government Printing Office, 1992. These data include revisions in health expenditures back to 1985 and differ from those published in *Health, United States* editions published prior to 1992.

★ 603 ★

Expenditures

National Health Expenditures, by Type

In millions of dollars, except percent. Includes Puerto Rico and outlying areas.

TYPE OF EXPENDITURE	1980	1985	1989	1990	1991	1992	1993	1994
Total	247,245	428,204	622,027	697,453	761,258	833,559	892,267	949,419
Annual percent change[1]	14.9	9.9	11.2	12.1	9.1	9.5	7.0	6.4
Private expenditures	142,463	253,903	369,844	413,145	440,978	477,024	505,086	528,584
Health services and supplies	138,010	247,403	360,792	402,897	430,854	465,898	493,052	517,056
Out-of-pocket payments	60,254	100,595	136,186	148,390	155,098	164,382	169,376	174,879
Insurance premiums[2]	69,728	132,254	203,761	232,436	251,851	276,596	296,469	313,268
Other	8,028	14,554	20,846	22,071	23,905	24,920	27,207	28,909
Medical research	292	538	882	960	1,090	1,183	1,215	1,276
Medical facilities construction	4,161	5,962	8,170	9,288	9,034	9,942	10,819	10,252
Public expenditures	104,782	174,301	252,183	284,309	320,279	356,535	387,181	420,835
Percent Federal of public	68.7	70.7	69.3	68.9	70.1	71.5	71.9	72.1
Health services and supplies	97,599	164,430	239,012	270,033	305,469	340,100	370,036	402,163
Medicare[3]	37,519	72,186	102,484	112,091	122,986	138,723	151,717	169,246
Public assistance medical payments[4]	28,033	44,439	66,388	80,395	99,235	112,396	124,408	134,765
Temporary disability insurance[5]	52	51	64	62	66	70	54	53
Workers' compensation (medical)[5]	5,141	7,971	14,298	16,067	17,163	18,983	18,910	18,903
Defense Dept. hospital, medical	4,350	7,498	10,319	11,579	12,849	12,886	13,406	13,156
Maternal, child health programs	892	1,262	1,795	1,892	2,014	2,119	2,194	2,286
Public health activities	6,732	11,618	18,060	19,613	21,408	23,417	25,675	28,849
Veterans' hospital, medical care	5,934	8,713	10,640	11,424	12,366	13,205	14,267	15,140
Medical vocational rehabilitation	298	401	523	555	595	635	619	705
State and local hospitals[6]	5,589	7,030	10,583	11,346	11,030	11,134	11,841	11,784
Other[7]	3,059	3,263	3,859	5,009	5,758	6,531	6,944	7,277

[Continued]

★ 603 ★

National Health Expenditures, by Type

[Continued]

TYPE OF EXPENDITURE	1980	1985	1989	1990	1991	1992	1993	1994
Medical research	5,169	7,302	10,377	11,254	11,827	12,995	13,278	14,650
Medical facilities construction	2,014	2,569	2,793	3,022	2,983	3,440	3,866	4,021

Source: 1996 Statistical Abstract of the United States on CD-ROM [machine-readable datafiles]. CD-8A-97. Washington, DC: U.S. Department of Commerce, Economics and Statistics Administration, Bureau of the Census, Data User Services Division, January 1997. Primary source: U.S. Health Care Financing Administration, *Health Care Financing Review,* spring 1996. *Notes:* 1. Change from immediate prior year. 2. Covers insurance benefits and amount retained by insurance companies for expenses, additions to reserves, and profits (net cost of insurance). 3. Represents expenditures for benefits and administrative cost from Federal hospital and medical insurance trust funds under old-age, survivors, disability, and health insurance programs. 4. Payments made directly to suppliers of medical care (primarily Medicaid). 5. Includes medical benefits paid under public law by private insurance carriers, state governments, and self-insurers. 6. Expenditures not offset by other revenues. 7. Covers expenditures for Substance Abuse and Mental Health Services Administration, Indian Health Service; school health and other programs.

★ 604 ★

Expenditures

Per Capita Federal Government Expenditures on Health Care, by Type: 1996

| Cancer - 203 |
| Multiple sclerosis - 161 |
| Heart disease - 130 |
| Schizophrenia - 14 |
| Tooth decay - 11 |
| Depressive disorders - 10 |

Type of health care	Amount
Muscular dystrophy	$1,000
Cancer	203
Multiple sclerosis	161
Heart disease	130
Schizophrenia	14
Tooth decay	11
Depressive disorders	10

Source: Carter, J.P. "By the Numbers." *Journal of Psychosocial Nursing* 1996, vol. 34, no. 3, p. 11.

★ 605 ★

Expenditures

Personal Health Care Expenditures (PHCE), by Source of Funds, Selected Calendar Years - I

[Amounts are in billions of dollars]

Year	Total PHCE[1]			Direct Patient Payments		All third parties		Private		Government	
	Amount	Percent of GDP	Per Capita	Amount	Percent of PHCE	Amount	Percent of PHCE	Amount	Percent of PHCE	Amount	Percent of PHCE
1960	23.9	4.7	124	13.4	56.0	10.5	44.0	5.4	22.6	5.1	21.4
1970	64.8	6.4	302	25.4	39.2	39.4	60.8	16.9	26.1	22.5	34.6
1980	220.1	8.1	923	61.3	27.9	158.8	72.1	71.8	32.6	87.0	39.5
1981	255.7	8.4	1,077	69.6	27.2	186.1	72.8	84.8	33.2	101.3	39.6
1982	287.6	9.1	1,199	76.5	26.6	211.0	73.4	97.8	34.0	113.2	39.4
1983	316.0	9.3	1,305	83.0	26.3	233.0	73.7	108.0	34.2	125.0	39.6
1984	345.6	9.2	1,414	90.4	26.2	255.2	73.8	118.8	34.4	136.4	39.5
1985	380.5	9.4	1,542	98.8	26.0	281.7	74.0	133.7	35.1	148.0	38.9
1986	414.5	9.7	1,664	105.0	25.3	309.5	74.7	147.4	35.6	162.1	40.5
1987	453.8	10.0	1,804	111.6	24.6	342.2	75.4	165.8	36.5	176.4	38.9
1988	500.2	10.2	1,970	123.0	24.6	377.3	75.4	186.2	37.2	191.1	38.2
1989	550.5	10.5	2,147	127.8	23.2	422.7	76.8	208.4	37.9	214.3	38.9
1990	612.4	11.0	2,362	138.3	22.6	474.2	77.4	230.7	37.7	243.5	39.8
1991	670.8	11.7	2,558	143.3	21.4	527.6	78.7	250.0	37.3	277.6	41.4
1992	730.0	12.1	2,755	150.6	20.6	579.1	79.3	269.8	37.0	309.3	42.4
1993	782.5	12.3	2,920	157.5	20.1	625.1	79.9	288.1	36.8	337.0	43.1
1994	832.5	12.4	3,074	163.7	19.7	668.8	80.3	302.2	36.3	366.6	44.0

Average Annual Rate of Change											
1960-94	11.0	-	-	7.6	-	13.0	-	12.6	-	13.4	-
1970-94	11.2	-	-	8.1	-	12.5	-	12.8	-	12.3	-
1980-94	10.0	-	-	73	-	10.8	-	10.8	-	10.8	-
1970-80	13.0	-	-	9.2	-	15.0	-	15.6	-	14.5	-
1980-90	10.8	-	-	8.5	-	11.6	-	12.4	-	10.8	-
1990-94	8.0	-	-	4.3	-	9.0	-	7.0	-	10.8	-

Source: U.S. Department of Health and Human Services. Health Care Financing Administration. Office of Research and Demonstrations. *Health Care Financing Review, Medicare and Medicaid Statistical Supplement, 1996,* pp. 188-189. Primary source: The Personal Health Care Expenditures estimates are available in *Health Care Financing Review* (Summer 1995 and Spring 1996); historical estimates for selected calendar years 1960-93 have been revised. *Notes:* GDP represents "gross domestic product." Numbers may not add to totals because of rounding. 1. Represents benefit payments aggregated on an incurred basis and 100-percent estimates. Because of differences in methodology and completeness, the benefit payments are somewhat higher than the corresponding program payments shown.

★ 606 ★

Expenditures

Personal Health Care Expenditures (PHCE), by Source of Funds, Selected Calendar Years - II

This table shows more detail on the private and government third party payments for health care.

[Amounts in billions of dollars]

Year	All Third Parties		Private		Government								
	Amount	Percent of PHCE	Amount	Percent of PHCE	Amount	Percent of PHCE	Federal	State and Local	Medicare[1]		Medicaid[2]	
									Amount	Percent of PHCE	Amount	Percent of PHCE
1960	10.5	44.0	5.4	22.6	5.1	21.4	2.1	3.0	-	-	-	-
1970	39.4	60.8	16.9	26.1	22.5	34.6	14.7	7.8	7.3	11.3	5.1	7.9
1980	158.8	72.1	71.8	32.6	87.0	39.5	63.4	23.6	36.4	16.5	24.7	11.2
1981	186.1	72.8	84.8	33.2	101.3	39.6	74.6	26.7	43.6	18.9	28.9	11.3
1982	211.0	73.4	97.8	34.0	113.2	39.4	83.8	29.5	51.2	17.8	30.6	10.6
1983	233.0	73.7	108.0	34.2	125.0	39.6	93.3	31.7	58.3	18.4	33.6	10.6
1984	255.2	73.8	118.8	34.4	136.4	39.5	102.4	34.0	64.9	18.8	36.2	10.5
1985	281.7	74.0	133.7	35.1	148.0	38.9	111.3	36.7	70.3	18.5	39.2	10.3
1986	309.5	74.7	147.4	35.6	162.1	40.5	120.2	41.9	75.1	18.1	43.3	10.4
1987	342.2	75.4	165.8	36.5	176.4	38.9	129.4	47.0	80.4	17.7	47.9	10.6
1988	377.3	75.4	186.2	37.2	191.1	38.2	140.4	50.6	87.1	17.4	52.3	10.5
1989	422.7	76.8	208.4	37.9	214.3	38.9	158.6	55.7	100.1	18.2	59.2	10.8
1990	474.2	77.4	230.7	37.7	243.5	39.8	178.1	65.3	109.6	17.9	71.7	11.7
1991	527.6	78.7	250.0	37.3	277.6	41.4	206.0	71.6	120.5	18.0	89.9	13.4
1992	579.1	79.3	269.8	37.0	309.3	42.4	234.0	75.3	135.4	18.5	103.6	14.2
1993	625.1	79.9	288.1	36.8	337.0	43.1	259.0	78.1	151.1	19.3	112.8	14.4
1994	668.8	80.3	302.2	36.3	366.6	44.0	283.8	82.9	168.1	20.2	123.6	14.8
Average Annual Rate of Change												
1960-94	13.0	-	12.6	-	13.4	-	15.5	10.3	-	-	-	-
1970-94	12.5	-	12.8	-	12.3	-	13.1	10.3	14.0	-	14.2	-
1980-94	10.8	-	10.8	-	10.8	-	11.3	9.4	11.5	-	12.2	-
1970-80	15.0	-	15.6	-	14.5	-	15.7	11.7	17.4	-	17.1	-
1980-90	11.6	-	12.4	-	10.8	-	10.9	10.7	11.7	-	11.2	-
1990-94	9.0	-	7.0	-	10.8	-	12.4	6.1	11.3	-	14.6	-

Source: U.S. Department of Health and Human Services. Health Care Financing Administration. Office of Research and Demonstrations. *Health Care Financing Review, Medicare and Medicaid Statistical Supplement, 1996,* pp 188-189. Primary source: The Personal Health Care Expenditures estimates are available in *Health Care Financing Review* (Summer 1996 and Spring 1996); historical estimates for selected calendar years 1960-93 have been revised. *Notes:* GDP represents "gross domestic product." Numbers may not add to totals because of rounding. 1. Subset of Federal Funds. 2. Subset of Federal and State and local funds.

★ 607 ★

Expenditures

Physicians' Services Expenditures: 1991-1994

Data in the table show expenditures for physicians' services and the percent distribution by source of funds for the years shown. Data were compiled by the Health Care Financing Administration.

Service and year	Total in billions	Out-of-pocket payments	Private health insurance	Other private funds	Government		
					Total[1]	Medicaid	Medicare
1991	158.6	22.4	45.0	1.6	31.0	5.8	19.4
1992	174.7	21.7	46.6	1.5	30.2	6.4	18.2
1993	181.1	20.4	47.1	1.5	30.9	7.0	18.7
1994	189.4	18.9	47.3	1.6	32.1	7.1	20.1

Source: U.S. Department of Health and Human Services. Public Health Service. Centers for Disease Control and Prevention. National Center for Health Statistics. *Health, United States, 1995.* Hyattsville, MD: Public Health Service, 1996. p. 250. Primary source: Office of National Health Statistics, Office of the Actuary. National Health Expenditures, 1994. *Health Care Financing Review,* vol. 17, no. 3. *Notes:* These data include revisions in health expenditures and in population back to 1960 and differ from previous editions of *Health, United States.* 1. Includes other government expenditures for these health care services, for example, care funded by the Department of Veterans Affairs and State and locally financed subsidies to hospitals.

Medical Prices

★ 608 ★

Coronary-Artery Bypass Fees, 1995: A Comparison

The table shows typical fees charged by heart surgeons for bypass surgery, vein only, three grafts. Hospital charges are not included.

City	Customary fee	Typical managed care	Percent Discount
Philadelphia, PA	$10,452	$3,525	66
San Francisco, CA	9,991	3,600	64
Chicago, IL	9,720	3,859	60
New York City, NY	10,136	4,286	58
Atlanta, GA	8,085	4,346	56
Los Angeles, CA	8,675	3,962	54
Boston, MA	8,257	3,934	52

Source: Anders, George. "Who Pays Cost of Cut-Rate Heart Care?" *Wall Street Journal,* 15 October 1996, p. B9.

★ 609 ★

Medical Prices

Index Levels of Medical Prices: 1992-1996

Item	Calendar year				1996	
	1992	1993	1994	1995	Q1	Q2
Consumer Price Indexes, All Urban Consumers[1]						
Medical Care Services[2]	190.5	202.9	213.4	224.2	230.1	231.5
Professional Services	175.8	184.7	192.5	201.0	205.9	207.5
Physicians' Services	181.2	191.3	199.8	208.8	214.3	215.8
Dental Services	178.7	188.1	197.1	206.8	212.5	215.1
Hospital and Related Services	214.0	231.9	245.6	257.8	266.1	267.7
Hospital Room	208.7	226.4	239.2	251.2	257.9	259.0
Other Inpatient Services (1986=100)	172.3	185.7	197.1	206.8	214.3	215.5
Outpatient Services (1986=100)	168.7	184.3	195.0	204.6	211.7	213.9
Medical Care Commodities	188.1	195.0	200.7	204.5	208.4	209.9
Prescription Drugs	214.7	223.0	230.6	235.0	240.1	242.3
Non-Prescription Drugs and Medical Supplies (1986=100)	131.2	135.5	138.1	140.5	142.5	142.9
Internal and Respiratory Over-the-Counter Drugs	158.2	163.5	165.9	167.0	169.3	169.5
Non-Prescription Medical Equipment and Supplies	150.9	155.9	160.0	166.3	168.7	169.3
Producer Price Indexes[3]						
Industry Groupings:[4]						
Health Services (12/94=100)	-	-	-	102.4	104.1	104.4
Offices and Clinics of Doctors of medicine (12/93=100)	-	-	102.8	106.8	107.4	107.5
Medicare Treatments (12/93=100)	-	-	104.7	109.6	105.5	105.5
Non-Medicare Treatments (12/93=100)	-	-	102.3	105.9	107.5	107.7
Hospitals (12/92=100)	-	102.5	106.2	110.0	112.2	112.3
General Medical and Surgical Hospitals (12/92=100)	-	102.4	106.0	109.9	112.2	112.2
Inpatient Treatments (12/92=100)	-	102.5	106.0	109.2	111.5	111.6
Medicare Patients (12/92=100)	-	100.6	102.6	104.7	107.8	107.8
Medicaid Patients (12/92=100)	-	102.3	107.1	109.8	111.7	112.5
All Other Patients (12/92=100)	-	103.5	107.7	111.7	113.6	113.4
Outpatient Treatments (12/92=100)	-	102.5	106.7	113.3	115.6	115.8
Medicare Patients (12/92=100)	-	103.7	107.0	111.2	112.3	112.5
Medicaid Patients (12/92=100)	-	101.6	103.3	106.4	107.1	107.1
All Other Patients (12/92=100)	-	102.4	106.9	114.2	116.9	117.1
Skilled and Intermediate Care Facilities (12/94=100)	-	-	-	103.6	108.2	109.5
Public Payors (12/94=100)	-	-	-	103.8	108.6	110.1
Private Payors (12/94=100)	-	-	-	103.6	108.2	109.1
Medical Laboratories (6/94=100)	-	-	-	104.0	105.3	105.2
Commodity Groupings:						
Drugs and Pharmaceuticals	192.2	200.9	206.0	210.9	213.8	214.6
Ethical (Prescription) Preparations	231.7	242.2	250.0	257.0	262.5	265.1
Proprietary (Over-the-Counter) Preparations	173.6	180.0	183.2	186.6	188.3	184.5
Medical, Surgical, and Personal Aid Devices	133.9	137.8	140.4	141.3	143.5	143.4
Personal Aid Equipment	120.2	122.3	130.1	133.7	136.8	139.8
Medical Instruments and Equipment (6/82=100)	123.4	126.0	126.7	128.3	130.3	130.1
Surgical Appliances and Supplies (6/83=100)	145.0	151.0	155.7	154.8	157.4	158.1

[Continued]

★ 609 ★

Index Levels of Medical Prices: 1992-1996
[Continued]

Item	Calendar year				1996	
	1992	1993	1994	1995	Q1	Q2
Ophthalmic Goods (12/83 = 100)	118.0	119.0	119.6	122.2	122.2	119.7
Dental Equipment and Supplies (6/85 = 100)	126.6	131.5	135.2	137.5	140.7	140.7

Source: U.S. Department of Labor. Bureau of Labor Statistics. *CPI Detailed Report.* Washington, DC: U.S. Government Printing Office. *Notes:* Q designates quarter of year. Quarterly data are not seasonally adjusted. 1. Unless otherwise noted, base year is 1982-84 = 100 2. Includes the net cost of private health insurance, not shown separately. 3. Unless otherwise noted, base year is 1982 = 100. Producer price indexes are classified by industry (price changes received for the industry's output sold outside the industry) and commodity (price changes by similarity of end use or material composition). 4. Further detail for Producer Price Industry groupings, such as types of physician practices, hospital DRG groupings, etc., are available from BLS.

★ 610 ★

Medical Prices

Percent Change in Medical Prices from Same Period a Year Ago: 1992-1996

Table shows percentage change from year to year or from one period to the same period of a year before.

Item	Calendar year				1996	
	1992	1993	1994	1995	Q1	Q2
Consumer Price Indexes, All Urban Consumers[1]						
Medical Care Services[2]	7.6	6.5	5.2	5.0	4.1	3.8
Professional Services	6.1	5.1	4.3	4.4	3.8	3.7
Physicians' Services	6.3	5.6	4.4	4.5	4.2	3.7
Dental Services	6.7	5.3	4.8	4.9	4.2	4.6
Hospital and Related Services	9.1	8.4	5.9	5.0	4.7	4.7
Hospital Room	8.8	8.5	5.7	5.0	4.1	3.9
Other Inpatient Services (1986 = 100)	9.1	7.8	6.1	5.0	5.0	5.0
Outpatient Services (1986 = 100)	10.0	9.3	5.8	4.9	5.0	5.7
Medical Care Commodities	6.4	3.7	2.9	1.9	2.4	3.1
Prescription Drugs	7.6	3.9	3.4	1.9	2.9	3.6
Non-Prescription Drugs and Medical Supplies (1986 = 100)	3.9	3.3	1.9	1.8	1.5	2.0
Internal and Respiratory Over-the-Counter Drugs	3.8	3.3	1.5	0.6	1.3	2.1
Non-Prescription Medical Equipment and Supplies	4.1	3.3	2.7	3.9	1.7	1.8
Producer Price Indexes[3]						
Industry Groupings:[4]						
Health Services (12/94 = 100)	-	-	-	2.5	2.4	-
Offices and Clinics of Doctors of Medicine (12/93 = 100)	-	-	-	3.9	1.0	0.7
Medicare Treatments (12/93 = 100)	-	-	-	4.7	-3.7	-3.7
Non-Medicare Treatments (12/93 = 100)	-	-	-	3.6	1.9	1.5
Hospitals (12/92 = 100)	-	-	3.6	3.5	2.7	2.7
General Medical and Surgical Hospitals (12/92 = 100)	-	-	3.5	3.7	2.9	2.8
Inpatient Treatments (12/92 = 100)	-	-	3.5	3.1	2.8	2.8
Medicare Patients (12/92 = 100)	-	-	2.0	2.0	4.1	4.1
Medicaid Patients (12/92 = 100)	-	-	4.6	2.5	2.1	2.6
All Other Patients (12/92 = 100)	-	-	4.0	3.7	2.3	2.0

[Continued]

★ 610 ★

Percent Change in Medical Prices from Same Period a Year Ago: 1992-1996

[Continued]

Item	Calendar year				1996	
	1992	1993	1994	1995	Q1	Q2
Outpatient Treatments (12/92=100)	-	-	4.1	6.2	3.3	2.9
Medicare Patients (12/92=100)	-	-	3.1	4.0	1.9	1.3
Medicaid Patients (12/92=100)	-	-	1.7	2.9	1.3	1.2
All Other Patients (12/92=100)	-	-	4.4	6.9	3.7	3.4
Skilled and Intermediate Care Facilities (12/94=100)	-	-	-	-	6.1	6.5
Public Payors (12/94=100)	-	-	-	-	6.6	7.2
Private Payors (12/94=100)	-	-	-	-	5.9	5.8
Medical Laboratories (6/94=100)	-	-	-	-	3.7	1.8
Commodity Groupings:						
Drugs and Pharmaceuticals	5.3	4.5	2.5	2.4	2.5	2.0
Ethical (Prescription) Preparations	6.5	4.5	3.2	2.8	3.9	3.6
Proprietary (Over-the-Counter) Preparations	5.0	3.7	1.8	1.8	1.5	-1.1
Medical, Surgical, and Personal Aid Devices	2.7	3.0	1.8	0.7	2.0	1.8
Personal Aid Equipment	2.6	1.7	6.4	2.7	4.3	6.1
Medical Instruments and Equipment (6/82=100)	2.2	2.1	0.5	1.3	2.0	1.6
Surgical Appliances and Supplies (6/83=100)	3.1	4.1	3.1	-0.6	2.0	2.6
Ophthalmic Goods (12/83=100)	1.7	0.9	0.6	2.2	0.4	-1.8
Dental Equipment and Supplies (6/85=100)	4.5	3.8	2.9	1.7	3.2	2.0

Source: U.S. Department of Labor. Bureau of Labor Statistics. *CPI Detailed Report.* Washington, DC: U.S. Government Printing Office. Monthly reports for January 1991-June 1996. *Notes:* Q designates quarter of year. Quarterly data are not seasonally adjusted. 1. Unless otherwise noted, base year is 1982-84 = 100 2. Includes the net cost of private health insurance, not shown separately. 3. Unless otherwise noted, base year is 1982 = 100. Producer price indexes are classified by industry (price changes received for the industry's output sold outside the industry) and commodity (price changes by similarity of end use or material composition). 4. Further detail for Producer Price Industry groupings, such as types of physician practices, hospital DRG groupings, etc., are available from BLS.

★ 611 ★

Medical Prices

Prices of Newer and Older Psychiatric Medications

Medications	Pill Strength	Avg. Wholesale Price Per Pill	Typical Daily Dose for Adult Outpatients
Paxil	20 mg.	$1.90	20 mg.
Prozac	20 mg.	2.24	20 mg.
Zoloft	50 mg.	2.02	50 mg.
Tricyclics			
Amitriptyline	25 mg.	$0.07	75-150 mg.

[Continued]

★ 611 ★

Prices of Newer and Older Psychiatric Medications
[Continued]

Medications	Pill Strength	Avg. Wholesale Price Per Pill	Typical Daily Dose for Adult Outpatients
Desipramine	50 mg.	0.11	100-200 mg.
Imipramine	50 mg.	0.06	75-150 mg.

Source: *Wall Street Journal,* 1 December 1995, p. A4. Primary source: SmithKline Beecham, Eli Lilly, Pfizer, and Schein Pharmaceuticals.

Mental Health

★ 612 ★

Treatment Costs for Mental Disorders, 1990

This table shows the direct costs of treating all mental disorders, a $67 billion expenditure, 11.4 percent of all medical spending. Data are shown by categories.

[In billions of dollars]

Category	$ billion
Mental health institutions[1]	19.5
Hospital care, short-term	13.4
Physician's office visits	3.7
Other mental health professionals	6.6
Nursing homes	16.5
Drugs	2.2
Administration	5.2

Source: "Mental Disorders: The Toll." *USA TODAY,* 28 May 1996. Primary sources: National Institute of Mental Health; Dorothy Rice, University of California, San Francisco; *Psychotherapy Finances. Note:* 1. Includes psychiatric hospitals, treatment centers, and prisons.

Trends and Projections

★ 613 ★

Average Annual Percent Change in Consumer Price Index for Medical Care and Selected Items: 1992-1995

Data are based on reporting by samples of providers and other retail outlets.

Year	All items	Medical care	Food	Apparel and upkeep	Housing	Energy	Personal care
1992-93	3.0	5.9	2.2	1.4	2.7	1.2	2.3
1993-94	2.6	4.8	2.4	-0.2	2.5	0.4	2.2
1994-95	2.8	4.5	2.8	-1.0	2.6	0.6	1.7

Source: U.S. Department of Health and Human Services. Public Health Service. Centers for Disease Control and Prevention. National Center for Health Statistics. *Health, United States, 1995.* Hyattsville, MD: Public Health Service, 1996. p. 241. Primary source: U.S. Department of Labor, Bureau of Labor Statistics, Consumer Price Index (various releases). *Note:* 1982-84 = 100.

★ 614 ★

Trends and Projections

Average Annual Percent Change in Consumer Price Index for Medical Care Components: 1992-1995

Data are based on reporting by samples of providers and other retail outlets.

Item and medical care component	1992-93	1993-94	1994-95
Average annual percent change			
CPI, all items	3.0	2.6	2.8
Less medical care	2.7	2.5	2.7
CPI, all services	3.9	3.3	3.4
All medical care	5.9	4.8	4.5
Medical care services	6.5	5.2	5.1
Professional medical services	5.1	4.2	4.4
Physicians' services	5.6	4.4	4.5
Dental services	5.3	4.8	4.9
Eye care[1]	2.7	2.0	3.0
Services by other medical professionals[1]	3.2	4.0	1.8
Hospital and related services	8.4	5.9	5.0
Hospital rooms	8.5	5.7	5.0
Other inpatient services[1]	7.8	6.1	4.9
Outpatient services[1]	9.2	5.8	4.9
Medical care commodities	3.7	2.9	1.9

[Continued]

★ 614 ★

Average Annual Percent Change in Consumer Price Index for Medical Care Components: 1992-1995

[Continued]

Item and medical care component	1992-93	1993-94	1994-95
Prescription drugs	3.9	3.4	1.9
Nonprescription drugs and medical supplies[1]	3.3	1.9	1.7
Internal and respiratory over-the-counter drugs	3.4	1.5	0.7
Nonprescription medical equipment and supplies	3.3	2.6	3.9

Source: U.S. Department of Health and Human Services. Public Health Service. Centers for Disease Control and Prevention. National Center for Health Statistics. *Health, United States, 1995.* Hyattsville, MD: Public Health Service, 1996. p. 242. Primary source: U.S. Department of Labor, Bureau of Labor Statistics, Consumer Price Index (various releases). *Notes:* 1982-84=100, except where noted. 1. Dec. 1986=100.

★ 615 ★

Trends and Projections

Consumer Price Index for Medical Care and Selected Items: 1992-1995

Data are based on reporting by samples of providers and other retail outlets.

Year	All items	Medical care	Food	Apparel and upkeep	Housing	Energy	Personal care
1992	140.3	190.1	137.9	131.9	137.5	103.0	138.3
1993	144.5	201.4	140.9	133.7	141.2	104.2	141.5
1994	148.2	211.0	144.3	133.4	144.8	104.6	144.6
1995	152.4	220.5	148.4	132.0	148.5	105.2	147.1

Source: U.S. Department of Health and Human Services. Public Health Service. Centers for Disease Control and Prevention. National Center for Health Statistics. *Health, United States, 1995.* Hyattsville, MD: Public Health Service, 1996. p. 241. Primary source: U.S. Department of Labor, Bureau of Labor Statistics, Consumer Price Index (various releases). *Note:* 1982-84=100.

★ 616 ★

Trends and Projections

Consumer Price Index for Medical Care Components: 1992-1995

Data are based on reporting by samples of providers and other retail outlets.

Item and medical care component	1992	1993	1994	1995
Consumer Price Index				
CPI, all items	140.3	144.5	148.2	152.4
Less medical care	137.5	141.2	144.7	148.6
CPI, all services	152.0	157.9	163.1	168.7
All medical care	190.1	201.4	211.0	220.5
Medical care services	190.5	202.9	213.4	224.2
Professional medical services	175.8	184.7	192.5	201.0
Physicians' services	181.2	191.3	199.8	208.8
Dental services	178.7	188.1	197.1	206.8
Eye care[1]	127.0	130.4	133.0	137.0
Services by other medical professionals[1]	131.7	135.9	141.3	143.9
Hospital and related services	214.0	231.9	245.6	257.8
Hospital rooms	208.7	226.4	239.2	251.2
Other inpatient services[1]	172.3	185.7	197.1	206.8
Outpatient services[1]	168.7	184.3	195.0	204.6
Medical care commodities	188.1	195.0	200.7	204.5
Prescription drugs	214.7	223.0	230.6	235.0
Nonprescription drugs and medical supplies[1]	131.2	135.5	138.1	140.5
Internal and respiratory over-the-counter drugs	158.2	163.5	165.9	167.0
Nonprescription medical equipment and supplies	150.9	155.9	160.0	166.3

Source: U.S. Department of Health and Human Services. Public Health Service. Centers for Disease Control and Prevention. National Center for Health Statistics. *Health, United States, 1995.* Hyattsville, MD: Public Health Service, 1996. p. 242. Primary source: U.S. Department of Labor, Bureau of Labor Statistics, Consumer Price Index (various releases). *Notes:* 1982-84 = 100, except where noted. 1. Dec. 1986 = 100.

★ 617 ★

Trends and Projections

National Health Care Expenditures Average Annual Percent Change, by Source of Funds: 1991-1994

Data in the table include revisions in health expenditures and differ from previous editions. They reflect Social Security Administration revisions as of July 1995.

Year	All health expenditures in billions	Private funds		Public funds	
		Amount in billions	Amount per capita	Amount in billions	Amount per capita
1991-92	9.5	8.2	7.0	11.3	10.1
1992-93	7.0	5.9	4.8	8.6	7.5
1993-94	6.4	4.7	3.6	8.7	7.6

Source: U.S. Department of Health and Human Services. Public Health Service. Centers for Disease Control and Prevention. National Center for Health Statistics. *Health, United States, 1995.* Hyattsville, MD: Public Health Service, 1996. p. 243. Primary source: Office of National Health Statistics, Office of the Actuary. National Health Expenditures, 1994. *Health Care Financing Review,* vol. 17, no. 3.

★ 618 ★

Trends and Projections

National Health Care Expenditures, by Source of Funds: 1992-1994

Data in the table include revisions in health expenditures and differ from previous editions. They reflect Social Security Administration revisions as of July 1995.

Year	All health expenditures in billions	Private funds			Public funds		
		Amount in billions	Amount per capita	Percent of total	Amount in billions	Amount per capita	Percent of total
1992	833.6	477.0	1,799	57.2	356.5	1,345	42.8
1993	892.3	505.1	1,886	56.6	387.2	1,445	43.4
1994	949.4	528.6	1,954	55.7	420.8	1,556	44.3

Source: U.S. Department of Health and Human Services. Public Health Service. Centers for Disease Control and Prevention. National Center for Health Statistics. *Health, United States, 1995.* Hyattsville, MD: Public Health Service, 1996. p. 243. Primary source: Office of National Health Statistics, Office of the Actuary. National Health Expenditures, 1994. *Health Care Financing Review,* vol. 17, no. 3.

Chapter 7
HEALTH CARE PROGRAMS

Tables that present information on health insurance and other forms of health programs are brought together in this chapter. Data on major programs (HMOs, Medicare, Medicaid) are presented along with information on health insurance coverage and special topics. For a profiling of the health care delivery system, please see Chapter 3 - Health Care Establishment. For additional data on costs and expenditures, see Chapter 6 - Health Expenditures and Funding. International comparisons are shown in Chapter 11.

Children

★ 619 ★

Estimated Number of U.S. Children Under 19, by Health Insurance, Family Income, and Race/Ethnicity: 1982-91

[In thousands]

| Year and Race/Ethnicity | Total children | Family income as percent of Federal Poverty Level (FPL) | | | | 200% FPL & above non-Medicaid insured and uninsured |
| | | Below 200% FPL | | | | |
		Medicaid only	Medicaid plus non-Medicaid insurance	Uninsured	Non-Medicaid insurance	
1982						
Total	57,914	6,014	772	6,910	16,483	27,736
White	41,580	2,213	347	3,925	11,681	23,413
African-American	8,270	2,442	343	1,271	2,524	1,690
Hispanic	6,401	1,107	53	1,465	1,864	1,912
Other	1,663	253	29	249	412	720
1988						
Total	56,232	6,731	2,243	5,245	13,012	29,001
White	38,594	2,410	1,039	2,643	9,069	23,433
African-American	8,389	2,645	633	944	2,108	2,059
Hispanic	7,369	1,387	428	1,406	1,509	2,639

[Continued]

★ 619 ★

Estimated Number of U.S. Children Under 19, by Health Insurance, Family Income, and Race/Ethnicity: 1982-91
[Continued]

Year and Race/Ethnicity	Total children	Family income as percent of Federal Poverty Level (FPL)				200% FPL & above non-Medicaid insured and uninsured
		Below 200% FPL				
		Medicaid only	Medicaid plus non-Medicaid insurance	Uninsured	Non-Medicaid insurance	
Other	1,880	289	144	252	325	870
1991						
Total	57,765	9,286	815	6,433	13,797	27,434
White	38,460	3,306	430	3,011	9,520	22,194
African-American	8,470	3,269	226	1,164	1,945	1,866
Hispanic	8,844	2,294	118	2,059	1,932	2,442
Other	1,992	418	42	199	400	933
Percent change 1982-91						
Total	-0.3	54.4	5.6	-6.9	-16.3	-1.1
White	-7.5	49.4	23.6	-23.3	-18.5	-5.2
African-American	2.4	33.9	-34.1	-8.4	-22.9	10.4
Hispanic	38.2	107.3	121.8	40.5	3.6	27.7
Other	19.8	65.4	45.5	-19.8	-3.0	29.5
Percent						
1982						
Total	100.0	10.4	1.3	11.9	28.5	47.8
White	100.0	5.3	0.8	9.4	28.1	56.3
African-American	100.0	29.5	4.1	15.4	30.5	20.4
Hispanic	100.0	17.3	0.8	22.9	29.1	29.9
Other	100.0	15.2	1.7	15.0	24.8	43.3
1988						
Total	100.0	12.0	4.0	9.3	23.1	51.6
White	100.0	6.2	2.7	6.8	23.5	60.7
African-American	100.0	31.5	7.5	11.3	25.1	24.5
Hispanic	100.0	18.8	5.8	19.1	20.5	35.8
Other	100.0	15.4	7.6	13.4	17.3	46.3
1992						
Total	100.0	16.1	1.4	11.1	23.9	47.5
White	100.0	8.6	1.1	7.8	24.8	57.7
African-American	100.0	38.6	2.7	13.7	23.0	22.0
Hispanic	100.0	25.9	1.3	23.3	21.8	27.6
Other	100.0	21.0	2.1	10.0	20.1	46.8

Source: U.S. Department of Health and Human Services. Health Care Financing Administration. Office of Research and Demonstrations. *Health Care Financing Review, Medicare and Medicaid Statistical Supplement, 1996,* pp. 438-439. Primary source: DHHS, NCHS, National Health Interview Survey, 1982, 1988, 1991.

★ 620 ★

Children

Estimated Number of U.S. Children Under 19, by Health Insurance, Family Income and Region: 1982-91

| Year and Region | Total Children | Family Income as Percent of Federal Poverty Level (FPL) | | | | 200% FPL & Above Non-Medicaid Insured and Uninsured |
| | | Below 200% FPL | | | | |
		Medicaid Only	Medicaid Plus Other Insurance	Uninsured	Non-Medicaid Insurance	
In Thousands						
1982						
Total	57,903	6,014	772	6,910	16,499	27,708
Northeast	12,047	1,726	139	898	3,382	5,902
Midwest	15,308	1,510	263	1,278	4,471	7,786
South	19,194	1,630	193	3,040	5,824	8,506
West	11,354	1,149	177	1,693	2,821	5,514
1988						
Total	56,233	6,738	2,243	5,240	13,012	29,001
Northeast	10,178	1,205	482	509	2,095	5,887
Midwest	14,869	1,885	733	745	3,617	7,888
South	19,192	2,221	451	2,675	4,971	8,874
West	11,995	1,427	576	1,311	2,329	6,351
1992						
Total	57,809	9,295	816	6,439	13,797	27,461
Northeast	11,255	1,801	85	836	2,414	6,118
Midwest	13,920	2,006	219	1,042	3,739	6,913
South	18,955	3,083	271	2,843	4,884	7,874
West	13,679	2,405	240	1,718	2,759	6,557
Percent Change 1982-91						
Total	-0.2	54.6	5.7	-6.8	-16.4	-0.9
Northeast	-6.6	4.4	-39.0	-6.9	-28.6	3.7
Midwest	-9.1	32.9	-16.7	-18.5	-16.4	-11.2
South	-1.2	89.2	40.6	-6.5	-16.1	-7.4
West	20.5	109.4	36.0	1.5	-2.2	18.9
Percent						
1982						
Total						
Northeast	100.0	14.63	1.2	7.5	28.1	49.0
Midwest	100.0	9.9	1.7	8.4	29.2	50.9
South	100.0	8.5	1.0	15.8	30.3	44.3
West	100.0	10.1	1.6	14.9	24.8	48.6
1988						
Total	100.0	12.0	4.0	9.3	23.1	51.6
Northeast	100.0	11.8	4.7	5.0	20.6	57.8
Midwest	100.0	12.7	4.9	5.0	24.3	53.1

[Continued]

★ 620 ★

Estimated Number of U.S. Children Under 19, by Health Insurance, Family Income and Region: 1982-91
[Continued]

Year and Region	Total Children	Family Income as Percent of Federal Poverty Level (FPL)				200% FPL & Above Non-Medicaid Insured and Uninsured
		Below 200% FPL				
		Medicaid Only	Medicaid Plus Other Insurance	Uninsured	Non-Medicaid Insurance	
South	100.0	11.6	2.3	13.9	25.9	46.2
West	100.0	11.9	4.8	10.9	19.4	52.9
1992						
Total	100.0	16.1	1.4	11.1	23.9	47.5
Northeast	100.0	16.0	0.8	7.4	21.5	54.4
Midwest	100.0	14.4	1.6	7.5	26.9	49.7
South	100.0	16.3	1.4	15.0	25.8	41.5
West	100.0	17.6	1.8	12.6	20.2	47.9

Source: U.S. Department of Health and Human Services. Health Care Financing Administration. Office of Research and Demonstrations. *Health Care Financing Review, Medicare and Medicaid Statistical Supplement, 1996,* pp. 441-442. Primary source: DHHS, NCHS, National Health Interview Survey, 1982, 1988, 1991.

★ 621 ★
Children

Percent Distribution of Health Insurance Coverage of U.S. Children Under 19 Living in Families With Family Income Less Than 200 Percent of the Federal Poverty Level: 1982-91

Year and Race/Ethnicity	Children Below 200% Federal Poverty Level (000)	Insurance Coverage				
		Percent				
		Children Below 200% FPL as Percent of All U.S. Children	Children Below 200% FPL With Medicaid Only	Children Below 200% FPL With Medicaid Plus Other Insurance	Children Below 200% FPL With No Health Insurance	Children Below 200% FPL With Private Health Insurance
1982						
Total	30,179	52.1	19.9	2.6	22.9	54.6
White	18,167	43.7	12.2	1.9	21.6	64.3
African-American	6,580	79.6	37.1	5.2	19.3	38.4
Hispanic	4,489	70.1	24.7	1.2	32.6	41.5
Other	942	56.7	26.8	3.0	26.4	43.8
1988						
Total	27,231	48.4	24.7	8.2	19.3	47.8
White	15,161	39.3	15.9	6.8	17.4	59.8
African-American	6,330	75.5	41.8	10.0	14.9	33.3
Hispanic	4,730	64.2	29.3	9.1	29.7	31.9
Other	1,010	53.7	28.7	14.2	24.9	32.2

[Continued]

★ 621 ★

Percent Distribution of Health Insurance Coverage of U.S. Children Under 19 Living in Families With Family Income Less Than 200 Percent of the Federal Poverty Level: 1982-91

[Continued]

Year and Race/Ethnicity	Children Below 200% Federal Poverty Level (000)	Insurance Coverage				
		Percent				
		Children Below 200% FPL as Percent of All U.S. Children	Children Below 200% FPL With Medicaid Only	Children Below 200% FPL With Medicaid Plus Other Insurance	Children Below 200% FPL With No Health Insurance	Children Below 200% FPL With Private Health Insurance
1992						
Total	30,331	52.5	30.6	2.7	21.2	45.5
White	16,266	42.3	20.3	2.6	18.5	58.5
African-American	6,604	78.0	49.5	3.4	17.6	29.5
Hispanic	6,402	72.4	35.8	1.8	32.2	30.2
Other	1,059	53.2	39.5	3.9	18.8	37.8

Source: U.S. Department of Health and Human Services. Health Care Financing Administration. Office of Research and Demonstrations. *Health Care Financing Review, Medicare and Medicaid Statistical Supplement, 1996,* p. 440. Primary source: DHHS, NCHS, National Health Interview Survey, 1982, 1988, 1991.

★ 622 ★

Children

Percent Distribution of Health Insurance Coverage of U.S. Children Under 19 Living in Families With Family Income Less Than 200 Percent of the Federal Poverty Level, by Region:

Year and Region	Children Below 200% Federal Poverty Level (FPL) (000)	Percent				
		Children Below 200% FPL as Percent of All Children	Health Insurance coverage			
			Children Below 200% FPL With Medicaid Only	Children Below 200% FPL With Medicaid Plus Other Insurance	Children Below 200% FPL With No Health Insurance	Children Below 200% FPL With Private Health Insurance
1982						
Total	30,195	100.0	19.9	2.6	22.9	54.6
Northeast	6,146	100.0	28.1	2.3	14.6	55.0
Midwest	7,522	100.0	20.1	3.5	17.0	59.4
South	10,687	100.0	15.2	1.8	28.4	54.5
West	5,840	100.0	19.7	3.0	29.0	48.3
1988						
Total	27,232	100.0	24.7	8.2	19.2	47.8
Northeast	4,291	100.0	28.1	11.2	11.9	48.8
Midwest	6,980	100.0	27.0	10.5	10.7	51.8
South	10,318	100.0	21.5	4.4	25.9	48.2
West	5,644	100.0	25.3	10.2	23.2	41.3

[Continued]

★ 622 ★

Percent Distribution of Health Insurance Coverage of U.S. Children Under 19 Living in Families With Family Income Less Than 200 Percent of the Federal Poverty Level, by Region:

[Continued]

Year and Region	Children Below 200% Federal Poverty Level (FPL) (000)	Percent				
		Health Insurance coverage				
		Children Below 200% FPL as Percent of All Children	Children Below 200% FPL With Medicaid Only	Children Below 200% FPL With Medicaid Plus Other Insurance	Children Below 200% FPL With No Health Insurance	Children Below 200% FPL With Private Health Insurance
1992						
Total	30,384	52.5	30.6	2.7	21.2	45.5
Northeast	5,137	45.6	35.1	1.6	16.3	47.0
Midwest	7,006	50.3	28.6	3.1	14.9	53.4
South	11,082	58.5	27.8	2.4	25.7	44.1
West	7,123	52.1	33.8	3.4	24.1	38.7

Source: U.S. Department of Health and Human Services. Health Care Financing Administration. Office of Research and Demonstrations. *Health Care Financing Review, Medicare and Medicaid Statistical Supplement, 1996,* p. 443. Primary source: DHHS, NCHS, National Health Interview Survey, 1982, 1988, 1991.

Health Insurance Coverage

★ 623 ★

Coverage for Behavioral Health Care in the U.S. Population: 1994

This table shows health care coverage, by type of plan, for so-called behavioral disorders, i.e., those that include mental and addictive disorders.

[In millions]

Plan	Number covered (million)
Indemnity (conventional)	77
Managed Behavioral Health Care	108
Medicaid	30
No insurance	40

Source: SAMHSA News (Summer 1995), p. 12. Primary source: American Managed Care Review Association, 1994, and *Open Minds Newsletter,* 1995.

★ 624 ★

Health Insurance Coverage

Growth of Managed Care

This table shows employee health coverage by type for 1988 and 1993, illustrating the decline of conventional (indemnity) plans and the growth of managed care programs.

Type	Percent of coverage	
	1988	1993
Indemnity (conventional)	71.0	49.0
Health Maintenance Organizations (HMO)	18.0	22.0
Preferred Provider Organization (PPO)	11.0	20.0
Point of Service (POS)	11.0	9.0

Source: SAMHSA News (Summer 1995), p. 11. Primary source: Peat Marwick, 1993.

★ 625 ★

Health Insurance Coverage

Health Insurance Coverage by Selected Characteristics

This table shows health insurance coverage status of all persons by selected characteristics for 1995.

[Numbers in thousands]

Characteristic	Total Number	Total Covered Number	Total Covered Percent	Not Covered Number	Not Covered Percent
All persons	264,315	223,733	84.6	40,582	15.4
Sex:					
Male	129,144	107,496	83.2	21,648	16.8
Female	135,171	116,237	86.0	18,934	14.0
Age:					
Under 18 years	71,148	61,353	86.2	9,795	13.8
18 to 24 years	24,843	17,847	71.8	6,996	28.2
25 to 34 years	40,919	31,561	77.1	9,358	22.9
35 to 44 years	43,078	35,946	83.4	7,132	16.6
45 to 64 years	52,668	45,668	86.7	7,000	13.3
65 years and over	31,658	31,358	99.1	300	0.9
Race and Hispanic Origin:					
White	218,443	187,338	85.8	31,105	14.2
Black	33,889	26,782	79.0	7,107	21.0
Hispanic origin[1]	28,438	18,964	66.7	9,474	33.3
Education:					
(persons age 18+)					
No high school dipl	36,474	27,611	75.7	8,863	24.3
High sch grad, only	64,118	52,760	82.3	11,358	17.7
Some college, no deg	37,840	32,233	85.2	5,607	14.8

[Continued]

★ 625 ★

Health Insurance Coverage by Selected Characteristics
[Continued]

Characteristic	Total Number	Total Covered		Not Covered	
		Number	Percent	Number	Percent
Associate degree	13,159	11,603	88.2	1,556	11.8
Bachelor's degree +	41,575	38,174	91.8	3,401	8.2
Work Experience:					
(persons age 18 to 64)					
Worked during year	131,391	108,423	82.5	22,968	17.5
Full-time	107,314	89,728	83.6	17,586	16.4
Part-time	24,078	18,695	77.6	5,383	22.4
Did not work	30,117	22,598	75.0	7,519	25.0
Foreign-Born:					
Native	239,757	207,159	86.4	32,598	13.6
Foreign-born	24,557	16,573	67.5	7,984	32.5
Naturalized citizen	7,904	6,652	84.2	1,252	15.8
Not a citizen	16,653	9,921	59.6	6,732	40.4
Household Income:					
Less than $25,000	78,435	59,722	76.1	18,713	23.9
$25,000-$49,999	84,459	70,762	83.8	13,697	16.2
$50,000-$74,999	53,453	48,479	90.7	4,974	9.3
$75,000 or more	47,967	44,770	93.3	3,197	6.7
Firm Size:					
All firms	140,338	74,602	53.2	65,736	46.8
Under 25 persons	42,833	12,115	28.3	30,718	71.7
25 to 99 persons	17,777	9,541	53.7	8,236	46.3
100 to 499 persons	19,062	12,102	63.5	6,960	36.5
500 to 999 persons	8,091	5,269	65.1	2,822	34.9
1000 or more persons	52,575	35,575	67.7	17,000	32.3

Source: U.S. Department of Commerce. Bureau of the Census. *Current Population Survey,* March 1996.
Note: 1. Persons of Hispanic origin may be of any race.

★ 626 ★
Health Insurance Coverage

Health Insurance Coverage Status and Type of Coverage - All Races, Females: 1987 to 1995

Numbers in thousands. Persons as of March of the following year.

| Year | Total persons | Covered by private or government health insurance | | | | | | | Not covered |
| | | Total | Private health insurance | | Government health insurance | | | | |
			Total	Group health	Total	Medicaid	Medicare	Military health care[1]	
ALL RACES FEMALE NUMBERS									
1995	135,171	116,237	94,606	80,709	39,110	18,452	19,769	4,338	18,934
1994[2]	134,033	115,625	93,880	79,891	39,269	18,428	19,388	5,134	18,408
1993[3]	132,838	114,779	92,965	74,126	38,849	18,705	19,044	4,508	18,060
1992[4]	131,393	113,890	92,853	74,726	37,599	17,368	19,185	4,475	17,503
1991	128,919	112,873	92,964	75,411	36,298	16,072	18,969	4,588	16,046
1990	127,695	111,688	93,307	75,491	34,481	14,299	18,580	4,676	16,007
1989	126,380	110,673	93,919	75,941	32,487	12,657	18,072	4,654	15,707
1988	125,211	109,970	93,233	75,624	32,125	12,535	17,812	4,635	15,241
1987[5]	123,970	109,454	93,544	75,023	31,706	11,959	17,571	4,913	14,516
PERCENTS									
1995	100.0	86.0	70.0	59.7	28.9	13.7	14.6	3.2	14.0
1994[2]	100.0	86.3	70.0	59.6	29.3	13.7	14.5	3.8	13.7
1993[3]	100.0	86.4	70.0	55.8	29.2	14.1	14.3	3.4	13.6
1992[4]	100.0	86.7	70.7	56.9	28.6	13.2	14.6	3.4	13.3
1991	100.0	87.6	72.1	58.5	28.2	12.5	14.7	3.6	12.4
1990	100.0	87.5	73.1	59.1	27.0	11.2	14.6	3.7	12.5
1989	100.0	87.6	74.3	60.1	25.7	10.0	14.3	3.7	12.4
1988	100.0	87.8	74.5	60.4	25.7	10.0	14.2	3.7	12.2
1987[5]	100.0	88.3	75.5	60.5	25.6	9.6	14.2	4.0	11.7

Source: U.S. Department of Commerce, U.S. Bureau of the Census, Income Statistics Branch/HHES Division, Washington, D.C. Unpublished March Current Population Survey for data prior to 1989 and Current Population Reports, Series P-60 for 1989 forward. *Notes:* 1. Includes CHAMPUS (Comprehensive Health and Medical Plan for Uniformed Services), Veterans, and military health care. 2. Health insurance questions were redesigned, decreases in estimates of group health and military health care coverage may be partially due to questionnaire changes. Overall coverage estimates were not affected. 3. Data collection method changed from paper and pencil to computer-assisted interviewing. 4. Implementation of 1990 census population controls. 5. Implementation of a new March CPS processing system.

★ 627 ★
Health Insurance Coverage

Health Insurance Coverage Status and Type of Coverage - All Races, Males: 1987 to 1995

Numbers in thousands. Population count as of March of the following year.

| Year | Total persons | Covered by private or government health insurance | | | | | | | | Not covered |
| | | Total | Private health insurance | | Government health insurance | | | | | |
			Total	Group health	Total	Medicaid	Medicare	Military health care[1]		
ALL RACES MALE NUMBERS										
1995	129,143	107,496	91,275	80,744	30,666	13,425	14,886	5,038		21,647
1994[2]	128,072	106,762	90,438	79,743	30,894	13,218	14,513	6,032		21,310
1993[3]	126,914	105,261	89,385	74,192	29,705	13,043	14,053	5,052		21,653
1992[4]	125,437	104,300	88,613	74,069	28,645	12,048	14,045	5,035		21,337
1991	122,528	103,130	88,410	74,666	27,584	10,808	13,938	5,232		19,398
1990	121,191	102,478	88,828	74,724	26,483	9,962	13,680	5,246		18,712
1989	119,811	102,134	89,691	75,702	24,895	8,528	13,424	5,216		17,678
1988	118,474	101,035	88,786	75,316	24,725	8,192	13,113	5,470		17,439
1987[5]	117,217	100,707	88,616	74,716	24,576	8,251	12,886	5,629		16,510
PERCENTS										
1995	100.0	83.2	70.7	62.5	23.7	10.4	11.5	3.9		16.8
1994[2]	100.0	83.4	70.6	62.3	24.1	10.3	11.3	4.7		16.6
1993[3]	100.0	82.9	70.4	58.5	23.4	10.3	11.1	4.0		17.1
1992[4]	100.0	83.1	70.6	59.0	22.8	9.6	11.2	4.0		16.9
1991	100.0	84.2	72.2	60.9	22.5	8.8	11.4	4.3		15.8
1990	100.0	84.6	73.3	61.7	21.9	8.2	11.3	4.3		15.4
1989	100.0	85.2	74.9	63.2	20.8	7.1	11.2	4.4		14.8
1988	100.0	85.3	74.9	63.6	20.9	6.9	11.1	4.6		14.7
1987[5]	100.0	85.9	75.6	63.7	21.0	7.0	11.0	4.8		14.1

Source: U.S. Department of Commerce, U.S. Bureau of the Census, Income Statistics Branch/HHES Division, Washington, D.C. Unpublished March Current Population Survey for data prior to 1989 and Current Population Reports, Series P-60 for 1989 forward. *Notes:* 1. Includes CHAMPUS (Comprehensive Health and Medical Plan for Uniformed Services), Veterans, and military health care. 2. Health insurance questions were redesigned, decreases in estimates of group health and military health care coverage may be partially due to questionnaire changes. Overall coverage estimates were not affected. 3. Data collection method changed from paper and pencil to computer-assisted interviewing. 4. Implementation of 1990 census population controls. 5. Implementation of a new March CPS processing system.

★ 628 ★

Health Insurance Coverage

Health Insurance Coverage Status and Type of Coverage - Blacks, Both Sexes: 1987 to 1995

Numbers in thousands. Persons as of March of the following year.

| Year | Total persons | Covered by private or government health insurance | | | | | | | Not covered |
| | | Total | Private health insurance | | Government health insurance | | | | |
			Total	Group health	Total	Medicaid	Medicare	Military health care[1]	
BLACKS, BOTH SEXES NUMBERS									
1995	33,889	26,781	17,106	15,683	12,465	9,184	3,316	1,171	7,108
1994[2]	33,531	26,928	17,147	15,607	12,693	9,007	3,167	1,683	6,603
1993[3]	33,040	26,279	16,590	13,693	12,588	9,283	3,072	1,331	6,761
1992[4]	32,535	25,967	15,994	13,545	12,464	9,122	3,154	1,459	6,567
1991	31,439	24,932	15,466	13,297	11,776	8,352	3,248	1,482	6,507
1990	30,895	24,802	15,957	13,560	11,150	7,809	3,106	1,402	6,093
1989	30,392	24,550	16,520	14,187	10,443	7,123	3,043	1,340	5,843
1988	29,904	24,029	15,818	13,418	10,415	7,049	3,064	1,385	5,875
1987[5]	29,417	23,555	15,358	13,055	10,380	7,046	2,918	1,497	5,862
PERCENTS									
1995	100.0	79.0	50.5	46.3	36.8	27.1	9.8	3.5	21.0
1994[2]	100.0	80.3	51.1	46.5	37.9	26.9	9.4	5.0	19.7
1993[3]	100.0	79.5	50.2	41.4	38.1	28.1	9.3	4.0	20.5
1992[4]	100.0	79.8	49.2	41.6	38.3	28.0	9.7	4.5	20.2
1991	100.0	79.3	49.2	42.3	37.5	26.6	10.3	4.7	20.7
1990	100.0	80.3	51.6	43.9	36.1	25.3	10.1	4.5	19.7
1989	100.0	80.8	54.4	46.7	34.4	23.4	10.0	4.4	19.2
1988	100.0	80.4	52.9	44.9	34.8	23.6	10.2	4.6	19.6
1987[5]	100.0	80.1	52.2	44.4	35.3	24.0	9.9	5.1	19.9

Source: U.S. Department of Commerce, U.S. Bureau of the Census, Income Statistics Branch/HHES Division, Washington, D.C. Unpublished March Current Population Survey for data prior to 1989 and Current Population Reports, Series P-60 for 1989 forward. *Notes:* 1. Includes CHAMPUS (Comprehensive Health and Medical Plan for Uniformed Services), Veterans, and military health care. 2. Health insurance questions were redesigned, decreases in estimates of group health and military health care coverage may be partially due to questionnaire changes. Overall coverage estimates were not affected. 3. Data collection method changed from paper and pencil to computer-assisted interviewing. 4. Implementation of 1990 census population controls. 5. Implementation of a new March CPS processing system.

★ 629 ★

Health Insurance Coverage

Health Insurance Coverage Status and Type of Coverage - Blacks, Females: 1987 to 1995

Numbers in thousands. Persons as of March of the following year.

| Year | Total persons | Covered by private or government health insurance | | | | | | | Not covered |
| | | Total | Private health insurance | | Government health insurance | | | | |
			Total	Group health	Total	Medicaid	Medicare	Military health care[1]	
BLACKS, FEMALES NUMBERS									
1995	18,065	14,796	9,099	8,293	7,189	5,469	1,966	501	3,269
1994[2]	17,844	14,756	9,069	8,174	7,291	5,358	1,865	752	3,088
1993[3]	17,582	14,531	8,812	7,312	7,274	5,564	1,869	566	3,051
1992[4]	17,327	14,370	8,496	7,167	7,252	5,548	1,889	617	2,957
1991	16,658	13,736	8,115	6,984	6,861	5,148	1,897	648	2,923
1990	16,400	13,581	8,348	7,009	6,530	4,754	1,829	654	2,819
1989	16,137	13,372	8,594	7,310	6,123	4,379	1,762	646	2,766
1988	15,883	13,185	8,247	6,907	6,059	4,395	1,832	576	2,698
1987[5]	15,634	12,881	8,110	6,780	5,969	4,287	1,719	647	2,753
PERCENTS									
1995	100.0	81.9	50.4	45.9	39.8	30.3	10.9	2.8	18.1
1994[2]	100.0	82.7	50.8	45.8	40.9	30.0	10.5	4.2	17.3
1993[3]	100.0	82.6	50.1	41.6	41.4	31.6	10.6	3.2	17.4
1992[4]	100.0	82.9	49.0	41.4	41.9	32.0	10.9	3.6	17.1
1991	100.0	82.5	48.7	41.9	41.2	30.9	11.4	3.9	17.5
1990	100.0	82.8	50.9	42.7	39.8	29.0	11.2	4.0	17.2
1989	100.0	82.9	53.3	45.3	37.9	27.1	10.9	4.0	17.1
1988	100.0	83.0	51.9	43.5	38.1	27.7	11.5	3.6	17.0
1987[5]	100.0	82.4	51.9	43.4	38.2	27.4	11.0	4.1	17.6

Source: U.S. Department of Commerce, U.S. Bureau of the Census, Income Statistics Branch/HHES Division, Washington, D.C. Unpublished March Current Population Survey for data prior to 1989 and Current Population Reports, Series P-60 for 1989 forward. *Notes:* 1. Includes CHAMPUS (Comprehensive Health and Medical Plan for Uniformed Services), Veterans, and military health care. 2. Health insurance questions were redesigned, decreases in estimates of group health and military health care coverage may be partially due to questionnaire changes. Overall coverage estimates were not affected. 3. Data collection method changed from paper and pencil to computer-assisted interviewing. 4. Implementation of 1990 census population controls. 5. Implementation of a new March CPS processing system.

★ 630 ★
Health Insurance Coverage

Health Insurance Coverage Status and Type of Coverage - Blacks, Males: 1987 to 1995

Numbers in thousands. Persons as of March of the following year.

| Year | Total persons | Covered by private or government health insurance | | | | | | | Not covered |
| | | Total | Private health insurance | | Government health insurance | | | | |
			Total	Group health	Total	Medicaid	Medicare	Military health care[1]	
BLACKS, MALES NUMBERS									
1995	15,824	11,986	8,007	7,390	5,276	3,715	1,350	670	3,838
1994[2]	15,687	12,172	8,078	7,434	5,402	3,650	1,302	930	3,515
1993[3]	15,458	11,748	7,779	6,382	5,314	3,719	1,203	765	3,710
1992[4]	15,208	11,597	7,498	6,379	5,212	3,574	1,265	842	3,611
1991	14,781	11,196	7,351	6,313	4,915	3,204	1,350	834	3,585
1990	14,495	11,221	7,609	6,551	4,620	3,055	1,277	748	3,274
1989	14,255	11,178	7,925	6,877	4,320	2,745	1,281	694	3,077
1988	14,021	10,844	7,571	6,510	4,356	2,654	1,232	809	3,177
1987[5]	13,783	10,674	7,249	6,275	4,412	2,760	1,198	850	3,109
PERCENTS									
1995	100.0	75.7	50.6	46.7	33.3	23.5	8.5	4.2	24.3
1994[2]	100.0	77.6	51.5	47.4	34.4	23.3	8.3	5.9	22.4
1993[3]	100.0	76.0	50.3	41.3	34.4	24.1	7.8	4.9	24.0
1992[4]	100.0	76.3	49.3	41.9	34.3	23.5	8.3	5.5	23.7
1991	100.0	75.7	49.7	42.7	33.3	21.7	9.1	5.6	24.3
1990	100.0	77.4	52.5	45.2	31.9	21.1	8.8	5.2	22.6
1989	100.0	78.4	55.6	48.2	30.3	19.3	9.0	4.9	21.6
1988	100.0	77.3	54.0	46.4	31.1	18.9	8.8	5.8	22.7
1987[5]	100.0	77.4	52.6	45.5	32.0	20.0	8.7	6.2	22.6

Source: U.S. Department of Commerce, U.S. Bureau of the Census, Income Statistics Branch/HHES Division, Washington, D.C. Unpublished March Current Population Survey for data prior to 1989 and Current Population Reports, Series P-60 for 1989 forward. *Notes:* 1. Includes CHAMPUS (Comprehensive Health and Medical Plan for Uniformed Services), Veterans, and military health care. 2. Health insurance questions were redesigned, decreases in estimates of group health and military health care coverage may be partially due to questionnaire changes. Overall coverage estimates were not affected. 3. Data collection method changed from paper and pencil to computer-assisted interviewing. 4. Implementation of 1990 census population controls. 5. Implementation of a new March CPS processing system.

★ 631 ★

Health Insurance Coverage

Health Insurance Coverage Status and Type of Coverage - Hispanic Origin, Both Sexes: 1987 to 1995

Numbers in thousands. Persons as of March of the following year.

| Year | Total persons | Covered by private or government health insurance | | | | | | | Not covered |
| | | Total | Private health insurance | | Government health insurance | | | | |
			Total	Group health	Total	Medicaid	Medicare	Military health care[1]	
HISPANIC ORIGIN BOTH SEXES NUMBERS									
1995	28,438	18,964	12,187	11,309	8,027	6,478	1,732	516	9,474
1994[2]	27,521	18,244	11,743	10,729	7,829	6,226	1,677	630	9,277
1993[3]	26,646	18,235	12,021	9,981	7,873	6,328	1,613	530	8,411
1992[4]	25,682	17,242	11,330	9,786	7,099	5,703	1,578	523	8,441
1991	22,096	15,128	10,336	8,972	5,845	4,597	1,309	522	6,968
1990	21,437	14,479	10,281	8,948	5,169	3,912	1,269	519	6,958
1989	20,779	13,846	10,348	8,914	4,526	3,221	1,180	595	6,932
1988	20,076	13,684	10,188	8,831	4,414	3,125	1,114	594	6,391
1987[5]	19,428	13,456	9,845	8,490	4,482	3,214	1,029	631	5,972
PERCENTS									
1995	100.0	66.7	42.9	39.8	28.2	22.8	6.1	1.8	33.3
1994[2]	100.0	66.3	42.7	39.0	28.4	22.6	6.1	2.3	33.7
1993[3]	100.0	68.4	45.1	37.5	29.5	23.7	6.1	2.0	31.6
1992[4]	100.0	67.1	44.1	38.1	27.6	22.2	6.1	2.0	32.9
1991	100.0	68.5	46.8	40.6	26.5	20.8	5.9	2.4	31.5
1990	100.0	67.5	48.0	41.7	24.1	18.3	5.9	2.4	32.5
1989	100.0	66.6	49.8	42.9	21.8	15.5	5.7	2.9	33.4
1988	100.0	68.2	50.7	44.0	22.0	15.6	5.5	3.0	31.8
1987[5]	100.0	69.3	50.7	43.7	23.1	16.5	5.3	3.2	30.7

Source: U.S. Department of Commerce, U.S. Bureau of the Census, Income Statistics Branch/HHES Division, Washington, D.C. Unpublished March Current Population Survey for data prior to 1989 and Current Population Reports, Series P-60 for 1989 forward. *Notes:* 1. Includes CHAMPUS (Comprehensive Health and Medical Plan for Uniformed Services), Veterans, and military health care. 2. Health insurance questions were redesigned, decreases in estimates of group health and military health care coverage may be partially due to questionnaire changes. Overall coverage estimates were not affected. 3. Data collection method changed from paper and pencil to computer-assisted interviewing. 4. Implementation of 1990 census population controls. 5. Implementation of a new March CPS processing system.

★ 632 ★
Health Insurance Coverage

Health Insurance Coverage Status and Type of Coverage - Hispanic Origin, Females: 1987 to 1995

Numbers in thousands. Persons as of March of the following year.

Year	Total persons	Covered by private or government health insurance							Not covered
		Total	Private health insurance		Government health insurance				
			Total	Group health	Total	Medicaid	Medicare	Military health care[1]	
HISPANIC ORIGIN, FEMALES NUMBERS									
1995	14,060	9,840	5,896	5,454	4,582	3,771	982	264	4,219
1994[2]	13,606	9,401	5,754	5,201	4,332	3,554	890	294	4,205
1993[3]	13,157	9,451	5,968	4,881	4,366	3,585	881	269	3,707
1992[4]	12,676	8,920	5,552	4,757	3,978	3,256	889	264	3,756
1991	11,036	7,864	5,052	4,341	3,351	2,733	761	247	3,172
1990	10,677	7,518	5,119	4,446	2,915	2,270	714	266	3,160
1989	10,354	7,098	5,143	4,389	2,488	1,842	624	295	3,256
1988	10,005	7,120	5,080	4,366	2,526	1,893	601	281	2,885
1987[5]	9,676	6,929	4,856	4,138	2,514	1,880	573	308	2,747
PERCENTS									
1995	100.0	70.0	41.9	38.8	32.6	26.8	7.0	1.9	30.0
1994[2]	100.0	69.1	42.3	38.2	31.8	26.1	6.5	2.2	30.9
1993[3]	100.0	71.8	45.4	37.1	33.2	27.2	6.7	2.0	28.2
1992[4]	100.0	70.4	43.8	37.5	31.4	25.7	7.0	2.1	29.6
1991	100.0	71.3	45.8	39.3	30.4	24.8	6.9	2.2	28.7
1990	100.0	70.4	47.9	41.6	27.3	21.3	6.7	2.5	29.6
1989	100.0	68.6	49.7	42.4	24.0	17.8	6.0	2.8	31.4
1988	100.0	71.2	50.8	43.6	25.3	18.9	6.0	2.8	28.8
1987[5]	100.0	71.6	50.2	42.8	26.0	19.4	5.9	3.2	28.4

Source: U.S. Department of Commerce, U.S. Bureau of the Census, Income Statistics Branch/HHES Division, Washington, D.C. Unpublished March Current Population Survey for data prior to 1989 and Current Population Reports, Series P-60 for 1989 forward. *Notes:* 1. Includes CHAMPUS (Comprehensive Health and Medical Plan for Uniformed Services), Veterans, and military health care. 2. Health insurance questions were redesigned, decreases in estimates of group health and military health care coverage may be partially due to questionnaire changes. Overall coverage estimates were not affected. 3. Data collection method changed from paper and pencil to computer-assisted interviewing. 4. Implementation of 1990 census population controls. 5. Implementation of a new March CPS processing system.

★ 633 ★

Health Insurance Coverage

Health Insurance Coverage Status and Type of Coverage - Hispanic Origin, Males: 1987 to 1995

Numbers in thousands. Persons as of March of the following year.

Year	Total persons	Covered by private or government health insurance							Not covered
		Total	Private health insurance		Government health insurance				
			Total	Group health	Total	Medicaid	Medicare	Military health care[1]	
HISPANIC ORIGIN, MALES NUMBERS									
1995	14,378	9,123	6,291	5,855	3,446	2,707	750	253	5,255
1994[2]	13,915	8,842	5,988	5,528	3,497	2,673	787	336	5,073
1993[3]	13,489	8,784	6,054	5,100	3,507	2,742	732	261	4,704
1992[4]	13,006	8,322	5,778	5,029	3,121	2,447	689	259	4,685
1991	11,061	7,264	5,285	4,630	2,494	1,864	548	275	3,797
1990	10,760	6,961	5,162	4,502	2,254	1,643	555	253	3,798
1989	10,425	6,748	5,205	4,526	2,038	1,379	556	300	3,677
1988	10,071	6,565	5,108	4,465	1,888	1,232	512	313	3,506
1987[5]	9,751	6,526	4,989	4,353	1,968	1,334	455	323	3,225
PERCENTS									
1995	100.0	63.5	43.8	40.7	24.0	18.8	5.2	1.8	36.5
1994[2]	100.0	63.5	43.0	39.7	25.1	19.2	5.7	2.4	36.5
1993[3]	100.0	65.1	44.9	37.8	26.0	20.3	5.4	1.9	34.9
1992[4]	100.0	64.0	44.4	38.7	24.0	18.8	5.3	2.0	36.0
1991	100.0	65.7	47.8	41.9	22.5	16.9	5.0	2.5	34.3
1990	100.0	64.7	48.0	41.8	21.0	15.3	5.2	2.3	35.3
1989	100.0	64.7	49.9	43.4	19.6	13.2	5.3	2.9	35.3
1988	100.0	65.2	50.7	44.3	18.7	12.2	5.1	3.1	34.8
1987[5]	100.0	66.9	51.2	44.6	20.2	13.7	4.7	3.3	33.1

Source: U.S. Department of Commerce, U.S. Bureau of the Census, Income Statistics Branch/HHES Division, Washington, D.C. Unpublished March Current Population Survey for data prior to 1989 and Current Population Reports, Series P-60 for 1989 forward. *Notes:* 1. Includes CHAMPUS (Comprehensive Health and Medical Plan for Uniformed Services), Veterans, and military health care. 2. Health insurance questions were redesigned, decreases in estimates of group health and military health care coverage may be partially due to questionnaire changes. Overall coverage estimates were not affected. 3. Data collection method changed from paper and pencil to computer-assisted interviewing. 4. Implementation of 1990 census population controls. 5. Implementation of a new March CPS processing system.

★ 634 ★

Health Insurance Coverage

Health Insurance Coverage Status and Type of Coverage - Whites, Both Sexes: 1987 to 1995

Numbers in thousands. Persons as of March of the following year.

| Year | Total persons | Covered by private or government health insurance | | | | | | | Not covered |
| | | Total | Private health insurance | | Government health insurance | | | | |
			Total	Group health	Total	Medicaid	Medicare	Military health care[1]	
WHITE									
BOTH SEXES									
NUMBERS									
1995	218,442	187,337	161,303	139,151	54,141	20,528	30,580	7,656	31,105
1994[2]	216,751	186,447	160,414	137,966	54,288	20,464	29,978	8,845	30,305
1993[3]	215,221	184,732	158,586	128,855	53,222	20,642	29,297	7,689	30,489
1992[4]	213,198	183,479	158,612	129,685	51,195	18,659	29,341	7,556	29,719
1991	210,257	183,130	159,628	131,646	49,699	17,058	28,940	7,867	27,127
1990	208,754	181,795	160,146	131,836	47,589	15,078	28,530	8,022	26,959
1989	206,983	181,126	161,363	132,882	44,868	12,779	27,859	8,116	25,857
1988	205,333	180,122	160,753	133,050	44,477	12,504	27,293	8,305	25,211
1987[5]	203,745	179,845	161,338	132,264	44,028	12,163	27,044	8,482	23,900
PERCENTS									
1995	100.0	85.8	73.8	63.7	24.8	9.4	14.0	3.5	14.2
1994[2]	100.0	86.0	74.0	63.7	25.0	9.4	13.8	4.1	14.0
1993[3]	100.0	85.8	73.7	59.9	24.7	9.6	13.6	3.6	14.2
1992[4]	100.0	86.1	74.4	60.8	24.0	8.8	13.8	3.5	13.9
1991	100.0	87.1	75.9	62.6	23.6	8.1	13.8	3.7	12.9
1990	100.0	87.1	76.7	63.2	22.8	7.2	13.7	3.8	12.9
1989	100.0	87.5	78.0	64.2	21.7	6.2	13.5	3.9	12.5
1988	100.0	87.7	78.3	64.8	21.7	6.1	13.3	4.0	12.3
1987[5]	100.0	88.3	79.2	64.9	21.6	6.0	13.3	4.2	11.7

Source: U.S. Department of Commerce, U.S. Bureau of the Census, Income Statistics Branch/HHES Division, Washington, D.C. Unpublished March Current Population Survey for data prior to 1989 and Current Population Reports, Series P-60 for 1989 forward. *Notes:* 1. Includes CHAMPUS (Comprehensive Health and Medical Plan for Uniformed Services), Veterans, and military health care. 2. Health insurance questions were redesigned, decreases in estimates of group health and military health care coverage may be partially due to questionnaire changes. Overall coverage estimates were not affected. 3. Data collection method changed from paper and pencil to computer-assisted interviewing. 4. Implementation of 1990 census population controls. 5. Implementation of a new March CPS processing system.

★ 635 ★
Health Insurance Coverage

Health Insurance Coverage Status and Type of Coverage - Whites, Females: 1987 to 1995

Numbers in thousands. Persons as of March of the following year.

| Year | Total persons | Covered by private or government health insurance | | | | | | | Not covered |
| | | Total | Private health insurance | | Government health insurance | | | | |
			Total	Group health	Total	Medicaid	Medicare	Military health care[1]	
WHITES, FEMALES NUMBERS									
1995	110,951	96,424	81,678	69,066	30,190	11,815	17,374	3,511	14,527
1994[2]	110,231	96,208	81,419	68,686	30,230	11,892	17,105	4,011	14,023
1993[3]	109,382	95,490	80,440	63,837	30,037	12,119	16,759	3,636	13,892
1992[4]	108,457	95,032	80,897	64,747	28,933	10,938	16,884	3,567	13,425
1991	107,293	95,034	81,676	65,844	28,103	10,118	16,677	3,655	12,258
1990	106,537	94,142	81,899	66,071	26,661	8,780	16,391	3,697	12,395
1989	105,729	93,582	82,365	66,243	25,260	7,603	16,012	3,757	12,147
1988	105,011	93,229	82,185	66,442	25,014	7,500	15,708	3,820	11,782
1987[5]	104,224	93,075	82,667	66,011	24,688	7,106	15,583	3,942	11,149
PERCENTS									
1995	100.0	86.9	73.6	62.2	27.2	10.6	15.7	3.2	13.1
1994[2]	100.0	87.3	73.9	62.3	27.4	10.8	15.5	3.6	12.7
1993[3]	100.0	87.3	73.5	58.4	27.5	11.1	15.3	3.3	12.7
1992[4]	100.0	87.6	74.6	59.7	26.7	10.1	15.6	3.3	12.4
1991	100.0	88.6	76.1	61.4	26.2	9.4	15.5	3.4	11.4
1990	100.0	88.4	76.9	62.0	25.0	8.2	15.4	3.5	11.6
1989	100.0	88.5	77.9	62.7	23.9	7.2	15.1	3.6	11.5
1988	100.0	88.8	78.3	63.3	23.8	7.1	15.0	3.6	11.2
1987[5]	100.0	89.3	79.3	63.3	23.7	6.8	15.0	3.8	10.7

Source: U.S. Department of Commerce, U.S. Bureau of the Census, Income Statistics Branch/HHES Division, Washington, D.C. Unpublished March Current Population Survey for data prior to 1989 and Current Population Reports, Series P-60 for 1989 forward. *Notes;* 1. Includes CHAMPUS (Comprehensive Health and Medical Plan for Uniformed Services), Veterans, and military health care. 2. Health insurance questions were redesigned, decreases in estimates of group health and military health care coverage may be partially due to questionnaire changes. Overall coverage estimates were not affected. 3. Data collection method changed from paper and pencil to computer-assisted interviewing. 4. Implementation of 1990 census population controls. 5. Implementation of a new March CPS processing system.

★ 636 ★

Health Insurance Coverage

Health Insurance Coverage Status and Type of Coverage - Whites, Males: 1987 to 1995

Numbers in thousands. Persons as of March of the following year.

| Year | Total persons | Covered by private or government health insurance | | | | | | | Not covered |
| | | Total | Private health insurance | | Government health insurance | | | | |
			Total	Group health	Total	Medicaid	Medicare	Military health care[1]	
WHITES, MALES NUMBERS									
1995	107,491	90,913	79,625	70,085	23,951	8,713	13,206	4,145	16,578
1994[2]	106,520	90,238	78,996	69,279	24,058	8,572	12,873	4,835	16,282
1993[3]	105,840	89,243	78,146	65,018	23,185	8,523	12,539	4,054	16,597
1992[4]	104,741	88,447	77,716	64,938	22,261	7,721	12,458	3,989	16,294
1991	102,965	88,096	77,952	65,802	21,595	6,940	12,263	4,213	14,869
1990	102,217	87,653	78,247	65,765	20,928	6,298	12,139	4,325	14,564
1989	101,253	87,544	78,997	66,639	19,608	5,176	11,848	4,359	13,710
1988	100,322	86,893	78,568	66,608	19,463	5,004	11,585	4,486	13,429
1987[5]	99,521	86,770	78,671	66,253	19,340	5,057	11,460	4,541	12,751
PERCENTS									
1995	100.0	84.6	74.1	65.2	22.3	8.1	12.3	3.9	15.4
1994[2]	100.0	84.7	74.2	65.0	22.6	8.0	12.1	4.5	15.3
1993[3]	100.0	84.3	73.8	61.4	21.9	8.1	11.8	3.8	15.7
1992[4]	100.0	84.4	74.2	62.0	21.3	7.4	11.9	3.8	15.6
1991	100.0	85.6	75.7	63.9	21.0	6.7	11.9	4.1	14.4
1990	100.0	85.8	76.6	64.3	20.5	6.2	11.9	4.2	14.2
1989	100.0	86.5	78.0	65.8	19.4	5.1	11.7	4.3	13.5
1988	100.0	86.6	78.3	66.4	19.4	5.0	11.5	4.5	13.4
1987[5]	100.0	87.2	79.0	66.6	19.4	5.1	11.5	4.6	12.8

Source: U.S. Department of Commerce, U.S. Bureau of the Census, Income Statistics Branch/HHES Division, Washington, D.C. Unpublished March Current Population Survey for data prior to 1989 and Current Population Reports, Series P-60 for 1989 forward. *Notes:* 1. Includes CHAMPUS (Comprehensive Health and Medical Plan for Uniformed Services), Veterans, and military health care. 2. Health insurance questions were redesigned, decreases in estimates of group health and military health care coverage may be partially due to questionnaire changes. Overall coverage estimates were not affected. 3. Data collection method changed from paper and pencil to computer-assisted interviewing. 4. Implementation of 1990 census population controls. 5. Implementation of a new March CPS processing system.

★ 637 ★

Health Insurance Coverage

Health Insurance Coverage Status of Poor Persons, by Selected Characteristics: 1995

This table shows health insurance coverage status of all poverty-stricken persons by selected characteristics.

[Numbers in thousands]

Characteristic	Total Number	Total Covered		Not Covered	
		Number	Percent	Number	Percent
Poor persons	36,425	25,432	69.8	10,993	30.2
Sex:					
Male	15,683	10,232	65.2	5,451	34.8
Female	20,742	15,200	73.3	5,542	26.7
Age:					
Under 18 years	14,665	11,534	78.6	3,131	21.4
18 to 24 years	4,553	2,586	56.8	1,967	43.2
25 to 34 years	5,196	2,830	54.5	2,366	45.5
35 to 44 years	4,064	2,282	56.2	1,782	43.8
45 to 64 years	4,629	2,970	64.2	1,659	35.8
65 years and over	3,318	3,230	97.3	88	2.7
Race and Hispanic Origin:					
White	24,423	16,292	66.7	8,131	33.3
Black	9,872	7,552	76.5	2,320	23.5
Hispanic origin[1]	8,574	5,076	59.2	3,498	40.8
Education:					
No high school dipl	9,538	6,158	64.6	3,380	35.4
High sch grad, no deg	6,722	4,168	62.0	2,554	38.0
Some college, no deg	3,327	2,150	64.6	1,177	35.4
Associate degree	795	519	65.3	276	34.7
Bachelor's degree +	1,378	903	65.5	475	34.5
Work Experience:					
Worked during year	9,043	4,592	50.8	4,451	49.2
Full-time	5,558	2,675	48.1	2,883	51.9
Part-time	3,486	1,917	55.0	1,569	45.0
Did not work	9,398	6,076	64.7	3,322	35.3
Foreign-Born:					
Native	30,972	22,801	73.6	8,171	26.4
Foreign-born	5,452	2,631	48.3	2,821	51.7
Naturalized citizen	833	549	65.9	284	34.1
Not a citizen	4,619	2,082	45.1	2,537	54.9

Source: U.S. Department of Commerce. Bureau of the Census. *Current Population Survey,* March 1996.
Note: 1. Persons of Hispanic origin may be of any race.

★ 638 ★

Health Insurance Coverage

Health Insurance: Overview

Coverage	Number in category (million)	Percent of total
Total managed-care enrollees	115	44
Total indemnity/fee-for-service enrollees	108	41
Total uninsured	39	15

Source: Meyer, Harris. "Indemnity Insurance: Down But Not Out." *Medical Economics,* 12 August 1996, p. 212. Primary sources: Foster Higgins; Health Insurance Association of America; Blue Cross-Blue Shield Association; Employee Benefits Research Institute; Health Care Financing Administration; Kaiser Family Foundation.

★ 639 ★

Health Insurance Coverage

Health Insurance Status

This table shows health insurance status by program and by poverty status for 1995.

[Numbers in thousands]

	Total Number	% Dist.	Poor persons	
			Number	% Dist.
All persons	264,315	100.0	36,425	100.0
Total covered	223,733	84.6	25,432	69.8
Private	185,882	70.3	8,119	22.3
Employment-based	161,453	61.1	5,303	14.6
Government:				
Medicare	34,655	13.1	4,234	11.6
Medicaid	31,877	12.1	16,900	46.4
Military	9,376	3.5	758	2.1
Not covered	40,582	15.4	10,993	30.2

Source: U.S. Department of Commerce. Bureau of the Census. *Current Population Survey,* March 1996. *Notes:* The estimates by type of coverage are not mutually exclusive; in other words, persons can be covered by more than one type of health insurance during the year.

★ 640 ★

Health Insurance Coverage

Health Insurance Status by Type of Coverage

This table shows health insurance coverage status and type of coverage, all races, both sexes, for 1987 to 1995. Numbers in thousands. Population count as of March of the following year.

| Year | Total persons | Covered by private or government health insurance | | | | | | | Not covered |
| | | Total | Private health insurance | | Government health insurance | | | | |
			Total	Group health	Total	Medicaid	Medicare	Military health care[1]	
ALL RACES, BOTH SEXES									
NUMBER									
1995	264,314	223,733	185,881	161,453	69,776	31,877	34,655	9,375	40,582
1994[2]	262,105	222,387	184,318	159,634	70,163	31,645	33,901	11,165	39,718
1993[3]	259,753	220,040	182,351	148,318	68,554	31,749	33,097	9,560	39,713
1992[4]	256,830	218,189	181,466	148,796	66,244	29,416	33,230	9,510	38,641
1991	251,447	216,003	181,375	150,077	63,882	26,880	32,907	9,820	35,445
1990	248,886	214,167	182,135	150,215	60,965	24,261	32,260	9,922	34,719
1989	246,191	212,807	183,610	151,644	57,382	21,185	31,495	9,870	33,385
1988	243,685	211,005	182,019	150,940	56,850	20,728	30,925	10,105	32,680
1987[5]	241,187	210,161	182,160	149,739	56,282	20,211	30,458	10,542	31,026
PERCENT									
1995	100.0	84.6	70.3	61.1	26.4	12.1	13.1	3.5	15.4
1994[2]	100.0	84.8	70.3	60.9	26.8	12.1	12.9	4.3	15.2
1993[3]	100.0	84.7	70.2	57.1	26.4	12.2	12.7	3.7	15.3
1992[4]	100.0	85.0	70.7	57.9	25.8	11.5	12.9	3.7	15.0
1991	100.0	85.9	72.1	59.7	25.4	10.7	13.1	3.9	14.1
1990	100.0	86.1	73.2	60.4	24.5	9.7	13.0	4.0	13.9
1989	100.0	86.4	74.6	61.6	23.3	8.6	12.8	4.0	13.6
1988	100.0	86.6	74.7	61.9	23.3	8.5	12.7	4.1	13.4
1987[5]	100.0	87.1	75.5	62.1	23.3	8.4	12.6	4.4	12.9

Source: U.S. Department of Commerce. Bureau of the Census. Income Statistics Branch/HHES Division, Washington, D.C. Unpublished March Current Population Survey for data prior to 1989 and Current Population Reports, Series P-60 for 1989 forward. *Notes:* 1. Includes CHAMPUS (Comprehensive Health and Medical Plan for Uniformed Services), Veterans, and military health care. 2. Health insurance questions were redesigned, decreases in estimates of group health and military health care coverage may be partially due to questionnaire changes. Overall coverage estimates were not affected. 3. Data collection method changed from paper and pencil to computer-assisted interviewing. 4. Implementation of 1990 census population controls. 5. Implementation of a new March CPS processing system.

★ 641 ★

Health Insurance Coverage

Persons Not Covered by Health Insurance, by State: 1994

In percent. Based on the Current Population Survey and subject to sampling error.

STATE	1994
United States	15.2
Alabama	19.2
Alaska	13.3
Arizona	20.2
Arkansas	17.4
California	21.1
Colorado	12.4
Connecticut	10.4
Delaware	13.5
District of Columbia	16.4
Florida	17.2
Georgia	16.2
Hawaii	9.2
Idaho	14.0
Illinois	11.4
Indiana	10.5
Iowa	9.7
Kansas	12.9
Kentucky	15.2
Louisiana	19.2
Maine	13.1
Maryland	12.6
Massachusetts	12.5
Michigan	10.8
Minnesota	9.5
Mississippi	17.8
Missouri	12.2
Montana	13.6
Nebraska	10.7
Nevada	15.7
New Hampshire	11.9
New Jersey	13.0
New Mexico	23.1
New York	16.0
North Carolina	13.3
North Dakota	8.4
Ohio	11.0
Oklahoma	17.8
Oregon	13.1
Pennsylvania	10.6
Rhode Island	11.5
South Carolina	14.2
South Dakota	10.0
Tennessee	10.2
Texas	24.2

[Continued]

★ 641 ★

Persons Not Covered by Health Insurance, by State: 1994

[Continued]

STATE	1994
Utah	11.5
Vermont	8.6
Virginia	12.0
Washington	12.7
West Virginia	16.2
Wisconsin	8.9
Wyoming	15.4

Source: 1996 Statistical Abstract of the United States on CD-ROM [machine-readable datafiles]. CD-8A-97. Washington, DC: U.S. Department of Commerce, Economics and Statistics Administration, Bureau of the Census, Data User Services Division, January 1997. Primary source: U.S. Bureau of the Census, *Current Population Reports*, series P60-190.

★ 642 ★

Health Insurance Coverage

Pre-Existing Condition Restrictions, by Type of Health Plan: 1995

Health plans	Percentage
Conventional plans	59
PPOs	70
POS plans	56

Source: "Pre-Existing Restriction." *Workplace Vitality* (May 1995), p. 15. Primary sources: Survey of large employers by KPMG Peat Marwick; Council for Affordable Health Insurance. *Notes:* PPO represents "Preferred Provider Organization." POS represents "Point of Service" plan or "Point of Sale."

★ 643 ★

Health Insurance Coverage

Psychiatric Inpatient Admissions by Payer, 1994

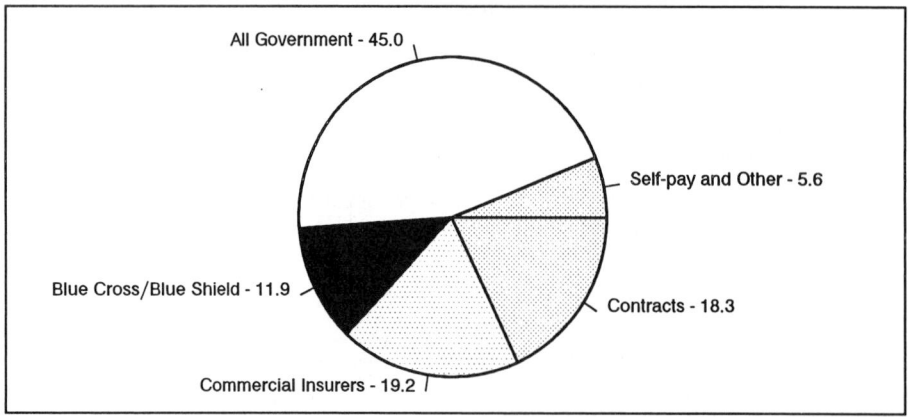

	Percent of admissions
All Government	45.0
Commercial Insurers	19.2
Contracts	18.3
Blue Cross/Blue Shield	11.9
Self-pay and Other	5.6

Source: Psychiatric Times (November 1995), p. 71. Primary source: National Association of Psychiatric Health Systems, *1995 Annual Survey: Final Report.*

★ 644 ★

Health Insurance Coverage

Trends in Indemnity Insurance by Size of Employer

Table shows companies offering coverage and employees enrolled for the years 1992-1995.

Year	Percent offering indemnity insurance		Percent of employees enrolled	
	Small companies[1]	Large companies[2]	Small companies	Large companies
1992	61	68	58	49
1993	57	68	54	43
1994	47	60	42	34
1995	38	54	33	27

Source: Meyer, Harris. "Indemnity Insurance: Down But Not Out." *Medical Economics,* 12 August 1996, p. 219. Primary source: Foster Higgins. *Notes:* 1. 10-499 employees. 2. 500 or more employees.

★ 645 ★

Health Insurance Coverage

Uninsured Population, by Age

Age group	Percentage uninsured
Under age 19	25.5
19-24	16.8
25-34	24.1
35-44	16.0
45-54	9.4
55-64	7.4
65 years and more	0.8

Source: "Sketch of the USA's Uninsured." *USA TODAY,* 8 August 1994, p. 8A. Primary sources: U.S. Census Bureau; Employee Benefit Research Institute; U.S. Treasury Department.

★ 646 ★

Health Insurance Coverage

Uninsured Population, by Earnings Income

Earnings income level	Percentage uninsured
Under $10,000	22.4
$10,000-$19,999	27.7
$20,000-$29,999	18.9
$30,000-$49,999	17.9
$50,000 and more	13.1

Source: "Sketch of the USA's Uninsured." *USA TODAY,* 8 August 1994, p. 8A. Primary sources: U.S. Census Bureau; Employee Benefit Research Institute; U.S. Treasury Department.

★ 647 ★

Health Insurance Coverage

Uninsured Population, by Educational Attainment

Educational attainment	Percentage uninsured
Less than high school diploma	31.9
High school graduate	36.7
Some college	20.1
Bachelor's degree and more	11.3

Source: "Sketch of the USA's Uninsured." *USA TODAY,* 8 August 1994, p. 8A. Primary sources: U.S. Census Bureau; Employee Benefit Research Institute; U.S. Treasury Department.

★ 648 ★

Health Insurance Coverage

Uninsured Population, by Job Status

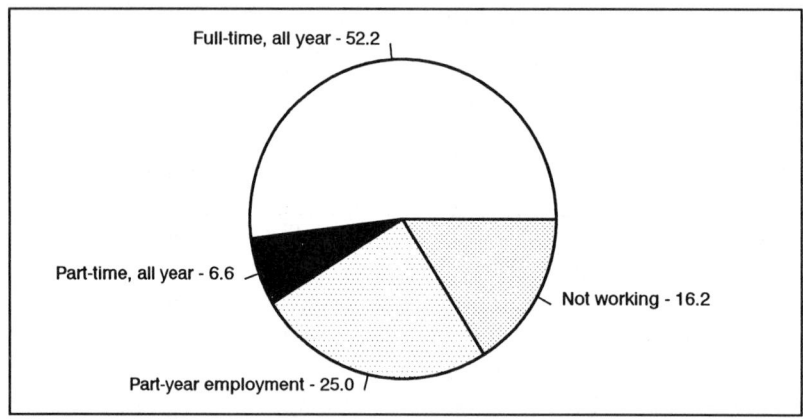

Job status of head of household	Percentage uninsured
Full-time, all year	52.2
Part-time, all year	6.6
Part-year employment	25.0
Not working	16.2

Source: "Sketch of the USA's Uninsured." *USA TODAY,* 8 August 1994, p. 8A. Primary sources: U.S. Census Bureau; Employee Benefit Research Institute; U.S. Treasury Department.

★ 649 ★

Health Insurance Coverage

Uninsured Population, by Length of Time Uninsured

Months without insurance	Percentage uninsured
1-8	15.1
9-16	17.9
17-24	13.0
25 months and more	54.0

Source: "Sketch of the USA's Uninsured." *USA TODAY,* 8 August 1994, p. 8A. Primary sources: U.S. Census Bureau; Employee Benefit Research Institute; U.S. Treasury Department.

★ 650 ★

Health Insurance Coverage

Uninsured Population, by Marital Status

Marital status	Percentage uninsured
Never married	54.5
Married	30.0
Divorced/separated	13.0
Widowed	2.5

Source: "Sketch of the USA's Uninsured." *USA TODAY,* 8 August 1994, p. 8A. Primary sources: U.S. Census Bureau; Employee Benefit Research Institute; U.S. Treasury Department.

★ 651 ★

Health Insurance Coverage

Uninsured Population, by Race and Ethnicity

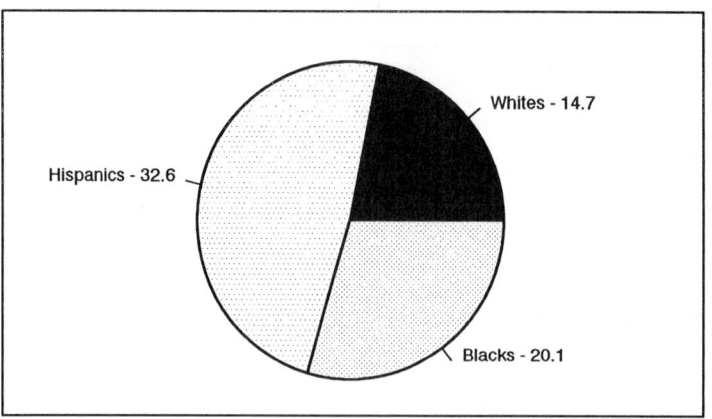

Race and ethnicity	Percentage uninsured
Hispanics	32.6
Blacks	20.1
Whites	14.7

Source: "Sketch of the USA's Uninsured." *USA TODAY,* 8 August 1994, p. 8A. Primary sources: U.S. Census Bureau; Employee Benefit Research Institute; U.S. Treasury Department. *Note:* Hispanics may be of any race.

★ 652 ★

Health Insurance Coverage

Uninsured Population, by Sex

Sex	Percentage uninsured
Men	54.7
Women	45.3

Source: "Sketch of the USA's Uninsured." *USA TODAY,* 8 August 1994, p. 8A. Primary sources: U.S. Census Bureau; Employee Benefit Research Institute; U.S. Treasury Department.

★ 653 ★

Health Insurance Coverage

Uninsured Population, by State: Highest Percentages

State	Percentage uninsured
Nevada	22.7
Texas	22.4
Louisiana	22.1
Oklahoma	21.6
District of Columbia	21.3

Source: "Sketch of the USA's Uninsured." *USA TODAY,* 8 August 1994, p. 8A. Primary sources: U.S. Census Bureau; Employee Benefit Research Institute; U.S. Treasury Department.

★ 654 ★

Health Insurance Coverage

Uninsured Population, by State: Lowest Percentages

State	Percentage uninsured
Hawaii	6.0
Connecticut	8.1
Minnesota	8.1
North Dakota	8.3
Pennsylvania	8.5

Source: "Sketch of the USA's Uninsured." *USA TODAY,* 8 August 1994, p. 8A. Primary sources: U.S. Census Bureau; Employee Benefit Research Institute; U.S. Treasury Department.

Health Maintenance Organizations

★ 655 ★

HMO Complaints

Percentage of consumers who said they are not satisfied with their health plan on each measure of care access. Data are based on a Sachs/Scarborough Health Plus survey of 85,000 consumers in 27 metropolitan areas.

Complaint	Percent
Wait time for appointment	
When sick	33.0
When well	30.0
Getting specialist referrals	30.0
Panel of doctors available	25.0
Panel of hospitals available	21.0

Source: "HMO Complaints." *New York Times,* 2 February 1997, p. 12Y.

★ 656 ★

Health Maintenance Organizations

Leading States in Medicaid Health Maintenance Organization Enrollment: 1996

Health maintenance organization	Medicaid enrollees	Percent of plan's enrollees
Tennessee Managed Care Network	249,116	100.0
Foundation Health, A California Health Plan	198,599	25.0
Keystone Health Plan East (Pennsylvania)	155,984	27.0
PCA Family Health Plan, Inc. (Florida)	145,992	61.0
Comprehensive Health Services, Inc. (Michigan)	139,071	92.0
HMO Oregon/Health Maintenance of Oregon	134,915	30.0
United HealthCare of Illinois, Inc.	128,871	37.0
CIGNA HealthCare of California	100,293	18.0
Optimum Choice, Inc. (Maryland)	96,806	16.0
Keystone Health Plan West, Inc. (Pennsylvania)	94,886	11.0

Source: "State Report: Managing Medicaid: How the Numbers Add Up." *Business & Health* (June 1997), p. 64. Primary sources: The InterStudy Competitive Edge; *HMO Industry Report 7.1;* Health Care Financing Administration.

★ 657 ★

Health Maintenance Organizations

Managed Care: States with Fewest Enrolled

State	Percent
Mississippi	1.2
North Dakota	1.2
South Dakota	2.8
Montana	2.9
Idaho	3.7
Iowa	4.9

Source: "States with Fewest in HMOs." *USA TODAY,* 5 March 1997, p. 1A. Primary source: *1997 Health Care Almanac and Yearbook.*

★ 658 ★

Health Maintenance Organizations

Managed Care: States with Most Enrolled

State	Percent
Oregon	44.8
California	40.3
Massachusetts	39.0
Maryland	30.9
Utah	30.1
Connecticut	29.8

Source: "Where HMOs Rule." *USA TODAY,* 4 March 1997, p. 1A. Primary source: *1997 Health Care Almanac and Yearbook.*

Medicaid

★ 659 ★

Distribution of Medicaid Payments by Eligibility Group: FY 1994

Eligibility group	Persons served		Payments	
	Number (million)	%	Value ($ bil.)	%
Total	35.1	100.0	108.3	100.0
Low Income Children	17.2	49.0	17.3	16.0
Low Income Adults	7.6	21.7	13.6	12.6
Low Income Disabled	5.5	15.7	42.3	39.0
Low Income Aged	4.0	11.4	33.6	31.0
Other	0.8	2.2	1.5	1.4

Source: U.S. Department of Health and Human Services. Health Care Financing Administration. Office of Research and Demonstrations. *Health Care Financing Review, Medicare and Medicaid Statistical Supplement, 1996,* p. 181. *Note:* FY represents "fiscal year."

★ 660 ★

Medicaid

Leading States in Medicaid Managed Care Enrollment: 1996

From the source: "Enrollment in Medicaid managed care plans has increased by more than 170 percent since 1993, including a 33 percent rise from 1995 to 1996. As of June 30, 1996 (the most recent data available), 35 percent of all Medicaid beneficiaries—13 million people— were in managed care. All but two states, Alaska and Wyoming, offer some form of managed care..."

State	Medicaid managed care enrollees	Percent of state's Medicaid pop.
California	1,251,791	23.0
Tennessee	1,180,449	100.0
Florida	980,371	64.0
Pennsylvania	852,265	53.0
Michigan	834,348	73.0
Puerto Rico	801,758	76.0
Washington	695,562	100.00
New York	645,570	23.0

[Continued]

★ 660 ★

Leading States in Medicaid Managed Care
Enrollment: 1996
[Continued]

State	Medicaid managed care enrollees	Percent of state's Medicaid pop.
Virginia	461,720	68.0
Massachusetts	456,289	70.0

Source: "State Report: Managing Medicaid: How the Numbers Add Up." *Business & Health* (June 1997), p. 64. Primary source: The InterStudy Competitive Edge; *HMO Industry Report 7.1;* Health Care Financing Administration.

★ 661 ★

Medicaid

Medicaid and Medicare Payments for the Aged
[Dollars in billions; percent of total]

Service	Medicaid	Medicare	Combined
Total outlays - in $ billion	$33.6	$128.1	$161.7
Physician Services	27.7	26.6	21.4
Outpatient Hospital	7.6	8.8	8.5
Inpatient Hospital	5.8	51.0	41.6
Nursing Facility	67.4	4.0	17.5
Home Health	7.9	9.1	8.9
ICF/MR[1]	1.7	na	na
Prescribed drugs	7.9	na	1.6

Source: U.S. Department of Health and Human Services. Health Care Financing Administration. Office of Research and Demonstrations. *Health Care Financing Review, Medicare and Medicaid Statistical Supplement, 1996,* p. 153. Data are for 1994 from HCFA Form 2082. *Notes:* na stands for "not available." 1. ICF/MR represents "intermediate care facility for the mentally retarded." Medicare does not cover ICF/MR, less than skilled level nursing care, or outpatient prescription drugs.

★ 662 ★

Medicaid

Medicaid: As Part of Federal Aid to States and Localities, 1975 and 1994

[Dollars in billions; percent]

Type of Aid	1975	1994
Total Aid - in $ billion	49.8	217.3
Components of Aid in %		
Medicaid	13.7	40.1
Education, Training, Social Services	24.4	15.8
Transportation	11.8	10.6
Family Support Payments	10.3	7.6
Housing and Urban Development	2.7	7.3
Child Nutrition	2.9	3.3
Other	34.3	15.2

Source: U.S. Department of Health and Human Services. Health Care Financing Administration. Office of Research and Demonstrations. *Health Care Financing Review, Medicare and Medicaid Statistical Supplement, 1996,* p. 175.

★ 663 ★

Medicaid

Medicaid Medical Assistance Payment and Administration Expenditures: FY 1975-94

Fiscal Year[1]	State reported expenditures, current expenditures								(%) Current expenditures
	1994 Inflation-adjusted Computable per benefi-ciary[3]	1994 inflation-adjusted total computable[3] (1,000)	Total computable[2] (1,000)	Federal share amount (1,000)	(%)	Net adjusted expenditures[4]			
						State share (1,000)	Federal share	(%) Annual increase	
1975	$2,343	$51,558,703	$12,635,543	$6,986,038	55.3	$5,649,505	$7,056,374	-	101.0
1976	2,399	54,723,943	14,641,774	8,109,360	55.4	6,532,414	8,306,296	17.7	102.4
1977	2,571	58,708,286	17,211,156	9,569,074	55.6	7,642,082	9,727,198	17.1	101.7
1978	2,712	59,560,735	19,136,864	10,578,607	55.3	8,558,257	10,763,863	10.7	101.8
1979	2,900	62,406,455	21,807,998	12,106,159	55.5	9,701,839	12,048,834	11.9	99.5
1980	3,032	65,497,716	25,221,795	13,987,330	55.5	11,234,465	14,069,421	16.8	100.6
1981	3,155	69,348,238	29,812,946	16,522,663	55.4	13,290,283	16,681,025	18.6	101.0
1982[5]	3,080	66,545,154	31,797,537	17,614,406	55.4	14,183,131	17,866,898	7.1	101.4
1983[5,6]	3,123	67,302,413	34,851,343	19,371,133	55.6	15,480,210	19,326,227	8.2	99.8
1984[5,6]	3,115	67,312,730	37,311,446	20,653,977	55.4	16,657,469	20,697,444	7.1	100.2
1985[6]	3,226	70,378,681	41,235,221	22,853,715	55.4	18,381,506	22,685,387	9.6	99.3
1986[6]	3,126	73,133,592	44,512,468	24,824,095	55.8	19,688,373	24,668,512	8.7	99.4
1987[6]	3,349	77,383,077	49,122,700	27,511,307	56.0	21,611,393	27,528,933	11.6	100.1
1988[6]	3,478	79,660,723	54,073,380	30,450,896	56.3	23,622,484	30,521,156	10.9	100.2
1989[6]	3,548	83,428,432	61,329,325	34,633,142	56.5	26,696,183	34,350,182	12.5	99.2
1990[6]	3,642	91,976,256	72,920,339	41,369,626	56.7	31,550,713	41,194,571	19.9	99.6
1991[6]	3,859	109,129,621	91,901,764	52,462,592	57.1	39,439,172	52,509,502	27.5	100.1
1992[6]	4,283	132,468,449	118,176,825	67,942,878	57.5	50,233,947	68,599,998	30.6	101.0
1993[6]	4,143	138,505,126	130,839,006	74,953,006	57.3	55,886,000	76,145,907	11.0	101.6
1994[6]	4,087	143,265,264	141,757,970	81,204,361	57.3	60,553,609	81,836,691	7.5	100.8

[Continued]

★ 663 ★

Medicaid Medical Assistance Payment and Administration Expenditures: FY 1975-94

[Continued]

Fiscal Year[1]	State reported expenditures, current expenditures								(%) Current expenditures
	1994 Inflation-adjusted Computable per benefi-ciary[3]	1994 inflation-adjusted total computable[3] (1,000)	Total computable[2] (1,000)	Federal share amount (1,000)	(%)	Net adjusted expenditures[4]			
						State share (1,000)	Federal share	(%) Annual increase	
Percent Change 1975-94	74.5	177.9	1,021.9	1,062.4	3.6	971.8	1,059.8	-	-

Source: U.S. Department of Health and Human Services. Health Care Financing Administration. Office of Research and Demonstrations. *Health Care Financing Review, Medicare and Medicaid Statistical Supplement, 1996,* p. 400. Primary source: State Reported Expenditures HCFA Form-64 and Predecessors, "Quarterly Medicaid Statement of Expenditures for the Medical Assistance Program." *Notes:* 1. Prior to 1976, the Federal fiscal year was June 1 through May 31; beginning on October 1, 1976, the Federal fiscal year became October 1 through September 30. The transition quarter (July 1-September 30, 1976) is omitted in this table. 2. Amounts do not include State Survey and certification and fraud Control Unit expenditures. 3. Dollar amounts adjusted using a personal consumption expenditure index for medical services, U.S. department of Commerce, Bureau of Economic Analysis, expressed in 1994 dollars. 4. States' net reported expenditures as adjusted by HCFA. 5. Section 2161 OBRA 1981 reductions are not included. 6. Arizona began reporting financial data in 1983.

★ 664 ★

Medicaid

Medicaid Medical Assistance Payment Expenditures: FY 1975-94

Numbers in thousands, except percent.

Fiscal year[1]	State Reported Expenditures current Expenditures				Net Adjusted Expenditures[4]		HCFA Form-20822 Medicaid vendor payments[5]	Claims payments as percent of HCFA-64 final Payments
	Total comput-able[2]	1994 inflation-adjusted total computable[3]	Federal share	State share	Federal share	Annual increase		
1975	$12,086,166	$49,316,998	$6,686,193	$5,399,973	$6,739,689	-	$12,142,000	100.5
1976	13,977,348	52,240,637	7,740,497	6,236,851	7,887,740	17.0	14,091,000	100.8
1977	16,354,599	55,786,519	9,090,431	7,264,168	9,181,522	16.4	16,239,000	99.3
1978	18,168,065	56,545,487	10,030,306	8,137,759	10,152,249	10.6	17,992,000	99.0
1979	20,736,011	59,338,823	11,477,292	9,258,719	11,385,227	12.1	20,472,000	98.7
1980	24,041,116	62,431,646	13,291,174	10,749,942	13,351,569	17.3	23,311,000	97.0
1981	28,485,289	66,259,959	15,739,472	12,745,817	15,854,390	18.7	27,204,000	95.5
1982[6]	30,330,765	63,475,527	16,743,303	13,587,462	16,905,605	6.6	29,399,000	96.9
1983[6]	33,298,880	64,304,408	18,442,095	14,856,785	18,378,777	8.7	32,391,000	97.3
1984[6]	35,671,888	64,354,840	19,681,391	15,990,497	19,614,400	6.7	33,891,000	95.0
1985	39,413,219	67,268,958	21,766,157	17,647,062	21,483,421	9.5	37,508,000	95.2
1986	42,525,605	69,869,193	23,651,806	18,873,799	23,417,441	9.0	41,005,000	96.4
1987	46,956,072	73,969,984	26,253,711	20,702,361	26,198,011	11.9	45,050,000	95.9
1988	51,645,666	76,084,223	29,054,102	22,591,564	29,012,189	10.7	48,710,000	94.3
1989	58,645,953	79,778,147	33,097,420	25,548,533	32,696,722	12.7	54,500,000	92.9
1990	69,754,495	87,983,097	39,559,671	30,194,824	39,189,976	19.9	64,859,000	93.0
1991	88,377,773	104,945,024	50,475,739	37,902,034	50,354,654	28.5	76,964,000	87.1
1992	114,365,915	128,196,669	65,808,335	48,557,580	66,235,131	31.5	91,480,000	80.0
1993	126,573,138	133,989,312	72,568,820	54,004,318	73,463,767	10.9	101,708,889	80.4
1994	136,886,366	138,341,861	78,494,472	58,391,894	78,772,198	7.2	108,270,147	79.1

[Continued]

★ 664 ★

Medicaid Medical Assistance Payment Expenditures: FY 1975-94
[Continued]

Fiscal year[1]	State Reported Expenditures current Expenditures				Net Adjusted Expenditures[4]		HCFA Form-20822 Medicaid vendor payments[5]	Claims payments as percent of HCFA-64 final Payments
	Total comput-able[2]	1994 inflation-adjusted total computable[3]	Federal share	State share	Federal share	Annual increase		
Percent change 1975-94	1,032.6	180.5	1,074.0	981.3	1,068.8	-	791.7	-

Source: U.S. Department of Health and Human Services. Health Care Financing Administration. Office of Research and Demonstrations. *Health Care Financing Review, Medicare and Medicaid Statistical Supplement, 1996,* p. 401. Primary source: State Reported Expenditures - Form HCFA-64 and Predecessors, "Quarterly Medicaid Statement of Expenditures for the Medical Assistance Program." *Notes:* 1. Prior to 1976, the Federal fiscal year was June 1 through May 31; beginning October 1, 1976, the Federal fiscal year became October 1 through September 30. The transition quarter (July 1-September 30, 1976) is omitted from this table. 2. Amounts do not include State Survey and Certification and Fraud Control Unit expenditures. 3. Dollar amounts adjusted using a personal consumption expenditure index for medical services, U.S. Department of Commerce, Bureau of Economic Analysis, expressed in calendar year 1994 dollars. 4. States' net reported expenditures as adjusted by HCFA, including final adjustments and disproportionate share payments. 5. The HCFA 2082 annual report from the state is generated from the Medicaid Management Information System and reports payments to claims from vendors and counts the number of recipients of health care services. The years 1993 and 1994 include Arizona, whereas the preceding years exclude Arizona. Arizona began reporting financial data in 1983. 6. Section 2161 OBRA 1981 reductions are not included.

★ 665 ★

Medicaid

Medicaid Payments, Adults, by Type of Service: Fiscal Years 1975-94
[Amount in millions of dollars]

Year	Total[1]	Inpatient Hospital	ICF/MR	Nursing Facility[2]	Physician	Outpatient Hospital	Home Health	Prescribed Drugs	Other
1975	2,062	1,009	-3	9	392	109	6	160	377
1976	2,288	1,153	4	8	429	157	9	154	374
1977	2,606	1,294	4	5	473	257	11	171	391
1978	2,673	1,369	1	5	484	244	13	181	376
1979	3,021	1,591	3	5	518	252	21	200	431
1980	3,231	1,672	8	27	587	314	10	208	405
1981	3,763	1,897	2	5	674	418	12	243	512
1982	4,093	2,117	4	5	701	446	13	258	549
1983	4,487	2,314	11	5	730	495	14	286	632
1984	4,420	2,243	8	8	727	496	15	303	620
1985	4,746	2,330	9	7	775	537	22	342	724
1986	4,880	2,271	2	9	877	534	26	374	787
1987	5,592	2,654	2	39	926	635	21	427	888
1988	5,883	2,771	5	23	991	671	21	443	958
1989	6,897	3,219	3	127	1,186	795	26	494	1,047
1990	8,590	4,209	8	23	1,453	977	34	571	1,314
1991	10,241	4,886	5	27	1,782	1,268	44	680	1,728
1992	12,403	5,555	14	46	2,150	1,532	56	817	2,233
1993	13,605	5,943	10	40	2,334	1,734	67	920	2,557
1994	13,585	5,768	2	24	2,290	1,674	74	961	2,792

[Continued]

★ 665 ★

Medicaid Payments, Adults, by Type of Service: Fiscal Years 1975-94
[Continued]

Year	Total[1]	Inpatient Hospital	ICF/MR	Nursing Facility[2]	Physician	Outpatient Hospital	Home Health	Prescribed Drugs	Other
Average Annual Rate of Change 1975-94	10.4	9.6	-	5.3	9.7	15.5	9.9	11.1	14.1

Source: U.S. Department of Health and Human Services. Health Care Financing Administration. Office of Research and Demonstrations. *Health Care Financing Review, Medicare and Medicaid Statistical Supplement, 1996,* p. 432. Primary source: Health Care Financing Administration: Statistical Report on Medical Care: Eligibles, Recipients, Payments, and Services, HCFA Form-2082. *Notes:* ICF/MR stands for intermediate care facility for the mentally retarded. 1. The total includes payments for all types of services reported on the HCFA Form-2082, not just the eight types of services listed here. 2. Data shown include services shown separately in earlier years as SNF and intermediate care facilities, other than for the mentally retarded (ICF-Other). Beginning in fiscal year 1991, the conditions of participation for SNFs and ICF-Other were unified, the distinction between them removed, and the services renamed nursing facility services. It is possible that the combined number of recipients includes some persons who used both types of nursing facility care during the reported fiscal year. This could somewhat inflate the number of users and lower the average payments per user.

★ 666 ★

Medicaid

Medicaid Payments, Aged, by Type of Service: Fiscal Years 1975-94
[Amount in millions of dollars]

Year	Total[1]	Inpatient Hospital	ICF/MR	Nursing Facility[2]	Physician	Outpatient Hospital	Home Health	Prescribed Drugs	Other
1975	4,358	205	20	3,325	133	25	27	297	326
1976	4,910	244	18	3,594	147	34	56	364	453
1977	5,499	300	18	4,091	166	44	72	387	421
1978	6,308	382	29	4,755	174	44	85	410	429
1979	7,046	454	33	5,370	184	58	78	449	420
1980	8,739	806	199	6,288	225	67	202	519	433
1981	9,926	941	167	6,959	259	81	267	611	641
1982	10,739	1,006	95	7,674	247	90	310	629	688
1983	11,954	1,482	161	8,233	257	106	378	692	645
1984	12,815	1,396	106	8,649	255	110	451	763	1,085
1985	14,096	1,450	175	9,409	264	105	639	883	1,171
1986	15,097	1,603	179	10,057	264	126	766	973	1,129
1987	16,037	1,375	226	10,687	249	145	982	1,075	1,298
1988	17,135	1,411	216	11,618	240	161	1,143	1,186	1,160
1989	18,558	1,263	264	12,559	272	181	1,441	1,282	1,296
1990	21,508	1,315	372	14,536	286	194	1,733	1,507	1,566
1991	25,444	1,634	430	17,121	343	255	2,026	1,823	1,812
1992	29,089	1,872	517	19,589	400	311	2,250	2,190	1,960
1993	31,554	2,023	590	21,191	489	406	2,370	2,441	2,046
1994	33,618	1,964	585	22,660	544	454	2,663	2,651	2,097
Average Annual Rate of Change 1975-94	11.4	12.6	19.4	10.6	7.7	16.5	27.3	12.2	10.3

Source: U.S. Department of Health and Human Services. Health Care Financing Administration. Office of Research and Demonstrations. *Health Care Financing Review, Medicare and Medicaid Statistical Supplement, 1996,* p. 434. Primary source: Health Care Financing Administration: Statistical Report on Medical Care: Eligibles, Recipients, Payments, and Services, HCFA Form-2082. *Notes:* ICF/MR stands for intermediate care facility for the mentally retarded. 1. The total includes payments for all types of services reported on the HCFA Form-2082, not just the eight types of services listed here. 2. Data shown include services shown separately in earlier years as SNF and intermediate care facilities, other than for the mentally retarded (ICF-Other). Beginning in fiscal year 1991, the conditions of participation for SNFs and ICF-Other were unified, the distinction between them removed, and the services renamed nursing facility services. It is possible that the combined number of recipients includes some persons who used both types of nursing facility care during the reported fiscal year. This could somewhat inflate the number of users and lower the average payments per user.

★ 667 ★
Medicaid

Medicaid Payments, Aged, By Type of Service: Fiscal Years 1987-94

[In millions of 1994 dollars]

Year	Total	Inpatient	ICF/MR	Nursing Facility	Physician	Outpatient	Home health	Prescribed drugs	Other
1987	24,987	2,142	352	16,651	388	2,248	1,530	1,675	2,022
1988	24,793	2,042	313	16,810	347	1,911	1,654	1,716	1,678
1989	24,751	1,685	352	16,750	363	1,970	1,922	1,710	1,729
1990	26,646	1,629	461	18,009	354	2,179	2,147	1,867	1,939
1991	29,801	1,914	504	20,053	402	2,421	2,373	2,135	2,122
1992	32,147	2,069	571	21,648	442	2,510	2,486	2,420	2,166
1993	32,941	2,112	616	22,122	510	2,558	2,474	2,548	2,134
1994	33,618	1,964	585	22,660	544	2,551	2,663	2,651	2,097
Average Annual Rate of Change									
1987-94	4.3	-1.2	7.5	4.5	4.9	1.8	8.2	6.8	0.5
1987-88	-0.8	-4.7	-11.2	1.0	-10.5	-15.0	8.1	2.5	-17.0
1989-92	9.1	7.1	17.5	8.9	6.8	8.4	9.0	12.3	7.8
1993-94	2.1	-7.0	-5.0	2.4	6.6	-0.3	7.6	4.0	-1.7

Source: U.S. Department of Health and Human Services. Health Care Financing Administration. Office of Research and Demonstrations. *Health Care Financing Review, Medicare and Medicaid Statistical Supplement, 1996,* p. 450. Primary source: Health Care Financing Administration: Statistical Report on Medical Care: Eligibles, Recipients, Payments, and Services, HCFA Form 2082. *Note:* ICF/MR stands for intermediate care facility for the mentally retarded.

★ 668 ★
Medicaid

Medicaid Payments, All Eligibility Groups, by Type of Service: Fiscal Years 1975-94

[Amount in millions of dollars]

Year	Total[1]	Inpatient Hospital	ICF/MR	Nursing Facility[2]	Physician	Outpatient Hospital	Home Health	Prescribed Drugs	Other
1975	12,242	3,374	380	4,319	1,225	373	70	815	1,686
1976	14,091	3,905	634	4,685	1,369	555	134	940	1,869
1977	16,239	4,562	917	5,328	1,505	877	180	1,018	1.852
1978	17,992	4,992	1,192	6,229	1,554	835	210	1,082	1,898
1979	20,472	5,655	1,488	7,152	1,635	847	263	1,196	2,236
1980	23,311	6,412	1,989	7,887	1,875	1,101	332	1,318	2,397
1981	27,204	7,194	2,996	8,542	2,101	1,409	428	1,535	2,999
1982	29,399	7,670	3,467	9,406	2,086	1,438	496	1,599	3,237
1983	32,391	8,813	4,079	10,002	2,175	1,574	597	1,771	3,380
1984	33,891	8,848	4,256	10,633	2,220	1,646	774	1,968	3,546
1985	37,508	9,453	4,731	11,587	2,346	1,789	1,120	2,315	4,167
1986	41,005	10,364	5,072	12,433	2,547	1,980	1,352	2,692	4,565
1987	45,050	11,302	5,591	13,247	2,776	2,226	1,690	2,988	5,230
1988	48,710	12,076	6,022	14,277	2,953	2,413	2,015	3,294	5,660
1989	54,500	13,378	6,649	15,531	3,408	2,837	2,572	3,689	6,436
1990	64,859	16,674	7,354	17,693	4,018	3,324	3,404	4,420	7,971
1991	76,964	19,851	7,680	20,699	4,946	4,280	4,101	5,424	9,983
1992	91,480	23,686	8,552	23,547	6,122	5,296	4,888	6,790	12,599
1993	101,709	25,734	8,831	25,431	6,952	6,215	5,601	7,970	14,975

[Continued]

★ 668 ★

Medicaid Payments, All Eligibility Groups, by Type of Service: Fiscal Years 1975-94
[Continued]

Year	Total[1]	Inpatient Hospital	ICF/MR	Nursing Facility[2]	Physician	Outpatient Hospital	Home Health	Prescribed Drugs	Other
1994	108,270	26,180	8,347	27,095	7,189	6,342	7,042	8,875	17,200
Average Annual Rate of Change									
1975-94	12.2	11.4	17.7	10.1	9.8	16.1	27.5	13.4	13.0

Source: U.S. Department of Health and Human Services. Health Care Financing Administration. Office of Research and Demonstrations. *Health Care Financing Review, Medicare and Medicaid Statistical Supplement, 1996,* p. 428. Primary source: Health Care Financing Administration: Statistical Report on Medical Care: Eligibles, Recipients, Payments, and Services, HCFA Form-2082. *Notes:* ICF/MR stands for intermediate care facility for the mentally retarded. 1. The total includes payments for all types of services reported on the HCFA Form-2082, not just the eight types of services listed here. 2. Data shown include services shown separately in earlier years as SNF and intermediate care facilities, other than for the mentally retarded (ICF-Other). Beginning in fiscal year 1991, the conditions of participation for SNFs and ICF-Other were unified, the distinction between them removed, and the services renamed nursing facility services. It is possible that the combined number of recipients includes some persons who used both types of nursing facility care during the reported fiscal year. This could somewhat inflate the number of users and lower the average payments per user.

★ 669 ★

Medicaid

Medicaid Payments, by Eligibility Group: FY 1975-94

Values have been inflated so that all years are expressed in the purchasing value of the dollar in 1994.

[In millions of 1994 dollars]

Year	Total	Low-Income Children	Low-Income Adults	Low-Income Aged	Low-Income Disabled	Other
1975	49,953	8,920	8,414	17,783	12,833	2,004
1976	52,665	9,086	8,551	18,351	14,651	2,026
1977	55,392	8,903	8,889	18,757	16,656	2,186
1978	55,998	8,553	8,319	19,633	17,491	2,001
1979	58,583	8,253	8,645	20,163	19,694	1,829
1980	60,536	8,110	8,390	22,694	19,791	1,550
1981	63,280	8,160	8,753	23,089	21,993	1,284
1982	61,526	7,268	8,566	22,474	21,775	1,442
1983	62,551	7,408	8,665	23,085	21,951	1,443
1984	61,142	7,178	7,974	23,119	21,607	1,263
1985	64,017	7,534	8,100	24,059	22,959	1,365
1986	67,371	8,437	8,018	24,804	24,502	1,610
1987	70,967	8,677	8,809	25,263	26,492	1,727
1988	71,759	8,614	8,667	25,243	27,393	1,843
1989	74,138	9,375	9,382	25,245	28,411	1,725
1990	81,808	11,478	10,835	27,129	30,781	1,585
1991	91,392	13,775	12,375	30,214	33,547	1,482
1992	102,543	16,543	13,903	32,607	38,116	1,374
1993	107,668	17,471	14,402	33,403	40,920	1,391
1994	109,421	17,486	13,729	33,975	42,748	1,467

[Continued]

★ 669 ★

Medicaid Payments, by Eligibility Group: FY 1975-94

[Continued]

Year	Total	Low-Income Children	Low-Income Adults	Low-Income Aged	Low-Income Disabled	Other
Average Annual Rate of Change 1975-94	4.2	3.6	2.6	3.5	6.4	-1.6

Source: U.S. Department of Health and Human Services. Health Care Financing Administration. Office of Research and Demonstrations. *Health Care Financing Review, Medicare and Medicaid Statistical Supplement, 1996,* p. 415. Primary source: Health Care Financing Administration: Statistical Report on Medical Care: Eligibles, Recipients, Payments, and Services HCFA Form-2082.

★ 670 ★

Medicaid

Medicaid Payments by Type of Service, 1975 and 1994

Service	1975		1994	
	Expenditure ($ bil.)	%	Expenditure ($ bil.)	%
Physician Services	7.2	6.6	1.2	10.0
Outpatient Hospital	6.3	5.9	0.4	3.0
Inpatient Hospital	26.2	24.2	3.4	27.6
Home Health	7.0	6.5	0.1	0.6
Nursing Homes	27.1	25.0	4.3	35.3
ICF/MR[1]	8.3	7.7	0.4	3.1
Prescription Drugs	8.9	8.2	0.8	6.7
Other Services	17.2	15.9	1.7	13.8

Source: U.S. Department of Health and Human Services. Health Care Financing Administration. Office of Research and Demonstrations. *Health Care Financing Review, Medicare and Medicaid Statistical Supplement, 1996,* p. 152. Primary source: Data derived from HCFA Form 2082. *Notes:* 1. ICF/MR represents "intermediate care facility for the mentally retarded." Covered only by Medicaid, not by Medicare.

★ 671 ★

Medicaid

Medicaid Payments, Children, by Type of Service: Fiscal Years 1975-94

[Amount in millions of dollars]

Year	Total[1]	Inpatient Hospital	ICF/MR	Nursing Facility[2]	Physician	Outpatient Hospital	Home Health	Prescribed Drugs	Other
1975	2,186	881	17	24	397	143	8	127	589
1976	2,431	1,012	11	19	442	219	13	126	589
1977	2,610	1,149	16	16	456	348	17	125	483
1978	2,748	1,260	14	13	471	332	24	135	499
1979	2,884	1,334	22	13	474	310	33	140	558

[Continued]

★ 671 ★

Medicaid Payments, Children, by Type of Service: Fiscal Years 1975-94
[Continued]

Year	Total[1]	Inpatient Hospital	ICF/MR	Nursing Facility[2]	Physician	Outpatient Hospital	Home Health	Prescribed Drugs	Other
1980	3,123	1,476	22	24	528	381	8	156	528
1981	3,508	1,595	14	4	586	493	9	171	636
1982	3,473	1,593	9	9	573	483	9	170	627
1983	3,836	1,771	8	4	592	523	10	183	745
1984	3,979	1,847	10	4	639	536	13	202	728
1985	4,414	2,028	12	4	651	576	22	217	904
1986	5,135	2,412	13	17	685	656	24	296	1,032
1987	5,508	2,544	40	17	785	657	22	285	1,158
1988	5,848	2,718	11	5	833	675	25	298	1,283
1989	6,892	3,270	20	6	950	793	38	343	1,472
1990	9,100	4,422	47	2	1,187	1,005	55	445	1,936
1991	11,600	5,376	38	20	1,518	1,333	93	590	2,631
1992	14,758	6,594	39	15	1,949	1,737	122	808	3,494
1993	16,504	6,950	44	27	2,216	1,928	154	965	4,220
1994	17,302	6,903	45	24	2,271	1,925	204	1,063	4,867
Average Annual Rate of Change									
1975-94	11.5	11.4	5.3	0.0	9.6	14.7	18.6	11.8	11.8

Source: U.S. Department of Health and Human Services. Health Care Financing Administration. Office of Research and Demonstrations. *Health Care Financing Review, Medicare and Medicaid Statistical Supplement, 1996,* p. 430. Primary source: Health Care Financing Administration: Statistical Report on Medical Care: Eligibles, Recipients, Payments, and Services, HCFA Form-2082. *Notes:* ICF/MR stands for intermediate care facility for the mentally retarded. 1. The total includes payments for all types of services reported on the HCFA Form-2082, not just the eight types of services listed here. 2. Data shown include services shown separately in earlier years as SNF and intermediate care facilities, other than for the mentally retarded (ICF-Other). Beginning in fiscal year 1991, the conditions of participation for SNFs and ICF-Other were unified, the distinction between them removed, and the services renamed nursing facility services. It is possible that the combined number of recipients includes some persons who used both types of nursing facility care during the reported fiscal year. This could somewhat inflate the number of users and lower the average payments per user.

★ 672 ★

Medicaid

Medicaid Payments, Disabled, by Type of Service: Fiscal Years 1975-94
[Amount in millions of dollars]

Year	Total[1]	Inpatient Hospital	ICF/MR	Nursing Facility[2]	Physician	Outpatient Hospital	Home Health	Prescribed Drugs	Other
1975	3,145	1,049	294	941	243	81	27	201	309
1976	3,920	1,247	545	1,052	286	121	55	258	356
1977	4,883	1,498	819	1,197	342	193	76	299	459
1978	5,620	1,652	1,086	1,426	358	190	87	321	500
1979	6,882	1,957	1,402	1,703	396	208	129	372	715
1980	7,621	2,207	1,699	1,506	475	275	111	424	924
1981	9,455	2,521	2,760	1,562	529	353	140	500	1,090
1982	10,405	2,691	3,296	1,683	512	349	162	531	1,181
1983	11,367	2,943	3,838	1,749	543	369	194	599	1,132
1984	11,977	3,064	4,073	1,962	540	429	292	687	930
1985	13,452	3,293	4,477	2,157	588	484	433	855	1,165
1986	14,913	3,636	4,817	2,337	637	566	531	1,025	1,364
1987	16,817	4,213	5,282	2,491	714	679	658	1,174	1,606
1988	18,594	4,588	5,748	2,615	779	803	815	1,336	1,910
1989	20,885	5,043	6,311	2,812	892	962	1,052	1,540	2,273
1990	24,404	6,130	6,878	3,075	1,001	1,039	1,559	1,864	2,858
1991	28,251	7,352	7,181	3,500	1,205	1,312	1,917	2,297	3,487

[Continued]

★ 672 ★

Medicaid Payments, Disabled, by Type of Service: Fiscal Years 1975-94
[Continued]

Year	Total[1]	Inpatient Hospital	ICF/MR	Nursing Facility[2]	Physician	Outpatient Hospital	Home Health	Prescribed Drugs	Other
1992	34,004	9,079	7,973	3,878	1,515	1,624	2,439	2,936	4,560
1993	38,655	10,230	8,170	4,149	1,774	2,044	2,988	3,572	5,728
1994	42,298	10,951	7,701	4,362	1,939	2,188	4,075	4,147	6,935
Average Annual Rate of Change									
1975-94	14.7	13.1	18.8	8.4	11.6	18.9	30.2	17.3	17.8

Source: U.S. Department of Health and Human Services. Health Care Financing Administration. Office of Research and Demonstrations. *Health Care Financing Review, Medicare and Medicaid Statistical Supplement, 1996,* p. 436. Primary source: Health Care Financing Administration: Statistical Report on Medical Care: Eligibles, Recipients, Payments, and Services, HCFA Form-2082. *Notes:* ICF/MR stands for intermediate care facility for the mentally retarded. 1. The total includes payments for all types of services reported on the HCFA Form-2082, not just the eight types of services listed here. 2. Data shown include services shown separately in earlier years as SNF and intermediate care facilities, other than for the mentally retarded (ICF-Other). Beginning in fiscal year 1991, the conditions of participation for SNFs and ICF-Other were unified, the distinction between them removed, and the services renamed nursing facility services. It is possible that the combined number of recipients includes some persons who used both types of nursing facility care during the reported fiscal year. This could somewhat inflate the number of users and lower the average payments per user.

★ 673 ★

Medicaid

Medicaid Payments per Person Served, Adults, by Type of Service: Fiscal Years 1975-94
[in 1994 dollars]

Year	Total[1]	Inpatient Hospital	ICF/MR	Nursing Facility[2]	Physician	Outpatient Hospital	Home Health	Prescribed Drugs
1975	1,857	4,427	-	-	473	233	494	208
1976	1,790	4,493	-	-	467	277	1,061	172
1977	1,859	4,441	-	-	450	403	1,078	171
1978	1,793	4,370	-	-	436	352	1,422	162
1979	1,892	4,693	-	-	435	363	2,189	175
1980	1,722	4,345	-	-	475	327	654	171
1981	1,686	4,264	-	-	449	365	705	161
1982	1,786	4,783	-	-	461	379	823	173
1983	1,678	4,491	-	-	414	356	841	163
1984	1,423	4,021	-	-	355	310	741	150
1985	1,468	4,018	-	-	364	312	824	164
1986	1,420	3,675	-	-	389	288	711	168
1987	1,574	3,918	-	-	394	326	723	184
1988	1,575	3,745	-	-	401	342	840	180
1989	1,641	3,512	-	-	415	339	846	175
1990	1,803	3,645	51,627	-	440	351	894	177
1991	1,846	3,576	50,923	-	462	379	676	175
1992	1,975	3,640	48,486	-	467	423	884	180
1993	1,919	3,592	52,879	9,501	448	429	810	180
1994	1,810	3,487	25,549	7,688	424	408	640	181

[Continued]

★ 673 ★

Medicaid Payments per Person Served, Adults, by Type of Service: Fiscal Years 1975-94

[Continued]

Year	Total[1]	Inpatient Hospital	ICF/MR	Nursing Facility[2]	Physician	Outpatient Hospital	Home Health	Prescribed Drugs
Average Annual Rate of Change 1975-94	-0.1	-1.2	-	-	-0.6	3.0	1.4	-0.7

Source: U.S. Department of Health and Human Services. Health Care Financing Administration. Office of Research and Demonstrations. *Health Care Financing Review, Medicare and Medicaid Statistical Supplement, 1996,* p. 423. Primary source: Health Care Financing Administration: Statistical Report on Medical Care: Eligibles, Recipients, Payments, and Services, HCFA Form-2082. *Notes:* Dollar amounts adjusted using a personal consumption expenditure index for medical services, U.S. Department of Commerce, Bureau of Economic Analysis, expressed in calendar year 1994 dollars. ICF/MR is intermediate care facility, mentally retarded. 1. The total includes payments for all types of services reported on the HCFA Form 2082, not just the eight types of services listed here. 2. Data shown include services shown separately in earlier years as SNF and intermediate care facilities, other than for the mentally retarded (ICF-Other). Beginning in fiscal year 1991, the conditions of participation for SNFs and ICF-Other were unified, the distinction between them removed, and the services renamed nursing facility services. It is possible that the combined number of recipients includes some persons who used both types of nursing facility care during the reported fiscal year. This could somewhat inflate the number of users and lower the average payments per user.

★ 674 ★

Medicaid

Medicaid Payments per Person Served, Aged, by Type of Service: Fiscal Years 1975-94

[In 1994 dollars]

Year	Total[1]	Inpatient Hospital	ICF/MR	Nursing Facility[2]	Physician	Outpatient Hospital	Home Health	Prescribed Drugs
1975	4,917	1,106	28,257	13,261	241	143	971	453
1976	5,079	1,159	33,455	12,438	243	157	1,843	501
1977	5,158	1,242	25,522	12,549	242	181	1,825	491
1978	5,817	1,388	30,190	13,539	243	149	2,493	492
1979	5,992	1,628	28,055	14,228	238	192	3,969	512
1980	6,596	2,519	42,448	14,911	262	192	4,864	514
1981	6,857	2,594	44,771	14,275	274	212	6,104	535
1982	7,749	2,901	26,799	16,235	269	236	6,882	582
1983	7,419	3,520	42,584	14,528	239	203	3,828	573
1984	7,139	3,208	42,113	13,404	215	189	4,083	563
1985	7,860	3,396	45,956	13,714	208	224	4,661	628
1986	7,900	3,661	53,115	13,944	196	233	4,954	647
1987	7,837	2,990	62,782	13,960	175	250	5,594	681
1988	7,992	2,854	67,179	13,714	171	258	6,400	698
1989	8,061	2,386	69,738	13,924	186	261	7,417	706
1990	8,472	2,352	66,778	14,853	176	259	7,584	733
1991	9,045	2,555	66,536	16,078	187	288	8,014	794
1992	8,697	2,412	48,293	16,399	189	291	7,784	855
1993	8,647	2,355	64,469	16,373	201	322	7,049	874
1994	8,421	2,203	54,557	16,381	205	323	6,814	889

[Continued]

★ 674 ★

Medicaid Payments per Person Served, Aged, by Type of Service: Fiscal Years 1975-94
[Continued]

Year	Total[1]	Inpatient Hospital	ICF/MR	Nursing Facility[2]	Physician	Outpatient Hospital	Home Health	Prescribed Drugs
Average Annual Rate of Change 1975-94	2.9	3.7	3.5	1.1	-0.8	4.4	10.8	3.6

Source: U.S. Department of Health and Human Services. Health Care Financing Administration. Office of Research and Demonstrations. *Health Care Financing Review, Medicare and Medicaid Statistical Supplement, 1996,* p. 425. Primary source: Health Care Financing Administration: Statistical Report on Medical Care: Eligibles, Recipients, Payments, and Services, HCFA Form-2082. *Notes:* Dollar amounts adjusted using a personal consumption expenditure index for medical services, U.S. Department of Commerce, Bureau of Economic Analysis, expressed in calendar year 1994 dollars. ICF/MR is intermediate care facility, mentally retarded. 1. The total includes payments for all types of services reported on the HCFA Form-2082, not just the eight types of services listed here. 2. Data shown include services shown separately in earlier years as SNF and intermediate care facilities, other than for the mentally retarded (ICF-Other). Beginning in fiscal year 1991, the conditions of participation for SNFs and ICF-Other were unified, the distinction between them removed, and the services renamed nursing facility services. It is possible that the combined number of recipients includes some persons who used both types of nursing facility care during the reported fiscal year. This could somewhat inflate the number of users and lower the average payments per user.

★ 675 ★

Medicaid

Medicaid Payments per Person Served, All Eligibility Groups, by Type of Service: Fiscal Years 1975-94

[In 1994 dollars]

Year	Total[1]	Inpatient hospital	ICF/MR	Nursing Facility[2]	Physician	Outpatient Hospital	Home Health	Prescribed Drugs
1975	2,269	4,011	22,598	13,433	331	204	832	237
1976	2,310	4,111	26,667	12,865	329	243	1,570	235
1977	2,425	4,131	29,096	13,027	321	348	1,654	225
1978	2,549	4,108	35,749	14,059	308	302	1,737	221
1979	2,721	4,487	37,264	14,875	309	315	2,100	240
1980	2,802	4,524	42,690	14,683	353	293	2,197	249
1981	2,880	4,520	46,085	14,482	340	328	2,477	251
1982	3,182	5,077	54,495	16,607	351	341	3,069	276
1983	3,145	4,989	56,518	15,313	324	326	2,963	270
1984	2,831	4,604	54,429	14,157	281	296	3,190	254
1985	2,934	4,699	55,023	14,383	278	304	3,571	283
1986	2,992	4,804	57,651	14,601	281	304	3,743	301
1987	3,070	4,726	59,058	14,685	285	320	4,375	312
1988	3,132	4,642	61,009	14,555	284	337	5,218	317
1989	3,153	4,422	61,214	14,550	295	340	5,747	316
1990	3,239	4,579	63,127	15,272	297	339	5,970	322
1991	3,268	4,701	62,687	16,497	307	362	6,020	329
1992	3,292	4,586	63,485	16,779	316	391	5,917	345
1993	3,220	4,622	62,622	16,724	310	400	5,558	353
1994	3,122	4,510	53,055	16,707	299	387	5,504	367

[Continued]

★ 675 ★

Medicaid Payments per Person Served, All Eligibility Groups, by Type of Service: Fiscal Years 1975-94

[Continued]

Year	Total[1]	Inpatient hospital	ICF/MR	Nursing Facility[2]	Physician	Outpatient Hospital	Home Health	Prescribed Drugs
Average Annual Rate of Change 1975-94	1.7	0.6	4.6	1.2	-0.5	3.4	10.5	2.3

Source: U.S. Department of Health and Human Services. Health Care Financing Administration. Office of Research and Demonstrations. *Health Care Financing Review, Medicare and Medicaid Statistical Supplement, 1996,* p. 419. Primary source: Health Care financing Administration: Statistical Report on Medical Care: Eligibles, Recipients, Payments, and Services, HCFA Form-2082. *Notes:* ICF/MR is intermediate care facility, mentally retarded. 1. The total includes payments for all types of services reported on the HCFA Form-2082, not just the eight types of services listed here. 2. Data shown include services shown separately in earlier years as SNF and intermediate care facilities, other than for the mentally retarded (ICF-Other). Beginning in fiscal year 1991, the conditions of participation for SNFs and ICF-Other were unified, the distinction between them removed, and the services renamed nursing facility services. It is possible that the combined number of recipients includes some persons who used both types of nursing facility care during the reported fiscal year. This could somewhat inflate the number of users and lower the average payments per user.

★ 676 ★

Medicaid

Medicaid Payments per Person Served, Children, by Type of Service: Fiscal Years 1975-94

[In 1994 dollars]

Year	Total[1]	Inpatient Hospital	ICF/MR	Nursing Facility[2]	Physician	Outpatient Hospital	Home Health	Prescribed Drugs
1975	930	3,652	-	-	245	163	584	94
1976	916	3,764	-	-	239	202	863	78
1977	921	3,848	-	-	225	293	959	72
1978	912	3,834	-	-	218	258	523	68
1979	907	4,043	-	-	209	252	515	72
1980	870	3,919	-	-	226	234	273	73
1981	851	3,887	-	-	209	268	219	67
1982	849	4,297	-	-	217	271	306	72
1983	841	4,204	-	-	203	264	525	69
1984	741	3,944	-	-	182	231	512	65
1985	771	4,006	-	-	178	230	579	67
1986	841	4,290	-	-	173	243	567	82
1987	854	3,986	-	-	186	228	588	74
1988	859	3,994	-	-	186	230	738	72
1989	909	3,910	-	-	188	231	869	72
1990	1,023	4,146	44,394	-	195	242	929	77
1991	1,072	4,337	51,360	-	202	257	1,078	81
1992	1,088	3,710	44,434	-	210	272	1,085	90
1993	1,072	3,861	52,941	28,170	206	267	1,092	93
1994	1,017	3,626	50,391	22,225	199	255	1,021	96

[Continued]

★ 676 ★

Medicaid Payments per Person Served, Children, by Type of Service: Fiscal Years 1975-94
[Continued]

Year	Total[1]	Inpatient Hospital	ICF/MR	Nursing Facility[2]	Physician	Outpatient Hospital	Home Health	Prescribed Drugs
Average Annual Rate of Change 1975-94	0.5	-0.0	-	-	-1.1	2.4	3.0	0.1

Source: U.S. Department of Health and Human Services. Health Care Financing Administration. Office of Research and Demonstrations. *Health Care Financing Review, Medicare and Medicaid Statistical Supplement, 1996,* p. 421. Primary source: Health Care Financing Administration: Statistical Report on Medical Care: Eligibles, Recipients, Payments, and Services, HCFA Form-2082. *Notes:* Dollar amounts adjusted using a personal consumption expenditure index for medical services, U.S. Department of Commerce, Bureau of Economic Analysis, expressed in calendar year 1994 dollars. ICF/MR is intermediate care facility, mentally retarded. 1. The total includes payments for all types of services reported on the HCFA Form-2082, not just the eight types of services listed here. 2. Data shown include services shown separately in earlier years as SNF and intermediate care facilities, other than for the mentally retarded (ICF-Other). Beginning in fiscal year 1991, the conditions of participation for SNFs and ICF-Other were unified, the distinction between them removed, and the services renamed nursing facility services. It is possible that the combined number of recipients includes some persons who used both types of nursing facility care during the reported fiscal year. This could somewhat inflate the number of users and lower the average payments per user.

★ 677 ★

Medicaid

Medicaid Payments per Person Served, Disabled, by Type of Service: Fiscal Years 1975-94
[In 1994 dollars]

Year	Total[1]	Inpatient Hospital	ICF/MR	Nursing Facility[2]	Physician	Outpatient Hospital	Home Health	Prescribed Drugs
1975	5,207	8,067	21,161	14,065	600	375	1,126	469
1976	5,490	7,744	25,938	14,509	591	426	1,839	505
1977	5,945	7,552	29,622	15,067	590	580	2,047	498
1978	6,436	7,445	37,118	16,082	570	514	2,779	489
1979	7,154	7,824	39,259	16,864	572	532	4,258	512
1980	6,801	7,656	43,246	13,257	608	564	1,693	501
1981	7,143	7,569	45,248	13,359	593	579	1,926	523
1982	8,415	8,584	53,917	15,737	589	636	2,258	575
1983	8,143	8,233	53,368	15,844	552	571	2,821	582
1984	7,418	7,570	52,955	15,389	473	568	3,271	563
1985	7,610	7,723	54,149	15,868	464	585	3,931	638
1986	7,701	7,954	56,621	16,550	455	593	4,259	687
1987	7,836	8,285	57,897	16,627	458	630	4,687	704
1988	7,855	8,106	60,268	16,750	455	667	5,551	719
1989	7,913	7,754	60,489	17,078	468	684	6,058	726
1990	8,279	8,472	63,372	17,913	462	661	6,625	778
1991	8,318	8,818	62,544	19,231	482	709	6,682	831
1992	8,494	9,319	64,762	19,670	507	738	6,904	897
1993	8,158	9,023	62,656	19,551	489	758	6,824	918
1994	7,832	8,925	53,308	19,335	470	717	7,289	946

[Continued]

★ 677 ★

Medicaid Payments per Person Served, Disabled, by Type of Service: Fiscal Years 1975-94

[Continued]

Year	Total[1]	Inpatient Hospital	ICF/MR	Nursing Facility[2]	Physician	Outpatient Hospital	Home Health	Prescribed Drugs
Average Annual Rate of Change 1975-94	2.2	0.5	5.0	1.7	-1.3	3.5	10.3	3.8

Source: U.S. Department of Health and Human Services. Health Care Financing Administration. Office of Research and Demonstrations. *Health Care Financing Review, Medicare and Medicaid Statistical Supplement, 1996,* p. 427. Primary source: Health Care Financing Administration: Statistical Report on Medical Care: Eligibles, Recipients, Payments, and Services, HCFA Form-2082. *Notes:* Dollar amounts adjusted using a personal consumption expenditure index for medical services, U.S. Department of Commerce, Bureau of Economic Analysis, expressed in calendar year 1994 dollars. ICF/MR is intermediate care facility, mentally retarded. 1. The total includes payments for all types of services reported on the HCFA Form-2082, not just the eight types of services listed here. 2. Data shown include services shown separately in earlier years as SNF and intermediate care facilities, other than for the mentally retarded (ICF-Other). Beginning in fiscal year 1991, the conditions of participation for SNFs and ICF-Other were unified, the distinction between them removed, and the services renamed nursing facility services. It is possible that the combined number of recipients includes some persons who used both types of nursing facility care during the reported fiscal year. This could somewhat inflate the number of users and lower the average payments per user.

★ 678 ★

Medicaid

Medicaid Payments per Person Served: FY 1975-94

Values have been inflated so that all years are expressed in the purchasing value of the dollar in 1994.

[In 1994 dollars]

Year[1]	Total	Low-Income Children	Low-Income Adults	Low-Income Aged	Low-Income Disabled
1975	2,269	930	1,857	4,917	5,207
1976	2,310	916	1,790	5,079	5,490
1977	2,425	921	1,859	5,158	5,945
1978	2,549	912	1,793	5,817	6,436
1979	2,721	907	1,892	5,992	7,154
1980	2,802	870	1,722	6,596	6,801
1981	2,880	851	1,686	6,857	7,143
1982	2,848	760	1,599	6,938	7,534
1983	2,902	776	1,549	6,846	7,514
1984	2,831	741	1,423	7,139	7,418
1985	2,934	771	1,468	7,860	7,610
1986	2,992	841	1,420	7,900	7,701
1987	3,070	854	1,574	7,837	7,836
1988	3,132	859	1,575	7,992	7,855
1989	3,153	909	1,641	8,061	7,913
1990	3,239	1,023	1,802	8,472	8,279
1991	3,628	1,071	1,846	9,045	8,318
1992	3,292	1,088	1,975	8,697	8,494
1993	3,220	1,072	1,919	8,647	8,158
1994	3,122	1,017	1,810	8,421	7,832
Percent Change 1975-94	37.6	9.63	-2.5	71.3	50.4

[Continued]

★ 678 ★

Medicaid Payments per Person Served: FY 1975-94
[Continued]

Year[1]	Total	Low-Income Children	Low-Income Adults	Low-Income Aged	Low-Income Disabled
1975-84	22.5	-19.0	-20.5	40.5	35.1
1985-94	6.4	31.8	23.3	7.1	2.9

Source: U.S. Department of Health and Human Services. Health Care Financing Administration. Office of Research and Demonstrations. *Health Care Financing Review, Medicare and Medicaid Statistical Supplement, 1996,* p. 417. Primary source: Health Care Financing Administration: Statistical Report on Medical Care: Eligibles, Recipients, Payments, and Services, HCFA Form-2082. *Notes:* Dollar amounts are adjusted using a personal consumption expenditure index for medical services, U.S. Department of Commerce, Bureau of Economic Analysis, expressed in calendar year 1994 dollars. 1. The total includes payments for all types of services on the HCFA Form-2082.

★ 679 ★

Medicaid

Medicare and Medicaid Payments, Aged, by Type of Service: Calendar Years 1987-94
[In millions of 1994 dollars]

Year	Total[1]	Inpatient Hospital	ICF/MR	Nursing Facility[2]	Physician	Outpatient Hospital	Home Health	Prescribed Drugs
1987	129,529	64,458	352	17,453	31,415	10,060	4,115	1,675
1988	129,243	63,578	313	17,981	31,058	10,292	4,281	1,716
1989	135,127	63,192	352	20,485	34,001	10,415	4,924	1,710
1990	137,677	63,427	461	20,345	34,194	10,863	6,461	1,867
1991	144,652	65,385	504	22,569	34,224	11,458	8,250	2,135
1992	149,555	66,201	571	25,065	32,839	12,209	10,065	2,420
1993	151,420	64,332	616	26,406	32,873	12,499	11,873	2,548
1994	161,687	67,296	585	28,352	34,658	13,487	14,348	2,651
Average Annual Rate of Change								
1987-94	3.2	0.6		7.2	1.4	4.3	19.5	
1987-88	-0.2	-1.4		3.0	-1.1	2.3	4.0	
1989-92	3.4	1.6		7.0	-1.2	5.4	26.9	
1993-94	6.8	4.6		7.4	5.4	7.9	20.8	

Source: U.S. Department of Health and Human Services. Health Care Financing Administration. Office of Research and Demonstrations. *Health Care Financing Review, Statistical Supplement, 1996,* p 454. Primary source: Health Care Financing Administration: Statistical Report on Medical Care: Eligibles, Recipients, Payments, and Services, HCFA Form-2082. Medicare data from the Medicare Decision Support system; data development by the Office of Research and Demonstrations. *Notes:* ICF/MR stands for intermediate care facility for the mentally retarded. 1. The total includes users for all types of services reported on the HCFA Form-2082. A person receiving multiple services (e.g., inpatient hospital, physician, and outpatient services) is included once in the user count for each type of service and once in the total. 2. Data shown include services shown separately in earlier years as skilled nursing facility (SNF) and intermediate care facilities, other than for the mentally retarded (ICF-Other). Beginning in fiscal year 1991, the conditions of participation for SNFs and ICF-Other were unified, the distinction between them removed, and the services renamed nursing facility services. It is possible that the combined number of recipients includes some persons who used both types of nursing facility care during the reported fiscal year. This could somewhat inflate the number of users and lower the average payments per recipient.

★ 680 ★

Medicaid

Number of Medicaid Persons Served, Aged, by Type of Service: FY 1975-94

Year	Total[1]	Inpatient Hospital	ICF/MR	Nursing Facility[2]	Physician	Outpatient Hospital	Home Health	Prescribed Drugs
Number in thousands								
1975	3,615	757	3	1,023	2,263	732	115	2,673
1976	3,612	786	2	1,080	2,275	816	113	2,718
1977	3,636	824	2	1,112	2,338	828	134	2,678
1978	3,376	858	3	1,093	2,245	908	106	2,595
1979	3,364	798	3	1,080	2,222	874	56	2,504
1980	3,440	831	12	1,095	2,221	903	108	2,524
1981	3,367	843	9	1,134	2,208	895	102	2,655
1982	3,240	811	8	1,105	2,148	885	105	2,523
1983	3,372	881	8	1,186	2,265	1,088	207	2,526
1984	3,238	785	5	1,164	2,140	1,041	199	2,444
1985	3,061	729	7	1,171	2,166	804	234	2,400
1986	3,140	720	6	1,185	2,216	884	254	2,468
1987	3,224	725	6	1,206	2,239	912	277	2,490
1988	3,159	728	5	1,248	2,066	918	263	2,504
1989	3,132	720	5	1,227	1,989	940	264	2,471
1990	3,202	705	7	1,234	2,056	944	288	2,591
1991	3,341	759	8	1,265	2,185	1,049	300	2,727
1992	3,749	870	12	1,339	2,366	1,196	324	2,872
1993	3,863	909	10	1,370	2,569	1,335	356	2,954
1994	4,035	901	11	1,398	2,681	1,420	395	3,012
Average Annual Rate of Change								
1975-94	0.6	0.9	7.1	1.7	0.9	3.5	6.7	0.6
Percent Distribution								
1975	100.0	20.9	0.1	28.3	62.6	20.2	3.2	73.9
1976	100.0	12.8	0.1	29.9	63.0	22.6	3.1	75.2
1977	100.0	22.7	0.1	30.6	64.3	22.8	3.7	73.7
1978	100.0	25.4	0.1	32.4	66.5	26.9	3.1	76.9
1979	100.0	23.7	0.1	32.1	66.1	26.0	1.7	74.4
1980	100.0	24.2	0.3	31.8	64.6	26.3	3.1	73.4
1981	100.0	25.0	0.3	33.7	65.6	26.6	3.0	78.9
1982	100.0	25.0	0.2	34.1	66.3	27.3	3.2	77.9
1983	100.0	26.1	0.2	35.2	67.2	32.3	6.1	74.9
1984	100.0	24.2	0.2	35.9	66.1	32.1	6.1	75.5
1985	100.0	23.8	0.2	38.3	70.8	26.3	7.6	78.4
1986	100.0	22.9	0.2	37.7	70.6	28.2	8.1	78.6
1987	100.0	22.5	0.2	37.4	69.4	28.3	8.6	77.2
1988	100.0	23.0	0.2	39.5	65.4	29.1	8.3	79.3
1989	100.0	23.0	0.2	39.2	63.5	30.0	8.4	78.9
1990	100.0	22.0	0.2	38.5	64.2	29.5	9.0	80.9
1991	100.0	22.7	0.2	37.9	65.4	31.4	9.0	81.6
1992	100.0	23.2	0.3	35.7	63.1	31.9	8.6	76.6

[Continued]

★ 680 ★

Number of Medicaid Persons Served, Aged, by Type of Service: FY 1975-94

[Continued]

Year	Total[1]	Inpatient Hospital	ICF/MR	Nursing Facility[2]	Physician	Outpatient Hospital	Home Health	Prescribed Drugs
1993	100.0	23.5	0.3	35.5	66.5	34.6	9.2	76.5
1994	100.0	22.3	0.3	34.6	66.4	35.2	9.8	74.6

Source: U.S. Department of Health and Human Services. Health Care Financing Administration. Office of Research and Demonstrations. *Health Care Financing Review, Medicare and Medicaid Statistical Supplement, 1996,* p. 410. Primary source: Health Care Financing Administration: Statistical Report on Medical Care: Eligibles, Recipients, Payments and Services, HCFA Form-2082. *Notes:* These totals for "all eligibility groups presented" (low-income aged, low-income disabled, children in low-income families, adults in low-income families), and the "Other Title XIX" group which is not presented separately. ICF/MR stands for Intermediate Care Facility for Mentally Retarded Persons. 1. The total includes users for all types of services reported on the HCFA Form-2082. A person receiving multiple services (e.g., inpatient hospital, physician, and outpatient services) is included once in the user count for each type of service and once in the total. 2. Data shown include services shown separately in earlier years as skilled nursing facility (SNF) and intermediate care facilities, other than for the mentally retarded (ICF-Other). Beginning in fiscal year 1991, the conditions of participation for SNFs and ICF-Other were unified, the distinction between them removed, and the services renamed nursing facility services. It is possible that the combined number of recipients includes some persons who used both types of nursing facility care during the reported fiscal year. This could somewhat inflate the number of users and lower the average payments per recipient.

★ 681 ★

Medicaid

Number of Medicaid Persons Served, All Categories, by Type of Service: FY 1975-94

Year	Total[1]	Inpatient Hospital	ICF/MR	Nursing Facility[2]	Physician	Outpatient Hospital	Home Health	Prescribed Drugs
Number in thousands								
1975	22,007	3,432	69	1,312	15,198	7,437	343	14,155
1976	22,815	3,551	89	1,361	15,624	8,482	319	14,883
1977	22,832	3,768	107	1,395	16,074	8,619	371	15,370
1978	21,965	3,782	104	1,379	15,668	8,628	376	15,188
1979	21,520	3,608	114	1,376	15,168	7,710	359	14,283
1980	21,605	3,680	121	1,395	13,765	9,705	392	13,707
1981	21,980	3,703	151	1,372	14,403	10,018	402	14,256
1982	21,603	3,530	149	1,324	13,894	9,853	377	13,547
1983	21,554	3,696	151	1,367	14,056	10,069	422	13,732
1984	21,607	3,467	141	1,355	14,195	10,035	438	13,935
1985	21,814	3,434	147	1,375	14,387	10,072	535	13,921
1986	22,515	3,544	145	1,399	14,894	10,702	593	14,704
1987	23,109	3,767	149	1,421	15,373	10,979	609	15,083
1988	22,907	3,832	145	1,445	15,265	10,533	569	15,323
1989	23,511	4,170	148	1,452	15,686	11,344	609	15,916
1990	25,255	4,593	147	1,461	17,078	12,370	719	17,294
1991	27,967	5,014	145	1,490	19,119	14,031	809	19,581
1992	31,150	5,790	151	1,573	21,683	15,167	926	22,070
1993	33,432	5,894	149	1,610	23,746	16,436	1,067	23,901
1994	35,053	5,866	159	1,639	24,267	16,567	1,293	24,471
Average Annual Rate of Change								
1975-94	2.5	2.9	4.5	1.2	2.5	4.3	7.2	2.9
Percent Distribution								
1975	100.0	15.6	0.3	6.0	69.1	33.8	1.6	64.3
1976	100.0	15.6	0.4	6.0	68.5	37.2	1.4	65.2
1977	100.0	16.5	0.5	6.1	70.4	37.7	1.6	67.3

[Continued]

★ 681 ★

Number of Medicaid Persons Served, All Categories, by Type of Service: FY 1975-94
[Continued]

Year	Total[1]	Inpatient Hospital	ICF/MR	Nursing Facility[2]	Physician	Outpatient Hospital	Home Health	Prescribed Drugs
1978	100.0	17.2	0.5	6.3	71.3	39.3	1.7	69.1
1979	100.0	16.8	0.5	6.4	70.5	35.8	1.7	66.4
1980	100.0	17.0	0.6	6.5	63.7	44.9	1.8	63.4
1981	100.0	16.8	0.7	6.2	65.5	45.6	1.8	64.9
1982	100.0	16.3	0.7	6.1	64.3	45.6	1.7	62.7
1983	100.0	17.1	0.7	6.3	65.2	46.7	2.0	63.7
1984	100.0	16.0	0.7	6.3	65.7	46.4	2.0	63.8
1985	100.0	15.7	0.7	6.3	66.0	46.2	2.5	63.8
1986	100.0	15.7	0.6	6.2	66.2	47.5	2.6	65.3
1987	100.0	16.3	0.6	6.1	66.5	47.5	2.6	65.3
1988	100.0	16.7	0.6	6.3	66.6	46.0	2.5	66.9
1989	100.0	17.7	0.6	6.2	66.7	48.2	2.6	67.7
1990	100.0	18.2	0.6	5.8	67.6	49.0	2.8	68.5
1991	100.0	17.9	0.5	5.3	68.4	50.2	2.9	70.0
1992	100.0	18.6	0.5	5.0	69.6	48.7	3.0	70.9
1993	100.0	17.6	0.4	4.8	71.0	49.2	3.2	71.5
1994	100.0	16.7	0.5	4.7	69.2	47.3	3.7	69.8

Source: U.S. Department of Health and Human Services. Health Care Financing Administration. Office of Research and Demonstrations. *Health Care Financing Review, Medicare and Medicaid Statistical Supplement, 1996,* p. 404. Primary source: Health Care Financing Administration: Statistical Report on Medical Care: Eligibles, Recipients, Payments and Services, HCFA Form-2082. *Notes:* These totals for "all eligibility groups" include the four eligibility groups presented (low-income aged, low-income disabled, children in low-income families, adults in low-income families), and the "Other Title XIX" group which is not presented separately. ICF/MR represents "Intermediate Care Facility for Mentally Retarded Persons." 1. The total includes users for all types of services reported on the HCFA Form-2082. A person receiving multiple services (e.g., inpatient hospital, physician, and outpatient services) is included once in the user count for each type of service and once in total. 2. Data shown include services shown separately in earlier years as skilled nursing facility (SNF) and intermediate care facilities, other than for the mentally retarded (ICF-Other). Beginning in fiscal year 1991, the conditions of participation for SNFs and ICF-Other were unified, the distinction between them removed, and the services renamed nursing facility services. It is possible that the combined number of recipients includes some persons who use both types of nursing facility care during the reported fiscal year. This could somewhat inflate the number of users and lower the average payments per recipient.

★ 682 ★

Medicaid

Number of Medicaid Persons Served, by Eligibility Group: FY 1975-94

Year	Total	Low-Income Children	Low-Income Adult	Low-Income Aged	Low-Income Disabled	Other
Number in thousands						
1975	22,007	9,598	4,529	3,615	2,464	1,801
1976	22,815	9,924	4,773	3,612	2,669	1,837
1977	22,832	9,651	4,785	3,636	2,802	1,958
1978	21,965	9,376	4,643	3,376	2,718	1,852
1979	21,520	9,106	4,570	3,364	2,753	1,727
1980	21,605	9,333	4,877	3,440	2,911	1,044
1981	21,980	9,581	5,187	3,367	3,079	766
1982	21,603	9,563	5,356	3,240	2,891	553
1983	21,554	9,535	5,592	3,372	2,921	134
1984	21,607	9,684	5,600	3,238	2,913	172
1985	21,814	9,757	5,518	3,061	3,012	466

[Continued]

★ 682 ★

Number of Medicaid Persons Served, by Eligibility Group: FY 1975-94
[Continued]

Year	Total	Low-Income Children	Low-Income Adult	Low-Income Aged	Low-Income Disabled	Other
1986	22,515	10,029	5,647	3,140	3,182	517
1987	23,109	10,168	5,599	3,224	3,381	737
1988	22,907	10,037	5,503	3,159	3,487	721
1989	23,511	10,318	5,717	3,132	3,590	754
1990	25,255	11,220	6,010	3,202	3,718	1,105
1991[1]	27,967	12,855	6,703	3,341	4,033	1,035
1992	31,150	15,200	7,040	3,749	4,487	674
1993	33,432	16,285	7,505	3,863	5,016	763
1994	35,053	17,194	7,586	4,035	5,458	780
Average Annual Rate of Change						
1975-80	-0.4	-0.6	1.5	-1.0	3.4	-10.3
1981-84	-0.4	0.3	1.9	-1.0	-1.4	-31.2
1985-88	1.2	0.7	-0.1	0.8	3.7	11.5
1989-92	7.3	10.2	5.3	4.6	5.7	-2.8
1993-94	2.4	2.8	0.5	2.2	4.3	1.1
1975-94	2.5	3.1	2.8	0.6	4.3	-4.3
Percent Distribution						
1975	100.0	43.6	20.6	16.4	11.2	8.2
1976	100.0	43.5	20.9	15.8	11.7	8.1
1977	100.0	42.3	21.0	15.9	12.3	8.6
1978	100.0	42.7	21.1	15.4	12.4	8.4
1979	100.0	42.3	21.2	15.6	12.8	8.0
1980	100.0	43.2	22.6	15.9	13.5	4.8
1981	100.0	43.6	23.6	15.3	14.0	3.5
1982	100.0	44.3	24.8	15.0	13.4	2.6
1983	100.0	44.2	25.9	15.6	13.6	0.6
1984	100.0	44.8	25.9	15.0	13.5	0.8
1985	100.0	44.7	25.3	14.0	13.8	2.1
1986	100.0	44.5	25.1	13.9	14.1	2.3
1987	100.0	44.0	24.2	14.0	14.6	3.2
1988	100.0	43.8	24.0	13.8	15.2	3.1
1989	100.0	43.9	24.3	13.3	15.3	3.2
1990	100.0	44.4	23.8	12.7	14.7	4.4
1991[1]	100.0	46.0	24.0	11.9	14.4	3.7
1992	100.0	48.8	22.6	12.0	14.4	2.2
1993	100.0	48.7	22.4	11.6	15.0	2.3
1994	100.0	49.1	21.6	11.5	15.6	2.2

Source: U.S. Department of Health and Human Services. Health Care Financing Administration. Office of Research and Demonstrations. *Health Care Financing Review, Medicare and Medicaid Statistical Supplement, 1996,* p. 402. Primary source: Health Care Financing Administration: Statistical Report on Medical Care: Eligibles, Recipients, Payments, and Services, HCFA Form-2082. *Notes:* SNF represents "skilled nursing facility." ICF represents "intermediate care facility." 1. Beginning in fiscal year 1991, the conditions of participation for SNFs and ICF-Other were unified, the distinction between them removed, and the services renamed nursing facility services. It is possible that the combined number of recipients includes some persons who use both types of nursing facility care during the reported fiscal year. This could somewhat inflate the number of users and lower the average payments per recipient.

★ 683 ★

Medicaid

Number of Medicaid Persons Served, Disabled, by Type of Service: FY 1975-94

Year	Total[1]	Inpatient Hospital	ICF/MR	Nursing Facility[2]	Physician	Outpatient Hospital	Home Health	Prescribed Drugs
Number in thousands								
1975	2,464	531	57	273	1,652	874	99	1,745
1976	2,669	602	78	271	1,816	1,064	112	1,912
1977	2,802	677	94	271	1,980	1,137	127	2,049
1978	2,718	691	91	276	1,956	1,150	97	2,046
1979	2,753	718	102	289	1,985	1,120	87	2,081
1980	2,911	749	102	295	2,032	1,269	170	2,193
1981	3,079	775	142	272	2,076	1,418	169	2,226
1982	2,891	733	143	250	2,030	1,284	168	2,156
1983	2,921	748	151	231	2,057	1,354	144	2,156
1984	2,913	730	139	230	2,056	1,361	161	2,200
1985	3,012	728	141	232	2,161	1,413	188	2,287
1986	3,182	751	140	232	2,298	1,569	205	2,451
1987	3,381	801	144	236	2,458	1,698	221	2,627
1988	3,487	834	140	230	2,521	1,772	216	2,738
1989	3,590	885	142	224	2,596	1,911	236	2,882
1990	3,718	913	137	217	2,735	1,982	297	3,022
1991	4,033	990	136	216	2,971	2,196	341	3,282
1992	4,487	1,092	138	221	3,353	2,467	396	3,671
1993	5,016	1,200	138	225	3,842	2,854	464	4,118
1994	5,458	1,240	146	228	4,167	3,088	565	4,429
Average Annual Rate of Change								
1975-94	4.3	4.6	5.1	-0.9	5.0	6.9	9.6	5.0
Percent Distribution								
1975	100.0	21.6	2.3	11.1	67.0	35.5	4.0	70.8
1976	100.0	22.6	2.9	10.2	68.0	39.9	4.2	71.6
1977	100.0	24.2	3.4	9.7	70.7	40.6	4.5	73.1
1978	100.0	25.4	3.3	10.2	72.0	42.3	3.6	75.3
1979	100.0	26.1	3.7	10.5	72.1	40.7	3.2	75.6
1980	100.0	25.7	3.5	10.1	69.8	43.6	5.8	75.3
1981	100.0	25.2	4.6	8.8	67.4	46.1	5.5	72.3
1982	100.0	25.4	4.9	8.6	70.2	44.4	5.8	74.6
1983	100.0	25.6	5.2	7.9	70.4	46.4	4.9	73.8
1984	100.0	25.1	4.8	7.9	70.6	46.7	5.5	75.5
1985	100.0	24.2	4.7	7.7	71.7	46.9	6.2	75.9
1986	100.0	23.6	4.4	7.3	72.2	49.3	6.4	77.0
1987	100.0	23.7	4.3	7.0	72.7	50.2	6.5	77.7
1988	100.0	23.9	4.0	6.6	72.3	50.8	6.2	78.5
1989	100.0	24.7	4.0	6.2	72.3	53.2	6.6	80.3
1990	100.0	24.5	3.7	5.8	73.6	53.3	8.0	81.3
1991	100.0	24.6	3.4	5.4	73.7	54.4	8.4	81.4
1992	100.0	24.4	3.1	4.9	74.7	55.0	8.8	81.8

[Continued]

★ 683 ★

Number of Medicaid Persons Served, Disabled, by Type of Service: FY 1975-94
[Continued]

Year	Total[1]	Inpatient Hospital	ICF/MR	Nursing Facility[2]	Physician	Outpatient Hospital	Home Health	Prescribed Drugs
1993	100.0	23.9	2.8	4.5	76.6	56.9	9.3	82.1
1994	100.0	22.7	2.7	4.2	76.3	56.6	10.4	81.1

Source: U.S. Department of Health and Human Services. Health Care Financing Administration. Office of Research and Demonstrations. Health Care Financing Review, Medicare and Medicaid Statistical Supplement, 1996, p. 412. Primary source: Health Care Financing Administration: Statistical Report on Medical Care: Eligibles, Recipients, Payments and Services, HCFA Form-2082. Notes: These totals for "all eligibility groups" presented (low-income aged, low-income disabled, children in low-income families, adults in low-income families), and the "Other Title XIX" group which is not presented separately. ICF/MR stands for Intermediate Care Facility for Mentally Retarded Persons 1. The total includes users for all types of services reported on the HCFA Form-2082. A person receiving multiple services (e.g., inpatient hospital, physician, and outpatient services) is included once in the user count for each type of service and once in the total. 2. Data shown include services shown separately in earlier years as skilled nursing facility (SNF) and intermediate care facilities, other than for the mentally retarded (ICF-Other). Beginning in fiscal year 1991, the conditions of participation for SNFs and ICF-Other were unified, the distinction between them removed, and the services renamed nursing facility services. It is possible that the combined number of recipients includes some persons who used both types of nursing facility care during the reported fiscal year. This could somewhat inflate the number of users and lower the average payments per recipient.

★ 684 ★

Medicaid

Selected State Characteristics by Region - Part I

State	Medicaid[1] Persons Served 1994	Medicaid Enrollees Per 1,000 Persons With Income Less Than 100% FPL[2]	1995 Federal Medicaid Match Rate[3] (FMAP) (%)	Medical Payments & Administration Per Medicaid User of Services, 1994[4] ($)	Rank of Medicaid Payments Per $ of State Tax Capacity, 1991[5]	Maximum Income for Medicaid: AFDC[6]
MIDWEST						
Minnesota	425,563	710	54.3	5,172	7	15
Wisconsin	473,740	810	59.8	4,257	16	17
Indiana	604,770	770	63.0	4,172	19	46
South Dakota	72,151	610	68.1	3,995	35	30
Nebraska	164,440	910	60.4	3,896	33	35
Missouri	668,765	680	59.9	3,755	30	44
Michigan	1,186,621	890	56.8	3,575	12	10
Kansas	251,742	820	58.9	3,543	28	23
Illinois	1,441,034	740	50.0	3,534	14	33
North Dakota	62,769	750	68.7	3,471	24	31
Ohio	1,523,296	1,060	60.7	3,457	8	40
Iowa	302,535	880	82.6	3,279	26	24
NORTHEAST						
New Hampshire	85,555	740	50.0	10,654	15	12
New York	2,907,963	920	50.0	7,063	1	7
Rhode Island	114,850	1,770	55.5	7,050	2	8
Connecticut	354,473	1,030	50.0	6,794	5	5
New Jersey	789,692	890	50.0	6,074	9	21

[Continued]

★ 684 ★

Selected State Characteristics by Region - Part I
[Continued]

State	Medicaid[1] Persons Served 1994	Medicaid Enrollees Per 1,000 Persons With Income Less Than 100% FPL[2]	1995 Federal Medicaid Match Rate[3] (FMAP) (%)	Medical Payments & Administration Per Medicaid User of Services, 1994[4] ($)	Rank of Medicaid Payments Per $ of State Tax Capacity, 1991[5]	Maximum Income for Medicaid: AFDC[6]
Maine	176,998	980	63.3	5,314	6	9
Pennsylvania	1,255,358	840	54.3	4,680	10	27
Massachusetts	710,490	1,114	50.0	4,353	4	6
Vermont	94,150	1,310	60.8	3,296	13	2
SOUTH						
Louisiana	778,223	680	72.7	5,362	22	49
District of Columbia	127,208	910	50.0	5,214	3	29
South Carolina	486,110	630	70.7	3,896	40	22
Delaware	74,800	700	50.0	3,865	23	41
Maryland	415,101	660	50.0	3,782	11	34
Texas	2,513,959	640	66.5	3,324	17	50
Alabama	543,537	660	70.5	3,199	46	51
Georgia	1,084,929	720	62.2	3,071	21	26
West Virginia	366,638	760	74.6	3,004	36	47
Oklahoma	390,628	610	70.1	2,921	38	19
North Carolina	985,273	730	64.7	2,890	29	14
Arkansas	339,920	770	73.8	2,829	34	48
Virginia	642,347	860	50.0	2,692	32	45
Florida	1,727,034	750	56.3	2,603	27	43
Mississippi	536,916	760	78.6	2,409	39	32
Kentucky	637,558	790	69.6	2,246	25	16
Tennessee	938,711	920	66.5	1,899	20	24
WEST						
Alaska	68,854	930	50.0	4,487	42	1
Hawaii	120,793	780	50.0	3,820	45	3
Nevada	95,411	410	50.0	3,606	48	38
Wyoming	50,544	880	42.9	3,224	50	36
Colorado	289,423	700	70.0	3,026	41	27
Idaho	110,043	540	70.0	2,972	44	42
California	5,007,635	920	50.0	2,902	18	4
Washington	668,363	1,010	52.0	2,776	31	13
Montana	96,206	530	70.8	2,743	43	18
Utah	157,099	810	63.3	2,464	49	10
Arizona	509,663	700	66.4	2,426	-	39

[Continued]

★ 684 ★

Selected State Characteristics by Region - Part I

[Continued]

State	Medicaid[1] Persons Served 1994	Medicaid Enrollees Per 1,000 Persons With Income Less Than 100% FPL[2]	1995 Federal Medicaid Match Rate[3] (FMAP) (%)	Medical Payments & Administration Per Medicaid User of Services, 1994[4] ($)	Rank of Medicaid Payments Per $ of State Tax Capacity, 1991[5]	Maximum Income for Medicaid: AFDC[6]
Oregon	411,311	880	62.4	2,351	37	20
New Mexico	268,204	640	73.3	2,078	47	37

Source: U.S. Department of Health and Human Services. Health Care Financing Administration. Office of Research and Demonstrations. *Health Care Financing Review, Medicare and Medicaid Statistical Supplement, 1996,* pp. 444-446. *Notes:* 1. Fiscal year 1994 Medicaid Recipients, HCFA Form 2082. Includes persons enrolled in Medicaid for whom services are billed by fee-for-service providers. 2. Ratio of the number of Fiscal Year 1992 Medicaid recipients and the number of persons living in families with incomes below 100 percent of the Federal Poverty Level. The figure overstates the percentage of persons living in poverty who are covered by Medicaid because of the eligibility expansions for persons with incomes over 100 percent of the Federal Poverty Level. 3. The Federal Medical Assistance Percentage is determined annually for each State by a formula that compares the State's average per capita income level to the national average. By law, the FMAP cannot be less than 50% nor greater than 83%, with the exception of 100% matching of State expenditures for services provided by Indian Health Service facilities and 90% matching for family planning services. 4. HCFA Form 64, total computable Medical Assistance payments plus total computable State and local administration payments, divided by HCFA Form 2082 reported recipients of billed services, plus two-thirds of the beneficiaries in managed care plans, (to estimate the number of beneficiaries in capitated plans for whom fee-for-service bills would not be filed). The HCFA Form 64 included Federal payments to disproportionate share hospitals (DSH) and mental health facilities. The high total payment in New Hampshire reflects DSH payments for multiple years, but were paid in 1994. 5. Cromwell, J., et al., *Examining The Medicaid Fiscal Crisis: Final Report.* Waltham, MA, October 20, 1994, pp. 8-10. 6. American Association of Retired Persons, *Reforming the Health Care System: State Profiles 1994.* Maximum income for Medicaid AFDC eligibility refers to the January 1994 annualized income limit for a family of 3 to be eligible to receive cash payments under the Aid to Families with Dependent Children program and, therefore, to be eligible for Medicaid coverage. The income amount is expressed as a percentage of the Federal poverty guidelines. Because specified amounts of personal income are disregarded in determining eligibility for AFDC, a family with income exceeding the payment standard in states where the payment standard drives program eligibility may still be eligible for Medicaid. National Governor's Association. "State Coverage of Pregnant Women and Children, January 1994," Maternal and Child Health Update. Washington, DC, 1994.

★ 685 ★

Medicaid

Selected State Characteristics by Region - Part II

State	1994, Number Medicaid Users in Managed Care[1]	1994 Percent Medicaid Users in Managed Care[2]	1992 Percent Population in Poverty[3]	Per Capita Income 1993[4]	Percent Under Age 12 1993[5]	Percent Over Age 65 1993[6]	Percent Rural Population 1992[7]	Percent Minority Population 1993[8]	Heart Disease Deaths per 100,000 Pop. 1991[9]	Violent Crime per 100,000 Pop. 1992[10]
MIDWEST										
Minnesota	116,539	23.1	12.8	21,063	0.2	0.1	0.3	0.1	241	338
Wisconsin	124,280	22.3	10.8	19,811	19.2	13.4	31.9	9.0	289.5	276
Indiana	0	0.0	11.7	19,203	18.5	12.7	28.4	13.0	299.4	508
South Dakota	3,066	4.1	14.8	17,666	21.0	14.7	67.5	9.0	331.2	195
Nebraska	0	0.0	10.3	19,726	19.7	14.2	49.4	7.0	322.4	349
Missouri	37,536	5.4	15.6	19,463	19.0	14.1	31.7	14.0	344.8	740
Michigan	413,176	28.2	13.5	20,453	19.2	12.4	17.3	18.0	294.7	770
Kansas	51,962	18.1	11	20,139	19.6	13.9	45.4	12.0	301.3	511
Illinois	159,433	10.3	15.3	22,582	19.3	12.6	16.0	27.0	309	977
North Dakota	29,100	35.4	11.9	17,488	19.4	14.8	58.5	8.0	285.5	83
Ohio	175,858	10.7	12.4	19,688	18.8	13.3	18.7	17.0	319.9	526
Iowa	46,358	13.9	11.3	18,315	18.5	15.5	56.2	5.0	345.7	278
NORTHEAST										
New Hampshire	8,253	9.1	8.6	22,659	18.9	11.9	38.0	0.0	246.4	126
New York	331,448	10.6	15.3	24,623	18.3	13.1	8.3	30.0	353.1	1,122
Rhode Island	2,077	1.8	12	21,096	17.5	15.5	8.7	10.0	323.4	395
Connecticut	0	0.0	9.4	28,110	17.7	14.1	8.5	16.0	290.6	495
New Jersey	25,842	3.2	10	26,967	17.9	13.6	0.0	26.0	301.1	626
Maine	0	0.0	13.4	18,895	17.9	13.7	60.0	0.0	299.8	131
Pennsylvania	407,409	26.7	11.7	21,351	17.4	15.8	15.2	11.0	363.3	427
Massachusetts	476,615	46.3	10	24,563	17.5	14.0	1.5	11.0	285.4	779
Vermont	0	0.0	10.4	19,467	18.4	12.0	68.3	0.0	258.7	109

[Continued]

★ 685 ★

Selected State Characteristics by Region - Part II
[Continued]

State	1994, Number Medicaid Users in Managed Care[1]	1994 Percent Medicaid Users in Managed Care[2]	1992 Percent Population in Poverty[3]	Per Capita Income 1993[4]	Percent Under Age 12 1993[5]	Percent Over Age 65 1993[6]	Percent Rural Population 1992[7]	Percent Minority Population 1993[8]	Heart Disease Deaths per 100,000 Pop. 1991[9]	Violent Crime per 100,000 Pop. 1992[10]
SOUTH										
Louisiana	26,867	3.4	24.2	16,667	20.8	11.3	25.0	31.0	292.6	985
District of Columbia	42,586	27.3	20.3	29,438	15.3	13.3	0.0	73.0	311.9	2,833
South Carolina	12,340	2.5	18.9	16,923	18.9	11.7	30.2	38.0	267.6	944
Delaware	2,600	3.4	7.6	21,481	18.7	12.4	17.4	25.0	283.2	621
Maryland	312,759	50.1	11.6	24,044	18.8	11.1	7.2	33.0	241.5	1,000
Texas	65,617	2.6	17.8	19,189	21.3	10.2	16.1	40.0	226.7	806
Alabama	36,487	6.4	17.1	17,234	18.4	13.0	32.6	33.0	322.2	872
Georgia	2,548	0.2	17.8	19,278	18.4	10.1	32.3	39.0	249.4	733
West Virginia	85,966	20.3	22.3	16,209	16.3	15.3	58.2	7.0	392.8	212
Oklahoma	0	0.0	18.4	17,020	19.4	13.6	39.9	21.0	340.4	623
North Carolina	196,562	17.6	15.7	18,702	17.9	12.5	33.7	32.0	281.4	681
Arkansas	76,784	19.6	17.4	16,143	18.7	15.0	55.3	20.0	346	577
Virginia	196,710	25.4	9.4	21,634	18.2	11.0	22.5	26.0	250	375
Florida	492,048	23.9	15.3	20,857	17.2	18.6	7.0	31.0	348.2	1,207
Mississippi	31,989	5.7	24.5	14,894	20.5	12.5	69.3	42.0	371.6	412
Kentucky	304,785	36.2	19.7	17,173	18.1	12.7	51.5	14.0	321.6	535
Tennessee	759,923	52.5	17	18,434	18.0	12.8	32.3	29.0	312.8	746
WEST										
Alaska	0	0.0	10	22,846	23.9	4.4	58.2	26.0	82.5	660
Hawaii	4,825	3.9	11	23,354	23.9	11.7	25.3	71.0	180.4	258
Nevada	22,882	20.7	14.4	22,729	19.3	11.1	15.2	20.0	249.8	697
Wyoming	0	0.0	10.3	19,539	20.7	10.9	70.3	6.0	197.8	320
Colorado	135,651	35.7	10.6	21,564	19.6	10.0	18.2	19.0	181.7	579
Idaho	3,086	2.8	15	17,646	20.4	11.8	70.0	10.0	225	281
California	816,048	14.7	15.8	21,821	20.9	10.6	3.3	43.0	222	1,120
Washington	471,993	47.9	11	21,887	19.6	10.9	17.0	12.0	223.1	535
Montana	45,000	35.6	13.7	17,322	19.8	13.4	76.0	10.0	240.5	170
Utah	94,196	42.8	9.3	16,180	25.5	8.9	22.5	7.0	157.2	291
Arizona	351,741	47.2	15.1	18,121	20.4	13.4	15.3	24.0	234.4	671
Oregon	192,348	35.6	11.3	19,443	18.6	13.8	29.9	1.0	246.4	510
New Mexico	106,120	31.3	21	16,297	21.8	11.0	44.0	45.0	199.9	935

Source: U.S. Department of Health and Human Services. Health Care Financing Administration. Office of Research and Demonstrations. *Health Care Financing Review, Medicare and Medicaid Statistical Supplement, 1996,* pp. 444-447. *Notes:* 1. Health Care Financing Administration, Office of Managed Care, June 30, 1994. 2. HCFA Form 2082. 3. U.S. Dept. of Commerce, Bureau of the Census. Current Population Reports, Consumer Income, Series P-60-185, Poverty in the United States. Percentage of total population with incomes below the Federal Poverty Level. 4. U.S. Dept. of Commerce, Economic and Statistics Administration, Bureau of Economic Analysis, Regional Economic Measurement Division. "Per Capita Personal Income by State and Region, 19890-1993" Washington, DC, 1994. Refers to the estimated average income received by state residents from all sources during the calendar year. 5. AARP, based on unpublished data from U.S. Dept. of Commerce, Bureau of the Census, Population Estimates Branch, December 1993. Refers to the projected total population, including Armed Forces stationed in the area, residing in each state as of July 1, 1993. 6. U.S. Dept. of Commerce, Economics and Statistics Administration, Bureau of the Census. *Statistical Abstract of the United States: 1994.* Washington, DC, 1994. 7. AARP calculations based on U.S. Dept. of Agriculture, Economic Research Service, Agriculture and Rural Economy Division. 1990-1992 Population Estimates File, "Population Change and Net Migration, 1990-1992" [Unpublished table] Refers to net population residing in nonmetropolitan areas as of 1992, using metropolitan area definition as of June 1993. 8. AARP calculations based on unpublished data from U.S. Dept. of Commerce, Bureau of the Census. Current Population Surveys March 1992, 1992-3 merged. Refers to noninstitutionalized population who identified racial origin as Black, American indian, or Asian/Pacific Islander or ethnic origin as Hispanic. 9. U.S. Dept. of Commerce, Economics and Statistics Administration, Bureau of the Census. *Statistical Abstract of the United States: 1994.* Washington DC, 1994. Table 129, Death Rates, by Cause—States: 1991. Refers to deaths per 100,000 resident population enumerated as of April 1, 1991. 10. U.S. Dept. of Commerce, Economics and Statistics Administration, Bureau of the Census. *Statistical Abstract of the United States: 1994.* Washington DC, 1994. Table 303, Crime Rates, by State, 1990 to 1992, and by Type, 1992. Offenses known to the police per 100,000 estimated resident population as of July 1. Source: U.S. Federal Bureau of Investigation, Crime in the United States, annual.

Medicaid: Disbursements

★ 686 ★

Annual Medicaid Spending, by Age Group: 1995

[In dollars spent per recipient]

Age	Amount
65 or older	8,704
21-64	1,717
Under 21	955

Source: Welch, William M. "Medicaid: The Bill-Payer of Last Resort." *USA TODAY,* 29 August 1995, p. 4A. Primary source: Kaiser Foundation.

★ 687 ★

Medicaid: Disbursements

Medicaid Recipients and Vendor, Medical Assistance, and Administrative Payments

Fiscal year	Recipients (millions) Total	Vendor payments ($ bil.) Total	Program payments ($ bil.)		Administrative payments ($ bil.)	
			Total	Federal	Total	Federal
1987	23.1	45.0	47.7	26.6	2.4	1.4
1988	22.9	48.7	51.6	29.0	2.6	1.5
1989	23.5	54.5	58.0	32.7	2.9	1.7
1990	25.3	64.9	68.7	38.9	3.5	2.0
1991	28.3	77.0	90.5	50.2	3.9	2.2
1992	31.2	91.5	115.9	66.1	4.3	2.4
1993	33.4	101.7	125.8	73.4	4.9	2.7
1994	35.1	108.0	137.6	78.6	6.2	3.1
1995	36.3	120.1	151.8	85.5	7.7	3.5

Source: Health Care Financing Administration, BDMS, OSM, Division of Program Systems, obtained electronically from http://www.hcfa.gov, March 21, 1997.

★ 688 ★

Medicaid: Disbursements

Medicaid Spending, by Type of Care: 1995

Type of care	Percentage
Long-term care	
Nursing facility	21
Mentally retarded care	7
Home health care	5
Mental health care	2
Other	19
Acute care	
Inpatient hospital	20
Physicians/outpatient	14
Drugs/other	12

Source: Welch, William M. "Medicaid: The Bill-Payer of Last Resort." *USA TODAY,* 29 August 1995, p. 4A. Primary source: Kaiser Foundation.

★ 689 ★

Medicaid: Disbursements

Medicaid Vendor Payments by Age of Recipient

Age	Vendor payments ($ bil.)			Percent of total			Vendor payments per recipient		
	1993	1994	1995	1993	1994	1995	1993	1994	1995
Total	101.7	108.3	120.1	100	100	100	3,042	3,089	3,311
0-5	11.3	11.8	12.2	11	11	10	1,322	1,347	1,404
6-14	5.9	6.6	7.8	6	6	6	996	1,042	1,150
15-20	6.3	6.7	7.4	6	6	6	2,136	2,178	2,297
21-44	28.3	29.6	32.7	28	27	27	3,506	3,543	3,799
45-64	15.0	16.4	19.4	15	15	16	6,373	6,475	6,896
65-74	8.4	8.9	10.1	8	8	8	5,163	5,274	5,767
75-84	12.0	12.6	13.9	12	12	12	8,266	8,534	9,195
85 and over	13.3	14.3	15.8	13	13	13	12,094	12,530	13,406
Unknown	1.3	1.3	0.8	1	1	1	875	764	476

Source: Health Care Financing Administration, BDMS, OSM, Division of Program Systems; obtained electronically from http:// www.hcfa.gov, March 21, 1997.

★ 690 ★

Medicaid: Disbursements

Medicaid Vendor Payments by Sex

Age	Vendor payments ($ bil.)			Percent of total			Vendor payments per recipient		
	1993	1994	1995	1993	1994	1995	1993	1994	1995
Total	101.7	108.3	120.1	100	100	100	3,042	3,089	3,311
Male	36.7	39.6	45.4	36	37	38	3,078	3,143	3,429
Female	63.6	67.2	73.8	62	62	61	3,185	3,249	3,478
Unknown	1.4	1.4	1.0	1	1	1	913	801	520

Source: Health Care Financing Administration, BDMS, OSM, Division of Program Systems; obtained electronically from http:// www.hcfa.gov, March 21, 1997.

Medicaid: Recipients

★ 691 ★

Managed Care Trends: 1991-1996

Year	1991	1992	1993	1994	1995	1996
Managed Care Trends						
Total Medicaid Population	28,280,000	30,926,390	33,430,051	33,634,000	33,373,000*	33,241,147
FFS Population	25,583,603	27,291,874	28,621,100	25,839,750	23,573,000*	19,911,028
Managed Care Population	2,696,397	3,634,516	4,808,951	7,794,250	9,800,000*	13,330,119
% Managed Care Enrollment	9.53	11.75	14.39	23.17	29.37*	40.10

Source: National Summary of Medicaid Managed Care Programs and Enrollment, June 30, 1996, HCFA, BDMS, OSM, Division of Program Systems; obtained electronically from http:// www.hcfa.gov, March 21, 1997. *Note:* * Indicates approximate numbers.

★ 692 ★

Medicaid: Recipients

Medicaid Recipients and Vendor Payments: By Eligibility

Category	Recipients (millions)			Percent of total			Vendor payments ($ bil.)			Percent of total		
	1993	1994	1995	1993	1994	1995	1993	1994	1995	1993	1994	1995
Total	33.4	35.1	36.3	100	100	100	101.7	108.3	120.1	100	100	100
Aged, blind, and disabled	8.9	9.5	10.0	27	27	27	70.2	75.9	85.9	69	70	72
Children under 21	16.3	17.2	17.2	49	49	47	16.5	17.3	18.0	16	16	15
Adults in FDC	7.5	7.6	7.6	22	22	21	13.6	13.6	13.5	13	13	11
Other	0.6	0.6	0.6	2	2	2	1.2	1.2	1.5	1	1	1
Unknown	0.1	0.2	0.9	0	1	2	0.2	0.2	1.2	0	0	1

Source: Health Care Financing Administration, BDMS, OSM, Division of Program Systems; obtained electronically from http:// www.hcfa.gov, March 21, 1997. FDC stands for Families with Dependent Children.

★ 693 ★

Medicaid: Recipients

Medicaid Recipients and Vendor Payments: By Maintenance Status

Category	Recipients (millions)			Percent of total			Vendor payments ($ bil.)			Percent of total		
	1993	1994	1995	1993	1994	1995	1993	1994	1995	1993	1994	1995
Total	33.4	35.1	36.3	100	100	100	101.7	108.3	120.1	100	100	100
Categorically needy	23.8	24.2	24.1	71	69	66	65.3	67.9	74.2	64	63	62
Medically needy	3.8	3.9	4.1	11	11	11	18.9	18.9	21.4	19	17	18
Other	5.7	6.7	7.2	17	19	20	17.3	21.3	23.3	17	20	19
Unknown	0.1	0.2	0.9	0	1	2	0.2	0.2	1.2	0	0	1

Source: Health Care Financing Administration, BDMS, OSM, Division of Program Systems; obtained electronically from http:// www.hcfa.gov, March 21, 1997.

★ 694 ★

Medicaid: Recipients

Medicaid Recipients as Percentage of Population, by Age

Age	Census population (millions)			Medicaid recipients (millions)			As % of population		
	1993	1994	1995	1993	1994	1995	1993	1994	1995
Total	257.9	260.3	262.8	33.4	35.1	36.3	13	13	14
0-5	23.5	23.6	23.6	8.5	8.8	8.7	36	37	37
6-14	33.3	33.7	34.1	5.9	6.4	6.8	18	19	20
15-20	20.8	21.1	21.6	2.9	3.1	3.2	14	15	15
21-44	97.9	97.9	97.7	8.1	8.4	8.6	8	9	9
45-64	49.6	50.9	52.2	2.4	2.5	2.8	5	5	5
65-74	18.7	18.7	18.8	1.6	1.7	1.7	9	9	9
75-84	10.8	10.9	11.1	1.4	1.5	1.5	13	14	14
85 and over	3.4	3.5	3.6	1.1	1.1	1.2	33	32	32
Unknown	NA	NA	NA	1.5	1.6	1.7	NA	NA	NA

Source: Health Care Financing Administration, BDMS, OSM, Division of Program Systems; obtained electronically from http:// www.hcfa.gov, March 21, 1997.

★ 695 ★

Medicaid: Recipients

Medicaid Recipients as Percentage of Population, by Sex

Sex	Medicaid Census Population (millions)			Recipients (millions)			As percentage of Population		
	1993	1994	1995	1993	1994	1995	1993	1994	1995
Total	257.9	260.3	262.8	33.4	35.1	36.3	13	13	14
Male	125.9	127.1	128.3	11.9	12.6	13.2	9	10	10
Female	132.0	133.3	134.4	20.0	20.7	21.2	15	16	16
Unknown	NA	NA	NA	1.5	1.7	1.8	NA	NA	NA

Source: Health Care Financing Administration, BDMS, OSM, Division of Program Systems; U.S. Bureau of the Census, Population Estimates Branch; obtained electronically from http:// www.hcfa.gov, March 21, 1997.

★ 696 ★

Medicaid: Recipients

Medicaid Recipients, by Race

Race	Medicaid Recipients by Race					
	Recipients (millions)			Percent of total		
	1993	1994	1995	1993	1994	1995
Total	33.4	35.1	36.3			
White	15.4	16.0	16.5	46	46	45
Black	8.4	8.7	9.0	25	25	25
American Indian or Alaskan Native	0.3	0.3	0.3	1	1	1
Asian	0.8	0.8	0.8	2	2	2
Hispanic	5.4	5.9	6.3	16	17	17
Unknown	3.2	3.3	3.5	9	9	10

Source: Health Care Financing Administration, BDMS, OSM, Division of Program Systems; obtained electronically from http://www.hcfa.gov, March 21, 1997.

★ 697 ★

Medicaid: Recipients

Medicaid Recipients, by Type of Service

Type of service	Recipients (millions)			% of recipients receiving service		
	1993	1994	1995	1993	1994	1995
Total	33.4	35.1	36.3	100	100	100
General hospital	5.9	5.9	5.6	18	17	15
Mental hospital	0.1	0.1	0.1	0	0	0
Nursing facilities	1.6	1.6	1.7	5	5	5
ICF mentally retarded	0.1	0.2	0.2	0	0	0
Physician services	23.7	24.3	23.8	71	69	66
Dental services	6.2	6.4	6.4	18	18	18
Other practitioner	5.2	5.4	5.5	16	15	15
Outpatient hospital	16.4	16.6	16.7	49	47	46
Clinic services	4.8	5.3	5.3	14	15	15
Lab & X-ray	13.0	13.4	13.1	39	38	36
Home health	1.1	1.3	1.6	3	4	5
Prescribed drugs	23.9	24.5	23.7	71	70	65
Family planning	2.5	2.6	2.5	8	7	7
EPSDT	5.9	6.5	6.6	18	18	18
Rural clinic	1.0	0.9	1.2	3	3	3

[Continued]

★ 697 ★

Medicaid Recipients, by Type of Service
[Continued]

Type of service	Recipients (millions)			% of recipients receiving service		
	1993	1994	1995	1993	1994	1995
Other care	8.1	9.9	11.4	24	28	31
Unknown	0.0	0.0	0.0	0.0	0.0	0.0

Source: Health Care Financing Administration, BDMS, OSM, Division of Program Systems; obtained electronically from http://www.hcfa.gov, March 21, 1997. *Notes:* ICF stands for intermediate care facility. EPSDT stands for Early and Periodic Screening, Diagnosis and Treatment.

★ 698 ★

Medicaid: Recipients

Medicaid Vendor Payments by Type of Service

Type of service	Payments ($ bil.)			Percent of total		
	1993	1994	1995	1993	1994	1995
Total	101.7	108.3	120.1	100	100	100
General hospital	25.7	26.2	26.3	25	24	22
Mental hospital	2.2	2.1	2.5	2	2	2
Nursing facilities	25.4	27.1	29.1	25	25	24
ICF mentally retarded	8.8	8.3	10.4	9	8	9
Physician services	7.0	7.2	7.4	7	7	6
Dental services	1.0	1.0	1.0	1	1	1
Other practitioner	0.9	1.0	1.0	1	1	1
Outpatient hospital	6.2	6.3	6.6	6	6	6
Clinic services	3.5	3.7	4.3	3	3	4
Lab & X-ray	1.1	1.2	1.2	1	1	1
Home health	5.6	7.0	9.4	6	7	8
Prescribed drugs	8.0	8.9	9.8	8	8	8
Family planning	0.5	0.5	0.5	1	0	0
EPSDT	0.9	1.0	1.2	1	1	1
Rural clinic	0.2	0.2	0.2	0	0	0
Other care	4.7	6.5	9.2	5	6	8
Unknown	0.0	0.0	0.1	0	0	0

Source: Health Care Financing Administration, BDMS, OSM, Division of Program Systems; obtained electronically from http://www.hcfa.gov, March 21, 1997. *Note:* EPSDT stands for Early and Periodic Screening, Diagnosis, and Treatment.

Medicare

★ 699 ★

Average Annual Growth Rate in Medicare Payments, by Type of Service: 1991 to 1996

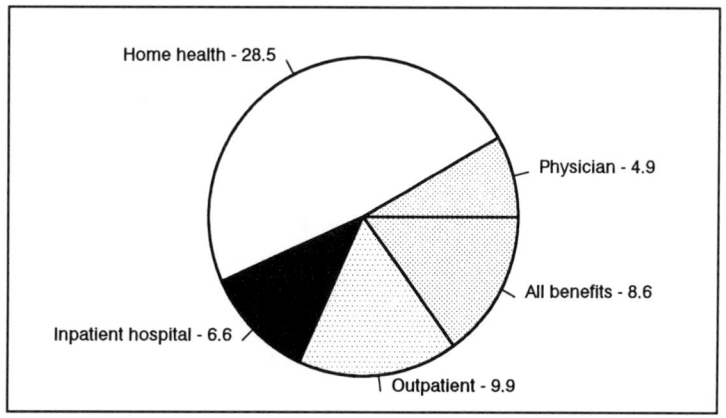

Service	Growth rate
Home health	28.5
Outpatient	9.9
Inpatient hospital	6.6
Physician	4.9
All benefits	8.6

Source: Ryan, Richard A. "Medicare Reform to Cost Seniors." *Detroit News,* 10 July 1997, p. 1A. Primary source: Medicare Chart Book, The Kaiser Medicare Policy Project, June 1997.

★ 700 ★

Medicare

Distribution of Medicare Enrollees, by Age, Gender, Race, and Residence: 1994

Characteristic	Percent
Age	
Under 65 years	12.2
65-74	45.9
75-84	29.2
85 and over	10.1
Gender	
Female	57.3

[Continued]

★ 700 ★

Distribution of Medicare Enrollees, by Age, Gender, Race, and Residence: 1994

[Continued]

Characteristic	Percent
Male	42.7
Race	
White	86.5
Black	8.9
Other	4.6
Residence	
Urban	76.3
Rural	23.7

Source: U.S. Department of Health and Human Services. Health Care Financing Administration. Office of Research and Demonstrations. *Health Care Financing Review, Medicare and Medicaid Statistical Supplement, 1996,* p. 23.

★ 701 ★

Medicare

Distribution of Medicare Physician Allowed Charges

This table shows changes in medical fees allowed by Medicare as a result of the introduction of the Medicare fee schedule (MFS) in January 1992. The objective of MFS is to ensure greater equity in payments between procedure-based services and primary care services.

Type of Service	1990	1994	Percent change
Surgery	27.6	23.5	-15
Anesthesia	3.5	2.6	-26
Diagnostic radiology	8.2	6.1	-26
Medical care	29.2	32.0	10
Consultation	3.0	3.9	30

Source: U.S. Department of Health and Human Services. Health Care Financing Administration. Office of Research and Demonstrations. *Health Care Financing Review, Medicare and Medicaid Statistical Supplement, 1996,* p. 94.

★ 702 ★

Medicare

Growth Rates of Total Health Care and Medicare Expenditures

This table shows the growth of all personal health care expenditures and Medicare, 1967 to 1983 and 1983 to 1994. Medicare growth is due to increasing life expectancy and Medicare coverage of catastrophic medical expenses (among other causes).

Expenditure type	Average annual rate growth (%)	
	1967-1983	1983-1994
Hospital		
Personal health care expenditures	13.9	7.9
Medicare	17.3	7.4
Physician		
Personal health care expenditures	12.4	9.9
Medicare	16.4	9.8

Source: U.S. Department of Health and Human Services. Health Care Financing Administration. Office of Research and Demonstrations. *Health Care Financing Review, Medicare and Medicaid Statistical Supplement, 1996,* p. 35.

★ 703 ★

Medicare

Hospital Insurance and Supplementary Medical Insurance Trust Fund Operations: 1992-1996

Item	Calendar year				1996	
	1992	1993	1994	1995	Q1	Q2
Total Medicare Outlays						
In Millions of Dollars	135,845	152,174	164,862	184,203	47,456	52,009
Hospital Insurance Trust Fund	85,015	94,391	104,545	117,604	31,288	34,526
Supplementary Medical Insurance	50,830	57,783	60,317	66,599	16,168	17,483
Hospital Insurance Trust Fund Operations: (in $ million)						
Income	93,836	98,187	109,570	115,027	26,293	39,365
Outlays	85,015	94,391	104,545	117,604	31,288	34,526
Difference	8,821	3,796	5,025	(2,577)	(4,995)	4,839
Assets at End of Period [1]	124,022	127,818	132,844	130,267	125,272	130,111
Supplementary Medical Insurance Trust Fund Operations: (in $ million)						
Income	57,237	57,679	55,608	60,306	26,596	19,654
Outlays	50,830	57,783	60,317	66,599	16,168	17,483

[Continued]

★ 703 ★

Hospital Insurance and Supplementary Medical Insurance Trust Fund Operations: 1992-1996
[Continued]

Item	Calendar year				1996	
	1992	1993	1994	1995	Q1	Q2
Difference	6,407	(104)	(4,709)	(6,293)	10,428	2,171
Assets at End of Period [1]	24,235	24,131	19,422	13,130	23,558	25,729
Percent change from previous period						
Total Medicare Outlays	11.9	12.0	8.3	11.7	7.0	11.3
Hospital Insurance Trust Fund	17.1	11.0	10.8	12.5	9.3	13.2
Supplementary Medical Insurance	4.0	13.7	4.4	10.4	2.9	7.8
Hospital Insurance Trust Fund Operations						
Income	5.6	4.6	11.6	5.0	4.3	10.7
Outlays	17.1	11.0	10.8	12.5	9.3	13.2
Assets at End of Period	7.7	3.1	3.9	-1.9	-3.2	-3.2
Supplementary Medical Insurance Trust Fund Operations						
Income	11.7	0.8	-3.6	8.5	61.4	14.3
Outlays	4.0	13.7	4.4	10.4	2.9	7.8
Assets at End of Period	35.9	-0.4	-19.5	-32.4	16.7	21.6

Source: Monthly Treasury Statement of Receipts and Outlays of the United States Government. Financial Management Service, U.S. Department of the Treasury. 1996 Annual Reports of the Board of Trustees of the HI and SMI Trust Funds. Office of the Actuary, Health Care Financing Administration. *Notes:* 1. As shown in the Monthly Treasury Statement. Excludes undisbursed balance.

★ 704 ★

Medicare

Medicare and Hospitals, 1994

This table shows percent distribution of providers, discharges, and payments for Medicare short-stay hospital beneficiaries, by type of hospital, in 1994.

Category	Number or billion $	Percent of total hospitals		
		Voluntary[1]	Government	Proprietary
Providers	5,235	58.1	28.7	13.2
Discharges	11,400,000	74.2	15.5	10.3
Payments	$70.4	75.6	14.4	10.0

Source: U.S. Department of Health and Human Services. Health Care Financing Administration. Office of Research and Demonstrations. *Health Care Financing Review, Medicare and Medicaid Statistical Supplement, 1996*, p. 59. *Notes:* 1. Non-profit hospitals operated by churches and other non-profit groups.

★ 705 ★

Medicare

Medicare and Medicaid: As Part of the U.S. Budget

This table shows a major shift in emphasis from defense expenditures to health, welfare, and retirement expenditures between 1955 and 1994.

	1955	1975	1990	1994
Total Budget - in billions	$68.4	$332.3	$1,252.7	$1,460.9
Components in % of total				
Medicare	-	4	8	11
Medicaid	-	2	3	6
AFDC	-	-	-	1
Social Security	6	20	21	22
National Defense	62	28	24	19
Other	25	41	29	27
National Debt	7	7	15	14

Source: U.S. Department of Health and Human Services. Health Care Financing Administration. Office of Research and Demonstrations. *Health Care Financing Review, Medicare and Medicaid Statistical Supplement, 1996,* p. 144. *Note:* AFDC represents "Aid to Families with Dependent Children."

★ 706 ★

Medicare

Medicare Cost Sharing by Beneficiaries, 1994

This table shows that, for instance, the 1.8 percent of Medicare beneficiaries with liabilities of $5,000 or more accounted for 19.6 percent of all costs shared ($24.3 billion). Conversely, 63 percent had liabilities of less than $500 and accounted for 16.6 percent of all costs shared.

Category	Cost sharing liability				
	Less than $500	$500-999	$1000-1999	$2000-4999	$5000 or more
Percent of persons (31.1 million)	63.0	12.6	15.2	7.4	1.8
Percent of cost-sharing liability ($24.3 billion)	16.6	11.4	26.2	26.2	19.6

Source: U.S. Department of Health and Human Services. Health Care Financing Administration. Office of Research and Demonstrations. *Health Care Financing Review, Medicare and Medicaid Statistical Supplement, 1996,* p. 45.

★ 707 ★

Medicare

Medicare: Expenditures on the Most Used Medical Services

The medical services shown are based on the Berenson/Eggers Type of Service Classification System (BETOS). The top 20 BETOS categories, based on allowed charges, accounted for 57 percent ($28.9 billion) of all Medicare physician and supplier allowed charges in 1994. This table shows the top 7 BETOS categories.

Category	Expenditures ($ bil.)
Office Visits-Established	5.50
Hospital Visits-Subsequent	3.52
Eye Procedures-Cataract Removal/Lens Insertion	1.97
Consultations	1.96
Ambulance	1.76
Lab Test, Other (Non-Medicare Fee Schedule)	1.63
Anesthesia	1.30

Source: U.S. Department of Health and Human Services. Health Care Financing Administration. Office of Research and Demonstrations. *Health Care Financing Review, Medicare and Medicaid Statistical Supplement, 1996,* p. 105.

★ 708 ★

Medicare

Medicare Managed Care Contracts and Terminations, 1985-1996

A managed care plan is traditionally an insurance company working in partnership with hospitals, doctors, and other health care professionals to provide a comprehensive, planned, and coordinated program of health care. Medicare managed care plans have the option of contracting with HCFA to provide services to Medicare enrollees and receive monthly payments on a risk or cost basis. Risk plans are called health maintenance organizations (HMOs) and cost plans can be HMOs or health care prepayment plans (HCPPs). Managed care plans can terminate their Medicare contracts. Terminations have disappeared, over time. They are also shown below.

Category	1985	1987	1988	1989	1990	1991	1992	1993	1994	1995	1996
Risk Contracts	87	161	155	131	96	93	96	110	154	183	219
Cost Contracts	87	68	64	58	66	74	77	85	86	87	85
Terminations	3	29	34	38	14	12	8	4	1	0	0

Source: U.S. Department of Health and Human Services. Health Care Financing Administration. Office of Research and Demonstrations. *Health Care Financing Review, Medicare and Medicaid Statistical Supplement, 1996,* p. 125. *Notes:* All data are as of December of the year indicated, except for 1996, which is as of June. Data not available for 1986. Risk plans include health maintenance organizations (HMOs). Cost Plans include HMOs and health care prepayment plans.

★ 709 ★
Medicare

Medicare Managed Care Enrollment, 1985-1996

Category	1985	1986	1987	1988	1989	1990	1991	1992	1993	1994	1995	1996
Enrollees (1,000)												
Risk Plans	441	814	1,013	1,069	1,134	1,264	1,389	1,566	1,815	2,268	3,089	3,636
Cost Plans	731	768	704	671	681	737	750	770	799	765	705	654
Percent of Medicare Population in Managed Care - %	3.5	5.0	5.2	5.1	5.3	5.8	6.0	6.4	7.1	8.1	10.1	11.2

Source: U.S. Department of Health and Human Services. Health Care Financing Administration. Office of Research and Demonstrations. *Health Care Financing Review, Medicare and Medicaid Statistical Supplement, 1996,* p. 127. *Notes:* All data are as of December of the year indicated, except for 1996, which is as of June. Data not available for 1986. Risk plans include health maintenance organizations (HMOs). Cost plans include HMOs and health care prepayment plans.

★ 710 ★
Medicare

Medicare Payments, Aged, By Type of Service: Calendar Years 1987-94

[In millions of 1994 dollars]

Year	Total	Inpatient Hospital	ICF/MR	Nursing Facility	Physician	Outpatient Hospital	Home Health	Prescribed Drugs
1987	104,542	62,316	0	802	31,028	7,812	2,585	0
1988	104,449	61,537	0	1,170	30,711	8,403	2,627	0
1989	110,375	61,507	0	3,735	33,638	8,493	3,003	0
1990	111,030	61,798	0	2,336	33,839	8,744	4,314	0
1991	114,851	63,471	0	2,515	33,822	9,166	5,877	0
1992	117,408	64,132	0	3,417	32,397	9,883	7,579	0
1993	118,479	62,220	0	4,283	32,363	10,214	9,398	0
1994	128,069	65,332	0	5,692	34,114	11,245	11,685	0
Average Annual Rate of Change								
1987-94	2.9	0.7	-	32.3	1.4	5.3	24.1	-
1987-88	-0.1	-1.2	-	45.9	-1.0	7.6	1.6	-
1989-92	2.1	1.4	-	-2.9	-1.2	5.2	36.2	-
1993-94	8.1	5.0	-	32.9	5.4	10.1	24.3	-

Source: U.S. Department of Health and Human Services. Health Care Financing Administration. Office of Research and Demonstrations. *Health Care Financing Review, Medicare and Medicaid Statistical Supplement, 1996,* p. 452. Primary source: Health Care Financing Administration, Bureau of Data Management and Strategy: Data from the Medicare Decision Support System. *Note:* ICF/MR stands for intermediate care facility for the mentally retarded.

★ 711 ★
Medicare

Medicare: Percent Distribution of Allowed Charges, by Place of Service, 1990 and 1994

[Dollars in billions; percent]

Category	1990	1994
Total Charges Allowed - $ bill.	37.4	51.0
Percent distribution - %		
Office Visit	32.6	34.5
Inpatient Hospital	35.3	28.2
Outpatient Hospital	13.2	10.3
Home	3.2	8.6
Ambulatory Surgical Center	3.2	3.2
Independent Laboratory	4.0	4.1
Skilled Nursing Facility	1.3	2.7
Other[1]	7.2	8.4

Source: U.S. Department of Health and Human Services. Health Care Financing Administration. Office of Research and Demonstrations. *Health Care Financing Review, Medicare and Medicaid Statistical Supplement, 1996*, p. 97. *Notes:* 1. Other includes hospital emergency rooms, custodial care facilities, comprehensive inpatient rehabilitation facilities, end stage renal disease treatment facilities, hospice, ambulance, nursing homes, community mental health centers, other medical services, etc.

★ 712 ★
Medicare

Medicare: Percent Distribution of Allowed Charges, by Type of Service, 1990 and 1994

[Dollars in billions; percent]

	1990	1994
Total Charges Allowed - $ bill.	37.4	46.4
Percent distribution - %		
Medical Care	29.2	32.0
Surgery	27.6	23.5
Diagnostic Laboratory	12.8	12.9
Durable Medical Equipment	5.1	7.1
Diagnostic X-ray	8.2	6.1
Other Medical Services	5.1	6.0
Consultation	3.0	3.9
Anesthesia	3.5	2.6
Other[1]	5.5	6.0

Source: U.S. Department of Health and Human Services. Health Care Financing Administration. Office of Research and Demonstrations. *Health Care Financing Review, Medicare and Medicaid Statistical Supplement, 1996*, p. 95. *Notes:* 1. Other includes ambulatory surgery center services, therapeutic radiology, psychological therapy assistance at surgery, monthly capitation dialysis services, etc.

★ 713 ★

Medicare

Medicare: Percent Distribution of Allowed Charges for Physician and Supplier Services, by Type of Specialty, 1994

[Dollars in billions; percent]

Specialty	Value
Total Allowed Charges - $ bil.	51.0
Percent of Total	
Supplier Services	17.8
Internal Medicine	10.5
Ophthalmology	7.6
Cardiology	6.9
Radiology	5.6
Family Practice	4.8
General Surgery	3.9
Orthopedic Surgery	3.8
Other	39.1
Thoracic surgery	1.3
Podiatry	1.7
Gastroenterology	2.2
General Practice	2.3
Clinic/Group Practice	2.6
Anesthesiology	2.4
Urology	3.2
Other	23.4

Source: U.S. Department of Health and Human Services. Health Care Financing Administration. Office of Research and Demonstrations. *Health Care Financing Review, Medicare and Medicaid Statistical Supplement, 1996,* p. 99.

★ 714 ★

Medicare

Medicare: Percent Distribution of Home Health Visits, 1988 and 1994

Visits, by number, do not correspond to visits, by charges, because different kinds of visits have different prices.

[Dollars in billions; percent]

Type of visit	1988		1994	
	Visits	Charges	Visits	Charges
Total - Million visits and $ bil. charges	37.7	$2.3	208.6	$17.2
Percentage distribution - %				
Nursing care	51.1%	56.0%	42.0%	51.1%
Physical therapy	11.5%	12.8%	7.2%	9.0%

[Continued]

★ 714 ★

Medicare: Percent Distribution of Home Health Visits, 1988 and 1994
[Continued]

Type of visit	1988		1994	
	Visits	Charges	Visits	Charges
Home Health Aide	33.8%	26.9%	48.2%	36.2%
Other	3.6%	4.3%	2.6%	2.7%

Source: U.S. Department of Health and Human Services. Health Care Financing Administration. Office of Research and Demonstrations. *Health Care Financing Review, Medicare and Medicaid Statistical Supplement, 1996,* p. 81.

★ 715 ★

Medicare

Medicare: Percent Distribution of Hospital Outpatient Charges, 1985 and 1994

Between 1985 and 1994, charges for hospital outpatient services to Medicare beneficiaries increased by a factor of nearly 5, from $6.5 billion to $36.7 billion. In 1985, nearly one-half of all Medicare hospital outpatient charges were for three services: radiology (22.2%), end stage renal disease (ESRD) (13.2%, primarily for renal dialysis), and laboratory (12.9%). In 1994, radiology (21.0%) and laboratory services (12.8%) accounted for the two largest shares of Medicare charges; however, charges for operating room services (11.5) displaced ESRD (8.1%) as one of the three leading types of service.

[Dollars in billions; percent]

Category	1985	1994
Covered charges - in $ bil.	6.5	36.2
Types of Services - %		
Clinic	3.6	1.7
Emergency Room	4.6	3.3
Laboratory	12.9	12.8
Radiology	22.2	21.0
Pharmacy	4.7	6.3
Physical therapy	3.0	2.0
Operating Room	6.8	11.5
End Stage Renal Disease[1]	13.2	8.1
Other[2]	29.0	33.3

Source: U.S. Department of Health and Human Services. Health Care Financing Administration. Office of Research and Demonstrations. *Health Care Financing Review, Medicare and Medicaid Statistical Supplement, 1996,* p. 113. *Notes:* 1. Services to end stage renal disease patients consists primarily of renal dialysis. 2. Includes charges for medical and surgical supplies, computerized axial tomography, durable medical equipment, blood, ambulance, etc.

★ 716 ★

Medicare

Medicare: Percent Distribution of Supplementary Medical Insurance Disbursements, 1970 and 1994

Supplementary Medical Insurance (also known as Medicare Part B) is a voluntary insurance program that provides insurance benefits for physicians, outpatient hospital services, ambulatory services, and other medical supplies and services to aged and disabled individuals who elect to enroll under the program in accordance with the provisions of title XVII of the Social Security Act. The SMI program is financed by enrollee premium payments and contributions from funds appropriated by the Federal Government.

[Dollars in billions; percent]

	1970	1994
Total Disbursements - $ bil.	$2.0	$58.6
Percentage distribution - %		
Physicians and suppliers	90.6	63.9
Independent laboratories	0.6	3.6
Home health agencies	1.7	0.2
Alternative payment systems	1.3	9.3
Outpatient facilities	5.8	23.0

Source: U.S. Department of Health and Human Services. Health Care Financing Administration. Office of Research and Demonstrations. *Health Care Financing Review, Medicare and Medicaid Statistical Supplement, 1996,* p 91.

★ 717 ★

Medicare

Medicare: Services Used and Charges Allowed per Person

"Services" include physicians visits, diagnostic tests, radiology and pathology services, physical and occupational therapy, etc. Allowed charges are the payments authorized by Medicare for the mix of services used. In 1994, charges per person were $1,656. Of this total, Medicare paid $1,335; the difference ($321) was paid by the patient in cost-sharing.

Demographic characteristic	Number of services per person served	Allowed charges per person served ($)
Sex		
Male	36.2	1,758
Female	36.2	1,586
Age		
65	38.8	1,822
65-74	31.8	1,454
75-84	39.5	1,828

[Continued]

★ 717 ★

Medicare: Services Used and Charges Allowed per Person
[Continued]

Demographic characteristic	Number of services per person served	Allowed charges per person served ($)
85 Years or Over	41.9	1,833
Race		
White	35.7	1,625
Other than White	38.4	1,822
Medicare Status		
Aged	35.4	1,611
Disabled	33.8	1,580
ESRD[1]	165.4	8,032

Source: U.S. Department of Health and Human Services. Health Care Financing Administration. Office of Research and Demonstrations. *Health Care Financing Review, Medicare and Medicaid Statistical Supplement, 1996,* p. 93. *Note:* 1. ESRD represents end stage renal disease.

★ 718 ★
Medicare

Medicare Short-Stay Hospital Receipts by Type, 1983 and 1994

This table shows where Medicare payments to short-stay hospitals went by type of service.

[Dollars in billions; percent]

Category	1983	1994	Change
Total Charges ($ billion)	$54.8	$148.5	$93.7
Type of Services (%)			
Routine care	35.9	23.3	-12.6
Intensive or coronary care	6.8	8.6	1.8
Operating room	6.1	7.0	0.9
Anesthesia	1.0	-	na
Cardiology	-	4.4	na
Pharmacy	11.3	14.6	3.3
Laboratory	11.6	11.3	-0.3
Radiology	4.7	5.6	0.9
Inhalation therapy	5.3	5.2	-0.1

[Continued]

★ 718 ★

Medicare Short-Stay Hospital Receipts by Type, 1983 and 1994

[Continued]

Category	1983	1994	Change
Supplies	7.5	12.8	5.3
Other	9.8	7.3	-2.5

Source: U.S. Department of Health and Human Services. Health Care Financing Administration. Office of Research and Demonstrations. *Health Care Financing Review, Medicare and Medicaid Statistical Supplement, 1996,* p. 63.

★ 719 ★

Medicare

Medicare Skilled Nursing Facility Charges by Type, 1990 and 1994

This table shows where Medicare payments to skilled nursing facilities went by type of service.

[Dollars in billions; percent]

Category	1990	1994	Change
Total Charges ($ billion)	$4.4	$13.1	$8.7
Type of Service (%)			
Accommodations	58.5	47.9	-10.6
Rehabilitation	18.5	29.3	10.8
Pharmacy	10.0	10.6	0.6
Radiology	0.7	0.7	0.0
Laboratory	2.1	1.9	-0.2
Inhalation therapy	2.7	3.9	1.2
Supplies	5.9	4.3	-1.6
Other	1.6	1.4	-0.2

Source: U.S. Department of Health and Human Services. Health Care Financing Administration. Office of Research and Demonstrations. *Health Care Financing Review, Medicare and Medicaid Statistical Supplement, 1996,* p. 67.

★ 720 ★

Medicare

Medicare Skilled Nursing Facility Utilization, 1994

Category	% of total Admissions	Average length of stay per Admissions (days)	Program payments per Admission ($)
Hospital-based	27.0	16.6	4,810
Non-hospital based	67.0	33.0	4,616
Swing-bed hospital[1]	6.0	11.3	1,685

Source: U.S. Department of Health and Human Services. Health Care Financing Administration. Office of Research and Demonstrations. *Health Care Financing Review, Medicare and Medicaid Statistical Supplement, 1996,* p. 71. *Notes:* 1. A swing-bed hospital is a small, rural hospital approved by HCFA to use its beds to furnish either acute-care services or skilled nursing facility services to medicare beneficiaries.

★ 721 ★

Medicare

Percent Distribution of Medicare Enrollees and Program Payments Under Medicare: 1994

Program payments	Percent of Persons Served	Percent of Program Payments
Total - millions and $ billions	37.0	146.5
$25,000 or more	3.9	43.6
$10,000-24,999	7.2	28.9
$5,000-9,999	6.7	12.0
$2,000-4,999	10.3	8.5
$500-1,999	20.6	5.4
$1-499	32.7	1.6
$0	18.6	

Source: U.S. Department of Health and Human Services. Health Care Financing Administration. Office of Research and Demonstrations. *Health Care Financing Review, Medicare and Medicaid Statistical Supplement, 1996,* p. 31.

★ 722 ★

Medicare

Percent Distribution of Medicare Program Payments by Type of Service: 1967 and 1994

[Dollars in billions; percent]

Service	1967	1994
Total - in $ billion	4.2	146.5
Inpatient Hospital	62.7	51.7
Skilled Nursing Care	6.5	4.1
Home Health Agency	1.1	8.6
Physician	28.9	26.3
Outpatient	0.9	9.3

Source: U.S. Department of Health and Human Services. Health Care Financing Administration. Office of Research and Demonstrations. *Health Care Financing Review, Medicare and Medicaid Statistical Supplement, 1996,* p. 29.

★ 723 ★

Medicare

Proposed Premium Hikes for Medicare

The table shows premium changes under the U.S. Senate proposal for "Part B" Medicare, which covers doctors' visits; inpatient and outpatient medical and surgical services and supplies; clinical laboratory services, such as blood tests and urinalyses; physical and speech therapy; diagnostic tests; and durable medical equipment, such as a wheelchair.

Under current law:	1988	2000	2002
Premium cost	$45.80	$48.50	$51.50
Singles income (Couples' income)			
$0-50,000 ($0-75,000)	$45.10	$54.20	$65.10
55,000 (80,000)	58.60	70.50	84.60
60,000 (85,000)	72.10	86.70	104.20
65,000 (90,000)	85.70	103.00	123.70
70,000 (95,000)	99.20	119.20	143.20
75,000 (100,000)	112.70	135.50	162.80
80,000 (105,000)	126.20	151.70	182.30
85,000 (110,000)	139.80	168.00	201.90
90,000 (115,000)	153.30	184.20	221.40
95,000 (120,000)	166.80	200.50	240.90
100,000 (125,000)	198.70	216.70	260.40

Source: Ryan, Richard A. "Medicare Reform to Cost Seniors." *Detroit News,* 10 July 1997, p. 1A. Primary source: Congressional Budget Office.

★ 724 ★

Medicare

Prospective Payment System and Non-PPS Hospitals

Under the Prospective Payment System, hospitals receive fixed reimbursements for diagnosis-related groupings of services. PPS differs from non-PPS, in which reimbursement is based on a "reasonable cost" basis. Certain types of hospitals are defined as non-PPS because the PPS is based on acute care (easier to define) diagnostic models. Non-PPS expenditures have grown very rapidly, suggesting the need for bringing non-PPS medical services into the PPS. Non-PPS hospitals include psychiatric (57%), rehabilitation (15.6%), children's (5.8%), long term (11.8%), and special exclusion status (9.8% - including demonstrations, cancer hospitals, others).

Category	Number of Hospitals	Percent of Hospitals	% of Medicare Payments 1984	% of Medicare Payments 1994
Prospective Payment System (PPS)	6,414	80.6	97.9	89.3
Non-PPS	1,244	19.4	2.1	10.7

Source: U.S. Department of Health and Human Services. Health Care Financing Administration. Office of Research and Demonstrations. *Health Care Financing Review, Medicare and Medicaid Statistical Supplement, 1996,* p. 61. *Note:* PPS represents "Prospective Payment System."

★ 725 ★

Medicare

Three Highest-Cost Medicare User Categories

Medicare program spending is concentrated on a relatively small percentage of enrollees with serious health problems. As a result, certain groups of beneficiaries account for a disproportionate share of Medicare program payments. In 1994, about 11 percent (4.1 million) of all Medicare enrollees had payments of $10,000 or more and accounted for 73 percent ($106.8 billion) of all Medicare payments. This distribution of payments has remained stable during the past two decades. This table shows the per capita payments to the highest categories and their equivalent low-cost categories.

Category	Payments per person
Died during Reporting Year	15,761
Alive during Reporting Year	4,131
End Stage Renal Disease	33,745
Non-ESRD	4,637
Hospitalized during Reporting Year	16,925
Not hospitalized during Reporting Year	1,301

Source: U.S. Department of Health and Human Services. Health Care Financing Administration. Office of Research and Demonstrations. *Health Care Financing Review, Medicare and Medicaid Statistical Supplement, 1996,* p. 33. *Note:* ESRD represents "end-stage renal disease.'

★ 726 ★

Medicare

Total Medicare Expenditures, by Type of Expenditure and Coverage, 1994

Type	Expenditures ($ bill.)	Cost Sharing (%)	Program Payments (%)
Total Expenditures	170.8	14.2	85.8
Hospital Insurance	102.3	7.9	92.1
Supplementary Medical Insurance	68.5	23.6	76.4

Source: U.S. Department of Health and Human Services. Health Care Financing Administration. Office of Research and Demonstrations. *Health Care Financing Review, Medicare and Medicaid Statistical Supplement, 1996,* p. 41.

Chapter 8
MEDICAL PROFESSIONS

This chapter presents information on health professionals, notably employment and compensation data and information on professional preparations and education. Somewhat related information bearing on the medical professional is presented in the next chapter on Medical Practices and Procedures. Data on the places where professionals practice are in Chapter 3 - Health Care Establishment. Information on special topics, including malpractice, assisted suicide, etc. may be found in Chapter 12 - Politics, Opinion, and Law.

Compensation

★ 727 ★

Average Base Salaries of Full-Time Health Field Faculty and Staff in Postsecondary Institutions: 1992-1993

Field of instruction	1992-93											
	All institu-tions	Total public	Total private	Public re-search	Private re-search	Public doc-toral	Private doc-toral	Public compre-hensive	Private compre-hensive	Private liberal	Public 2-year	Other
All fields	$46,833	$46,767	$46,993	$56,443	$63,967	$51,497	$56,011	$43,487	$43,255	$37,623	$39,351	$40,458
Health	55,624	54,097	59,720	73,467	73,080	63,839	66,120	38,311	45,678	42,363	35,790	41,900

Source: U.S. Department of Education. Office of Educational Research and Improvement. National Center for Education Statistics. *Digest of Education Statistics, 1996.* Washington, DC: U.S. Government Printing Office, 1996, p. 241. Primary source: U.S. Department of Education, National Center for Education Statistics, National Study of Postsecondary Faculty (NSOPF), 1992-93. Table prepared September 1996. *Note:* Because of rounding, details may not add to totals.

★ 728 ★

Compensation

Beginning and Average Compensation of Medical Laboratory Specialists, 1994

[In dollars per hour]

Occupation	Beginning	Average
Medical technologist		
Staff	12.08	14.76
Supervisor	14.75	17.97
Manager	17.00	21.00
Cytotechnologist		
Staff	13.74	17.56
Supervisor	16.28	20.56
Histology		
Technician	10.00	12.56
Technologist	11.90	14.93
Supervisor	13.99	17.97
Medical laboratory technician	9.70	11.80
Phlebotomist	6.75	8.00

Source: *Laboratory Medicine*, vol. 26, no. 2 (February 1995), p. 107.

★ 729 ★

Compensation

Medical Technologists: Pay Rates by Workplace Characteristics, 1994

[In dollars per hour]

Occupation	Workplace[1]				Hospital Bed Size			
	Total	Private C/L	Hospitals	Private group	Less than 100	100-299	300-499	More than 500
Medical technologist								
Staff								
Beginning	12.08	12.50	12.18	11.52	11.80	12.00	12.60	12.70
Top	17.00	17.00	17.32	14.63	15.90	17.60	17.90	18.90
Average	14.76	14.69	14.95	13.03	13.70	14.90	16.50	16.00
Supervisor								
Beginning	14.75	15.00	14.80	12.75	13.00	14.00	15.40	16.00
Top	20.00	20.50	20.40	16.40	17.40	20.20	22.40	23.60
Average	17.97	18.00	18.00	15.00	15.70	17.00	19.80	20.00
Manager								
Beginning	17.00	18.00	17.24	14.00	15.00	18.00	20.30	19.30
Top	24.00	24.00	24.49	18.00	20.00	25.00	30.20	27.00
Average	21.00	21.50	21.70	16.00	18.20	22.00	27.50	24.30
Cytotechnologist								
Staff								
Beginning	13.74	14.40	13.72	11.83	13.10	13.50	14.00	13.90
Top	20.00	19.06	20.04	17.16	17.50	19.40	19.20	20.90

[Continued]

★ 729 ★

Medical Technologists: Pay Rates by Workplace Characteristics, 1994

[Continued]

Occupation	Workplace[1]				Hospital Bed Size			
	Total	Private C/L	Hospitals	Private group	Less than 100	100-299	300-499	More than 500
Average	17.56	18.55	17.50	15.59	17.00	16.70	18.10	18.00
Supervisor								
Beginning	16.28	18.38	16.04	13.46	29.90	14.50	17.10	16.40
Top	22.68	25.22	22.68	19.25	32.90	19.50	22.30	24.90
Average	20.56	22.00	20.00	19.25	23.00	18.00	21.00	20.77
Histology								
Technician								
Beginning	10.00	9.68	10.00	10.75	9.70	9.70	10.70	10.10
Top	14.15	13.32	14.15	16.13	13.00	13.80	14.30	15.30
Average	12.56	11.04	12.56	12.70	13.10	11.70	13.50	12.80
Technologist								
Beginning	11.90	12.44	11.90	10.64	11.40	11.80	12.50	11.90
Top	17.09	15.56	17.24	15.43	15.90	16.60	17.10	17.80
Average	14.93	14.99	15.00	13.03	15.90	14.40	15.90	14.90
Supervisor								
Beginning	13.99	15.13	13.95	11.54	10.80	12.60	14.40	14.80
Top	20.29	22.24	20.25	13.00	15.10	18.30	20.30	22.60
Average	17.97	20.49	17.90	13.00	17.50	16.50	18.30	18.80
Medical Laboratory technician								
Beginning	9.70	9.50	9.76	9.00	9.40	9.70	10.20	10.20
Top	13.50	13.07	13.72	11.92	12.50	13.90	14.30	15.20
Average	11.80	11.95	11.89	10.57	11.00	11.80	12.90	13.00
Phlebotomist								
Beginning	6.75	6.50	6.81	6.32	6.00	6.70	7.60	7.40
Top	9.50	9.90	9.51	8.80	8.30	9.50	10.50	10.90
Average	8.00	8.00	8.13	7.30	7.30	7.90	9.60	9.00

Source: *Laboratory Medicine*, vol. 26, no. 2 (February 1995), p. 108. *Notes:* 1. Private C/L indicates private clinic/reference lab. A Private Group is a private doctors' practice group.

★ 730 ★

Compensation

Medical Technologists: Percent Increase or Decrease in Median Beginning Hourly Rates of Pay

	1988-1990	1990-1992	1992-1994
Medical technologist			
Staff	11.3	11.2	2.4
Supervisor	13.5	8.8	6.1
Manager	9.8	5.1	6.2
Cytotechnologist			
Staff	19.1	17.4	3.3
Supervisor	22.1	14.4	3.7

[Continued]

★ 730 ★

Medical Technologists: Percent Increase or Decrease in Median Beginning Hourly Rates of Pay
[Continued]

	1988-1990	1990-1992	1992-1994
Histology			
Technician	7.9	13.3	2.0
Technologist		11	7.2
Supervisor	13.8	10.9	2.9
Medical Laboratory technician	11.1	9.4	4.3
Phlebotomist	5.7	19.9	-7.5

Source: *Laboratory Medicine*, vol. 26, no. 2 (February 1995), p. 107.

★ 731 ★

Compensation

Occupational Compensation: Accountant 2, Health Services

Data show earnings by this occupation. Occupations followed by numerical ratings (2, 3, etc.) indicate grades in the occupation. The higher the number, the higher the skill level required.

[In dollars per week]

Location	Compensation			Survey date
	FQ[1]	Median	TQ[2]	
Health Services				
Anaheim, CA	630	679	714	02/01/96
Baltimore, MD	578	640	706	05/01/95
Bergen-Passaic, NJ	576	611	632	10/01/95
Boston, MA	538	601	645	10/01/95
Davenport-Rock Island-Moline, IA-IL	-	552	-	02/01/95
Gary-Hammond, IN	-	534	-	02/01/95
Lawrence-Haverhill, MA-NH	-	572	-	10/01/94
Memphis, TN-AR-MS	-	556	-	11/01/94
Miami-Hialeah, FL	519	582	615	10/01/94
Minneapolis-St. Paul, MN-WI	539	605	694	02/01/95
Monmouth-Ocean, NJ	587	619	651	09/01/94
New Orleans, LA	454	509	551	01/01/96
Newark, NJ	589	657	692	06/01/95
Oakland, CA	692	732	759	01/01/95
Philadelphia, PA-NJ	538	598	649	11/01/94
Portland, OR	520	569	616	11/09/95
Riverside-San Bernardino, CA	583	611	635	11/01/95
Salt Lake City, UT	534	599	660	08/01/95
San Jose, CA	692	714	758	07/01/94
South Bend-Mishawaka, IN	-	553	-	09/01/94
Health Services, Government				
Boston, MA	479	543	560	10/01/95
Minneapolis-St. Paul, MN-WI	-	727	-	02/01/95

[Continued]

★ 731 ★

Occupational Compensation: Accountant 2, Health Services
[Continued]

Location	Compensation			Survey date
	FQ[1]	Median	TQ[2]	
Health Services, Private				
Anaheim, CA	630	662	696	02/01/96
Augusta, GA-SC	-	531	-	06/01/94
Baltimore, MD	578	640	706	05/01/95
Bergen-Passaic, NJ	576	611	632	10/01/95
Boston, MA	544	608	645	10/01/95
Charlotte-Gastonia-Rock Hill, NC-SC	-	532	-	09/01/94
Gary-Hammond, IN	-	534	-	02/01/95
Lawrence-Haverhill, MA-NH	-	562	-	10/01/94
Memphis, TN-AR-MS	-	543	-	11/01/94
Miami-Hialeah, FL	519	585	615	10/01/94
Minneapolis-St. Paul, MN-WI	522	575	615	02/01/95
Monmouth-Ocean, NJ	577	605	651	09/01/94
New Orleans, LA	-	516	-	01/01/96
Newark, NJ	589	657	692	06/01/95
Oakland, CA	692	738	759	01/01/95
Philadelphia, PA-NJ	538	596	648	11/01/94
Portland, OR	-	579	-	11/09/95
Riverside-San Bernardino, CA	583	617	635	11/01/95
Saginaw-Bay City-Midland, MI	-	579	-	06/01/95
Salt Lake City, UT	549	607	660	08/01/95
San Jose, CA	692	714	758	07/01/94
Scranton-Wilkes Barre, PA	424	480	531	11/01/94
South Bend-Mishawaka, IN	-	553	-	09/01/94
Wilmington, DE-NJ-MD	475	553	654	12/01/94

Source: U.S. Department of Labor. Bureau of Labor Statistics. *Occupational Compensation Survey.* Tables were assembled from data downloaded from http:// stats.bls.gov. *Notes:* 1. FQ stands for First Quartile and means that 25% of the workers surveyed earned less than the dollar amount shown. 2. TQ stands for Third Quartile and means that 75% of workers earned less than the dollar amount shown and 25% earned more than the dollar amount shown.

★ 732 ★
Compensation

Occupational Compensation: Accountant 2, Hospitals

Data show earnings by this occupation. Occupations followed by numerical ratings (2, 3, etc.) indicate grades in the occupation. The higher the number, the higher the skill level required.

[In dollars per week]

Location	Compensation			Survey date
	FQ[1]	Median	TQ[2]	
Hospitals				
Anaheim, CA	-	679	-	02/01/96
Baltimore, MD	566	636	710	05/01/95
Bergen-Passaic, NJ	560	599	623	10/01/95
Boston, MA	532	605	663	10/01/95
Davenport-Rock Island-Moline, IA-IL	-	552	-	02/01/95
Gary-Hammond, IN	-	552	-	02/01/95
Memphis, TN-AR-MS	-	574	-	11/01/94
Miami-Hialeah, FL	557	592	645	10/01/94
Minneapolis-St. Paul, MN-WI	633	668	721	02/01/95
Monmouth-Ocean, NJ	-	608	-	09/01/94
New Orleans, LA	-	527	-	01/01/96
Oakland, CA	730	748	797	01/01/95
Philadelphia, PA-NJ	546	599	649	11/01/94
Portland, OR	514	579	616	11/09/95
Riverside-San Bernardino, CA	583	611	635	11/01/95
San Jose, CA	-	734	-	07/01/94
Scranton-Wilkes Barre, PA	424	480	531	11/01/94
South Bend-Mishawaka, IN	-	544	-	09/01/94
Hospitals, Government				
Boston, MA	-	530	-	10/01/95
Hospitals, Private				
Augusta, GA-SC	-	531	-	06/01/94
Baltimore, MD	566	636	710	05/01/95
Bergen-Passaic, NJ	560	599	623	10/01/95
Boston, MA	558	618	663	10/01/95
Charlotte-Gastonia-Rock Hill, NC-SC	-	512	-	09/01/94
Gary-Hammond, IN	-	552	-	02/01/95
Miami-Hialeah, FL	564	604	654	10/01/94
Monmouth-Ocean, NJ	-	608	-	09/01/94
New Orleans, LA	-	516	-	01/01/96
Oakland, CA	731	757	797	01/01/95
Philadelphia, PA-NJ	541	596	649	11/01/94
Portland, OR	-	614	-	11/09/95
Riverside-San Bernardino, CA	583	617	635	11/01/95
San Jose, CA	-	734	-	07/01/94
Scranton-Wilkes Barre, PA	424	480	531	11/01/94

[Continued]

★ 732 ★

Occupational Compensation: Accountant 2, Hospitals

[Continued]

Location	Compensation			Survey date
	FQ[1]	Median	TQ[2]	
South Bend-Mishawaka, IN	-	544	-	09/01/94
Wilmington, DE-NJ-MD	-	579	-	12/01/94

Source: U.S. Department of Labor. Bureau of Labor Statistics. *Occupational Compensation Survey.* Tables were assembled from data downloaded from http:// stats.bls.gov. *Notes:* 1. FQ stands for First Quartile and means that 25% of the workers surveyed earned less than the dollar amount shown. 2. TQ stands for Third Quartile and means that 75% of workers earned less than the dollar amount shown and 25% earned more than the dollar amount shown.

★ 733 ★

Compensation

Occupational Compensation: Accountant 4, Health Services

Data show earnings by this occupation. Occupations followed by numerical ratings (2, 3, etc.) indicate grades in the occupation. The higher the number, the higher the skill level required.

[In dollars per week]

Location	Compensation			Survey date
	FQ[1]	Median	TQ[2]	
Health Services				
Anaheim, CA	996	1,038	1,058	02/01/96
Baltimore, MD	830	1,034	1,268	05/01/95
Bergen-Passaic, NJ	-	1,018	-	10/01/95
Boston, MA	876	1,020	1,152	10/01/95
Jackson, MS	-	910	-	02/01/95
Miami-Hialeah, FL	938	1,105	1,442	10/01/94
Minneapolis-St. Paul, MN-WI	827	923	1,067	02/01/95
Newark, NJ	1,128	1,208	1,339	06/01/95
Oakland, CA	-	1,118	-	01/01/95
Philadelphia, PA-NJ	907	1,007	1,073	11/01/94
Riverside-San Bernardino, CA	-	1,088	-	11/01/95
Health Services, Government				
Minneapolis-St. Paul, MN-WI	-	936	-	02/01/95
Health Services, Private				
Anaheim, CA	-	1,040	-	02/01/96
Baltimore, MD	866	1,088	1,268	05/01/95
Bergen-Passaic, NJ	-	1,018	-	10/01/95
Boston, MA	885	1,022	1,154	10/01/95
Miami-Hialeah, FL	936	1,155	1,442	10/01/94
Minneapolis-St. Paul, MN-WI	-	907	-	02/01/95
Newark, NJ	1,185	1,232	1,341	06/01/95
Oakland, CA	-	1,118	-	01/01/95

[Continued]

★ 733 ★

Occupational Compensation: Accountant 4, Health Services
[Continued]

Location	Compensation			Survey date
	FQ[1]	Median	TQ[2]	
Philadelphia, PA-NJ	907	1,007	1,073	11/01/94
Riverside-San Bernardino, CA	-	1,102	-	11/01/95

Source: U.S. Department of Labor. Bureau of Labor Statistics. *Occupational Compensation Survey.* Tables were assembled from data downloaded from http:// stats.bls.gov. *Notes:* 1. FQ stands for First Quartile and means that 25% of the workers surveyed earned less than the dollar amount shown. 2. TQ stands for Third Quartile and means that 75% of workers earned less than the dollar amount shown and 25% earned more than the dollar amount shown.

★ 734 ★

Compensation

Occupational Compensation: Accountant 4, Hospitals

Data show earnings by this occupation. Occupations followed by numerical ratings (2, 3, etc.) indicate grades in the occupation. The higher the number, the higher the skill level required.

[In dollars per week]

Location	Compensation			Survey date
	FQ[1]	Median	TQ[2]	
Hospitals				
Anaheim, CA	-	1,045	-	02/01/96
Baltimore, MD	830	987	1,250	05/01/95
Boston, MA	923	1,024	1,140	10/01/95
Jackson, MS	-	910	-	02/01/95
Miami-Hialeah, FL	934	974	1,040	10/01/94
Minneapolis-St. Paul, MN-WI	-	937	-	02/01/95
Oakland, CA	-	1,118	-	01/01/95
Philadelphia, PA-NJ	890	987	1,134	11/01/94
Riverside-San Bernardino, CA	-	1,088	-	11/01/95
Hospitals, Private				
Baltimore, MD	-	1,043	-	05/01/95
Boston, MA	941	1,029	1,140	10/01/95
Miami-Hialeah, FL	-	989	-	10/01/94
Oakland, CA	-	1,118	-	01/01/95
Philadelphia, PA-NJ	890	987	1,134	11/01/94
Riverside-San Bernardino, CA	-	1,102	-	11/01/95

Source: U.S. Department of Labor. Bureau of Labor Statistics. *Occupational Compensation Survey.* Tables were assembled from data downloaded from http:// stats.bls.gov. *Notes:* 1. FQ stands for First Quartile and means that 25% of the workers surveyed earned less than the dollar amount shown. 2. TQ stands for Third Quartile and means that 75% of workers earned less than the dollar amount shown and 25% earned more than the dollar amount shown.

★ 735 ★
Compensation

Occupational Compensation: Accounting Clerk 2, Health Services

Data show earnings by this occupation. Occupations followed by numerical ratings (2, 3, etc.) indicate grades in the occupation. The higher the number, the higher the skill level required.

[In dollars per week]

Location	Compensation			Survey date
	FQ[1]	Median	TQ[2]	
Health Services				
Anaheim, CA	406	451	504	02/01/96
Appleton-Oshkosh-Neenah, WI	326	363	397	05/01/94
Baltimore, MD	340	378	402	05/01/95
Bergen-Passaic, NJ	388	422	443	10/01/95
Billings, MT	-	349	-	09/01/94
Boston, MA	368	411	441	10/01/95
Bradenton, FL	290	325	351	04/01/94
Davenport-Rock Island-Moline, IA-IL	324	347	368	02/01/95
Elkhart-Goshen, IN	-	367	-	11/01/94
Jackson, MS	320	331	350	02/01/95
Lawrence-Haverhill, MA-NH	-	395	-	10/01/94
Memphis, TN-AR-MS	298	324	355	11/01/94
Miami-Hialeah, FL	318	358	400	10/01/94
Minneapolis-St. Paul, MN-WI	380	407	451	02/01/95
Monmouth-Ocean, NJ	351	404	427	09/01/94
New Orleans, LA	308	345	378	01/01/96
Newark, NJ	400	449	480	06/01/95
Oakland, CA	440	500	584	01/01/95
Parkersburg-Marietta, WV-OH	-	356	-	08/01/95
Philadelphia, PA-NJ	385	415	452	11/01/94
Portland, OR	331	388	420	11/09/95
Poughkeepsie, NY	-	386	-	08/01/94
Riverside-San Bernardino, CA	352	396	423	11/01/95
Rochester, NY	297	316	333	11/01/94
Salt Lake City, UT	280	334	378	08/01/95
San Angelo, TX	-	276	-	10/01/94
San Jose, CA	-	373	-	07/01/94
San Luis Obispo County, CA	-	440	-	09/01/94
Scranton-Wilkes Barre, PA	284	373	440	11/01/94
South Bend-Mishawaka, IN	-	322	-	09/01/94
Visalia-Tulare-Porterville, CA	350	387	433	07/01/94
Health Services, Government				
Appleton-Oshkosh-Neenah, WI	-	407	-	05/01/94
Memphis, TN-AR-MS	355	363	382	11/01/94
Minneapolis-St. Paul, MN-WI	-	401	-	02/01/95
New Orleans, LA	318	342	380	01/01/96
Philadelphia, PA-NJ	383	473	540	11/01/94
Visalia-Tulare-Porterville, CA	380	415	498	07/01/94
Health Services, Private				
Anaheim, CA	406	451	504	02/01/96

[Continued]

★ 735 ★

Occupational Compensation: Accounting Clerk 2, Health Services

[Continued]

Location	Compensation			Survey date
	FQ[1]	Median	TQ[2]	
Augusta, GA-SC	-	354	-	06/01/94
Baltimore, MD	340	378	402	05/01/95
Bergen-Passaic, NJ	386	423	443	10/01/95
Billings, MT	-	349	-	09/01/94
Boston, MA	368	412	442	10/01/95
Bradenton, FL	290	325	351	04/01/94
Charlotte-Gastonia-Rock Hill, NC-SC	328	361	388	09/01/94
Davenport-Rock Island-Moline, IA-IL	-	352	-	02/01/95
Elkhart-Goshen, IN	-	367	-	11/01/94
Jackson, MS	320	335	356	02/01/95
Lawrence-Haverhill, MA-NH	-	395	-	10/01/94
Little Rock-North Little Rock, AR	268	305	327	12/01/94
Memphis, TN-AR-MS	296	316	331	11/01/94
Miami-Hialeah, FL	318	358	400	10/01/94
Minneapolis-St. Paul, MN-WI	380	408	455	02/01/95
Monmouth-Ocean, NJ	351	404	427	09/01/94
New Orleans, LA	307	345	376	01/01/96
Newark, NJ	400	449	480	06/01/95
Oakland, CA	440	500	584	01/01/95
Philadelphia, PA-NJ	385	412	435	11/01/94
Portland, OR	324	378	441	11/09/95
Poughkeepsie, NY	-	386	-	08/01/94
Riverside-San Bernardino, CA	352	391	422	11/01/95
Rochester, NY	297	316	333	11/01/94
Salt Lake City, UT	278	334	378	08/01/95
San Angelo, TX	-	276	-	10/01/94
San Jose, CA	-	373	-	07/01/94
Scranton-Wilkes Barre, PA	276	339	336	11/01/94
Wilmington, DE-NJ-MD	306	354	424	12/01/94

Source: U.S. Department of Labor. Bureau of Labor Statistics. *Occupational Compensation Survey.* Tables were assembled from data downloaded from http:// stats.bls.gov. *Notes:* 1. FQ stands for First Quartile and means that 25% of the workers surveyed earned less than the dollar amount shown. 2. TQ stands for Third Quartile and means that 75% of workers earned less than the dollar amount shown and 25% earned more than the dollar amount shown.

★ 736 ★
Compensation

Occupational Compensation: Accounting Clerk 2, Hospitals

Data show earnings by this occupation. Occupations followed by numerical ratings (2, 3, etc.) indicate grades in the occupation. The higher the number, the higher the skill level required.

[In dollars per week]

Location	Compensation			Survey date
	FQ[1]	Median	TQ[2]	
Hospitals				
Anaheim, CA	421	464	506	02/01/96
Appleton-Oshkosh-Neenah, WI	-	407	-	05/01/94
Baltimore, MD	360	391	430	05/01/95
Bergen-Passaic, NJ	393	416	429	10/01/95
Boston, MA	386	415	440	10/01/95
Davenport-Rock Island-Moline, IA-IL	-	346	-	02/01/95
Jackson, MS	318	336	350	02/01/95
Little Rock-North Little Rock, AR	268	320	380	12/01/94
Memphis, TN-AR-MS	322	344	374	11/01/94
Miami-Hialeah, FL	315	353	383	10/01/94
Minneapolis-St. Paul, MN-WI	349	384	416	02/01/95
Monmouth-Ocean, NJ	344	383	406	09/01/94
New Orleans, LA	311	349	380	01/01/96
Philadelphia, PA-NJ	400	427	461	11/01/94
Portland, OR	400	417	420	11/09/95
Riverside-San Bernardino, CA	352	397	418	11/01/95
Rochester, NY	300	315	326	11/01/94
Scranton-Wilkes Barre, PA	288	358	424	11/01/94
Visalia-Tulare-Porterville, CA	-	373	-	07/01/94
Hospitals, Government				
New Orleans, LA	-	353	-	01/01/96
Visalia-Tulare-Porterville, CA	-	378	-	07/01/94
Hospitals, Private				
Augusta, GA-SC	-	352	-	06/01/94
Baltimore, MD	360	391	430	05/01/95
Bergen-Passaic, NJ	-	420	-	10/01/95
Boston, MA	386	417	441	10/01/95
Charlotte-Gastonia-Rock Hill, NC-SC	388	403	416	09/01/94
Jackson, MS	-	346	-	02/01/95
Little Rock-North Little Rock, AR	-	332	-	12/01/94
Memphis, TN-AR-MS	316	331	353	11/01/94
Miami-Hialeah, FL	315	353	383	10/01/94
Monmouth-Ocean, NJ	344	383	406	09/01/94
New Orleans, LA	307	347	384	01/01/96
Philadelphia, PA-NJ	400	424	454	11/01/94
Portland, OR	-	433	-	11/09/95
Riverside-San Bernardino, CA	352	389	418	11/01/95
Rochester, NY	300	315	326	11/01/94

[Continued]

★ 736 ★

Occupational Compensation: Accounting Clerk 2,
Hospitals
[Continued]

Location	Compensation			Survey date
	FQ[1]	Median	TQ[2]	
Scranton-Wilkes Barre, PA	276	326	388	11/01/94
Wilmington, DE-NJ-MD	-	387	-	12/01/94

Source: U.S. Department of Labor. Bureau of Labor Statistics. *Occupational Compensation Survey.* Tables were assembled from data downloaded from http:// stats.bls.gov. *Notes:* 1. FQ stands for First Quartile and means that 25% of the workers surveyed earned less than the dollar amount shown. 2. TQ stands for Third Quartile and means that 75% of workers earned less than the dollar amount shown and 25% earned more than the dollar amount shown.

★ 737 ★

Compensation

Occupational Compensation: Accounting Clerk 4,
Health Services

Data show earnings by this occupation. Occupations followed by numerical ratings (2, 3, etc.) indicate grades in the occupation. The higher the number, the higher the skill level required.

[In dollars per week]

Location	Compensation			Survey date
	FQ[1]	Median	TQ[2]	
Health Services				
Minneapolis-St. Paul, MN-WI	470	534	577	02/01/95
San Jose, CA	-	646	-	07/01/94
Health Services, Private				
Minneapolis-St. Paul, MN-WI	470	516	577	02/01/95
San Jose, CA	-	646	-	07/01/94

Source: U.S. Department of Labor. Bureau of Labor Statistics. *Occupational Compensation Survey.* Tables were assembled from data downloaded from http:// stats.bls.gov. *Notes:* 1. FQ stands for First Quartile and means that 25% of the workers surveyed earned less than the dollar amount shown. 2. TQ stands for Third Quartile and means that 75% of workers earned less than the dollar amount shown and 25% earned more than the dollar amount shown.

★ 738 ★
Compensation

Occupational Compensation: Buyer & Contracting Specialist 2, Health Services

Data show earnings by this occupation. Occupations followed by numerical ratings (2, 3, etc.) indicate grades in the occupation. The higher the number, the higher the skill level required.

[In dollars per week]

Location	Compensation			Survey date
	FQ[1]	Median	TQ[2]	
Health Services				
Anaheim, CA	-	686	-	02/01/96
Baltimore, MD	-	679	-	05/01/95
Bergen-Passaic, NJ	-	703	-	10/01/95
Boston, MA	604	658	693	10/01/95
Miami-Hialeah, FL	557	610	666	10/01/94
Minneapolis-St. Paul, MN-WI	608	657	759	02/01/95
Newark, NJ	-	669	-	06/01/95
Oakland, CA	719	800	876	01/01/95
Philadelphia, PA-NJ	562	612	646	11/01/94
Portland, OR	-	669	-	11/09/95
Riverside-San Bernardino, CA	561	576	602	11/01/95
San Jose, CA	-	642	-	07/01/94
Health Services, Private				
Anaheim, CA	-	686	-	02/01/96
Baltimore, MD	-	695	-	05/01/95
Bergen-Passaic, NJ	-	703	-	10/01/95
Boston, MA	604	659	692	10/01/95
Miami-Hialeah, FL	-	608	-	10/01/94
Minneapolis-St. Paul, MN-WI	581	662	759	02/01/95
Newark, NJ	-	669	-	06/01/95
Philadelphia, PA-NJ	562	612	648	11/01/94
Portland, OR	-	670	-	11/09/95
Riverside-San Bernardino, CA	561	576	602	11/01/95
San Jose, CA	-	642	-	07/01/94
Wilmington, DE-NJ-MD	-	719	-	12/01/94

Source: U.S. Department of Labor. Bureau of Labor Statistics. *Occupational Compensation Survey.* Tables were assembled from data downloaded from http:// stats.bls.gov. *Notes:* 1. FQ stands for First Quartile and means that 25% of the workers surveyed earned less than the dollar amount shown. 2. TQ stands for Third Quartile and means that 75% of workers earned less than the dollar amount shown and 25% earned more than the dollar amount shown.

★ 739 ★

Compensation

Occupational Compensation: Buyer & Contracting Specialist 2, Hospitals

Data show earnings by this occupation. Occupations followed by numerical ratings (2, 3, etc.) indicate grades in the occupation. The higher the number, the higher the skill level required.

[In dollars per week]

Location	Compensation			Survey date
	FQ[1]	Median	TQ[2]	
Hospitals				
Baltimore, MD	-	679	-	05/01/95
Bergen-Passaic, NJ	-	695	-	10/01/95
Boston, MA	577	632	691	10/01/95
Miami-Hialeah, FL	557	610	666	10/01/94
Minneapolis-St. Paul, MN-WI	613	687	759	02/01/95
Oakland, CA	719	800	876	01/01/95
Philadelphia, PA-NJ	562	612	648	11/01/94
Hospitals, Private				
Baltimore, MD	-	695	-	05/01/95
Bergen-Passaic, NJ	-	695	-	10/01/95
Boston, MA	577	630	676	10/01/95
Miami-Hialeah, FL	-	608	-	10/01/94
Philadelphia, PA-NJ	562	612	648	11/01/94
Wilmington, DE-NJ-MD	-	719	-	12/01/94

Source: U.S. Department of Labor. Bureau of Labor Statistics. *Occupational Compensation Survey.* Tables were assembled from data downloaded from http:// stats.bls.gov. *Notes:* 1. FQ stands for First Quartile and means that 25% of the workers surveyed earned less than the dollar amount shown. 2. TQ stands for Third Quartile and means that 75% of workers earned less than the dollar amount shown and 25% earned more than the dollar amount shown.

★ 740 ★

Compensation

Occupational Compensation: Computer Operator 2, Health Services

Data show earnings by this occupation. Occupations followed by numerical ratings (2, 3, etc.) indicate grades in the occupation. The higher the number, the higher the skill level required.

[In dollars per week]

Location	Compensation			Survey date
	FQ[1]	Median	TQ[2]	
Health Services				
Anaheim, CA	387	475	520	02/01/96
Baltimore, MD	418	459	489	05/01/95
Bergen-Passaic, NJ	419	469	487	10/01/95

[Continued]

★ 740 ★

Occupational Compensation: Computer Operator 2, Health Services
[Continued]

Location	Compensation			Survey date
	FQ[1]	Median	TQ[2]	
Boston, MA	437	478	518	10/01/95
Gary-Hammond, IN	403	413	440	02/01/95
Jackson, MS	315	364	380	02/01/95
Memphis, TN-AR-MS	375	419	454	11/01/94
Miami-Hialeah, FL	350	383	404	10/01/94
Minneapolis-St. Paul, MN-WI	408	434	450	02/01/95
Monmouth-Ocean, NJ	365	424	478	09/01/94
New Orleans, LA	404	429	456	01/01/96
Newark, NJ	406	442	461	06/01/95
Oakland, CA	460	544	626	01/01/95
Philadelphia, PA-NJ	437	473	527	11/01/94
Portland, OR	399	452	495	11/09/95
Salt Lake City, UT	-	383	-	08/01/95
Scranton-Wilkes Barre, PA	326	364	394	11/01/94
South Bend-Mishawaka, IN	-	406	-	09/01/94
Health Services, Private				
Anaheim, CA	387	469	508	02/01/96
Baltimore, MD	418	459	489	05/01/95
Bergen-Passaic, NJ	463	473	487	10/01/95
Boston, MA	443	480	521	10/01/95
Gary-Hammond, IN	403	413	440	02/01/95
Memphis, TN-AR-MS	374	410	454	11/01/94
Miami-Hialeah, FL	350	383	404	10/01/94
Minneapolis-St. Paul, MN-WI	408	429	448	02/01/95
Monmouth-Ocean, NJ	365	424	478	09/01/94
New Orleans, LA	404	431	479	01/01/96
Newark, NJ	406	442	461	06/01/95
Oakland, CA	460	544	626	01/01/95
Philadelphia, PA-NJ	437	473	527	11/01/94
Saginaw-Bay City-Midland, MI	-	406	-	06/01/95
Salt Lake City, UT	-	383	-	08/01/95
Scranton-Wilkes Barre, PA	326	364	394	11/01/94
South Bend-Mishawaka, IN	-	406	-	09/01/94

Source: U.S. Department of Labor. Bureau of Labor Statistics. *Occupational Compensation Survey.* Tables were assembled from data downloaded from http:// stats.bls.gov. *Notes:* 1. FQ stands for First Quartile and means that 25% of the workers surveyed earned less than the dollar amount shown. 2. TQ stands for Third Quartile and means that 75% of workers earned less than the dollar amount shown and 25% earned more than the dollar amount shown.

★ 741 ★

Compensation

Occupational Compensation: Computer Operator 2, Hospitals

Data show earnings by this occupation. Occupations followed by numerical ratings (2, 3, etc.) indicate grades in the occupation. The higher the number, the higher the skill level required.

[In dollars per week]

Location	Compensation			Survey date
	FQ[1]	Median	TQ[2]	
Hospitals				
Baltimore, MD	411	458	490	05/01/95
Bergen-Passaic, NJ	-	490	-	10/01/95
Boston, MA	442	479	521	10/01/95
Gary-Hammond, IN	403	413	440	02/01/95
Jackson, MS	315	364	380	02/01/95
Little Rock-North Little Rock, AR	295	331	359	12/01/94
Memphis, TN-AR-MS	375	419	454	11/01/94
Miami-Hialeah, FL	350	383	404	10/01/94
Minneapolis-St. Paul, MN-WI	430	453	468	02/01/95
Monmouth-Ocean, NJ	365	424	478	09/01/94
New Orleans, LA	404	429	456	01/01/96
Oakland, CA	-	613	-	01/01/95
Philadelphia, PA-NJ	437	473	527	11/01/94
Portland, OR	388	447	495	11/09/95
Scranton-Wilkes Barre, PA	330	379	444	11/01/94
Hospitals, Private				
Baltimore, MD	411	458	490	05/01/95
Boston, MA	449	482	526	10/01/95
Gary-Hammond, IN	403	413	440	02/01/95
Memphis, TN-AR-MS	374	410	454	11/01/94
Miami-Hialeah, FL	350	383	404	10/01/94
Monmouth-Ocean, NJ	365	424	478	09/01/94
New Orleans, LA	404	431	479	01/01/96
Oakland, CA	-	613	-	01/01/95
Philadelphia, PA-NJ	437	473	527	11/01/94
Scranton-Wilkes Barre, PA	330	379	444	11/01/94

Source: U.S. Department of Labor. Bureau of Labor Statistics. *Occupational Compensation Survey.* Tables were assembled from data downloaded from http:// stats.bls.gov. *Notes:* 1. FQ stands for First Quartile and means that 25% of the workers surveyed earned less than the dollar amount shown. 2. TQ stands for Third Quartile and means that 75% of workers earned less than the dollar amount shown and 25% earned more than the dollar amount shown.

★ 742 ★

Compensation

Occupational Compensation: Computer Programmer 2, Health Services

Data show earnings by this occupation. Occupations followed by numerical ratings (2, 3, etc.) indicate grades in the occupation. The higher the number, the higher the skill level required.

[In dollars per week]

Location	Compensation			Survey date
	FQ[1]	Median	TQ[2]	
Health Services				
Baltimore, MD	544	603	645	05/01/95
Boston, MA	577	624	673	10/01/95
Philadelphia, PA-NJ	-	597	-	11/01/94
Health Services, Private				
Saginaw-Bay City-Midland, MI	-	609	-	06/01/95
Baltimore, MD	544	603	645	05/01/95
Boston, MA	577	624	673	10/01/95

Source: U.S. Department of Labor. Bureau of Labor Statistics. *Occupational Compensation Survey.* Tables were assembled from data downloaded from http:// stats.bls.gov. *Notes:* 1. FQ stands for First Quartile and means that 25% of the workers surveyed earned less than the dollar amount shown. 2. TQ stands for Third Quartile and means that 75% of workers earned less than the dollar amount shown and 25% earned more than the dollar amount shown.

★ 743 ★

Compensation

Occupational Compensation: Computer Programmer 2, Hospitals

Data show earnings by this occupation. Occupations followed by numerical ratings (2, 3, etc.) indicate grades in the occupation. The higher the number, the higher the skill level required.

[In dollars per week]

Location	Compensation			Survey date
	FQ[1]	Median	TQ[2]	
Hospitals				
Philadelphia, PA-NJ	-	597	-	11/01/94
Hospitals, Private				
Baltimore, MD	544	603	645	05/01/95
Boston, MA	560	613	654	10/01/95

Source: U.S. Department of Labor. Bureau of Labor Statistics. *Occupational Compensation Survey.* Tables were assembled from data downloaded from http:// stats.bls.gov. *Notes:* 1. FQ stands for First Quartile and means that 25% of the workers surveyed earned less than the dollar amount shown. 2. TQ stands for Third Quartile and means that 75% of workers earned less than the dollar amount shown and 25% earned more than the dollar amount shown.

★ 744 ★

Compensation

Occupational Compensation: General Clerk 2, General, Health Services

Data show earnings by this occupation. Occupations followed by numerical ratings (2, 3, etc.) indicate grades in the occupation. The higher the number, the higher the skill level required.

[In dollars per week]

Location	Compensation			Survey date
	FQ[1]	Median	TQ[2]	
Health Services				
Anaheim, CA	313	351	372	02/01/96
Appleton-Oshkosh-Neenah, WI	308	346	373	05/01/94
Boston, MA	309	350	366	10/01/95
Minneapolis-St. Paul, MN-WI	357	387	416	02/01/95
Philadelphia, PA-NJ	320	398	480	11/01/94
Portland, OR	298	326	361	11/09/95
Riverside-San Bernardino, CA	306	335	346	11/01/95
Salt Lake City, UT	283	295	315	08/01/95
San Jose, CA	360	424	511	07/01/94
Scranton-Wilkes Barre, PA	302	366	394	11/01/94
South Bend-Mishawaka, IN	-	270	-	09/01/94
Health Services, Government				
Boston, MA	-	373	-	10/01/95
Minneapolis-St. Paul, MN-WI	380	403	423	02/01/95
Health Services, Private				
Anaheim, CA	313	347	371	02/01/96
Appleton-Oshkosh-Neenah, WI	308	340	363	05/01/94
Boston, MA	307	341	361	10/01/95
Charlotte-Gastonia-Rock Hill, NC-SC	270	298	319	09/01/94
Minneapolis-St. Paul, MN-WI	357	368	416	02/01/95
Philadelphia, PA-NJ	319	399	483	11/01/94
Riverside-San Bernardino, CA	306	335	346	11/01/95
Saginaw-Bay City-Midland, MI	268	330	385	06/01/95
Salt Lake City, UT	302	304	319	08/01/95
San Jose, CA	345	425	511	07/01/94
South Bend-Mishawaka, IN	-	270	-	09/01/94

Source: U.S. Department of Labor. Bureau of Labor Statistics. *Occupational Compensation Survey.* Tables were assembled from data downloaded from http:// stats.bls.gov. *Notes:* 1. FQ stands for First Quartile and means that 25% of the workers surveyed earned less than the dollar amount shown. 2. TQ stands for Third Quartile and means that 75% of workers earned less than the dollar amount shown and 25% earned more than the dollar amount shown.

★ 745 ★

Compensation

Occupational Compensation: General Clerk 2, General, Hospitals

Data show earnings by this occupation. Occupations followed by numerical ratings (2, 3, etc.) indicate grades in the occupation. The higher the number, the higher the skill level required.

[In dollars per week]

Location	Compensation			Survey date
	FQ[1]	Median	TQ[2]	
Hospitals				
Anaheim, CA	313	352	371	02/01/96
Appleton-Oshkosh-Neenah, WI	317	350	373	05/01/94
Boston, MA	307	347	366	10/01/95
Memphis, TN-AR-MS	251	304	343	11/01/94
Philadelphia, PA-NJ	368	424	485	11/01/94
San Jose, CA	360	429	525	07/01/94
Scranton-Wilkes Barre, PA	299	354	380	11/01/94
Hospitals, Private				
Boston, MA	307	341	361	10/01/95
Philadelphia, PA-NJ	375	425	485	11/01/94
San Jose, CA	360	429	525	07/01/94

Source: U.S. Department of Labor. Bureau of Labor Statistics. *Occupational Compensation Survey.* Tables were assembled from data downloaded from http:// stats.bls.gov. *Notes:* 1. FQ stands for First Quartile and means that 25% of the workers surveyed earned less than the dollar amount shown. 2. TQ stands for Third Quartile and means that 75% of workers earned less than the dollar amount shown and 25% earned more than the dollar amount shown.

★ 746 ★

Compensation

Occupational Compensation: General Clerk 4, General, Health Services

Data show earnings by this occupation. Occupations followed by numerical ratings (2, 3, etc.) indicate grades in the occupation. The higher the number, the higher the skill level required.

[In dollars per week]

Location	Compensation			Survey date
	FQ[1]	Median	TQ[2]	
Health Services				
Boston, MA	470	510	570	10/01/95
Minneapolis-St. Paul, MN-WI	457	486	520	02/01/95
Health Services, Government				
Boston, MA	470	463	486	10/01/95
Minneapolis-St. Paul, MN-WI	468	490	520	02/01/95

[Continued]

★ 746 ★

Occupational Compensation: General Clerk 4, General, Health Services
[Continued]

Location	Compensation			Survey date
	FQ[1]	Median	TQ[2]	
Health Services, Private				
Minneapolis-St. Paul, MN-WI	-	450	-	02/01/95

Source: U.S. Department of Labor. Bureau of Labor Statistics. *Occupational Compensation Survey.* Tables were assembled from data downloaded from http:// stats.bls.gov. *Notes:* 1. FQ stands for First Quartile and means that 25% of the workers surveyed earned less than the dollar amount shown. 2. TQ stands for Third Quartile and means that 75% of workers earned less than the dollar amount shown and 25% earned more than the dollar amount shown.

★ 747 ★

Compensation

Occupational Compensation: General Clerk 4, General, Hospitals

Data show earnings by this occupation. Occupations followed by numerical ratings (2, 3, etc.) indicate grades in the occupation. The higher the number, the higher the skill level required.

[In dollars per week]

Location	Compensation			Survey date
	FQ[1]	Median	TQ[2]	
Hospitals				
Boston, MA	470	519	586	10/01/95
Minneapolis-St. Paul, MN-WI	457	486	520	02/01/95
Philadelphia, PA-NJ	-	482	-	11/01/94
Hospitals, Government				
Boston, MA	470	466	498	10/01/95
Hospitals, Private				
Philadelphia, PA-NJ	-	482	-	11/01/94

Source: U.S. Department of Labor. Bureau of Labor Statistics. *Occupational Compensation Survey.* Tables were assembled from data downloaded from http:// stats.bls.gov. *Notes:* 1. FQ stands for First Quartile and means that 25% of the workers surveyed earned less than the dollar amount shown. 2. TQ stands for Third Quartile and means that 75% of workers earned less than the dollar amount shown and 25% earned more than the dollar amount shown.

★ 748 ★

Compensation

Occupational Compensation: Guard 2, Health Services

Data show earnings by this occupation. Occupations followed by numerical ratings (2, 3, etc.) indicate grades in the occupation. The higher the number, the higher the skill level required.

[In dollars per hour]

Location	Compensation			Survey date
	FQ[1]	Median	TQ[2]	
Health Services				
Baltimore, MD	8.77	9.15	9.37	05/01/95
Boston, MA	10.60	12.04	13.75	10/01/95
Miami-Hialeah, FL	7.25	10.08	12.20	10/01/94
Portland, OR	11.19	12.20	13.11	11/09/95
Health Services, Private				
Baltimore, MD	8.77	9.15	9.37	05/01/95
Boston, MA	10.60	12.04	13.75	10/01/95
Miami-Hialeah, FL	7.04	7.78	8.60	10/01/94
Portland, OR	11.68	12.44	13.54	11/09/95

Source: U.S. Department of Labor. Bureau of Labor Statistics. *Occupational Compensation Survey.* Tables were assembled from data downloaded from http:// stats.bls.gov. *Notes:* 1. FQ stands for First Quartile and means that 25% of the workers surveyed earned less than the dollar amount shown. 2. TQ stands for Third Quartile and means that 75% of workers earned less than the dollar amount shown and 25% earned more than the dollar amount shown.

★ 749 ★

Compensation

Occupational Compensation: Guard 2, Hospitals

Data show earnings by this occupation. Occupations followed by numerical ratings (2, 3, etc.) indicate grades in the occupation. The higher the number, the higher the skill level required.

[In dollars per hour]

Location	Compensation			Survey date
	FQ[1]	Median	TQ[2]	
Hospitals				
Baltimore, MD	8.77	9.15	9.37	05/01/95
Boston, MA	10.60	12.04	13.75	10/01/95
Miami-Hialeah, FL	7.25	10.08	12.20	10/01/94
Portland, OR	11.18	12.20	13.17	11/09/95
Hospitals, Private				
Baltimore, MD	8.77	9.15	9.37	05/01/95
Boston, MA	10.60	12.04	13.75	10/01/95

[Continued]

★ 749 ★

Occupational Compensation: Guard 2, Hospitals

[Continued]

Location	Compensation			Survey date
	FQ[1]	Median	TQ[2]	
Miami-Hialeah, FL	7.04	7.78	8.60	10/01/94
Portland, OR	11.35	12.44	13.65	11/09/95

Source: U.S. Department of Labor. Bureau of Labor Statistics. *Occupational Compensation Survey.* Tables were assembled from data downloaded from http:// stats.bls.gov. *Notes:* 1. FQ stands for First Quartile and means that 25% of the workers surveyed earned less than the dollar amount shown. 2. TQ stands for Third Quartile and means that 75% of workers earned less than the dollar amount shown and 25% earned more than the dollar amount shown.

★ 750 ★

Compensation

Occupational Compensation: Janitor, Health Services

Data show earnings by this occupation. Occupations followed by numerical ratings (2, 3, etc.) indicate grades in the occupation. The higher the number, the higher the skill level required.

[In dollars per hour]

Location	Compensation			Survey date
	FQ[1]	Median	TQ[2]	
Health Services				
Anaheim, CA	6.38	7.72	9.14	02/01/96
Appleton-Oshkosh-Neenah, WI	6.63	7.51	7.91	05/01/94
Baltimore, MD	6.60	7.32	8.15	05/01/95
Beaufort County, SC	-	6.08	-	09/01/94
Bergen-Passaic, NJ	7.76	9.14	9.93	10/01/95
Billings, MT	6.07	6.68	7.27	09/01/94
Boston, MA	7.70	8.70	9.80	10/01/95
Bradenton, FL	5.03	5.54	5.93	04/01/94
Butler County, MO	4.65	5.25	5.64	06/01/94
Carroll County, IA	5.54	5.82	6.00	11/01/94
Carroll County, NH	6.02	6.81	7.56	05/01/94
Danbury, CT	7.79	9.05	10.02	02/01/94
Davenport-Rock Island-Moline, IA-IL	5.98	6.74	7.41	02/01/95
Elkhart-Goshen, IN	5.50	6.69	8.39	11/01/94
Gary-Hammond, IN	5.95	7.41	9.02	02/01/95
Jackson, MS	4.80	5.50	6.10	02/01/95
Lawrence-Haverhill, MA-NH	6.75	7.68	8.67	10/01/94
Memphis, TN-AR-MS	5.66	6.52	7.44	11/01/94
Miami-Hialeah, FL	5.75	6.59	7.23	10/01/94
Minneapolis-St. Paul, MN-WI	7.45	9.12	10.46	02/01/95
Monmouth-Ocean, NJ	7.08	7.90	8.97	09/01/94
New Orleans, LA	4.74	5.41	6.10	01/01/96
Newark, NJ	8.03	9.29	10.28	06/01/95
Oakland, CA	8.33	11.42	13.63	01/01/95
Parkersburg-Marietta, WV-OH	5.59	6.46	7.57	08/01/95

[Continued]

★ 750 ★

Occupational Compensation: Janitor, Health Services
[Continued]

Location	Compensation			Survey
	FQ[1]	Median	TQ[2]	date
Philadelphia, PA-NJ	7.07	8.79	10.60	11/01/94
Portland, OR	7.12	8.65	10.13	11/09/95
Poughkeepsie, NY	8.03	8.88	10.03	08/01/94
Riverside-San Bernardino, CA	5.50	7.06	8.36	11/01/95
Rochester, NY	6.46	7.73	8.68	11/01/94
Salt Lake City, UT	5.53	6.18	6.54	08/01/95
San Angelo, TX	4.55	4.81	5.00	10/01/94
San Jose, CA	8.00	10.61	13.31	07/01/94
San Luis Obispo County, CA	5.83	7.84	10.51	09/01/94
Scioto County, OH	5.75	6.90	8.05	O1/01/95
Scranton-Wilkes Barre, PA	6.59	7.70	8.25	11/01/94
South Bend-Mishawaka, IN	5.80	7.00	8.38	09/01/94
St. Cloud, MN	6.60	7.09	7.70	03/01/94
Visalia-Tulare-Porterville, CA	5.50	6.55	7.97	07/01/94
Health Services, Government				
Boston, MA	9.00	9.50	10.06	10/01/95
Memphis, TN-AR-MS	5.70	7.30	8.80	11/01/94
Minneapolis-St. Paul, MN-WI	10.45	11.13	12.23	02/01/95
New Orleans, LA	5.10	5.62	6.20	01/01/96
Philadelphia, PA-NJ	7.95	9.71	11.86	11/01/94
Riverside-San Bernardino, CA	7.60	8.91	9.81	11/01/95
Rochester, NY	8.68	9.77	10.91	11/01/94
Visalia-Tulare-Porterville, CA	6.72	7.62	8.18	07/01/94
Health Services, Private				
Anaheim, CA	6.10	7.42	8.44	02/01/96
Appleton-Oshkosh-Neenah, WI	6.58	7.08	7.66	05/01/94
Augusta, GA-SC	5.25	5.75	6.12	06/01/94
Baltimore, MD	6.50	7.25	8.10	05/01/95
Bergen-Passaic, NJ	7.47	8.85	9.83	10/01/95
Billings, MT	6.07	6.68	7.27	09/01/94
Boise City, ID	6.08	6.93	7.42	11/01/94
Boston, MA	7.50	8.53	9.49	10/01/95
Bradenton, FL	5.03	5.54	5.93	04/01/94
Butler County, MO	4.64	5.24	5.62	06/01/94
Carroll County, NH	6.02	6.81	7.56	05/01/94
Charlotte-Gastonia-Rock Hill, NC-SC	5.55	6.32	6.96	09/01/94
Danbury, CT	7.65	8.47	9.28	02/01/94
Davenport-Rock Island-Moline, IA-IL	6.03	6.82	7.48	02/01/95
Elkhart-Goshen, IN	5.50	6.69	8.39	11/01/94
Gary-Hammond, IN	5.95	7.41	9.02	02/01/95
Jackson, MS	4.80	5.40	6.00	02/01/95
Lawrence-Haverhill, MA-NH	6.75	7.56	8.13	10/01/94
Little Rock-North Little Rock, AR	4.40	4.98	5.25	12/01/94
Memphis, TN-AR-MS	5.66	6.37	7.37	11/01/94
Miami-Hialeah, FL	5.66	6.37	7.13	10/01/94
Middlesex-Somerset-Hunterdon, NJ	7.70	8.54	9.15	03/01/95

[Continued]

★ 750 ★

Occupational Compensation: Janitor, Health Services
[Continued]

Location	Compensation			Survey date
	FQ[1]	Median	TQ[2]	
Minneapolis-St. Paul, MN-WI	7.00	8.33	9.52	02/01/95
Monmouth-Ocean, NJ	7.08	7.90	8.97	09/01/94
New Orleans, LA	4.70	5.38	6.05	01/01/96
Newark, NJ	8.03	9.19	10.12	06/01/95
Oakland, CA	8.24	11.27	13.97	01/01/95
Parkersburg-Marietta, WV-OH	5.59	6.46	7.57	08/01/95
Philadelphia, PA-NJ	7.03	8.77	10.41	11/01/94
Portland, OR	7.00	8.69	10.13	11/09/95
Poughkeepsie, NY	6.42	7.24	8.04	08/01/94
Riverside-San Bernardino, CA	5.25	6.82	7.97	11/01/95
Rochester, NY	6.29	7.45	8.58	11/01/94
Saginaw-Bay City-Midland, MI	6.90	7.62	8.33	06/01/95
Salt Lake City, UT	5.40	6.16	6.84	08/01/95
San Angelo, TX	4.55	4.81	5.00	10/01/94
San Jose, CA	8.00	10.61	13.31	07/01/94
San Luis Obispo County, CA	5.58	6.41	7.26	09/01/94
Scioto County, OH	5.55	5.84	6.05	O1/01/95
Scranton-Wilkes Barre, PA	6.50	7.53	8.25	11/01/94
South Bend-Mishawaka, IN	5.78	7.02	8.38	09/01/94
St. Cloud, MN	6.55	7.05	7.70	03/01/94
Visalia-Tulare-Porterville, CA	4.99	5.52	5.88	07/01/94
Wilmington, DE-NJ-MD	7.46	8.39	9.28	12/01/94

Source: U.S. Department of Labor. Bureau of Labor Statistics. *Occupational Compensation Survey.* Tables were assembled from data downloaded from http:// stats.bls.gov. *Notes:* 1. FQ stands for First Quartile and means that 25% of the workers surveyed earned less than the dollar amount shown. 2. TQ stands for Third Quartile and means that 75% of workers earned less than the dollar amount shown and 25% earned more than the dollar amount shown.

★ 751 ★

Compensation

Occupational Compensation: Janitor, Hospitals

Data show earnings by this occupation. Occupations followed by numerical ratings (2, 3, etc.) indicate grades in the occupation. The higher the number, the higher the skill level required.

[In dollars per hour]

Location	Compensation			Survey date
	FQ[1]	Median	TQ[2]	
Hospitals				
Anaheim, CA	7.37	8.62	9.74	02/01/96
Appleton-Oshkosh-Neenah, WI	6.59	7.47	7.86	05/01/94
Baltimore, MD	6.67	7.53	8.24	05/01/95
Bergen-Passaic, NJ	9.00	10.01	10.50	10/01/95
Boston, MA	7.77	8.77	9.83	10/01/95

[Continued]

★ 751 ★

Occupational Compensation: Janitor, Hospitals
[Continued]

Location	Compensation			Survey date
	FQ[1]	Median	TQ[2]	
Danbury, CT	8.34	9.65	11.54	02/01/94
Davenport-Rock Island-Moline, IA-IL	6.13	6.92	7.51	02/01/95
Gary-Hammond, IN	7.84	8.36	9.25	02/01/95
Jackson, MS	4.86	5.57	6.24	02/01/95
Lawrence-Haverhill, MA-NH	7.10	8.00	8.67	10/01/94
Little Rock-North Little Rock, AR	4.55	5.24	5.75	12/01/94
Memphis, TN-AR-MS	5.70	6.54	7.39	11/01/94
Miami-Hialeah, FL	5.83	6.67	7.54	10/01/94
Minneapolis-St. Paul, MN-WI	9.52	10.42	10.97	02/01/95
Monmouth-Ocean, NJ	7.22	8.14	8.82	09/01/94
New Orleans, LA	5.12	5.78	6.36	01/01/96
Oakland, CA	12.95	12.87	13.97	01/01/95
Parkersburg-Marietta, WV-OH	5.81	6.71	7.75	08/01/95
Philadelphia, PA-NJ	8.64	10.09	11.86	11/01/94
Portland, OR	8.98	9.43	10.17	11/09/95
Riverside-San Bernardino, CA	6.98	8.18	9.35	11/01/95
Rochester, NY	6.50	7.71	8.58	11/01/94
San Jose, CA	11.86	12.30	13.31	07/01/94
Scranton-Wilkes Barre, PA	6.31	7.58	8.59	11/01/94
South Bend-Mishawaka, IN	6.90	7.71	8.38	09/01/94
St. Cloud, MN	7.15	7.74	8.68	03/01/94
Visalia-Tulare-Porterville, CA	6.08	7.16	8.18	07/01/94
Hospitals, Government				
Boston, MA	9.11	9.65	10.25	10/01/95
Minneapolis-St. Paul, MN-WI	10.19	11.09	12.68	02/01/95
Riverside-San Bernardino, CA	7.60	8.91	9.81	11/01/95
Visalia-Tulare-Porterville, CA	6.72	7.62	8.18	07/01/94
Hospitals, Private				
Appleton-Oshkosh-Neenah, WI	6.54	7.06	7.69	05/01/94
Augusta, GA-SC	5.33	5.99	6.57	06/01/94
Baltimore, MD	6.67	7.44	8.10	05/01/95
Boston, MA	7.59	8.62	9.70	10/01/95
Charlotte-Gastonia-Rock Hill, NC-SC	6.19	6.94	7.49	09/01/94
Davenport-Rock Island-Moline, IA-IL	6.26	7.05	7.51	02/01/95
Gary-Hammond, IN	7.84	8.36	9.25	02/01/95
Jackson, MS	4.80	5.46	6.30	02/01/95
Lawrence-Haverhill, MA-NH	6.94	7.76	8.42	10/01/94
Little Rock-North Little Rock, AR	4.46	5.09	5.51	12/01/94
Memphis, TN-AR-MS	5.73	6.55	7.39	11/01/94
Miami-Hialeah, FL	5.74	6.42	7.00	10/01/94
Middlesex-Somerset-Hunterdon, NJ	7.75	8.66	9.24	03/01/95
Minneapolis-St. Paul, MN-WI	9.21	9.66	10.37	02/01/95
Monmouth-Ocean, NJ	7.22	8.14	8.82	09/01/94
New Orleans, LA	5.11	5.79	6.43	01/01/96
Oakland, CA	13.10	12.88	13.97	01/01/95
Parkersburg-Marietta, WV-OH	5.81	6.71	7.75	08/01/95

[Continued]

★ 751 ★

Occupational Compensation: Janitor, Hospitals
[Continued]

Location	Compensation			Survey date
	FQ[1]	Median	TQ[2]	
Philadelphia, PA-NJ	8.68	10.09	11.86	11/01/94
Portland, OR	9.22	9.67	10.29	11/09/95
Riverside-San Bernardino, CA	6.90	7.97	9.05	11/01/95
Rochester, NY	6.43	7.66	8.58	11/01/94
Saginaw-Bay City-Midland, MI	7.44	7.83	8.33	06/01/95
San Jose, CA	11.86	12.30	13.31	07/01/94
Scranton-Wilkes Barre, PA	6.29	7.44	8.45	11/01/94
South Bend-Mishawaka, IN	7.09	7.79	8.43	09/01/94

Source: U.S. Department of Labor. Bureau of Labor Statistics. *Occupational Compensation Survey.* Tables were assembled from data downloaded from http:// stats.bls.gov. *Notes:* 1. FQ stands for First Quartile and means that 25% of the workers surveyed earned less than the dollar amount shown. 2. TQ stands for Third Quartile and means that 75% of workers earned less than the dollar amount shown and 25% earned more than the dollar amount shown.

★ 752 ★

Compensation

Occupational Compensation: Key Entry Operator 2, Health Services

Data show earnings by this occupation. Occupations followed by numerical ratings (2, 3, etc.) indicate grades in the occupation. The higher the number, the higher the skill level required.

[In dollars per week]

Location	Compensation			Survey date
	FQ[1]	Median	TQ[2]	
Health Services				
Anaheim, CA	410	427	443	02/01/96
Boston, MA	378	424	464	10/01/95
Memphis, TN-AR-MS	-	343	-	11/01/94
Miami-Hialeah, FL	369	401	444	10/01/94
Newark, NJ	381	429	480	06/01/95
Oakland, CA	340	436	493	01/01/95
Philadelphia, PA-NJ	360	396	412	11/01/94
Health Services, Government				
Boston, MA	-	419	-	10/01/95
Health Services, Private				
Anaheim, CA	410	427	443	02/01/96
Boston, MA	378	425	465	10/01/95
Memphis, TN-AR-MS	-	348	-	11/01/94
Miami-Hialeah, FL	320	372	420	10/01/94
Newark, NJ	381	429	480	06/01/95

[Continued]

★ 752 ★

Occupational Compensation: Key Entry Operator 2, Health Services
[Continued]

Location	Compensation			Survey date
	FQ[1]	Median	TQ[2]	
Oakland, CA	340	436	493	01/01/95
Philadelphia, PA-NJ	360	385	406	11/01/94

Source: U.S. Department of Labor. Bureau of Labor Statistics. *Occupational Compensation Survey.* Tables were assembled from data downloaded from http:// stats.bls.gov. *Notes:* 1. FQ stands for First Quartile and means that 25% of the workers surveyed earned less than the dollar amount shown. 2. TQ stands for Third Quartile and means that 75% of workers earned less than the dollar amount shown and 25% earned more than the dollar amount shown.

★ 753 ★

Compensation

Occupational Compensation: Key Entry Operator 2, Hospitals

Data show earnings by this occupation. Occupations followed by numerical ratings (2, 3, etc.) indicate grades in the occupation. The higher the number, the higher the skill level required.

[In dollars per week]

Location	Compensation			Survey date
	FQ[1]	Median	TQ[2]	
Hospitals				
Bergen-Passaic, NJ	-	469	-	10/01/95
Boston, MA	386	428	465	10/01/95
Miami-Hialeah, FL	360	399	444	10/01/94
Philadelphia, PA-NJ	396	421	459	11/01/94
Riverside-San Bernardino, CA	-	460	-	11/01/95
Hospitals, Government				
Boston, MA	-	419	-	10/01/95
Hospitals, Private				
Boston, MA	386	430	474	10/01/95
Philadelphia, PA-NJ	396	402	422	11/01/94
Riverside-San Bernardino, CA	-	460	-	11/01/95

Source: U.S. Department of Labor. Bureau of Labor Statistics. *Occupational Compensation Survey.* Tables were assembled from data downloaded from http:// stats.bls.gov. *Notes:* 1. FQ stands for First Quartile and means that 25% of the workers surveyed earned less than the dollar amount shown. 2. TQ stands for Third Quartile and means that 75% of workers earned less than the dollar amount shown and 25% earned more than the dollar amount shown.

★ 754 ★

Compensation

Occupational Compensation: Maintenance Electrician, Health Services

Data show earnings by this occupation. Occupations followed by numerical ratings (2, 3, etc.) indicate grades in the occupation. The higher the number, the higher the skill level required.

[In dollars per hour]

Location	Compensation			Survey date
	FQ[1]	Median	TQ[2]	
Health Services				
Anaheim, CA	-	18.67	-	02/01/96
Baltimore, MD	13.50	14.53	15.65	05/01/95
Bergen-Passaic, NJ	17.72	18.05	18.26	10/01/95
Boston, MA	16.69	17.75	18.73	10/01/95
Gary-Hammond, IN	-	16.45	-	02/01/95
Memphis, TN-AR-MS	12.57	13.96	14.29	11/01/94
Miami-Hialeah, FL	13.50	15.02	16.86	10/01/94
Minneapolis-St. Paul, MN-WI	17.31	20.89	22.24	02/01/95
Monmouth-Ocean, NJ	13.82	14.79	15.74	09/01/94
New Orleans, LA	12.51	13.40	14.36	01/01/96
Newark, NJ	14.37	16.09	17.01	06/01/95
Philadelphia, PA-NJ	14.78	15.77	17.10	11/01/94
Portland, OR	-	16.23	-	11/09/95
Poughkeepsie, NY	-	14.67	-	08/01/94
Riverside-San Bernardino, CA	-	17.27	-	11/01/95
Salt Lake City, UT	-	14.79	-	08/01/95
San Jose, CA	-	21.30	-	07/01/94
Scranton-Wilkes Barre, PA	12.85	13.57	15.28	11/01/94
Health Services, Government				
Boston, MA	13.90	14.69	15.83	10/01/95
Philadelphia, PA-NJ	11.86	14.28	16.30	11/01/94
Health Services, Private				
Baltimore, MD	14.25	15.43	15.72	05/01/95
Bergen-Passaic, NJ	17.84	18.10	18.28	10/01/95
Boston, MA	17.43	18.39	19.20	10/01/95
Gary-Hammond, IN	-	16.45	-	02/01/95
Memphis, TN-AR-MS	-	14.19	-	11/01/94
Miami-Hialeah, FL	12.04	13.44	14.22	10/01/94
New Orleans, LA	12.79	13.58	14.25	01/01/96
Newark, NJ	14.37	16.22	17.40	06/01/95
Philadelphia, PA-NJ	14.83	16.03	17.20	11/01/94
Riverside-San Bernardino, CA	-	16.57	-	11/01/95
Scranton-Wilkes Barre, PA	-	13.80	-	11/01/94

Source: U.S. Department of Labor. Bureau of Labor Statistics. *Occupational Compensation Survey.* Tables were assembled from data downloaded from http:// stats.bls.gov. *Notes:* 1. FQ stands for First Quartile and means that 25% of the workers surveyed earned less than the dollar amount shown. 2. TQ stands for Third Quartile and means that 75% of workers earned less than the dollar amount shown and 25% earned more than the dollar amount shown.

★ 755 ★
Compensation

Occupational Compensation: Maintenance Electrician, Hospitals

Data show earnings by this occupation. Occupations followed by numerical ratings (2, 3, etc.) indicate grades in the occupation. The higher the number, the higher the skill level required.

[In dollars per hour]

Location	Compensation			Survey date
	FQ[1]	Median	TQ[2]	
Hospitals				
Anaheim, CA	-	18.56	-	02/01/96
Baltimore, MD	13.50	14.21	15.45	05/01/95
Bergen-Passaic, NJ	17.72	18.05	18.26	10/01/95
Boston, MA	16.99	18.07	18.89	10/01/95
Gary-Hammond, IN	-	16.45	-	02/01/95
Memphis, TN-AR-MS	12.57	13.96	14.29	11/01/94
Miami-Hialeah, FL	13.50	15.02	16.86	10/01/94
Minneapolis-St. Paul, MN-WI	17.31	20.89	22.24	02/01/95
New Orleans, LA	12.51	13.40	14.36	01/01/96
Philadelphia, PA-NJ	14.78	15.78	17.10	11/01/94
Portland, OR	-	16.23	-	11/09/95
Riverside-San Bernardino, CA	-	17.27	-	11/01/95
Scranton-Wilkes Barre, PA	-	14.04	-	11/01/94
Hospitals, Government				
Boston, MA	-	15.47	-	10/01/95
Philadelphia, PA-NJ	10.89	14.23	16.60	11/01/94
Hospitals, Private				
Baltimore, MD	14.25	15.06	15.66	05/01/95
Bergen-Passaic, NJ	17.84	18.10	18.28	10/01/95
Boston, MA	17.43	18.35	19.19	10/01/95
Gary-Hammond, IN	-	16.45	-	02/01/95
Memphis, TN-AR-MS	-	14.19	-	11/01/94
Miami-Hialeah, FL	12.04	13.44	14.22	10/01/94
New Orleans, LA	12.79	13.58	14.25	01/01/96
Philadelphia, PA-NJ	14.83	16.03	17.20	11/01/94
Riverside-San Bernardino, CA	-	16.57	-	11/01/95
Scranton-Wilkes Barre, PA	-	13.80	-	11/01/94

Source: U.S. Department of Labor. Bureau of Labor Statistics. *Occupational Compensation Survey.* Tables were assembled from data downloaded from http:// stats.bls.gov. *Notes:* 1. FQ stands for First Quartile and means that 25% of the workers surveyed earned less than the dollar amount shown. 2. TQ stands for Third Quartile and means that 75% of workers earned less than the dollar amount shown and 25% earned more than the dollar amount shown.

★ 756 ★
Compensation

Occupational Compensation: Maintenance Electronics Technician 2, Health Services

Data show earnings by this occupation. Occupations followed by numerical ratings (2, 3, etc.) indicate grades in the occupation. The higher the number, the higher the skill level required.

[In dollars per hour]

Location	Compensation			Survey date
	FQ[1]	Median	TQ[2]	
Health Services				
Anaheim, CA	16.19	18.01	20.16	02/01/96
Appleton-Oshkosh-Neenah, WI	13.51	16.01	18.63	05/01/94
Baltimore, MD	14.20	14.93	15.69	05/01/95
Boston, MA	14.70	16.85	18.99	10/01/95
Gary-Hammond, IN	13.32	15.24	16.50	02/01/95
Jackson, MS	-	12.51	-	02/01/95
Memphis, TN-AR-MS	11.83	13.43	14.95	11/01/94
Miami-Hialeah, FL	13.01	14.67	16.13	10/01/94
Minneapolis-St. Paul, MN-WI	15.63	16.99	19.01	02/01/95
Newark, NJ	-	18.10	-	06/01/95
Philadelphia, PA-NJ	14.39	16.23	18.47	11/01/94
Portland, OR	-	16.89	-	11/09/95
Riverside-San Bernardino, CA	15.92	17.39	18.44	11/01/95
Salt Lake City, UT	-	14.43	-	08/01/95
San Jose, CA	-	21.65	-	07/01/94
South Bend-Mishawaka, IN	15.35	16.11	16.92	09/01/94
Health Services, Private				
Anaheim, CA	16.76	18.76	20.16	02/01/96
Appleton-Oshkosh-Neenah, WI	13.51	16.14	18.63	05/01/94
Baltimore, MD	14.20	14.93	15.69	05/01/95
Boston, MA	14.70	16.85	18.99	10/01/95
Charlotte-Gastonia-Rock Hill, NC-SC	-	15.03	-	09/01/94
Gary-Hammond, IN	13.32	15.24	16.50	02/01/95
Jackson, MS	-	12.62	-	02/01/95
Miami-Hialeah, FL	12.55	13.27	14.29	10/01/94
Newark, NJ	-	18.21	-	06/01/95
Philadelphia, PA-NJ	14.39	16.23	18.47	11/01/94
Portland, OR	-	16.89	-	11/09/95
Riverside-San Bernardino, CA	17.10	17.48	18.45	11/01/95
Saginaw-Bay City-Midland, MI	-	13.95	-	06/01/95
San Jose, CA	-	21.65	-	07/01/94
South Bend-Mishawaka, IN	15.35	16.11	16.92	09/01/94
Wilmington, DE-NJ-MD	13.98	15.88	17.77	12/01/94

Source: U.S. Department of Labor. Bureau of Labor Statistics. *Occupational Compensation Survey.* Tables were assembled from data downloaded from http:// stats.bls.gov. *Notes:* 1. FQ stands for First Quartile and means that 25% of the workers surveyed earned less than the dollar amount shown. 2. TQ stands for Third Quartile and means that 75% of workers earned less than the dollar amount shown and 25% earned more than the dollar amount shown.

★ 757 ★
Compensation

Occupational Compensation: Maintenance Electronics Technician 2, Hospitals

Data show earnings by this occupation. Occupations followed by numerical ratings (2, 3, etc.) indicate grades in the occupation. The higher the number, the higher the skill level required.

[In dollars per hour]

Location	Compensation			Survey date
	FQ[1]	Median	TQ[2]	
Hospitals				
Anaheim, CA	16.51	18.12	20.16	02/01/96
Appleton-Oshkosh-Neenah, WI	13.51	16.01	18.63	05/01/94
Baltimore, MD	14.20	14.93	15.69	05/01/95
Boston, MA	14.70	16.85	18.99	10/01/95
Gary-Hammond, IN	13.32	15.24	16.50	02/01/95
Jackson, MS	-	12.51	-	02/01/95
Memphis, TN-AR-MS	11.83	13.43	14.95	11/01/94
Miami-Hialeah, FL	13.01	14.67	16.13	10/01/94
Minneapolis-St. Paul, MN-WI	15.63	16.99	19.01	02/01/95
Philadelphia, PA-NJ	14.39	16.23	18.47	11/01/94
Portland, OR	-	18.61	-	11/09/95
Riverside-San Bernardino, CA	15.92	17.39	18.44	11/01/95
San Jose, CA	-	21.65	-	07/01/94
Hospitals, Private				
Appleton-Oshkosh-Neenah, WI	13.51	16.14	18.63	05/01/94
Baltimore, MD	14.20	14.93	15.69	05/01/95
Boston, MA	14.70	16.85	18.99	10/01/95
Charlotte-Gastonia-Rock Hill, NC-SC	-	15.03	-	09/01/94
Gary-Hammond, IN	13.32	15.24	16.50	02/01/95
Jackson, MS	-	12.62	-	02/01/95
Miami-Hialeah, FL	12.55	13.27	14.29	10/01/94
Philadelphia, PA-NJ	14.39	16.23	18.47	11/01/94
Portland, OR	-	18.61	-	11/09/95
Riverside-San Bernardino, CA	17.10	17.48	18.45	11/01/95
Saginaw-Bay City-Midland, MI	-	13.95	-	06/01/95
San Jose, CA	-	21.65	-	07/01/94
Wilmington, DE-NJ-MD	13.98	15.88	17.77	12/01/94

Source: U.S. Department of Labor. Bureau of Labor Statistics. *Occupational Compensation Survey.* Tables were assembled from data downloaded from http:// stats.bls.gov. *Notes:* 1. FQ stands for First Quartile and means that 25% of the workers surveyed earned less than the dollar amount shown. 2. TQ stands for Third Quartile and means that 75% of workers earned less than the dollar amount shown and 25% earned more than the dollar amount shown.

★ 758 ★
Compensation

Occupational Compensation: Maintenance Worker, General, Health Services

Data show earnings by this occupation. Occupations followed by numerical ratings (2, 3, etc.) indicate grades in the occupation. The higher the number, the higher the skill level required.

[In dollars per hour]

Location	Compensation			Survey date
	FQ[1]	Median	TQ[2]	
Health Services				
Anaheim, CA	8.84	11.36	13.83	02/01/96
Appleton-Oshkosh-Neenah, WI	8.18	9.33	10.18	05/01/94
Baltimore, MD	8.65	9.87	11.33	05/01/95
Beaufort County, SC	-	8.94	-	09/01/94
Bergen-Passaic, NJ	9.61	12.01	14.09	10/01/95
Boston, MA	10.30	11.68	13.08	10/01/95
Bradenton, FL	7.25	8.67	9.36	04/01/94
Butler County, MO	-	8.96	-	06/01/94
Danbury, CT	-	9.84	-	02/01/94
Davenport-Rock Island-Moline, IA-IL	7.25	8.83	10.69	02/01/95
Gary-Hammond, IN	7.09	8.42	9.50	02/01/95
Jackson, MS	7.98	8.49	9.22	02/01/95
Lawrence-Haverhill, MA-NH	9.45	10.89	12.50	10/01/94
Memphis, TN-AR-MS	7.82	8.93	9.93	11/01/94
Miami-Hialeah, FL	7.04	9.07	10.35	10/01/94
Minneapolis-St. Paul, MN-WI	8.65	9.71	10.82	02/01/95
Monmouth-Ocean, NJ	9.88	11.57	12.84	09/01/94
New Orleans, LA	8.37	10.08	12.30	01/01/96
Newark, NJ	9.91	12.17	13.32	06/01/95
Oakland, CA	7.95	10.44	12.60	01/01/95
Philadelphia, PA-NJ	9.95	11.22	12.55	11/01/94
Portland, OR	6.02	8.29	10.06	11/09/95
Poughkeepsie, NY	10.66	11.73	12.95	08/01/94
Riverside-San Bernardino, CA	9.50	11.53	13.84	11/01/95
Rochester, NY	8.95	10.09	11.44	11/01/94
Salt Lake City, UT	7.50	10.50	13.61	08/01/95
San Angelo, TX	-	7.54	-	10/01/94
San Jose, CA	8.45	10.10	12.00	07/01/94
San Luis Obispo County, CA	9.88	11.92	14.71	09/01/94
Scioto County, OH	-	9.35	-	O1/01/95
Scranton-Wilkes Barre, PA	8.25	8.94	9.54	11/01/94
South Bend-Mishawaka, IN	7.53	8.18	8.73	09/01/94
St. Cloud, MN	10.59	10.80	11.25	03/01/94
Visalia-Tulare-Porterville, CA	8.87	10.28	12.06	07/01/94
Health Services, Government				
Boston, MA	11.50	11.37	11.50	10/01/95
Memphis, TN-AR-MS	7.51	8.83	9.75	11/01/94
Minneapolis-St. Paul, MN-WI	-	13.39	-	02/01/95
Riverside-San Bernardino, CA	-	14.44	-	11/01/95
Rochester, NY	11.44	12.23	13.23	11/01/94

[Continued]

★ 758 ★

Occupational Compensation: Maintenance Worker, General, Health Services
[Continued]

Location	Compensation			Survey date
	FQ[1]	Median	TQ[2]	
Visalia-Tulare-Porterville, CA	9.60	11.38	12.12	07/01/94
Health Services, Private				
Anaheim, CA	8.84	11.17	13.35	02/01/96
Appleton-Oshkosh-Neenah, WI	8.00	8.95	9.82	05/01/94
Augusta, GA-SC	8.96	9.82	11.00	06/01/94
Baltimore, MD	8.65	9.87	11.33	05/01/95
Bergen-Passaic, NJ	9.61	12.01	14.09	10/01/95
Boise City, ID	-	9.26	-	11/01/94
Boston, MA	10.00	11.73	13.67	10/01/95
Bradenton, FL	7.25	8.67	9.36	04/01/94
Butler County, MO	-	8.96	-	06/01/94
Charlotte-Gastonia-Rock Hill, NC-SC	8.42	9.28	10.01	09/01/94
Danbury, CT	-	9.84	-	02/01/94
Davenport-Rock Island-Moline, IA-IL	7.20	8.67	10.09	02/01/95
Gary-Hammond, IN	7.09	8.42	9.50	02/01/95
Jackson, MS	8.40	8.62	9.24	02/01/95
Lawrence-Haverhill, MA-NH	9.35	10.77	11.52	10/01/94
Memphis, TN-AR-MS	7.82	8.97	10.48	11/01/94
Miami-Hialeah, FL	7.00	9.02	10.22	10/01/94
Middlesex-Somerset-Hunterdon, NJ	9.00	10.74	12.70	03/01/95
Minneapolis-St. Paul, MN-WI	8.65	9.42	10.45	02/01/95
Monmouth-Ocean, NJ	9.88	11.57	12.84	09/01/94
New Orleans, LA	8.35	10.15	12.41	01/01/96
Newark, NJ	9.46	12.12	15.07	06/01/95
Oakland, CA	7.95	10.44	12.60	01/01/95
Philadelphia, PA-NJ	9.95	11.20	12.55	11/01/94
Portland, OR	5.35	7.31	8.84	11/09/95
Poughkeepsie, NY	10.66	11.69	13.15	08/01/94
Riverside-San Bernardino, CA	9.50	11.20	13.25	11/01/95
Rochester, NY	8.48	9.14	9.55	11/01/94
Salt Lake City, UT	7.50	10.50	13.61	08/01/95
San Angelo, TX	-	7.54	-	10/01/94
San Jose, CA	8.45	10.10	12.00	07/01/94
San Luis Obispo County, CA	-	10.80	-	09/01/94
Scranton-Wilkes Barre, PA	8.25	8.94	9.54	11/01/94
South Bend-Mishawaka, IN	7.40	8.20	8.85	09/01/94
St. Cloud, MN	-	10.35	-	03/01/94
Visalia-Tulare-Porterville, CA	-	7.82	-	07/01/94
Wilmington, DE-NJ-MD	10.13	10.53	11.55	12/01/94

Source: U.S. Department of Labor. Bureau of Labor Statistics. *Occupational Compensation Survey.* Tables were assembled from data downloaded from http:// stats.bls.gov. *Notes:* 1. FQ stands for First Quartile and means that 25% of the workers surveyed earned less than the dollar amount shown. 2. TQ stands for Third Quartile and means that 75% of workers earned less than the dollar amount shown and 25% earned more than the dollar amount shown.

★ 759 ★
Compensation

Occupational Compensation: Maintenance Worker, General, Hospitals

Data show earnings by this occupation. Occupations followed by numerical ratings (2, 3, etc.) indicate grades in the occupation. The higher the number, the higher the skill level required.

[In dollars per hour]

Location	Compensation			Survey date
	FQ[1]	Median	TQ[2]	
Hospitals				
Anaheim, CA	12.25	13.45	15.00	02/01/96
Appleton-Oshkosh-Neenah, WI	-	10.09	-	05/01/94
Baltimore, MD	9.59	10.84	11.77	05/01/95
Bergen-Passaic, NJ	11.84	13.94	16.12	10/01/95
Boston, MA	11.13	12.38	13.98	10/01/95
Davenport-Rock Island-Moline, IA-IL	9.35	10.35	11.35	02/01/95
Jackson, MS	8.02	8.70	9.24	02/01/95
Lawrence-Haverhill, MA-NH	-	11.99	-	10/01/94
Little Rock-North Little Rock, AR	6.32	7.40	8.59	12/01/94
Memphis, TN-AR-MS	8.66	9.66	10.71	11/01/94
Miami-Hialeah, FL	9.20	9.75	10.62	10/01/94
Minneapolis-St. Paul, MN-WI	-	12.81	-	02/01/95
Monmouth-Ocean, NJ	11.92	12.61	13.42	09/01/94
New Orleans, LA	9.64	11.08	12.52	01/01/96
Philadelphia, PA-NJ	11.56	12.64	14.03	11/01/94
Riverside-San Bernardino, CA	10.46	11.99	13.80	11/01/95
Rochester, NY	9.54	9.90	10.00	11/01/94
San Luis Obispo County, CA	-	12.41	-	09/01/94
Scranton-Wilkes Barre, PA	8.47	9.35	10.09	11/01/94
South Bend-Mishawaka, IN	-	8.02	-	09/01/94
Hospitals, Government				
Minneapolis-St. Paul, MN-WI	-	13.15	-	02/01/95
Riverside-San Bernardino, CA	-	14.44	-	11/01/95
Hospitals, Private				
Appleton-Oshkosh-Neenah, WI	-	9.66	-	05/01/94
Augusta, GA-SC	8.96	9.72	10.62	06/01/94
Baltimore, MD	9.59	10.84	11.77	05/01/95
Bergen-Passaic, NJ	11.84	13.94	16.12	10/01/95
Boston, MA	10.64	12.48	14.06	10/01/95
Davenport-Rock Island-Moline, IA-IL	9.35	10.37	11.80	02/01/95
Lawrence-Haverhill, MA-NH	-	11.87	-	10/01/94
Miami-Hialeah, FL	9.30	9.74	10.62	10/01/94
Monmouth-Ocean, NJ	11.92	12.61	13.42	09/01/94
New Orleans, LA	10.46	11.44	12.61	01/01/96
Philadelphia, PA-NJ	11.56	12.64	14.03	11/01/94
Riverside-San Bernardino, CA	10.46	11.20	12.48	11/01/95
Rochester, NY	9.54	9.78	10.00	11/01/94

[Continued]

★ 759 ★

Occupational Compensation: Maintenance Worker, General, Hospitals

[Continued]

Location	Compensation			Survey date
	FQ[1]	Median	TQ[2]	
Scranton-Wilkes Barre, PA	8.47	9.35	10.09	11/01/94
Wilmington, DE-NJ-MD	-	11.55	-	12/01/94

Source: U.S. Department of Labor. Bureau of Labor Statistics. *Occupational Compensation Survey.* Tables were assembled from data downloaded from http:// stats.bls.gov. *Notes:* 1. FQ stands for First Quartile and means that 25% of the workers surveyed earned less than the dollar amount shown. 2. TQ stands for Third Quartile and means that 75% of workers earned less than the dollar amount shown and 25% earned more than the dollar amount shown.

★ 760 ★

Compensation

Occupational Compensation: Nurse 2, Licensed Practical

Data show earnings by this occupation. Occupations followed by numerical ratings (2, 3, etc.) indicate grades in the occupation. The higher the number, the higher the skill level required.

[In dollars per week]

Location	Compensation			Survey date
	FQ[1]	Median	TQ[2]	
Anaheim, CA	520	573	631	02/01/96
Baltimore, MD	495	531	571	05/01/95
Bergen-Passaic, NJ	560	631	695	10/01/95
Boston, MA	598	635	675	10/01/95
Butler County, MO	310	339	360	06/01/94
Carroll County, NH	-	407	-	05/01/94
Lawrence-Haverhill, MA-NH	514	570	612	10/01/94
Memphis, TN-AR-MS	400	432	475	11/01/94
Miami-Hialeah, FL	427	466	510	10/01/94
Minneapolis-St. Paul, MN-WI	431	473	510	02/01/95
New Orleans, LA	417	463	501	01/01/96
New York, NY	541	575	601	05/01/95
Newark, NJ	542	599	632	06/01/95
Oakland, CA	593	653	712	01/01/95
Parkersburg-Marietta, WV-OH	347	409	487	08/01/95
Philadelphia, PA-NJ	515	557	595	11/01/94
Portland, OR	475	528	562	11/09/95
Riverside-San Bernardino, CA	447	489	529	11/01/95

[Continued]

★ 760 ★

Occupational Compensation: Nurse 2, Licensed Practical
[Continued]

Location	Compensation			Survey date
	FQ[1]	Median	TQ[2]	
Saginaw-Bay City-Midland, MI	437	462	497	06/01/95
Salt Lake City, UT	350	406	450	08/01/95

Source: U.S. Department of Labor. Bureau of Labor Statistics. *Occupational Compensation Survey.* Tables were assembled from data downloaded from http:// stats.bls.gov. *Notes:* 1. FQ stands for First Quartile and means that 25% of the workers surveyed earned less than the dollar amount shown. 2. TQ stands for Third Quartile and means that 75% of workers earned less than the dollar amount shown and 25% earned more than the dollar amount shown.

★ 761 ★
Compensation

Occupational Compensation: Nurse 2, Licensed Practical, Government

Data show earnings by this occupation. Occupations followed by numerical ratings (2, 3, etc.) indicate grades in the occupation. The higher the number, the higher the skill level required.

[In dollars per week]

Location	Compensation			Survey date
	FQ[1]	Median	TQ[2]	
Anaheim, CA	545	575	636	02/01/96
Augusta, GA-SC	357	384	413	06/01/94
Baltimore, MD	502	498	502	05/01/95
Bergen-Passaic, NJ	560	609	674	10/01/95
Boston, MA	611	625	642	10/01/95
Lawrence-Haverhill, MA-NH	578	600	624	10/01/94
Little Rock-North Little Rock, AR	352	414	452	12/01/94
Memphis, TN-AR-MS	430	440	483	11/01/94
Minneapolis-St. Paul, MN-WI	551	573	605	02/01/95
Monmouth-Ocean, NJ	565	608	632	09/01/94
New Orleans, LA	421	462	495	01/01/96
New York, NY	512	579	607	05/01/95
Oakland, CA	627	656	701	01/01/95
Philadelphia, PA-NJ	522	575	632	11/01/94
Riverside-San Bernardino, CA	483	501	537	11/01/95
Rochester, NY	456	492	536	11/01/94
Salt Lake City, UT	403	452	501	08/01/95

[Continued]

★ 761 ★

Occupational Compensation: Nurse 2, Licensed Practical, Government
[Continued]

Location	Compensation			Survey date
	FQ[1]	Median	TQ[2]	
Visalia-Tulare-Porterville, CA	470	501	537	07/01/94
Wilmington, DE-NJ-MD	447	477	515	12/01/94

Source: U.S. Department of Labor. Bureau of Labor Statistics. *Occupational Compensation Survey.* Tables were assembled from data downloaded from http:// stats.bls.gov. *Notes:* 1. FQ stands for First Quartile and means that 25% of the workers surveyed earned less than the dollar amount shown. 2. TQ stands for Third Quartile and means that 75% of workers earned less than the dollar amount shown and 25% earned more than the dollar amount shown.

★ 762 ★
Compensation

Occupational Compensation: Nurse 2, Licensed Practical, Health Services

Data show earnings by this occupation. Occupations followed by numerical ratings (2, 3, etc.) indicate grades in the occupation. The higher the number, the higher the skill level required.

[In dollars per week]

Location	Compensation			Survey date
	FQ[1]	Median	TQ[2]	
Anaheim, CA	521	575	634	02/01/96
Appleton-Oshkosh-Neenah, WI	406	432	460	05/01/94
Baltimore, MD	495	530	570	05/01/95
Beaufort County, SC	360	418	490	09/01/94
Bergen-Passaic, NJ	560	639	715	10/01/95
Billings, MT	366	403	428	09/01/94
Boston, MA	599	636	675	10/01/95
Bradenton, FL	378	409	433	04/01/94
Butler County, MO	310	338	359	06/01/94
Danbury, CT	568	623	662	02/01/94
Davenport-Rock Island-Moline, IA-IL	392	415	448	02/01/95
Elkhart-Goshen, IN	478	515	556	11/01/94
Gary-Hammond, IN	423	471	514	02/01/95
Jackson, MS	374	407	442	02/01/95
Lawrence-Haverhill, MA-NH	517	573	622	10/01/94
Memphis, TN-AR-MS	404	433	475	11/01/94
Miami-Hialeah, FL	440	474	520	10/01/94
Minneapolis-St. Paul, MN-WI	431	477	514	02/01/95
Monmouth-Ocean, NJ	480	537	608	09/01/94
New Orleans, LA	420	466	507	01/01/96
Newark, NJ	542	598	632	06/01/95
Oakland, CA	593	656	744	01/01/95
Parkersburg-Marietta, WV-OH	349	410	487	08/01/95
Philadelphia, PA-NJ	517	559	600	11/01/94

[Continued]

★ 762 ★

Occupational Compensation: Nurse 2, Licensed Practical, Health Services

[Continued]

Location	Compensation			Survey date
	FQ[1]	Median	TQ[2]	
Portland, OR	475	528	560	11/09/95
Poughkeepsie, NY	425	467	495	08/01/94
Riverside-San Bernardino, CA	445	489	529	11/01/95
Rochester, NY	420	460	506	11/01/94
Salt Lake City, UT	372	415	450	08/01/95
San Angelo, TX	341	370	400	10/01/94
San Jose, CA	580	645	700	07/01/94
San Luis Obispo County, CA	437	484	524	09/01/94
Scioto County, OH	398	425	450	O1/01/95
Scranton-Wilkes Barre, PA	392	447	502	11/01/94
South Bend-Mishawaka, IN	430	470	509	09/01/94
St. Cloud, MN	361	409	446	03/01/94
Visalia-Tulare-Porterville, CA	436	478	514	07/01/94

Source: U.S. Department of Labor. Bureau of Labor Statistics. *Occupational Compensation Survey.* Tables were assembled from data downloaded from http:// stats.bls.gov. *Notes:* 1. FQ stands for First Quartile and means that 25% of the workers surveyed earned less than the dollar amount shown. 2. TQ stands for Third Quartile and means that 75% of workers earned less than the dollar amount shown and 25% earned more than the dollar amount shown.

★ 763 ★

Compensation

Occupational Compensation: Nurse 2, Licensed Practical, Health Services, Government

Data show earnings by this occupation. Occupations followed by numerical ratings (2, 3, etc.) indicate grades in the occupation. The higher the number, the higher the skill level required.

[In dollars per week]

Location	Compensation			Survey date
	FQ[1]	Median	TQ[2]	
Boston, MA	611	620	642	10/01/95
Lawrence-Haverhill, MA-NH	578	600	624	10/01/94
Memphis, TN-AR-MS	430	440	483	11/01/94
Minneapolis-St. Paul, MN-WI	551	563	589	02/01/95
New Orleans, LA	433	478	523	01/01/96
Newark, NJ	542	583	624	06/01/95
Philadelphia, PA-NJ	554	585	632	11/01/94

[Continued]

★ 763 ★

Occupational Compensation: Nurse 2, Licensed Practical, Health Services, Government

[Continued]

Location	Compensation			Survey date
	FQ[1]	Median	TQ[2]	
Riverside-San Bernardino, CA	457	500	556	11/01/95
Visalia-Tulare-Porterville, CA	486	509	537	07/01/94

Source: U.S. Department of Labor. Bureau of Labor Statistics. *Occupational Compensation Survey.* Tables were assembled from data downloaded from http:// stats.bls.gov. *Notes:* 1. FQ stands for First Quartile and means that 25% of the workers surveyed earned less than the dollar amount shown. 2. TQ stands for Third Quartile and means that 75% of workers earned less than the dollar amount shown and 25% earned more than the dollar amount shown.

★ 764 ★

Compensation

Occupational Compensation: Nurse 2, Licensed Practical, Health Services, Private

Data show earnings by this occupation. Occupations followed by numerical ratings (2, 3, etc.) indicate grades in the occupation. The higher the number, the higher the skill level required.

[In dollars per week]

Location	Compensation			Survey date
	FQ[1]	Median	TQ[2]	
Anaheim, CA	522	577	640	02/01/96
Appleton-Oshkosh-Neenah, WI	402	429	453	05/01/94
Augusta, GA-SC	399	433	480	06/01/94
Baltimore, MD	492	534	572	05/01/95
Beaufort County, SC	382	445	510	09/01/94
Bergen-Passaic, NJ	560	641	710	10/01/95
Billings, MT	366	403	428	09/01/94
Boise City, ID	416	443	463	11/01/94
Boston, MA	597	638	682	10/01/95
Bradenton, FL	378	409	433	04/01/94
Butler County, MO	310	338	359	06/01/94
Charlotte-Gastonia-Rock Hill, NC-SC	444	473	504	09/01/94
Danbury, CT	568	623	662	02/01/94
Davenport-Rock Island-Moline, IA-IL	394	417	448	02/01/95
Elkhart-Goshen, IN	478	515	556	11/01/94
Gary-Hammond, IN	423	471	514	02/01/95
Jackson, MS	378	418	454	02/01/95
Lawrence-Haverhill, MA-NH	514	571	615	10/01/94
Little Rock-North Little Rock, AR	320	371	418	12/01/94
Memphis, TN-AR-MS	400	431	475	11/01/94
Miami-Hialeah, FL	427	466	510	10/01/94
Middlesex-Somerset-Hunterdon, NJ	530	588	630	03/01/95
Minneapolis-St. Paul, MN-WI	430	473	510	02/01/95
Monmouth-Ocean, NJ	474	525	580	09/01/94

[Continued]

★ 764 ★

Occupational Compensation: Nurse 2, Licensed Practical, Health Services, Private

[Continued]

Location	Compensation			Survey date
	FQ[1]	Median	TQ[2]	
New Orleans, LA	416	463	502	01/01/96
Newark, NJ	540	601	646	06/01/95
Oakland, CA	590	652	734	01/01/95
Parkersburg-Marietta, WV-OH	349	411	487	08/01/95
Philadelphia, PA-NJ	517	557	600	11/01/94
Portland, OR	474	530	562	11/09/95
Poughkeepsie, NY	425	467	495	08/01/94
Riverside-San Bernardino, CA	445	488	527	11/01/95
Rochester, NY	415	453	483	11/01/94
Saginaw-Bay City-Midland, MI	437	462	497	06/01/95
Salt Lake City, UT	371	412	448	08/01/95
San Angelo, TX	341	370	400	10/01/94
San Jose, CA	618	662	720	07/01/94
San Luis Obispo County, CA	437	484	524	09/01/94
Scioto County, OH	398	418	434	O1/01/95
Scranton-Wilkes Barre, PA	386	445	498	11/01/94
South Bend-Mishawaka, IN	430	470	509	09/01/94
St. Cloud, MN	360	405	445	03/01/94
Wilmington, DE-NJ-MD	503	551	616	12/01/94

Source: U.S. Department of Labor. Bureau of Labor Statistics. *Occupational Compensation Survey.* Tables were assembled from data downloaded from http://stats.bls.gov. *Notes:* 1. FQ stands for First Quartile and means that 25% of the workers surveyed earned less than the dollar amount shown. 2. TQ stands for Third Quartile and means that 75% of workers earned less than the dollar amount shown and 25% earned more than the dollar amount shown.

★ 765 ★

Compensation

Occupational Compensation: Nurse 2, Licensed Practical, Hospitals

Data show earnings by this occupation. Occupations followed by numerical ratings (2, 3, etc.) indicate grades in the occupation. The higher the number, the higher the skill level required.

[In dollars per week]

Location	Compensation			Survey date
	FQ[1]	Median	TQ[2]	
Anaheim, CA	494	549	616	02/01/96
Appleton-Oshkosh-Neenah, WI	431	440	450	05/01/94
Baltimore, MD	502	523	560	05/01/95
Bergen-Passaic, NJ	580	670	741	10/01/95
Boston, MA	594	630	678	10/01/95
Davenport-Rock Island-Moline, IA-IL	421	433	459	02/01/95
Gary-Hammond, IN	444	496	524	02/01/95

[Continued]

★ 765 ★

Occupational Compensation: Nurse 2, Licensed Practical, Hospitals
[Continued]

Location	Compensation			Survey date
	FQ[1]	Median	TQ[2]	
Jackson, MS	366	402	440	02/01/95
Lawrence-Haverhill, MA-NH	566	613	684	10/01/94
Little Rock-North Little Rock, AR	317	372	426	12/01/94
Memphis, TN-AR-MS	401	441	481	11/01/94
Miami-Hialeah, FL	434	478	521	10/01/94
Minneapolis-St. Paul, MN-WI	480	519	548	02/01/95
Monmouth-Ocean, NJ	471	526	588	09/01/94
New Orleans, LA	441	484	533	01/01/96
Oakland, CA	616	702	777	01/01/95
Parkersburg-Marietta, WV-OH	377	429	490	08/01/95
Philadelphia, PA-NJ	512	547	587	11/01/94
Portland, OR	495	514	544	11/09/95
Poughkeepsie, NY	-	481	-	08/01/94
Riverside-San Bernardino, CA	440	485	532	11/01/95
Rochester, NY	416	466	536	11/01/94
San Jose, CA	622	674	736	07/01/94
Scranton-Wilkes Barre, PA	420	481	543	11/01/94
South Bend-Mishawaka, IN	427	474	515	09/01/94
Visalia-Tulare-Porterville, CA	444	482	514	07/01/94

Source: U.S. Department of Labor. Bureau of Labor Statistics. *Occupational Compensation Survey.* Tables were assembled from data downloaded from http:// stats.bls.gov. *Notes:* 1. FQ stands for First Quartile and means that 25% of the workers surveyed earned less than the dollar amount shown. 2. TQ stands for Third Quartile and means that 75% of workers earned less than the dollar amount shown and 25% earned more than the dollar amount shown.

★ 766 ★

Compensation

Occupational Compensation: Nurse 2, Licensed Practical, Hospitals, Government

Data show earnings by this occupation. Occupations followed by numerical ratings (2, 3, etc.) indicate grades in the occupation. The higher the number, the higher the skill level required.

[In dollars per week]

Location	Compensation			Survey date
	FQ[1]	Median	TQ[2]	
Boston, MA	618	619	642	10/01/95
Minneapolis-St. Paul, MN-WI	546	551	582	02/01/95
New Orleans, LA	440	486	530	01/01/96
Philadelphia, PA-NJ	563	594	632	11/01/94

[Continued]

★ 766 ★

Occupational Compensation: Nurse 2, Licensed Practical, Hospitals, Government
[Continued]

Location	Compensation			Survey date
	FQ[1]	Median	TQ[2]	
Riverside-San Bernardino, CA	457	500	556	11/01/95
Visalia-Tulare-Porterville, CA	486	508	537	07/01/94

Source: U.S. Department of Labor. Bureau of Labor Statistics. *Occupational Compensation Survey.* Tables were assembled from data downloaded from http://stats.bls.gov. *Notes:* 1. FQ stands for First Quartile and means that 25% of the workers surveyed earned less than the dollar amount shown. 2. TQ stands for Third Quartile and means that 75% of workers earned less than the dollar amount shown and 25% earned more than the dollar amount shown.

★ 767 ★

Compensation

Occupational Compensation: Nurse 2, Licensed Practical, Hospitals, Private

Data show earnings by this occupation. Occupations followed by numerical ratings (2, 3, etc.) indicate grades in the occupation. The higher the number, the higher the skill level required.

[In dollars per week]

Location	Compensation			Survey date
	FQ[1]	Median	TQ[2]	
Appleton-Oshkosh-Neenah, WI	431	440	450	05/01/94
Baltimore, MD	494	531	572	05/01/95
Bergen-Passaic, NJ	596	683	791	10/01/95
Boston, MA	588	634	683	10/01/95
Charlotte-Gastonia-Rock Hill, NC-SC	450	464	487	09/01/94
Gary-Hammond, IN	444	496	524	02/01/95
Jackson, MS	384	420	456	02/01/95
Lawrence-Haverhill, MA-NH	558	611	684	10/01/94
Memphis, TN-AR-MS	397	438	475	11/01/94
Miami-Hialeah, FL	410	460	518	10/01/94
Middlesex-Somerset-Hunterdon, NJ	530	586	639	03/01/95
Minneapolis-St. Paul, MN-WI	470	514	548	02/01/95
Monmouth-Ocean, NJ	471	526	588	09/01/94
New Orleans, LA	442	483	533	01/01/96
Oakland, CA	616	698	777	01/01/95
Parkersburg-Marietta, WV-OH	377	429	490	08/01/95
Philadelphia, PA-NJ	510	543	581	11/01/94
Portland, OR	496	520	544	11/09/95
Poughkeepsie, NY	-	481	-	08/01/94
Riverside-San Bernardino, CA	438	481	529	11/01/95
Rochester, NY	406	454	492	11/01/94
Saginaw-Bay City-Midland, MI	424	460	497	06/01/95
San Jose, CA	622	674	736	07/01/94
Scranton-Wilkes Barre, PA	420	478	540	11/01/94

[Continued]

★ 767 ★

Occupational Compensation: Nurse 2, Licensed Practical, Hospitals, Private

[Continued]

| Location | Compensation | | | Survey |
	FQ[1]	Median	TQ[2]	date
South Bend-Mishawaka, IN	427	476	515	09/01/94
Wilmington, DE-NJ-MD	479	552	621	12/01/94

Source: U.S. Department of Labor. Bureau of Labor Statistics. *Occupational Compensation Survey.* Tables were assembled from data downloaded from http:// stats.bls.gov. *Notes:* 1. FQ stands for First Quartile and means that 25% of the workers surveyed earned less than the dollar amount shown. 2. TQ stands for Third Quartile and means that 75% of workers earned less than the dollar amount shown and 25% earned more than the dollar amount shown.

★ 768 ★

Compensation

Occupational Compensation: Nurse 2, Licensed Practical, Service Producing Industry

Data show earnings by this occupation. Occupations followed by numerical ratings (2, 3, etc.) indicate grades in the occupation. The higher the number, the higher the skill level required.

[In dollars per week]

| Location | Compensation | | | Survey |
	FQ[1]	Median	TQ[2]	date
Anaheim, CA	520	573	630	02/01/96
Baltimore, MD	492	536	574	05/01/95
Bergen-Passaic, NJ	560	641	710	10/01/95
Boston, MA	594	637	681	10/01/95
Lawrence-Haverhill, MA-NH	514	570	612	10/01/94
Memphis, TN-AR-MS	400	433	475	11/01/94
Miami-Hialeah, FL	427	466	510	10/01/94
Minneapolis-St. Paul, MN-WI	431	473	510	02/01/95
New Orleans, LA	416	463	502	01/01/96
New York, NY	541	575	601	05/01/95
Oakland, CA	590	652	734	01/01/95
Philadelphia, PA-NJ	515	556	594	11/01/94
Portland, OR	475	530	562	11/09/95
Riverside-San Bernardino, CA	445	487	523	11/01/95
Salt Lake City, UT	349	403	446	08/01/95

Source: U.S. Department of Labor. Bureau of Labor Statistics. *Occupational Compensation Survey.* Tables were assembled from data downloaded from http:// stats.bls.gov. *Notes:* 1. FQ stands for First Quartile and means that 25% of the workers surveyed earned less than the dollar amount shown. 2. TQ stands for Third Quartile and means that 75% of workers earned less than the dollar amount shown and 25% earned more than the dollar amount shown.

★ 769 ★

Compensation

Occupational Compensation: Nurse 2, Registered

Data show earnings by this occupation. Occupations followed by numerical ratings (2, 3, etc.) indicate grades in the occupation. The higher the number, the higher the skill level required.

[In dollars per week]

Location	Compensation			Survey date
	FQ[1]	Median	TQ[2]	
Anaheim, CA	732	827	903	02/01/96
Appleton-Oshkosh-Neenah, WI	583	649	711	05/01/94
Austin, TX	680	722	800	12/01/95
Baltimore, MD	636	735	827	05/01/95
Bergen-Passaic, NJ	810	914	1,002	10/01/95
Boston, MA	785	919	1,051	10/01/95
Butler County, MO	440	509	567	06/01/94
Carroll County, IA	436	481	513	11/01/94
Davenport-Rock Island-Moline, IA-IL	496	570	626	02/01/95
Eau Claire-La Crosse-Rochester, WI-MN	-	716	-	06/01/95
Gary-Hammond, IN	606	691	791	02/01/95
Kalamazoo-Battle Creek, MI	-	672	-	05/01/95
Kokomo-Logansport, IN	-	655	-	04/01/94
Lawrence-Haverhill, MA-NH	666	757	888	10/01/94
Little Rock-North Little Rock, AR	528	617	687	12/01/94
Memphis, TN-AR-MS	538	604	660	11/01/94
Miami-Hialeah, FL	640	711	782	10/01/94
Middlesex-Somerset-Hunterdon, NJ	750	820	887	03/01/95
Minneapolis-St. Paul, MN-WI	680	783	902	02/01/95
Monmouth-Ocean, NJ	687	754	800	09/01/94
New Orleans, LA	664	758	845	01/01/96
New York, NY	871	980	1,070	05/01/95
Newark, NJ	734	823	911	06/01/95
Oakland, CA	954	1,034	1,132	01/01/95
Parkersburg-Marietta, WV-OH	516	592	670	08/01/95
Philadelphia, PA-NJ	710	774	833	11/01/94
Portland, OR	688	749	831	11/09/95
Portsmouth-Chillicothe-Gallipolis, OH	640	668	694	04/01/95
Poughkeepsie, NY	684	730	774	08/01/94
Riverside-San Bernardino, CA	623	711	783	11/01/95
Rochester, NY	576	650	714	11/01/94
Saginaw-Bay City-Midland, MI	636	705	764	06/01/95
Salt Lake City, UT	576	664	744	08/01/95
San Jose, CA	856	982	1,108	07/01/94
South Bend-Mishawaka, IN	603	662	731	09/01/94
Visalia-Tulare-Porterville, CA	735	784	838	07/01/94
Wilmington, DE-NJ-MD	687	760	829	12/01/94

Source: U.S. Department of Labor. Bureau of Labor Statistics. *Occupational Compensation Survey.* Tables were assembled from data downloaded from http:// stats.bls.gov. *Notes:* 1. FQ stands for First Quartile and means that 25% of the workers surveyed earned less than the dollar amount shown. 2. TQ stands for Third Quartile and means that 75% of workers earned less than the dollar amount shown and 25% earned more than the dollar amount shown.

★ 770 ★

Compensation

Occupational Compensation: Nurse 2, Registered, Government

Data show earnings by this occupation. Occupations followed by numerical ratings (2, 3, etc.) indicate grades in the occupation. The higher the number, the higher the skill level required.

[In dollars per week]

Location	Compensation			Survey date
	FQ[1]	Median	TQ[2]	
Anaheim, CA	774	848	904	02/01/96
Augusta, GA-SC	570	634	682	06/01/94
Baltimore, MD	662	670	675	05/01/95
Boston, MA	823	872	951	10/01/95
Davenport-Rock Island-Moline, IA-IL	499	553	593	02/01/95
Lawrence-Haverhill, MA-NH	780	808	844	10/01/94
Little Rock-North Little Rock, AR	521	588	647	12/01/94
Memphis, TN-AR-MS	508	597	673	11/01/94
Minneapolis-St. Paul, MN-WI	771	843	906	02/01/95
New Orleans, LA	687	751	801	01/01/96
New York, NY	822	838	871	05/01/95
Oakland, CA	1,064	1,091	1,132	01/01/95
Philadelphia, PA-NJ	722	750	773	11/01/94
Portland, OR	736	788	839	11/09/95
Poughkeepsie, NY	744	758	774	08/01/94
Riverside-San Bernardino, CA	735	775	808	11/01/95
Rochester, NY	655	679	722	11/01/94
Salt Lake City, UT	573	675	767	08/01/95
St. Cloud, MN	655	704	736	03/01/94
Visalia-Tulare-Porterville, CA	748	801	852	07/01/94
Wilmington, DE-NJ-MD	601	643	692	12/01/94

Source: U.S. Department of Labor. Bureau of Labor Statistics. *Occupational Compensation Survey.* Tables were assembled from data downloaded from http:// stats.bls.gov. *Notes:* 1. FQ stands for First Quartile and means that 25% of the workers surveyed earned less than the dollar amount shown. 2. TQ stands for Third Quartile and means that 75% of workers earned less than the dollar amount shown and 25% earned more than the dollar amount shown.

★ 771 ★

Compensation

Occupational Compensation: Nurse 2, Registered, Health Services

Data show earnings by this occupation. Occupations followed by numerical ratings (2, 3, etc.) indicate grades in the occupation. The higher the number, the higher the skill level required.

[In dollars per week]

Location	Compensation			Survey date
	FQ[1]	Median	TQ[2]	
Anaheim, CA	729	831	909	02/01/96
Appleton-Oshkosh-Neenah, WI	592	650	711	05/01/94
Baltimore, MD	638	731	822	05/01/95
Beaufort County, SC	560	631	700	09/01/94
Bergen-Passaic, NJ	813	919	1,015	10/01/95
Boston, MA	785	920	1,052	10/01/95
Butler County, MO	440	508	567	06/01/94
Carroll County, IA	436	481	513	11/01/94
	490	543	575	05/01/94
Davenport-Rock Island-Moline, IA-IL	496	566	626	02/01/95
Gary-Hammond, IN	606	692	792	02/01/95
Jackson, MS	552	647	735	02/01/95
Lawrence-Haverhill, MA-NH	678	764	861	10/01/94
Memphis, TN-AR-MS	538	604	660	11/01/94
Miami-Hialeah, FL	660	739	823	10/01/94
Minneapolis-St. Paul, MN-WI	682	787	906	02/01/95
Monmouth-Ocean, NJ	687	755	800	09/01/94
New Orleans, LA	666	761	843	01/01/96
Newark, NJ	734	824	912	06/01/95
Oakland, CA	934	1,033	1,133	01/01/95
Parkersburg-Marietta, WV-OH	516	593	670	08/01/95
Philadelphia, PA-NJ	713	775	834	11/01/94
Portland, OR	694	751	826	11/09/95
Poughkeepsie, NY	670	726	774	08/01/94
Riverside-San Bernardino, CA	647	721	808	11/01/95
Rochester, NY	575	648	710	11/01/94
Salt Lake City, UT	578	661	739	08/01/95
San Angelo, TX	496	581	644	10/01/94
San Jose, CA	852	991	1,113	07/01/94
San Luis Obispo County, CA	766	810	852	09/01/94
Scranton-Wilkes Barre, PA	568	635	700	11/01/94
South Bend-Mishawaka, IN	603	662	731	09/01/94
Visalia-Tulare-Porterville, CA	741	787	847	07/01/94

Source: U.S. Department of Labor. Bureau of Labor Statistics. *Occupational Compensation Survey.* Tables were assembled from data downloaded from http:// stats.bls.gov. *Notes:* 1. FQ stands for First Quartile and means that 25% of the workers surveyed earned less than the dollar amount shown. 2. TQ stands for Third Quartile and means that 75% of workers earned less than the dollar amount shown and 25% earned more than the dollar amount shown.

★ 772 ★

Compensation

Occupational Compensation: Nurse 2, Registered, Health Services, Government

Data show earnings by this occupation. Occupations followed by numerical ratings (2, 3, etc.) indicate grades in the occupation. The higher the number, the higher the skill level required.

[In dollars per week]

Location	Compensation			Survey date
	FQ[1]	Median	TQ[2]	
Boston, MA	823	874	951	10/01/95
Davenport-Rock Island-Moline, IA-IL	499	553	593	02/01/95
Memphis, TN-AR-MS	508	597	673	11/01/94
Minneapolis-St. Paul, MN-WI	788	856	913	02/01/95
New Orleans, LA	691	768	826	01/01/96
Philadelphia, PA-NJ	758	767	792	11/01/94
Riverside-San Bernardino, CA	702	770	808	11/01/95
Rochester, NY	655	680	722	11/01/94
Visalia-Tulare-Porterville, CA	751	805	852	07/01/94

Source: U.S. Department of Labor. Bureau of Labor Statistics. *Occupational Compensation Survey.* Tables were assembled from data downloaded from http:// stats.bls.gov. *Notes:* 1. FQ stands for First Quartile and means that 25% of the workers surveyed earned less than the dollar amount shown. 2. TQ stands for Third Quartile and means that 75% of workers earned less than the dollar amount shown and 25% earned more than the dollar amount shown.

★ 773 ★

Compensation

Occupational Compensation: Nurse 2, Registered, Health Services, Private

Data show earnings by this occupation. Occupations followed by numerical ratings (2, 3, etc.) indicate grades in the occupation. The higher the number, the higher the skill level required.

[In dollars per week]

Location	Compensation			Survey date
	FQ[1]	Median	TQ[2]	
Anaheim, CA	722	828	911	02/01/96
Appleton-Oshkosh-Neenah, WI	583	649	711	05/01/94
Augusta, GA-SC	581	676	777	06/01/94
Baltimore, MD	636	735	827	05/01/95
Bergen-Passaic, NJ	810	914	1,002	10/01/95
Boston, MA	784	924	1,068	10/01/95
Butler County, MO	440	509	567	06/01/94
Carroll County, NH	490	543	575	05/01/94
Charlotte-Gastonia-Rock Hill, NC-SC	600	675	746	09/01/94
Davenport-Rock Island-Moline, IA-IL	496	568	626	02/01/95

[Continued]

★ 773 ★

Occupational Compensation: Nurse 2, Registered, Health Services, Private

[Continued]

Location	Compensation			Survey date
	FQ[1]	Median	TQ[2]	
Gary-Hammond, IN	606	692	792	02/01/95
Jackson, MS	562	656	744	02/01/95
Lawrence-Haverhill, MA-NH	665	757	889	10/01/94
Little Rock-North Little Rock, AR	530	625	695	12/01/94
Memphis, TN-AR-MS	545	605	660	11/01/94
Miami-Hialeah, FL	640	710	781	10/01/94
Minneapolis-St. Paul, MN-WI	660	770	890	02/01/95
Monmouth-Ocean, NJ	687	755	800	09/01/94
New Orleans, LA	664	759	846	01/01/96
Newark, NJ	736	827	916	06/01/95
Oakland, CA	899	1,019	1,133	01/01/95
Parkersburg-Marietta, WV-OH	516	598	677	08/01/95
Philadelphia, PA-NJ	711	775	836	11/01/94
Portland, OR	688	749	831	11/09/95
Riverside-San Bernardino, CA	622	711	783	11/01/95
Rochester, NY	573	645	700	11/01/94
Saginaw-Bay City-Midland, MI	636	705	764	06/01/95
Salt Lake City, UT	578	652	727	08/01/95
San Angelo, TX	496	581	644	10/01/94
San Jose, CA	911	1,013	1,126	07/01/94
Scranton-Wilkes Barre, PA	562	631	697	11/01/94
South Bend-Mishawaka, IN	603	662	731	09/01/94
Visalia-Tulare-Porterville, CA	600	665	714	07/01/94
Wilmington, DE-NJ-MD	687	760	829	12/01/94

Source: U.S. Department of Labor. Bureau of Labor Statistics. *Occupational Compensation Survey.* Tables were assembled from data downloaded from http:// stats.bls.gov. *Notes:* 1. FQ stands for First Quartile and means that 25% of the workers surveyed earned less than the dollar amount shown. 2. TQ stands for Third Quartile and means that 75% of workers earned less than the dollar amount shown and 25% earned more than the dollar amount shown.

★ 774 ★
Compensation

Occupational Compensation: Nurse 2, Registered, Hospitals

Data show earnings by this occupation. Occupations followed by numerical ratings (2, 3, etc.) indicate grades in the occupation. The higher the number, the higher the skill level required.

[In dollars per week]

Location	Compensation			Survey date
	FQ[1]	Median	TQ[2]	
Anaheim, CA	748	847	926	02/01/96
Appleton-Oshkosh-Neenah, WI	609	666	711	05/01/94
Baltimore, MD	635	735	828	05/01/95
Bergen-Passaic, NJ	846	951	1,024	10/01/95
Boston, MA	791	926	1,066	10/01/95
Davenport-Rock Island-Moline, IA-IL	515	577	626	02/01/95
Gary-Hammond, IN	606	711	804	02/01/95
Jackson, MS	552	646	736	02/01/95
Lawrence-Haverhill, MA-NH	700	777	894	10/01/94
Little Rock-North Little Rock, AR	528	620	691	12/01/94
Memphis, TN-AR-MS	534	602	667	11/01/94
Miami-Hialeah, FL	664	748	831	10/01/94
Minneapolis-St. Paul, MN-WI	788	852	917	02/01/95
Monmouth-Ocean, NJ	694	760	810	09/01/94
New Orleans, LA	666	762	845	01/01/96
Oakland, CA	1,078	1,099	1,156	01/01/95
Parkersburg-Marietta, WV-OH	516	600	684	08/01/95
Philadelphia, PA-NJ	717	775	832	11/01/94
Portland, OR	736	786	840	11/09/95
Riverside-San Bernardino, CA	647	721	808	11/01/95
Rochester, NY	567	642	697	11/01/94
San Angelo, TX	496	583	655	10/01/94
San Jose, CA	956	1,049	1,137	07/01/94
San Luis Obispo County, CA	779	822	852	09/01/94
Scranton-Wilkes Barre, PA	575	639	700	11/01/94
Visalia-Tulare-Porterville, CA	748	793	831	07/01/94

Source: U.S. Department of Labor. Bureau of Labor Statistics. *Occupational Compensation Survey.* Tables were assembled from data downloaded from http:// stats.bls.gov. *Notes:* 1. FQ stands for First Quartile and means that 25% of the workers surveyed earned less than the dollar amount shown. 2. TQ stands for Third Quartile and means that 75% of workers earned less than the dollar amount shown and 25% earned more than the dollar amount shown.

★ 775 ★

Compensation

Occupational Compensation: Nurse 2, Registered, Hospitals, Government

Data show earnings by this occupation. Occupations followed by numerical ratings (2, 3, etc.) indicate grades in the occupation. The higher the number, the higher the skill level required.

[In dollars per week]

Location	Compensation			Survey date
	FQ[1]	Median	TQ[2]	
Boston, MA	823	874	951	10/01/95
Minneapolis-St. Paul, MN-WI	789	859	914	02/01/95
New Orleans, LA	702	773	833	01/01/96
Riverside-San Bernardino, CA	702	770	808	11/01/95
Visalia-Tulare-Porterville, CA	751	802	838	07/01/94

Source: U.S. Department of Labor. Bureau of Labor Statistics. *Occupational Compensation Survey.* Tables were assembled from data downloaded from http:// stats.bls.gov. *Notes:* 1. FQ stands for First Quartile and means that 25% of the workers surveyed earned less than the dollar amount shown. 2. TQ stands for Third Quartile and means that 75% of workers earned less than the dollar amount shown and 25% earned more than the dollar amount shown.

★ 776 ★

Compensation

Occupational Compensation: Nurse 2, Registered, Hospitals, Private

Data show earnings by this occupation. Occupations followed by numerical ratings (2, 3, etc.) indicate grades in the occupation. The higher the number, the higher the skill level required.

[In dollars per week]

Location	Compensation			Survey date
	FQ[1]	Median	TQ[2]	
Appleton-Oshkosh-Neenah, WI	606	666	711	05/01/94
Augusta, GA-SC	581	676	777	06/01/94
Baltimore, MD	634	737	831	05/01/95
Bergen-Passaic, NJ	844	946	1,015	10/01/95
Boise City, ID	598	660	711	11/01/94
Boston, MA	788	931	1,069	10/01/95
Charlotte-Gastonia-Rock Hill, NC-SC	608	691	780	09/01/94
Davenport-Rock Island-Moline, IA-IL	520	583	632	02/01/95
Gary-Hammond, IN	606	711	804	02/01/95
Jackson, MS	560	655	744	02/01/95
Lawrence-Haverhill, MA-NH	684	770	903	10/01/94
Little Rock-North Little Rock, AR	528	629	706	12/01/94
Memphis, TN-AR-MS	534	603	668	11/01/94
Miami-Hialeah, FL	640	715	800	10/01/94

[Continued]

★ 776 ★

Occupational Compensation: Nurse 2, Registered, Hospitals, Private

[Continued]

Location	Compensation			Survey date
	FQ[1]	Median	TQ[2]	
Minneapolis-St. Paul, MN-WI	788	850	917	02/01/95
Monmouth-Ocean, NJ	694	760	810	09/01/94
New Orleans, LA	660	759	850	01/01/96
Oakland, CA	1,076	1,095	1,156	01/01/95
Parkersburg-Marietta, WV-OH	516	600	684	08/01/95
Philadelphia, PA-NJ	714	775	833	11/01/94
Portland, OR	736	787	840	11/09/95
Riverside-San Bernardino, CA	622	709	783	11/01/95
Rochester, NY	565	643	700	11/01/94
Saginaw-Bay City-Midland, MI	650	712	772	06/01/95
San Angelo, TX	496	583	655	10/01/94
San Jose, CA	956	1,049	1,137	07/01/94
Scranton-Wilkes Barre, PA	571	637	700	11/01/94

Source: U.S. Department of Labor. Bureau of Labor Statistics. *Occupational Compensation Survey.* Tables were assembled from data downloaded from http:// stats.bls.gov. *Notes:* 1. FQ stands for First Quartile and means that 25% of the workers surveyed earned less than the dollar amount shown. 2. TQ stands for Third Quartile and means that 75% of workers earned less than the dollar amount shown and 25% earned more than the dollar amount shown.

★ 777 ★

Compensation

Occupational Compensation: Nurse 2, Registered, Service Producing Industry

Data show earnings by this occupation. Occupations followed by numerical ratings (2, 3, etc.) indicate grades in the occupation. The higher the number, the higher the skill level required.

[In dollars per week]

Location	Compensation			Survey date
	FQ[1]	Median	TQ[2]	
Anaheim, CA	721	822	903	02/01/96
Appleton-Oshkosh-Neenah, WI	583	649	711	05/01/94
Baltimore, MD	636	735	827	05/01/95
Bergen-Passaic, NJ	810	914	1,002	10/01/95
Boston, MA	783	923	1,067	10/01/95
Davenport-Rock Island-Moline, IA-IL	496	569	626	02/01/95
Gary-Hammond, IN	606	692	792	02/01/95
Lawrence-Haverhill, MA-NH	665	757	889	10/01/94
Little Rock-North Little Rock, AR	530	625	695	12/01/94
Memphis, TN-AR-MS	545	605	660	11/01/94
Miami-Hialeah, FL	640	711	782	10/01/94
Minneapolis-St. Paul, MN-WI	659	766	890	02/01/95
Monmouth-Ocean, NJ	687	755	800	09/01/94

[Continued]

★ 777 ★

Occupational Compensation: Nurse 2, Registered, Service Producing Industry

[Continued]

Location	Compensation			Survey date
	FQ[1]	Median	TQ[2]	
New Orleans, LA	664	758	846	01/01/96
New York, NY	914	1,001	1,087	05/01/95
Oakland, CA	900	1,017	1,133	01/01/95
Philadelphia, PA-NJ	710	775	835	11/01/94
Portland, OR	688	749	831	11/09/95
Riverside-San Bernardino, CA	623	711	783	11/01/95
Rochester, NY	573	645	700	11/01/94
Salt Lake City, UT	577	660	740	08/01/95
San Jose, CA	911	1,013	1,126	07/01/94
South Bend-Mishawaka, IN	603	662	731	09/01/94
Visalia-Tulare-Porterville, CA	600	665	714	07/01/94
Wilmington, DE-NJ-MD	687	760	829	12/01/94

Source: U.S. Department of Labor. Bureau of Labor Statistics. *Occupational Compensation Survey.* Tables were assembled from data downloaded from http:// stats.bls.gov. *Notes:* 1. FQ stands for First Quartile and means that 25% of the workers surveyed earned less than the dollar amount shown. 2. TQ stands for Third Quartile and means that 75% of workers earned less than the dollar amount shown and 25% earned more than the dollar amount shown.

★ 778 ★

Compensation

Occupational Compensation: Nurse Specialist 2, Registered

Data show earnings by this occupation. Occupations followed by numerical ratings (2, 3, etc.) indicate grades in the occupation. The higher the number, the higher the skill level required.

[In dollars per week]

Location	Compensation			Survey date
	FQ[1]	Median	TQ[2]	
Anaheim, CA	800	901	1,019	02/01/96
Baltimore, MD	834	924	969	05/01/95
Boston, MA	882	995	1,044	10/01/95
Memphis, TN-AR-MS	640	701	764	11/01/94
Miami-Hialeah, FL	732	787	840	10/01/94
Minneapolis-St. Paul, MN-WI	843	897	951	02/01/95
New Orleans, LA	735	807	879	01/01/96
Newark, NJ	840	911	1,018	06/01/95

[Continued]

★ 778 ★

Occupational Compensation: Nurse Specialist 2, Registered

[Continued]

Location	Compensation			Survey date
	FQ[1]	Median	TQ[2]	
Philadelphia, PA-NJ	798	840	892	11/01/94
Riverside-San Bernardino, CA	769	807	847	11/01/95

Source: U.S. Department of Labor. Bureau of Labor Statistics. *Occupational Compensation Survey.* Tables were assembled from data downloaded from http:// stats.bls.gov. *Notes:* 1. FQ stands for First Quartile and means that 25% of the workers surveyed earned less than the dollar amount shown. 2. TQ stands for Third Quartile and means that 75% of workers earned less than the dollar amount shown and 25% earned more than the dollar amount shown.

★ 779 ★

Compensation

Occupational Compensation: Nurse Specialist 2, Registered, Health Services

Data show earnings by this occupation. Occupations followed by numerical ratings (2, 3, etc.) indicate grades in the occupation. The higher the number, the higher the skill level required.

[In dollars per week]

Location	Compensation			Survey date
	FQ[1]	Median	TQ[2]	
Anaheim, CA	800	901	1,019	02/01/96
Appleton-Oshkosh-Neenah, WI	-	699	-	05/01/94
Baltimore, MD	834	924	969	05/01/95
Boston, MA	882	995	1,044	10/01/95
Memphis, TN-AR-MS	640	701	764	11/01/94
Miami-Hialeah, FL	730	785	835	10/01/94
Minneapolis-St. Paul, MN-WI	842	893	951	02/01/95
New Orleans, LA	760	828	893	01/01/96
Newark, NJ	840	911	1,018	06/01/95
Philadelphia, PA-NJ	799	841	893	11/01/94
Salt Lake City, UT	564	638	716	08/01/95
Scranton-Wilkes Barre, PA	561	627	684	11/01/94

Source: U.S. Department of Labor. Bureau of Labor Statistics. *Occupational Compensation Survey.* Tables were assembled from data downloaded from http:// stats.bls.gov. *Notes:* 1. FQ stands for First Quartile and means that 25% of the workers surveyed earned less than the dollar amount shown. 2. TQ stands for Third Quartile and means that 75% of workers earned less than the dollar amount shown and 25% earned more than the dollar amount shown.

★ 780 ★

Compensation

Occupational Compensation: Nurse Specialist 2, Registered, Health Services, Government

Data show earnings by this occupation. Occupations followed by numerical ratings (2, 3, etc.) indicate grades in the occupation. The higher the number, the higher the skill level required.

[In dollars per week]

Location	Compensation			Survey date
	FQ[1]	Median	TQ[2]	
Minneapolis-St. Paul, MN-WI	844	907	951	02/01/95
New Orleans, LA	818	879	948	01/01/96

Source: U.S. Department of Labor. Bureau of Labor Statistics. *Occupational Compensation Survey.* Tables were assembled from data downloaded from http:// stats.bls.gov. *Notes:* 1. FQ stands for First Quartile and means that 25% of the workers surveyed earned less than the dollar amount shown. 2. TQ stands for Third Quartile and means that 75% of workers earned less than the dollar amount shown and 25% earned more than the dollar amount shown.

★ 781 ★

Compensation

Occupational Compensation: Nurse Specialist 2, Registered, Health Services, Private

Data show earnings by this occupation. Occupations followed by numerical ratings (2, 3, etc.) indicate grades in the occupation. The higher the number, the higher the skill level required.

[In dollars per week]

Location	Compensation			Survey date
	FQ[1]	Median	TQ[2]	
Anaheim, CA	800	901	1,019	02/01/96
Appleton-Oshkosh-Neenah, WI	-	704	-	05/01/94
Baltimore, MD	834	924	969	05/01/95
Boston, MA	851	1,039	1,289	10/01/95
Memphis, TN-AR-MS	640	701	764	11/01/94
Miami-Hialeah, FL	730	785	835	10/01/94
Minneapolis-St. Paul, MN-WI	842	880	962	02/01/95
New Orleans, LA	735	807	879	01/01/96
Newark, NJ	840	910	1,016	06/01/95
Philadelphia, PA-NJ	799	841	893	11/01/94
Salt Lake City, UT	564	638	716	08/01/95

[Continued]

★ 781 ★

Occupational Compensation: Nurse Specialist 2, Registered, Health Services, Private

[Continued]

Location	Compensation			Survey date
	FQ[1]	Median	TQ[2]	
Scranton-Wilkes Barre, PA	561	627	684	11/01/94
Wilmington, DE-NJ-MD	691	817	902	12/01/94

Source: U.S. Department of Labor. Bureau of Labor Statistics. *Occupational Compensation Survey.* Tables were assembled from data downloaded from http:// stats.bls.gov. *Notes:* 1. FQ stands for First Quartile and means that 25% of the workers surveyed earned less than the dollar amount shown. 2. TQ stands for Third Quartile and means that 75% of workers earned less than the dollar amount shown and 25% earned more than the dollar amount shown.

★ 782 ★

Compensation

Occupational Compensation: Nurse Specialist 2, Registered, Hospitals

Data show earnings by this occupation. Occupations followed by numerical ratings (2, 3, etc.) indicate grades in the occupation. The higher the number, the higher the skill level required.

[In dollars per week]

Location	Compensation			Survey date
	FQ[1]	Median	TQ[2]	
Anaheim, CA	709	844	940	02/01/96
Baltimore, MD	834	927	988	05/01/95
Boston, MA	882	995	1,044	10/01/95
Memphis, TN-AR-MS	630	687	728	11/01/94
Miami-Hialeah, FL	730	785	835	10/01/94
Minneapolis-St. Paul, MN-WI	877	919	951	02/01/95
New Orleans, LA	761	831	895	01/01/96
Philadelphia, PA-NJ	799	841	893	11/01/94
Scranton-Wilkes Barre, PA	561	627	684	11/01/94

Source: U.S. Department of Labor. Bureau of Labor Statistics. *Occupational Compensation Survey.* Tables were assembled from data downloaded from http:// stats.bls.gov. *Notes:* 1. FQ stands for First Quartile and means that 25% of the workers surveyed earned less than the dollar amount shown. 2. TQ stands for Third Quartile and means that 75% of workers earned less than the dollar amount shown and 25% earned more than the dollar amount shown.

★ 783 ★

Compensation

Occupational Compensation: Nurse Specialist 2, Registered, Hospitals, Private

Data show earnings by this occupation. Occupations followed by numerical ratings (2, 3, etc.) indicate grades in the occupation. The higher the number, the higher the skill level required.

[In dollars per week]

Location	Compensation			Survey date
	FQ[1]	Median	TQ[2]	
Baltimore, MD	834	927	988	05/01/95
Boston, MA	851	1,039	1,289	10/01/95
Memphis, TN-AR-MS	630	687	728	11/01/94
Miami-Hialeah, FL	730	785	835	10/01/94
Minneapolis-St. Paul, MN-WI	864	925	967	02/01/95
New Orleans, LA	734	807	878	01/01/96
Philadelphia, PA-NJ	799	841	893	11/01/94
Scranton-Wilkes Barre, PA	561	627	684	11/01/94
Wilmington, DE-NJ-MD	-	887	-	12/01/94

Source: U.S. Department of Labor. Bureau of Labor Statistics. *Occupational Compensation Survey.* Tables were assembled from data downloaded from http:// stats.bls.gov. *Notes:* 1. FQ stands for First Quartile and means that 25% of the workers surveyed earned less than the dollar amount shown. 2. TQ stands for Third Quartile and means that 75% of workers earned less than the dollar amount shown and 25% earned more than the dollar amount shown.

★ 784 ★

Compensation

Occupational Compensation: Nurse Specialist 2, Registered, Service Producing Industry

Data show earnings by this occupation. Occupations followed by numerical ratings (2, 3, etc.) indicate grades in the occupation. The higher the number, the higher the skill level required.

[In dollars per week]

Location	Compensation			Survey date
	FQ[1]	Median	TQ[2]	
Anaheim, CA	800	901	1,019	02/01/96
Baltimore, MD	834	924	969	05/01/95
Memphis, TN-AR-MS	640	701	764	11/01/94
Minneapolis-St. Paul, MN-WI	-	880	-	02/01/95
New Orleans, LA	735	807	879	01/01/96

[Continued]

★ 784 ★

Occupational Compensation: Nurse Specialist 2, Registered, Service Producing Industry

[Continued]

Location	Compensation			Survey date
	FQ[1]	Median	TQ[2]	
Philadelphia, PA-NJ	799	841	893	11/01/94
Riverside-San Bernardino, CA	769	807	847	11/01/95

Source: U.S. Department of Labor. Bureau of Labor Statistics. *Occupational Compensation Survey.* Tables were assembled from data downloaded from http:// stats.bls.gov. *Notes:* 1. FQ stands for First Quartile and means that 25% of the workers surveyed earned less than the dollar amount shown. 2. TQ stands for Third Quartile and means that 75% of workers earned less than the dollar amount shown and 25% earned more than the dollar amount shown.

★ 785 ★

Compensation

Occupational Compensation: Nursing Assistant 2

Data show earnings by this occupation. Occupations followed by numerical ratings (2, 3, etc.) indicate grades in the occupation. The higher the number, the higher the skill level required.

[In dollars per week]

Location	Compensation			Survey date
	FQ[1]	Median	TQ[2]	
Anaheim, CA	260	298	322	02/01/96
Baltimore, MD	246	290	335	05/01/95
Bergen-Passaic, NJ	310	357	391	10/01/95
Boston, MA	322	374	410	10/01/95
Butler County, MO	180	199	210	06/01/94
Carroll County, IA	240	252	264	11/01/94
	230	280	305	05/01/94
Lawrence-Haverhill, MA-NH	300	334	367	10/01/94
Memphis, TN-AR-MS	218	243	260	11/01/94
Miami-Hialeah, FL	250	274	292	10/01/94
Minneapolis-St. Paul, MN-WI	298	334	363	02/01/95
New Orleans, LA	180	218	254	01/01/96
New York, NY	381	409	465	05/01/95
Newark, NJ	320	368	400	06/01/95
Oakland, CA	280	367	427	01/01/95
Parkersburg-Marietta, WV-OH	210	263	330	08/01/95
Philadelphia, PA-NJ	266	309	339	11/01/94
Portland, OR	288	326	351	11/09/95
Riverside-San Bernardino, CA	221	265	299	11/01/95

[Continued]

★ 785 ★

Occupational Compensation: Nursing Assistant 2
[Continued]

Location	Compensation			Survey date
	FQ[1]	Median	TQ[2]	
Saginaw-Bay City-Midland, MI	268	284	304	06/01/95
Salt Lake City, UT	250	266	276	08/01/95

Source: U.S. Department of Labor. Bureau of Labor Statistics. *Occupational Compensation Survey.* Tables were assembled from data downloaded from http:// stats.bls.gov. *Notes:* 1. FQ stands for First Quartile and means that 25% of the workers surveyed earned less than the dollar amount shown. 2. TQ stands for Third Quartile and means that 75% of workers earned less than the dollar amount shown and 25% earned more than the dollar amount shown.

★ 786 ★

Compensation

Occupational Compensation: Nursing Assistant 2, Government

Data show earnings by this occupation. Occupations followed by numerical ratings (2, 3, etc.) indicate grades in the occupation. The higher the number, the higher the skill level required.

[In dollars per week]

Location	Compensation			Survey date
	FQ[1]	Median	TQ[2]	
Anaheim, CA	346	404	467	02/01/96
Augusta, GA-SC	266	285	328	06/01/94
Baltimore, MD	409	400	409	05/01/95
Boston, MA	433	457	482	10/01/95
Lawrence-Haverhill, MA-NH	375	378	375	10/01/94
Memphis, TN-AR-MS	358	348	358	11/01/94
Minneapolis-St. Paul, MN-WI	394	418	452	02/01/95
New Orleans, LA	221	248	281	01/01/96
New York, NY	378	429	480	05/01/95
Oakland, CA	513	513	513	01/01/95
Philadelphia, PA-NJ	378	411	426	11/01/94
Riverside-San Bernardino, CA	314	342	372	11/01/95
Visalia-Tulare-Porterville, CA	269	299	325	07/01/94
Wilmington, DE-NJ-MD	308	317	324	12/01/94

Source: U.S. Department of Labor. Bureau of Labor Statistics. *Occupational Compensation Survey.* Tables were assembled from data downloaded from http:// stats.bls.gov. *Notes:* 1. FQ stands for First Quartile and means that 25% of the workers surveyed earned less than the dollar amount shown. 2. TQ stands for Third Quartile and means that 75% of workers earned less than the dollar amount shown and 25% earned more than the dollar amount shown.

★ 787 ★
Compensation

Occupational Compensation: Nursing Assistant 2, Health Services

Data show earnings by this occupation. Occupations followed by numerical ratings (2, 3, etc.) indicate grades in the occupation. The higher the number, the higher the skill level required.

[In dollars per week]

Location	Compensation			Survey date
	FQ[1]	Median	TQ[2]	
Anaheim, CA	260	298	323	02/01/96
Appleton-Oshkosh-Neenah, WI	274	306	342	05/01/94
Baltimore, MD	251	308	360	05/01/95
Beaufort County, SC	200	234	260	09/01/94
Bergen-Passaic, NJ	310	359	394	10/01/95
Billings, MT	220	252	284	09/01/94
Boston, MA	330	385	428	10/01/95
Bradenton, FL	242	271	288	04/01/94
Butler County, MO	180	199	210	06/01/94
Carroll County, IA	240	252	264	11/01/94
Danbury, CT	313	346	367	02/01/94
Davenport-Rock Island-Moline, IA-IL	225	254	278	02/01/95
Elkhart-Goshen, IN	234	269	312	11/01/94
Gary-Hammond, IN	199	251	302	02/01/95
Jackson, MS	215	242	263	02/01/95
Lawrence-Haverhill, MA-NH	300	336	375	10/01/94
Memphis, TN-AR-MS	222	258	302	11/01/94
Miami-Hialeah, FL	246	273	290	10/01/94
Minneapolis-St. Paul, MN-WI	300	338	367	02/01/95
Monmouth-Ocean, NJ	304	336	356	09/01/94
New Orleans, LA	176	214	247	01/01/96
Newark, NJ	320	368	400	06/01/95
Oakland, CA	280	363	415	01/01/95
Parkersburg-Marietta, WV-OH	210	263	330	08/01/95
Philadelphia, PA-NJ	262	310	342	11/01/94
Portland, OR	290	326	353	11/09/95
Poughkeepsie, NY	290	326	346	08/01/94
Riverside-San Bernardino, CA	216	255	282	11/01/95
Rochester, NY	277	309	327	11/01/94
Salt Lake City, UT	246	263	273	08/01/95
San Angelo, TX	190	211	230	10/01/94
San Jose, CA	260	343	404	07/01/94
San Luis Obispo County, CA	225	256	270	09/01/94
Scioto County, OH	222	257	274	O1/01/95
Scranton-Wilkes Barre, PA	256	316	361	11/01/94
South Bend-Mishawaka, IN	201	243	254	09/01/94

[Continued]

★ 787 ★

Occupational Compensation: Nursing Assistant 2, Health Services

[Continued]

Location	Compensation			Survey date
	FQ[1]	Median	TQ[2]	
St. Cloud, MN	237	272	312	03/01/94
Visalia-Tulare-Porterville, CA	224	255	276	07/01/94

Source: U.S. Department of Labor. Bureau of Labor Statistics. *Occupational Compensation Survey.* Tables were assembled from data downloaded from http:// stats.bls.gov. *Notes:* 1. FQ stands for First Quartile and means that 25% of the workers surveyed earned less than the dollar amount shown. 2. TQ stands for Third Quartile and means that 75% of workers earned less than the dollar amount shown and 25% earned more than the dollar amount shown.

★ 788 ★

Compensation

Occupational Compensation: Nursing Assistant 2, Health Services, Government

Data show earnings by this occupation. Occupations followed by numerical ratings (2, 3, etc.) indicate grades in the occupation. The higher the number, the higher the skill level required.

[In dollars per week]

Location	Compensation			Survey date
	FQ[1]	Median	TQ[2]	
Boston, MA	425	456	482	10/01/95
Lawrence-Haverhill, MA-NH	375	378	375	10/01/94
Memphis, TN-AR-MS	358	348	358	11/01/94
Minneapolis-St. Paul, MN-WI	394	417	452	02/01/95
New Orleans, LA	220	240	254	01/01/96
Riverside-San Bernardino, CA	284	304	329	11/01/95
Visalia-Tulare-Porterville, CA	269	299	325	07/01/94

Source: U.S. Department of Labor. Bureau of Labor Statistics. *Occupational Compensation Survey.* Tables were assembled from data downloaded from http:// stats.bls.gov. *Notes:* 1. FQ stands for First Quartile and means that 25% of the workers surveyed earned less than the dollar amount shown. 2. TQ stands for Third Quartile and means that 75% of workers earned less than the dollar amount shown and 25% earned more than the dollar amount shown.

★ 789 ★
Compensation

Occupational Compensation: Nursing Assistant 2, Health Services, Private

Data show earnings by this occupation. Occupations followed by numerical ratings (2, 3, etc.) indicate grades in the occupation. The higher the number, the higher the skill level required.

[In dollars per week]

Location	Compensation			Survey date
	FQ[1]	Median	TQ[2]	
Anaheim, CA	260	293	318	02/01/96
Appleton-Oshkosh-Neenah, WI	262	286	310	05/01/94
Augusta, GA-SC	206	238	262	06/01/94
Baltimore, MD	244	290	334	05/01/95
Beaufort County, SC	200	230	256	09/01/94
Bergen-Passaic, NJ	300	351	388	10/01/95
Billings, MT	220	252	284	09/01/94
Boise City, ID	233	259	281	11/01/94
Boston, MA	325	376	414	10/01/95
Bradenton, FL	242	271	288	04/01/94
Butler County, MO	180	199	210	06/01/94
Charlotte-Gastonia-Rock Hill, NC-SC	233	273	304	09/01/94
Danbury, CT	313	346	367	02/01/94
Davenport-Rock Island-Moline, IA-IL	225	253	277	02/01/95
Elkhart-Goshen, IN	234	269	312	11/01/94
Gary-Hammond, IN	199	251	302	02/01/95
Jackson, MS	201	240	270	02/01/95
Lawrence-Haverhill, MA-NH	300	334	367	10/01/94
Little Rock-North Little Rock, AR	182	218	246	12/01/94
Memphis, TN-AR-MS	213	243	262	11/01/94
Miami-Hialeah, FL	245	269	290	10/01/94
Middlesex-Somerset-Hunterdon, NJ	331	365	386	03/01/95
Minneapolis-St. Paul, MN-WI	300	336	364	02/01/95
Monmouth-Ocean, NJ	304	336	356	09/01/94
New Orleans, LA	176	211	245	01/01/96
Newark, NJ	316	351	378	06/01/95
Oakland, CA	280	361	407	01/01/95
Parkersburg-Marietta, WV-OH	210	263	330	08/01/95
Philadelphia, PA-NJ	262	308	340	11/01/94
Portland, OR	286	325	350	11/09/95
Poughkeepsie, NY	290	326	346	08/01/94
Riverside-San Bernardino, CA	216	254	278	11/01/95
Rochester, NY	274	305	325	11/01/94
Saginaw-Bay City-Midland, MI	268	284	304	06/01/95
Salt Lake City, UT	244	259	272	08/01/95
San Angelo, TX	190	211	230	10/01/94
San Jose, CA	260	343	404	07/01/94
San Luis Obispo County, CA	225	256	270	09/01/94
Scioto County, OH	220	247	270	O1/01/95
Scranton-Wilkes Barre, PA	250	287	340	11/01/94
South Bend-Mishawaka, IN	200	243	254	09/01/94

[Continued]

★ 789 ★

Occupational Compensation: Nursing Assistant 2, Health Services, Private

[Continued]

Location	Compensation			Survey date
	FQ[1]	Median	TQ[2]	
St. Cloud, MN	237	268	312	03/01/94
Visalia-Tulare-Porterville, CA	216	242	263	07/01/94
Wilmington, DE-NJ-MD	250	291	323	12/01/94

Source: U.S. Department of Labor. Bureau of Labor Statistics. *Occupational Compensation Survey.* Tables were assembled from data downloaded from http:// stats.bls.gov. *Notes:* 1. FQ stands for First Quartile and means that 25% of the workers surveyed earned less than the dollar amount shown. 2. TQ stands for Third Quartile and means that 75% of workers earned less than the dollar amount shown and 25% earned more than the dollar amount shown.

★ 790 ★

Compensation

Occupational Compensation: Nursing Assistant 2, Hospitals

Data show earnings by this occupation. Occupations followed by numerical ratings (2, 3, etc.) indicate grades in the occupation. The higher the number, the higher the skill level required.

[In dollars per week]

Location	Compensation			Survey date
	FQ[1]	Median	TQ[2]	
Anaheim, CA	320	348	372	02/01/96
Appleton-Oshkosh-Neenah, WI	306	326	343	05/01/94
Baltimore, MD	317	357	409	05/01/95
Bergen-Passaic, NJ	366	414	438	10/01/95
Boston, MA	360	415	465	10/01/95
Davenport-Rock Island-Moline, IA-IL	251	279	304	02/01/95
Gary-Hammond, IN	326	348	368	02/01/95
Jackson, MS	224	254	277	02/01/95
Lawrence-Haverhill, MA-NH	320	356	383	10/01/94
Memphis, TN-AR-MS	243	280	312	11/01/94
Miami-Hialeah, FL	255	289	322	10/01/94
Minneapolis-St. Paul, MN-WI	364	395	424	02/01/95
Monmouth-Ocean, NJ	315	365	394	09/01/94
New Orleans, LA	236	258	281	01/01/96
Oakland, CA	354	464	548	01/01/95
Parkersburg-Marietta, WV-OH	294	320	334	08/01/95
Philadelphia, PA-NJ	350	393	438	11/01/94
Portland, OR	354	386	416	11/09/95
Riverside-San Bernardino, CA	277	313	341	11/01/95
Rochester, NY	294	331	376	11/01/94
San Jose, CA	417	480	547	07/01/94
Scranton-Wilkes Barre, PA	259	294	318	11/01/94
South Bend-Mishawaka, IN	274	323	380	09/01/94

[Continued]

★ 790 ★

Occupational Compensation: Nursing Assistant 2, Hospitals

[Continued]

Location	Compensation			Survey date
	FQ[1]	Median	TQ[2]	
St. Cloud, MN	277	299	331	03/01/94
Visalia-Tulare-Porterville, CA	250	278	296	07/01/94

Source: U.S. Department of Labor. Bureau of Labor Statistics. *Occupational Compensation Survey.* Tables were assembled from data downloaded from http:// stats.bls.gov. *Notes:* 1. FQ stands for First Quartile and means that 25% of the workers surveyed earned less than the dollar amount shown. 2. TQ stands for Third Quartile and means that 75% of workers earned less than the dollar amount shown and 25% earned more than the dollar amount shown.

★ 791 ★

Compensation

Occupational Compensation: Nursing Assistant 2, Hospitals, Government

Data show earnings by this occupation. Occupations followed by numerical ratings (2, 3, etc.) indicate grades in the occupation. The higher the number, the higher the skill level required.

[In dollars per week]

Location	Compensation			Survey date
	FQ[1]	Median	TQ[2]	
Boston, MA	416	445	482	10/01/95
Minneapolis-St. Paul, MN-WI	402	425	452	02/01/95
New Orleans, LA	222	242	254	01/01/96
Riverside-San Bernardino, CA	284	304	329	11/01/95
Visalia-Tulare-Porterville, CA	269	299	325	07/01/94

Source: U.S. Department of Labor. Bureau of Labor Statistics. *Occupational Compensation Survey.* Tables were assembled from data downloaded from http:// stats.bls.gov. *Notes:* 1. FQ stands for First Quartile and means that 25% of the workers surveyed earned less than the dollar amount shown. 2. TQ stands for Third Quartile and means that 75% of workers earned less than the dollar amount shown and 25% earned more than the dollar amount shown.

★ 792 ★

Compensation

Occupational Compensation: Nursing Assistant 2, Hospitals, Private

Data show earnings by this occupation. Occupations followed by numerical ratings (2, 3, etc.) indicate grades in the occupation. The higher the number, the higher the skill level required.

[In dollars per week]

Location	Compensation			Survey date
	FQ[1]	Median	TQ[2]	
Appleton-Oshkosh-Neenah, WI	282	314	343	05/01/94
Baltimore, MD	302	331	356	05/01/95
Bergen-Passaic, NJ	364	413	437	10/01/95
Boise City, ID	278	298	312	11/01/94
Boston, MA	353	409	458	10/01/95
Charlotte-Gastonia-Rock Hill, NC-SC	265	309	356	09/01/94
Davenport-Rock Island-Moline, IA-IL	252	281	304	02/01/95
Gary-Hammond, IN	326	348	368	02/01/95
Jackson, MS	240	269	300	02/01/95
Lawrence-Haverhill, MA-NH	320	353	383	10/01/94
Memphis, TN-AR-MS	242	280	312	11/01/94
Miami-Hialeah, FL	252	281	308	10/01/94
Middlesex-Somerset-Hunterdon, NJ	332	380	422	03/01/95
Minneapolis-St. Paul, MN-WI	363	386	424	02/01/95
Monmouth-Ocean, NJ	315	365	394	09/01/94
New Orleans, LA	240	264	283	01/01/96
Oakland, CA	354	461	548	01/01/95
Parkersburg-Marietta, WV-OH	294	320	334	08/01/95
Philadelphia, PA-NJ	350	393	438	11/01/94
Portland, OR	374	400	419	11/09/95
Riverside-San Bernardino, CA	276	315	344	11/01/95
Rochester, NY	287	322	348	11/01/94
Saginaw-Bay City-Midland, MI	292	317	331	06/01/95
San Jose, CA	417	480	547	07/01/94
Scranton-Wilkes Barre, PA	259	294	318	11/01/94
South Bend-Mishawaka, IN	288	335	382	09/01/94
Wilmington, DE-NJ-MD	295	332	387	12/01/94

Source: U.S. Department of Labor. Bureau of Labor Statistics. *Occupational Compensation Survey.* Tables were assembled from data downloaded from http:// stats.bls.gov. *Notes:* 1. FQ stands for First Quartile and means that 25% of the workers surveyed earned less than the dollar amount shown. 2. TQ stands for Third Quartile and means that 75% of workers earned less than the dollar amount shown and 25% earned more than the dollar amount shown.

★ 793 ★

Compensation

Occupational Compensation: Nursing Assistant 2, Service Producing Industry

Data show earnings by this occupation. Occupations followed by numerical ratings (2, 3, etc.) indicate grades in the occupation. The higher the number, the higher the skill level required.

[In dollars per week]

Location	Compensation			Survey date
	FQ[1]	Median	TQ[2]	
Anaheim, CA	260	293	317	02/01/96
Baltimore, MD	246	290	335	05/01/95
Bergen-Passaic, NJ	300	348	382	10/01/95
Boston, MA	322	374	410	10/01/95
Lawrence-Haverhill, MA-NH	300	334	367	10/01/94
Memphis, TN-AR-MS	218	243	260	11/01/94
Miami-Hialeah, FL	245	269	290	10/01/94
Minneapolis-St. Paul, MN-WI	298	334	363	02/01/95
New Orleans, LA	176	211	245	01/01/96
New York, NY	381	409	465	05/01/95
Oakland, CA	280	361	407	01/01/95
Philadelphia, PA-NJ	266	309	339	11/01/94
Portland, OR	288	326	351	11/09/95
Riverside-San Bernardino, CA	216	258	287	11/01/95
Salt Lake City, UT	250	263	272	08/01/95

Source: U.S. Department of Labor. Bureau of Labor Statistics. *Occupational Compensation Survey.* Tables were assembled from data downloaded from http:// stats.bls.gov. *Notes:* 1. FQ stands for First Quartile and means that 25% of the workers surveyed earned less than the dollar amount shown. 2. TQ stands for Third Quartile and means that 75% of workers earned less than the dollar amount shown and 25% earned more than the dollar amount shown.

★ 794 ★

Compensation

Occupational Compensation: Personnel Clerk & Assistant 2, Health Services

Data show earnings by this occupation. Occupations followed by numerical ratings (2, 3, etc.) indicate grades in the occupation. The higher the number, the higher the skill level required.

[In dollars per week]

Location	Compensation			Survey date
	FQ[1]	Median	TQ[2]	
Health Services				
Baltimore, MD	-	440	-	05/01/95
Bergen-Passaic, NJ	-	412	-	10/01/95
Boston, MA	-	395	-	10/01/95

[Continued]

★ 794 ★

Occupational Compensation: Personnel Clerk & Assistant 2, Health Services
[Continued]

Location	Compensation			Survey date
	FQ[1]	Median	TQ[2]	
Jackson, MS	-	367	-	02/01/95
Memphis, TN-AR-MS	-	410	-	11/01/94
Miami-Hialeah, FL	-	373	-	10/01/94
Minneapolis-St. Paul, MN-WI	-	416	-	02/01/95
Monmouth-Ocean, NJ	410	449	487	09/01/94
Philadelphia, PA-NJ	430	455	483	11/01/94
Health Services, Private				
Saginaw-Bay City-Midland, MI	364	414	455	06/01/95
Baltimore, MD	-	440	-	05/01/95
Bergen-Passaic, NJ	-	412	-	10/01/95
Boston, MA	-	395	-	10/01/95
Jackson, MS	-	370	-	02/01/95
Miami-Hialeah, FL	-	373	-	10/01/94
Monmouth-Ocean, NJ	-	442	-	09/01/94
Philadelphia, PA-NJ	430	455	483	11/01/94
Saginaw-Bay City-Midland, MI	-	374	-	06/01/95

Source: U.S. Department of Labor. Bureau of Labor Statistics. *Occupational Compensation Survey.* Tables were assembled from data downloaded from http:// stats.bls.gov. *Notes:* 1. FQ stands for First Quartile and means that 25% of the workers surveyed earned less than the dollar amount shown. 2. TQ stands for Third Quartile and means that 75% of workers earned less than the dollar amount shown and 25% earned more than the dollar amount shown.

★ 795 ★

Compensation

Occupational Compensation: Personnel Clerk & Assistant 2, Hospitals

Data show earnings by this occupation. Occupations followed by numerical ratings (2, 3, etc.) indicate grades in the occupation. The higher the number, the higher the skill level required.

[In dollars per week]

Location	Compensation			Survey date
	FQ[1]	Median	TQ[2]	
Hospitals				
Baltimore, MD	-	440	-	05/01/95
Boston, MA	-	395	-	10/01/95
Jackson, MS	-	367	-	02/01/95
Memphis, TN-AR-MS	-	412	-	11/01/94
Monmouth-Ocean, NJ	-	450	-	09/01/94
Hospitals, Private				
Baltimore, MD	-	440	-	05/01/95
Boston, MA	-	395	-	10/01/95

[Continued]

★ 795 ★

Occupational Compensation: Personnel Clerk & Assistant 2, Hospitals

[Continued]

Location	Compensation			Survey date
	FQ[1]	Median	TQ[2]	
Jackson, MS	-	370	-	02/01/95
Monmouth-Ocean, NJ	-	450	-	09/01/94
Saginaw-Bay City-Midland, MI	375	419	455	06/01/95

Source: U.S. Department of Labor. Bureau of Labor Statistics. *Occupational Compensation Survey.* Tables were assembled from data downloaded from http:// stats.bls.gov. *Notes:* 1. FQ stands for First Quartile and means that 25% of the workers surveyed earned less than the dollar amount shown. 2. TQ stands for Third Quartile and means that 75% of workers earned less than the dollar amount shown and 25% earned more than the dollar amount shown.

★ 796 ★

Compensation

Occupational Compensation: Personnel Specialist 2, Health Services

Data show earnings by this occupation. Occupations followed by numerical ratings (2, 3, etc.) indicate grades in the occupation. The higher the number, the higher the skill level required.

[In dollars per week]

Location	Compensation			Survey date
	FQ[1]	Median	TQ[2]	
Health Services				
Anaheim, CA	-	668	-	02/01/96
Baltimore, MD	560	605	656	05/01/95
Bergen-Passaic, NJ	529	609	646	10/01/95
Boston, MA	537	619	666	10/01/95
Jackson, MS	-	545	-	02/01/95
Lawrence-Haverhill, MA-NH	-	551	-	10/01/94
Memphis, TN-AR-MS	385	488	596	11/01/94
Miami-Hialeah, FL	500	574	654	10/01/94
Minneapolis-St. Paul, MN-WI	577	597	620	02/01/95
Monmouth-Ocean, NJ	576	613	676	09/01/94
New Orleans, LA	486	518	539	01/01/96
Newark, NJ	577	634	635	06/01/95
Philadelphia, PA-NJ	474	544	619	11/01/94
Riverside-San Bernardino, CA	-	608	-	11/01/95
Rochester, NY	481	518	544	11/01/94
Salt Lake City, UT	-	549	-	08/01/95
San Jose, CA	-	674	-	07/01/94
Scranton-Wilkes Barre, PA	469	561	649	11/01/94
Health Services, Government				
Boston, MA	-	656	-	10/01/95

[Continued]

★ 796 ★

Occupational Compensation: Personnel Specialist 2, Health Services
[Continued]

Location	Compensation			Survey date
	FQ[1]	Median	TQ[2]	
Health Services, Private				
Anaheim, CA	-	668	-	02/01/96
Baltimore, MD	560	605	656	05/01/95
Bergen-Passaic, NJ	529	609	646	10/01/95
Boston, MA	537	615	659	10/01/95
Charlotte-Gastonia-Rock Hill, NC-SC	-	564	-	09/01/94
Jackson, MS	-	557	-	02/01/95
Lawrence-Haverhill, MA-NH	-	551	-	10/01/94
Memphis, TN-AR-MS	385	480	600	11/01/94
Miami-Hialeah, FL	500	571	654	10/01/94
Minneapolis-St. Paul, MN-WI	577	592	587	02/01/95
Monmouth-Ocean, NJ	576	609	665	09/01/94
New Orleans, LA	486	524	539	01/01/96
Newark, NJ	577	634	635	06/01/95
Philadelphia, PA-NJ	449	534	615	11/01/94
Riverside-San Bernardino, CA	-	617	-	11/01/95
Rochester, NY	481	518	544	11/01/94
Saginaw-Bay City-Midland, MI	585	735	844	06/01/95
Salt Lake City, UT	-	549	-	08/01/95
San Jose, CA	-	674	-	07/01/94
Scranton-Wilkes Barre, PA	442	519	647	11/01/94

Source: U.S. Department of Labor. Bureau of Labor Statistics. *Occupational Compensation Survey.* Tables were assembled from data downloaded from http:// stats.bls.gov. *Notes:* 1. FQ stands for First Quartile and means that 25% of the workers surveyed earned less than the dollar amount shown. 2. TQ stands for Third Quartile and means that 75% of workers earned less than the dollar amount shown and 25% earned more than the dollar amount shown.

★ 797 ★

Compensation

Occupational Compensation: Personnel Specialist 2, Hospitals

Data show earnings by this occupation. Occupations followed by numerical ratings (2, 3, etc.) indicate grades in the occupation. The higher the number, the higher the skill level required.

[In dollars per week]

Location	Compensation			Survey date
	FQ[1]	Median	TQ[2]	
Hospitals				
Baltimore, MD	577	629	671	05/01/95
Bergen-Passaic, NJ	-	655	-	10/01/95
Boston, MA	577	641	702	10/01/95
Jackson, MS	-	555	-	02/01/95

[Continued]

★ 797 ★

Occupational Compensation: Personnel Specialist 2, Hospitals

[Continued]

Location	Compensation			Survey date
	FQ[1]	Median	TQ[2]	
Memphis, TN-AR-MS	515	550	600	11/01/94
Miami-Hialeah, FL	500	577	654	10/01/94
Monmouth-Ocean, NJ	576	617	676	09/01/94
New Orleans, LA	-	508	-	01/01/96
Philadelphia, PA-NJ	532	595	640	11/01/94
Riverside-San Bernardino, CA	-	608	-	11/01/95
Rochester, NY	466	532	614	11/01/94
Scranton-Wilkes Barre, PA	449	535	647	11/01/94
Hospitals, Private				
Baltimore, MD	577	629	671	05/01/95
Bergen-Passaic, NJ	-	655	-	10/01/95
Boston, MA	580	646	702	10/01/95
Memphis, TN-AR-MS	-	552	-	11/01/94
Miami-Hialeah, FL	500	573	654	10/01/94
Monmouth-Ocean, NJ	576	617	676	09/01/94
New Orleans, LA	-	508	-	01/01/96
Philadelphia, PA-NJ	532	584	635	11/01/94
Riverside-San Bernardino, CA	-	617	-	11/01/95
Rochester, NY	466	532	614	11/01/94
Scranton-Wilkes Barre, PA	442	519	647	11/01/94
Saginaw-Bay City-Midland, MI	709	844	956	06/01/95

Source: U.S. Department of Labor. Bureau of Labor Statistics. *Occupational Compensation Survey.* Tables were assembled from data downloaded from http:// stats.bls.gov. *Notes:* 1. FQ stands for First Quartile and means that 25% of the workers surveyed earned less than the dollar amount shown. 2. TQ stands for Third Quartile and means that 75% of workers earned less than the dollar amount shown and 25% earned more than the dollar amount shown.

★ 798 ★

Compensation

Occupational Compensation: Personnel Specialist 4, Health Services

Data show earnings by this occupation. Occupations followed by numerical ratings (2, 3, etc.) indicate grades in the occupation. The higher the number, the higher the skill level required.

[In dollars per week]

Location	Compensation			Survey date
	FQ[1]	Median	TQ[2]	
Health Services				
Anaheim, CA	904	1,056	1,164	02/01/96
Baltimore, MD	799	985	1,138	05/01/95
Bergen-Passaic, NJ	995	1,066	1,137	10/01/95

[Continued]

★ 798 ★

Occupational Compensation: Personnel Specialist 4, Health Services

[Continued]

Location	Compensation			Survey date
	FQ[1]	Median	TQ[2]	
Boston, MA	894	1,011	1,104	10/01/95
Memphis, TN-AR-MS	-	848	-	11/01/94
Miami-Hialeah, FL	1,000	1,048	1,111	10/01/94
Minneapolis-St. Paul, MN-WI	841	867	932	02/01/95
New Orleans, LA	-	909	-	01/01/96
Newark, NJ	1,007	1,112	1,184	06/01/95
Oakland, CA	1,000	1,093	1,173	01/01/95
Philadelphia, PA-NJ	904	967	1,038	11/01/94
Riverside-San Bernardino, CA	-	948	-	11/01/95
Rochester, NY	865	928	1,039	11/01/94
Scranton-Wilkes Barre, PA	-	871	-	11/01/94
Health Services, Private				
Anaheim, CA	904	1,056	1,164	02/01/96
Baltimore, MD	920	1,071	1,154	05/01/95
Bergen-Passaic, NJ	995	1,066	1,137	10/01/95
Boston, MA	894	1,011	1,104	10/01/95
Miami-Hialeah, FL	1,000	1,048	1,111	10/01/94
Minneapolis-St. Paul, MN-WI	-	814	-	02/01/95
New Orleans, LA	-	909	-	01/01/96
Newark, NJ	1,032	1,124	1,188	06/01/95
Oakland, CA	1,000	1,093	1,173	01/01/95
Philadelphia, PA-NJ	904	968	1,040	11/01/94
Rochester, NY	-	911	-	11/01/94
Saginaw-Bay City-Midland, MI	-	976	-	06/01/95
Scranton-Wilkes Barre, PA	-	871	-	11/01/94

Source: U.S. Department of Labor. Bureau of Labor Statistics. *Occupational Compensation Survey.* Tables were assembled from data downloaded from http:// stats.bls.gov. *Notes:* 1. FQ stands for First Quartile and means that 25% of the workers surveyed earned less than the dollar amount shown. 2. TQ stands for Third Quartile and means that 75% of workers earned less than the dollar amount shown and 25% earned more than the dollar amount shown.

★ 799 ★
Compensation

Occupational Compensation: Personnel Specialist 4, Hospitals

Data show earnings by this occupation. Occupations followed by numerical ratings (2, 3, etc.) indicate grades in the occupation. The higher the number, the higher the skill level required.

[In dollars per week]

Location	Compensation			Survey date
	FQ[1]	Median	TQ[2]	
Hospitals				
Anaheim, CA	-	974	-	02/01/96
Baltimore, MD	783	991	1,140	05/01/95
Bergen-Passaic, NJ	-	1,088	-	10/01/95
Boston, MA	894	1,029	1,136	10/01/95
Memphis, TN-AR-MS	-	848	-	11/01/94
Miami-Hialeah, FL	-	1,025	-	10/01/94
Minneapolis-St. Paul, MN-WI	-	917	-	02/01/95
New Orleans, LA	-	909	-	01/01/96
Philadelphia, PA-NJ	894	990	1,040	11/01/94
Riverside-San Bernardino, CA	-	948	-	11/01/95
Rochester, NY	-	954	-	11/01/94
Scranton-Wilkes Barre, PA	-	953	-	11/01/94
Hospitals, Private				
Baltimore, MD	1,031	1,084	1,154	05/01/95
Bergen-Passaic, NJ	-	1,088	-	10/01/95
Boston, MA	894	1,029	1,136	10/01/95
Miami-Hialeah, FL	-	1,025	-	10/01/94
New Orleans, LA	-	909	-	01/01/96
Philadelphia, PA-NJ	913	992	1,040	11/01/94
Saginaw-Bay City-Midland, MI	-	976	-	06/01/95
Scranton-Wilkes Barre, PA	-	953	-	11/01/94

Source: U.S. Department of Labor. Bureau of Labor Statistics. *Occupational Compensation Survey.* Tables were assembled from data downloaded from http:// stats.bls.gov. *Notes:* 1. FQ stands for First Quartile and means that 25% of the workers surveyed earned less than the dollar amount shown. 2. TQ stands for Third Quartile and means that 75% of workers earned less than the dollar amount shown and 25% earned more than the dollar amount shown.

★ 800 ★

Compensation

Occupational Compensation: Secretary 2, Health Services

Data show earnings by this occupation. Occupations followed by numerical ratings (2, 3, etc.) indicate grades in the occupation. The higher the number, the higher the skill level required.

[In dollars per week]

Location	Compensation			Survey
	FQ[1]	Median	TQ[2]	date
Health Services				
Anaheim, CA	462	489	510	02/01/96
Appleton-Oshkosh-Neenah, WI	434	460	481	05/01/94
Baltimore, MD	436	457	482	05/01/95
Boston, MA	480	532	573	10/01/95
Jackson, MS	334	358	374	02/01/95
Lawrence-Haverhill, MA-NH	393	430	458	10/01/94
Memphis, TN-AR-MS	380	433	487	11/01/94
Miami-Hialeah, FL	434	464	494	10/01/94
Minneapolis-St. Paul, MN-WI	413	442	477	02/01/95
New Orleans, LA	333	389	437	01/01/96
Newark, NJ	405	449	490	06/01/95
Oakland, CA	536	541	600	01/01/95
Philadelphia, PA-NJ	440	484	530	11/01/94
Poughkeepsie, NY	376	433	478	08/01/94
Riverside-San Bernardino, CA	405	448	480	11/01/95
Rochester, NY	404	422	441	11/01/94
San Jose, CA	530	578	631	07/01/94
Scranton-Wilkes Barre, PA	329	369	421	11/01/94
Health Services, Government				
Boston, MA	490	507	518	10/01/95
New Orleans, LA	316	356	400	01/01/96
Health Services, Private				
Anaheim, CA	462	489	510	02/01/96
Appleton-Oshkosh-Neenah, WI	434	456	480	05/01/94
Baltimore, MD	438	466	490	05/01/95
Boston, MA	479	533	576	10/01/95
Charlotte-Gastonia-Rock Hill, NC-SC	394	469	526	09/01/94
Lawrence-Haverhill, MA-NH	393	428	454	10/01/94
Little Rock-North Little Rock, AR	-	404	-	12/01/94
Newark, NJ	405	449	490	06/01/95
Oakland, CA	536	541	600	01/01/95
Philadelphia, PA-NJ	440	484	530	11/01/94
Poughkeepsie, NY	376	433	478	08/01/94
Riverside-San Bernardino, CA	400	446	480	11/01/95
Rochester, NY	404	422	441	11/01/94
Saginaw-Bay City-Midland, MI	460	491	510	06/01/95

[Continued]

★ 800 ★

Occupational Compensation: Secretary 2, Health Services

[Continued]

Location	Compensation			Survey date
	FQ[1]	Median	TQ[2]	
San Jose, CA	530	578	631	07/01/94
Scranton-Wilkes Barre, PA	329	369	421	11/01/94

Source: U.S. Department of Labor. Bureau of Labor Statistics. *Occupational Compensation Survey.* Tables were assembled from data downloaded from http:// stats.bls.gov. *Notes:* 1. FQ stands for First Quartile and means that 25% of the workers surveyed earned less than the dollar amount shown. 2. TQ stands for Third Quartile and means that 75% of workers earned less than the dollar amount shown and 25% earned more than the dollar amount shown.

★ 801 ★

Compensation

Occupational Compensation: Secretary 2, Hospitals

Data show earnings by this occupation. Occupations followed by numerical ratings (2, 3, etc.) indicate grades in the occupation. The higher the number, the higher the skill level required.

[In dollars per week]

Location	Compensation			Survey date
	FQ[1]	Median	TQ[2]	
Hospitals				
Anaheim, CA	464	501	513	02/01/96
Appleton-Oshkosh-Neenah, WI	-	481	-	05/01/94
Baltimore, MD	435	454	482	05/01/95
Boston, MA	482	536	579	10/01/95
Jackson, MS	334	358	374	02/01/95
Lawrence-Haverhill, MA-NH	390	428	454	10/01/94
Memphis, TN-AR-MS	381	439	488	11/01/94
New Orleans, LA	350	408	453	01/01/96
Oakland, CA	561	589	615	01/01/95
Philadelphia, PA-NJ	443	486	532	11/01/94
Riverside-San Bernardino, CA	420	461	497	11/01/95
San Jose, CA	532	579	631	07/01/94
Scranton-Wilkes Barre, PA	329	369	421	11/01/94
Hospitals, Government				
Boston, MA	490	507	518	10/01/95
Hospitals, Private				
Appleton-Oshkosh-Neenah, WI	-	478	-	05/01/94
Baltimore, MD	437	464	489	05/01/95
Boston, MA	481	537	583	10/01/95
Lawrence-Haverhill, MA-NH	390	426	453	10/01/94
Oakland, CA	561	589	615	01/01/95
Philadelphia, PA-NJ	443	486	532	11/01/94
Riverside-San Bernardino, CA	420	459	497	11/01/95

[Continued]

★ 801 ★

Occupational Compensation: Secretary 2, Hospitals

[Continued]

Location	Compensation			Survey date
	FQ[1]	Median	TQ[2]	
San Jose, CA	532	579	631	07/01/94
Scranton-Wilkes Barre, PA	329	369	421	11/01/94

Source: U.S. Department of Labor. Bureau of Labor Statistics. *Occupational Compensation Survey.* Tables were assembled from data downloaded from http:// stats.bls.gov. *Notes:* 1. FQ stands for First Quartile and means that 25% of the workers surveyed earned less than the dollar amount shown. 2. TQ stands for Third Quartile and means that 75% of workers earned less than the dollar amount shown and 25% earned more than the dollar amount shown.

★ 802 ★

Compensation

Occupational Compensation: Secretary 4, Health Services

Data show earnings by this occupation. Occupations followed by numerical ratings (2, 3, etc.) indicate grades in the occupation. The higher the number, the higher the skill level required.

[In dollars per week]

Location	Compensation			Survey date
	FQ[1]	Median	TQ[2]	
Health Services				
Anaheim, CA	635	673	734	02/01/96
Baltimore, MD	553	581	600	05/01/95
Boston, MA	577	633	688	10/01/95
Lawrence-Haverhill, MA-NH	-	575	-	10/01/94
Miami-Hialeah, FL	578	625	675	10/01/94
Minneapolis-St. Paul, MN-WI	565	607	626	02/01/95
New Orleans, LA	-	537	-	01/01/96
Newark, NJ	593	680	714	06/01/95
Oakland, CA	692	721	769	01/01/95
Philadelphia, PA-NJ	544	589	632	11/01/94
Portland, OR	-	684	-	11/09/95
Poughkeepsie, NY	669	694	712	08/01/94
Riverside-San Bernardino, CA	641	676	704	11/01/95
San Jose, CA	633	685	698	07/01/94
Scranton-Wilkes Barre, PA	-	525	-	11/01/94
Health Services, Government				
Rochester, NY	-	692	-	11/01/94
Health Services, Private				
Anaheim, CA	635	674	734	02/01/96
Baltimore, MD	553	581	600	05/01/95
Boston, MA	577	633	691	10/01/95
Lawrence-Haverhill, MA-NH	-	578	-	10/01/94

[Continued]

★ 802 ★

Occupational Compensation: Secretary 4, Health Services

[Continued]

Location	Compensation			Survey date
	FQ[1]	Median	TQ[2]	
Miami-Hialeah, FL	-	606	-	10/01/94
Minneapolis-St. Paul, MN-WI	579	610	634	02/01/95
Newark, NJ	593	678	714	06/01/95
Oakland, CA	679	728	773	01/01/95
Philadelphia, PA-NJ	544	584	627	11/01/94
Portland, OR	-	684	-	11/09/95
Riverside-San Bernardino, CA	641	677	704	11/01/95
San Jose, CA	640	688	699	07/01/94
Scranton-Wilkes Barre, PA	-	525	-	11/01/94

Source: U.S. Department of Labor. Bureau of Labor Statistics. *Occupational Compensation Survey.* Tables were assembled from data downloaded from http:// stats.bls.gov. *Notes:* 1. FQ stands for First Quartile and means that 25% of the workers surveyed earned less than the dollar amount shown. 2. TQ stands for Third Quartile and means that 75% of workers earned less than the dollar amount shown and 25% earned more than the dollar amount shown.

★ 803 ★

Compensation

Occupational Compensation: Secretary 4, Hospitals

Data show earnings by this occupation. Occupations followed by numerical ratings (2, 3, etc.) indicate grades in the occupation. The higher the number, the higher the skill level required.

[In dollars per week]

Location	Compensation			Survey date
	FQ[1]	Median	TQ[2]	
Hospitals				
Anaheim, CA	622	651	673	02/01/96
Boston, MA	583	640	700	10/01/95
Lawrence-Haverhill, MA-NH	-	596	-	10/01/94
Miami-Hialeah, FL	578	625	675	10/01/94
Minneapolis-St. Paul, MN-WI	593	615	670	02/01/95
Oakland, CA	692	729	773	01/01/95
Philadelphia, PA-NJ	537	590	634	11/01/94
Portland, OR	-	665	-	11/09/95
Riverside-San Bernardino, CA	641	676	704	11/01/95
San Jose, CA	-	725	-	07/01/94
Scranton-Wilkes Barre, PA	-	525	-	11/01/94
Hospitals, Private				
Boston, MA	583	640	705	10/01/95
Lawrence-Haverhill, MA-NH	-	603	-	10/01/94
Miami-Hialeah, FL	-	603	-	10/01/94
Minneapolis-St. Paul, MN-WI	616	625	679	02/01/95

[Continued]

★ 803 ★

Occupational Compensation: Secretary 4, Hospitals
[Continued]

Location	Compensation			Survey date
	FQ[1]	Median	TQ[2]	
Oakland, CA	679	756	773	01/01/95
Philadelphia, PA-NJ	537	586	634	11/01/94
Portland, OR	-	665	-	11/09/95
Riverside-San Bernardino, CA	641	677	704	11/01/95
San Jose, CA	-	725	-	07/01/94
Scranton-Wilkes Barre, PA	-	525	-	11/01/94

Source: U.S. Department of Labor. Bureau of Labor Statistics. *Occupational Compensation Survey.* Tables were assembled from data downloaded from http:// stats.bls.gov. *Notes:* 1. FQ stands for First Quartile and means that 25% of the workers surveyed earned less than the dollar amount shown. 2. TQ stands for Third Quartile and means that 75% of workers earned less than the dollar amount shown and 25% earned more than the dollar amount shown.

★ 804 ★
Compensation

Occupational Compensation: Secretary 5, Health Services

Data show earnings by this occupation. Occupations followed by numerical ratings (2, 3, etc.) indicate grades in the occupation. The higher the number, the higher the skill level required.

[In dollars per week]

Location	Compensation			Survey date
	FQ[1]	Median	TQ[2]	
Health Services, Private				
Anaheim, CA	-	789	-	02/01/96
Boston, MA	764	785	784	10/01/95
Philadelphia, PA-NJ	653	685	740	11/01/94

Source: U.S. Department of Labor. Bureau of Labor Statistics. *Occupational Compensation Survey.* Tables were assembled from data downloaded from http:// stats.bls.gov. *Notes:* 1. FQ stands for First Quartile and means that 25% of the workers surveyed earned less than the dollar amount shown. 2. TQ stands for Third Quartile and means that 75% of workers earned less than the dollar amount shown and 25% earned more than the dollar amount shown.

★ 805 ★

Compensation

Occupational Compensation: Secretary 5, Hospitals

Data show earnings by this occupation. Occupations followed by numerical ratings (2, 3, etc.) indicate grades in the occupation. The higher the number, the higher the skill level required.

[In dollars per week]

Location	Compensation			Survey date
	FQ[1]	Median	TQ[2]	
Hospitals				
Anaheim, CA	-	776	-	02/01/96
Boston, MA	-	792	-	10/01/95
Philadelphia, PA-NJ	653	685	740	11/01/94
Hospitals, Private				
Boston, MA	-	792	-	10/01/95
Philadelphia, PA-NJ	653	685	740	11/01/94

Source: U.S. Department of Labor. Bureau of Labor Statistics. *Occupational Compensation Survey.* Tables were assembled from data downloaded from http:// stats.bls.gov. *Notes:* 1. FQ stands for First Quartile and means that 25% of the workers surveyed earned less than the dollar amount shown. 2. TQ stands for Third Quartile and means that 75% of workers earned less than the dollar amount shown and 25% earned more than the dollar amount shown.

★ 806 ★

Compensation

Occupational Compensation: Shipping & Receiving Clerk, Health Services

Data show earnings by this occupation. Occupations followed by numerical ratings (2, 3, etc.) indicate grades in the occupation. The higher the number, the higher the skill level required.

[In dollars per hour]

Location	Compensation			Survey date
	FQ[1]	Median	TQ[2]	
Health Services				
Anaheim, CA	8.28	9.55	10.45	02/01/96
Baltimore, MD	7.51	8.50	9.64	05/01/95
Bergen-Passaic, NJ	8.62	10.21	12.39	10/01/95
Boston, MA	9.71	10.78	11.90	10/01/95
Davenport-Rock Island-Moline, IA-IL	-	8.29	-	02/01/95
Memphis, TN-AR-MS	-	7.84	-	11/01/94
Miami-Hialeah, FL	-	7.86	-	10/01/94
Newark, NJ	-	11.27	-	06/01/95
Philadelphia, PA-NJ	9.61	10.36	11.08	11/01/94
Riverside-San Bernardino, CA	7.20	8.33	9.63	11/01/95
Salt Lake City, UT	-	7.38	-	08/01/95

[Continued]

★ 806 ★

Occupational Compensation: Shipping & Receiving Clerk, Health Services
[Continued]

Location	Compensation			Survey date
	FQ[1]	Median	TQ[2]	
Health Services, Government				
Boston, MA	-	10.72	-	10/01/95
Health Services, Private				
Anaheim, CA	8.28	9.55	10.45	02/01/96
Baltimore, MD	7.51	8.50	9.64	05/01/95
Bergen-Passaic, NJ	8.62	10.21	12.39	10/01/95
Boston, MA	9.73	10.79	11.90	10/01/95
Charlotte-Gastonia-Rock Hill, NC-SC	6.56	7.45	7.96	09/01/94
Davenport-Rock Island-Moline, IA-IL	-	8.29	-	02/01/95
Memphis, TN-AR-MS	-	7.84	-	11/01/94
Miami-Hialeah, FL	-	7.86	-	10/01/94
Newark, NJ	-	11.27	-	06/01/95
Philadelphia, PA-NJ	9.61	10.36	11.08	11/01/94
Riverside-San Bernardino, CA	7.20	8.33	9.63	11/01/95
Salt Lake City, UT	-	7.38	-	08/01/95

Source: U.S. Department of Labor. Bureau of Labor Statistics. *Occupational Compensation Survey.* Tables were assembled from data downloaded from http:// stats.bls.gov. *Notes:* 1. FQ stands for First Quartile and means that 25% of the workers surveyed earned less than the dollar amount shown. 2. TQ stands for Third Quartile and means that 75% of workers earned less than the dollar amount shown and 25% earned more than the dollar amount shown.

★ 807 ★

Compensation

Occupational Compensation: Shipping & Receiving Clerk, Hospitals

Data show earnings by this occupation. Occupations followed by numerical ratings (2, 3, etc.) indicate grades in the occupation. The higher the number, the higher the skill level required.

[In dollars per hour]

Location	Compensation			Survey date
	FQ[1]	Median	TQ[2]	
Hospitals				
Anaheim, CA	8.04	9.37	10.15	02/01/96
Baltimore, MD	7.51	8.50	9.64	05/01/95
Boston, MA	9.70	10.78	11.90	10/01/95
Davenport-Rock Island-Moline, IA-IL	-	8.29	-	02/01/95
Memphis, TN-AR-MS	-	7.84	-	11/01/94
Miami-Hialeah, FL	-	8.02	-	10/01/94
Philadelphia, PA-NJ	9.10	10.29	11.34	11/01/94
Riverside-San Bernardino, CA	7.20	8.33	9.63	11/01/95
Rochester, NY	-	9.40	-	11/01/94

[Continued]

★ 807 ★

Occupational Compensation: Shipping & Receiving Clerk, Hospitals
[Continued]

Location	Compensation			Survey date
	FQ[1]	Median	TQ[2]	
Hospitals, Government				
Boston, MA	-	10.72	-	10/01/95
Hospitals, Private				
Baltimore, MD	7.51	8.50	9.64	05/01/95
Boston, MA	9.73	10.79	11.90	10/01/95
Charlotte-Gastonia-Rock Hill, NC-SC	6.56	7.41	7.95	09/01/94
Davenport-Rock Island-Moline, IA-IL	-	8.29	-	02/01/95
Memphis, TN-AR-MS	-	7.84	-	11/01/94
Miami-Hialeah, FL	-	8.02	-	10/01/94
Philadelphia, PA-NJ	9.10	10.29	11.34	11/01/94
Riverside-San Bernardino, CA	7.20	8.33	9.63	11/01/95
Rochester, NY	-	9.40	-	11/01/94

Source: U.S. Department of Labor. Bureau of Labor Statistics. *Occupational Compensation Survey.* Tables were assembled from data downloaded from http:// stats.bls.gov. *Notes:* 1. FQ stands for First Quartile and means that 25% of the workers surveyed earned less than the dollar amount shown. 2. TQ stands for Third Quartile and means that 75% of workers earned less than the dollar amount shown and 25% earned more than the dollar amount shown.

★ 808 ★

Compensation

Occupational Compensation: Switchboard Operator-Receptionist, Health Services

Data show earnings by this occupation. Occupations followed by numerical ratings (2, 3, etc.) indicate grades in the occupation. The higher the number, the higher the skill level required.

[In dollars per week]

Location	Compensation			Survey date
	FQ[1]	Median	TQ[2]	
Health Services				
Anaheim, CA	311	348	378	02/01/96
Appleton-Oshkosh-Neenah, WI	-	288	-	05/01/94
Baltimore, MD	269	313	346	05/01/95
Bergen-Passaic, NJ	397	424	453	10/01/95
Billings, MT	-	317	-	09/01/94
Boston, MA	346	375	406	10/01/95
Bradenton, FL	226	246	260	04/01/94
Gary-Hammond, IN	229	276	373	02/01/95
Lawrence-Haverhill, MA-NH	329	354	358	10/01/94
Memphis, TN-AR-MS	272	287	296	11/01/94
Minneapolis-St. Paul, MN-WI	330	345	364	02/01/95
Monmouth-Ocean, NJ	297	376	477	09/01/94
New Orleans, LA	221	255	277	01/01/96

[Continued]

★ 808 ★

Occupational Compensation: Switchboard Operator-Receptionist, Health Services
[Continued]

Location	Compensation			Survey date
	FQ[1]	Median	TQ[2]	
Newark, NJ	325	371	400	06/01/95
Oakland, CA	372	411	442	01/01/95
Philadelphia, PA-NJ	301	357	392	11/01/94
Portland, OR	320	370	412	11/09/95
Poughkeepsie, NY	280	319	350	08/01/94
Rochester, NY	306	333	370	11/01/94
Salt Lake City, UT	268	300	317	08/01/95
San Angelo, TX	-	226	-	10/01/94
San Jose, CA	340	365	412	07/01/94
Scranton-Wilkes Barre, PA	314	332	340	11/01/94
South Bend-Mishawaka, IN	280	322	380	09/01/94
Health Services, Government				
Boston, MA	396	396	406	10/01/95
Health Services, Private				
Anaheim, CA	311	348	378	02/01/96
Appleton-Oshkosh-Neenah, WI	-	288	-	05/01/94
Augusta, GA-SC	280	304	337	06/01/94
Baltimore, MD	263	310	332	05/01/95
Bergen-Passaic, NJ	397	424	453	10/01/95
Billings, MT	-	317	-	09/01/94
Boise City, ID	-	316	-	11/01/94
Boston, MA	346	369	387	10/01/95
Bradenton, FL	226	246	260	04/01/94
Charlotte-Gastonia-Rock Hill, NC-SC	280	313	336	09/01/94
Gary-Hammond, IN	229	276	373	02/01/95
Lawrence-Haverhill, MA-NH	329	354	358	10/01/94
Little Rock-North Little Rock, AR	242	276	300	12/01/94
Memphis, TN-AR-MS	272	281	296	11/01/94
Middlesex-Somerset-Hunterdon, NJ	-	363	-	03/01/95
Minneapolis-St. Paul, MN-WI	330	345	364	02/01/95
Monmouth-Ocean, NJ	297	376	477	09/01/94
New Orleans, LA	220	254	277	01/01/96
Newark, NJ	325	371	400	06/01/95
Oakland, CA	372	411	442	01/01/95
Philadelphia, PA-NJ	301	357	392	11/01/94
Portland, OR	320	370	412	11/09/95
Poughkeepsie, NY	280	319	350	08/01/94
Rochester, NY	306	333	370	11/01/94
Saginaw-Bay City-Midland, MI	228	240	257	06/01/95
Salt Lake City, UT	268	300	317	08/01/95
San Angelo, TX	-	226	-	10/01/94
San Jose, CA	340	365	412	07/01/94
Scranton-Wilkes Barre, PA	314	332	340	11/01/94

[Continued]

★ 808 ★

Occupational Compensation: Switchboard Operator-Receptionist, Health Services
[Continued]

Location	Compensation			Survey date
	FQ[1]	Median	TQ[2]	
South Bend-Mishawaka, IN	291	325	380	09/01/94
Wilmington, DE-NJ-MD	254	307	328	12/01/94

Source: U.S. Department of Labor. Bureau of Labor Statistics. *Occupational Compensation Survey.* Tables were assembled from data downloaded from http:// stats.bls.gov. *Notes:* 1. FQ stands for First Quartile and means that 25% of the workers surveyed earned less than the dollar amount shown. 2. TQ stands for Third Quartile and means that 75% of workers earned less than the dollar amount shown and 25% earned more than the dollar amount shown.

★ 809 ★

Compensation

Occupational Compensation: Switchboard Operator-Receptionist, Hospitals

Data show earnings by this occupation. Occupations followed by numerical ratings (2, 3, etc.) indicate grades in the occupation. The higher the number, the higher the skill level required.

[In dollars per week]

Location	Compensation			Survey date
	FQ[1]	Median	TQ[2]	
Hospitals				
Anaheim, CA	373	396	412	02/01/96
Baltimore, MD	266	316	360	05/01/95
Boston, MA	372	400	410	10/01/95
Little Rock-North Little Rock, AR	215	257	300	12/01/94
Memphis, TN-AR-MS	250	281	296	11/01/94
Miami-Hialeah, FL	250	293	338	10/01/94
New Orleans, LA	223	257	267	01/01/96
Philadelphia, PA-NJ	316	374	408	11/01/94
Portland, OR	376	415	456	11/09/95
Riverside-San Bernardino, CA	300	317	347	11/01/95
Rochester, NY	297	312	335	11/01/94
Scranton-Wilkes Barre, PA	-	344	-	11/01/94
South Bend-Mishawaka, IN	-	318	-	09/01/94
Hospitals, Government				
Boston, MA	406	398	408	10/01/95
Hospitals, Private				
Baltimore, MD	258	304	355	05/01/95
Boston, MA	367	401	418	10/01/95
Memphis, TN-AR-MS	250	281	296	11/01/94
Miami-Hialeah, FL	250	293	338	10/01/94
New Orleans, LA	223	256	265	01/01/96
Philadelphia, PA-NJ	316	374	408	11/01/94
Portland, OR	376	415	456	11/09/95

[Continued]

★ 809 ★

Occupational Compensation: Switchboard Operator-Receptionist, Hospitals

[Continued]

Location	Compensation			Survey date
	FQ[1]	Median	TQ[2]	
Rochester, NY	297	312	335	11/01/94
Scranton-Wilkes Barre, PA	-	344	-	11/01/94
South Bend-Mishawaka, IN	-	323	-	09/01/94

Source: U.S. Department of Labor. Bureau of Labor Statistics. *Occupational Compensation Survey.* Tables were assembled from data downloaded from http:// stats.bls.gov. *Notes:* 1. FQ stands for First Quartile and means that 25% of the workers surveyed earned less than the dollar amount shown. 2. TQ stands for Third Quartile and means that 75% of workers earned less than the dollar amount shown and 25% earned more than the dollar amount shown.

★ 810 ★

Compensation

Occupational Compensation: Systems Analyst 2, Health Services

Data show earnings by this occupation. Occupations followed by numerical ratings (2, 3, etc.) indicate grades in the occupation. The higher the number, the higher the skill level required.

[In dollars per week]

Location	Compensation			Survey date
	FQ[1]	Median	TQ[2]	
Health Services				
Anaheim, CA	774	900	1,020	02/01/96
Baltimore, MD	867	971	1,058	05/01/95
Boston, MA	865	936	1,010	10/01/95
Memphis, TN-AR-MS	707	804	881	11/01/94
Miami-Hialeah, FL	802	913	1,064	10/01/94
Minneapolis-St. Paul, MN-WI	796	868	932	02/01/95
Monmouth-Ocean, NJ	-	853	-	09/01/94
New Orleans, LA	673	794	950	01/01/96
Newark, NJ	983	1,037	1,132	06/01/95
Oakland, CA	1,027	1,061	1,097	01/01/95
Philadelphia, PA-NJ	754	824	908	11/01/94
Riverside-San Bernardino, CA	-	882	-	11/01/95
Rochester, NY	-	808	-	11/01/94
San Jose, CA	-	980	-	07/01/94
Visalia-Tulare-Porterville, CA	-	935	-	07/01/94
Health Services, Government				
Visalia-Tulare-Porterville, CA	-	935	-	07/01/94
Health Services, Private				
Anaheim, CA	774	895	1,020	02/01/96
Baltimore, MD	867	971	1,058	05/01/95
Boston, MA	865	936	1,010	10/01/95
Memphis, TN-AR-MS	701	793	880	11/01/94

[Continued]

★ 810 ★

Occupational Compensation: Systems Analyst 2, Health Services

[Continued]

Location	Compensation			Survey date
	FQ[1]	Median	TQ[2]	
Miami-Hialeah, FL	-	897	-	10/01/94
Minneapolis-St. Paul, MN-WI	798	887	965	02/01/95
Monmouth-Ocean, NJ	-	853	-	09/01/94
Newark, NJ	983	1,037	1,132	06/01/95
Oakland, CA	1,022	1,053	1,080	01/01/95
Philadelphia, PA-NJ	754	824	908	11/01/94
Riverside-San Bernardino, CA	-	882	-	11/01/95
Rochester, NY	-	808	-	11/01/94
Saginaw-Bay City-Midland, MI	-	794	-	06/01/95

Source: U.S. Department of Labor. Bureau of Labor Statistics. *Occupational Compensation Survey.* Tables were assembled from data downloaded from http:// stats.bls.gov. *Notes:* 1. FQ stands for First Quartile and means that 25% of the workers surveyed earned less than the dollar amount shown. 2. TQ stands for Third Quartile and means that 75% of workers earned less than the dollar amount shown and 25% earned more than the dollar amount shown.

★ 811 ★

Compensation

Occupational Compensation: Systems Analyst 2, Hospitals

Data show earnings by this occupation. Occupations followed by numerical ratings (2, 3, etc.) indicate grades in the occupation. The higher the number, the higher the skill level required.

[In dollars per week]

Location	Compensation			Survey date
	FQ[1]	Median	TQ[2]	
Hospitals				
Anaheim, CA	-	820	-	02/01/96
Baltimore, MD	865	926	998	05/01/95
Boston, MA	857	937	1,010	10/01/95
Memphis, TN-AR-MS	707	804	881	11/01/94
Miami-Hialeah, FL	802	913	1,064	10/01/94
Minneapolis-St. Paul, MN-WI	795	842	896	02/01/95
Monmouth-Ocean, NJ	-	853	-	09/01/94
New Orleans, LA	673	794	950	01/01/96
Oakland, CA	1,027	1,061	1,097	01/01/95
Philadelphia, PA-NJ	754	824	908	11/01/94
Portland, OR	757	786	875	11/09/95
Riverside-San Bernardino, CA	-	882	-	11/01/95
Rochester, NY	-	808	-	11/01/94
Visalia-Tulare-Porterville, CA	-	930	-	07/01/94
Hospitals, Government				
Visalia-Tulare-Porterville, CA	-	930	-	07/01/94

[Continued]

★ 811 ★

Occupational Compensation: Systems Analyst 2, Hospitals
[Continued]

Location	Compensation			Survey date
	FQ[1]	Median	TQ[2]	
Hospitals, Private				
Baltimore, MD	865	926	998	05/01/95
Boston, MA	856	937	1,010	10/01/95
Memphis, TN-AR-MS	701	793	880	11/01/94
Miami-Hialeah, FL	-	897	-	10/01/94
Monmouth-Ocean, NJ	-	853	-	09/01/94
Oakland, CA	1,022	1,053	1,080	01/01/95
Philadelphia, PA-NJ	754	824	908	11/01/94
Riverside-San Bernardino, CA	-	882	-	11/01/95
Rochester, NY	-	808	-	11/01/94

Source: U.S. Department of Labor. Bureau of Labor Statistics. *Occupational Compensation Survey.* Tables were assembled from data downloaded from http:// stats.bls.gov. *Notes:* 1. FQ stands for First Quartile and means that 25% of the workers surveyed earned less than the dollar amount shown. 2. TQ stands for Third Quartile and means that 75% of workers earned less than the dollar amount shown and 25% earned more than the dollar amount shown.

★ 812 ★

Compensation

Occupational Compensation: Truck Driver, Light Truck, Health Services

Data show earnings by this occupation. Occupations followed by numerical ratings (2, 3, etc.) indicate grades in the occupation. The higher the number, the higher the skill level required.

[In dollars per hour]

Location	Compensation			Survey date
	FQ[1]	Median	TQ[2]	
Health Services				
Anaheim, CA	7.98	8.34	9.19	02/01/96
Boston, MA	7.06	9.64	10.14	10/01/95
Memphis, TN-AR-MS	6.33	7.42	8.72	11/01/94
Minneapolis-St. Paul, MN-WI	-	9.39	-	02/01/95
Riverside-San Bernardino, CA	7.05	7.34	7.56	11/01/95
Rochester, NY	-	9.33	-	11/01/94
Health Services, Private				
Anaheim, CA	7.98	8.34	9.19	02/01/96
Boston, MA	7.06	9.54	10.00	10/01/95
Charlotte-Gastonia-Rock Hill, NC-SC	-	8.35	-	09/01/94

[Continued]

★ 812 ★

Occupational Compensation: Truck Driver, Light Truck, Health Services

[Continued]

Location	Compensation			Survey date
	FQ[1]	Median	TQ[2]	
Riverside-San Bernardino, CA	7.05	7.34	7.56	11/01/95
Rochester, NY	-	9.33	-	11/01/94

Source: U.S. Department of Labor. Bureau of Labor Statistics. *Occupational Compensation Survey.* Tables were assembled from data downloaded from http://stats.bls.gov. *Notes:* 1. FQ stands for First Quartile and means that 25% of the workers surveyed earned less than the dollar amount shown. 2. TQ stands for Third Quartile and means that 75% of workers earned less than the dollar amount shown and 25% earned more than the dollar amount shown.

★ 813 ★

Compensation

Occupational Compensation: Warehouse Specialist, Health Services

Data show earnings by this occupation. Occupations followed by numerical ratings (2, 3, etc.) indicate grades in the occupation. The higher the number, the higher the skill level required.

[In dollars per hour]

Location	Compensation			Survey date
	FQ[1]	Median	TQ[2]	
Health Services				
Anaheim, CA	10.17	11.17	10.95	02/01/96
Boston, MA	10.73	11.56	12.66	10/01/95
Lawrence-Haverhill, MA-NH	-	9.72	-	10/01/94
Memphis, TN-AR-MS	-	7.59	-	11/01/94
Minneapolis-St. Paul, MN-WI	11.21	11.96	12.98	02/01/95
Portland, OR	-	10.45	-	11/09/95
Riverside-San Bernardino, CA	11.31	12.69	14.07	11/01/95
Salt Lake City, UT	6.63	7.41	8.25	08/01/95
San Jose, CA	12.24	12.73	14.04	07/01/94
Health Services, Government				
Minneapolis-St. Paul, MN-WI	11.21	11.96	12.98	02/01/95
Health Services, Private				
Boston, MA	9.85	10.97	11.61	10/01/95
Riverside-San Bernardino, CA	-	11.18	-	11/01/95

Source: U.S. Department of Labor. Bureau of Labor Statistics. *Occupational Compensation Survey.* Tables were assembled from data downloaded from http://stats.bls.gov. *Notes:* 1. FQ stands for First Quartile and means that 25% of the workers surveyed earned less than the dollar amount shown. 2. TQ stands for Third Quartile and means that 75% of workers earned less than the dollar amount shown and 25% earned more than the dollar amount shown.

★ 814 ★

Compensation

Occupational Compensation: Warehouse Specialist, Hospitals

Data show earnings by this occupation. Occupations followed by numerical ratings (2, 3, etc.) indicate grades in the occupation. The higher the number, the higher the skill level required.

[In dollars per hour]

Location	Compensation			Survey date
	FQ[1]	Median	TQ[2]	
Hospitals				
Anaheim, CA	9.97	10.53	10.95	02/01/96
Boston, MA	10.73	11.56	12.66	10/01/95
Lawrence-Haverhill, MA-NH	-	9.72	-	10/01/94
Riverside-San Bernardino, CA	-	13.07	-	11/01/95
Hospitals, Private				
Boston, MA	9.85	10.97	11.61	10/01/95
Riverside-San Bernardino, CA	-	11.51	-	11/01/95

Source: U.S. Department of Labor. Bureau of Labor Statistics. *Occupational Compensation Survey.* Tables were assembled from data downloaded from http:// stats.bls.gov. *Notes:* 1. FQ stands for First Quartile and means that 25% of the workers surveyed earned less than the dollar amount shown. 2. TQ stands for Third Quartile and means that 75% of workers earned less than the dollar amount shown and 25% earned more than the dollar amount shown.

★ 815 ★

Compensation

Physicians: Median Compensation in 1993 and 1994

Field	Compensation ($000)	
	1993	1994
Family practice	120	122
Internal medicine	129	134
Cardiology (invasive)	301	313
Obstetrics and gynecology	205	211
Pediatrics	125	126
Orthopedic surgery	289	292

Source: Medical Tribune, 21 September 1995, p. 18. Primary source: 1995 CEJKA & Company/ MGMA *Physician Compensation and Production Survey.*

★ 816 ★

Compensation

Salaries and Wages in Leading Occupations: Information Specialist in the Health Care Industry

Profession	Entry level $	Midlevel $	Top $
Information specialist	27,500	47,500	82,500

Source: "Career Guide: 20 Hot Job Tracks." *U.S. News & World Report,* 30 October 1995, p. 104. Primary source: American Health Information Management Association; American Hospital Association; Bureau of Labor Statistics.

★ 817 ★

Compensation

Salaries and Wages in Selected Leading Health Care Occupations

Profession	Median salary $
Medical technician	19,000-20,000
Medical technologist	23,000-24,000
Dietitian	27,924
Staff nurse, (Registered)	35,464
Speech therapist	36,036
Pharmacist	49,608
Physician assistant	50,000-55,000
Nurse practitioner, (Registered)	50,000-55,000

Source: "Career Guide: 20 Hot Job Tracks." *U.S. News & World Report,* 30 October 1995, p. 104. Primary source: American Health Information Management Association; American Hospital Association; Bureau of Labor Statistics.

★ 818 ★

Compensation

Salaries and Wages of CEOs in the Managed Care Industry: 1996

Names of managed care companies are shown in parentheses.

[In millions of dollars]

CEO compensation	Amount
Norman C. Payson, MD (Healthsource)	14.3
Daniel D. Crowley (Foundation Health Corp.)	12.1
William Wayne McGuire (United Healthcare Corp.)	6.1
George T. Jochum (Mid-Atlantic Medical Services)	4.8
Leonard Abramson (U.S. Healthcare)	3.9
Stephen F. Wiggins (Oxford Health Plans)	2.8
David A. Jones (Humana)	2.2

Source: "Snapshots of the Workplace Health Industry: Extra Pocket Money." *Workplace Vitality* (July/August 1996), p. 15. Primary source: Crystal Report: Hospitals & Health Networks.

Education

★ 819 ★

Associate Degrees Conferred in the Health Field, by Sex, Race, and Ethnicity: 1993-1994

Race/ethnicity/sex	All fields, total[1]	Health professions and related sciences
Total	540,923	95,832
White, non-Hispanic	428,273	81,747
Black, non-Hispanic	46,451	6,758
Hispanic	32,438	3,469
Asian/Pacific Islander	18,659	2,293
American Indian/Alaskan Native	4,975	761
Non-resident alien	10,127	804
Men		
Total	220,191	15,476
White, non-Hispanic	174,947	12,616
Black, non-Hispanic	17,379	1,140
Hispanic	13,395	826
Asian/Pacific Islander	8,403	571

[Continued]

★ 819 ★

Associate Degrees Conferred in the Health Field, by Sex, Race, and Ethnicity: 1993-1994

[Continued]

Race/ethnicity/sex	All fields, total[1]	Health professions and related sciences
American Indian/Alaskan Native	1,895	153
Non-resident alien	4,172	170
Women		
Total	320,732	80,356
White, non-Hispanic	253,326	69,131
Black, non-Hispanic	29,072	5,618
Hispanic	19,043	2,643
Asian/Pacific Islander	10,256	1,722
American Indian/Alaskan Native	3,080	608
Non-resident alien	5,955	634

Source: U.S. Department of Education. Office of Educational Research and Improvement. National Center for Education Statistics. *Digest of Education Statistics, 1996.* Washington, D.C.: U.S. Government Printing Office, 1996, p. 284. Primary source: U.S. Department of Education, National Center for Education Statistics, Integrated Postsecondary Education Data System (IPEDS), "Completions" survey. Table prepared May 1996. *Notes:* 1. Reported racial/ethnic distributions of students by level of degree, field of degree, and sex were used to estimate race/ethnicity for students whose race/ethnicity was not reported. Excludes 799 men and 727 women whose racial/ethnic group and field of study were not available.

★ 820 ★

Education

Associate/Subbaccalaureate Degrees Conferred, by Length of Curriculum and Sex of Student: 1993-1994

Field of study	Less than 1-year awards			1- to less than 4-year awards			Associate degrees		
	Total	Men	Women	Total	Men	Women	Total	Men	Women
Total	71,748	34,732	37,016	152,849	63,886	88,963	542,449	220,990	321,459
Health professions and related sciences	24,909	7,140	17,769	42,569	6,805	35,764	95,832	15,476	80,356
Dental assisting	283	16	267	2,552	126	2,426	4,325	284	4,041
Emergency medical technician-ambulance and paramedic	6,551	4,293	2,258	1,863	1,327	536	514	357	157
Medical lab technician	39	5	34	207	91	116	2,570	665	1,905
Medical assisting	1,707	205	1,502	3,410	105	3,305	2,785	113	2,672
Nursing assisting	8,046	1,010	7,036	295	35	260	6	1	5
Practical nursing	519	63	456	19,431	2,124	17,307	740	68	672
Nursing, R.N. and other	2,355	280	2,075	3,529	384	3,145	57,531	6,679	50,852
Health sciences, other	5,409	1,268	4,141	11,282	2,613	8,669	27,361	7,309	20,052

Source: U.S. Department of Education. Office of Educational Research and Improvement. National Center for Education Statistics. *Digest of Education Statistics, 1996.* Washington, D.C.: U.S. Government Printing Office, 1996, p. 256. Primary source: U.S. Department of Education, National Center for Education Statistics, Integrated Postsecondary Education Data System (IPEDS), "Completions" survey. Table prepared May 1996.

★ 821 ★

Education

Average GPAs of Applicants and Matriculants to Medical Schools: 1995

According to the source, the difference in GPAs between medical school applicants and medical school matriculants was .2.

Subject areas	Appli-cants	Matric-ulants
Sciences	3.22	3.47
Non-sciences	3.43	3.58
Total	3.31	3.51

Source: "Monitor: Head of the Class." *New Physician* (January/February 1996), p. 8. Primary source: Association of American Medical Colleges. *Notes:* Note: "GPA" stands for "Grade point average." Standard deviation for all applicants' GPAs ranges from 0.38 to 0.49. Standard deviation for all matriculants' GPAs ranges from 0.32 to 0.39.

★ 822 ★

Education

Average MCAT Scores of Applicants and Matriculants to Medical Schools: 1995

According to the source, the average medical school applicant scored an 8.5 on the physical sciences portion of the MCAT, while the average matriculant scored a 9.7.

Test subject	Appli-cants	Matric-ulants
Verbal reasoning	8.5	9.5
Physical sciences	8.6	9.7
Writing sample	O	P
Biological sciences	8.7	9.8

Source: "Monitor: Head of the Class." *New Physician* (January/February 1996), p. 8. Primary source: Association of American Medical Colleges. *Notes:* Note: "MCAT" stands for "Medical College Admission Test" or "Medical College Aptitude Test." Note: Writing samples are graded on a scale from "A" to "R," with "R" being the highest score. Note: Standard deviation for all applicants' scores in verbal reasoning, physical sciences, and biological sciences is 2.2. Standard deviation for all matriculants' scores in verbal reasoning, physical sciences, and biological sciences is 2.0.

★ 823 ★

Education

Bachelor's Degrees Conferred in the Health Field: 1970-1994

Year	Total degrees (All fields)	Health professions and related sciences
1970-71	839,730	25,226
1975-76	925,746	53,958
1980-81	935,140	63,649
1981-82	952,998	63,653
1982-83	969,510	64,685
1983-84	974,309	64,288
1984-85	979,477	64,422
1985-86	987,823	64,396
1986-87	991,264	63,103
1987-88	994,829	60,644
1988-89	1,018,755	59,005
1989-90	1,051,344	58,302
1990-91	1,094,538	59,070
1991-92	1,136,553	61,720
1992-93	1,165,178	67,089
1993-94	1,169,275	74,421

Source: U.S. Department of Education. Office of Educational Research and Improvement. National Center for Education Statistics. *Digest of Education Statistics, 1996.* Washington, D.C.: U.S. Government Printing Office, 1996, p. 274. Primary source: U.S. Department of Education, National Center for Education Statistics, "Degrees and Other Formal Awards Conferred" surveys, and Integrated Postsecondary Education Data System (IPEDS), "Completions" surveys. Table prepared February 1996.

★ 824 ★

Education

Bachelor's Degrees Conferred in the Health Field, by Sex, Race, and Ethnicity: 1993-1994

Race/ethnicity/sex	All fields, total[1]	Health professions and related sciences
Total	1,165,973	74,421
White, non-Hispanic	936,227	62,756
Black, non-Hispanic	83,576	4,896
Hispanic	50,241	2,274
Asian/Pacific Islander	55,660	3,070
American Indian/Alaskan Native	6,189	398
Non-resident alien	34,080	1,027

[Continued]

★ 824 ★

Bachelor's Degrees Conferred in the Health Field, by Sex, Race, and Ethnicity: 1993-1994

[Continued]

Race/ethnicity/sex	All fields, total[1]	Health professions and related sciences
Men		
Total	530,804	13,062
White, non-Hispanic	429,121	10,861
Black, non-Hispanic	30,648	674
Hispanic	21,807	469
Asian/Pacific Islander	26,938	709
American Indian/Alaskan Native	2,616	82
Non-resident alien	19,674	267
Women		
Total	635,169	61,359
White, non-Hispanic	507,106	51,895
Black, non-Hispanic	52,928	4,222
Hispanic	28,434	1,805
Asian/Pacific Islander	28,722	2,361
American Indian/Alaskan Native	3,573	316
Non-resident alien	14,406	760

Source: U.S. Department of Education. Office of Educational Research and Improvement. National Center for Education Statistics. *Digest of Education Statistics, 1996.* Washington, D.C.: U.S. Government Printing Office, 1996, p. 287. Primary source: U.S. Department of Education, National Center for Education Statistics, Integrated Postsecondary Education Data System (IPEDS), "Completions" survey. Table prepared May 1996. *Notes:* 1. Reported racial/ethnic distribution of students by level of degree, field of degree, and sex were used to estimate race/ethnicity for students whose race/ethnicity was not reported. Excludes 1,618 men and 1,684 women whose racial/ethnic group and field of study were not available.

★ 825 ★

Education

Degrees Conferred, by Sex of Student: 1993-1994

Field of study	Bachelor's degrees requiring 4 or 5 years			Master's degrees			Doctoral degrees (Ph.D., Ed.D., etc.)		
	Total	Men	Women	Total	Men	Women	Total	Men	Women
Health professions and related sciences, total	74,421	13,062	61,359	28,025	5,814	22,211	1,902	789	1,113
Communication disorders sciences and services	5,405	270	5,135	4,176	211	3,965	94	21	73
Community health liaison	586	120	466	176	41	135	0	0	0
Dentistry	0	0	0	346	251	95	42	32	10
Dental services	915	27	888	42	20	22	0	0	0

[Continued]

★ 825 ★

Degrees Conferred, by Sex of Student: 1993-1994
[Continued]

Field of study	Bachelor's degrees requiring 4 or 5 years			Master's degrees			Doctoral degrees (Ph.D., Ed.D., etc.)		
	Total	Men	Women	Total	Men	Women	Total	Men	Women
Epidemiology	0	0	0	271	106	165	111	43	68
Health services administration, total	3,635	899	2,736	3,525	1,219	2,306	80	30	50
Health services administration	1,815	474	1,341	1,807	683	1,124	47	18	29
Medical records administration	699	93	606	0	0	0	0	0	0
Medical records technology/technician	1	0	1	3	2	1	2	2	0
Health and medical administrative services, other	1,120	332	788	1,715	534	1,181	31	10	21
Health and medical assistants, total	1,015	497	518	178	54	124	0	0	0
Medical assistant	1	0	1	0	0	0	0	0	0
Physician assistant	924	479	445	160	49	111	0	0	0
Health and medical assistants, other	90	18	72	18	5	13	0	0	0
Health and medical diagnostic and treatment services, total	1,459	553	906	95	68	27	2	2	0
Respiratory therapy technology/technician	417	184	233	0	0	0	0	0	0
Health and medical diagnostic and treatment services, other	1,042	369	673	95	68	27	2	2	0
Medical laboratory technologies, total	2,763	856	1,907	481	185	296	80	33	47
Medical technology	2,393	725	1,668	75	26	49	4	3	1
Health and medical laboratory technologies/technicians, other	370	131	239	406	159	247	76	30	46
Pre-dentistry studies	70	46	24	0	0	0	0	0	0
Pre-medicine studies	756	438	318	23	5	18	0	0	0
Pre-pharmacy studies	52	25	27	0	0	0	0	0	0
Pre-veterinary studies	314	101	213	3	1	2	0	0	0
Medical basic sciences	245	94	151	261	136	125	335	201	134
Mental health services, total	546	103	443	384	89	295	31	7	24
Alcohol/drug abuse counseling	69	22	47	62	18	44	1	0	1
Psychiatric/mental health services technician	127	26	101	36	11	25	0	0	0
Clinical and medical social work	119	22	97	103	31	72	30	7	23
Mental health services, other	231	33	198	183	29	154	0	0	0
Nursing	39,076	3,735	35,341	8,991	599	8,392	382	24	358
Optometry	221	95	126	18	4	14	1	1	0
Pharmacy	6,044	2,235	3,809	243	134	109	278	144	134
Rehabilitation/therapeutic services, total	7,169	1,531	5,638	4,433	1,084	3,349	34	15	19
Art therapy	74	1	73	164	9	155	0	0	0
Dance therapy	2	0	2	30	1	29	0	0	0
Music therapy	144	21	123	18	4	14	0	0	0
Occupational therapy	2,652	305	2,347	619	58	561	4	0	4
Orthotics/prosthetics	58	46	12	0	0	0	0	0	0
Physical therapy	3,265	903	2,362	2,583	734	1,849	4	1	3
Recreational therapy	137	28	109	22	2	20	1	0	1
Vocational rehabilitation counseling	155	45	110	640	175	465	8	6	2
Rehabilitative services, other	682	182	500	357	101	256	17	8	9
Veterinary medicine	87	33	54	178	95	83	117	75	42
Miscellaneous health professions	436	205	231	249	122	127	35	23	12

[Continued]

★ 825 ★

Degrees Conferred, by Sex of Student: 1993-1994

[Continued]

Field of study	Bachelor's degrees requiring 4 or 5 years			Master's degrees			Doctoral degrees (Ph.D., Ed.D., etc.)		
	Total	Men	Women	Total	Men	Women	Total	Men	Women
Health professions and related sciences, other	3,627	1,199	2,428	3,952	1,390	2,562	280	138	142

Source: U.S. Department of Education. Office of Educational Research and Improvement. National Center for Education Statistics. *Digest of Education Statistics, 1996.* Washington, D.C.: U.S. Government Printing Office, 1996, p. 262. Primary source: U.S. Department of Education, National Center for Education Statistics, National Study of Postsecondary Faculty (NSOPF), 1992-93. Table prepared September 1996.

★ 826 ★

Education

Degrees Conferred in the Health Field, by Type of Institution and Degree Level: 1993-1994

Discipline division	Public institutions				Private institutions			
	Associate degrees	Bachelor's degrees	Master's degrees	Doctoral degrees	Associate degrees	Bachelor's degrees	Master's degrees	Doctoral degrees
Total	456,190	789,148	221,428	28,524	86,259	380,127	165,642	14,661
Health professions and related sciences	83,889	50,641	17,009	1,356	11,943	23,780	11,016	546

Source: U.S. Department of Education. Office of Educational Research and Improvement. National Center for Education Statistics. *Digest of Education Statistics, 1996.* Washington, D.C.: U.S. Government Printing Office, 1996, p. 277. Primary source: U.S. Department of Education, National Center for Education Statistics, Integrated Postsecondary Education Data System (IPEDS), "Completions" survey, 1993-94, and "Consolidated" survey 1994. Table prepared May 1996.

★ 827 ★

Education

Degrees Conferred in the Health Professions and Related Sciences, by Level of Degree and Sex of Student: 1970-1994

Year	Bachelor's degrees			Master's degrees			Doctoral degrees		
	Total	Men	Women	Total	Men	Women	Total	Men	Women
1970-71	25,226	5,788	19,438	5,749	2,567	3,182	466	389	77
1971-72	28,611	7,005	21,606	7,207	3,141	4,066	442	362	80
1972-73	33,564	7,754	25,810	8,362	3,567	4,795	646	485	161
1973-74	41,459	9,388	32,071	9,599	3,819	5,780	578	447	131
1974-75	49,090	10,930	38,160	10,692	4,092	6,600	618	441	177
1975-76	53,958	11,456	42,502	12,556	4,217	8,339	577	411	166
1976-77	57,328	11,947	45,381	12,951	4,163	8,788	538	366	172

[Continued]

★ 827 ★

Degrees Conferred in the Health Professions and Related Sciences, by Level of Degree and Sex of Student: 1970-1994
[Continued]

Year	Bachelor's degrees			Master's degrees			Doctoral degrees		
	Total	Men	Women	Total	Men	Women	Total	Men	Women
1977-78	59,434	11,593	47,841	14,325	4,265	10,060	654	402	252
1978-79	62,085	11,205	50,880	15,485	4,494	10,991	718	454	264
1979-80	63,920	11,391	52,529	15,704	4,357	11,347	786	435	351
1980-81	63,649	10,519	53,130	16,515	4,316	12,199	842	475	367
1981-82	63,653	10,105	53,548	16,503	4,006	12,497	925	503	422
1982-83	64,685	10,218	54,467	17,047	4,235	12,812	1,155	649	506
1983-84	64,288	10,040	54,248	17,411	4,251	13,160	1,164	574	590
1984-85	64,422	9,741	54,681	17,385	4,119	13,266	1,199	565	634
1985-86	64,396	9,630	54,766	18,573	4,428	14,145	1,241	604	637
1986-87	63,103	9,134	53,969	18,394	3,874	14,250	1,213	564	649
1987-88	60,644	8,929	51,715	18,657	4,047	14,610	1,261	548	713
1988-89	59,005	8,872	50,133	19,268	4,226	15,042	1,437	609	828
1989-90	58,302	9,118	49,184	20,321	4,534	15,787	1,536	704	832
1990-91	59,070	9,596	49,474	21,200	4,444	16,756	1,613	694	919
1991-92	61,720	10,189	51,531	23,065	4,691	18,374	1,661	698	963
1992-93	67,089	11,347	55,742	25,718	5,227	20,491	1,767	753	1,014
1993-94	74,421	13,062	61,359	28,025	5,814	22,211	1,902	789	1,113

Source: U.S. Department of Education. Office of Educational Research and Improvement. National Center for Education Statistics. *Digest of Education Statistics, 1996.* Washington, D.C.: U.S. Government Printing Office, 1996, p. 303. Primary source: U.S. Department of Education, National Center for Education Statistics, "Degrees and Other Formal Awards Conferred" surveys, and Integrated Postsecondary Education Data System (IPEDS), "Completions" survey. Table prepared November 1995.

★ 828 ★

Education

Doctoral Degrees Conferred in the Health Field, by Sex, Race, and Ethnicity: 1993-1994

Race/ethnicity/sex	All fields, total[1]	Health professions and related sciences
Total	43,149	1,902
White, non-Hispanic	27,156	1,282
Black, non-Hispanic	1,393	59
Hispanic	903	26
Asian/Pacific Islander	2,025	104
American Indian/Alaskan Native	134	7
Non-resident alien	11,538	424
Men		
Total	26,531	789
White, non-Hispanic	15,126	465

[Continued]

★ 828 ★

Doctoral Degrees Conferred in the Health Field, by Sex, Race, and Ethnicity: 1993-1994

[Continued]

Race/ethnicity/sex	All fields, total[1]	Health professions and related sciences
Black, non-Hispanic	631	14
Hispanic	465	10
Asian/Pacific Islander	1,373	58
American Indian/Alaskan Native	66	1
Non-resident alien	8,870	241
Women		
Total	16,618	1,113
White, non-Hispanic	12,030	817
Black, non-Hispanic	762	45
Hispanic	438	16
Asian/Pacific Islander	652	46
American Indian/Alaskan Native	68	6
Non-resident alien	2,668	183

Source: U.S. Department of Education. Office of Educational Research and Improvement. National Center for Education Statistics. *Digest of Education Statistics, 1996.* Washington, D.C.: U.S. Government Printing Office, 1996, p. 293. Primary source: U.S. Department of Education, National Center for Education Statistics, Integrated Postsecondary Education Data System (IPEDS), "Completions" survey. Table prepared May 1996. *Notes:* 1. Reported racial/ethnic distribution of students by level of degree, field of degree, and sex were used to estimate race/ethnicity for students whose race/ethnicity was not reported. Excludes 21 men and 15 women whose racial/ethnic group and field of study were not available.

★ 829 ★

Education

Doctoral Degrees Conferred in the Health Fields: 1970-1994

Year	All fields, total	Health professions and related sciences
1970-71	32,107	466
1975-76	34,064	577
1980-81	32,958	842
1981-82	32,707	925
1982-83	32,775	1,155
1983-84	33,209	1,164
1984-85	32,943	1,199
1985-86	33,653	1,241
1986-87	34,041	1,213
1987-88	34,870	1,261

[Continued]

★ 829 ★

Doctoral Degrees Conferred in the Health Fields:
1970-1994
[Continued]

Year	All fields, total	Health professions and related sciences
1988-89	35,720	1,437
1989-90	38,371	1,536
1990-91	39,294	1,613
1991-92	40,659	1,661
1992-93	42,132	1,767
1993-94	43,185	1,902

Source: U.S. Department of Education. Office of Educational Research and Improvement. National Center for Education Statistics. *Digest of Education Statistics, 1996.* Washington, D.C.: U.S. Government Printing Office, 1996, p. 276. Primary source: U.S. Department of Education, National Center for Education Statistics, "Degrees and Other Formal Awards Conferred" surveys, and Integrated Postsecondary Education Data System (IPEDS), "Completions" surveys. Table prepared February 1996.

★ 830 ★

Education

Enrollment in Postsecondary Institutions, by Selected Characteristics: 1992-1993 - Part I

Field of study	All students				Undergraduate 2-year institutions			
	Total, in thousands	Percentage distribution, by age			Total, in thousands	Percentage distribution, by age		
		Under 25	25 to 34	Over 35		Under 25	25 to 34	Over 35
Total	21,096	54.1	25.0	20.9	9,881	48.5	26.9	24.6
Health	2,809	47.3	30.6	22.2	1,735	44.1	32.4	23.5
Medical doctor	147	51.1	41.9	7.0	38	51.9	36.0	12.1
Nursing	1,286	38.8	33.9	27.3	872	35.6	37.6	26.7
Other	1,375	54.7	26.2	19.0	825	52.7	26.8	20.6

Source: U.S. Department of Education. Office of Educational Research and Improvement. National Center for Education Statistics. *Digest of Education Statistics, 1996.* Washington, D.C.: U.S. Government Printing Office, 1996, p. 214. Primary source: U.S. Department of Education, National Center for Education Statistics, "The 1992-93 National Postsecondary Student Aid Study," unpublished data. Table prepared July 1995. *Notes:* Because of different survey editing and processing procedures, enrollment data in this table may differ from those appearing in other tables. Because of rounding, details may not add to totals. Includes students who enrolled at any time during the 1992-93 academic year.

★ 831 ★

Education

Enrollment in Postsecondary Institutions, by Selected Characteristics: 1992-1993 - Part II

| Field of study | Undergraduate 4-year institutions | | | | Graduate and first-professional | | | |
| | Total, in thousands | Percentage distribution, by age | | | Total, in thousands | Percentage distribution, by age | | |
		Under 25	25 to 34	Over 35		Under 25	25 to 34	Over 35
Total	8,558	71.7	16.7	11.7	2,657	18.6	45.0	36.4
Health	766	62.0	20.5	17.4	307	28.2	45.0	26.8
Medical doctor	27	76.5	17.7	5.9	81	42.1	52.9	5.0
Nursing	355	51.7	23.9	24.4	59	8.1	38.9	53.1
Other	384	70.1	17.9	12.0	157	30.9	41.2	27.9

Source: U.S. Department of Education. Office of Educational Research and Improvement. National Center for Education Statistics. *Digest of Education Statistics, 1996.* Washington, D.C.: U.S. Government Printing Office, 1996, p. 214. Primary source: U.S. Department of Education, National Center for Education Statistics, "The 1992-93 National Postsecondary Student Aid Study," unpublished data. Table prepared July 1995. *Notes:* Because of different survey editing and processing procedures, enrollment data in this table may differ from those appearing in other tables. Because of rounding, details may not add to totals. Includes students who enrolled at any time during the 1992-93 academic year.

★ 832 ★

Education

First Professional Degrees Conferred, by Field of Study, Race, Ethnicity: 1993-1994

| Major field of study | Total | | | | | | |
	Total	White, Non-Hispanic	Black, Non-Hispanic	Hispanic	Asian/ Pacific Islander	American Indian/ Alaskan Native	Non-resident alien
All fields[1]	75,418	60,140	4,444	3,134	5,892	371	1,437
Dentistry (D.D.S. or D.M.D.)	3,787	2,559	171	218	538	17	284
Medicine (M.D.)	15,368	11,287	937	613	2,282	68	181
Optometry (O.D.)	1,103	818	36	38	153	3	55
Osteopathic medicine (D.O.)	1,798	1,478	48	70	182	8	12
Pharmacy (Pharm.D.)	1,936	1,297	155	54	347	1	82
Podiatry (Pod.D. or D.P.) or podiatric medicine (D.P.M.)	465	339	32	41	43	2	8
Veterinary medicine (D.V.M.)	2,089	1,923	39	66	40	14	7
Chiropractic medicine (D.C. or D.C.M.)	2,806	2,370	40	80	115	18	182
Law (LL.B. or J.D.)	40,044	33,420	2,472	1,842	1,816	223	271

[Continued]

★ 832 ★

First Professional Degrees Conferred, by Field of Study, Race, Ethnicity: 1993-1994
[Continued]

Major field of study	Total						
	Total	White, Non-Hispanic	Black, Non-Hispanic	Hispanic	Asian/ Pacific Islander	American Indian/ Alaskan Native	Non-resident alien
Theology (M.Div., M.H.L., B.D., or Ord.)	5,967	4,607	513	109	375	16	347
Other	55	42	1	3	1	0	8

Source: U.S. Department of Education. Office of Educational Research and Improvement. National Center for Education Statistics. *Digest of Education Statistics, 1996.* Washington, D.C.: U.S. Government Printing Office, 1996, p. 296. Primary source: U.S. Department of Education, National Center for Education Statistics, Integrated Postsecondary Education Data System (IPEDS), "Completions" survey. Table prepared January 1995. *Notes:* 1. Reported racial/ethnic distributions of students by level of degree, field of degree, and sex were used to estimate race/ethnicity for students whose race/ethnicity was not reported.

★ 833 ★

Education

First-Year Enrollment and Graduates of Health Professions Schools

First-year enrollment and graduates of health professions schools and number of schools, according to profession, United States, selected years 1950-93, and projections for year 2000.

Year	Medi-cine	Osteo-pathy	Registered nursing				Licensed prac-tical nur-sing	Den-tis-try	Op-tom-etry	Phar-ma-cy	Chi-roprac-tic
			Total	Bac-calau-reate	Asso-ciate degree	Di-plo-ma					
First-year enrollment											
1980	16,930	1,426	105,952	35,414	53,633	16,905	56,316	6,066	1,185	7,905	---
1981	17,186	1,496	110,201	35,808	56,899	17,494	58,479	5,964	1,174	7,442	---
1982	17,268	1,582	115,279	35,928	60,423	18,928	60,426	5,789	1,162	6,617	---
1983	17,254	1,682	120,579	37,264	63,947	19,368	61,453	5,498	1,120	6,280	---
1984	17,150	1,746	123,824	39,400	66,576	17,848	57,865	5,207	1,187	6,598	1,025
1985	16,997	1,750	118,224	39,573	63,776	14,875	47,043	4,983	1,177	6,749	1,383
1986[2]	16,963	1,737	100,791	34,310	56,635	9,846	44,477	4,777	1,154	6,584	1,712
1987[3]	16,819	1,724	90,693	28,026	54,330	8,337	42,452	4,494	1,210	7,081	1,598
1988[3]	16,713	1,692	94,269	28,505	57,376	8,389	43,776	4,316	1,234	7,309	1,507
1989[3]	16,868	1,780	103,025	29,042	63,973	10,010	47,602	4,148	1,271	8,067	1,531
1990	16,756	1,884	108,580	29,858	68,634	10,088	52,969	3,938	1,258	8,009	1,485
1991	16,876	1,950	113,526	33,437	69,869	10,220	56,176	3,961	1,207	---	1,467
1992	17,071	1,974	122,656	37,886	74,079	10,691	58,245	4,006	1,321	8,264	1,411
1993	17,079	2,035	---	---	---	---	---	4,029	---	8,664	1,743
Graduates											
1950[4]	5,553	373	25,790	---	---	---	2,828	2,565	961	---	---
1960	7,081	427	30,113	4,136	789	25,188	16,491	3,253	364	3,497	660
1970	8,367	432	43,103	9,069	11,483	22,551	36,456	3,749	445	4,758	642

[Continued]

★ 833 ★

First-Year Enrollment and Graduates of Health Professions Schools
[Continued]

| Year | Medi-cine | Osteo-pathy | Registered nursing | | | | Licensed prac-tical nur-sing | Den-tis-try | Op-tom-etry | Phar-ma-cy | Chi-roprac-tic |
			Total	Bac-calau-reate	Asso-ciate degree	Di-plo-ma					
1975	12,714	702	73,915	20,170	32,183	21,562	45,375	4,969	806	6,712	1,093
1980	15,135	1,059	75,523	24,994	36,034	14,495	41,892	5,256	1,073	7,432	2,049
1981	15,667	1,151	73,985	24,370	36,712	12,903	41,002	5,550	1,092	7,323	2,526
1982	15,985	1,017	74,052	24,081	38,289	11,682	43,299	5,371	1,106	6,859	2,631
1983	15,824	1,317	77,408	23,855	41,849	11,704	45,174	5,756	1,168	6,374	2,948
1984	16,327	1,287	80,312	23,718	44,394	12,200	44,654	5,337	1,188	5,963	---
1985	16,319	1,474	82,075	24,975	45,208	11,892	36,955	5,353	1,114	5,724	---
1986	16,125	1,560	77,027	25,170	41,333	10,524	29,599	4,957	1,085	5,800	1,924
1987	15,836	1,587	70,561	23,761	38,528	8,272	27,285	4,717	1,081	5,854	1,429
1988	15,887	1,572	64,839	21,504	37,397	5,938	26,912	4,581	1,106	6,171	1,650
1989[5]	15,620	1,609	61,660	18,997	37,837	4,826	30,368	4,312	1,143	6,557	1,753
1990	15,336	1,529	66,088	18,571	42,318	5,199	35,417	4,233	1,115	6,956	1,661
1991	15,481	1,534	72,230	19,264	46,794	6,172	38,100	3,995	1,136	7,122	1,631
1992	15,386	1,532	80,839	21,415	52,896	6,528	41,951	3,918	1,150	7,113	1,664
1993[6]	15,554	1,609	88,144	24,442	56,770	6,932	---	3,744	---	---	1,591
2000[7]	16,112	1,934	68,800	20,580	43,450	4,770	---	3,242	1,200	7,120	2,950
Schools[8]											
1950[4]	79	6	1,170	---	---	---	85	42	10	---	20
1960	86	6	1,137	172	57	908	661	47	10	76	12
1970	103	7	1,340	267	437	636	1,233	53	11	74	11
1975	114	9	1,362	326	608	428	1,315	59	12	73	12
1980	126	14	1,385	377	697	311	1,299	60	15	72	14
1981	126	15	1,401	383	715	303	1,309	60	16	72	16
1982	127	15	1,432	402	742	288	1,295	60	16	72	16
1983	127	15	1,466	421	764	281	1,297	60	16	72	17
1984	127	15	1,477	427	777	273	1,254	60	16	72	17
1985	127	15	1,473	441	776	256	1,165	60	16	72	17
1986	127	15	1,469	455	776	238	1,087	59	16	73	17
1987	127	15	1,465	467	789	209	1,068	58	16	74	17
1988	127	15	1,442	479	792	171	1,095	58	16	72	17
1989	127	15	1,457	488	812	157	1,171	58	16	74	17
1990	126	15	1,470	489	829	152	1,154	56	16	74	17
1991	126	15	1,484	501	838	145	1,125	55	16	74	17

[Continued]

★ 833 ★

First-Year Enrollment and Graduates of Health Professions Schools
[Continued]

Year	Medi-cine	Osteo-pathy	Registered nursing				Licensed prac-tical nur-sing	Den-tis-try	Op-tom-etry	Phar-ma-cy	Chi-roprac-tic
			Total	Bac-calau-reate	Asso-ciate degree	Di-plo-ma					
1992	126	15	1,484	501	848	135	1,154	55	16	74	17
1993	126	15	---	---	---	---	---	54	16	74	17

Source: U.S. Department of Health and Human Services. Public Health Service. Centers for Disease Control and Prevention. National Center for Health Statistics. *Health, United States, 1994.* Hyattsville, MD: Public Health Service, 1995, p. 207. *Notes:* Data on the number of schools are reported as of the beginning of the academic year while data on first-year enrollment and number of graduates are reported as of the end of the academic year. 1. Chiropractic first-year enrollment data are partial data from 8 reporting schools. 2. First-year enrollment data for optometry exclude Ohio State University. 3. First-year enrollment data for pharmacy include the University of Puerto Rico. 4. Data for total registered nursing are for 1951. 5. Data for chiropractic medicine are estimated. 6. Nursing data are preliminary estimates. 7. Projected. 8. Some nursing schools offer more than 1 type of program. Numbers shown for nursing are number of nursing programs.

★ 834 ★
Education

International Medical Graduates

"The original House [of Representatives] Medicare bill phased out and eliminated residency slots for foreign IMGs by 1999. (Medicare is the primary source of funding for residency positions.) The final version of the bill reduces funding by 75 percent over three years. The bill will reduce the number of residency slots to 126 percent of U.S. medical school graduates, down from the current 146 percent, but above the 110 percent advocated by some physician work-force experts..."

Source: "Follow Up: Good News for Off-Shore." *New Physician* (January/February 1996), p. 8.

★ 835 ★
Education

Master's Degrees Conferred in the Health Field:
1970-1994

Year	Total	Health professions and related sciences
1970-71	230,509	5,749
1975-76	311,771	12,556
1980-81	295,739	16,515
1981-82	295,546	16,503

[Continued]

★ 835 ★

Master's Degrees Conferred in the Health Field: 1970-1994
[Continued]

Year	Total	Health professions and related sciences
1982-83	289,921	17,047
1983-84	284,263	17,411
1984-85	286,251	17,385
1985-86	288,567	18,573
1986-87	289,349	18,394
1987-88	299,317	18,657
1988-89	310,621	19,268
1989-90	324,301	20,321
1990-91	337,168	21,200
1991-92	352,838	23,065
1992-93	369,585	25,718
1993-94	387,070	28,025

Source: U.S. Department of Education. Office of Educational Research and Improvement. National Center for Education Statistics. *Digest of Education Statistics, 1996.* Washington, D.C.: U.S. Government Printing Office, 1996, p. 275. Primary source: U.S. Department of Education, National Center for Education Statistics, "Degrees and Other Formal Awards Conferred" surveys, and Integrated Postsecondary Education Data System (IPEDS), "Completions" surveys. Table prepared February 1996.

★ 836 ★

Education

Master's Degrees Conferred in the Health Field, by Sex, Race, and Ethnicity: 1993-1994

Race/ethnicity/sex	All fields, total[1]	Health professions and related sciences
Total	385,419	28,025
White, non-Hispanic	288,288	23,175
Black, non-Hispanic	21,937	1,496
Hispanic	11,913	710
Asian/Pacific Islander	15,267	1,007
American Indian/Alaskan Native	1,697	137
Non-resident alien	46,317	1,500
Men		
Total	175,355	5,814
White, non-Hispanic	123,854	4,446
Black, non-Hispanic	7,413	232
Hispanic	5,113	200

[Continued]

★ 836 ★

Master's Degrees Conferred in the Health Field, by Sex, Race, and Ethnicity: 1993-1994

[Continued]

Race/ethnicity/sex	All fields, total[1]	Health professions and related sciences
Asian/Pacific Islander	8,225	311
American Indian/Alaskan Native	691	27
Non-resident alien	30,059	598
Women		
Total	210,064	22,211
White, non-Hispanic	164,434	18,729
Black, non-Hispanic	14,524	1,264
Hispanic	6,800	510
Asian/Pacific Islander	7,042	696
American Indian/Alaskan Native	1,006	110
Non-resident alien	16,258	902

Source: U.S. Department of Education. Office of Educational Research and Improvement. National Center for Education Statistics. *Digest of Education Statistics, 1996.* Washington, D.C.: U.S. Government Printing Office, 1996, p. 290. Primary source: U.S. Department of Education, National Center for Education Statistics, Integrated Postsecondary Education Data System (IPEDS), "Completions" survey. Table prepared May 1996. *Notes:* 1. Reported racial/ethnic distribution of students by level of degree, field of degree, and sex were used to estimate race/ethnicity for students whose race/ethnicity was not reported. Excludes 730 men and 921 women whose racial/ethnic group and field of study were not available.

★ 837 ★

Education

Minority Enrollment

Total enrollment of minorities in schools for selected health occupations, according to detailed race and Hispanic origin, United States, academic years 1970-71, 1980-81, 1990-91, 1992-93. Data are based on reporting by health professions associations.

Occupation, detailed race, and Hispanic origin	Total enrollment							
	Number of students				Percent of students			
	1970-71[1]	1980-81	1990-91	1992-93[2]	1970-71[1]	1980-81	1990-91	1992-93[2]
Allopathic medicine								
All races[3]	40,238	65,189	65,163	66,142	100.0	100.0	100.0	100.0
Non-Hispanic white	37,944	55,434	47,893	46,465	94.3	85.0	73.5	70.3
Non-Hispanic black	1,509	3,708	4,241	4,638	3.8	5.7	6.5	7.0
Hispanic	196	2,761	3,538	3,810	0.5	4.2	5.4	5.8
Mexican American	---	951	1,109	1,332	---	1.5	1.7	2.0
Mainland Puerto Rican	---	329	457	484	---	0.5	0.7	0.7
Other Hispanic[4]	---	1,481	1,972	1,994	---	2.3	3.0	3.0
American Indian	18	221	277	333	*	0.3	0.4	0.5

[Continued]

★ 837 ★

Minority Enrollment
[Continued]

Occupation, detailed race, and Hispanic origin	Total enrollment							
	Number of students				Percent of students			
	1970-71[1]	1980-81	1990-91	1992-93[2]	1970-71[1]	1980-81	1990-91	1992-93[2]
Asian	571	1,924	8,436	9,994	1.4	3.0	12.9	15.1
Osteopathic medicine								
All races	2,304	4,940	6,792	7,375	100.0	100.0	100.0	100.0
Non-Hispanic white[3]	2,241	4,688	5,680	6,063	97.3	94.9	83.6	82.2
Non-Hispanic black	27	94	217	231	1.2	1.9	3.2	3.1
Hispanic	19	52	277	293	0.8	1.1	4.1	4.0
American Indian	6	19	36	45	0.3	0.4	0.5	0.6
Asian	11	87	582	743	0.5	1.8	8.6	10.1
Podiatry								
All races	1,268	2,577	2,226	2,438	100.0	100.0	100.0	100.0
Non-Hispanic white[3]	1,228	2,353	1,671	1,795	96.8	91.3	75.1	73.6
Non-Hispanic black	27	110	237	226	2.1	4.3	10.6	9.3
Hispanic	5	39	148	162	0.4	1.5	6.6	6.6
American Indian	1	6	7	9	0.1	0.2	0.3	0.4
Asian	7	69	163	246	0.6	2.7	7.3	10.1
Dentistry[5]								
All races	19,187	22,842	15,770	15,813	100.0	100.0	100.0	100.0
Non-Hispanic white[3]	17,531	20,208	11,185	11,187	91.4	88.5	70.9	70.7
Non-Hispanic black	872	1,022	940	943	4.5	4.5	6.0	6.0
Hispanic	185	519	1,073	985	1.0	2.3	6.8	6.2
American Indian	28	53	53	48	0.1	0.2	0.3	0.3
Asian	490	1,040	2,519	2,650	2.6	4.6	16.0	16.8
Optometry[5]								
All races	3,094	4,540	4,650	4,743	100.0	100.0	100.0	100.0
Non-Hispanic white[3]	2,913	4,148	3,706	3,751	94.1	91.4	79.7	79.1
Non-Hispanic black	32	57	134	140	1.0	1.3	2.9	3.0
Hispanic	30	80	186	178	1.0	1.8	4.0	3.8
American Indian	2	12	21	22	0.1	0.3	0.5	0.5
Asian	117	243	603	652	3.8	5.4	13.0	13.7
Pharmacy[5,6]								
All races	17,909	21,628	22,764	23,266	100.0	100.0	100.0	100.0

[Continued]

★ 837 ★

Minority Enrollment
[Continued]

| Occupation, detailed race, and Hispanic origin | Total enrollment | | | | | | | |
| | Number of students | | | | Percent of students | | | |
	1970-71[1]	1980-81	1990-91	1992-93[2]	1970-71[1]	1980-81	1990-91	1992-93[2]
Non-Hispanic white[3]	16,222	19,153	18,325	18,242	90.6	88.6	80.5	78.4
Non-Hispanic black	659	945	1,301	1,531	3.7	4.4	5.7	6.6
Hispanic	254	459	945	651	1.4	2.1	4.2	2.8
American Indian	29	36	63	87	0.2	0.2	0.3	0.4
Asian	672	1,035	2,130	2,755	3.8	4.8	9.4	11.8
Registered nurses[5,7]								
All races	211,239	230,966	221,170	257,983	100.0	100.0	100.0	100.0
Non-Hispanic white[3]	---	---	183,102	218,178	---	---	82.8	84.6
Non-Hispanic black	---	---	23,094	22,147	---	---	10.4	8.6
Hispanic	---	---	6,580	7,667	---	---	3.0	3.0
American Indian	---	---	1,803	1,685	---	---	0.8	0.7
Asian	---	---	6,591	8,306	---	---	3.0	3.2

Source: U.S. Department of Health and Human Services. Public Health Service. Centers for Disease Control and Prevention. National Center for Health Statistics. *Health, United States, 1994.* Hyattsville, MD: Public Health Service, 1995, p. 208-209. *Notes:* Total enrollment data are collected at the beginning of the academic year. * indicates that the figure did not meet standards of reliability or precision.— means data not available. 1. Data for osteopathic medicine, podiatry, and optometry are for 1971-72. Data for pharmacy and registered nurses are for 1972-73. 2. Data for optometry and pharmacy are for 1991-92. 3. Includes race and ethnicity unspecified. 4. Includes Puerto Rican Commonwealth students. 5. Excludes Puerto Rican schools. 6. Pharmacy total enrollment data are the students in the final 3 years of pharmacy education. 7. In 1990, the National League for Nursing developed a new system for analyzing minority data. In evaluating the former system, much underreporting was noted. Therefore, any data prior to 1989 would not be comparable.

★ 838 ★

Education

Women in Medical Schools

First-year and total enrollment of women in schools for selected health occupations, according to detailed race and Hispanic origin: United States, academic years 1971-1993. Data are based on reporting by health professions associations.

| Enrollment, occupation, detailed race, and Hispanic origin | Number of students | | | | Percent of students | | | |
| | Both sexes | | | | Women | | | |
	1971-72[1]	1980-81	1990-91	1992-93[2]	1971-72[1]	1980-81	1990-91	1992-93[2]
First-year enrollment								
Allopathic medicine[3]	12,361	17,186	16,876	17,079	13.7	28.9	38.8	41.9
Non-Hispanic white	---	14,262	11,830	11,562	---	27.4	37.7	39.8
Non-Hispanic black	881	1,128	1,263	1,425	22.7	45.5	55.3	60.8
Hispanic	---	818	933	1,103	---	31.5	42.0	45.2
Mexican American	118	258	185	447	8.5	30.6	39.3	44.3
Mainland Puerto Rican	40	95	120	126	15.0	43.2	43.3	51.6
Other Hispanic[4]	---	465	528	530	---	29.7	43.3	44.5

[Continued]

★ 838 ★

Women in Medical Schools
[Continued]

Enrollment, occupation, detailed race, and Hispanic origin	Number of students				Percent of students			
	Both sexes				Women			
	1971-72[1]	1980-81	1990-91	1992-93[2]	1971-72[1]	1980-81	1990-91	1992-93[2]
American Indian	23	67	76	123	34.8	35.8	40.8	43.9
Asian	217	72	2,527	2,615	19.4	31.5	40.3	40.2
Podiatry	399	695	622	802	---	---	---	---
Osteopathy medicine	670	1,496	1,950	2,035	4.3	22.0	34.2	35.1
Dentistry[5]	4,705	5,964	3,961	4,029	3.1	19.8	37.9	35.0
Optometry[5]	906	1,174	1,207	1,321	5.3	25.3	50.6	53.1
Pharmacy[5,6]	6,532	7,442	8,009	8,664	25.8	48.4	---	63.1
Registered nurses[5]	93,344	110,201	113,526	122,656	94.5	92.7	89.3	88.0
Total enrollment								
Allopathic medicine[3]	43,650	65,189	65,163	66,142	10.9	26.5	37.3	39.4
Non-Hispanic white	---	55,434	47,893	46,465	---	25.0	35.4	37.5
Non-Hispanic black	2,055	3,708	4,241	4,638	20.4	44.3	55.8	57.9
Hispanic	---	2,761	3,538	3,810	---	30.1	39.0	41.0
Mexican American	252	951	1,109	1,332	9.5	26.4	38.5	39.9
Mainland Puerto Rican	76	329	457	484	17.1	35.9	43.1	43.2
Other Hispanic[4]	---	1,481	1,972	1,994	---	31.1	38.4	41.2
American Indian	42	221	277	333	23.8	28.5	42.6	45.9
Asian	647	1,924	8,436	9,994	17.9	340.4	37.7	39.5
Dentistry[5]	16,553	22,842	15,770	15,813	---	17.0	34.2	36.1
Osteopathic medicine	2,304	4,940	6,792	7,375	3.4	19.7	32.7	34.1
Podiatry	1,268	2,577	2,226	2,438	1.2	11.9	---	---
Optometry[5]	3,094	4,540	2,650	4,743	---	---	47.3	49.5
Registered nurses[5]	211,239	230,966	221,170	257,983	95.5	94.3	---	88.9

Source: U.S. Department of Health and Human Services. Public Health Service. Centers for Disease Control and Prevention. National Center for Health Statistics. *Health, United States, 1994.* Hyattsville, MD: Public Health Service, 1995, p. 210. *Notes:*— indicates that the figure did not meet standards of reliability or precision. Data not available on total enrollment of women in schools of pharmacy. Total enrollment data are collected at the beginning of the academic year while first-year enrollment data are collected at the end of the academic year. 1. Total enrollments for registered nurse students are for 1972-73. 2. First-year enrollments for optometry and nursing students are for 1991-92. Total enrollments for optometry are for 1991-92. 3. Includes race and ethnicity unspecified. 4. Includes Puerto Rican Commonwealth students. 5. Excludes Puerto Rican schools. 6. Pharmacy first-year enrollment data for students in the first year of the final 3 years of pharmacy education.

Employment

★ 839 ★

Employment in the Health Service Industries: 1980 to 1995

In thousands.

INDUSTRY	1987 SIC Code[1]	1980	1985	1990	1993	1994	1995
Health services[2]	80	5,278	6,293	7,814	8,756	8,992	9,257
Offices and clinics of MDs	801	802	1,028	1,338	1,506	1,545	1,606
Offices and clinics of Dentists	802	(NA)	439	513	556	574	597
Offices and clinics of other practitioners	804	96	165	277	353	378	407
Nursing and personal care facilities	805	997	1,198	1,415	1,585	1,649	1,693
Skilled nursing care facilities	8051	(NA)	791	989	1,147	1,221	1,252
Intermediate care facilities	8052	(NA)	(NA)	200	215	206	213
Other, n.e.c.[3]	8059	(NA)	(NA)	227	224	222	229
Hospitals	806	2,750	2,997	3,549	3,779	3,763	3,784
General medical and surgical hospitals	8062	(NA)	2,811	3,268	3,475	3,459	3,484
Psychiatric hospitals	8063	(NA)	59	104	99	97	91
Specialty hospitals, exc. psychiatric	8069	(NA)	126	176	205	207	208
Medical and dental laboratories	807	(NA)	119	166	187	189	193
Home health care services	808	(NA)	(NA)	291	469	559	626

Source: 1996 Statistical Abstract of the United States on CD-ROM [machine-readable datafiles]. CD-8A-97. Washington, DC: U.S. Department of Commerce, Economics and Statistics Administration, Bureau of the Census, Data User Services Division, January 1997. Primary source: U.S. Bureau of Labor Statistics, Bulletins 2445 and 2481, and *Employment and Earnings*, March and June issues. *Notes:* NA indicates not available. 1. Based on the 1987 Standard Industrial Classification code. 2. Includes other industries not shown separately. 3. N.e.c. means not elsewhere classified.

★ 840 ★
Employment

Persons Employed in Health Service Sites: United States, Selected Years 1987-1993

Data are based on household interviews of a sample of the civilian noninstitutionalized population.

Site	1987	1988	1989	1990	1991	1992	1993
Number of persons in thousands							
All employed civilians	112,440	114,968	117,342	117,914	116,877	117,598	119,306
All health service sites	8,478	8,781	9,110	9,447	9,817	10,271	10,553
Offices and clinics of physicians	950	985	1,039	1,098	1,128	1,434	1,450
Offices and clinics of dentists	552	521	560	580	574	583	567

[Continued]

★ 840 ★

Persons Employed in Health Service Sites: United States, Selected Years 1987-1993

[Continued]

Site	1987	1988	1989	1990	1991	1992	1993
Offices and clinics of chiropractors[1]	72	77	97	90	105	122	116
Hospitals	4,444	4,520	4,568	4,690	4,839	4,915	5,032
Nursing and personal care facilities	1,337	1,467	1,521	1,543	1,626	1,750	1,752
Other health service sites	1,123	1,211	1,325	1,446	1,545	1,467	1,635
Percent of employed civilians							
All health service sites	7.5	7.6	7.8	8.0	8.4	8.7	8.8
Percent distribution							
All health service sites	100.0	100.0	100.0	100.0	100.0	100.0	100.0
Offices and clinics of physicians	11.2	11.2	11.4	11.6	11.5	14.0	13.7
Offices and clinics of dentists	6.5	5.9	6.1	6.1	5.8	5.7	5.4
Offices and clinics of chiropractors[1]	0.8	0.9	1.1	1.0	1.1	1.2	1.1
Hospitals	52.4	51.5	50.1	49.6	49.3	47.9	47.7
Nursing and personal care facilities	15.8	16.7	16.7	16.3	16.6	17.0	16.6
Other health service sites	13.2	13.8	14.5	15.3	15.7	14.3	15.5

Source: U.S. Department of Health and Human Services. Public Health Service. Centers for Disease Control and Prevention. National Center for Health Statistics. *Health, United States, 1994.* Hyattsville, MD: Public Health Service, 1995, p. 197. *Notes:* Totals exclude persons in health-related occupations who are working in nonhealth industries, as classified by the U.S. Bureau of the Census, such as pharmacists employed in drugstores, school nurses, and nurses working in private households. Totals include Federal, State, and county health workers. 1983-91, persons were classified according to the system used in the 1980 Census of Population. Beginning in 1992 persons were classified according to the system used in the 1990 Census of Population. 1. Data are from the U.S. Bureau of Labor Statistics.

Employment by Occupation

★ 841 ★

Ambulance Drivers and Attendants, Except EMTs: 1994 and 2005

Data for 1994 are based on BLS surveys. Data for 2005 are BLS projections using a variety of methods and statistical tools.

Industry	1994		2005 employment			% change 1994-2005 (Mid)
	Total employ-ment	% of industry empl.	Low	Mid	High	
Total, all industries	17,935	100	19,737	20,610	21,446	14.91
Local and interurban passenger transit	10,689	59.6	12,064	12,476	12,715	16.72
Hospitals, public and private	2,590	14.44	2,820	2,913	3,084	12.47
Funeral service and crematories	524	2.92	628	641	654	22.33

[Continued]

★ 841 ★

Ambulance Drivers and Attendants, Except EMTs: 1994 and 2005
[Continued]

Industry	1994		2005 employment			% change 1994-2005
	Total employ- ment	% of industry empl.	Low	Mid	High	(Mid)
Nursing and personal care facilities	145	0.81	216	219	225	51.03
Health and allied services, nec	102	0.57	145	147	149	44.12

Source: National Industry Occupation Matrix, 1994, acquired on electronic media. Prepared by Bureau of Labor Statistics, Washington, DC: U.S. Department of Labor, 1994.

★ 842 ★

Employment by Occupation

Cardiology Technologists: 1994 and 2005

Data for 1994 are based on BLS surveys. Data for 2005 are BLS projections using a variety of methods and statistical tools.

Industry	1994		2005 employment			% change 1994-2005
	Total employ- ment	% of industry empl.	Low	Mid	High	(Mid)
Hospitals, public and private	14,247	100	16,868	17,425	18,445	22.31
Total, all industries	14,247	100	16,868	17,425	18,445	22.31

Source: National Industry Occupation Matrix, 1994, acquired on electronic media. Prepared by Bureau of Labor Statistics, Washington, DC: U.S. Department of Labor, 1994.

★ 843 ★

Employment by Occupation

Chiropractors: 1994 and 2005

Data for 1994 are based on BLS surveys. Data for 2005 are BLS projections using a variety of methods and statistical tools.

Industry	1994		2005 employment			% change 1994-2005
	Total employ- ment	% of industry empl.	Low	Mid	High	(Mid)
Total, all industries	17,563	100	22,827	22,607	22,273	28.72
Offices of other health practitioners	17,154	97.67	22,249	22,032	21,702	28.44
Offices of physicians including osteopaths	333	1.9	464	460	453	38.14

Source: National Industry Occupation Matrix, 1994, acquired on electronic media. Prepared by Bureau of Labor Statistics, Washington, DC: U.S. Department of Labor, 1994.

★ 844 ★

Employment by Occupation

Clinical Laboratory Technologists and Technicians: 1994 and 2005

Data for 1994 are based on BLS surveys. Data for 2005 are BLS projections using a variety of methods and statistical tools.

Industry	1994		2005 employment			% change 1994-2005
	Total employ-ment	% of industry empl.	Low	Mid	High	(Mid)
Total, all industries	272,251	100	298,485	304,972	315,148	12.02
Hospitals, public and private	150,204	55.17	139,593	144,197	152,641	-4.00
Offices of physicians including osteopaths	42,379	15.57	47,229	46,770	46,069	10.36
Medical and dental laboratories	38,733	14.23	59,254	60,099	60,877	55.16
Health and allied services, nec	10,128	3.72	18,291	18,552	18,792	83.18
Federal government	9,284	3.41	8,649	8,622	8,597	-7.13
Research and testing services	4,687	1.72	5,937	5,950	5,964	26.95
State government, except education and hospitals	4,277	1.57	4,097	4,476	4,914	4.65
Education, public and private	4,236	1.56	5,014	5,456	5,960	28.80
Local government, except education and hospitals	3,899	1.43	3,852	4,209	4,620	7.95
Management and public relations	1,201	0.44	1,801	1,822	1,844	51.71
Offices of other health practitioners	943	0.35	1,529	1,514	1,492	60.55
Chemicals and allied products	774	0.28	910	957	992	23.64
Nursing and personal care facilities	708	0.26	1,054	1,065	1,097	50.42
Offices and clinics of dentists	390	0.14	514	509	501	30.51
Home health care services	255	0.09	561	569	577	123.14

Source: National Industry Occupation Matrix, 1994, acquired on electronic media. Prepared by Bureau of Labor Statistics, Washington, DC: U.S. Department of Labor, 1994.

★ 845 ★

Employment by Occupation

Dental Assistants: 1994 and 2005

Data for 1994 are based on BLS surveys. Data for 2005 are BLS projections using a variety of methods and statistical tools.

Industry	1994		2005 employment			% change 1994-2005
	Total employ-ment	% of industry empl.	Low	Mid	High	(Mid)
Total, all industries	189,717	100	271,474	269,201	265,681	41.90
Offices and clinics of dentists	179,600	94.67	260,218	257,689	253,829	43.48
Federal government	2,781	1.47	2,591	2,583	2,575	-7.12
Hospitals, public and private	2,259	1.19	2,460	2,541	2,690	12.48
Offices of physicians including osteopaths	2,045	1.08	2,849	2,821	2,779	37.95
State government, except education and hospitals	1,184	0.62	1,134	1,239	1,360	4.65
Local government, except education and hospitals	1,084	0.57	1,070	1,170	1,284	7.93
Health and allied services, nec	305	0.16	432	438	444	43.61

[Continued]

★ 845 ★

Dental Assistants: 1994 and 2005

[Continued]

Industry	1994		2005 employment			% change 1994-2005
	Total employ-ment	% of industry empl.	Low	Mid	High	(Mid)
Offices of other health practitioners	255	0.13	413	409	403	60.39
Nursing and personal care facilities	53	0.03	79	80	83	50.94

Source: National Industry Occupation Matrix, 1994, acquired on electronic media. Prepared by Bureau of Labor Statistics, Washington, DC: U.S. Department of Labor, 1994.

★ 846 ★

Employment by Occupation

Dental Hygienists: 1994 and 2005

Data for 1994 are based on BLS surveys. Data for 2005 are BLS projections using a variety of methods and statistical tools.

Industry	1994		2005 employment			% change 1994-2005
	Total employ-ment	% of industry empl.	Low	Mid	High	(Mid)
Total, all industries	124,701	100	179,580	178,002	175,568	42.74
Offices and clinics of dentists	120,488	96.62	174,572	172,876	170,286	43.48
Offices of physicians including osteopaths	1,267	1.02	1,765	1,748	1,722	37.96
Hospitals, public and private	962	0.77	1,048	1,082	1,146	12.47
Local government, except education and hospitals	577	0.46	570	623	684	7.97
State government, except education and hospitals	533	0.43	510	558	612	4.69
Federal government	377	0.3	352	350	349	-7.16
Offices of other health practitioners	194	0.16	314	311	307	60.31
Medical and dental laboratories	113	0.09	157	159	161	40.71
Nursing and personal care facilities	73	0.06	109	110	113	50.68

Source: National Industry Occupation Matrix, 1994, acquired on electronic media. Prepared by Bureau of Labor Statistics, Washington, DC: U.S. Department of Labor, 1994.

★ 847 ★

Employment by Occupation

Dental Laboratory Technicians, Precision: 1994 and 2005

Data for 1994 are based on BLS surveys. Data for 2005 are BLS projections using a variety of methods and statistical tools.

| Industry | 1994 | | 2005 employment | | | % change 1994- 2005 |
	Total employ- ment	% of industry empl.	Low	Mid	High	(Mid)
Total, all industries	39,412	100	36,730	37,066	37,332	-5.95
Medical and dental laboratories	31,751	80.56	28,703	29,112	29,489	-8.31
Offices and clinics of dentists	6,837	17.35	7,204	7,134	7,027	4.34
Federal government	727	1.84	677	675	673	-7.15

Source: National Industry Occupation Matrix, 1994, acquired on electronic media. Prepared by Bureau of Labor Statistics, Washington, DC: U.S. Department of Labor, 1994.

★ 848 ★

Employment by Occupation

Dentists: 1994 and 2005

Data for 1994 are based on BLS surveys. Data for 2005 are BLS projections using a variety of methods and statistical tools.

| Industry | 1994 | | 2005 employment | | | % change 1994- 2005 |
	Total employ- ment	% of industry empl.	Low	Mid	High	(Mid)
Total, all industries	84,452	100	89,779	89,018	87,884	5.41
Offices and clinics of dentists	78,801	93.31	83,035	82,228	80,997	4.35
Hospitals, public and private	1,816	2.15	1,977	2,042	2,162	12.44
Offices of physicians including osteopaths	1,741	2.06	2,425	2,402	2,366	37.97
Federal government	1,404	1.66	1,307	1,303	1,300	-7.19
Nursing and personal care facilities	324	0.38	483	487	502	50.31
Health and allied services, nec	224	0.27	317	321	325	43.30
Offices of other health practitioners	102	0.12	166	164	162	60.78

Source: National Industry Occupation Matrix, 1994, acquired on electronic media. Prepared by Bureau of Labor Statistics, Washington, DC: U.S. Department of Labor, 1994.

★ 849 ★

Employment by Occupation

EKG Technicians: 1994 and 2005

Data for 1994 are based on BLS surveys. Data for 2005 are BLS projections using a variety of methods and statistical tools.

Industry	1994		2005 employment			% change 1994-2005
	Total employ-ment	% of industry empl.	Low	Mid	High	(Mid)
Total, all industries	16,126	100	11,049	11,331	11,844	-29.73
Hospitals, public and private	14,073	87.27	8,718	9,005	9,532	-36.01
Offices of physicians including osteopaths	1,466	9.09	1,609	1,593	1,569	8.66
Medical and dental laboratories	365	2.27	445	451	457	23.56
Health and allied services, nec	182	1.13	225	228	231	25.27

Source: National Industry Occupation Matrix, 1994, acquired on electronic media. Prepared by Bureau of Labor Statistics, Washington, DC: U.S. Department of Labor, 1994.

★ 850 ★

Employment by Occupation

Electromedical and Biomedical Equipment Repairers: 1994 and 2005

Data for 1994 are based on BLS surveys. Data for 2005 are BLS projections using a variety of methods and statistical tools.

Industry	1994		2005 employment			% change 1994-2005
	Total employ-ment	% of industry empl.	Low	Mid	High	(Mid)
Total, all industries	9,542	100	10,901	11,191	11,695	17.28
Hospitals, public and private	7,167	75.11	7,804	8,061	8,533	12.47
Federal government	526	5.51	490	488	487	-7.22
Electrical repair shops	469	4.92	626	637	649	35.82
Repair shops and related services, nec	462	4.85	663	675	689	46.10
Medical and dental laboratories	353	3.7	491	498	505	41.08
Health and allied services, nec	316	3.31	447	453	459	43.35
Offices of physicians including osteopaths	162	1.69	225	223	220	37.65

Source: National Industry Occupation Matrix, 1994, acquired on electronic media. Prepared by Bureau of Labor Statistics, Washington, DC: U.S. Department of Labor, 1994.

★ 851 ★

Employment by Occupation

Electroneurodiagnostic Technologists: 1994 and 2005

Data for 1994 are based on BLS surveys. Data for 2005 are BLS projections using a variety of methods and statistical tools.

Industry	1994		2005 employment			% change 1994-2005
	Total employment	% of industry empl.	Low	Mid	High	(Mid)
Total, all industries	6,479	100	8,097	8,302	8,678	28.14
Hospitals, public and private	5,357	82.67	6,416	6,627	7,015	23.71
Offices of physicians including osteopaths	825	12.73	1,264	1,251	1,233	51.64
Medical and dental laboratories	176	2.71	244	248	251	40.91

Source: National Industry Occupation Matrix, 1994, acquired on electronic media. Prepared by Bureau of Labor Statistics, Washington, DC: U.S. Department of Labor, 1994.

★ 852 ★

Employment by Occupation

Emergency Medical Technicians: 1994 and 2005

Data for 1994 are based on BLS surveys. Data for 2005 are BLS projections using a variety of methods and statistical tools.

Industry	1994		2005 employment			% change 1994-2005
	Total employment	% of industry empl.	Low	Mid	High	(Mid)
Total, all industries	138,276	100	178,435	187,487	197,177	35.59
Local and interurban passenger transit	59,481	43.02	80,565	83,319	84,918	40.08
Local government, except education and hospitals	45,863	33.17	54,365	59,404	65,207	29.52
Hospitals, public and private	28,883	20.89	37,738	38,983	41,265	34.97
Offices of physicians including osteopaths	1,953	1.41	2,720	2,694	2,653	37.94
Offices of other health practitioners	806	0.58	1,307	1,294	1,275	60.55
Health and allied services, nec	539	0.39	762	773	783	43.41
State government, except education and hospitals	400	0.29	383	418	459	4.50
Nursing and personal care facilities	233	0.17	347	351	361	50.64
Home health care services	104	0.07	228	231	234	122.12

Source: National Industry Occupation Matrix, 1994, acquired on electronic media. Prepared by Bureau of Labor Statistics, Washington, DC: U.S. Department of Labor, 1994.

★ 853 ★

Employment by Occupation

Full-Time Equivalent Employment in Selected Occupations for Community Hospitals: United States, Selected Years 1983-92

Data are based on reporting by a census of registered hospitals.

Occupation	1983	1989	1990	1991	1992	Average annual percent change	
						1983-89	1989-92
All hospital personnel[1]	3,130,131	3,328,509	3,439,820	3,554,962	3,635,530	1.0	3.0
Administrators and assistant administrators[2]	28,805	37,269	37,015	39,505	52,575	4.4	12.2
Physicians	25,520	33,850	36,451	37,091	38,079	4.8	4.0
Physician assistants	2,222	3,313	3,543	3,940	4,320	6.9	9.2
Registered nurses	698,151	791,521	809,920	840,493	853,789	2.1	2.6
Licensed practical nurses	229,735	172,143	167,945	165,871	157,208	-4.7	-3.0
Ancillary nursing personnel	294,180	252,500	268,113	278,125	274,015	-2.5	2.8
Medical records administrators and technicians	39,115	47,834	50,723	51,380	53,033	3.4	3.5
Licensed pharmacists and pharmacy technicians	52,077	60,984	64,004	65,735	67,585	2.7	3.5
Medical technologists and other laboratory personnel	149,949	152,122	157,880	161,087	163,323	0.2	2.4
Dietitians and dietetic technicians	36,623	34,416	35,553	35,294	33,232	-1.0	-1.2
Radiologic service personnel	92,509	104,494	111,298	114,455	117,401	2.1	4.0
Occupational therapists, occupational therapy assistants, and recreational therapists	9,078	13,604	15,144	16,290	17,294	7.0	8.3
Physical therapists and physical therapy assistants and aides	28,759	33,104	35,455	38,004	38,956	2.4	5.6
Speech pathologists and audiologists	2,684	4,608	4,909	5,550	5,910	9.4	8.6
Respiratory therapists and respiratory therapy technicians	51,490	57,355	60,403	62,969	64,337	1.8	3.9
Medical social workers	14,489	19,698	21,389	23,077	23,515	5.3	6.1
Total trainee personnel[3]	66,515	68,641	69,111	71,570	73,324	0.5	2.2

Source: U.S. Department of Health and Human Services. Public Health Service. Centers for Disease Control and Prevention. National Center for Health Statistics. *Health, United States, 1994.* Hyattsville, MD: Public Health Service, 1995, p. 204. *Notes:* 1. Includes occupational categories not shown. 2. Beginning in 1992, the occupational definition of assistant was expanded to include additional administrative job titles in more areas of the facility. 3. This category is primarily composed of medical residents and interns.

★ 854 ★

Employment by Occupation

Home Health Aides: 1994 and 2005

Data for 1994 are based on BLS surveys. Data for 2005 are BLS projections using a variety of methods and statistical tools.

| Industry | 1994 | | 2005 employment | | | % change 1994-2005 |
	Total employ-ment	% of industry empl.	Low	Mid	High	(Mid)
Total, all industries	405,624	100	806,795	822,775	838,236	102.84
Home health care services	172,311	42.48	384,835	390,320	395,374	126.52
Individual and miscellaneous social services	79,456	19.59	130,815	135,070	137,238	69.99
Personnel supply services	64,900	16	101,323	102,958	105,009	58.64
Residential care	28,582	7.05	84,183	85,575	86,407	199.40
Hospitals, public and private	19,293	4.76	52,517	54,249	57,425	181.18
Nursing and personal care facilities	13,924	3.43	20,721	20,923	21,567	50.27
Local government, except education and hospitals	11,223	2.77	11,087	12,114	13,297	7.94
State government, except education and hospitals	5,293	1.3	5,070	5,539	6,081	4.65
Job training and related services	4,143	1.02	6,605	6,341	6,133	53.05
Health and allied services, nec	1,551	0.38	2,193	2,225	2,253	43.46
Management and public relations	687	0.17	1,030	1,042	1,055	51.67
Miscellaneous equipment rental and leasing	319	0.08	465	475	485	48.90
Services to buildings	79	0.02	149	152	155	92.41

Source: National Industry Occupation Matrix, 1994, acquired on electronic media. Prepared by Bureau of Labor Statistics, Washington, DC: U.S. Department of Labor, 1994.

★ 855 ★

Employment by Occupation

Human Services Workers: 1994 and 2005

Data for 1994 are based on BLS surveys. Data for 2005 are BLS projections using a variety of methods and statistical tools.

| Industry | 1994 | | 2005 employment | | | % change 1994-2005 |
	Total employ-ment	% of industry empl.	Low	Mid	High	(Mid)
Total, all industries	168,129	100	283,741	293,444	302,611	74.54
Individual and miscellaneous social services	45,192	26.88	89,285	92,189	93,669	103.99
Local government, except education and hospitals	33,052	19.66	39,180	42,811	46,993	29.53
Residential care	30,182	17.95	71,115	72,291	72,994	139.52
State government, except education and hospitals	19,418	11.55	20,458	22,353	24,538	15.11
Health and allied services, nec	9,304	5.53	15,790	16,015	16,223	72.13
Hospitals, public and private	9,239	5.5	11,065	11,430	12,100	23.71
Job training and related services	9,208	5.48	17,613	16,909	16,356	83.63
Nursing and personal care facilities	3,658	2.18	5,444	5,497	5,666	50.27
Home health care services	2,417	1.44	5,312	5,388	5,458	122.92
Civic and social associations	1,477	0.88	1,686	1,826	1,945	23.63
Child day care services	1,415	0.84	2,544	2,424	2,321	71.31

[Continued]

★ 855 ★

Human Services Workers: 1994 and 2005

[Continued]

Industry	1994		2005 employment			% change 1994-2005 (Mid)
	Total employ-ment	% of industry empl.	Low	Mid	High	
Federal government	1,265	0.75	1,179	1,175	1,172	-7.11
Offices of physicians including osteopaths	1,041	0.62	1,451	1,436	1,415	37.94
Offices of other health practitioners	354	0.21	574	568	560	60.45

Source: National Industry Occupation Matrix, 1994, acquired on electronic media. Prepared by Bureau of Labor Statistics, Washington, DC: U.S. Department of Labor, 1994.

★ 856 ★

Employment by Occupation

Licensed Practical Nurses: 1994 and 2005

Data for 1994 are based on BLS surveys. Data for 2005 are BLS projections using a variety of methods and statistical tools.

Industry	1994		2005 employment			% change 1994-2005 (Mid)
	Total employ-ment	% of industry empl.	Low	Mid	High	
Total, all industries	698,038	100	878,342	894,579	923,299	28.16
Hospitals, public and private	262,238	37.57	256,974	265,450	280,994	1.22
Nursing and personal care facilities	182,116	26.09	271,011	273,656	282,071	50.26
Offices of physicians including osteopaths	84,303	12.08	117,436	116,294	114,552	37.95
Personnel supply services	39,780	5.7	36,215	36,800	37,533	-7.49
Home health care services	39,774	5.7	87,413	88,659	89,807	122.91
Local government, except education and hospitals	16,237	2.33	16,039	17,526	19,238	7.94
State government, except education and hospitals	14,973	2.14	15,768	17,229	18,913	15.07
Residential care	14,872	2.13	23,361	23,747	23,978	59.68
Federal government	13,901	1.99	12,949	12,908	12,872	-7.14
Health and allied services, nec	8,392	1.2	11,869	12,038	12,194	43.45
Education, public and private	5,252	0.75	6,216	6,765	7,389	28.81
Individual and miscellaneous social services	3,869	0.55	6,370	6,577	6,682	69.99
Religious organizations	3,335	0.48	3,795	4,111	4,378	23.27
Offices of other health practitioners	2,966	0.42	4,808	4,762	4,690	60.55
Management and public relations	1,489	0.21	2,233	2,259	2,287	51.71
Job training and related services	1,072	0.15	1,708	1,640	1,586	52.99
Offices and clinics of dentists	893	0.13	1,176	1,165	1,147	30.46
Research and testing services	297	0.04	377	378	378	27.27
Miscellaneous equipment rental and leasing	221	0.03	322	329	336	48.87
Child day care services	209	0.03	375	357	342	70.81
Civic and social associations	146	0.02	167	181	192	23.97
Personal services, nec	144	0.02	222	210	200	45.83

Source: National Industry Occupation Matrix, 1994, acquired on electronic media. Prepared by Bureau of Labor Statistics, Washington, DC: U.S. Department of Labor, 1994.

★ 857 ★

Employment by Occupation

Medical Assistants: 1994 and 2005

Data for 1994 are based on BLS surveys. Data for 2005 are BLS projections using a variety of methods and statistical tools.

Industry	1994		2005 employment			% change 1994-2005
	Total employment	% of industry empl.	Low	Mid	High	(Mid)
Total, all industries	205,537	100	328,571	326,868	324,494	59.03
Offices of physicians including osteopaths	143,330	69.73	239,595	237,266	233,712	65.54
Offices of other health practitioners	25,647	12.48	41,579	41,175	40,558	60.55
Hospitals, public and private	12,281	5.98	13,372	13,813	14,622	12.47
Nursing and personal care facilities	11,992	5.83	17,846	18,020	18,574	50.27
Health and allied services, nec	6,264	3.05	8,859	8,985	9,102	43.44
Offices and clinics of dentists	1,619	0.79	2,132	2,111	2,080	30.39
Medical and dental laboratories	791	0.38	1,100	1,115	1,130	40.96
Home health care services	449	0.22	987	1,001	1,014	122.94
Federal government	87	0.04	81	81	81	-6.90

Source: National Industry Occupation Matrix, 1994, acquired on electronic media. Prepared by Bureau of Labor Statistics, Washington, DC: U.S. Department of Labor, 1994.

★ 858 ★

Employment by Occupation

Medical Records Technicians: 1994 and 2005

Data for 1994 are based on BLS surveys. Data for 2005 are BLS projections using a variety of methods and statistical tools.

Industry	1994		2005 employment			% change 1994-2005
	Total employment	% of industry empl.	Low	Mid	High	(Mid)
Total, all industries	81,089	100	124,507	126,309	129,551	55.77
Hospitals, public and private	35,444	43.71	46,310	47,838	50,639	34.97
Offices of physicians including osteopaths	18,747	23.12	35,256	34,913	34,390	86.23
Nursing and personal care facilities	8,771	10.82	17,621	17,793	18,341	102.86
Federal government	3,753	4.63	3,496	3,485	3,475	-7.14
Health and allied services, nec	2,673	3.3	3,780	3,834	3,884	43.43
Home health care services	2,426	2.99	5,331	5,407	5,477	122.88
Offices of other health practitioners	1,633	2.01	2,647	2,621	2,582	60.50
Offices and clinics of dentists	1,436	1.77	1,892	1,873	1,845	30.43
Residential care	1,216	1.5	2,389	2,428	2,452	99.67
Local government, except education and hospitals	1,151	1.42	1,137	1,243	1,364	7.99
State government, except education and hospitals	1,145	1.41	1,097	1,198	1,316	4.63
Individual and miscellaneous social services	624	0.77	1,028	1,061	1,078	70.03
Education, public and private	492	0.61	582	633	692	28.66
Medical and dental laboratories	384	0.47	534	541	548	40.89

[Continued]

★ 858 ★

Medical Records Technicians: 1994 and 2005
[Continued]

Industry	1994		2005 employment			% change 1994-2005 (Mid)
	Total employ-ment	% of industry empl.	Low	Mid	High	
Business and professional organizations	227	0.28	237	257	274	13.22
Fire, marine, and casualty insurance	167	0.21	183	187	191	11.98
Life insurance	149	0.18	160	164	168	10.07
Job training and related services	121	0.15	193	186	180	53.72
Medical service and health insurance	96	0.12	104	106	109	10.42
Child day care services	73	0.09	131	125	119	71.23

Source: National Industry Occupation Matrix, 1994, acquired on electronic media. Prepared by Bureau of Labor Statistics, Washington, DC: U.S. Department of Labor, 1994.

★ 859 ★

Employment by Occupation

Medical Scientists: 1994 and 2005

Data for 1994 are based on BLS surveys. Data for 2005 are BLS projections using a variety of methods and statistical tools.

Industry	1994		2005 employment			% change 1994-2005 (Mid)
	Total employ-ment	% of industry empl.	Low	Mid	High	
Total, all industries	34,780	100	43,674	45,910	48,425	32.00
State government, except education and hospitals	6,977	20.06	6,682	7,301	8,015	4.64
Education, public and private	5,843	16.8	8,989	9,783	10,686	67.43
Research and testing services	5,689	16.36	9,369	9,389	9,411	65.04
Chemicals and allied products	4,349	12.51	6,094	6,406	6,642	47.30
Local government, except education and hospitals	3,709	10.66	3,664	4,003	4,394	7.93
Hospitals, public and private	3,677	10.57	3,203	3,308	3,502	-10.04
Federal government	1,311	3.77	1,466	1,461	1,457	11.44
Medical and dental laboratories	1,036	2.98	1,441	1,462	1,481	41.12
Instruments and related products	632	1.82	688	697	713	10.28
Offices of physicians including osteopaths	324	0.93	452	448	441	38.27
Health and allied services, nec	170	0.49	241	245	248	44.12
Wholesale trade, nec	135	0.39	153	157	162	16.30

Source: National Industry Occupation Matrix, 1994, acquired on electronic media. Prepared by Bureau of Labor Statistics, Washington, DC: U.S. Department of Labor, 1994.

★ 860 ★

Employment by Occupation

Medical Secretaries: 1994 and 2005

Data for 1994 are based on BLS surveys. Data for 2005 are BLS projections using a variety of methods and statistical tools.

Industry	1994		2005 employment			% change 1994-2005 (Mid)
	Total employment	% of industry empl.	Low	Mid	High	
Total, all industries	225,551	100	280,309	280,747	281,898	24.47
Offices of physicians including osteopaths	113,903	50.5	142,803	141,415	139,297	24.15
Hospitals, public and private	53,200	23.59	57,924	59,835	63,338	12.47
Offices and clinics of dentists	19,494	8.64	23,109	22,884	22,541	17.39
Offices of other health practitioners	16,800	7.45	24,513	24,275	23,911	44.49
Home health care services	5,404	2.4	10,689	10,842	10,982	100.63
Health and allied services, nec	4,729	2.1	6,019	6,105	6,184	29.10
Nursing and personal care facilities	4,614	2.05	6,179	6,240	6,432	35.24
Medical and dental laboratories	4,119	1.83	5,156	5,229	5,297	26.95
Agricultural services	3,289	1.46	3,917	3,923	3,916	19.28

Source: National Industry Occupation Matrix, 1994, acquired on electronic media. Prepared by Bureau of Labor Statistics, Washington, DC: U.S. Department of Labor, 1994.

★ 861 ★

Employment by Occupation

Nuclear Medicine Technologists: 1994 and 2005

Data for 1994 are based on BLS surveys. Data for 2005 are BLS projections using a variety of methods and statistical tools.

Industry	1994		2005 employment			% change 1994-2005 (Mid)
	Total employment	% of industry empl.	Low	Mid	High	
Total, all industries	13,004	100	15,898	16,332	17,125	25.59
Hospitals, public and private	11,129	85.58	13,329	13,769	14,575	23.72
Offices of physicians including osteopaths	1,170	8.99	1,629	1,613	1,589	37.86
Medical and dental laboratories	269	2.07	374	379	384	40.89
Health and allied services, nec	230	1.77	325	330	334	43.48
Federal government	157	1.21	146	146	146	-7.01

Source: National Industry Occupation Matrix, 1994, acquired on electronic media. Prepared by Bureau of Labor Statistics, Washington, DC: U.S. Department of Labor, 1994.

★ 862 ★

Employment by Occupation

Nursing Aides, Orderlies, and Attendants: 1994 and 2005

Data for 1994 are based on BLS surveys. Data for 2005 are BLS projections using a variety of methods and statistical tools.

| Industry | 1994 | | 2005 employment | | | % change 1994-2005 |
	Total employ-ment	% of industry empl.	Low	Mid	High	(Mid)
Total, all industries	1,243,870	100	1,596,427	1,624,257	1,681,489	30.58
Nursing and personal care facilities	643,080	51.7	956,981	966,322	996,037	50.26
Hospitals, public and private	306,009	24.6	333,185	344,174	364,328	12.47
Private households	60,375	4.85	48,210	47,178	45,963	-21.86
Residential care	57,105	4.59	72,883	74,088	74,809	29.74
Local government, except education and hospitals	42,255	3.4	33,569	36,680	40,263	-13.19
Personnel supply services	33,984	2.73	30,939	31,438	32,064	-7.49
State government, except education and hospitals	27,232	2.19	16,946	18,516	20,325	-32.01
Home health care services	23,243	1.87	40,866	41,448	41,985	78.32
Federal government	15,390	1.24	14,337	14,292	14,251	-7.13
Individual and miscellaneous social services	6,086	0.49	10,021	10,346	10,513	70.00
Education, public and private	5,216	0.42	6,173	6,718	7,339	28.80
Health and allied services, nec	4,607	0.37	6,515	6,608	6,693	43.43
Offices of other health practitioners	3,857	0.31	6,253	6,192	6,099	60.54
Job training and related services	1,491	0.12	2,377	2,282	2,207	53.05
Civic and social associations	296	0.02	338	366	390	23.65
Miscellaneous equipment rental and leasing	161	0.01	234	239	244	48.45
Child day care services	149	0.01	267	254	244	70.47
Medical and dental laboratories	103	0.01	143	145	146	40.78

Source: National Industry Occupation Matrix, 1994, acquired on electronic media. Prepared by Bureau of Labor Statistics, Washington, DC: U.S. Department of Labor, 1994.

★ 863 ★

Employment by Occupation

Occupational Therapists: 1994 and 2005

Data for 1994 are based on BLS surveys. Data for 2005 are BLS projections using a variety of methods and statistical tools.

| Industry | 1994 | | 2005 employment | | | % change 1994-2005 |
	Total employ-ment	% of industry empl.	Low	Mid	High	(Mid)
Total, all industries	50,755	100	86,645	88,554	91,323	74.47
Hospitals, public and private	16,918	33.33	27,631	28,543	30,214	68.71
Offices of other health practitioners	8,380	16.51	20,380	20,182	19,880	140.84
Education, public and private	8,003	15.77	8,945	9,735	10,634	21.64
Health and allied services, nec	3,735	7.36	7,715	7,825	7,926	109.50
Home health care services	3,626	7.14	7,970	8,083	8,188	122.92

[Continued]

★ 863 ★

Occupational Therapists: 1994 and 2005
[Continued]

Industry	1994		2005 employment			% change 1994-2005
	Total employ-ment	% of industry empl.	Low	Mid	High	(Mid)
Nursing and personal care facilities	3,442	6.78	5,122	5,172	5,331	50.26
Offices of physicians including osteopaths	1,606	3.16	2,237	2,215	2,182	37.92
State government, except education and hospitals	1,048	2.07	1,004	1,097	1,204	4.68
Job training and related services	958	1.89	1,527	1,466	1,418	53.03
Local government, except education and hospitals	819	1.61	809	884	970	7.94
Federal government	751	1.48	699	697	695	-7.19
Residential care	683	1.35	1,341	1,363	1,377	99.56
Individual and miscellaneous social services	553	1.09	910	940	955	69.98
Child day care services	125	0.25	225	215	206	72.00
Civic and social associations	62	0.12	71	77	82	24.19

Source: National Industry Occupation Matrix, 1994, acquired on electronic media. Prepared by Bureau of Labor Statistics, Washington, DC: U.S. Department of Labor, 1994.

★ 864 ★

Employment by Occupation

Occupational Therapy Assistants and Aides: 1994 and 2005

Data for 1994 are based on BLS surveys. Data for 2005 are BLS projections using a variety of methods and statistical tools.

Industry	1994		2005 employment			% change 1994-2005
	Total employ-ment	% of industry empl.	Low	Mid	High	(Mid)
Total, all industries	15,717	100	28,283	28,624	29,306	82.12
Hospitals, public and private	6,180	39.32	10,094	10,427	11,037	68.72
Nursing and personal care facilities	3,949	25.13	5,877	5,934	6,117	50.27
Offices of other health practitioners	3,198	20.35	8,295	8,215	8,092	156.88
Residential care	651	4.14	1,278	1,299	1,311	99.54
Offices of physicians including osteopaths	532	3.39	741	734	723	37.97
Health and allied services, nec	402	2.56	568	576	583	43.28
Individual and miscellaneous social services	277	1.77	457	472	479	70.40
Home health care services	229	1.46	504	512	518	123.58
Job training and related services	173	1.1	276	265	256	53.18
Child day care services	77	0.49	138	132	126	71.43

Source: National Industry Occupation Matrix, 1994, acquired on electronic media. Prepared by Bureau of Labor Statistics, Washington, DC: U.S. Department of Labor, 1994.

★ 865 ★

Employment by Occupation

Optical Goods Workers, Precision: 1994 and 2005

Data for 1994 are based on BLS surveys. Data for 2005 are BLS projections using a variety of methods and statistical tools.

Industry	1994		2005 employment			% change 1994-2005 (Mid)
	Total employ-ment	% of industry empl.	Low	Mid	High	
Total, all industries	19,222	100	20,834	21,583	22,354	12.28
Instruments and related products	10,025	52.16	9,553	9,942	10,337	-0.83
General merchandise stores	167	0.87	167	173	179	3.59

Source: National Industry Occupation Matrix, 1994, acquired on electronic media. Prepared by Bureau of Labor Statistics, Washington, DC: U.S. Department of Labor, 1994.

★ 866 ★

Employment by Occupation

Opticians, Dispensing and Measuring: 1994 and 2005

Data for 1994 are based on BLS surveys. Data for 2005 are BLS projections using a variety of methods and statistical tools.

Industry	1994		2005 employment			% change 1994-2005 (Mid)
	Total employ-ment	% of industry empl.	Low	Mid	High	
Total, all industries	58,539	100	71,060	71,852	72,485	22.74
Offices of other health practitioners	27,104	46.3	31,779	31,470	30,998	16.11
Miscellaneous retail stores	24,198	41.34	31,151	32,186	33,235	33.01
Offices of physicians including osteopaths	4,049	6.92	4,513	4,469	4,402	10.37
General merchandise stores	1,675	2.86	1,949	2,014	2,080	20.24
Instruments and related products	558	0.95	547	567	585	1.61
Wholesale trade, nec	387	0.66	439	450	464	16.28
Hospitals, public and private	293	0.5	319	329	349	12.29
Health and allied services, nec	167	0.29	237	240	243	43.71

Source: National Industry Occupation Matrix, 1994, acquired on electronic media. Prepared by Bureau of Labor Statistics, Washington, DC: U.S. Department of Labor, 1994.

★ 867 ★

Employment by Occupation

Optometrists: 1994 and 2005

Data for 1994 are based on BLS surveys. Data for 2005 are BLS projections using a variety of methods and statistical tools.

Industry	1994		2005 employment			% change 1994-2005 (Mid)
	Total employ-ment	% of industry empl.	Low	Mid	High	
Total, all industries	23,286	100	26,921	26,837	26,652	15.25
Offices of other health practitioners	16,068	69	17,783	17,611	17,347	9.60
Offices of physicians including osteopaths	3,198	13.74	4,500	4,456	4,390	39.34
Miscellaneous retail stores	2,837	12.18	3,266	3,375	3,485	18.96
Federal government	283	1.22	267	266	265	-6.01
General merchandise stores	243	1.05	245	253	261	4.12
Hospitals, public and private	221	0.95	244	252	266	14.03
Health and allied services, nec	84	0.36	120	121	123	44.05

Source: National Industry Occupation Matrix, 1994, acquired on electronic media. Prepared by Bureau of Labor Statistics, Washington, DC: U.S. Department of Labor, 1994.

★ 868 ★

Employment by Occupation

Personal and Home Care Aides: 1994 and 2005

Data for 1994 are based on BLS surveys. Data for 2005 are BLS projections using a variety of methods and statistical tools.

Industry	1994		2005 employment			% change 1994-2005 (Mid)
	Total employ-ment	% of industry empl.	Low	Mid	High	
Total, all industries	178,569	100	382,179	390,581	396,943	118.73
Home health care services	69,980	39.19	156,292	158,520	160,572	126.52
Individual and miscellaneous social services	46,200	25.87	114,093	117,804	119,695	154.99
Residential care	31,010	17.37	73,066	74,275	74,997	139.52
Local government, except education and hospitals	8,904	4.99	8,796	9,611	10,550	7.94
Job training and related services	6,649	3.72	10,599	10,175	9,842	53.03
Hospitals, public and private	2,945	1.65	3,848	3,975	4,208	34.97
Nursing and personal care facilities	2,929	1.64	4,359	4,401	4,537	50.26
State government, except education and hospitals	2,730	1.53	2,615	2,857	3,136	4.65
Education, public and private	2,328	1.3	2,602	2,832	3,094	21.65
Federal government	991	0.56	923	920	918	-7.16
Health and allied services, nec	613	0.34	867	879	890	43.39

Source: National Industry Occupation Matrix, 1994, acquired on electronic media. Prepared by Bureau of Labor Statistics, Washington, DC: U.S. Department of Labor, 1994.

★ 869 ★

Employment by Occupation

Pharmacists: 1994 and 2005

Data for 1994 are based on BLS surveys. Data for 2005 are BLS projections using a variety of methods and statistical tools.

Industry	1994		2005 employment			% change 1994-2005
	Total employ-ment	% of industry empl.	Low	Mid	High	(Mid)
Total, all industries	160,678	100	183,487	189,198	196,490	17.75
Hospitals, public and private	45,846	28.53	54,909	56,720	60,041	23.72
Federal government	4,810	2.99	5,278	5,262	5,247	9.40
General merchandise stores	3,391	2.11	3,856	3,984	4,114	17.49
Offices of physicians including osteopaths	2,397	1.49	3,339	3,307	3,257	37.96
Wholesale trade, nec	1,839	1.14	2,288	2,349	2,423	27.73
State government, except education and hospitals	1,326	0.83	1,270	1,388	1,523	4.68
Home health care services	1,202	0.75	2,641	2,679	2,713	122.88
Nursing and personal care facilities	718	0.45	1,068	1,079	1,112	50.28
Health and allied services, nec	471	0.29	666	675	684	43.31
Chemicals and allied products	416	0.26	489	514	533	23.56
Individual and miscellaneous social services	269	0.17	443	457	464	69.89
Residential care	248	0.15	488	496	501	100.00
Offices of other health practitioners	115	0.07	187	185	183	60.87
Religious organizations	57	0.04	65	71	75	24.56
Medical and dental laboratories	51	0.03	71	72	73	41.18

Source: National Industry Occupation Matrix, 1994, acquired on electronic media. Prepared by Bureau of Labor Statistics, Washington, DC: U.S. Department of Labor, 1994.

★ 870 ★

Employment by Occupation

Pharmacy Assistants: 1994 and 2005

Data for 1994 are based on BLS surveys. Data for 2005 are BLS projections using a variety of methods and statistical tools.

Industry	1994		2005 employment			% change 1994-2005
	Total employ-ment	% of industry empl.	Low	Mid	High	(Mid)
Total, all industries	52,228	100	62,442	64,369	67,559	23.25
Hospitals, public and private	38,650	74	45,529	47,031	49,785	21.68
Miscellaneous retail stores	7,948	15.22	8,836	9,130	9,427	14.87
Food stores	2,516	4.82	3,530	3,647	3,766	44.95
Offices of physicians including osteopaths	1,494	2.86	2,081	2,061	2,030	37.95
Nursing and personal care facilities	542	1.04	807	815	840	50.37
General merchandise stores	305	0.58	303	313	323	2.62

[Continued]

★ 870 ★

Pharmacy Assistants: 1994 and 2005
[Continued]

Industry	1994		2005 employment			% change 1994-2005
	Total employment	% of industry empl.	Low	Mid	High	(Mid)
Health and allied services, nec	259	0.5	367	372	377	43.63
Offices of other health practitioners	69	0.13	111	110	109	59.42

Source: National Industry Occupation Matrix, 1994, acquired on electronic media. Prepared by Bureau of Labor Statistics, Washington, DC: U.S. Department of Labor, 1994.

★ 871 ★

Employment by Occupation

Pharmacy Technicians: 1994 and 2005

Data for 1994 are based on BLS surveys. Data for 2005 are BLS projections using a variety of methods and statistical tools.

Industry	1994		2005 employment			% change 1994-2005
	Total employment	% of industry empl.	Low	Mid	High	(Mid)
Total, all industries	81,313	100	97,987	101,085	104,244	24.32
Miscellaneous retail stores	68,383	84.1	81,492	84,199	86,944	23.13
Federal government	4,072	5.01	3,793	3,781	3,770	-7.15
Food stores	3,685	4.53	6,460	6,674	6,892	81.11
General merchandise stores	2,988	3.68	3,523	3,640	3,759	21.82
Wholesale trade, nec	2,164	2.66	2,695	2,767	2,854	27.87

Source: National Industry Occupation Matrix, 1994, acquired on electronic media. Prepared by Bureau of Labor Statistics, Washington, DC: U.S. Department of Labor, 1994.

★ 872 ★

Employment by Occupation

Physical and Corrective Therapy Assistants and Aides: 1994 and 2005

Data for 1994 are based on BLS surveys. Data for 2005 are BLS projections using a variety of methods and statistical tools.

Industry	1994		2005 employment			% change 1994-2005 (Mid)
	Total employ-ment	% of industry empl.	Low	Mid	High	
Total, all industries	77,538	100	141,382	141,970	143,073	83.10
Offices of other health practitioners	32,231	41.57	70,543	69,857	68,811	116.74
Hospitals, public and private	19,363	24.97	25,299	26,133	27,663	34.96
Health and allied services, nec	11,058	14.26	22,844	23,169	23,469	109.52
Nursing and personal care facilities	7,568	9.76	11,262	11,372	11,722	50.26
Offices of physicians including osteopaths	3,459	4.46	4,819	4,772	4,701	37.96
Federal government	922	1.19	859	856	854	-7.16
Residential care	649	0.84	1,273	1,295	1,307	99.54
Job training and related services	502	0.65	800	768	743	52.99
Individual and miscellaneous social services	132	0.17	217	224	228	69.70
Civic and social associations	66	0.08	75	81	87	22.73

Source: National Industry Occupation Matrix, 1994, acquired on electronic media. Prepared by Bureau of Labor Statistics, Washington, DC: U.S. Department of Labor, 1994.

★ 873 ★

Employment by Occupation

Physical Therapists: 1994 and 2005

Data for 1994 are based on BLS surveys. Data for 2005 are BLS projections using a variety of methods and statistical tools.

Industry	1994		2005 employment			% change 1994-2005 (Mid)
	Total employ-ment	% of industry empl.	Low	Mid	High	
Total, all industries	95,796	100	172,047	173,227	175,199	80.83
Offices of other health practitioners	31,878	33.28	69,771	69,093	68,058	116.74
Hospitals, public and private	29,611	30.91	38,689	39,965	42,305	34.97
Health and allied services, nec	9,495	9.91	19,614	19,893	20,151	109.51
Home health care services	9,378	9.79	20,611	20,905	21,176	122.92
Offices of physicians including osteopaths	6,455	6.74	9,891	9,795	9,649	51.74
Nursing and personal care facilities	6,137	6.41	9,133	9,222	9,506	50.27
Residential care	755	0.79	1,483	1,507	1,522	99.60
Federal government	650	0.68	605	603	602	-7.23
Job training and related services	581	0.61	927	890	860	53.18
Individual and miscellaneous social services	481	0.5	791	817	830	69.85

[Continued]

★ 873 ★

Physical Therapists: 1994 and 2005
[Continued]

Industry	1994		2005 employment			% change 1994-2005 (Mid)
	Total employ-ment	% of industry empl.	Low	Mid	High	
Civic and social associations	155	0.16	177	191	204	23.23
Child day care services	140	0.15	252	240	230	71.43

Source: *National Industry Occupation Matrix, 1994,* acquired on electronic media. Prepared by Bureau of Labor Statistics, Washington, DC: U.S. Department of Labor, 1994.

★ 874 ★

Employment by Occupation

Physician Assistants: 1994 and 2005

Data for 1994 are based on BLS surveys. Data for 2005 are BLS projections using a variety of methods and statistical tools.

Industry	1994		2005 employment			% change 1994-2005 (Mid)
	Total employ-ment	% of industry empl.	Low	Mid	High	
Total, all industries	56,343	100	69,333	69,494	69,759	23.34
Offices of physicians including osteopaths	31,435	55.79	40,173	39,782	39,186	26.55
Hospitals, public and private	8,860	15.73	10,612	10,962	11,604	23.72
Offices of other health practitioners	5,163	9.16	6,696	6,631	6,532	28.43
Local government, except education and hospitals	2,520	4.47	1,992	2,176	2,389	-13.65
Federal government	2,076	3.69	2,279	2,272	2,265	9.44
Offices and clinics of dentists	1,944	3.45	2,049	2,029	1,998	4.37
Nursing and personal care facilities	1,339	2.38	1,595	1,610	1,660	20.24
Home health care services	1,150	2.04	2,022	2,051	2,077	78.35
Health and allied services, nec	1,129	2	1,278	1,296	1,313	14.79
Education, public and private	303	0.54	286	312	340	2.97
State government, except education and hospitals	229	0.41	176	192	211	-16.16
Local and interurban passenger transit	123	0.22	111	115	117	-6.50

Source: *National Industry Occupation Matrix, 1994,* acquired on electronic media. Prepared by Bureau of Labor Statistics, Washington, DC: U.S. Department of Labor, 1994.

★ 875 ★

Employment by Occupation

Physicians: 1994 and 2005

Data for 1994 are based on BLS surveys. Data for 2005 are BLS projections using a variety of methods and statistical tools.

Industry	1994		2005 employment			% change 1994-2005
	Total employment	% of industry empl.	Low	Mid	High	(Mid)
Total, all industries	428,642	100	561,794	562,701	564,791	31.28
Offices of physicians including osteopaths	259,489	60.54	370,500	366,898	361,403	41.39
Hospitals, public and private	99,042	23.11	107,838	111,394	117,917	12.47
Federal government	38,550	8.99	43,093	42,958	42,837	11.43
Health and allied services, nec	8,307	1.94	9,398	9,532	9,655	14.75
State government, except education and hospitals	4,324	1.01	4,142	4,525	4,967	4.65
Medical and dental laboratories	3,873	0.9	5,387	5,464	5,534	41.08
Local government, except education and hospitals	3,542	0.83	3,499	3,824	4,197	7.96
Offices of other health practitioners	2,776	0.65	4,501	4,457	4,391	60.55
Nursing and personal care facilities	2,627	0.61	3,909	3,947	4,068	50.25
Home health care services	1,308	0.31	2,874	2,915	2,953	122.86
Offices and clinics of dentists	1,273	0.3	1,677	1,661	1,636	30.48
Individual and miscellaneous social services	1,150	0.27	1,893	1,954	1,986	69.91
Residential care	497	0.12	976	992	1,001	99.60
Medical service and health insurance	485	0.11	525	537	548	10.72
Life insurance	447	0.1	481	492	502	10.07
Business and professional organizations	422	0.1	442	479	510	13.51
Job training and related services	120	0.03	191	184	178	53.33

Source: National Industry Occupation Matrix, 1994, acquired on electronic media. Prepared by Bureau of Labor Statistics, Washington, DC: U.S. Department of Labor, 1994.

★ 876 ★

Employment by Occupation

Physicians: How They Are Employed: 1994

Category	Percentage
Self-employed as solo practitioners	29.3
Self-employed as group practitioners	28.4
Employed by others	42.3

Source: "A System for Docs, Pols, and Mobs." *U.S. News & World Report,* 2 September 1996, p. 14. Primary source: *Journal of the American Medical Association.*

★ 877 ★

Employment by Occupation

Psychiatric Aides: 1994 and 2005

Data for 1994 are based on BLS surveys. Data for 2005 are BLS projections using a variety of methods and statistical tools.

Industry	1994		2005 employment			% change 1994-2005 (Mid)
	Total employ-ment	% of industry empl.	Low	Mid	High	
Total, all industries	105,410	100	113,108	118,223	125,655	12.16
Hospitals, public and private	56,373	53.48	57,350	59,242	62,711	5.09
State government, except education and hospitals	26,898	25.52	25,751	28,137	30,886	4.61
Nursing and personal care facilities	10,458	9.92	15,563	15,715	16,198	50.27
Local government, except education and hospitals	6,459	6.13	6,380	6,971	7,652	7.93
Residential care	1,783	1.69	2,801	2,848	2,875	59.73
Health and allied services, nec	1,408	1.34	1,991	2,019	2,045	43.39
Individual and miscellaneous social services	672	0.64	1,106	1,142	1,160	69.94
Offices of other health practitioners	613	0.58	994	985	970	60.69
Offices of physicians including osteopaths	429	0.41	597	591	582	37.76
Home health care services	142	0.13	312	316	320	122.54
Job training and related services	136	0.13	218	209	202	53.68

Source: National Industry Occupation Matrix, 1994, acquired on electronic media. Prepared by Bureau of Labor Statistics, Washington, DC: U.S. Department of Labor, 1994.

★ 878 ★

Employment by Occupation

Psychiatric Technicians: 1994 and 2005

Data for 1994 are based on BLS surveys. Data for 2005 are BLS projections using a variety of methods and statistical tools.

Industry	1994		2005 employment			% change 1994-2005 (Mid)
	Total employ-ment	% of industry empl.	Low	Mid	High	
Total, all industries	72,051	100	78,068	80,195	83,914	11.30
Hospitals, public and private	59,718	82.88	57,557	59,455	62,937	-0.44
Residential care	4,588	6.37	9,009	9,158	9,247	99.61
Health and allied services, nec	2,885	4	4,081	4,139	4,192	43.47
Nursing and personal care facilities	2,720	3.77	4,047	4,087	4,212	50.26
Job training and related services	670	0.93	1,068	1,025	991	52.99
Individual and miscellaneous social services	652	0.9	1,073	1,108	1,126	69.94
Offices of physicians including osteopaths	507	0.7	707	700	689	38.07
Offices of other health practitioners	265	0.37	429	425	419	60.38

Source: National Industry Occupation Matrix, 1994, acquired on electronic media. Prepared by Bureau of Labor Statistics, Washington, DC: U.S. Department of Labor, 1994.

★ 879 ★

Employment by Occupation

Psychologists: 1994 and 2005

Data for 1994 are based on BLS surveys. Data for 2005 are BLS projections using a variety of methods and statistical tools.

Industry	1994		2005 employment			% change 1994-2005
	Total employ-ment	% of industry empl.	Low	Mid	High	(Mid)
Total, all industries	81,293	100	100,718	105,475	110,983	29.75
Education, public and private	32,153	39.55	38,148	41,518	45,351	29.13
Hospitals, public and private	11,364	13.98	12,404	12,813	13,564	12.75
Offices of other health practitioners	6,152	7.57	9,999	9,902	9,753	60.96
State government, except education and hospitals	5,866	7.22	5,632	6,154	6,756	4.91
Individual and miscellaneous social services	4,208	5.18	6,251	6,454	6,558	53.37
Federal government	4,172	5.13	3,896	3,884	3,873	-6.90
Health and allied services, nec	3,653	4.49	5,179	5,253	5,321	43.80
Offices of physicians including osteopaths	3,546	4.36	4,952	4,904	4,830	38.30
Local government, except education and hospitals	2,861	3.52	2,833	3,096	3,398	8.21
Management and public relations	1,910	2.35	2,872	2,905	2,941	52.09
Residential care	1,777	2.19	3,498	3,556	3,590	100.11
Research and testing services	1,690	2.08	2,146	2,151	2,156	27.28
Job training and related services	629	0.77	1,006	965	934	53.42
Nursing and personal care facilities	608	0.75	907	916	944	50.66
Child day care services	192	0.24	346	329	315	71.35
Civic and social associations	60	0.07	69	74	79	23.33

Source: National Industry Occupation Matrix, 1994, acquired on electronic media. Prepared by Bureau of Labor Statistics, Washington, DC: U.S. Department of Labor, 1994.

★ 880 ★

Employment by Occupation

Radiologic Technologists and Technicians: 1994 and 2005

Data for 1994 are based on BLS surveys. Data for 2005 are BLS projections using a variety of methods and statistical tools.

Industry	1994		2005 employment			% change 1994-2005
	Total employ-ment	% of industry empl.	Low	Mid	High	(Mid)
Total, all industries	166,915	100	222,274	225,601	231,632	35.16
Hospitals, public and private	95,215	57.04	114,038	117,799	124,697	23.72
Offices of physicians including osteopaths	52,352	31.36	72,928	72,219	71,137	37.95
Medical and dental laboratories	8,582	5.14	21,093	21,394	21,671	149.29
Federal government	3,480	2.08	3,242	3,232	3,222	-7.13
Offices of other health practitioners	2,982	1.79	4,835	4,788	4,716	60.56
Health and allied services, nec	2,152	1.29	3,044	3,087	3,127	43.45
Offices and clinics of dentists	1,759	1.05	2,316	2,294	2,260	30.42

[Continued]

★ 880 ★

Radiologic Technologists and Technicians: 1994 and 2005

[Continued]

Industry	1994		2005 employment			% change 1994-2005 (Mid)
	Total employ- ment	% of industry empl.	Low	Mid	High	
Home health care services	273	0.16	599	608	616	122.71
Nursing and personal care facilities	120	0.07	179	181	186	50.83

Source: National Industry Occupation Matrix, 1994, acquired on electronic media. Prepared by Bureau of Labor Statistics, Washington, DC: U.S. Department of Labor, 1994.

★ 881 ★

Employment by Occupation

Recreation Therapists: 1994 and 2005

Data for 1994 are based on BLS surveys. Data for 2005 are BLS projections using a variety of methods and statistical tools.

Industry	1994		2005 employment			% change 1994-2005 (Mid)
	Total employ- ment	% of industry empl.	Low	Mid	High	
Total, all industries	27,531	100	33,647	34,371	35,721	24.84
Hospitals, public and private	12,534	45.53	16,377	16,917	17,908	34.97
Nursing and personal care facilities	10,173	36.95	9,840	9,936	10,241	-2.33
Residential care	1,298	4.72	2,549	2,591	2,616	99.61
Health and allied services, nec	1,282	4.66	1,813	1,839	1,863	43.45
Federal government	817	2.97	761	759	756	-7.10
Individual and miscellaneous social services	509	1.85	838	865	879	69.94
Offices of other health practitioners	259	0.94	420	416	410	60.62
Job training and related services	250	0.91	399	383	370	53.20
Home health care services	133	0.48	293	297	301	123.31

Source: National Industry Occupation Matrix, 1994, acquired on electronic media. Prepared by Bureau of Labor Statistics, Washington, DC: U.S. Department of Labor, 1994.

★ 882 ★

Employment by Occupation

Registered Nurses: 1994 and 2005

Data for 1994 are based on BLS surveys. Data for 2005 are BLS projections using a variety of methods and statistical tools.

Industry	1994 Total employment	% of industry empl.	2005 employment Low	2005 employment Mid	2005 employment High	% change 1994-2005 (Mid)
Total, all industries	1,887,055	100	2,294,270	2,355,863	2,457,912	24.84
Hospitals, public and private	1,203,161	63.76	1,310,011	1,353,218	1,432,460	12.47
Offices of physicians including osteopaths	138,838	7.36	174,065	172,373	169,791	24.15
Home health care services	112,217	5.95	250,982	254,560	257,855	126.85
Nursing and personal care facilities	109,146	5.78	191,002	192,866	198,797	76.70
Personnel supply services	62,505	3.31	73,975	75,169	76,666	20.26
Education, public and private	51,879	2.75	61,397	66,821	72,991	28.80
Federal government	48,983	2.6	45,630	45,487	45,358	-7.14
Local government, except education and hospitals	36,881	1.95	32,962	36,017	39,535	-2.34
State government, except education and hospitals	35,481	1.88	33,983	37,131	40,760	4.65
Health and allied services, nec	22,976	1.22	32,494	32,957	33,383	43.44
Residential care	14,186	0.75	18,105	18,405	18,584	29.74
Individual and miscellaneous social services	9,653	0.51	15,893	16,410	16,674	70.00
Offices of other health practitioners	6,778	0.36	10,989	10,882	10,719	60.55
Private households	5,939	0.31	4,742	4,640	4,521	-21.87
Medical service and health insurance	5,523	0.29	8,895	9,094	9,292	64.66
Religious organizations	4,046	0.21	4,603	4,987	5,311	23.26
Management and public relations	3,643	0.19	5,464	5,527	5,595	51.72
Job training and related services	2,328	0.12	3,710	3,562	3,445	53.01
Research and testing services	1,472	0.08	1,865	1,869	1,874	26.97
Life insurance	1,384	0.07	1,488	1,521	1,554	9.90
Real estate operators and lessors	1,249	0.07	1,154	1,291	1,474	3.36
Chemicals and allied products	1,127	0.06	1,117	1,157	1,182	2.66
Business and professional organizations	1,123	0.06	1,176	1,274	1,357	13.45
Miscellaneous equipment rental and leasing	1,112	0.06	1,619	1,652	1,689	48.56
Offices and clinics of dentists	984	0.05	1,296	1,284	1,264	30.49
Medical and dental laboratories	736	0.04	1,023	1,038	1,051	41.03
Fire, marine, and casualty insurance	410	0.02	448	459	468	11.95
Child day care services	385	0.02	691	659	631	71.17
Personal services, nec	336	0.02	516	489	465	45.54
Accounting, auditing, and bookeeping	287	0.02	382	389	398	35.54
Civic and social associations	275	0.01	314	340	362	23.64
U.S. Postal Service	227	0.01	196	206	216	-9.25
Real estate agents and managers	164	0.01	163	183	208	11.59
Miscellaneous business services	102	0.01	182	186	190	82.35
Legal services	90	0	138	142	145	57.78

Source: National Industry Occupation Matrix, 1994, acquired on electronic media. Prepared by Bureau of Labor Statistics, Washington, DC: U.S. Department of Labor, 1994.

★ 883 ★

Employment by Occupation

Respiratory Therapists: 1994 and 2005

Data for 1994 are based on BLS surveys. Data for 2005 are BLS projections using a variety of methods and statistical tools.

Industry	1994		2005 employment			% change 1994-2005 (Mid)
	Total employment	% of industry empl.	Low	Mid	High	
Total, all industries	72,565	100	96,023	98,963	104,337	36.38
Hospitals, public and private	67,657	93.24	88,399	91,315	96,662	34.97
Offices of other health practitioners	1,306	1.8	2,117	2,097	2,065	60.57
Health and allied services, nec	936	1.29	1,324	1,343	1,360	43.48
Home health care services	822	1.13	1,806	1,832	1,855	122.87
Nursing and personal care facilities	634	0.87	944	953	982	50.32
Offices of physicians including osteopaths	594	0.82	827	819	807	37.88
Federal government	546	0.75	508	507	505	-7.14
Medical and dental laboratories	70	0.1	97	99	100	41.43

Source: National Industry Occupation Matrix, 1994, acquired on electronic media. Prepared by Bureau of Labor Statistics, Washington, DC: U.S. Department of Labor, 1994.

★ 884 ★

Employment by Occupation

Surgical Technologists: 1994 and 2005

Data for 1994 are based on BLS surveys. Data for 2005 are BLS projections using a variety of methods and statistical tools.

Industry	1994		2005 employment			% change 1994-2005 (Mid)
	Total employment	% of industry empl.	Low	Mid	High	
Total, all industries	45,605	100	63,509	65,007	67,786	42.54
Hospitals, public and private	41,051	90.02	49,166	50,788	53,762	23.72
Offices of physicians including osteopaths	3,806	8.35	13,254	13,125	12,929	244.85
Health and allied services, nec	329	0.72	466	473	479	43.77
Offices and clinics of dentists	281	0.62	370	367	361	30.60
Home health care services	63	0.14	138	140	142	122.22

Source: National Industry Occupation Matrix, 1994, acquired on electronic media. Prepared by Bureau of Labor Statistics, Washington, DC: U.S. Department of Labor, 1994.

Health Personnel

★ 885 ★

Active Health Personnel and Number Per 100,000 Population, by Occupation and Geographic Region: United States, 1970, 1980, and 1992

Data are compiled by the Bureau of Health Professions.

Year and occupation	Number of active health personnel	Number per 100,000 population[1]				
		United States	Geographic region			
			Northeast	Midwest	South	West
1970						
Physicians	---	---	---	---	---	---
Federal[2]	---	---	---	---	---	---
Non-Federal	290,862	142.7	185.0	127.5	114.8	158.2
Doctors of medicine[2,3]	279,212	137.0	178.7	118.2	111.5	154.8
Doctors of osteopathy[2]	11,650	5.7	6.3	9.3	3.3	3.4
Dentists[4]	95,700	47.0	58.9	46.3	35.3	54.9
Optometrists	18,400	9.0	9.7	10.3	6.6	10.5
Pharmacists	112,570	55.4	60.1	57.5	50.6	52.9
Podiatrists	7,110	3.5	6.0	3.6	1.6	3.0
Registered nurses	750,000	368.9	491.2	367.5	281.8	355.9
1980						
Physicians	427,122	189.8	---	---	---	---
Federal[2]	17,642	7.8	---	---	---	---
Doctors of medicine[2,3]	16,585	7.4	---	---	---	---
Doctors of osteopathy[2]	1,057	0.5	---	---	---	---
Non-Federal	409,480	182.0	224.5	165.2	157.0	200.0
Doctors of medicine[2,3]	393,407	174.9	216.1	153.3	152.8	195.8
Doctors of osteopathy[2]	16,073	7.1	8.4	11.9	4.2	4.2
Dentists[4]	121,240	53.5	66.2	52.7	42.6	59.2
Optometrists	22,330	9.8	9.9	10.9	7.7	11.6
Pharmacists	142,780	62.5	66.5	67.8	62.1	51.8
Podiatrists	8,880	4.0	6.3	3.9	2.5	4.1
Registered nurses	1,272,900	560.0	736.0	583.6	443.4	533.7
Associate and diploma	908,300	399.9	536.0	429.2	316.5	351.1
Baccalaureate	297,300	130.9	161.0	127.8	103.8	148.1
Masters and doctorate	67,300	29.6	39.0	26.7	23.0	34.6
1992						
Physicians	614,050	242.2	---	---	---	---
Federal	21,715	8.6	---	---	---	---
Doctors of medicine[3,5]	20,439	8.1	---	---	---	---

[Continued]

★ 885 ★

Active Health Personnel and Number Per 100,000 Population, by Occupation and Geographic Region: United States, 1970, 1980, and 1992

[Continued]

Year and occupation	Number of active health personnel	Number per 100,000 population[1]				
		United States	Geographic region			
			Northeast	Midwest	South	West
Doctors of osteopathy[2]	29,869	11.8	14.7	17.8	7.3	6.5
Non-Federal	592,335	233.7	306.8	217.6	205.5	225.1
Doctors of medicine[3,5]	562,466	221.9	292.1	199.8	198.2	218.6
Doctors of osteopathy[2]	29,869	11.8	14.7	17.8	7.3	6.5
Dentists[4]	153,800	61.4	---	---	---	---
Optometrists	27,000	10.6	---	---	---	---
Pharmacists	165,300	64.7	---	---	---	---
Podiatrists[6]	12,500	4.9	---	---	---	---
Registered nurses	1,893,400	742.3	923.4	806.4	660.6	634.2
Associate and diploma	1,143,300	448.2	558.9	503.5	404.0	355.3
Baccalaureate	587,700	230.3	276.6	241.0	200.0	224.5
Masters and doctorate	162,400	63.7	87.8	61.9	56.6	54.4

Source: U.S. Department of Health and Human Services. Public Health Service. Centers for Disease Control and Prevention. National Center for Health Statistics. *Health, United States, 1994.* Hyattsville, MD: Public Health Service, 1995, p. 203. *Notes:* 1. Ratios for physicians and dentists are based on civilian population; ratios for all other health occupations are based on resident population. 2. Starting in 1989 data for doctors of medicine are as of January 1; for earlier years these data are as of December 31. Data for doctors of osteopathy are as of December 31. 3. Excludes physicians not classified according to activity status from the number of active health personnel. 4. Excludes dentists in military service, U.S. Public Health Service, and Veterans Administration. 5. Data for doctors of medicine are as of January 1, 1993. 6. 1991 data.

★ 886 ★

Health Personnel

Mental Health Patient Care Staff

Full-time equivalent patient care staff in mental health organizations, according to type of organization and staff discipline: United States, selected years, 1984-90. Data are based on inventories of mental health organizations.

Organization and discipline	Number				Percent distribution			
	1984	1986	1988	1990	1984	1986	1988	1990
All organizations								
All patient care staff	313,243	346,630	381,216	416,282	100.0	100.0	100.0	100.0
Professional patient care staff	202,474	232,481	248,430	273,758	64.6	67.1	65.2	65.8
Psychiatrists	18,482	17,874	18,132	18,846	5.9	5.2	4.8	4.5
Psychologists	21,052	20,210	23,131	22,888	6.7	5.8	6.1	5.5
Social workers	36,397	40,951	46,218	53,487	11.6	11.8	12.1	12.8
Registered nurses	54,406	66,180	73,387	77,686	17.4	19.1	19.3	18.7
Other professional staff[1]	72,137	87,266	87,562	100,851	23.0	25.2	23.0	24.2
Other mental health workers	110,769	114,149	132,786	142,524	35.4	32.9	34.8	34.2

[Continued]

★ 886 ★

Mental Health Patient Care Staff
[Continued]

Organization and discipline	Number				Percent distribution			
	1984	1986	1988	1990	1984	1986	1988	1990
State and county mental hospitals								
All patient care staff	117,630	119,073	116,527	114,198	100.0	100.0	100.0	100.0
Professional patient care staff	51,290	54,853	49,184	50,035	43.6	46.1	42.2	43.8
Psychiatrists	4,108	3,762	3,830	3,849	3.5	3.2	3.3	3.4
Psychologists	3,239	3,412	3,536	3,324	2.8	2.9	3.0	2.9
Social workers	6,175	6,238	7,164	7,013	5.2	5.2	6.1	6.1
Registered nurses	16,051	19,425	20,292	20,848	13.6	16.3	17.4	18.3
Other professional staff[1]	21,717	22,016	14,362	15,001	18.5	18.5	12.3	13.1
Other mental health workers	66,340	64,220	67,343	64,163	56.4	53.9	57.8	56.2
Private psychiatric hospitals								
All patient care staff	26,359	35,480	55,658	57,200	100.0	100.0	100.0	100.0
Professional patient care staff	19,524	27,246	42,965	45,669	74.1	76.8	77.2	79.8
Psychiatrists	1,447	1,554	1,843	1,582	5.5	4.4	3.3	2.8
Psychologists	1,461	1,557	1,833	1,977	5.5	4.4	3.3	3.5
Social workers	2,179	2,893	4,067	4,044	8.3	8.2	7.3	7.1
Registered nurses	6,818	10,147	14,710	14,819	25.9	28.6	26.4	25.9
Other professional staff[1]	7,619	11,095	20,512	23,247	28.9	31.3	36.9	40.6
Other mental health workers	6,835	8,234	12,693	11,531	25.9	23.2	22.8	20.2
Non-Federal general hospitals' psychiatric services								
All patient care staff	59,848	61,148	62,066	72,214	100.0	100.0	100.0	100.0
Professional patient care staff	46,335	50,233	48,490	57,019	77.4	82.1	78.1	79.0
Psychiatrists	6,679	6,009	5,276	6,500	11.2	9.8	8.5	9.0
Psychologists	3,283	2,983	3,707	3,951	5.5	4.9	6.0	5.5
Social workers	4,898	5,634	5,568	7,241	8.2	9.2	9.0	10.0
Registered nurses	20,454	23,454	24,490	28,473	34.2	38.4	39.5	39.4
Other professional staff[1]	11,021	12,153	9,449	10,854	18.4	19.9	15.2	15.0
Other mental health workers	13,513	10,915	13,576	15,195	22.6	17.9	21.9	21.0
Department of Veterans Affairs psychiatric services								
All patient care staff	22,948	23,559	22,074	22,080	100.0	100.0	100.0	100.0
Professional patient care staff	16,265	17,782	15,061	14,619	70.9	75.5	68.2	66.2
Psychiatrists	2,463	2,245	2,132	2,103	10.7	9.5	9.7	9.5
Psychologists	1,247	1,439	1,340	1,476	5.4	6.1	6.1	6.7
Social workers	1,545	1,680	1,424	1,855	6.7	7.1	6.5	8.4
Registered nurses	5,699	6,761	6,514	5,888	24.8	28.7	29.5	26.7
Other professional staff[1]	5,311	5,647	3,651	3,297	23.1	24.0	16.5	14.9
Other mental health workers	6,683	5,777	7,013	7,461	29.1	24.5	31.8	33.8

[Continued]

★ 886 ★

Mental Health Patient Care Staff

[Continued]

Organization and discipline	Number				Percent distribution			
	1984	1986	1988	1990	1984	1986	1988	1990
Residential treatment centers for emotionally disturbed children								
All patient care staff	15,297	25,146	30,139	40,969	100.0	100.0	100.0	100.0
Professional patient care staff	10,551	17,599	19,688	26,032	69.0	70.0	65.3	63.5
Psychiatrists	240	335	449	498	1.6	1.3	1.5	1.2
Psychologists	820	911	1,274	1,492	5.4	3.6	4.2	3.6
Social workers	2,283	4,585	4,211	5,636	14.9	18.2	14.0	13.8
Registered nurses	485	746	821	1,238	3.2	3.0	2.7	3.0
Other professional staff[1]	6,723	11,022	12,933	17,168	43.9	43.8	42.9	41.9
Other mental health workers	4,746	7,547	10,451	14,937	31.0	30.0	34.7	36.5
All other organizations[2]								
All patient care staff	71,161	82,224	94,749	109,621	100.0	100.0	100.0	100.0
Professional patient care staff	58,509	64,768	73,039	80,384	82.2	78.8	77.1	73.3
Psychiatrists	3,545	3,969	4,601	4,314	5.0	4.8	4.9	3.9
Psychologists	11,002	9,908	11,444	10,668	15.5	12.1	12.1	9.7
Social workers	19,317	19,921	23,784	27,698	27.1	24.2	25.1	25.3
Registered nurses	4,899	5,647	6,559	6,420	6.9	6.9	6.9	5.9
Other professional staff[1]	19,746	25,323	26,651	31,284	27.7	30.8	28.1	28.5
Other mental health workers	12,652	17,456	21,710	29,237	17.8	21.2	22.9	26.7

Source: U.S. Department of Health and Human Services. Public Health Service. Centers for Disease Control and Prevention. National Center for Health Statistics. *Health, United States, 1994.* Hyattsville, MD: Public Health Service, 1995, p. 205-206. *Notes:* Figures for nonpatient care staff (administrative, clerical, and maintenance staff) are not shown. 1. Includes occupational therapists, recreation therapists, vocational rehabilitation counselors, and teachers. 2. Includes freestanding outpatient clinics, freestanding day-night organizations, multiservice organizations, and other residential organizations.

Physicians

★ 887 ★

Active Non-Federal Physicians of Medicine

Active non-federal physicians and doctors of medicine in patient care per 10,000 civilian population, according to geographic division and state, United States, 1975, 1985, 1990, 1993. Data are based on reporting by physicians.

Geographic division and State	Total physicians[1]				Doctors of medicine in patient care[2]			
	1975	1985	1990	1993[3]	1975	1985	1990	1993
Number per 10,000 civilian population								
United States	15.3	20.7	22.2	23.4	13.5	18.0	19.5	20.7
New England	19.1	26.7	29.0	31.0	16.9	22.9	25.5	27.6
Maine	12.8	18.7	20.1	21.4	10.7	15.6	16.6	17.6
New Hampshire	14.3	18.1	20.1	21.3	13.1	16.7	18.6	19.7
Vermont	18.2	23.8	25.4	26.2	15.5	20.3	22.4	23.6
Massachusetts	20.8	30.2	32.8	35.3	18.3	25.4	28.6	31.4
Rhode Island	17.8	23.3	26.0	27.8	16.1	20.2	22.6	24.5
Connecticut	19.8	27.6	30.1	31.7	17.7	24.3	26.8	28.6
Middle Atlantic	19.5	26.1	28.4	30.9	17.0	22.2	24.5	26.7
New York	22.7	29.0	31.1	33.6	20.2	25.2	27.6	30.1
New Jersey	16.2	23.4	25.9	28.5	14.0	19.8	22.2	24.3
Pennsylvania	16.6	23.6	26.0	28.3	13.9	19.2	21.3	23.2
East North Central	13.9	19.3	20.6	22.2	12.0	16.4	17.6	18.9
Ohio	14.1	19.9	21.4	22.8	12.2	16.8	18.0	19.2
Indiana	10.6	14.7	16.0	17.4	9.6	13.2	14.6	15.8
Illinois	14.5	20.5	21.6	23.8	13.1	18.2	19.3	21.1
Michigan	15.4	20.8	22.1	23.5	12.0	16.0	16.9	18.0
Wisconsin	12.5	17.7	19.1	20.3	11.4	15.9	17.4	18.5
West North Central	13.3	18.3	19.8	21.1	11.4	15.6	17.1	18.4
Minnesota	14.9	20.5	22.0	23.3	13.7	18.5	20.1	21.6
Iowa	11.4	15.6	17.2	18.3	9.4	12.4	13.8	14.4
Missouri	15.0	20.5	22.0	23.2	11.6	16.3	17.7	19.1
North Dakota	9.7	15.8	17.0	18.9	9.2	14.9	16.0	17.7
South Dakota	8.2	13.4	14.2	15.8	7.7	12.3	13.2	14.8
Nebraska	12.1	15.7	17.0	18.9	10.9	14.4	15.9	17.6
Kansas	12.8	17.3	18.6	19.8	11.2	15.1	16.3	17.2
South Atlantic	14.0	19.7	21.7	22.7	12.6	17.6	19.3	20.4
Delaware	14.3	19.7	21.3	22.7	12.7	17.1	18.3	19.3
Maryland	18.6	30.4	32.5	33.4	16.5	24.9	27.8	29.0
District of Columbia	39.6	55.3	60.0	63.9	34.6	45.6	50.1	53.8
Virginia	12.9	19.5	21.2	21.8	11.9	17.8	19.5	20.2
West Virginia	11.0	16.3	17.7	19.8	10.0	14.6	15.4	16.9
North Carolina	11.7	16.9	18.9	19.9	10.6	15.0	17.2	18.3
South Carolina	10.0	14.7	16.0	17.5	9.3	13.6	15.0	16.4

[Continued]

★ 887 ★

Active Non-Federal Physicians of Medicine
[Continued]

Geographic division and State	Total physicians[1]				Doctors of medicine in patient care[2]			
	1975	1985	1990	1993[3]	1975	1985	1990	1993
Georgia	11.5	16.2	17.6	18.8	10.6	14.7	16.2	17.3
Florida	15.2	20.2	21.6	22.5	13.4	17.8	19.2	20.1
East South Central	10.5	15.0	16.8	18.1	9.7	14.0	15.7	16.8
Kentucky	10.9	15.1	16.8	18.1	10.1	13.9	15.7	16.9
Tennessee	12.4	17.7	19.5	21.4	11.3	16.2	18.1	19.9
Alabama	9.2	14.2	15.7	17.2	8.6	13.1	14.6	15.9
Mississippi	8.4	11.8	13.3	13.3	8.0	11.1	12.6	12.4
West South Central	11.9	16.4	17.8	18.7	10.5	14.5	15.8	16.6
Arkansas	9.1	13.8	15.1	16.6	8.5	12.8	14.1	15.4
Louisiana	11.4	17.3	18.6	20.0	10.5	16.1	17.4	18.7
Oklahoma	11.6	16.1	17.1	18.1	9.4	12.9	13.6	14.3
Texas	12.5	16.8	18.1	18.8	11.0	14.7	16.0	16.6
Mountain	14.3	17.8	19.3	20.0	12.6	15.7	17.0	17.7
Montana	10.6	14.0	16.0	17.3	10.1	13.2	15.2	16.3
Idaho	9.5	12.1	12.7	13.7	8.9	11.4	12.0	12.7
Wyoming	9.5	12.9	13.9	14.2	8.9	12.0	13.1	13.1
Colorado	17.3	20.7	22.1	23.8	15.0	17.7	19.2	20.8
New Mexico	12.2	17.0	18.9	19.9	10.1	14.7	16.7	17.7
Arizona	16.7	20.2	21.5	21.4	14.1	17.1	18.4	18.4
Utah	14.1	17.2	18.5	19.2	13.0	15.5	16.9	17.6
Nevada	11.9	16.0	16.6	16.4	10.9	14.5	14.9	14.5
Pacific	17.9	22.5	23.4	23.5	16.3	20.5	21.3	21.5
Washington	15.3	20.2	21.5	22.7	13.6	17.9	19.3	20.6
Oregon	15.6	19.7	21.1	21.8	13.8	17.6	19.1	19.7
California	18.8	23.7	24.1	23.9	17.3	21.5	21.9	21.9
Alaska	8.4	13.0	14.8	15.0	7.8	12.1	13.7	13.7
Hawaii	16.2	21.5	23.8	24.8	14.7	19.8	21.9	22.8

Source: U.S. Department of Health and Human Services. Public Health Service. Centers for Disease Control and Prevention. National Center for Health Statistics. *Health, United States, 1994.* Hyattsville, MD: Public Health Service, 1995, p. 198-199. *Notes:* Starting in 1989 data for doctors of medicine are as of January 1; in earlier years these data are as of December 31. Data for doctors of osteopathy are as of December 31. 1. Includes active non-Federal doctors of medicine and active doctors of osteopathy. 2. Excludes doctors of osteopathy; states with large numbers are Florida, Michigan, Missouri, New Jersey, Ohio, Pennsylvania, and Texas. Excludes doctors of medicine in medical teaching, administration, research, and other nonpatient care activities. 3. Data for doctors of osteopathy are as of December 31, 1992.

★ 888 ★

Physicians

Active Physicians by Type and Number

Active physicians, according to type of physician and number per 10,000 population: United States and outlying U.S. areas, selected years 1950-93 and projections for the year 2000. Data are based on reporting by physicians and medical schools.

| Year | Number of physicians | | | Active physicians per 10,000 population |
	All active physicians	Doctors of medicine	Doctors of osteopathy[1]	
1950	219,900	209,000	10,900	14.1
1960	259,500	247,300	12,200	14.0
1970	326,500	312,400	12,300	15.6
1971	337,400	325,000	12,400	16.1
1972	348,300	335,500	12,800	16.4
1973	355,700	342,500	13,200	16.4
1974	370,000	356,400	13,600	16.9
1975	384,500	370,400	14,100	17.4
1976	399,500	385,000	14,500	17.9
1977	405,900	390,800	15,100	18.0
1978	424,000	408,300	15,700	18.6
1979	440,400	424,000	16,400	19.1
1980	457,500	440,400	17,100	19.7
1981	466,700	448,700	18,000	20.0
1982	483,700	465,000	18,700	20.5
1983	501,200	481,500	19,700	21.0
1984	---	---	20,800	---
1985	534,800	512,900	21,900	22.0
1986	544,100	520,900	23,200	22.2
1987	560,300	536,200	24,100	22.6
1988	---	---	25,300	---
1989	577,200	550,700	26,500	23.3
1990	589,500	561,400	28,100	23.4
1991[2]	603,400	574,200	29,200	23.8
1992	626,800	595,700	31,100	24.5
1993	638,200	605,800	32,400	24.6

[Continued]

★ 888 ★

Active Physicians by Type and Number
[Continued]

| Year | Number of physicians | | | Active physicians per 10,000 population |
	All active physicians	Doctors of medicine	Doctors of osteopathy[1]	
Projections 2000	724,200	682,400	41,800	26.2

Source: U.S. Department of Health and Human Services. Public Health Service. Centers for Disease Control and Prevention. National Center for Health Statistics. *Health, United States, 1994.* Hyattsville, MD: Public Health Service, 1995, p. 200. *Notes:*— indicates that the figure does not meet standards of reliability or precision. Starting in 1989 data for doctors of medicine are as of January 1; in earlier years these data are as of December 31. Data for doctors of osteopathy are as of December 31. Population estimates include residents in the United States, Puerto Rico, and other U.S. outlying areas; U.S. citizens in foreign countries; and the Armed Forces in the United States and abroad. For the year 2000, the Series II projections of the total population from the U.S. Bureau of the Census are used. Estimation and projection methods are from the Bureau of Health Professions. The numbers of doctors of medicine presented in this table differ from American Medical Association figures because approximately 90 percent of physicians not classified by activity status and whose addresses are unknown are included in this tabulation. 1. Beginning in 1992, doctors of osteopathy data are from the American Osteopathic Association. Data prior to 1992 are Bureau of Health Professions estimates. 2. Doctors of medicine data are unpublished from the American Medical Association.

★ 889 ★

Physicians

Physicians, According to Activity and Place of Medical Education: United States and Outlying U.S. Areas, Selected Years 1975-93

Data are based on reporting by physicians.

Activity and place of medical education	1975	1980	1985	1989	1990	1992	1993
Number of physicians							
Doctors of medicine	393,742	467,679	552,716	600,789	615,421	653,062	670,336
Professionally active[1]	340,280	414,916	497,140	536,755	547,310	578,108	591,017
Place of medical education:							
U.S. medical graduates	---	333,325	392,007	423,172	432,884	451,712	458,528
International medical graduates[2]	---	81,591	105,133	113,583	114,426	126,396	132,489
Activity:[3]							
Non-Federal	312,089	397,129	475,573	516,396	526,835	558,892	569,343
Patient care	287,837	361,915	431,527	468,902	479,547	513,427	525,771
Office-based practice	213,334	271,268	329,041	350,066	359,932	387,903	398,804
General and family practice	46,347	47,772	53,862	56,318	57,571	58,603	58,075
Cardiovascular diseases	5,046	6,725	9,054	10,235	10,670	11,449	12,095
Dermatology	3,442	4,372	5,325	5,721	5,996	5,723	6,539
Gastroenterology	1,696	2,735	4,135	4,942	5,200	5,723	6,293
Internal medicine	28,188	40,514	52,712	56,946	57,799	65,073	67,329

[Continued]

★ 889 ★

Physicians, According to Activity and Place of Medical Education: United States and Outlying U.S. Areas, Selected Years 1975-93

[Continued]

Activity and place of medical education	1975	1980	1985	1989	1990	1992	1993
Pediatrics	12,687	17,436	22,392	24,692	26,494	28,984	30,825
Pulmonary diseases	1,166	2,040	3,035	3,578	3,659	4,005	4,386
General surgery	19,710	22,409	24,708	24,737	24,498	24,902	24,337
Obstetrics and gynecology	15,613	19,503	23,525	25,161	25,475	27,072	27,603
Ophthalmology	8,795	10,598	12,212	12,847	13,055	13,730	13,906
Orthopedic surgery	8,148	10,719	13,033	14,071	14,187	15,814	16,309
Otolaryngology	4,297	5,262	5,751	6,223	6,360	6,633	6,721
Plastic surgery	1,706	2,437	3,299	3,648	3,835	4,042	4,130
Urological surgery	5,025	6,222	7,081	7,338	7,392	7,682	7,770
Anesthesiology	8,970	11,336	15,285	16,720	17,789	19,974	20,646
Diagnostic radiology	1,978	4,190	7,735	9,012	9,806	10,888	11,877
Emergency medicine	---	---	---	8,041	8,402	9,355	9,876
Neurology	1,862	3,245	4,691	5,374	5,587	6,316	6,806
Pathology anatomical/clinical	4,195	5,952	6,877	7,022	7,269	7,920	8,542
Psychiatry	12,173	15,946	18,521	19,625	20,048	21,826	22,261
Radiology	6,970	7,791	7,355	6,164	6,056	5,850	5,748
Other specialty	15,320	24,064	28,453	21,651	22,784	25,754	26,730
Hospital-based practice	74,503	90,647	102,486	118,836	119,615	125,524	126,967
Residents and interns	53,527	59,615	72,159	80,019	81,664	85,432	83,097
Full-time hospital staff	20,976	31,032	30,327	38,817	37,951	40,092	43,870
Other professional activity[4]	24,252	35,214	44,046	47,494	47,288	45,465	43,572
Federal[5]	28,191	17,787	21,567	20,359	20,475	19,216	21,674
Patient care	24,100	14,597	17,293	15,570	15,632	14,665	18,098
Office-based practice	2,095	732	1,156	1,135	1,063	1,461	50
Hospital-based practice	22,005	13,865	16,137	14,435	14,569	13,204	18,048
Residents and interns	4,275	2,427	3,252	2,084	1,725	1,036	3,954
Full-time hospital staff	17,730	11,438	12,885	12,351	12,844	12,168	14,094
Other professional activity[4]	4,091	3,190	4,274	4,789	4,843	4,551	3,576
Inactive	21,449	25,744	38,646	48,804	52,653	55,656	62,997
Not classified	26,145	20,629	13,950	12,405	12,678	16,589	14,668
Unknown address	5,868	6,390	2,980	2,825	2,780	2,709	1,654

Source: U.S. Department of Health and Human Services. Public Health Service. Centers for Disease Control and Prevention. National Center for Health Statistics. *Health, United States, 1994.* Hyattsville, MD: Public Health Service, 1995, p. 201. *Notes:* Starting in 1989 data for doctors of medicine are as of January 1; in earlier years these data are as of December 31. Data for doctors of osteopathy are as of December 31. 1. Excludes inactive, not classified, and address unknown. 2. International medical graduates received their medical education in schools outside the United States and Canada. 3. Specialty information based on the physician's self-designated primary area of practice. Categories include generalists and specialists. 4. Includes medical teaching, administration, research, clinical fellows, and other. 5. Beginning in 1993 data collection for Federal physicians was revised.

★ 890 ★

Physicians

Physicians: Private Doctors per 100,000 Population

This table shows areas with the highest and lowest number of physicians per 100,000 persons.

Location	Number per 100,000 population
United States	252
Lowest	
Idaho	154
Alaska	151
Mississippi	145
Highest	
District of Columbia	693
Massachusetts	400
New York	369

Source: "Too Many, Too Few." *American Medical News,* 26 February 1996, p. 24.

★ 891 ★

Physicians

Primary Care Doctors of Medicine by Specialty and School

Primary care doctors of medicine, according to specialty and medical school seniors according to specialty certification plans, United States and outlying U.S. areas, selected years.

Specialty	1985	1990	1992	1993
Total[1]	552,716	615,421	653,062	670,336
Active doctors of medicine[2]	497,140	547,310	578,108	591,017
Primary care generalists	170,741	183,294	197,719	198,607
General/family practice	67,051	70,480	71,687	71,677
Internal medicine	70,691	76,295	85,839	86,102
Pediatrics	32,999	36,519	40,193	40,828
Primary care specialists	22,011	27,434	27,906	30,850
Internal medicine	18,171	22,054	23,178	24,481
Pediatrics	3,840	5,380	5,728	6,369
Percent active doctors of medicine				
Primary care generalists	34.3	33.5	34.2	33.6
General/family practice	13.5	12.9	12.4	12.1
Internal medicine	14.2	13.9	14.8	14.6
Pediatrics	6.6	6.7	7.0	6.9
Primary care specialists	4.4	5.0	5.0	5.2

[Continued]

★ 891 ★

Primary Care Doctors of Medicine by Specialty and School

[Continued]

Specialty	1985	1990	1992	1993
Internal medicine	3.7	4.0	4.0	4.1
Pediatrics	0.8	1.0	1.0	1.1
Medical school seniors' certification plans	1991[3]	1992	1993	1994
All respondents	11,434	12,096	12,131	12,892
Total with certification plans[4]	7,749	8,062	8,128	8,410
Percent of medical school seniors with certification plans				
Primary care generalists	14.9	14.6	19.3	22.8
General/family practice	9.4	9.0	11.8	13.1
Internal medicine	2.9	3.2	4.5	6.2
Pediatrics	2.6	2.4	3.0	3.5
Primary care specialists	23.3	23.6	21.9	19.2
General/family practice	2.0	1.9	2.3	2.5
Internal medicine	16.0	16.4	14.2	12.2
Pediatrics	5.3	5.3	5.4	4.5

Source: U.S. Department of Health and Human Services. Public Health Service. Centers for Disease Control and Prevention. National Center for Health Statistics. *Health, United States, 1994.* Hyattsville, MD: Public Health Service, 1995, p. 202. *Notes:* 1. Includes MDs engaged in Federal and non-Federal patient care (office-based or hospital-based) and professional activities. 2. Beginning in 1970, MDs who are inactive, have unknown address, or primary specialty not classified are excluded. 3. In 1991 the medical school graduation questionnaire was revised to allow respondents to indicate they were undecided on an area of certification. 4. Excludes medical school seniors who are not planning certification, undecided on area of certification, or did not respond to certification question.

Workplace Issues

★ 892 ★

Nonphysicians Prescribing Drugs

This table shows the growth in the number of prescriptions written by physician assistants and nurse practitioners. These nonphysicians write almost 1 million prescriptions per month.

Year	Prescriptions by non-physicians (% of total)
1992	0.22
1993	0.24
1994	0.24
1995	0.40

[Continued]

★ 892 ★

Nonphysicians Prescribing Drugs
[Continued]

Year	Prescriptions by non-physicians (% of total)
Jan. 1996	0.50
April 1996	0.57

Source: "The Week in Medicine: Nonphysician Prescribing Doubles." *American Medical News,* 17 June 1996, p. 2. Primary source: : IMS America, Totowa, NJ.

★ 893 ★

Workplace Issues

Vacancy Rates for Laboratory Positions, Selected Years: 1988-1994

Rates were calculated by dividing the number of vacant positions by the number of budgeted full-time equivalent employees.

Occupation	1988	1990	1992	1994
Medical technologist: staff	9.3	11.6	13.8	9.6
Medical technologist: supervisor	5.0	10.2	9.3	10.3
Medical technologist: manager	5.2	7.1	15.0	15.4
Cytotechnologist: staff	13.6	27.3	21.2	19.2
Cytotechnologist: supervisor	5.0	10.0	20.0	11.1
Histologic technician: staff	6.2	9.5	12.0	8.7
Histologic supervisor	11.7	10.0	10.0	10.0
Histologic technologist	NA	14.3	12.0	17.4
Medical laboratory technician	6.5	11.1	14.6	14.8
Phlebotomist	8.2	12.2	15.4	14.8

Source: Laboratory Medicine, vol. 26, no. 2 (February 1995), p. 111. *Note:* NA indicates "not available."

★ 894 ★

Workplace Issues

Violence in the Workplace

This table reports on registered nurses' experiences with physical violence in the workplace.

Subjected to	Patients/ clients	Family/ visitors	Other employees	Doctors	Other Nurses	Supervisors
Threats of physical harm (n = 143)	84.4	22.0	5.0	2.8	2.8	0.0
Actually been physically assaulted (n = 87)	93.5	0.0	0.0	5.5	1.1	0.0
Sexual assault (n = 13)	36.4	0.0	0.0	54.5	0.0	9.1

Source: Williams, Margie Ford. "Violence and Sexual Harassment." *AAOHN Journal,* vol. 44, no. 2 (February 1996), p. 75.

★ 895 ★

Workplace Issues

Why Registered Nurses Find Job More Difficult

Based on a survey of 303 readers of *RN.* Percentages represent multiple answers from the registered nurses surveyed.

Factor	% of nurses who cite it
Loss of RN/LPN staff	50
Reorganization of the nursing department	38
Decreases in average length of stay	21
Cross-training of RNs for different units	19
Drop in inpatient census	15
Hiring of UAPs[1] to handle nursing tasks	14
Cross-training of staff from other departments to handle nursing tasks	12
Other factors[2]	33

Source: RN (September 1996), p. 45. Primary source: Medical Economics Research Group (March 1996), Montvale, NJ, *Unlicensed Nursing Personnel. Notes:* 1. Unlicensed assistive personnel 2. Includes increases in patient workload/census, heightened patient acuity, and new or additional responsibilities.

Chapter 9
MEDICAL PRACTICES AND PROCEDURES

Cosmetic Procedures

★ 896 ★

Cosmetic Surgery in 1994: By Procedure

Procedure	Number of Patients
Liposuction	51,072
Eyelid surgery	50,838
Breast augmentation	39,247
Breast implant removal	37,853
Nose reshaping	35,927
Face-lift	32,283
Chemical peel	29,072
Collagen injection	27,052
Retin-A treatment	20,875
Tummy tuck	16,829

Source: "Looking Good: Top Cosmetic Procedures." *American Health* (November 1995), p. 50.

Inpatient Discharges

★ 897 ★

Procedures for Inpatients Discharged From Short-Stay Hospitals: 1980 to 1993

Excludes newborn infants and discharges from Federal hospitals.

SEX AND TYPE OF PROCEDURE	NUMBER OF PROCEDURES (1,000)				RATE PER 1,000 POPULATION[2]			
	1980	1985	1990[1]	1993[1]	1980	1985	1990[1]	1993[1]
Surgical procedures, total [3,4]	24,494	24,799	23,051	22,767	108.6	104.6	92.4	88.8
MALE								
Total [3,4]	8,505	8,805	8,538	8,355	78.1	76.8	70.6	67.1
Cardiac catheterization	228	439	620	613	2.1	3.8	5.1	4.9
Prostatectomy	335	367	364	317	3.1	3.2	3.0	2.5
Reduction of fracture[5]	325	339	300	294	3.0	3.0	2.5	2.4
Repair of inguinal hernia	483	370	181	96	4.4	3.2	1.5	0.8
FEMALE								
Total [3,4]	15,989	15,994	14,513	14,411	137.1	130.6	113.0	109.3
Procedures to assist delivery[4]	2,391	2,494	2,491	2,428	20.5	20.4	19.4	18.4
Cesarean section	619	877	945	917	5.3	7.2	7.4	7.0
Repair of current obstetric laceration	355	548	795	860	3.0	4.5	6.2	6.5
Hysterectomy	649	670	591	562	5.6	5.5	4.6	4.3
Diagnostic and other nonsurgical procedures [4,6]	6,918	11,961	17,455	18,842	30.7	50.5	70.0	73.5
MALE								
Total [4,6]	3,386	5,889	7,378	7,787	31.1	51.4	61.0	62.5
Angiocardiography and arteriography[7]	355	693	1,051	1,024	3.3	6.0	8.7	8.2
CAT scan[8]	152	671	736	565	1.4	5.9	6.1	4.5
FEMALE								
Total [4,6]	3,532	6,072	10,077	11,055	30.3	49.6	78.5	83.8
Diagnostic ultrasound	204	756	941	848	1.7	6.2	7.3	6.4
CAT scan[8]	154	707	770	594	1.3	5.8	6.0	4.5

Source: 1996 Statistical Abstract of the United States on CD-ROM [machine-readable datafiles]. CD-8A-97. Washington, DC: U.S. Department of Commerce, Economics and Statistics Administration, Bureau of the Census, Data User Services Division, January 1997. Primary source: U.S. National Center for Health Statistics, *Vital Health Statistics*, series 13; and unpublished data. *Notes:* 1. Comparisons beginning 1988 with data for earlier years should be made with caution as estimates of change may reflect improvements in the design rather than true changes in hospital use. 2. Based on Bureau of the Census estimated civilian population as of July 1. Population estimates for the 1980's do not reflect revised estimates based on the 1990 Census of Population. 3. Includes other types of surgical procedures not shown separately. 4. Beginning in 1989, the definition of some surgical and diagnostic and other non-surgical procedures was revised, causing a discontinuity in the trends for some totals. 5. Excluding skull, nose, and jaw. 6. Includes other nonsurgical procedures not shown separately. 7. Using contrast material. 8. Computerized axial tomography.

Medication Errors

★ 898 ★

Problems in Administering Drugs

This table shows a breakdown of types of errors encountered in administering medication. Findings are based on 9,399 medication errors reported by 25 hospitals between October 1993 and November 1994.

Error	%
Dose omitted	29.4
Miscellaneous errors[1]	23.3
Wrong dose	14.0
Wrong drug	10.7
Extra dose	9.6
Wrong time	6.7
Wrong rates	6.3

Source: RN (October 1995), p. 13. Primary source: Premier Health Alliance, Westchester, Illinois, 1995. *Notes:* 1. For example, wrong patient, wrong form of drug, administered despite documented drug allergy, medication given but not charted.

Organ Transplants

★ 899 ★

Number of Organ Transplants in the U.S., 1988-1994

This table shows the number of organ transplants performed in the 1988-1994 period.

Organ	1988	1989	1990	1991	1992	1993	1994
Kidney	9,041	8,988	9,879	10,124	10,230	11,021	11,390
Liver	1,713	2,201	2,690	2,953	3,064	3,440	3,653
Pancreas	249	417	528	531	557	774	844
Heart	1,676	1,705	2,108	2,125	2,171	2,298	2,340
Heart-lung	74	67	52	51	48	59	70
Lung	33	93	203	405	535	675	737

Source: Levy, Doug. "Matchmaking at the Heart of Transplant Process." *USA TODAY,* 19 October 1995, p. 6D. Primary source: United Network for Organ Sharing.

★ 900 ★

Organ Transplants

Organ Donors: Bone Marrow

This table shows the number of donors registered with the National Marrow Donor Program.

As of date:	Number registered
Dec. 31, 1992	740,906
Dec. 31, 1993	1,100,000
Dec. 31, 1994	1,500,000
Nov. 11, 1995	1,900,000

Source: Wojciechowski, Gene. "An Appeal from Heart of Baseball." *Chicago Tribune,* 29 November 1995, p. 12. Primary sources: National Marrow Transplant Program; *The American Medical Encyclopedia of Medicine.*

★ 901 ★

Organ Transplants

Organ Donors: Bone Marrow, by Race and Ethnicity

This table shows the number of donors registered with the National Marrow Donor Program (reachable by dialing 1-800-627-7692).

Race/ethnicity	1992	1995	Percent increase
White	546,459	1,125,200	106
Black	34,248	129,359	278
Hispanic	35,453	115,589	226
Asian	28,203	89,153	216
Other[1]	14,780	34,836	136
Unknown[2]	81,763	391,802	379

Source: Wojciechowski, Gene. "An Appeal from Heart of Baseball." *Chicago Tribune,* 29 November 1995, p. 12. Primary sources: National Marrow Transplant Program; *The American Medical Encyclopedia of Medicine. Notes:* 1. Other usually denotes donors of mixed race or those who did not provide racial information; the values include data for American Indians. 2. Primarily white donors from foreign donor centers.

★ 902 ★

Organ Transplants

Organ Registrations: 1996

The table shows the number of requests received for each organ listed.

Organ	Number of registrations
Kidney	29,753
Liver	5,039
Heart	3,371
Lung	1,836
Kidney/pancreas	1,220
Pancreas	255
Heart/lung	214
Intestine	78

Source: "Which Organs Do People Need?" *Safety & Health* (May 1996), p. 75. Primary source: United Network for Organ Sharing.

★ 903 ★

Organ Transplants

Organ Transplants by Type of Organ and Ethnicity, 1994

Since only 25 percent of organ donors are minorities, minority recipients often wait twice as long as whites to get a compatible organ.

Organ	Number of transplants		
	Whites	Blacks	Hispanics[1]
Kidney	6,503	2,447	1,046
Liver	2,803	297	339
Heart	1,898	269	84
Lung	648	28	23

Source: Sabir, Nadirah Z. "Newspoints: A Second Chance." *Black Enterprise* (February 1996), p. 26. Primary source: United Network Organ Sharing, 1995. *Note:* 1. Hispanics may be of any race.

★ 904 ★

Organ Transplants

Organ Transplants: How Long Organs Remain Usable After Death of Donor

Organ	Time
Bone	5 years
Skin	5 years
Kidney	48-72 hours
Liver	16-32 hours
Pancreas	12-24 hours
Heart	4-6 hours
Lung	4-6 hours

Source: Sabir, Nadirah Z. "Newspoints: A Second Chance." *Black Enterprise* (February 1996), p. 26. Primary source: Center for Organ Recovery and Education, 1995.

★ 905 ★

Organ Transplants

Organ Transplants: Survival Rates

This table shows three-year patient survival rates for all U.S. transplants between October 1, 1987 and December 31, 1991. The highest survival rate is associated with kidney transplants, the lowest with lungs. A value of 80 percent means that 80 percent of those receiving a transplant survived three years after the operation.

Organ	Three-year survival rate (%)
Kidney	87.0
Liver	67.0
Heart	74.0
Pancreas	82.0
Heart/lung	42.0
Lung	39.0

Source: Auerbach, Stuart. "Organ Donations by Minorities Rise." *Washington Post,* 27 February 1996, p. 7. Primary source: Health Resources and Services Administration.

★ 906 ★

Organ Transplants

Waiting for Organs: Cases for the 1988-1995 Period

This table shows the number of people waiting for the organs shown, for the years 1988 through 1995.

Organ	1988	1989	1990	1991	1992	1993	1994	1995
Kidney	13,943	16,294	17,883	19,352	22,376	24,973	27,498	30,181
Liver	616	827	1,237	1,676	2,323	2,997	4,059	5,149
Pancreas	163	320	473	600	126	183	222	256
Heart	1,030	1,320	1,788	2,267	2,690	2,834	2,933	3,359
Heart-lung	205	240	225	154	180	202	205	208
Lung	69	94	308	670	942	1,240	1,625	1,887

Source: Levy, Doug. "Matchmaking at the Heart of Transplant Process." *USA TODAY,* 19 October 1995, p. 6D. Primary source: United Network for Organ Sharing.

Surgery

★ 907 ★

Back Surgery Rates in Selected Cities: 1995

[Surgeries per 1,000 people]

City	Rate
Salt Lake City, UT	4.0
Tucson, AZ	4.0
Seattle, WA	3.5
Denver, CO	3.2
Los Angeles, CA	3.0
Washington, DC	2.9
Houston, TX	2.8
St. Louis, MO	2.8
San Francisco, CA	2.5
Atlanta, GA	2.4
Boston, MA	1.9
Chicago, IL	1.7
Miami, FL	1.4
New York, NY	1.2

Source: Chang, Trina. "Health Care Compared: Back Surgery." *American Health* (May 1996), p. 25.

★ 908 ★

Surgery

Outpatient Surgeries, by Setting: 1996 and 2001

[In millions of surgeries]

Surgery setting	1996	2001
Hospital outpatient	13.8	14.7
Freestanding surgery	4.9	6.8
Physician's office	3.4	5.3

Source: "Outpatient Surgery Settings, 1991-2001." *Medical Tribune,* 20 June 1996, p. 9. Primary source: SMG Marketing Group, Inc., 1995.

★ 909 ★

Surgery

Risk of Death for Persons Over 65

Data show rates of death per 1,000 operations within 30 days for Medicare beneficiaries over 65.

Procedure	Deaths[1] per 1,000 operations
Coronary bypass	40
Coronary angioplasty	23
Hernia repair	17
Spinal fusion	14
Hip replacement	13
Prostate removal	9
Hysterectomy	7
Disc removal	5
Knee replacement	4

Source: Ross, Philip E. "First, Do No Harm." *Forbes,* 21 October 1996, p. 298. Primary source: Medicare. *Notes:* 1. Deaths occurring within 30 days of the operation on individuals over 65 years of age.

Technology

★ 910 ★

Breast Tumor Detection Technology

"A new method of high-resolution magnetic resonance imaging (MRI) has pinpointed exactly where tiny tumors of the breast's milk duct are located in 95% of the women studied. Using MRI, doctors can with greater confidence treat malignancies by removing a small amount of tissue in a lumpectomy, rather than performing a more invasive mastectomy."

Source: Cronin, Brian. "Health Report: The Good News." *Time,* 6 May 1996, p. 21. Primary source: American College of Radiology National Conference on Breast Cancer.

★ 911 ★

Technology

Hospital Staff Who Use Computers

Table shows computer use during a typical week at Beth Israel Hospital in Boston, by function and position. Data are for 1994.

Reason	Physicians	Residents	Medical students	Nurses and others	Total
Patient lookup	7,857	18,374	1,301	23,542	51,074
Utilities	579	1,127	16	1,396	3,118
Decision support	538	908	70	801	2,317
Order entry	248	1,353	0	115	1,716
Scheduling	395	582	22	645	1,644
Other	452	310	10	2,047	2,819
Total	10,069	22,654	1,419	28,546	62,688

Source: Borzo, Greg. "Physicians *Will* Use Computers." *American Medical News,* 23-30 October 1995, p. 3.

★ 912 ★

Technology

Repetitive Motion Injury Treatment

A new option is now available to treat the symptoms associated with repetitive motion injuries.

[Continued]

★ 912 ★

Repetitive Motion Injury Treatment
[Continued]

The treatment, called CTDx Electrostimulation System, uses a battery-operated unit to send mild electrical stimulation to the affected area through electrodes placed on the skin. The electrical impulses reduce pain, increase blood circulation, and improve motor nerve conduction through the carpal tunnel. The treatment is non-invasive, pain-free, and there are no side effects.

Source: Pipp, Tracy L. "Growing Pains." *Detroit News,* 10 July 1997, p. 1E.

★ 913 ★

Technology

Uses of Expensive Technology: Comparisons

This table shows how the U.S. and other nations use expensive medical devices such as magnetic resonance imagers (MRI) and computerized axial tomography (CT) scanners. Data show units installed per million people, in 1991.

Country	CT scanners	MRI scanners
Canada	7.0	1.0
West Germany	12.0	3.0
Sweden	10.0	2.5
United Kingdom	5.0	2.0
United States	27.0	10.0

Source: "Runaway Technology." *Workplace Vitality* (July/August 1995), p. 15. Primary source: Office of Technology Assessment.

Treatment Options and Alternatives

★914★

Common Cold Treatment Strategies

"Soothing music may help combat the common cold. In a recent survey Carl Charnetski and Francis Brennan, Jr., of Wilkes University measured levels of immunoglobulin A (IgA—an antibody) in volunteers' saliva before and after they listened to 30 minutes of Muzak, radio jazz, silence, or tones and clicks. They found that levels of IgA rose on average in the Muzak listeners by 14.1 percent and in jazz listeners by 7.2 percent. In contrast, IgA levels dropped by less than 1 percent in volunteers hearing silence and by a whopping 19.7 percent in those hearing tones and clicks."

Source: "In Brief: Making Music and Immunity." *Scientific American* (July 1997), p. 24.

Chapter 10
POLITICS, OPINION, AND LAW

Controversies

★ 915 ★

Doctor-Assisted Suicides

"A group led by clinical psychologist Lee Slome reports that in a survey of 118 San Francisco-area physicians working with AIDS patients, 53% indicated that they had knowingly prescribed a deadly dose of narcotics to patients who wanted to die. Most of the doctors who provided such aid, says Slome, did so from one to three times. One doctor admitted to 100 instances, a tally far outstripping that of Dr. Jack Kevorkian."

Source: Van Biema, David. "Fatal Doses: Assisted Suicide Soars in An Afflicted Community." *Time* 17 February 1997, p. 72.

★ 916 ★
Controversies

The Tobacco Industry Resolution: 1997

"On June 20, 1997, attorneys general of 40 states forced the tobacco industry to concede that cigarettes are deadly, to pay $368.5 billion in compensation over the next 25 years, and to submit to regulation by the federal Food and Drug Administration."

Source: Smolowe, Jill. "Sorry, Pardner: Big Tobacco Fesses Up and Pays Up—$368.5 Billion, but Congress Must Approve the Deal." *Time,* 30 June 1997, p. 26.

Disciplinary Actions

★ 917 ★

Disciplinary Actions Against Physicians, by State: 1996

[In number of actions per 1000 physicians]

State	Number
Mississippi	10.83
North Dakota	9.16
Iowa	8.57
Colorado	8.29
Arizona	8.18
Alaska	7.33
Oklahoma	7.14
Ohio	5.97
Nevada	5.92
Vermont	5.42
West Virginia	5.32
Kansas	4.94
Montana	4.87
Kentucky	4.70
Arkansas	4.61
Utah	4.51
Maine	4.48
New York	4.42
Georgia	4.39
New Jersey	4.38
Idaho	4.26
Florida	4.21
New Mexico	4.19
Nebraska	4.18
Rhode Island	4.02
Delaware	3.99
California	3.93
Michigan	3.75
Oregon	3.70
Missouri	3.67
Wyoming	3.59
Pennsylvania	3.58
Indiana	3.53
Wisconsin	3.51
Texas	3.47
District of Columbia	3.32
Connecticut	3.30
Alabama	3.27
Hawaii	3.11
Washington	3.09
Maryland	3.07
South Dakota	2.95

[Continued]

★ 917 ★

Disciplinary Actions Against Physicians, by State: 1996

[Continued]

State	Number
Massachusetts	2.87
Louisiana	2.69
South Carolina	2.46
Illinois	2.43
Minnesota	2.36
North Carolina	2.24
Tennessee	2.24
Virginia	2.20
New Hampshire	1.76

Source: Levy, Doug. "Disciplining Bad Doctors: Medical Boards Have Spotty Record." *USA TODAY,* 26 March 1996, p. 1D.

Discrimination

★ 918 ★

Complaints Filed Under the Americans With Disabilities Act, by Impairment: 1992-1995

Impairment involved	Number of complaints	% of total
Back	10,346	19
Emotional/mental	6,521	12
Neurological	6,329	12
Extremities	4,535	8
Heart	4,372	4
Substance abuse	1,934	4
Diabetes	1,926	4

Source: "News & Trends: A Close-Up of ADA Infractions." *Business & Health* (April 1996), p. 16.

Family and Medical Leave Act

★ 919 ★

Family and Medical Leave Act (FMLA) - Covered and Non-Covered Worksites: 1995

Changes	FMLA covered	FMLA not-covered
Before 1993	38.7	17.4
In 1993	40.0	4.5
After 1993	3.3	0.9
No policies	8.8	73.5
Don't know	9.1	3.7

Source: Commission on Family and Medical Leave. "A Workable Balance: Report to Congress on Family and Medical Leave Policies." 30 April 1996, p. 68.

★ 920 ★

Family and Medical Leave Act

Family and Medical Leave Act (FMLA): Additional Job Guarantee Benefits Provided to Employees

[In percentages]

Employee coverage	FMLA covered	FMLA non-covered
For more than 12 weeks a year	25.5	25.6
For employees who have worked less than 12 months	37.3	25.9
For employees who have worked less than 1,250 hours/year	31.1	33.0

Source: Commission on Family and Medical Leave. "A Workable Balance: Report to Congress on Family and Medical Leave Policies." 30 April 1996, p. 73.

★ 921 ★

Family and Medical Leave Act

Health Benefits Under the Family and Medical Leave Act (FMLA): Covered and Non-Covered Worksites

Data refer to continuation of health benefits during employee's leave from work.

Reason for leave	FMLA covered	FMLA non-covered
Employee's own serious health condition	93.5	77.9
Maternity disability	96.3	86.3
Parents to care for a newborn	95.7	72.5
Parents to care for adopted or foster child	95.8	75.9
Care of ill child, spouse, or parent	95.2	69.0

Source: Commission on Family and Medical Leave. "A Workable Balance: Report to Congress on Family and Medical Leave Policies," 30 April 1996, p. 71.

★ 922 ★

Family and Medical Leave Act

Job Guarantees Under the Family and Medical Leave Act (FMLA): Covered and Non-Covered Worksites

Reason for leave	FMLA covered	FMLA non-covered
Employee's own serious health condition	94.7	86.8
Maternity disability	99.2	87.3
Parents to care for a newborn	99.2	83.8
Parents to care for adopted or foster child	99.0	85.5
Care of ill child, spouse, or parent	98.9	86.0

Source: Commission on Family and Medical Leave. "A Workable Balance: Report to Congress on Family and Medical Leave Policies." 30 April 1996, p. 72.

★ 923 ★

Family and Medical Leave Act

Leave of Absence From Work Under Family and Medical Leave Act (FMLA), 1995: Covered and Non-Covered Worksites

Data refer to availability of up to 12 weeks' leave of absence.

Reason for leave	FMLA covered	FMLA non-covered
Employee's own serious health condition	92.6	45.7
Maternity disability	96.9	42.3
Parents to care for a newborn	92.5	32.3
Parents to care for adopted or foster child	91.3	29.0
Care of ill child, spouse, or parent	94.2	41.7
All of the FMLA reasons	80.0	20.7

Source: Commission on Family and Medical Leave. "A Workable Balance: Report to Congress on Family and Medical Leave Policies." 30 April 1996, p. 69.

★ 924 ★

Family and Medical Leave Act

Worksites Changing Family and Medical Leave Policies, by Type of Change: 1995

Table shows the percentage of businesses that have instituted each type of benefit.

Changes	Percentage
Leave is now job guaranteed	54.8
Health insurance continued during leave	52.9
Leave can be taken for more reasons	76.9
Leave can be taken for longer time	66.4
Males can take leave to care for ill/newborn children	69.3
Eligibility requirements eased	46.7

Source: Commission on Family and Medical Leave. "A Workable Balance: Report to Congress on Family and Medical Leave Policies." 30 April 1996, p. 67.

Lost Work Time

★ 925 ★

Employees Who Did Not Take Leave of Absence, by Reason: 1995

Reason	Percentage
Might lose job	29.2
Might hurt job advancement	22.0
Might lose seniority	14.1
Not eligible	13.9
Employer denied request	9.9
Couldn't afford	63.9
Wanted to save leave time	27.5
Work too important	39.4

Source: Commission on Family and Medical Leave. "A Workable Balance: Report to Congress on Family and Medical Leave Policies." 30 April 1996, p. 100.

★ 926 ★

Lost Work Time

Employees Who Needed But Did Not Take Leave of Absence, by Reason: 1995

Reason	Percentage
Own health	43.7
Maternity	0.5
Care of newborn, adopted or, foster child	8.4
Care for ill child, spouse, or parent	44.7
Care for ill relative, or other	10.2

Source: Commission on Family and Medical Leave. "A Workable Balance: Report to Congress on Family and Medical Leave Policies." 30 April 1996, p. 99.

★ 927 ★

Lost Work Time

Likelihood of Employee Requesting Leave of Absence During Next 5 Years: 1995

Response	Percentage
Very unlikely	34.1
Somewhat unlikely	36.0
Very likely	17.9
Somewhat likely	21.5

Source: Commission on Family and Medical Leave. "A Workable Balance: Report to Congress on Family and Medical Leave Policies." 30 April 1996, p. 101.

Malpractice

★ 928 ★

Average Malpractice Payment for Breast Cancer Diagnosis Delays: 1995

According to the source, delay in diagnosing breast cancer tops the list for medical malpractice claims. In addition, the most frequent claims included failure of the physician to recognize the implications of the physical findings, follow up with the patient, and/or to read a mammogram correctly.

Type	Cost
Overall	$217,500
Hospitals	117,500
Radiologists	182,000
Obstetricians/gynecologists	277,500
Pathologists	345,500

Source: "News Pulse: Expensive Delays." *Nursing95* (August 1995), p. 12. Primary source: Physician Insurance Association of America; *Modern Healthcare,* 5 June 1995.

★ 929 ★

Malpractice

Fines and Settlements Paid by Health Care Providers Charged With Fraud: 1996-1997

[In millions of dollars]

Company	Fines/settlement
SmithKline Beecham Clinical Labs	325
Horizon/CMS Healthcare Corp.	5.8
Spectra Laboratories, Inc.	10.1
Laboratory Corp. of America	187
First American Health Care of Georgia	255
FHP, Inc.	12
Damon Clinical Laboratories, Inc.	119

Source: "Feds Intensify Fraud Scrutiny, Hone Tactics." *American Medical News,* 9 June 1997, p. 7.

★ 930 ★

Malpractice

Heart-Attack Related Malpractice Payments by Internists, by Field: 1995

Field	Claims	Average indemnity
Family/general practice	160	162,138
Internal medicine	109	252,151
Emergency medicine	75	180,844
Other specialties	35	148,947
Cardiology	34	155,074
Surgical specialty	9	173,194
Physician extenders	4	51,139
Corporations	12	352,284
Hospitals	57	133,285

Source: Prager, Linda O. "Heart Attacks A Costly Liability Risk, Insurer Study Finds." *American Medical News,* 17 June 1996, p. 3. Primary source: Study of 349 heart-attack related cases by the Physician Insurers Association of America.

★ 931 ★

Malpractice

Malpractice Claims Made, Paid, and Average Payout

Data are for the period 1985 through 1995 derived from Physician Insurers Association of America data. The organization insures 25 percent of the nation's doctors.

Reason	Total claims made since 1985	Number of claims paid	Average payout ($)
Breast cancer	2,986	1,039	204,436
Brain-damaged infant	2,613	934	449,486
Pregnancy	1,953	530	128,978
Heart attack	1,770	563	190,347
Intervertebral-disc displacement	1,662	402	172,041
Lung cancer	1,639	504	149,823
Appendicitis	1,296	368	83,100
Femur fracture	1,290	365	85,255
Cataracts	1,151	269	96,603
Sterilization	1,119	349	46,770

Source: "The Cutting Edge: Vital Statistics." *Washington Post,* 12 September 1995, p. 5.

★ 932 ★

Malpractice

Percent of Doctors Sued for Malpractice

Data are as of 1994 and show the percent of doctors sued.

Field	Percent of doctors sued
General/family practice	37.3
Internal medicine	32.0
Surgery	54.1
Pediatrics	31.9
Obstetrics/gynecology	64.4
Radiology	39.0
Psychiatry	18.7
Anesthesiology	34.8
Pathology	23.9
Other	39.3

Source: St. Louis Post-Dispatch, 9 September 1996, p. 10BP. Primary source: American Medical Association.

Opinion

★ 933 ★

Health Advice in Women's Magazines, 1995: Best

Data refer to a *Ladies' Home Journal* article that listed tobacco as a risk factor in seven of the top ten causes of death in women. Dr. Elizabeth Whelan, president of the American Council on Science and Health, applauds the magazine for highlighting the risks of using tobacco.

Leading causes of death of women	Total deaths
Heart disease	360,161
Cancer	245,740
Stroke	87,124
Chronic lung disease	41,473
Pneumonia and influenza	40,254
Accidents	28,915
Diabetes	28,395
Kidney disease	11,346
Infections	11,140
Hardening of the arteries	10,503

Source: Whelan, Elizabeth. "Opinion USA: Tobacco Rules in Too Many Woman's Magazines." *USA TODAY,* 14 November 1995, p. 13A.

★ 934 ★
Opinion

Health Advice in Women's Magazines, 1995: Worst

"According to Dr. Elizabeth Whelan, president of the American Council on Science and Health, an article in the May 1995 issue of *Redbook* magazine offered the worst in health advice for women. The editors of the magazine ran a list of ways to lower cancer risk, but quitting smoking was not among them."

Source: Whelan, Elizabeth. "Opinion USA: Tobacco Rules in Too Many Woman's Magazines." *USA TODAY,* 14 November 1995, p. 13A.

★ 935 ★

Opinion

Importance of Well-Being, by Generational Group

Table shows how each generational group answered the question, "which form of well-being is most important to you?"

Form	Gen Xers	Baby boomers	Matures
Mental	45	39	32
Physical	29	30	33
Spiritual	26	31	35

Source: "Mind, Body, Sole: Mapping the Hierarchy of Modern Well-Being." *Adweek,* 24 March 1997, p. 19. Primary source: Based on a poll by Yankelovich Partners.

★ 936 ★

Opinion

Patients' Complaints About Hospitals

Issue	Percent complaining about
Continuity and transition	29
Emotional support	27
Information and education	23
Involvement of family/friends	22
Coordination of care	23
Respect for patients' preferences	22
Physical comfort	10

Source: "News & Trends: What We Have Here Is A Failure to Communicate." *Business & Health* (March 1997), p. 13. Primary source: Picker Institute poll of 24,000 patients.

★ 937 ★

Opinion

Pharmacists' Beliefs

"A recent survey of 625 pharmacists showed that 82% of them believe they have the right to refuse to fill a prescription for a drug such as RU-486 that would facilitate abortions."

Source: Lafferty, Elaine. "Beware the Counterpunch: What Happens When A Prescription Offends A Pharmacist's Beliefs?" *Time,* 28 April 1997, p. 66.

★ 938 ★

Opinion

Physicians Treating Minorities

Table shows the percentage of each minority group treated by physicians, by selected characteristics.

Characteristic	Black	Hispanic	Poor	Uninsured
All physicians (under age 45)	18.6	10.0	28.8	12.3
Race-ethnicity				
White	17.3	8.9	27.7	11.8
Black	45.8	10.2	40.0	13.2
Hispanic	20.2	30.5	36.5	17.0
Other (includes Asians and American Indians)	22.1	11.9	32.9	14.3

Source: "Who Treats Whom." *American Medical News,* 26 August 1996, p. 23. Primary source: Robert Wood Johnson Foundation Surveys of Young Physicians appearing in "Physician Service to the Underserved: Implications for Affirmative Action in Medical Education." *Inquiry* (Summer 1996).

Chapter 11
INTERNATIONAL COMPARISONS

This chapter presents a selection of tables that compare countries with one another. A variety of other tables, relating to the subject matter of this book but in an international context are also included.

Health Expenditures

★ 939 ★

Health Spending as Percent of Gross Domestic Product

Total health expenditures as a percent of gross domestic product and per capita health expenditures in dollars: Selected countries and years 1980-93.

[Data compiled by the Organization for Economic Cooperation and Development]

Country	Percent of Gross Domestic Product						
	1980	1985	1989	1990	1991	1992	1993[1]
Australia	7.3	7.7	7.8	8.2	8.5	8.5	8.5
Austria	7.9	8.1	8.5	8.4	8.6	9.0	9.3
Belgium	6.6	7.4	7.6	7.6	8.0	8.1	8.3
Canada	7.4	8.5	9.0	9.4	10.0	10.2	10.2
Denmark	6.8	6.3	6.5	6.5	6.6	6.6	6.7
Finland	6.5	7.3	7.4	8.0	9.1	9.4	8.8
France	7.6	8.5	8.7	8.9	9.1	9.4	9.8
Germany	8.4	8.7	8.3	8.3	8.4	8.6	8.6
Greece	4.3	4.9	5.1	5.3	5.3	5.5	5.7
Iceland	6.2	7.3	8.5	7.9	8.1	8.1	8.3
Ireland	8.7	7.8	6.6	6.7	7.1	6.8	6.7
Italy	6.9	7.0	7.6	8.1	8.4	8.5	8.5
Japan	6.6	6.6	6.8	6.8	6.7	7.0	7.3
Luxembourg	6.3	6.2	6.6	6.5	6.5	6.7	6.9
Netherlands	7.9	7.9	7.9	8.0	8.3	8.5	8.7

[Continued]

★ 939 ★

Health Spending as Percent of Gross Domestic Product

[Continued]

Country	Percent of Gross Domestic Product						
	1980	1985	1989	1990	1991	1992	1993[1]
New Zealand	7.2	6.4	7.2	7.4	7.8	7.7	7.7
Norway	6.6	6.4	7.4	7.5	8.0	8.3	8.2
Portugal	5.8	6.3	6.6	6.6	7.0	7.1	7.3
Spain	5.7	5.7	6.5	6.9	7.1	7.2	7.3
Sweden	9.4	8.9	8.6	8.6	8.4	7.6	7.5
Switzerland	7.3	8.1	8.4	8.4	9.0	9.4	9.9
Turkey	3.4	2.2	2.9	2.9	3.4	2.9	2.7
United Kingdom	5.6	5.9	5.8	6.0	6.5	7.0	7.1
United States	8.9	10.2	11.4	12.1	12.9	13.3	13.6

Source: U.S. Department of Health and Human Services. Public Health Service. Centers for Disease Control and Prevention. National Center for Health Statistics. *Health, United States, 1995.* Hyattsville, MD: Public Health Service, 1996, p. 240. Primary source: Some numbers in this table have been revised and differ from previous editions of *Health, United States. Note:* 1. Preliminary figures.

★ 940 ★

Health Expenditures

Per Capita Health Expenditures: Selected Countries, 1980-1993

Total health expenditures as a percent of gross domestic product and per capita health expenditures in dollars: Selected countries and years 1980-93.

[Data compiled by the Organization for Economic Cooperation and Development]

Country	Per capita health expenditures[2]						
	1980	1985	1989	1990	1991	1992	1993[1]
Australia	671	995	1,238	1,315	1,384	1,415	1,493
Austria	697	992	1,316	1,395	1,490	1,672	1,777
Belgium	586	887	1,160	1,247	1,377	1,532	1,601
Canada	739	1,215	1,601	1,716	1,846	1,912	1,971
Denmark	595	815	1,019	1,068	1,151	1,211	1,296
Finland	521	852	1,151	1,291	1,416	1,406	1,363
France	711	1,090	1,423	1,538	1,649	1,798	1,835
Germany	819	1,175	1,413	1,520	1,650	1,831	1,815
Greece	187	284	371	395	414	469	500
Iceland	588	949	1,403	1,372	1,450	1,513	1,564
Ireland	451	569	652	749	846	906	922
Italy	581	827	1,170	1,317	1,440	1,553	1,523
Japan	526	796	1,098	1,188	1,273	1,411	1,495
Luxembourg	693	1,008	1,442	1,532	1,616	1,817	1,993
Netherlands	702	934	1,172	1,279	1,358	1,494	1,531
New Zealand	556	714	949	996	1,059	1,109	1,179

[Continued]

★ 940 ★

Per Capita Health Expenditures: Selected Countries, 1980-1993

[Continued]

Country	Per capita health expenditures[2]						
	1980	1985	1989	1990	1991	1992	1993[1]
Norway	558	816	1,128	1,202	1,339	1,531	1,592
Portugal	263	386	573	616	730	815	866
Spain	332	455	711	813	907	963	972
Sweden	867	1,159	1,396	1,464	1,423	1,300	1,266
Switzerland	851	1,300	1,698	1,761	1,949	2,133	2,283
Turkey	76	73	120	133	164	148	146
United Kingdom	452	671	887	955	1,016	1,181	1,213
United States	1,052	1,735	2,422	2,688	2,902	3,144	3,331

Source: U.S. Department of Health and Human Services. Public Health Service. Centers for Disease Control and Prevention. National Center for Health Statistics. *Health, United States, 1995.* Hyattsville, MD: Public Health Service, 1996, p. 240. *Notes:* Some numbers in this table have been revised and differ from previous editions of *Health, United States.* 1. Preliminary figures. 2. Per capita health expenditures for each country have been adjusted to U.S. dollars using gross domestic product purchasing power parities for each year.

Health Status: Children

★ 941 ★

Malnourished Children by World Region: 1995

Data refer to children under 5 years of age.

[In millions]

Region	Number of malnourished
Americas	4
Middle East/North Africa	7
Sub-Saharan Africa	32
East Asia/Pacific	36
South Asia	86

Source: "Nutrition: A Tale of Two Statistics." *Progress of Nations 1996.* UNICEF, 1996. Data are available from the World Wide Web at http://www.unicef.org/pon96/nutale.htm. Primary source: Preliminary estimates for *Third World Report on the World Nutrition Situation 1996.*

Health Status: Diseases

★ 942 ★

HIV/AIDS Cases in Persons Age 15-45, by World Region: 1996

[In percentages]

Country, region, area	% age 15-45 with HIV/AIDS
North America	0.5
Latin America	0.6
Caribbean	1.7
Sub-Saharan Africa	5.6
North Africa/Middle East	0.1
Western Europe	0.2
Central and Eastern Europe and Central Asia	0.015
South and Southeast Asia	0.6
East Asia and Pacific	0.001
Australia and New Zealand	0.1

Source: Purvis, Andrew. "The Global Epidemic." *Time,* 30 December 1996-6 January 1997, p. 76. Primary source: UNAIDS.

★ 943 ★

Health Status: Diseases

How Persons Contracted AIDS in 1996: U.S. Compared to Rest of World

Cause	World percentage	U.S. percentage
Mode of transmission		
Heterosexual sex	70-75	8
Homosexual sex	5-10	51
Intravenous drug use	5-10	25
Blood transfusions	3-5	1
Other	0-17	8
Homosexual sex and intravenous drug use	NA	7

Source: Nash, J. Madeleine. "The Enemy Within." *Time* (Fall 1996), p. 19.

★ 944 ★

Health Status: Diseases

Percentage Change in HIV/AIDS Cases, by World Region: 1992-1996

Country, region, area	% change 1992 to 1996
East Asia and Pacific	658
South and Southeast Asia	261
Central and Eastern Europe and Central Asia	238
Caribbean	47
North Africa/Middle East	46
Latin America	43
Sub-Saharan Africa	37
Western Europe	2
North America	-13
Australia and New Zealand	-14

Source: Purvis, Andrew. "The Global Epidemic." *Time,* 30 December 1996 to 6 January 1997, p. 76. Primary source: UNAIDS.

★ 945 ★

Health Status: Diseases

Persons Who Died of HIV/AIDS, by World Region: 1996

Country, region, area	Number of deaths
Sub-Saharan Africa	783,700
South and Southeast Asia	143,700
Latin America	70,900
North America	61,300
Western Europe	21,000
Caribbean	14,500
North Africa/Middle East	10,800
East Asia and Pacific	1,200
Australia and New Zealand	1,000
Central and Eastern Europe and Central Asia	1,000

Source: Purvis, Andrew. "The Global Epidemic." *Time,* 30 December 1996 to 6 January 1997, p. 76. Primary source: UNAIDS.

★ 946 ★

Health Status: Diseases

Persons Who Get AIDS Worldwide

	Total
HIV infections, children	
New in 1996	400,000
Current total	830,000
HIV infections, adults and children	
New in 1996	3,100,000
Current total	22,600,000
Deaths in 1996	1,500,000
Cumulative numbers	
Infections	29,400,000
AIDS cases	8,400,000
Deaths	6,400,000

Source: Nash, J. Madeleine. "The Enemy Within." *Time* (Fall 1996), p. 19.

★ 947 ★

Health Status: Diseases

Persons Who Have HIV/AIDS, by World Region: 1996

Country, region, area	Persons with HIV/AIDS
Sub-Saharan Africa	14,000,000
South and Southeast Asia	5,200,000
Latin America	1,300,000
North America	750,000
Western Europe	510,000
Caribbean	270,000
North Africa/Middle East	200,000
East Asia and Pacific	100,000
Central and Eastern Europe and Central Asia	50,000
Australia and New Zealand	13,000

Source: Purvis, Andrew. "The Global Epidemic." *Time,* 30 December 1996 to 6 January 1997, p. 76. Primary source: UNAIDS.

★ 948 ★

Health Status: Diseases

Women Who Have HIV/AIDS, by World Region: 1996

[In percentages]

Country, region, area	% of women with HIV/AIDS
Sub-Saharan Africa	>50
Caribbean	>40
South and Southeast Asia	>30
Australia and New Zealand	20
Central and Eastern Europe and Central Asia	20
East Asia and Pacific	20
Latin America	20
North Africa/Middle East	20
North America	20
Western Europe	20

Source: Purvis, Andrew. "The Global Epidemic." *Time,* 30 December 1996 to 6 January 1997, p. 76. Primary source: UNAIDS *Note:* > stands for "more than".

Health Status: Women

★ 949 ★

Daily Deaths Caused by Pregnancy and Childbirth, by World Region: 1995

From the source: "The toll of injury and disability from pregnancy related causes is arguably the most neglected health problem in the world. For every woman who dies in childbirth, probably about 30 incur injuries and infections—many of which are often painful, disabling, embarrassing, and lifelong."

Region	Deaths per day
Asia and Pacific	818
Sub-Saharan Africa	615
Middle East and North Africa	98
Americas	65

[Continued]

★ 949 ★

Daily Deaths Caused by Pregnancy and Childbirth, by World Region: 1995
[Continued]

Region	Deaths per day
Central Asia	39
Europe	8

Source: "Women: New Estimates Put Toll at 585,000." *Progress of Nations 1996.* UNICEF, 1996. Data are available from the World Wide Web at http:// www.unicef.org/pon96/ woestima.htm#15. Primary source: WHO; UNICEF.

★ 950 ★

Health Status: Women

Maternal Deaths Worldwide: 1995

Region	Maternal deaths per year
Europe	3,000
Central Asia	14,000
Americas	23,000
Middle East and North Africa	35,000
Sub-Saharan Africa	219,000
Asia and Pacific	291,000
World	585,000

Source: "Women: New Estimates Put Toll at 585,000." *Progress of Nations 1996.* UNICEF, 1996. Data are available from the World Wide Web at http:// www.unicef.org/pon96/ woestima.htm#15. Primary source: WHO; UNICEF.

Sources

Thousands of statistics are produced by a variety of reliable sources each year in the field of health and medicine. Data were selected for inclusion in *Statistical Record of Health and Medicine* on the basis of their timeliness, interest or value to researchers and the general public, and their ability to contribute to the comprehensive coverage of the field. This list contains complete bibliographic citations for material from which tables were compiled or from which data were selected. Tables appear in the list by table number. Tables can be accessed by reference number or by page number using the Table of Contents or the Keyword Index.

1993 TAPS II, The Maxwell Consumer Report 1994, Ad $ Summary 1993. Table: 519.

1996 Statistical Abstract of the United States on CD-ROM [machine-readable datafiles]. CD-8A-97. Washington, DC: U.S. Department of Commerce, Economics and Statistics Administration, Bureau of the Census, Data User Services Division, January 1997. Tables: 15-16, 36-42, 54-56, 61, 93, 95, 103, 105, 208-209, 211, 251, 283, 439, 444-445, 447, 492-494, 595, 597, 599, 603, 641, 839, 897.

"A Good Gene Gone Bad." *Newsweek,* 23 December 1996. Table: 127.

"A System for Docs, Pols, and Mobs." *U.S. News & World Report,* 2 September 1996. Table: 876.

Abma, J.C., A. Chandra, W.D. Mosher, L. Peterson, and L. Piccinino. *Fertility, Family Planning, and Women's Health: New Data from the 1995 National Survey of Family Growth.* National Center for Health Statistics. Vital Health Statistics 23(19), 1997. Tables: 504-518.

"AJNNewsline: Many Aren't Reporting Exposures to Blood." *American Journal of Nursing* (May 1995). Table: 571.

Amado, Anthony J., Virginia Grow, and James Nofziger. "An Evaluation of Hospice Care with Terminally Ill Cancer Patients." *Caring Magazine* (November 1995). Tables: 48-49, 576-577.

American Hospital Association; Trend Analysis Group: National Hospital Panel Survey Reports. Chicago. Monthly reports for January 1992 - June 1996. Tables: 446, 467.

"American Pie: Teen Moms." *U.S. News & World Report,* 11 November 1996. Table: 14.

"Americans With Disabilities." *USA TODAY,* 28 August 1995. Table: 90.

Anders, George. "Who Pays Cost of Cut-Rate Heart Care?" *Wall Street Journal,* 15 October 1996. Table: 608.

Armstrong, Larry. "Besting AIDS—and the Drug Giants." *Business Week,* 9 June 1997. Table: 301.

Auerbach, Stuart. "Organ Donations by Minorities Rise." *Washington Post,* 27 February 1996. Table: 905.

Bates, Karl Leif. "Most Doctors Don't Know When to Bench a Player." *Detroit News,* 28 May 1997. Table: 228.

"Big-Ticket Sports Injuries." *USA TODAY,* 8 August 1996. Table: 229.

Borzo, Greg. "Physicians *Will* Use Computers." *American Medical News,* 23-30 October 1995. Table: 911.

"Breaking News: Lung Cancer Mortality Highs and Lows." *Patient Care,* 15 June 1997. Tables: 52-53.

Cancer Research Funding, Cancer Facts, U.S. Department of Health and Human Services, Public Health Service, National Institutes of Health, National Cancer Institute, September 1996. Table: 586.

"Career Guide: 20 Hot Job Tracks." *U.S. News & World Report,* 30 October 1995. Tables: 816-817.

Carter, J.P. "By the Numbers." *Journal of Psychosocial Nursing* 1996, vol. 34, no. 3. Table: 604.

"Cervical Cancer Screening by Age, 1987 and 1992." *Primary Care & Cancer* (April 1996). Table: 277.

Chang, Trina. "Health Care Compared: Back Surgery." *American Health* (May 1996). Table: 907.

Chang, Trina. "Health Care Compared: Breast Cancer Surgery." *American Health* (May 1996). Tables: 275-276.

Church, George J. "Backlash Against HMOs." *Time,* 14 April 1997. Table: 587.

Cohen, R.A., and J.F. Van Nostrand. *Trends in the Health of Older Americans: United States, 1994.* National Center for Health Statistics. Vital and Health Statistics 3(30). 1995. U.S. Department of Health and Human Services, Public Health Service, Centers for Disease Control and Prevention. Primary source: National Center for Health Statistics: *Health, United States, 1992.* Data are from the Office of National Health Statistics, Office of the Actuary: National Health Expenditures, 1991. *Health Care Financing Review.* Vol. 14, Number 2. HCFA Pub. No. 03335. Health Care Financing Administration. Washington: DC: U.S. Government Printing Office, 1992. Tables: 449-463, 594, 602.

Commission on Family and Medical Leave. "A Workable Balance: Report to Congress on Family and Medical Leave Policies." 30 April 1996. Tables: 919-927.

Conkling, Winifred. "Women, Men and Illness." *American Health* (July/August 1996). Table: 94.

"Continuum of Care: Home Health's Growth Spurt." *Hospitals & Health Networks,* 20 June 1996. Table: 440.

"Coping with Unwellcome News." *Economist,* 26 April 1997. Table: 306.

"Cosmetic Dental Work." *Consumer Reports* (December 1996). Table: 58.

"Cost of Rehabilitation." *USA TODAY,* 18 September 1995. Table: 578.

Cronin, Brian. "Health Report: The Bad News." *Time,* 2 December 1996. Tables: 144, 178.

Cronin, Brian. "Health Report: The Bad News." *Time,* 23 June 1997. Table: 11.

Cronin, Brian. "Health Report: The Bad News." *Time,* 28 April 1997. Tables: 20, 258, 539.

Cronin, Brian. "Health Report: The Bad News." *Time,* 3 February 1997. Table: 296.

Cronin, Brian. "Health Report: The Bad News." *Time,* 6 May 1996. Table: 12.

Cronin, Brian. "Health Report: The Bad News." *Time,* 7 July 1997. Table: 143.

Cronin, Brian. "Health Report: The Good News." *Time,* 14 July 1997. Tables: 253, 279.

Cronin, Brian. "Health Report: The Good News." *Time,* 2 December 1996. Table: 123.

Cronin, Brian. "Health Report: The Good News." *Time,* 23 June 1997. Tables: 290, 292.

Cronin, Brian. "Health Report: The Good News." *Time,* 3 February 1997. Table: 294.

Cronin, Brian. "Health Report: The Good News." *Time,* 6 May 1996. Table: 910.

Current Population Survey (CPS), 1992-1993. Obtained from the Centers for Disease Control and Prevention Tobacco Information & Prevention Sourcepage. See http://www.cdc.gov. Table: 524.

"The Cutting Edge: Vital Statistics." *Washington Post,* 12 September 1995. Table: 931.

"The Cutting Edge: Vital Statistics." *Washington Post,* 27 February 1996. Table: 503.

Detroit Free Press, 9 April 1996. Table: 91.

"Diabetes by Ethnicity." *Hispanic* (August 1996). Table: 147.

"Diabetes' Complications." *USA TODAY,* 6 February 1997. Table: 146.

"Direct Costs for GI Disorder Treatment Regimens." *Business & Health* (August 1996). Tables: 582-583.

Drug Topics, 20 November 1995. Table: 101.

"Equipped for Fitness." *Workplace Vitality* (May 1995). Table: 495.

"Feds Intensify Fraud Scrutiny, Hone Tactics." *American Medical News,* 9 June 1997. Table: 929.

Flynn, Julia. "A Hepatitis Drug That May Cure Glaxo." *Business Week*, 12 May 1997. Table: 298.

"Follow Up: Good News for Off-Shore." *New Physician* (January/February 1996). Table: 834.

Freudenheim, Milt. "A Bitter Pill for the HMOs." *New York Times,* 28 April 1995. Table: 596.

Gallagher, John. "Fast-Forward." *Advocate,* 19 March 1996. Table: 121.

Garner, Rochelle. "Painful Lessons." *Computerworld,* 20 January 1997. Table: 568.

Georges, Christopher. "Costly New AIDS Drug Therapy Finds Support in Congress, Due to Efforts of Unlikely Alliance." *Wall Street Journal,* 11 July 1996. Tables: 289, 291.

"'Gesundheit' Cities." *USA TODAY,* 20 March 1997. Table: 13.

"Going Natural." *American Health* (November 1995). Table: 264.

Gorman, Christine. "If the Condom Breaks." *Time,* 23 June 1997. Table: 120.

Graff, James L. "High Times At New Trier High." *Time,* 9 December 1996. Table: 562.

"Health Care Finance. The Nation's Health Dollar: Calendar Year 1995." *Missouri Medicine,* vol. 94, no. 5 (May 1997). Table: 585.

Health Care Financing Administration. BDMS. OSM. Division of Program Systems. Obtained electronically from http://www.hcfa.gov, March 21, 1997. Tables: 598, 600-601, 687, 689-690, 692-698.

"Heart Attacks and Cigarettes." *American Health* (November 1995). Table: 533.

Heinlein, Gary. "No Pursuit Without Risks, Police Driving School Teaches." *Detroit News,* 16 January 1997. Table: 217.

"Here's One to Think About." *Risk Management* (July 1996). Table: 569.

"HMO Complaints." *New York Times,* 2 February 1997. Table: 655.

Hobica, George. "Flying the Lowfat Skies: Special Order." *American Health* (November 1995). Table: 491.

"Home Health Care Update 95." *Nursing95* (July 1995). Table: 309.

"How Areas' Obese Weigh In." *USA TODAY,* 4 March 1997. Table: 499.

"How Health Care Bills Are Paid." *USA TODAY,* 13-15 January 1995. Table: 592.

"How Hospital Stays Differ." *USA TODAY,* 5 September 1995. Table: 443.

"How Teens Get AIDS." *Current Health* (February 1996). Table: 116.

"The Human Condition: Hearing Loss." *Time* (Fall 1996). Table: 206.

"Imaging News: Diagnostic Imaging Centers in the U.S., 1984-1994." *Diagnostic Imaging* (February 1996). Table: 286.

"In Brief: Making Music and Immunity." *Scientific American* (July 1997). Table: 914.

"The Invisible Worm." *Economist,* 17 May 1997. Table: 175.

"It's Red Ink for Health Care Investors." *Business & Health* (May 1997). Tables: 470-471.

Katzenstein, Larry. "Race and Breast Cancer Risk." *American Health* (July/August 1996). Table: 126.

Kluger, Jeffrey. "Distress Calls: A New Study Links Car Phones with Accidents." *Time,* 24 February 1997. Table: 219.

Kraus, Lewis E., Susan Stoddard, and David Gilmartin. *Chartbook on Disability in the United States, 1996.* Washington, DC: U.S. National Institute on Disability and Rehabilitation Research. Tables: 62-89.

Laboratory Medicine, vol. 26, no. 2 (February 1995). Tables: 728-730, 893.

Lafferty, Elaine. "Beware the Counterpunch: What Happens When A Prescription Offends A Pharmacist's Beliefs?" *Time,* 28 April 1997. Table: 937.

"Latest Statistics." *USA TODAY,* 5 June 1996. Table: 122.

Leukemia, Research Report, U.S. Department of Health and Human Services, Public Health Service, National Institutes of Health, National Cancer Institute, PHS 94-329, November 1993, modified October 1995. Table: 100.

Leutwyler, Kristin. "In Brief: Bad News Bugs." *Scientific American* (July 1997). Table: 17.

Levy, Doug. "Disciplining Bad Doctors: Medical Boards Have Spotty Record." *USA TODAY,* 26 March 1996. Table: 917.

Levy, Doug. "Matchmaking at the Heart of Transplant Process." *USA TODAY,* 19 October 1995. Tables: 899, 906.

Levy, Doug. "The Toll Smoking Will Take on Today's Youth: 16.6M Will Get Hooked and 5M Will Die." *USA TODAY,* 8 November 1996. Tables: 522, 537-538.

Light, Larry. "Up Front: Walk, Don't Run." *Business Week,* 23 October 1995. Table: 496.

"The List: Health Check." *Business Week,* 19 August 1996. Table: 98.

"Looking Good: Top Cosmetic Procedures." *American Health* (November 1995). Table: 896.

"The Mad Pace of Health Care Mergers." *Business & Health* (April 1996). Table: 473.

"Managed Care: Where It's At." *Hospitals & Health Networks,* 20 January 1997. Table: 472.

Manning, Anita. "TB Cases in USA Continue to Drop." *USA TODAY,* 24 March 1997. Table: 200.

Marosy, John Paul. "Elder Caregiving in the 21st Century." *CARING Magazine* (May 1997). Table: 207.

Mathias, Robert. "NIDA Survey Provides First National Data on Drug Use During Pregnancy." *NIDA Notes* (January/February 1995). Table: 543.

McGinley, Laurie, and Elyse Tanouye. "FDA to Assess Drugs to Treat Hypertension." *Wall Street Journal,* 25 January 1996. Table: 293.

Medical Tribune, 21 September 1995. Table: 815.

"Mental Disorders: The Toll." *USA TODAY,* 28 May 1996. Tables: 259, 262, 612.

"Mental Health: Does Therapy Help?" Consumer Reports (November 1995). Table: 260.

Merrill, PhD, Ray M. "Trends in Prostate Cancer Incidence and Surgery." *Primary Care & Cancer* (June 1996). Tables: 256-257.

Meyer, Harris. "Indemnity Insurance: Down But Not Out." *Medical Economics,* 12 August 1996. Tables: 638, 644.

Miller, William H. "Clean-Air Contention: EPA's proposed stricter air-quality standards stir heated controversy — and vehement industry opposition." *Industry Week,* 5 May 1997. Table: 203.

"Mind, Body, Sole: Mapping the Hierarchy of Modern Well-Being." *Adweek,* 24 March 1997. Table: 935.

"Missing Teeth: Comparing Your Options." *Consumer Reports* (December 1996). Table: 59.

"Money Machines: HMOs Pile Up Billions in Cash As Analysts Wonder What They Will Do With It." *Wall Street Journal,* 21 December 1994. Table: 437.

"Monitor: Head of the Class." *New Physician* (January/February 1996). Tables: 821-822.

Monitoring the Future Project. University of Michigan Survey Research Center, 1995. Table: 536.

Montague, Jim. "Currents: Drinking, Drugs and Rock 'n' Roll." *Hospitals & Health Networks,* 5 September 1996. Table: 541.

Montague, Jim. "Currents: The Most Dangerous Games." *Hospitals & Health Networks,* 5 September 1996. Table: 226.

Monthly Treasury Statement of Receipts and Outlays of the United States Government. Financial Management Service, U.S. Department of the Treasury. 1996 Annual Reports of the Board of Trustees of the HI and SMI Trust Funds. Office of the Actuary, Health Care Financing Administration. Table: 703.

"More Than 200 Cancer Medicines Now in Development." *Medical Marketing & Media* (July 1995). Table: 295.

Nash, J. Madeleine. "Addicted." *Time,* 5 May 1997. Table: 565.

Nash, J. Madeleine. "The Enemy Within." *Time* (Fall 1996). Tables: 131-132, 943, 946.

Nasser, Haya Ed. "Snowmobiles Skid Into Danger." *USA TODAY,* 28 February 1997. Table: 218.

National Center for Injury Prevention and Control. Centers for Disease Control and Prevention. State Injury Mortality Statistics. Downloaded from http://www.cdc.gov.ncip/ncipchm.htm on March 10, 1995. Tables: 232-250.

National Health Interview Surveys: 1965, 1970, 1974, 1979, 1983, 1988, 1992, 1993, 1994. Updated table, Surveillance for Selected Tobacco-Use Behaviors—United States, 1900-1994. Obtained from the Centers for Disease Control and Prevention Tobacco Information & Prevention Sourcepage. See http://www.cdc.gov. Table: 535.

National Health Interview Surveys: 1970, 1987, and 1991. Surveillance for Selected Tobacco-Use Behaviors—United States, 1900-1994. Obtained from the Centers for Disease Control and Prevention Tobacco Information & Prevention Sourcepage. See http://www.cdc.gov. Table: 530.

National Health Interview Surveys: 1980, 1983, 1985, 1987, 1988, 1990, 1991, 1992, 1993. Surveillance for Selected Tobacco-Use Behaviors—United States, 1900-1994. Obtained from the Centers for Disease Control and Prevention Tobacco Information & Prevention Sourcepage. See http://www.cdc.gov. Tables: 526-527, 529, 531.

National Health Interview Surveys: 1987 and 1991 (combined). Surveillance for Selected Tobacco-Use Behaviors—United States, 1900-1994. Obtained from the Centers for Disease Control and Prevention Tobacco Information & Prevention Sourcepage. See http://www.cdc.gov. Table: 520.

"National Hospice Usage, by Client Age, Gender, and Race." *Caring Magazine* (November 1995). Table: 441.

National Industry Occupation Matrix, 1994. Acquired on electronic media. Prepared by Bureau of Labor Statistics, Washington, DC: U.S. Department of Labor, 1994. Tables: 841-852, 854-875, 877-884.

National Summary of Medicaid Managed Care Programs and Enrollment, June 30, 1996. HCFA. BDMS. OSM. Division of Program Systems. Obtained electronically from http://www.hcfa.gov, March 21, 1997. Table: 691.

"The National Unintentional-Injury Fatality Toll." *Safety & Health* (May 1996). Table: 223.

NCI Surveillance Program. Extracted from *Lifetime Probability of Breast Cancer in American Women.* Cancer Facts. U.S. Department of Health and Human Services. Public Health Service. National Institutes of Health. National Cancer Institute. August 1993. Table: 129.

Neuborne, Ellen. "Work Rules Stir Debate on Mental Health." *USA TODAY,* 21 May 1997. Table: 570.

"News & Trends: A Close-Up of ADA Infractions." *Business & Health* (April 1996). Table: 918.

"News & Trends: Addressing the High Cost of Birth Defects." *Business & Health* (November 1995). Tables: 574-575.

"News & Trends: Brands on Top, No Matter Who Pays." *Business & Health* (November 1995). Tables: 304-305.

"News & Trends: What We Have Here Is A Failure to Communicate." *Business & Health* (March 1997). Table: 936.

"News Pulse: Affairs of the Heart." *Nursing95* (March 1995). Table: 204.

"News Pulse: Expensive Delays." *Nursing95* (August 1995). Table: 928.

"News You Can Use: The Top 10 Pregnancy Drugs." *U.S. News & World Report,* 27 March 1995. Table: 265.

"Notebook: The Belt and the Buckle." *Time,* 26 May 1997. Table: 145.

"Notebook: Blood Sports." *Time,* 17 June 1996. Table: 227.

"Notebook: The Fat of the Land." *Time,* 23 December 1996. Table: 501.

"Notebook: Implant Insights." *Time,* 9 June 1997. Table: 285.

"Notebook: Mail Handlers." *Time,* 24 June 1996. Table: 573.

"Number of Killings Declines." *USA TODAY,* 24 October 1995. Table: 44.

"Nutrition: A Tale of Two Statistics." *Progress of Nations 1996.* UNICEF, 1996. Data are available from the World Wide Web at http://www.unicef.org/pon96/nutale.htm. Table: 941.

Office on Smoking and Health. National Center for Chronic Disease Prevention and Health Promotion. Centers for Disease Control and Prevention, July 1996. The following references are cited: (1) Data compiled by the Centers for Disease Control and Prevention, Office on Smoking and Health, from the Current Population Survey, 1955, and the National Health Interview Surveys, 1965-1994. (2) Centers for Disease Control and Prevention. Cigarette smoking among adults—United States, 1994. Morbidity and Mortality Weekly Report 1996; 45(27):588-590. Table: 534.

Ostrovsky, Arkady. "Birthrate Down, Hardship Up." *Financial Times,* 29 May 1997. Tables: 176, 274.

"Outpatient Surgery Settings, 1991-2001." *Medical Tribune,* 20 June 1996. Table: 908.

"Paying for Health Care." *USA TODAY,* 12 January 1995. Table: 593.

"Paying for Psychiatric Care." *American Medical News,* 27 May 1996. Table: 263.

Pipp, Tracy L. "Growing Pains." *Detroit News,* 10 July 1997. Tables: 97, 912.

"POS Takes A Big Slice of Every Pie." *Business & Health* (August 1996). Table: 469.

Prager, Linda O. "Heart Attacks A Costly Liability Risk, Insurer Study Finds." *American Medical News,* 17 June 1996. Table: 930.

"Pre-Existing Restriction." *Workplace Vitality* (May 1995). Table: 642.

"Prozac Prescription Growth." *USA TODAY,* 9 July 1997. Table: 302.

Psychiatric Times (November 1995). Table: 643.

"Public Health News & Notes: Anxiety Disorders Lead Mental Ills in United States." *Public Health Records,* vol. III, no. 4 (July/August 1996). Table: 261.

"Public Health News & Notes: TB Deaths Reach Historic Levels." *Public Health Reports,* vol. III, no. 4 (July/August 1996). Table: 198.

Purvis, Andrew. "The Global Epidemic." *Time,* 30 December 1996-6 January 1997. Tables: 942, 944-945, 947-948.

"Recent Locations: Top U.S. States." *Site Selection* (February 1996). Table: 303.

Research Activities, AHCPR, Rockville, MD (November/December 1995). Table: 579.

"The Risks of Racing the Reproductive Clock." *Business Week,* 5 May 1997. Tables: 280-281.

RN (October 1995). Table: 898.

RN (September 1996). Table: 895.

"Road Sign." *Time,* 2 June 1997. Tables: 230-231.

"Rollover Fatality Rates." *Automotive News,* 10 June 1996. Tables: 222, 224.

Ross, Philip E. "First, Do No Harm." *Forbes,* 21 October 1996. Table: 909.

Rubin, Rita. "Rating the HMOs." *U.S. News & World Report,* 2 September 1996. Table: 438.

"Runaway Technology." *Workplace Vitality* (July/August 1995). Table: 913.

Ryan, Richard A. "Medicare Reform to Cost Seniors." *Detroit News,* 10 July 1997. Tables: 699, 723.

Sabir, Nadirah Z. "Newspoints: A Second Chance." *Black Enterprise* (February 1996). Tables: 903-904.

SAMHSA News (Summer 1995). Tables: 623-624.

"Science & Society: Rethinking Eyeglasses for Kids." *U.S. News & World Report,* 14 August 1995. Table: 18.

Scientific American (September 1996). Tables: 124-125, 128, 130, 133-140.

"Seat Belts Save Lives—and Money." *USA TODAY,* 25 March 1996. Table: 502.

SEER Cancer Statistics Review 1973-1991. Cancer Facts. U.S. Department of Health and Human Services. Public Health Service. National Institutes of Health. National Cancer Institute. June 1995. SEER stands for Surveillance, Epidemiology, and End Results. Table: 141.

Sexton, Kevin J. "The Ministry Change Imperative." *Health Progress* (March/April 1996). Table: 465.

"Shrinking Hospital Stays." *USA TODAY,* 5 September 1995. Table: 468.

"Sketch of the USA's Uninsured." *USA TODAY,* 8 August 1994. Tables: 645-654.

"Smoking status of high school seniors—United States." Monitoring the Future Project, 1976-1996, University of Michigan. Obtained from the Centers for Disease Control and Prevention Tobacco Information & Prevention Sourcepage. See http://www.cdc.gov. Table: 528.

Smolowe, Jill. "A Healthy Merger?" *Time,* 15 April 1996. Table: 474.

Smolowe, Jill. "Sorry, Pardner: Big Tobacco Fesses Up and Pays Up — $368.5 Billion, but Congress Must Approve the Deal." *Time,* 30 June 1997. Table: 916.

"Snapshots of the Workplace Health Industry: Extra Pocket Money." *Workplace Vitality* (July/August 1996). Table: 818.

"Snapshots of the Workplace Health Industry: Risk Takers." *Workplace Vitality* (July/August 1996). Table: 572.

"Snapshots of the Workplace Health Industry: What the Doctor Found." *Workplace Vitality* (July/August 1996). Table: 104.

"Special Report: Annual Rx Survey." *Drug Topics,* 7 April 1997. Table: 299.

"Speed Traps Focus on Fines, Not Keeping Public Safe." (editorial). *USA TODAY,* 27 November 1996. Tables: 46-47.

"Spotlight: Adults with Diabetes, by Race, Ethnicity." *Medical Tribune,* 11 January 1996. Table: 148.

"Spotlight: Medicines in Testing for Mental Illness." *Medical Tribune,* (Family Physician Edition), 23 May 1996. Table: 297.

Squires, Sally. "High Seas: The Hazards of Drunk Boating." *Washington Post,* 2 July 1996. Table: 220.

St. Louis Post-Dispatch, 9 September 1996. Table: 932.

"State Report: Managing Medicaid: How the Numbers Add Up." *Business & Health* (June 1997). Tables: 656, 660.

"States with Fewest in HMOs." *USA TODAY,* 5 March 1997. Table: 657.

"Stats on Bags & Belts." *Current Health* (April 1996). Table: 225.

Stephenson, Michelle. "Hospital Cost Shifting: Surgeon Found Items Marked Up As Much As 14,000%." *Today's O.R. Nurse* (September/October 1995). Table: 464.

Strahan, Genevieve. "An Overview of Nursing Homes and Their Current Residents: Data from the 1995 National Nursing Home Survey," Advance Data, Vital and Health Statistics, Centers for Disease Control and Prevention, National Center for Health Statistics, Number 280, January 23, 1997. Tables: 475-480, 482, 485-490.

"TB Cases Decline in U.S." *USA TODAY,* 12 May 1997. Table: 199.

"Teenagers and the 'Madness' of Drugs." *U.S. News & World Report,* 13 November 1995. Table: 557.

Thompson, Dick. "America's Deadliest Cities." *Time,* 9 December 1996. Table: 202.

Thompson, Dick. "Cancer: the Good News." *Time,* 25 November 1996. Table: 142.

Tobacco Situation and Outlook Report. U.S.D.A., April 1996 and September 1987. Miller, R. *U.S. cigarette consumption, 1900 to date.* In: Harr W, ed. Tobacco yearbook, 1981, page 53. Table: 532.

"Too Many, Too Few." *American Medical News,* 26 February 1996. Table: 890.

"Top Centers." *Detroit News,* 8 July 1996. Table: 287.

"The Torture of Second-Class Travel." *Economist,* 14 June 1997. Table: 96.

"Trends: Health Benefits Most Costly." *Corporate Cashflow* (January 1996). Table: 580.

U.S. Department of Commerce. Bureau of Economic Analysis: Survey of Current Business. Washington, DC: U.S. Government Printing Office. Monthly reports for January 1992-March 1996. Table: 584.

U.S. Department of Commerce. Bureau of the Census. *1992 Economic Census Report Series,* CD-ROM 1i, Washington, DC, October 1996. Tables: 310-436.

U.S. Department of Commerce. Bureau of the Census. *Current Population Survey*, March 1996. Tables: 625, 637, 639.

U.S. Department of Commerce. Bureau of the Census. Income Statistics Branch/HHES Division, Washington, D.C. Unpublished March Current Population Survey for data prior to 1989 and Current Population Reports, Series P-60 for 1989 forward. Tables: 626-631, 633-636.

U.S. Department of Education. Office of Educational Research and Improvement. National Center for Education Statistics. *Digest of Education Statistics, 1996.* Washington, DC: U.S. Government Printing Office, 1996. Tables: 727, 819-820, 823-832, 835-836.

U.S. Department of Health and Human Services. Health Care Financing Administration. Office of Research and Demonstrations. *Health Care Financing Review, Medicare and Medicaid Statistical Supplement, 1996.* Tables: 605-606, 619-622, 659, 661-685, 700-702, 704-722, 724-726.

U.S. Department of Health and Human Services. Public Health Service. Centers for Disease Control and Prevention. Division of STD Prevention. *Sexually Transmitted Disease Surveillance, 1995.* U.S. Department of Health and Human Services, Public Health Service, September 1996. Tables: 152-174, 177, 179-197.

U.S. Department of Health and Human Services. Public Health Service. Centers for Disease Control and Prevention. *HIV/AIDS Surveillance Report, 1996* vol. 8, no. 1. The HIV/AIDS Surveillance Report is now accessible via Internet: www.cdc.gov. Tables: 106, 108-114, 117-119.

U.S. Department of Health and Human Services. Public Health Service. Centers for Disease Control and Prevention. *Morbidity and Mortality Weekly Report,* vol. 44, no. 3, 27 January 1995. Table: 102.

U.S. Department of Health and Human Services. Public Health Service. Centers for Disease Control and Prevention. National Center for Health Statistics. Division of Health Examination Statistics. Hyattsville, MD: Public Health Service, 1995. Unpublished data. Tables: 150-151, 500.

U.S. Department of Health and Human Services. Public Health Service. Centers for Disease Control and Prevention. National Center for Health Statistics. Fluoridation Fact Sheet (FL-141), December 1993. Table: 60.

U.S. Department of Health and Human Services. Public Health Service. Centers for Disease Control and Prevention. National Center for Health Statistics. *Health, United States, 1994.* Hyattsville, MD: Public Health Service, 1995. Tables: 833, 837-838, 840, 853, 885-889, 891.

U.S. Department of Health and Human Services. Public Health Service. Centers for Disease Control and Prevention. National Center for Health Statistics. *Health, United States, 1995.* Hyattsville, MD: Public Health Service, 1996. Tables: 19, 21-35, 45, 50-51, 57, 92, 107, 115, 205, 210, 252, 254-255, 269-270, 278, 282, 284, 442, 466, 481, 483-484, 521, 525, 563-564, 589-590, 607, 613-618, 939-940.

U.S. Department of Health and Human Services. Public Health Service. Centers for Disease Control and Prevention. National Center for Health Statistics. "International Notes: Dengue Type 3 Infection — Nicaragua and Panama, October-November 1994." *CDC Surveillance Summaries. Morbidity and Mortality Weekly Report* vol. 44, no. 2, 20 January 1995. Table: 212.

U.S. Department of Health and Human Services. Public Health Service. Centers for Disease Control and Prevention. National Center for Health Statistics. "Vaccination Coverage Levels." *Morbidity and Mortality Weekly Report,* vol. 45, no. 7, 23 February 1996. Tables: 213-216.

U.S. Department of Health and Human Services. Public Health Service. Substance Abuse and Mental Health Services Administration. Office of Applied Studies. *Drug Use Among U.S. Workers: Prevalence and Trends by Occupation and Industry Categories.* Rockville, Maryland: SAMHSA, May 1996, DHHS pub. no. (SMA) 96-3089. Tables: 540, 542, 556, 558-561.

U.S. Department of Health and Human Services. Public Health Service. Substance Abuse and Mental Health Services Administration. Office of Applied Studies. *National Household Survey on Drug Abuse: Main Findings 1994. Tables: 544-555, 566.*

U.S. Department of Labor. Bureau of Labor Statistics. *CPI Detailed Report.* Washington, DC: U.S. Government Printing Office. Monthly reports for January 1991-June 1996. Tables: 609-610.

U.S. Department of Labor. Bureau of Labor Statistics. *Employment and Earnings.* Washington, DC: U.S. Government Printing Office. Monthly reports for January 1992-June 1996. Tables: 288, 307-308.

U.S. Department of Labor. Bureau of Labor Statistics. *Occupational Compensation Survey.* Tables were assembled from data downloaded from http://stats.bls. gov. Tables: 731-814.

U.S. Department of Labor. Press Release. December 20, 1993. The data presented are from a special survey of expenditures on health care plans conducted by the U.S. Department of Labor's Bureau of Labor Statistics for the Department of Health and Human Services' Health Care Financing Administration. Expenditures included employer and employee costs for health care plans, typically insurance premiums. Table: 588.

Van Biema, David. "Fatal Doses: Assisted Suicide Soars in An Afflicted Community." *Time* 17 February 1997. Table: 915.

Ventura, S.J., J.A. Martin, T.J. Mathews, and S.C. Clarke. "Advance Report of Final Natality Statistics, 1994." Monthly Vital Statistics Report, vol. 44, no. 11, supp.: National Center for Health Statistics, 1996. Tables: 266-268, 271.

Wall Street Journal, 1 December 1995. Table: 611.

Wall Street Journal, 24 June 1997. Tables: 149, 498.

Wallis, Claudia. "Healing." *Time,* 24 June 1996. Tables: 272-273.

"Washington Not Working Out." *USA TODAY,* 29 August 1996. Table: 497.

"The Week in Medicine: Incredible Shrinking Indemnity Coverage." *American Medical News,* 23-30 September 1996. Table: 581.

"The Week in Medicine: Nonphysician Prescribing Doubles." *American Medical News,* 17 June 1996. Table: 892.

"The Week in Medicine: Shorter Stays." *American Medical News,* 7 October 1996. Table: 448.

Welch, William M. "Medicaid: The Bill-Payer of Last Resort." *USA TODAY,* 29 August 1995. Tables: 686, 688.

Whelan, Elizabeth. "Opinion USA: Tobacco Rules in Too Many Woman's Magazines." *USA TODAY,* 14 November 1995. Tables: 933-934.

"Where HMOs Rule." *USA TODAY,* 4 March 1997. Table: 658.

"Which Organs Do People Need?" *Safety & Health* (May 1996). Table: 902.

"Who Treats Whom." *American Medical News,* 26 August 1996. Table: 938.

Wilke, Michael. "3 Agencies Vie for Colestid OTC Biz." *Advertising Age,* 7 July 1997. Table: 300.

Williams, Margie Ford. "Violence and Sexual Harassment." *AAOHN Journal,* vol. 44, no. 2 (February 1996). Table: 894.

Wojciechowski, Gene. "An Appeal from Heart of Baseball." *Chicago Tribune,* 29 November 1995. Tables: 900-901.

"Women: New Estimates Put Toll at 585,000." *Progress of Nations 1996.* UNICEF, 1996. Data are available from the World Wide Web at http://www.unicef. org/pon96/woestima.htm#15. Tables: 949-950.

"Workplace Notebook: In-Hospital Infections." *Workplace Vitality* (May 1996). Table: 99.

Wright, Andrew G. "Battling A Bad Bug." *ENR,* 2 June 1997. Table: 201.

Wulf, Steve. "Man's Best Friend?" *Time,* 23 June 1997. Tables: 43, 221.

"WV List: Who Ordered the Medical Errors?" *Workplace Vitality* (July/August 1996). Table: 591.

Youth Risk Behavior Survey (YRBS), 1993. Obtained from the Centers for Disease Control and Prevention Tobacco Information & Prevention Sourcepage. See http://www.cdc.gov. Table: 523.

Zack Figura, Susannah. "Carpal Tunnel Syndrome: The Facts Behind the Hype." *Managing Office Technology* (March 1997). Table: 567.

Keyword Index

This index provides access to all subjects covered in *Statistical Record of Health and Medicine*, including topics, geographical locations, occupations, company names, etc. Page references are provided; table references are also given inside brackets, e.g., [14]. Page references do not necessarily identify the page on which a table begins. In the cases where tables span two or more pages, references point to the page on which the index term appears—which may be the second or subsequent page of a table. Frequent cross-references have been added to index citations to facilitate the location of related topics and tables.

Numbers following p. or pp. are page references. Numbers in [ ] are table references.

962

Numbers following p. or pp. are page references. Numbers in [ ] are table references.

Keyword Index

Allentown – Bethlehem – Easton, PA continued:
— clinics, p. 265 [310]
— medical facilities, pp. 265, 269, 279, 294, 301, 303, 314, 321, 329, 334, 339, 346, 354, 359, 363, 367, 371, 376, 382, 392, 396, 411, 419, 421 [310, 312, 318, 328, 332-333, 340, 344, 348-349, 352, 356, 360, 362, 364, 366, 368, 370, 374, 380, 382, 392, 396-397]

Allergies
— and children, p. 10 [12]
— and prescriptions written, p. 10 [13]

Altoona, PA
— medical facilities, p. 329 [348]

Alzheimer's disease
See also: Diseases; Specific types of disease (e.g., Lyme disease)
— and insurance claims, p. 74 [98]
— and long-term care, p. 74 [98]

Amarillo, TX
— medical facilities, p. 329 [348]

Ambulatory surgical center
— and Medicare allowed charges, p. 762 [711]

American Indian females
— deaths, p. 23 [26]

American Indian males
— deaths, p. 24 [27]

American Indian or Alaskan Native females
— and prenatal care, pp. 235-236 [269-270]

American Indians
— and fertility rates, p. 245 [283]

Americans with Disabilities Act
See also: Disabilities; Work disabilities
— complaints, p. 932 [918]

Amitriptyline
— prices, p. 684 [611]

Amoxicillin
— and pregnancy, p. 233 [265]
— prescriptions written, pp. 260-261 [304-305]

Amoxil
— prescriptions written, pp. 260-261 [304-305]

Amphetamines
See also: Alcohol; Drug use (illicit); Marijuana and hashish; Substance abuse
— effects of, p. 649 [565]

Ampicillin
— and pregnancy, p. 233 [265]

Amputation
— and diabetes complications, p. 115 [146]

Anal atresia *See:* Colorectal or anal atresia

Analgesics
See also: Alcohol; Drug use (illicit); Marijuana and hashish; Substance abuse
— abuse, pp. 633-641, 650 [544-555, 566]

Anchorage, AK
— gonorrhea cases, p. 144 [170]
— medical facilities, pp. 269, 279, 294, 301, 314, 322, 329, 340, 347, 354, 359, 367, 371, 376, 382, 396, 411, 419 [312, 318, 328, 332, 340, 344, 348, 352, 356,

Anchorage, AK continued:
360, 362, 366, 368, 370, 374, 382, 392, 396]

Anderson, SC *See:* Greenville – Spartanburg – Anderson, SC

Anemias
See also: Chronic conditions; Diseases
— and death rates, p. 35 [40]

Anesthesia
— and Medicare allowed charges, pp. 756, 762-763 [701, 712-713]

Angiocardiography
— and men, pp. 225-226 [254]
— and women, pp. 240-241 [278]

Angioplasty, balloon *See:* Balloon angioplasty

Ann Arbor, MI
See also: Detroit – Ann Arbor – Flint, MI CMSA
— AIDS cases, p. 83 [108]

Anniston, AL
— medical facilities, p. 329 [348]

Antidepressants
See also: Drugs and medicines
— Prozac, p. 259 [302]

Antiulcer drugs
See also: Drugs and medicines
— Zantac, p. 261 [306]

Anxiety disorders, p. 231 [262]
— and drug research, p. 257 [297]
— and mental illness, p. 231 [261]

Apparel industry
— Consumer price index, pp. 686-687 [613, 615]

Appendectomies
— and hospital stays, p. 565 [468]
— and malpractice claims, p. 939 [931]
— and men, p. 227 [255]
— and women, p. 244 [282]

Appleton – Oshkosh – Neenah, WI
— medical facilities, pp. 269, 279, 294, 301, 314, 322, 329, 340, 347, 354, 359, 367, 371, 376, 382, 396, 411, 419 [312, 318, 328, 332, 340, 344, 348, 352, 356, 360, 362, 366, 368, 370, 374, 382, 392, 396]

Arizona
— active physicians, p. 911 [887]
— adult obesity rate, p. 595 [501]
— AIDS cases, pp. 82, 90, 99 [107, 112, 119]
— bicyclist fatalities, p. 208 [230]
— and births to teenagers, p. 11 [14]
— and disciplinary actions against physicians, p. 931 [917]
— and Medicaid, pp. 745, 747 [684-685]
— and motor-vehicle fatalities, p. 42 [46]
— chancroid cases, p. 119 [152]
— chlamydia cases, pp. 122, 124-125 [154-156]
— clinics, pp. 267, 320 [311, 343]
— deaths, pp. 37, 39, 609 [41, 522]
— dental clinics, p. 292 [327]
— diseases, p. 184 [200]
— expenditures, pp. 665, 667 [589-590]
— gonorrhea cases, pp. 136, 139-141 [164-167]
— health industry ratios, pp. 438-439, 441-442, 444-445, 447-448, 450-451, 453-454, 456-457, 459-460, 462-463, 465-

Numbers following p. or pp. are page references. Numbers in [ ] are table references.

964

Numbers following p. or pp. are page references. Numbers in [ ] are table references.

965

Keyword Index

Numbers following p. or pp. are page references. Numbers in [ ] are table references.

Numbers following p. or pp. are page references. Numbers in [ ] are table references.

Numbers following p. or pp. are page references. Numbers in [ ] are table references.

Keyword Index

Numbers following p. or pp. are page references. Numbers in [ ] are table references.

Numbers following p. or pp. are page references. Numbers in [ ] are table references.

970

Numbers following p. or pp. are page references. Numbers in [ ] are table references.

Numbers following p. or pp. are page references. Numbers in [ ] are table references.

Numbers following p. or pp. are page references. Numbers in [ ] are table references.

Keyword Index

973

Numbers following p. or pp. are page references. Numbers in [ ] are table references.

Numbers following p. or pp. are page references. Numbers in [ ] are table references.

Numbers following p. or pp. are page references. Numbers in [ ] are table references.

976

Numbers following p. or pp. are page references. Numbers in [ ] are table references.

977

Keyword Index

Numbers following p. or pp. are page references. Numbers in [ ] are table references.

Numbers following p. or pp. are page references. Numbers in [ ] are table references.

Keyword Index

Emergency medicine
— malpractice claims, p. 938 [930]
Emergency rooms
— and Medicare allowed charges, p. 764 [715]
Emotional and mental health
— and ADA complaints, p. 932 [918]
— and menopause, p. 242 [279]
Emphysema
See also: Diseases
— deaths, p. 35 [40]
Employment, pp. 878, 886 [840, 853]
— health care, pp. 438-439, 441-442, 444-445, 447-448, 450-451, 453-454, 456-457, 459-460, 462-463, 465-466, 468-469, 471-472, 474-475, 477-478, 480 [408-436]
— in health care facilities| 251, 262-263, 269, 272-273,
— projections, pp. 879-885, 887-905 [841-852, 854-875, 877-884]
End stage renal disease
— and Medicare allowed charges, p. 764 [715]
Endoscopies
— and men, pp. 225-226 [254]
— and women, pp. 240-241 [278]
Energy
— Consumer Price Index, pp. 686-687 [613, 615]
Engineers
— and alcohol use, p. 645 [560]
— and drug use, p. 645 [560]
English ivy
— poisonings, p. 76 [102]
Enid, OK
— medical facilities, p. 330 [348]
Enrollment
— health maintenance organizations, p. 720 [656]
— postsecondary institutions, pp. 868-869 [830-831]
Entertainment and recreation industry
— and alcohol use, pp. 631-632, 642 [540, 542, 556]
— and drug use, pp. 631-632, 642 [540, 542, 556]
Environmental Protection Agency
— and air quality standards, p. 187 [203]
Epidemiology
— degrees conferred, p. 864 [825]
Erie, PA
— medical facilities, p. 330 [348]
Erythromycin
— and pregnancy, p. 233 [265]
Eskimos
— and fertility rates, p. 245 [283]
Esophageal cancer, p. 112 [141]
See also: Cancer; Diseases; Specific types of cancer (e.g., Bladder cancer)
— and drugs, p. 255 [295]
Ethicon bone wax
— hospital prices, p. 561 [464]
Ethnicity
— and AIDS, p. 94 [115]
— and associate degrees conferred, p. 859 [819]
— and bachelor's degrees conferred, p. 862 [824]
— and birth control pills, p. 600 [510]

Ethnicity continued:
— and breast cancer, p. 104 [126]
— and contraception, pp. 597, 600 [505, 510]
— and deaths, pp. 27-28 [32-33]
— and dental visits, p. 49 [57]
— and diabetes, p. 115 [147]
— and doctoral degrees conferred, p. 866 [828]
— and fertility rates, p. 245 [283]
— and hypertension, p. 118 [151]
— and mammograms, p. 246 [284]
— and master's degrees conferred, p. 873 [836]
— and organ transplants, p. 923 [903]
— and prenatal care, pp. 235-236 [269-270]
— and sex education, p. 604 [517]
— and sexual intercourse, pp. 597, 600-602 [505, 510, 512, 514]
— and smoking, p. 607 [521]
— uninsured population, p. 718 [651]
Eucalyptus
— poisonings, p. 76 [102]
Eugene – Springfield, OR
— medical facilities, pp. 269, 279, 295, 301, 315, 322, 330, 340, 347, 354, 359, 368, 372, 376, 383, 396, 412, 419 [312, 318, 328, 332, 340, 344, 348, 352, 356, 360, 362, 366, 368, 370, 374, 382, 392, 396]
Europe
— and abortions, p. 238 [274]
— and deaths, p. 950 [949]
— and sexually transmitted diseases, p. 152 [176]
European Association for the Study of the Liver
— and drug testing, p. 257 [298]
Evansville – Henderson, IN – KY
— medical facilities, p. 330 [348]
Exercise
— by city, p. 591 [497]
— equipment, p. 589 [495]
Exercise videos
— ownership, p. 589 [495]
— use, p. 589 [495]
Expenditures, pp. 661, 669, 676 [585, 594, 602]
— by type, p. 669 [593]
— health care, pp. 663, 667, 673-675 [588, 591, 598, 600-601]
— hospital care, pp. 485, 661 [442, 585]
— Medicaid, pp. 724-725 [663-664]
— national, pp. 672, 677 [597, 603]
— nursing home care, pp. 575, 661 [481, 585]
— per capita, p. 678 [604]
— personal health care, p. 679 [605]
— physicians' services, pp. 661, 681 [585, 607]
Eye diseases
See also: Cataracts; Diabetes; Diseases
— diabetes complications, p. 115 [146]
— surgeries, pp. 228, 244-245 [255, 282]
Facial injuries
See also: Accidents; Injuries
— and car crashes, p. 205 [225]
Faculty, health
— salaries of, p. 772 [727]
Fall River, MA *See:* Providence – Fall River – Warwick, RI – MA
Family and general practice physicians
See also: Doctors; Internists; Physicians; Physicians by

Numbers following p. or pp. are page references. Numbers in [ ] are table references.

Numbers following p. or pp. are page references. Numbers in [ ] are table references.

Keyword Index

Numbers following p. or pp. are page references. Numbers in [ ] are table references.

Numbers following p. or pp. are page references. Numbers in [ ] are table references.

Keyword Index

Numbers following p. or pp. are page references. Numbers in [ ] are table references.

984

Numbers following p. or pp. are page references. Numbers in [ ] are table references.

985

Numbers following p. or pp. are page references. Numbers in [ ] are table references.

Numbers following p. or pp. are page references. Numbers in [ ] are table references.

Keyword Index

987

Numbers following p. or pp. are page references. Numbers in [ ] are table references.

Numbers following p. or pp. are page references. Numbers in [ ] are table references.

Numbers following p. or pp. are page references. Numbers in [ ] are table references.

990

Numbers following p. or pp. are page references. Numbers in [ ] are table references.

991

Keyword Index

Numbers following p. or pp. are page references. Numbers in [ ] are table references.

Kansas City, MO – KS continued:

360, 362, 364, 366, 368, 370, 372, 374, 376, 378, 380, 382, 384-385, 388, 390, 392-393, 396-397, 400-401, 404, 406]

— syphilis cases, pp. 159-160, 162, 175, 177-178, 180, 182 [183-185, 193-197]

Kennewick, WA *See:* Richland – Kennewick – Pasco, WA

Kenosha, WI *See:* Chicago – Gary – Kenosha, IL – IN – WI CMSA

Kentucky

— active physicians, p. 911 [887]

— adult obesity rate, p. 594 [501]

— AIDS cases, pp. 82, 91 [107, 112]

— and births to teenagers, p. 11 [14]

— and disciplinary actions against physicians, p. 931 [917]

— and exercise, p. 591 [497]

— and Medicaid, pp. 745, 747 [684-685]

— chancroid cases, p. 119 [152]

— chlamydia cases, pp. 122, 124, 126 [154-156]

— clinics, pp. 267, 320 [311, 343]

— deaths, pp. 37-38, 609 [41, 522]

— dental clinics, p. 293 [327]

— diseases, p. 184 [200]

— expenditures, pp. 665, 667 [589-590]

— gonorrhea cases, pp. 136, 138, 140-141 [164-167]

— health industry ratios, pp. 438, 440-442, 444-445, 447-448, 450-451, 453-454, 456-457, 459-460, 462-463, 465-466, 468-469, 471-472, 474-475, 477-478, 480 [408-436]

— health insurance, p. 712 [641]

— influenza cases, p. 195 [212]

— medical facilities, pp. 273, 275, 277, 283, 285, 287, 291, 293, 297, 300, 306, 308, 311, 313, 319-320, 326-327, 337-338, 344-345, 351-352, 358, 362, 366, 370, 375, 379, 381, 386, 388, 390, 394, 399, 403, 405, 408, 410, 416-417, 424, 426, 430-431, 434, 437-438, 440-442, 444-445, 447-448, 450-451, 453-454, 456-457, 459-460, 462-463, 465-466, 468-469, 471-472, 474-475, 477-478, 480 [314-315, 317, 320-321, 323, 326-327, 329, 331, 334-335, 337, 339, 342-343, 346-347, 350-351, 354-355, 358-359, 361, 363, 365, 367, 369, 371, 373, 375, 377, 379, 381, 383, 386-387, 389, 391, 394-395, 398-399, 402-403, 405, 407-436]

— nursing care facilities, p. 366 [365]

— nursing homes, pp. 577, 579 [483-484]

— physical fitness, p. 591 [497]

— physicians, p. 931 [917]

— smokers, p. 609 [522]

— syphilis cases, pp. 164-165, 167-168, 170-171, 173 [186-192]

— tuberculosis cases, p. 184 [200]

— vaccinations, p. 195 [212]

Key entry operators

— compensation for, pp. 797-798 [752-753]

Keystone Health Plan East, Inc.

— managed care enrollment, p. 720 [656]

— Medicaid enrollment, p. 720 [656]

Keystone Health Plan West, Inc.

— managed care enrollment, p. 720 [656]

— Medicaid enrollment, p. 720 [656]

Kidney diseases

See also: Diseases

— and advice in women's magazines, p. 940 [933]

— and cancer drugs, p. 255 [295]

— and deaths, p. 35 [40]

— and diabetes complications, p. 115 [146]

— and transplants, p. 923 [902]

Killeen – Temple, TX

— medical facilities, p. 331 [348]

Kingsport, TN *See:* Johnson City – Kingsport – Bristol, TN – VA

Knee prostheses

— hospital prices, p. 561 [464]

— risks in surgery, p. 926 [909]

Knee splints

— hospital prices, p. 561 [464]

Knoxville, TN

— AIDS cases, p. 84 [108]

— clinics, p. 265 [310]

— medical facilities, pp. 265, 270, 280, 295, 302, 304, 316, 323, 331, 335, 341, 348, 355, 360, 364, 368, 372, 377, 384, 392, 397, 413, 420, 422 [310, 312, 318, 328, 332-333, 340, 344, 348-349, 352, 356, 360, 362, 364, 366, 368, 370, 374, 380, 382, 392, 396-397]

Kokomo, IN

— medical facilities, p. 331 [348]

La Crosse, WI – MN

— medical facilities, p. 331 [348]

Laboratories

— and Medicare allowed charges, p. 764 [715]

— mergers and acquisitions, p. 568 [473]

Laboratory Corp. of America

— and fraud, p. 938 [929]

Laboratory technicians

— and AIDS infections, p. 98 [118]

Laborers *See:* Helpers and laborers

Lafayette, IN

— medical facilities, p. 331 [348]

Lafayette, LA

— medical facilities, pp. 270, 280, 295, 302, 316, 323, 331, 341, 348, 355, 360, 368, 372, 377, 384, 397, 413, 420 [312, 318, 328, 332, 340, 344, 348, 352, 356, 360, 362, 366, 368, 370, 374, 382, 392, 396]

Lake Charles, LA

— medical facilities, p. 331 [348]

Lakeland – Winter Haven, FL

— medical facilities, pp. 270, 280, 295, 302, 316, 323, 331, 341, 348, 355, 360, 368, 373, 377, 384, 397, 413, 420 [312, 318, 328, 332, 340, 344, 348, 352, 356, 360, 362, 366, 368, 370, 374, 382, 392, 396]

Lamivudine (drug)

— and AIDS treatment, p. 257 [298]

— and hepatitis B treatment, p. 257 [298]

Lancaster, PA

— medical facilities, pp. 270, 280, 295, 302, 316, 323, 331, 341, 348, 355, 360, 368, 373, 377, 384, 397, 413, 420 [312,

---

Numbers following p. or pp. are page references. Numbers in [ ] are table references.

Lancaster, PA continued:
318, 328, 332, 340, 344, 348, 352, 356, 360, 362, 366, 368, 370, 374, 382, 392, 396]

Lanoxin
— prescriptions written, pp. 260-261 [304-305]

Lansing – East Lansing, MI
— clinics, p. 265 [310]
— medical facilities, pp. 265, 270, 280, 295, 302, 304, 316, 323, 331, 335, 341, 348, 355, 360, 364, 368, 373, 377, 384, 392, 397, 413, 420, 422 [310, 312, 318, 328, 332-333, 340, 344, 348-349, 352, 356, 360, 362, 364, 366, 368, 370, 374, 380, 382, 392, 396-397]

Lansoprazole
— and gastrointestinal illnesses, p. 659 [583]
— costs, p. 659 [583]

Laparoscopies, pp. 240-241 [278]

Laredo, TX
— medical facilities, p. 331 [348]

Las Cruces, NM
— medical facilities, p. 331 [348]

Las Vegas, NV
— AIDS cases, p. 84 [108]
— medical facilities, pp. 270, 280, 295, 302, 316, 323, 331, 341, 348, 355, 360, 368, 373, 377, 384, 397, 413, 420 [312, 318, 328, 332, 340, 344, 348, 352, 356, 360, 362, 366, 368, 370, 374, 382, 392, 396]

Latin America and Caribbean
— and abortions, p. 238 [274]
— and sexually transmitted diseases, p. 152 [176]
— AIDS cases, pp. 946-949 [942, 944-945, 947-948]
— HIV cases, pp. 946-949 [942, 944-945, 947-948]

Lawrence, KS
— medical facilities, p. 331 [348]

Lawrence, MA See: Boston – Worcester – Lawrence, MA – NH – ME – CT CMSA

Lawton, OK
— medical facilities, p. 331 [348]

Lebanon, PA See: Harrisburg – Lebanon – Carlisle, PA

Legal services
— registered nurses employed, p. 904 [882]

Legislation
— Medicare, p. 769 [723]

Leukemia, p. 75 [100]
See also: Cancer; Diseases
— and P53 gene, p. 104 [127]
— deaths, pp. 35, 107 [40, 131]
— drugs, p. 255 [295]

Lewiston – Auburn, ME
— medical facilities, p. 331 [348]

Lexington, KY
— clinics, p. 266 [310]
— medical facilities, pp. 266, 270, 280, 295, 302, 304, 316, 323, 331, 335, 341, 348, 355, 360, 364, 368, 373, 377, 384, 393, 397, 413, 420, 422 [310, 312, 318, 328, 332-333, 340, 344, 348-349, 352, 356, 360, 362, 364, 366, 368, 370, 374, 380, 382, 392, 396-397]

Life expectancy
— by age, p. 224 [252]
— by race, pp. 223-224 [251-252]
— by sex, pp. 223-224 [251-252]

Life insurance
— medical records technicians employed, p. 890 [858]
— physicians employed, p. 900 [875]
— registered nurses employed, p. 904 [882]

Lima, OH
— medical facilities, p. 331 [348]

Lincoln, NE
— medical facilities, p. 331 [348]

Liquor
See also: Alcohol; Beer; Binge drinking; Drug use (illicit); Substance abuse
— and teenagers, p. 642 [557]

Little Rock – North Little Rock, AR
— AIDS cases, p. 84 [108]
— clinics, p. 266 [310]
— medical facilities, pp. 266, 270, 280, 295, 302, 304, 316, 323, 331, 335, 341, 348, 355, 360, 364, 368, 373, 377, 384, 393, 397, 413, 420, 422 [310, 312, 318, 328, 332-333, 340, 344, 348-349, 352, 356, 360, 362, 364, 366, 368, 370, 374, 380, 382, 392, 396-397]

Liver diseases
See also: Cancer; Diseases
— and P53 gene, p. 104 [127]
— cancer drugs, pp. 104, 112, 256 [127, 141, 295]
— death rates, p. 41 [44]
— transplants, pp. 921, 923-925 [899, 902-906]

Living Centers (company)
— profit growth, p. 567 [470]

Local governments
— dental assistants employed, p. 881 [845]
— dental hygienists employed, p. 882 [846]
— emergency medical technicians employed, p. 885 [852]
— home health aides employed, p. 887 [854]
— human services workers employed, p. 887 [855]
— licensed practical nurses employed, p. 888 [856]
— medical records technicians employed, p. 889 [858]
— medical scientists employed, p. 890 [859]
— nursing aides, orderlies, and attendants employed, p. 892 [862]
— occupational therapists employed, p. 893 [863]
— personal and home care aides employed, p. 895 [868]
— physician assistants employed, p. 899 [874]
— physicians employed, p. 900 [875]
— psychiatric aides employed, p. 901 [877]
— psychologists employed, p. 902 [879]
— registered nurses employed, p. 904 [882]

Lodi, CA See: Stockton – Lodi, CA

Lompoc, CA See: Santa Barbara – Santa Maria – Lompoc, CA

Long Beach, CA
— gonorrhea cases, p. 144 [170]

Long Island, NY See: New York – Northern New Jersey – Long Island, NY – NJ – CT CMSA

Longview – Marshall, TX
— medical facilities, p. 331 [348]

Numbers following p. or pp. are page references. Numbers in [ ] are table references.

Numbers following p. or pp. are page references. Numbers in [ ] are table references.

Numbers following p. or pp. are page references. Numbers in [ ] are table references.

Numbers following p. or pp. are page references. Numbers in [ ] are table references.

Keyword Index

Numbers following p. or pp. are page references. Numbers in [ ] are table references.

998

Numbers following p. or pp. are page references. Numbers in [ ] are table references.

999

Keyword Index

Numbers following p. or pp. are page references. Numbers in [ ] are table references.

1000

Numbers following p. or pp. are page references. Numbers in [ ] are table references.

1001

Numbers following p. or pp. are page references. Numbers in [ ] are table references.

Numbers following p. or pp. are page references. Numbers in [ ] are table references.

Keyword Index

1003

Numbers following p. or pp. are page references. Numbers in [ ] are table references.

Numbers following p. or pp. are page references. Numbers in [ ] are table references.

Keyword Index

Numbers following p. or pp. are page references. Numbers in [ ] are table references.

Numbers following p. or pp. are page references. Numbers in [ ] are table references.

Numbers following p. or pp. are page references. Numbers in [ ] are table references.

Numbers following p. or pp. are page references. Numbers in [ ] are table references.

Pacific Islander males
— deaths, p. 25 [29]
Pacific Islanders
— fertility rates, p. 245 [283]
Pacific Islands, U.S.
— AIDS cases, p. 92 [112]
PacifiCare Health Systems (company)
— finances, p. 481 [437]
— revenues, pp. 567, 671 [471, 596]
Pain
— and aging persons, p. 9 [11]
Painters, plasterers, and plumbers
— and alcohol use, p. 644 [559]
— and drug use, p. 644 [559]
Palate *See:* Cleft lip or palate
Palm Bay, FL *See:* Melbourne – Titusville – Palm Bay, Fl
Panama City, FL
— medical facilities, p. 332 [348]
Pancreatic diseases
— cancer, p. 112 [141]
— deaths, p. 107 [131-132]
— drugs, p. 256 [295]
— transplants, pp. 921, 923-925 [899, 902, 904-906]
Panic disorders
— prevalence, by sex, p. 71 [94]
Paradise, CA *See:* Chico – Paradise, CA
Paramedic *See:* Emergency medical technician and paramedic
Parkersburg – Marietta, WV – OH
— medical facilities, p. 332 [348]
Pascagoula, MS *See:* Biloxi – Gulfport – Pascagoula, MS
Pasco, WA *See:* Richland – Kennewick – Pasco, WA
Paso Robles, CA *See:* San Luis Obispo – Atascadero – Paso Robles, CA
Passaic, NJ *See:* Bergen – Passaic, NJ
Paterson, NJ
— breast cancer surgeries, p. 239 [275]
Pathologists
See also: Doctors; Physicians; Physicians by specialty (e.g., Cardiologists)
— malpractice claims against, p. 937 [928]
Paxil
— prices, p. 684 [611]
Payson, MD, Norman C.
— compensation for, p. 859 [818]
PCA Family Health Plan, Inc.
— managed care enrollment, p. 720 [656]
— Medicaid enrollment, p. 720 [656]
PCP
See also: Drug use (illicit); Marijuana and hashish; Substance abuse
— abuse, p. 650 [566]
Peace lily
— poisonings, p. 76 [102]
Pedestrians
— and motor vehicle-related deaths, p. 214 [239]
Pediatricians
See also: Doctors; Physicians; Physicians by specialty (e.g., Cardiologists)
— compensation for, p. 857 [815]

Pekin, IL *See:* Peoria – Pekin, IL
Pennsylvania
— active physicians, p. 910 [887]
— adult obesity rate, p. 594 [501]
— AIDS cases, pp. 81, 91, 99 [107, 112, 119]
— and births to teenagers, p. 11 [14]
— and disciplinary actions against physicians, p. 931 [917]
— and Medicaid, pp. 745-746 [684-685]
— and motor-vehicle fatalities, p. 42 [47]
— and police pursuits, p. 202 [217]
— and snowmobile-related deaths, p. 202 [218]
— cancer deaths, p. 47 [53]
— chancroid cases, p. 119 [152]
— chlamydia cases, pp. 123-124, 126 [154-156]
— clinics, pp. 268, 321 [311, 343]
— deaths, pp. 36, 38, 202, 609 [41, 218, 522]
— dental clinics, p. 293 [327]
— diseases, p. 185 [200]
— expenditures, pp. 664, 666 [589-590]
— gonorrhea cases, pp. 137, 139-140, 142 [164-167]
— health industry ratios, pp. 439-441, 443-444, 446-447, 449-450, 452-453, 455-456, 458-459, 461-462, 464-465, 467-468, 470-471, 473-474, 476-477, 479-480 [408-436]
— health insurance, p. 712 [641]
— influenza cases, p. 195 [212]
— lung cancer deaths, p. 47 [53]
— managed care enrollment, p. 722 [660]
— medical facilities, pp. 274-275, 278, 284-285, 288, 292-293, 297, 300, 307-308, 311, 314, 319, 321, 326, 328, 337, 339, 344, 346, 351, 353, 358, 362, 366, 371, 375, 379, 382, 386, 388, 391, 395, 400, 404-405, 408, 411, 416, 418, 425-426, 430-431, 434, 437, 439-441, 443-444, 446-447, 449-450, 452-453, 455-456, 458-459, 461-462, 464-465, 467-468, 470-471, 473-474, 476-477, 479-480 [314-315, 317, 320-321, 323, 326-327, 329, 331, 334-335, 337, 339, 342-343, 346-347, 350-351, 354-355, 358-359, 361, 363, 365, 367, 369, 371, 373, 375, 377, 379, 381, 383, 386-387, 389, 391, 394-395, 398-399, 402-403, 405, 407-436]
— nursing care facilities, p. 366 [365]
— nursing homes, pp. 576, 578 [483-484]
— physicians, p. 931 [917]
— smokers, p. 609 [522]
— syphilis cases, pp. 164, 166-167, 169-170, 172-173 [186-192]
— tuberculosis cases, p. 185 [200]
— uninsured population, p. 719 [654]
— vaccinations, p. 195 [212]
Pensacola, FL
— medical facilities, pp. 270, 280, 296, 302, 316, 323, 332, 341, 348, 356, 360, 369, 373, 377, 384, 398, 413, 420 [312, 318, 328, 332, 340, 344, 348, 352, 356, 360, 362, 366, 368, 370, 374, 382, 392, 396]
Peoria – Pekin, IL
— medical facilities, pp. 270, 280, 296, 302, 316, 323, 332, 341, 348, 356, 360, 369, 373, 377, 384, 398, 413, 420 [312, 318, 328, 332, 340, 344, 348, 352, 356, 360, 362, 366, 368, 370, 374, 382, 392, 396]
Pepcid AC
— and gastrointestinal illnesses, p. 659 [583]

Numbers following p. or pp. are page references. Numbers in [ ] are table references.

Numbers following p. or pp. are page references. Numbers in [ ] are table references.

Numbers following p. or pp. are page references. Numbers in [ ] are table references.

1013

Numbers following p. or pp. are page references. Numbers in [ ] are table references.

Numbers following p. or pp. are page references. Numbers in [ ] are table references.

Keyword Index

Numbers following p. or pp. are page references. Numbers in [ ] are table references.

1016

Numbers following p. or pp. are page references. Numbers in [ ] are table references.

Numbers following p. or pp. are page references. Numbers in [ ] are table references.

Numbers following p. or pp. are page references. Numbers in [ ] are table references.

Numbers following p. or pp. are page references. Numbers in [ ] are table references.

1020

Numbers following p. or pp. are page references. Numbers in [ ] are table references.

Numbers following p. or pp. are page references. Numbers in [ ] are table references.

Technicians, surgical
— and AIDS infections, p. 98 [118]
Technologists
— compensation for, pp. 773-775 [728-730]
Teenage mothers
— and birth rates, p. 11 [14]
Teenagers
— and AIDS cases, p. 96 [116]
— and contraception, pp. 597-599 [504-508]
— and crime, p. 646 [562]
— and drugs, p. 646 [562]
— and sex education, pp. 603-605 [515-518]
— and sexual intercourse, pp. 597-602 [504-508, 511-514]
— and sexual issues, p. 646 [562]
— and social pressures, p. 646 [562]
Temple, TX *See:* Killeen – Temple, TX
Tenet Healthcare (company)
— profit growth, p. 567 [470]
— revenues, p. 567 [471]
Tennessee
— active physicians, p. 911 [887]
— adult obesity rate, p. 594 [501]
— AIDS cases, pp. 82, 91 [107, 112]
— and births to teenagers, p. 11 [14]
— and disciplinary actions against physicians, p. 932 [917]
— and Medicaid, pp. 745, 747 [684-685]
— and motor-vehicle fatalities, p. 42 [46]
— chancroid cases, p. 120 [152]
— chlamydia cases, pp. 123-124, 126 [154-156]
— clinics, pp. 268, 321 [311, 343]
— deaths, pp. 37-38, 609 [41, 522]
— dental clinics, p. 293 [327]
— diseases, p. 184 [200]
— expenditures, pp. 665, 667 [589-590]
— gonorrhea cases, pp. 137-138, 140, 142 [164-167]
— health industry ratios, pp. 439-440, 442-443, 445-447, 449-450, 452-453, 455-456, 458-459, 461, 463-464, 466-468, 470-471, 473-474, 476-477, 479-480 [408-436]
— health insurance, p. 712 [641]
— influenza cases, p. 195 [212]
— managed care enrollment, p. 722 [660]
— medical facilities, pp. 274-275, 278, 284-285, 288, 292-293, 297, 300, 307-308, 311, 314, 319, 321, 326, 328, 337, 339, 344, 346, 351, 353, 358, 362, 366, 371, 375, 379, 382, 386, 388, 391, 395, 400, 404-405, 408, 411, 416, 418, 425-426, 430-431, 434, 437, 439-440, 442-443, 445-447, 449-450, 452-453, 455-456, 458-459, 461, 463-464, 466-468, 470-471, 473-474, 476-477, 479-480 [314-315, 317, 320-321, 323, 326-327, 329, 331, 334-335, 337, 339, 342-343, 346-347, 350-351, 354-355, 358-359, 361, 363, 365, 367, 369, 371, 373, 375, 377, 379, 381, 383, 386-387, 389, 391, 394-395, 398-399, 402-403, 405, 407-436]
— nursing care facilities, p. 366 [365]
— nursing homes, pp. 577, 579 [483-484]
— physicians, p. 932 [917]

Tennessee continued:
— smokers, pp. 609, 629 [522, 537]
— syphilis cases, pp. 164, 166-167, 169-170, 172-173 [186-192]
— tuberculosis cases, p. 184 [200]
— vaccinations, p. 195 [212]
Tennessee Managed Care Network
— managed care enrollment, p. 720 [656]
— Medicaid enrollment, p. 720 [656]
Terconazole
— and pregnancy, p. 233 [265]
Terre Haute, IN
— medical facilities, p. 333 [348]
Test scores
— medical colleges, p. 861 [822]
Tetanus
See also: Diphtheria; DTP; Pertussis
— vaccinations, pp. 196-197, 199-200 [213-216]
Texarkana, TX – AR
— medical facilities, p. 333 [348]
Texas
— accidental deaths, p. 202 [217]
— active physicians, p. 911 [887]
— adult obesity rate, p. 594 [501]
— AIDS cases, pp. 82, 91, 100, 253-254 [107, 112, 119, 289, 291]
— and births to teenagers, p. 11 [14]
— and Medicaid, pp. 745, 747 [684-685]
— and police pursuits, p. 202 [217]
— cancer deaths, p. 47 [53]
— chancroid cases, p. 120 [152]
— chlamydia cases, pp. 123-124, 126 [154-156]
— clinics, pp. 268, 321 [311, 343]
— deaths, pp. 37-38, 609 [41, 522]
— dental clinics, p. 293 [327]
— and disciplinary actions against physicians, p. 931 [917]
— diseases, p. 184 [200]
— expenditures, pp. 665, 667 [589-590]
— gonorrhea cases, pp. 137-138, 140, 142 [164-167]
— health industry ratios, pp. 439-440, 442-443, 445-447, 449-450, 452-453, 455-456, 458-459, 461, 463-464, 466-468, 470-471, 473-474, 476-477, 479-480 [408-436]
— health insurance, p. 712 [641]
— influenza cases, p. 195 [212]
— medical facilities, pp. 274, 276, 278, 284-285, 288, 292-293, 297, 300, 307-308, 311, 314, 319, 321, 326, 328, 337, 339, 344, 346, 351, 353, 358, 362, 366, 371, 375, 379, 382, 386, 388, 391, 395, 400, 404-405, 408, 411, 416, 418, 425-426, 430, 432, 434, 437, 439-440, 442-443, 445-447, 449-450, 452-453, 455-456, 458-459, 461, 463-464, 466-468, 470-471, 473-474, 476-477, 479-480 [314-315, 317, 320-321, 323, 326-327, 329, 331, 334-335, 337, 339, 342-343, 346-347, 350-351, 354-355, 358-359, 361, 363, 365, 367, 369, 371, 373, 375, 377, 379, 381, 383, 386-387, 389, 391, 394-395, 398-399, 402-403, 405, 407-436]
— nursing care facilities, p. 366 [365]
— nursing homes, pp. 577, 579 [483-484]
— pharmaceutical companies, p. 260 [303]
— physicians, p. 931 [917]

Numbers following p. or pp. are page references. Numbers in [ ] are table references.

1023

Texas continued:
— smokers, p. 609 [522]
— syphilis cases, pp. 164, 166-167, 169-170, 172-173 [186-192]
— tuberculosis cases, p. 184 [199-200]
— uninsured population, p. 719 [653]
— vaccinations, p. 195 [212]
Therapists
— and alcohol use, p. 645 [560]
— and drug use, p. 645 [560]
Thoracic surgeries
— and Medicare allowed charges, p. 763 [713]
Thyroid gland
— and cancer, p. 112 [141]
Titusville, FL See: Melbourne – Titusville – Palm Bay, FL
Tobacco industry
— compensation to states, p. 930 [916]
Toga space suit
— hospital price, p. 561 [464]
Toledo, OH
— AIDS cases, p. 85 [108]
— chancroid cases, p. 121 [153]
— chlamydia cases, pp. 128, 130, 132 [157-159]
— clinics, p. 267 [310]
— gonorrhea cases, pp. 146, 148-149, 151 [171-174]
— medical facilities, pp. 267, 271, 281, 296, 303, 305, 317, 324, 333, 336, 342, 349, 357, 361, 365, 369, 374, 378, 385, 394, 399, 414, 421, 423 [310, 312, 318, 328, 332-333, 340, 344, 348-349, 352, 356, 360, 362, 364, 366, 368, 370, 374, 380, 382, 392, 396-397]
— syphilis cases, pp. 159, 161, 163, 175, 177, 179, 181-182 [183-185, 193-197]
Tonsillectomies
— and hospital stays, p. 565 [468]
— by sex, pp. 227, 244 [255, 282]
Tooth decay
— per capita expenditures, p. 678 [604]
Topeka, KS
— medical facilities, p. 333 [348]
Traffic-related deaths
— by age, pp. 213, 215 [238, 241]
— by sex, pp. 213, 215 [238, 241]
Training specialists See: Personnel and training specialists
Tranquilizers
See also: Alcohol; Drug use (illicit); Marijuana and hashish; Substance abuse
— abuse, pp. 633-641, 650 [544-555, 566]
Transplants
— by type, p. 923 [902]
Treadmills
— ownership, p. 589 [495]
— use, p. 589 [495]
Tricyclics
— prices, p. 684 [611]
Trimox
— prescriptions written, pp. 260-261 [304-305]

Troy, NY See: Albany – Schenectady – Troy, NY
Truck drivers
— and alcohol use, p. 644 [559]
— and drug use, p. 644 [559]
— compensation for, pp. 855-856 [812]
Tuberculosis cases, pp. 184, 657 [199, 579]
— by state, p. 184 [200]
— deaths, pp. 35, 183 [40, 198]
Tucson, AZ
— AIDS cases, p. 85 [108]
— back surgeries, p. 925 [907]
— chancroid cases, p. 121 [153]
— chlamydia cases, pp. 128, 130, 132 [157-159]
— clinics, p. 267 [310]
— gonorrhea cases, pp. 146, 148-149, 151 [171-174]
— medical facilities, pp. 267, 271, 281, 296, 303, 305, 317, 324, 333, 336, 342, 349, 357, 361, 365, 369, 374, 378, 385, 394, 399, 414, 421, 423 [310, 312, 318, 328, 332-333, 340, 344, 348-349, 352, 356, 360, 362, 364, 366, 368, 370, 374, 380, 382, 392, 396-397]
— surgeries, p. 925 [907]
— syphilis cases, pp. 159, 161, 163, 175, 177, 179, 181, 183 [183-185, 193-197]
Tulare, CA See: Visalia – Tulare – Porterville, CA
Tulsa, OK
— AIDS cases, p. 85 [108]
— chancroid cases, p. 122 [153]
— chlamydia cases, pp. 128, 130, 132 [157-159]
— clinics, p. 267 [310]
— gonorrhea cases, pp. 146, 148-150 [171-174]
— medical facilities, pp. 267, 271, 281, 296, 303, 305, 317, 324, 333, 336, 342, 349, 357, 361, 365, 369, 374, 378, 385, 394, 399, 414, 421, 423 [310, 312, 318, 328, 332-333, 340, 344, 348-349, 352, 356, 360, 362, 364, 366, 368, 370, 374, 380, 382, 392, 396-397]
— syphilis cases, pp. 159, 161, 163, 175, 177, 179, 181-182 [183-185, 193-197]
Tumors
— and magnetic resonance imaging, p. 927 [910]
Tums
— and gastrointestinal illnesses, p. 659 [582]
— costs, p. 659 [582]
Turkey
— expenditures, pp. 944-945 [939-940]
Tuscaloosa, AL
— medical facilities, p. 333 [348]
Tyler, TX
— medical facilities, p. 333 [348]
Typists See: Secretaries and typists
Ulcers
— and deaths, p. 35 [40]
Ultrasound procedures, p. 250 [286]
Umbrella tree
— poisonings, p. 76 [102]
Uninsured populations
— by age, p. 715 [645]
— by earnings income, p. 715 [646]
— by educational attainment, p. 716 [647]

Numbers following p. or pp. are page references. Numbers in [ ] are table references.

Numbers following p. or pp. are page references. Numbers in [ ] are table references.

Numbers following p. or pp. are page references. Numbers in [ ] are table references.

Keyword Index

Numbers following p. or pp. are page references. Numbers in [ ] are table references.

Numbers following p. or pp. are page references. Numbers in [ ] are table references.

Numbers following p. or pp. are page references. Numbers in [ ] are table references.